a LANGE medical book

Behavioral Medicine

A Guide for Clinical Practice

Fifth Edition

Editors

Mitchell D. Feldman, MD, MPhil, FACP
Professor of Medicine
Chief, Division of General Internal Medicine
Associate Vice Provost, Faculty Mentoring
University of California, San Francisco
San Francisco, California

John F. Christensen, PhD
Healthcare Consultant
Corbett, Oregon

Associate Editors

Jason M. Satterfield, PhD
Professor of Medicine
University of California, San Francisco
San Francisco, California

Ryan Laponis, MD, MS
Associate Professor of Medicine
University of California, San Francisco
San Francisco, California

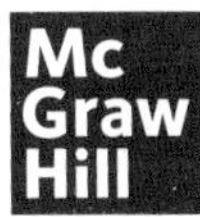

New York Chicago San Francisco Athens London Madrid
Mexico City Milan New Delhi Singapore Sydney Toronto

Behavioral Medicine: A Guide for Clinical Practice, Fifth Edition

1 2 3 4 5 6 7 8 9 LCR 24 23 22 21 20 19

ISBN 978-1-260-14268-6
MHID 1-260-14268-X

Notice

Medicine is an ever-changing science. As new research and clinical experience broaden our knowledge, changes in treatment and drug therapy are required. The authors and the publisher of this work have checked with sources believed to be reliable in their efforts to provide information that is complete and generally in accord with the standards accepted at the time of publication. However, in view of the possibility of human error or changes in medical sciences, neither the authors nor the publisher nor any other party who has been involved in the preparation or publication of this work warrants that the information contained herein is in every respect accurate or complete, and they disclaim all responsibility for any errors or omissions or for the results obtained from use of the information contained in this work. Readers are encouraged to confirm the information contained herein with other sources. For example and in particular, readers are advised to check the product information sheet included in the package of each drug they plan to administer to be certain that the information contained in this work is accurate and that changes have not been made in the recommended dose or in the contraindications for administration. This recommendation is of particular importance in connection with new or infrequently used drugs.

This book was set in Adobe Garamond Pro by Cenveo® Publisher Services.
The editors were Kay Conerly and Kim J. Davis.
The production supervisor was Richard Ruzycka.
Production management was provided by Revathi Viswanathan, Cenveo Publisher Services.
The cover designer was W2 Design.

This book is printed on acid-free paper.

Library of Congress Cataloging-in-Publication Data

Names: Feldman, Mitchell D., editor. | Christensen, John F., editor. | Satterfield, Jason M., editor. | Laponis, Ryan, editor.
Title: Behavioral medicine : a guide for clinical practice / editors, Mitchell D. Feldman, John F. Christensen ; associate editors, Jason M. Satterfield, Ryan Laponis.
Other titles: Behavioral medicine (Feldman)
Description: Fifth edition. | New York : McGraw-Hill Education, [2020] | "A Lange medical book." | Includes bibliographical references and index. | Summary: "This fifth edition of Behavioral Medicine: A Guide for Clinical Practice features important revisions of chapters from the previous editions to reflect advances in pharmacotherapy and evidence on the relationship between psychosocial factors and disease"— Provided by publisher.
Identifiers: LCCN 2019033369 (print) | LCCN 2019033370 (ebook) | ISBN 9781260142686 (pbk. ; alk. paper) | ISBN 9781260142693 (ebook)
Subjects: MESH: Primary Health Care | Behavioral Medicine | Behavior Therapy
Classification: LCC RC467 (print) | LCC RC467 (ebook) | NLM W 84.61 | DDC 616.89—dc23
LC record available at https://lccn.loc.gov/2019033369
LC ebook record available at https://lccn.loc.gov/2019033370

Contents

Videos

To access the collection of videos that accompany the text, please scan the QR code below or visit mhprofessional.com/feldman5evideos

SECTION II: GLOBAL HEALTH

SECTION III: WORKING WITH SPECIFIC POPULATIONS

SECTION IV: HEALTH-RELATED BEHAVIOR

Authors

Erin C. Accurso, PhD
Department of Psychiatry, Weill Institute for Neurosciences
University of California, San Francisco
San Francisco, California
Erin.Accurso@ucsf.edu
Chapter 23: Eating Disorders

Jonathan Amiel, MD
Associate Professor of Psychiatry
Columbia University Vagelos College of Physicians and Surgeons
New York State Psychiatric Institute, NewYork-Presbyterian Hospital
New York, New York
jma2106@cumc.columbia.edu
Chapter 47: Narrative Medicine

Anne Armstrong-Coben, MD
Associate Professor of Pediatrics at Columbia University Irving Medical Center
Columbia University Vagelos College of Physicians and Surgeons
NewYork-Presbyterian Hospital, Morgan Stanley Children's Hospital of New York
New York, New York
Aha2@cumc.columbia.edu
Chapter 47: Narrative Medicine

Robert B. Baron, MD, MS
Professor of Medicine
Associate Dean for Graduate and Continuing Medical Education
Vice Chief, Division of General Internal Medicine
University of California, San Francisco
San Francisco, California
Bobby.Baron@ucsf.edu
Chapter 22: Obesity

Melanie Bernitz, MD, MPH
Associate Vice President and Medical Director
Columbia Health
Associate Clinical Professor of Medicine
Columbia University
Columbia University Irving Medical Center
New York, New York
mjb239@cumc.columbia.edu
Chapter 47: Narrative Medicine

Adam L. Braddock, MD, MPhil
Assistant Clinical Professor of Pediatrics
Division of Academic General Pediatrics, Child Development, and Community Health
University of California, San Diego School of Medicine
San Diego, California
abraddock@ucsd.edu
Chapter 12: Children

David G. Bullard, PhD
Clinical Professor of Medicine
Clinical Professor of Medical Psychology (Psychiatry)
Consultant, Symptom Management Service
Helen Diller Family Comprehensive Cancer Center
Member, Professional Advisory Group, Spiritual Care Services
UCSF Medical Center and UCSF Benioff Children's Hospital
Private Clinical Practice of Individual and Couples Therapy
San Francisco, California
dgbullard@yahoo.com
Chapter 33: Sexual Problems

Bethany C. Calkins, MS, MD
Palliative Care Physician
VA Western New York Health Care System
Buffalo, New York
Bethany.Calkins@va.gov
Chapter 3: Delivering Serious News
Chapter 42: Palliative Care, Hospice, & Care of the Dying

Patricia A. Carney, PhD
Professor of Family Medicine
Oregon Health & Science University
Portland, Oregon
carneyp@ohsu.edu
Chapter 45: Assessing Learners & Curricula in the Behavioral & Social Sciences

Selena Chan, DO
Health Sciences Clinical Instructor, School of Medicine
Osher Center for Integrative Medicine
University of California, San Francisco
San Francisco, California
Selena.Chan@ucsf.edu
Chapter 35: Integrative Medicine

Rita Charon, MD, PhD
Professor and Chair, Medical Humanities and Ethics
Professor of Medicine at Columbia University Irving Medical Center
Columbia University Vagelos College of Physicians and Surgeons
Columbia University Irving Medical Center
New York, New York
rac5@cumc.columbia.edu
Chapter 47: Narrative Medicine

John F. Christensen, PhD
Healthcare Consultant
Corbett, Oregon
nagarkot247@gmail.com
Chapter 5: Suggestion & Hypnosis
Chapter 9: Environment, Health, and Behavior
Chapter 26: Depression
Chapter 36: Stress & Disease
Chapter 39: Errors in Medical Practice
Chapter 49: Trainee Well-Being

David Claman, MD
Director, UCSF Sleep Disorders Center
UCSF Professor of Medicine
San Francisco, California
David.Claman@ucsf.edu
Chapter 32: Sleep Disorders

Tiffany E. Cook, BGS
New York University School of Medicine
New York, New York
Tiffany.Cook@nyulangone.org
Chapter 17: Lesbian, Gay, Bisexual, Transgender, & Queer Patients

Ann Cottingham, MAR, MA
Director, Research in Health Professions Practice and Education
Center for Health Services Research
Regenstrief Institute
Indiana University School of Medicine
Indianapolis, Indiana
ancottin@iu.edu
Chapter 44: Teaching Behavioral Medicine: Theory & Practice

Hetty Cunningham, MD
Assistant Professor of Pediatrics at Columbia University Irving Medical Center
Columbia University Vagelos College of Physicians and Surgeons
NewYork-Presbyterian Hospital, Morgan Stanley Children's Hospital of New York
New York, New York
hc451@cumc.columbia.edu
Chapter 47: Narrative Medicine

Thomas Denberg, MD, PhD
Senior Medical Director
Medical Operations and Healthcare Strategy
Pinnacol Assurance
Denver, Colorado
tom.denberg@pinnacol.com
Chapter 15: Cross-Cultural Communication

Christine Derzko, MD
Associate Professor
Department of Obstetrics & Gynecology
Department of Internal Medicine (Endocrinology)
University of Toronto
St. Michael's Hospital
Toronto, Ontario, Canada
derzkoc@smh.ca
Chapter 33: Sexual Problems

Mark DiCorcia, PhD
Assistant Dean for Medical Education and Academic Affairs
Associate Professor of Integrated Medical Science
Charles E. Schmidt College of Medicine at Florida Atlantic University
Boca Raton, Florida
mdicorcia@health.fau.edu
Chapter 44: Teaching Behavioral Medicine: Theory & Practice

M. Robin DiMatteo, PhD
Distinguished Emerita Professor of Psychology
University of California
Riverside, California
robin.dimatteo@ucr.edu
Chapter 20: Patient Adherence

Elizabeth Eckstrom, MD, MPH
Professor and Chief, Geriatrics
Division of General Internal Medicine and Geriatrics
Oregon Health & Science University
Portland, Oregon
eckstrom@ohsu.edu
Chapter 14: Older Patients
Chapter 34: Dementia & Delirium

E. Jennifer Edelman, MD, MHS
Associate Professor of Medicine and Public Health
Yale Schools of Medicine and Public Health
New Haven, Connecticut
eva.edelman@yale.edu
Chapter 24: Unhealthy Alcohol & Other Substance Use

Michael Eisman, MD
eismanm@schuylerhospital.org
Chapter 42: Palliative Care, Hospice, & Care of the Dying

Ronald Epstein, MD
Professor of Family Medicine, Psychiatry, Oncology and Medicine (Palliative Care)
American Cancer Society Clinical Research Professor
University of Rochester School of Medicine and Dentistry
Rochester, New York
Ronald_Epstein@URMC.Rochester.edu
Chapter 7: Mindful Practice

Nate L. Ewigman, PhD, MPH
Staff Psychologist and Associate Director, IMPACT Team
San Francisco VA Health Care System
Clinical Assistant Professor of Psychiatry
University of California, San Francisco
San Francisco, California
newigman@gmail.com
Chapter 41: Trauma

Mitchell D. Feldman, MD, MPhil, FACP
Professor of Medicine
Chief, Division of General Internal Medicine
Associate Vice Provost, Faculty Mentoring
University of California, San Francisco
San Francisco, California
Mitchell.Feldman@ucsf.edu
Chapter 4: Difficult Patients/Difficult Situations
Chapter 11: Families
Chapter 15: Cross-Cultural Communication
Chapter 26: Depression
Chapter 27: Anxiety
Chapter 37: HIV/AIDS
Chapter 40: Intimate Partner Violence
Chapter 49: Trainee Well-Being

Sarah Forsberg, PsyD
Department of Psychiatry
Weill Institute for Neurosciences
University of California, San Francisco
San Francisco, California
drsarahforsberg@gmail.com
Chapter 23: Eating Disorders

Auguste H. Fortin, VI, MD, MPH
Professor of Medicine
Division of General Internal Medicine
Yale School of Medicine
Director of Psychosocial Communication
Yale Primary Care Internal Medicine Residency Program
New Haven, Connecticut
auguste.fortin@yale.edu
Chapter 2: Empathy

Richard M. Frankel, PhD
Professor of Medicine and Geriatrics
Indiana University School of Medicine
Director: Advanced Scholars Program for Internists in Research and Education
Indianapolis, Indiana
Education Institute
Cleveland Clinic
Cleveland, Ohio
rfrankel@iu.edu
Chapter 48: Educating for Professionalism

Lawrence S. Friedman, MD
Associate Dean for Clinical Affairs
Professor of Clinical Pediatrics and Medicine
University of California, San Diego Health System and School of Medicine
San Diego, California
lsfriedman@ucsd.edu
Chapter 13: Adolescents

Jennifer Gafford, PhD
Licensed Psychologist
Behavioral Health Consultant at Family Care Health Centers
Director of Behavioral Medicine Education
Saint Louis University Family Medicine Residency at SSM St. Mary's Health Center
St. Louis, Missouri
jengafford@aol.com
Chapter 10: Training of International Medical Graduates

Julie Glickstein, MD
Professor of Pediatrics
Columbia University Irving Medical Center
Department of Pediatrics / Division of Pediatric Cardiology
Columbia University Vagelos College of Physicians and Surgeons
NewYork-Presbyterian Hospital, Morgan Stanley Children's Hospital of New York
New York, New York
Jg2065@cumc.columbia.edu
Chapter 47: Narrative Medicine

Deepthiman Gowda, MD, MPH, MS
Assistant Dean for Medical Education
Kaiser Permanente School of Medicine
Pasadena, California
deepthiman.gowda@kp.org
Chapter 47: Narrative Medicine

Gillian Graham, MS, PMHNP-BC
Psychiatric Nurse Practitioner
Behavioral Health Network
Northampton, Massachusetts
gillian.graham87@gmail.com
Chapter 47: Narrative Medicine

Richard E. Greene, MD, MHPE, FACP
Associate Professor, Department of Medicine
New York University School of Medicine
New York, New York
Richard.Greene@nyumc.org
Chapter 17: Lesbian, Gay, Bisexual, Transgender, & Queer Patients

Frederic W. Hafferty, PhD
Professor of Medical Education
Mayo Clinic
Rochester, Minnesota
fredhafferty@mac.com
Chapter 48: Educating for Professionalism

Steven R. Hahn, MD
steven.hahn@nychhc.org
Chapter 11: Families

Frederick M. Hecht, MD
Professor of Medicine, Division of General Internal Medicine
Osher Center for Integrative Medicine
University of California, San Francisco
San Francisco, California
Rick.Hecht@ucsf.edu
Chapter 35: Integrative Medicine

Stephen G. Henry, MD, MSc
Associate Professor of Medicine
University of California, Davis School of Medicine
Sacramento, California
sghenry@ucdavis.edu
Chapter 25: Opioids

Nellie Hermann, MFA
Creative Director, Columbia Narrative Medicine
Department of Medical Humanities and Ethics
Columbia Vagelos College of Physicians and Surgeons
New York, New York
nellie.hermann@gmail.com
Chapter 47: Narrative Medicine

J. Carlo Hojilla, RN, PhD
Postdoctoral Fellow, Traineeship in Drug Abuse Treatment and Services Research
Department of Psychiatry
University of California, San Francisco
San Francisco, California
Carlo.hojilla@ucsf.edu
Chapter 24: Unhealthy Alcohol & Other Substance Use

Eric S. Holmboe, MD
Chief, Research, Milestones Development and Evaluation Officer
Accreditation Council for Graduate Medical Education
Adjunct Professor, Yale University School of Medicine
New Haven, Connecticut
Adjunct Professor
Uniformed Services University of the Health Sciences
Bethesda, Maryland
Adjunct Professor, Feinberg School of Medicine
Northwestern University
Chicago, Illinois
eholmboe@acgme.org
Chapter 43: Competency-Based Education for Behavioral Medicine

Elizabeth Imbert, MD, MPH
Assistant Professor
Division of HIV, Infectious Diseases and Global Medicine
Department of Medicine
Zuckerberg San Francisco General Hospital
University of California, San Francisco
San Francisco, California
elizabeth.imbert@ucsf.edu
Chapter 37: HIV/AIDS

Thomas S. Inui, ScM, MD, MACP
Director of Research, IU Center for Global Research
Professor of Medicine, IU School of Medicine
Investigator, Regenstrief Institute
Indianapolis, Indiana
tinui@iupui.edu
Chapter 44: Teaching Behavioral Medicine: Theory & Practice

Leah Kalin, MD
Geriatric Fellow
Oregon Health & Science University
Portland, Oregon
kalin@ohsu.edu
Chapter 14: Older Patients
Chapter 34: Dementia & Delirium

Sara Kalkhoran, MD, MAS
Assistant Professor of Medicine, Harvard Medical School
Investigator, Tobacco Research and Treatment Center and Assistant in Medicine
Division of General Internal Medicine, Massachusetts General Hospital
Boston, Massachusetts
skalkhoran@partners.org
Chapter 21: Tobacco Use

Nicholas Kinder, MSN, APN, AGNP-C
Assistant Professor
Division of General Internal Medicine & Geriatrics
Oregon Health & Science University
Portland, Oregon
kindern@ohsu.edu
Chapter 14: Older Patients
Chapter 34: Dementia & Delirium

Coleen Kivlahan, MD, MSPH
Executive Director Primary Care
Professor, Family and Community Medicine
University of California, San Francisco
San Francisco, California
Coleen.Kivlahan@ucsf.edu
Chapter 41: Trauma

Kavitha Kolappa, MD, MPH
The Chester M. Pierce, MD Division of Global Psychiatry
Department of Psychiatry, Massachusetts General Hospital
Boston, Massachusetts
kavitha.kolappa@gmail.com
Chapter 8: Global Health and Behavioral Medicine

Timothy R. Kreider, MD, PhD
Assistant Professor
Department of Psychiatry
Donald and Barbara Zucker School of Medicine at Hofstra/Northwell
Hempstead, New York
tkreider@northwell.edu
Chapter 30: Personality Disorders

Ryan Laponis, MD, MS
Associate Professor of Medicine
University of California, San Francisco
San Francisco, California
Ryan.Laponis@ucsf.edu
Chapter 4: Difficult Patients/Difficult Situations

Patrick T. Lee, MD, DTM&H
Chair of Medicine, North Shore Medical Center
Salem, Massachusetts
PTLEE@PARTNERS.ORG
Chapter 8: Global Health and Behavioral Medicine

Mack Lipkin, Jr., MD
Professor of Medicine
New York University School of Medicine
New York, New York
Mack.Lipkin@nyulangone.org
Chapter 1: The Medical Interview

Debra K. Litzelman, MA, MD
D. Craig Brater Professor of Medicine
Director of Education and Workforce Development
Indiana University Center for Global Health
Associate Director of Health Services Research
Regenstrief Institute
Indianapolis, Indiana
dklitzel@iu.edu
Chapter 44: Teaching Behavioral Medicine: Theory & Practice

Edward L. Machtinger, MD
Professor of Medicine
Director, Women's HIV Program
University of California, San Francisco
San Francisco, California
Edward.Machtinger@ucsf.edu
Chapter 41: Trauma

Felise Milan, MD
Professor of Medicine
Director, Ruth L. Gottesman Clinical Skills Center
Director, Introduction to Clinical Medicine Program
Albert Einstein College of Medicine
Bronx, New York
felise.milan@einstein.yu.edu
Chapter 45: Assessing Learners & Curricula in the Behavioral & Social Sciences

Vishnu Mohan, MD, MBI, FACP, FAMIA
Associate Professor, OHSU School of Medicine
Department of Medical Informatics and Clinical Epidemiology
Portland, Oregon
mohanv@ohsu.edu
Chapter 10: Training of International Medical Graduates

Gina Moreno-John, MD
Attending Physician and Professor of Medicine
University of California, San Francisco Medical Center
Department of General Internal Medicine
San Francisco, California
Gina.Moreno-John@ucsf.edu
Chapter 40: Intimate Partner Violence

Diane S. Morse, MD
Associate Professor of Psychiatry and Medicine
University of Rochester School of Medicine
Department of Psychiatry
Director, Women's Initiative Supporting Health
Center for Community Health
Rochester, New York
Diane_Morse@urmc.rochester.edu
Chapter 16: Women

Daniel O'Connell, PhD
Training, Coaching and Consultation
Clinical Instructor, University of Washington
Seattle, Washington
danoconn@me.com
Chapter 19: Behavior Change

Karli Okeson, DO
Pediatric Emergency Medicine Fellow
Emory University
Atlanta, Georgia
karlisinger@gmail.com
Chapter 32: Sleep Disorders

Steven Z. Pantilat, MD
Alan M. Kates and John M. Burnard Endowed Chair in Palliative Care
Director, Palliative Care Program, Division of Hospital Medicine
Department of Medicine
University of California, San Francisco
San Francisco, California
Steve.Pantilat@ucsf.edu
Chapter 38: Pain

Constance Molino Park, MD, PhD
Retired Associate Clinical Professor of Medicine
Columbia University Irving Medical Center
New York, New York
constancepark@gmail.com
Chapter 47: Narrative Medicine

Misa Perron-Burdick, MD, MAS
She Her Hers
Medical Director
Women's Health Center
Zuckerberg San Francisco General
Assistant Clinical Professor
Department of Obstetrics, Gynecology, and Reproductive Sciences
University of California, San Francisco
San Francisco, California
Misa.Perron-burdick@ucsf.edu
Chapter 16: Women

Stephen D. Persell, MD, MPH
Associate Professor of Medicine, Division of General Internal Medicine and Geriatrics
Director, Center for Primary Care Innovation, Institute for Public Health and Medicine
Feinberg School of Medicine, Northwestern University
Chicago, Illinois
SPersell@nm.org
Chapter 46: Evidence-Based Behavioral Practice

Olesya Pokorna, MD
PGY4 Resident Physician, Department of Psychiatry
University of California, San Francisco
San Francisco, California
olesya.pokorna@ucsf.edu
Chapter 31: Psychosis

Timothy E. Quill, MD, MACP, FAAHPM
Professor of Medicine, Psychiatry, Medical Humanities and Nursing
Palliative Care Division, Department of Medicine
University of Rochester School of Medicine
Rochester, New York
timothy_quill@urmc.rochester.edu
Chapter 3: Delivering Serious News
Chapter 42: Palliative Care, Hospice, & Care of the Dying

Michael W. Rabow, MD
Helen Diller Family Chair in Palliative Care
Director, the Symptom Management Service
Associate Chief for Education
Division of Palliative Medicine
University of California, San Francisco
San Francisco, California
Mike.Rabow@ucsf.edu
Chapter 38: Pain

Y. Pritham Raj, MD
Associate Professor,
Departments of Internal Medicine & Psychiatry
Oregon Health & Science University
Medical Director,
Emotional Wellness Center
Adventist Health Portland
Portland, Oregon
pritham.raj@duke.edu
Chapter 26: Depression
Chapter 29: Somatic Symptom & Related Disorders

Gita Ramamurthy, MD
Assistant Professor,
Department of Psychiatry and Family Medicine SUNY
Upstate Medical Center
Syracuse, New York
agramam@gmail.com
Chapter 6: Practitioner Well-Being

Neda Ratanawongsa, MD, MPH
Associate Chief Health Informatics Officer for Ambulatory Services
San Francisco Health Network
Associate Professor
Division of General Internal Medicine
UCSF Center for Vulnerable Populations
Zuckerberg San Francisco General Hospital
San Francisco, California
Neda.Ratanawongsa@ucsf.edu
Chapter 18: Vulnerable Patients

Giuseppe J. Raviola, MD, MPH
Assistant Professor of Psychiatry, and Global Health and Social Medicine
Harvard Medical School
Department of Psychiatry, Massachusetts General Hospital
Boston, Massachusetts
Giuseppe.Raviola@childrens.harvard.edu
Chapter 8: Global Health and Behavioral Medicine

Nancy A. Rigotti, MD
Professor of Medicine, Harvard Medical School
Director, Tobacco Research and Treatment Center, Massachusetts General Hospital
Associate Chief, Division of General Internal Medicine, Massachusetts General Hospital
Boston, Massachusetts
nrigotti@partners.org
Chapter 21: Tobacco Use

George W. Saba, PhD
Associate Program Director
Family and Community Medicine Residency
Department of Family and Community Medicine
University of California, San Francisco
San Francisco General Hospital
San Francisco, California
George.Saba@ucsf.edu
Chapter 18: Vulnerable Patients

Emma Samelson-Jones, MD
Assistant Clinical Professor
Department of Psychiatry
University of California, San Francisco
San Francisco, California
Emma.SamelsonJones@ucsf.edu
Chapter 31: Psychosis

Veronica J. Sanchez, PhD
Cerritos College
Department of Psychology
Norwalk, California
vsanc006@ucr.edu
Chapter 20: Patient Adherence

Derek D. Satre, PhD
Professor, Department of Psychiatry
Weill Institute for Neurosciences
University of California, San Francisco
San Francisco, California
Derek.Satre@ucsf.edu
Chapter 24: Unhealthy Alcohol & Other Substance Use

Jason M. Satterfield, PhD
Professor of Medicine
University of California, San Francisco
San Francisco, California
Jason.Satterfield@ucsf.edu
Chapter 27: Anxiety
Chapter 43: Competency-Based Education for Behavioral Medicine
Chapter 45: Assessing Learners & Curricula in the Behavioral & Social Sciences

Dean Schillinger, MD
UCSF Professor of Medicine in Residence
Chief, UCSF Division of General Internal Medicine
Zuckerberg San Francisco General Hospital
Director, Health Communication Research Program
UCSF Center for Vulnerable Populations
San Francisco, California
dean.schillinger@ucsf.edu
Chapter 18: Vulnerable Patients

Jason Schneider, MD, FACP
Associate Professor, Department of Medicine
Emory University School of Medicine
Atlanta, Georgia
jsschne@emory.edu
Chapter 17: Lesbian, Gay, Bisexual, Transgender, & Queer Patients

Antoinette Schoenthaler, EdD
Associate Professor of Population Health
Center for Healthful Behavior Change
Division of Health and Behavior
NYU School of Medicine
New York, New York
Antoinette.Schoenthaler@nyumc.org
Chapter 1: The Medical Interview

H. Russell Searight, PhD, MPH
Professor of Psychology
Lake Superior State University
Sault Sainte Marie, Michigan
hsearight@lssu.edu
Chapter 10: Training of International Medical Graduates
Chapter 28: Attention Deficit Hyperactivity Disorder

Taylor Severance, BS
Department of Psychology and Biological Sciences
Lake Superior State University
Sault Sainte Marie, Michigan
tseverance@lssu.edu
Chapter 28: Attention Deficit Hyperactivity Disorder

Ann C. Shah, MD
Assistant Clinical Professor
Pain Management Center
Department of Anesthesia and Perioperative Care
University of California, San Francisco
San Francisco, California
Ann.Shah@ucsf.edu
Chapter 38: Pain

Clifford Singer, MD
Chief, Geriatric Mental Health and Neuropsychiatry
Principal Investigator, Alzheimer's Disease Clinical Trials
Acadia Hospital and Eastern Maine Medical Center
Bangor, Maine
csinger@emhs.org
Chapter 32: Sleep Disorders

Gregory T. Smith, PhD
Director
Progressive Rehabilitation Associates
Portland, Oregon
Vancouver, Washington
greg@progrehab.com
Chapter 38: Pain

Bonnie Spring, PhD, ABPP
Professor of Preventive Medicine, Psychology, and Public Health
Director, Institute for Public Health and Medicine—Center for Behavior and Health
Co-Program Leader for Cancer Prevention
Team Science Director, NUCATS CTSA
Northwestern University Feinberg School of Medicine
Chicago, Illinois
bspring@northwestern.edu
Chapter 46: Evidence-Based Behavioral Practice

Anthony L. Suchman, MD
Senior Consultant, Relationship Centered Health Care
Clinical Professor
University of Rochester School of Medicine and Dentistry
Rochester, New York
asuchman@rchcweb.com
Chapter 6: Practitioner Well-Being

Howard L. Taras, MD
Professor of Pediatrics
University of California, San Diego
La Jolla, California
htaras@ucsd.edu
Chapter 12: Children

Delphine Taylor, MD
Associate Professor of Medicine at Columbia University Irving Medicine Center
Columbia University Vagelos College of Physician and Surgeons
Columbia University Irving Medical Center
New York, New York
Dst4@cumc.columbia.edu
Chapter 47: Narrative Medicine

Teresa Villela, MD
Professor and Chief of Family and Community Medicine
UCSF and Zuckerberg San Francisco General Hospital
San Francisco, California
Teresa.Villela@ucsf.edu
Chapter 18: Vulnerable Patients

Judith Walsh, MD, MPH
Professor of Clinical Medicine
University of California, San Francisco
Women's Health Clinical Research Center
University of California, San Francisco
San Francisco, California
Judith.Walsh@ucsf.edu
Chapter 16: Women

John Q. Young, MD, MPP, PhD
Professor and Vice Chair for Education
Department of Psychiatry
Donald and Barbara Zucker School of Medicine
Hofstra/Northwell
Hempstead, New York
JYoung9@northwell.edu
Chapter 30: Personality Disorders

Kelly C. Young-Wolff, PhD, MPH
Research Scientist
Division of Research
Kaiser Permanente Northern California
Oakland, California
Kelly.C.Young-Wolff@kp.org
Chapter 24: Unhealthy Alcohol & Other Substance Use

Foreword

The heart of health care is the relationship between clinician and patient. What happens in the clinical encounter substantially affects health outcomes for patients and families. Highly effective encounters amplify the effectiveness of advances in medical technologies, pharmaceuticals, and systems of healthcare delivery. The quality of this core relationship also impacts the well-being of clinicians, whose calling to serve in their profession is rooted in a desire to make a difference in people's lives.

The challenges for clinicians to maintain healing relationships with their patients are enormous. Increasingly, healthcare professionals are called upon to relate to patients with more diverse lifestyles, cultures, ethnicities, sexual orientations, gender identities, national origins, economic status, and beliefs. Intertwined with these social complexities are the mental health and behavioral problems with which many patients struggle.

Behavioral Medicine: A Guide for Clinical Practice, now in its 5th edition, gives practitioners useful clinical tools to address a wide range of patient care challenges. It also provides guidance about how to manage common situations, such as developing rapport, delivering serious news, or motivating patients to change health-risk behaviors. New chapters discuss the care of patients dealing with trauma or addiction to opioids. This book is also useful to those who teach behavioral medicine. It includes topics related to developing an evidence-based curriculum in the behavioral and social sciences, assessing the competencies of trainees, and educating for professionalism. These topics are particularly important in the context of an ever evolving healthcare system constantly buffeted by change.

One of the significant elements of the book is the recognition that the well-being of health professionals is critically important to caring for patients. As a profession, we often do not pay sufficient attention to the clinicians, many of whom become burned out doing the work they love. Chapters on mindful practice and the well-being of practitioners and trainees enhance the book.

With much new and evidenced-based content, this edition of the book provides insight and information not available anywhere else for those who seek to provide holistic, high-quality care for patients.

Eric S. Holmboe, MD MACP FRCP FAoME(hon) FRCPSCanada(hon) CAPT, MC, USNR-R
Chief, Research, Milestone Development and Evaluation Officer
Accreditation Council for Graduate Medical Education
Adjunct Professor, Yale University School of Medicine
Adjunct Professor, Uniformed Services University of the Health Sciences
Adjunct Professor, Feinberg School of Medicine at Northwestern University

Preface

Since the publication of the fourth edition of *Behavioral Medicine: A Guide for Clinical Practice*, there have been considerable advances in medical diagnosis and treatment, as well as changes in the ways in which health care is organized and delivered. The science of genetics has revolutionized the understanding of disease, and we have entered the era of personalized medicine in which therapies are not only targeted to specific diseases, but increasingly, to specific individuals. New medications, therapies, and technologies are continually emerging for the treatment of a variety of behavioral health problems, such as mood and anxiety disorders and substance use. Collaborative models of care for patients with mental and behavioral disorders have been shown to improve clinical outcomes and are increasingly being integrated into medical settings. The rapid adoption of electronic medical records as the standard in most treatment settings continues to pose challenges for establishing and maintaining rapport in the clinician–patient relationship. Health care organizations are now compelled to pay greater attention to the importance of clinician well-being in reducing burnout and error and in maximizing the performance of the organization, including financial outcomes.

This fifth edition addresses these and other new developments in the clinical practice and teaching of behavioral medicine. Although the term "behavioral medicine" is used widely in both medical and social science literature, there is little agreement as to its exact definition. We broadly define it as an interdisciplinary field that aims to integrate the biological and psychosocial perspectives on human behavior and to apply them to the practice of medicine. Our perspective includes a behavioral approach to somatic disease, the mental disorders as they commonly appear in medical practice, issues in the clinician–patient relationship, and other important topics that affect the delivery of medical care, such as motivating behavior change, maximizing adherence to medical treatment, integrative medicine, and care of the dying.

This edition features important revisions of chapters from the previous editions to reflect advances in pharmacotherapy and evidence on the relationship between psychosocial factors and disease. New chapters have been added to reflect emerging issues in clinical care. For example, with the continued growth of the opioid epidemic, there was a need for a chapter dedicated to working with patients on these agents. Likewise, the increased recognition of the importance of trauma and its impact on our patients' health and well-being prompted us to add a chapter dedicated to that important topic.

Untreated behavioral and mental illness contributes to the global burden of disease, and there are marked disparities among nations and regions in recognition of these problems and treatment availability. The chapter on global health and behavioral medicine addresses the cultural and economic determinants of these disparities and offers new models for behavioral medicine practice and training to reduce the treatment gaps. Health outcomes globally are also influenced by environmental factors such as climate change, and human behavior is deemed responsible for a growing stress to the earth and its natural functions. The chapter on environment, health, and behavior examines these interrelationships and suggests behavior change models on a societal scale to promote the health of the planet.

The training of physicians and other health professionals has continued to evolve. Greater clarity in defining and assessing competencies, including that in behavioral medicine, has warranted an extensive expansion of the section on teaching and assessment with an emphasis on new approaches to training for behavioral competencies. Among these are more precise descriptions of behavioral competencies, advances in evaluation, novel teaching strategies such as the use of narrative medicine, and evidence-based behavioral practice. Finally, helping trainees in the health professions to find balance in their lives and to develop the life skills for a sustainable career has challenged medical schools and residencies to create curricula and educational experiences to promote well-being. These concepts are addressed in the final chapter of the book.

We hope that general internists, hospitalists, family practitioners, pediatricians, nurse practitioners, physician assistants, pharmacists, and other clinicians will find that this book helps them to better understand and care for persons with a wide variety of mental and behavioral problems. For residents and students in health care settings, *Behavioral Medicine: A Guide for Clinical Practice* can function as a valuable resource for understanding the psychosocial dimensions of medicine.

It is our intent that medical educators will find this book to be a clinically relevant text that forms a basis for developing a comprehensive curriculum in behavioral medicine. Training in the core competencies required by the Accreditation Council for Graduate Medical Education (ACGME) will be enhanced by inclusion of topics covered thoroughly in this book, including clinician–patient communication, professionalism, and cultural competence. For faculty and students who wish to explore a topic in greater depth, the suggestions for further reading and web-based resources provided at the end of each chapter will be helpful.

The principles of behavior change discussed in this book apply not only to individuals but also to whole societies as they move through the "stages of change" to alter lifestyles that adversely impact the environment and human health. The health and well-being of our personal lives and of the organizations in which we work are intertwined with the health of our planet. Restoring the proper relationship of humans with the earth in a way that promotes sustainability in the whole system is what Thomas Berry has called "the great work" of our generation. Physicians and other health professionals have a vital role to play in this work, for our own health and well-being will only be as good as the health of the planet.

Acknowledgments

This book would not have been possible without the support and mentorship of several people. We are forever indebted to Stephen J. McPhee, MD, for recognizing the need for such a book and for continually providing encouragement and advice. Our deep appreciation is offered to Jason Satterfield, PhD, and to Ryan Laponis, MD, MS, for their invaluable assistance as associate editors for this edition. We thank Kay Conerly, Kim Davis, James Shanahan, and Leah Carton at McGraw-Hill for providing expert guidance, and we are very grateful to our contributing authors who, despite busy schedules as clinicians, researchers, and educators, have been generous and conscientious in going the distance with us.

Countless friends and colleagues at our own institutions, as well as the residents we have been privileged to teach and mentor, have contributed to our own learning and the selection of material for this book. We are especially indebted to our colleagues in the Society of General Internal Medicine and the American Academy on Communication in Healthcare, many of whom have contributed chapters for this book, for being the learning community that has helped us grow professionally.

Jane Kramer and Julie Burns Christensen and our children, Nina Mason and Jonathan Kramer-Feldman and Jake and Hank Christensen, as well as Hank's wife Kerry, Jake's wife Nancy, Nina's husband Adam, and their son Isaac, have continued to be a renewing and cherished presence in our lives. This book would not have been possible without their love and support.

Mitchell D. Feldman, MD, MPhil, FACP
John F. Christensen, PhD
San Francisco, California and Corbett, Oregon

SECTION I
The Doctor & Patient

The Medical Interview

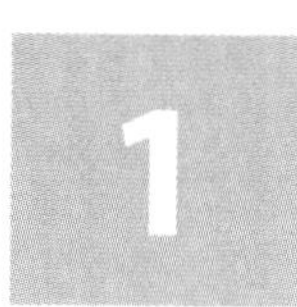

Mack Lipkin, Jr., MD & Antoinette Schoenthaler, EdD

INTRODUCTION

The medical interview is both the major medium of patient care and the core care element for patients and practitioners. A successful interview elicits accurate and complete data. Its dialogue determines whether patients agree to take a medication, undergo a test, actively participate in care, or change their lives. More than 80% of diagnoses are derived from the interview. The doctor–patient interaction is the keystone of patient satisfaction. Interview-related factors impact major outcomes of care, including physiologic responses, symptom resolution, pain control, functional status, propensity to sue in the event of an adverse outcome, and emotional health. The medical interview influences the quality of care, including malpractice suits and their resolution; the amount of patient disclosure of difficult or stigmatized information; time efficiency; and the elimination of "doorknob" questions at interview's end.

Although the interview is a major determinant of professional success, less than 10% of medical practitioners have spent time since medical school working on their interviewing ability. When asked, most physicians indicate that they have no plan or approach to monitoring, maintaining, or improving this critical skill. Can you imagine a professional musician, athlete, or pilot not practicing? One would question their commitment, competence, and chances of remaining successful.

The interview is also key to each practitioner's sense of professional well-being, being the factor that most influences satisfaction with each encounter. Physicians with high career dissatisfaction most often attribute this to unsatisfying communication and relationships with patients. Physicians with high job satisfaction have a significant interest in the psychosocial aspects of care, relate effectively with patients, and are able to manage difficult patient situations.

The Ubiquitous Interview

The central role of the interview derives from its epidemiology as well as its "one-on-one" impact. For most physicians, it is more prevalent than any other activity in their work or their lives. The average length of time per ambulatory patient visit for internists, family practitioners, and pediatricians is about 20 minutes, and these groups account for 75% of doctor visits. The average visit time for *all* physicians is 6 minutes, a rate curiously constant in the United States, the United Kingdom, the Netherlands, and elsewhere. Physicians who bring the average down to 6 minutes are moving scarily fast.

Making conservative estimates about how many hours a practitioner will work over a 40-year professional lifetime, a generalist will have around 250,000 patient encounters. Each interview can be the source of satisfaction or frustration, of learning or apathy, of efficiency or wasted effort, of personal growth and inspiration or dispiriting discouragement (Table 1-1). Despite the importance of performing this complex skill expertly, few trainees or physicians plan, or even contemplate, how to improve patient encounters to reach the desirable goals of satisfaction, learning, and efficiency.

Each discipline or special interest, such as psychiatry, occupational health, women's health, or domestic violence support has a specialized set of questions that must be asked of every patient for the interview to be complete

Table 1-1. Gains from improved interviewing techniques.

- Increased efficiency in use of time
- Increased accuracy and completeness of data
- Improved diagnosis
- Fewer tests and procedures
- Increased compliance
- Increased physician satisfaction
- Increased patient satisfaction
- Decreased dissatisfaction
- Increased mutual learning from each encounter

and to elicit that patient's particular problems. (If an interviewer were to ask every question recommended by each specialty, the interview would take hours.) In most cases, these questionnaires have neither been validated nor shown to be sensitive or specific. Notable exceptions include the CAGE questionnaire (Table 1-2), which is a highly specific, sensitive, and efficient screening test for alcoholism (see Chapter 24); the two-question depression screen (see Chapter 26); and the one-question domestic violence screen (see Chapter 40).

Rather than the use of a series of overspecific, narrowly focused questions, it is more effective to use a patient-centered approach. First, elicit the patient's complete set of concerns and questions. Then explore the priority, *negotiated* problem by asking open- to closed-ended cones of questions to encourage elaboration on the information and elicit the needed data about each concern. Open-ended questions elicit information more efficiently than lists of closed-ended questions. A patient-centered approach ensures that the patient's concerns are understood and accepted—a predictor of increased compliance. Because open-ended questions allow the patient to frame the response, the nature of framing reveals how the patient is processing the issue under discussion, information that is unavailable from closed-ended questions.

This approach is efficient for several reasons. First, patients usually have a sense of what is relevant and will include key information and data not thought of by the interviewer. A physician who is thinking of the next question rather than listening to what is being said loses the ability to attend and to listen on multiple levels. If the interviewer is talking and the patient is not, the flow of data is interrupted. The physician can always elaborate on specific items to round out the data once the patient's story is spontaneously roughed out and framed. If the same format is used for each interview, the variations in responses can be attributed to the patient, providing added insight.

Table 1-2. The CAGE questionnaire.

C: Have you ever tried to **C**ut down on your drinking?
A: Do you feel **A**nnoyed when asked about your drinking?
G: Do you feel **G**uilty about your drinking?
E: Do you ever take an **E**ye opener in the morning?

The evidence favoring a patient-centered approach goes beyond the practical advantages: outcomes of care are also improved. More complete and higher-quality information—with an attendant reduction in procedures and tests—reduces cost, side effects, and complications. Increased patient adherence to diagnostic and therapeutic plans leads to greater clinical efficiency and effectiveness, and patients take a more active role in their own care.

Efficiency & Active Listening

A number of factors enhance interview efficiency, which is increasingly valued as the corporatization, regulation, and digitization of health care cause doctors and patients to experience medical visits as more rushed and cramped. Although actual visit lengths have remained the same, the tasks to accomplish in a given visit have multiplied—more diseases and risks to evaluate, more treatments to choose among and explain, and more computer screens and bureaucratic hoops to negotiate. These trends will undoubtedly prove counterproductive: when the visit is jammed with too much to do, psychosocial discussion drops first. The result is in unnecessary testing, patient dissatisfaction, and hazardous or needless procedures and treatments. Challenges to efficiency and effectiveness are exacerbated when behavioral medicine is removed from the medical visit by outsourcing to an external "behavioral management" company. Then both sides compete not to care for the patient, and predictably the relationship and quality of care deteriorate.

Specific techniques enhance cost-effectiveness and efficiency. Open-ended questions allow patients to elaborate on responses, provide additional information, and make interviews shorter. "Active listening" involves listening to what is said on multiple levels—how it is said; what is included and what is left out; and how what is said reflects the person's culture, personality, mental status, affect, conscious and unconscious motivation, and cognitive style. Getting some or all of this provides layers of time-free rich added data. Active listening also involves acknowledging or repeating the essence of the information shared, whether clinical or emotional, which allows the patient to feel understood and to correct misperceptions. A skilled active listener acquires data quickly and continuously. Like a jazz musician, an active skilled practitioner creates a harmonious flow in sync with the patient's themes, rhythms, and style to enhance the ability of each to contribute to the complex, shifting improvisation of the interview. The experienced listener distinguishes his or her observations as clear data, hypotheses, or biases. This creates a complex and textured portrait of the patient that can be used in generating hypotheses, crafting replies, giving information, managing affective responses and nonverbal behaviors, and questioning further.

THE STRUCTURE OF THE INTERVIEW

Recent literature on the medical interview runs to more than 50,000 articles, chapters, and books. Although only a modest portion of these are derived from empirical studies, sufficient work has been done to describe the interview as having "structure" and "functions." Behavioral observations and detailed, reproducible analyses of interviews have related specific behaviors and skills to both structural elements and functions; performance of these behaviors and skills improves clinical outcomes. The following description of essential structural elements and their associated behaviors or techniques, although comprehensive, is complete yet practical. Key behaviors are summarized in Table 1-3. One comprehensive model of this approach is shown in Figure 1-1.

Preparing the Physical Environment

Architects and designers believe that form follows function. Similarly, how practitioners organize their physical environment reveals core characteristics of their practice: how they view the importance of the patient's comfort and ease; how they want to be regarded; and how they as practitioners control their own environment. Does the patient have a choice of seating? Do both the patient and provider sit at comparable eye level? Is the room accessible, quiet, and private? Optimal environments reduce anxiety and instill calm and a sense of well-being.

Preparing Oneself

Humans can process 7 bits of information plus or minus 2 simultaneously. Given this, it is advisable to consider how many of these bits are consumed by distractions or trivia in a clinical encounter. The hypnotic concept of focus or the recently accepted psychological concepts of centering or flow apply to the clinical encounter (see Chapter 5). Thoughts about the last or next patient, yesterday's mistake, last night's argument, passion, or movie can affect concentration; information and opportunity are lost. In contrast, a focused practitioner, without external or internal distractions, can expect the interview to be a challenging, fascinating, and unique experience.

Achieving a focused state of mind is personal and related to each situation. Nevertheless, successful centering includes eliminating outside intrusion by beepers and phone calls, tuning out extraneous sound, eliminating internal distraction and intrusive thoughts by resolving not to work on other matters, letting intrusive thoughts simply pass through your mind for the moment, and controlling distracting reactions within the interview by noting them, considering their origins, and putting them aside.

Such skills do not just happen. We teach our residents self-hypnosis; practitioners are routinely and efficiently able to get to a place of heightened, alert, and energetic focus. Using this skill together with the suggestions in Table 1-4, practitioners can enhance the opportunity for something profound to happen in each patient encounter.

Observing the Patient

A great deal can be learned by thoughtfully observing the patient's behavior and body language before and during the encounter. Although initial behavioral observations are purely heuristic—used to generate testable hypotheses about the patient—nonverbal behaviors can reveal as much about the patient's state of mind as verbal behavior. Physicians who are unaware of being influenced by initial reactions and observations in the patient interview may note that when they themselves get on a bus or an airplane, they instantly recognize the person next to whom they would prefer—or not—to sit. Such responses integrate multiple nonverbal cues. Similar input from patients relates to their overall health, vital signs, cardiac and pulmonary compensation, neurologic and liver function, and more. Observations about grooming, state-of-rest, alertness, and style of presentation reveal the patient's self-confidence; presence of psychosis, depression, or anxiety; chronic disease; personality style, culture, or subculture; and important changes from prior visits. The physician may also detect signs of possible alcohol or drug use. Escorting patients from the waiting area, letting them walk slightly ahead into the office, allows the physician to observe gait, how patients use their waiting time, companions, and clues to the relationship with companions. Often, especially with new patients, the very first words spoken by the patient may be epigraphic or may foreshadow the encounter.

Maximizing clinical observation skills starts with the commitment to do so. Developing the habit of systematically retaining and integrating initial observations will provide the physician with important data typically overlooked. Asking pertinent questions about behavioral cues will increase observation speed and comprehensiveness. Practicing in crowds, at rounds or lectures, on the airplane, or at parties helps train us to become more astute observers. It is the physician's equivalent of practicing scales on the piano or practicing an athletic stroke.

Table 1-3. Structural elements of the medical interview.

Element	Technique or Behavior
Prepare the environment	Create a private area. Eliminate noise and distractions. Provide comfortable seating at equal eye level. Provide easy physical access.

Prepare oneself	Eliminate distractions and interruptions.
	Focus through:
	  Self-hypnosis
	  Meditation
	  Constructive imaging
	Let intrusive thoughts pass.

Observe the patient	Create a personal list of categories of observation. Practice in a variety of settings. Notice physical signs. Notice patient's presentation and affect. Notice what is said and not said.
Greet the patient	Create a flexible personal opening. Introduce oneself. Check the patient's name and how it is pronounced. Create a positive social setting.
Begin the interview	Explain one's role and purpose. Check patient's expectations. Negotiate about differences in perspective. Be sure your expectations are congruent with patient's expectations.

Detect and overcome barriers to communication	Be aware of and look for potential barriers:
	  Language
	  Physical impediments such as deafness, delirium
	  Cultural differences
	  Psychological obstacles such as shame, fear, and paranoia

Survey problems	Develop personal methods to elicit problems. Ask "what else" until problems are described.
Negotiate priorities	Ask patient for his or her priorities. State your own priorities. Establish mutual interests. Reach agreement on the order of addressing issues.

Develop a narrative thread	Develop personal ways of asking patients to tell their story:
	  When did patient last feel healthy?
	  Describe entire course of illness.
	  Describe recent episode or typical episode.

Establish the life context of the patient	Use first opportunity to inquire about personal and social details. Flesh out developmental history. Learn about patient's support system. Learn about home, work, neighborhood, and safety issues.
Establish a safety net	Memorize complete review of systems. Review issues as appropriate to specific problems.
Present findings and options	Be succinct. Ascertain patient's level of understanding and cognitive style. Ask patient to review and state understanding. Summarize and check. Record interview and give copy of recording to patient. Ask patient's perspectives.
Negotiate plans	Involve patient actively. Agree on what is feasible. Respect patient's choices whenever possible.
Close the interview	Ask patient to review plans and arrangements. Schedule next encounter. Clarify what patient should do in the interim. Say good-bye.

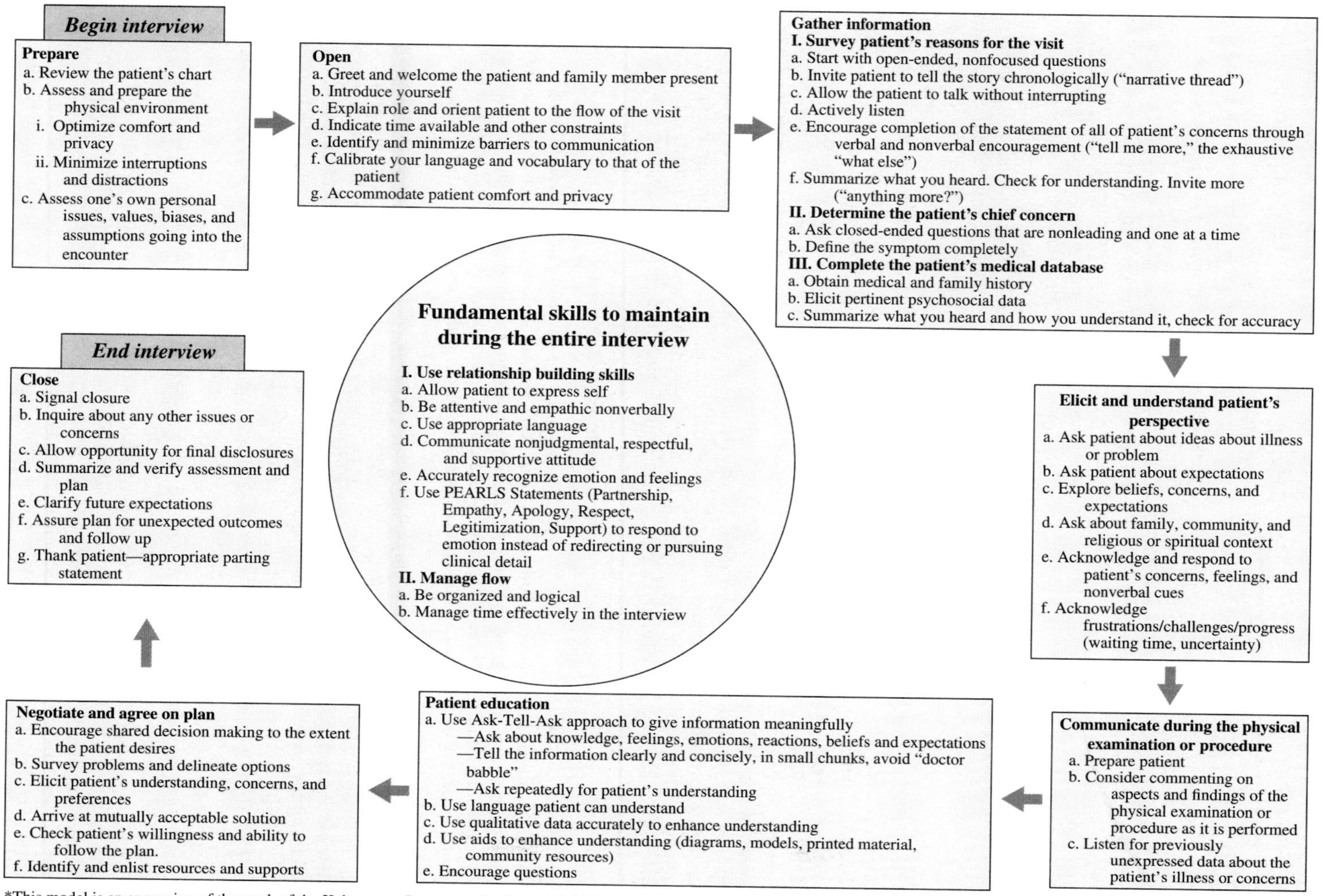

Begin interview

Prepare
- a. Review the patient's chart
- b. Assess and prepare the physical environment
  - i. Optimize comfort and privacy
  - ii. Minimize interruptions and distractions
- c. Assess one's own personal issues, values, biases, and assumptions going into the encounter

Open
- a. Greet and welcome the patient and family member present
- b. Introduce yourself
- c. Explain role and orient patient to the flow of the visit
- d. Indicate time available and other constraints
- e. Identify and minimize barriers to communication
- f. Calibrate your language and vocabulary to that of the patient
- g. Accommodate patient comfort and privacy

Gather information

I. Survey patient's reasons for the visit
- a. Start with open-ended, nonfocused questions
- b. Invite patient to tell the story chronologically ("narrative thread")
- c. Allow the patient to talk without interrupting
- d. Actively listen
- e. Encourage completion of the statement of all of patient's concerns through verbal and nonverbal encouragement ("tell me more," the exhaustive "what else")
- f. Summarize what you heard. Check for understanding. Invite more ("anything more?")

II. Determine the patient's chief concern
- a. Ask closed-ended questions that are nonleading and one at a time
- b. Define the symptom completely

III. Complete the patient's medical database
- a. Obtain medical and family history
- b. Elicit pertinent psychosocial data
- c. Summarize what you heard and how you understand it, check for accuracy

Elicit and understand patient's perspective
- a. Ask patient about ideas about illness or problem
- b. Ask patient about expectations
- c. Explore beliefs, concerns, and expectations
- d. Ask about family, community, and religious or spiritual context
- e. Acknowledge and respond to patient's concerns, feelings, and nonverbal cues
- f. Acknowledge frustrations/challenges/progress (waiting time, uncertainty)

Communicate during the physical examination or procedure
- a. Prepare patient
- b. Consider commenting on aspects and findings of the physical examination or procedure as it is performed
- c. Listen for previously unexpressed data about the patient's illness or concerns

Patient education
- a. Use Ask-Tell-Ask approach to give information meaningfully
  - —Ask about knowledge, feelings, emotions, reactions, beliefs and expectations
  - —Tell the information clearly and concisely, in small chunks, avoid "doctor babble"
  - —Ask repeatedly for patient's understanding
- b. Use language patient can understand
- c. Use qualitative data accurately to enhance understanding
- d. Use aids to enhance understanding (diagrams, models, printed material, community resources)
- e. Encourage questions

Negotiate and agree on plan
- a. Encourage shared decision making to the extent the patient desires
- b. Survey problems and delineate options
- c. Elicit patient's understanding, concerns, and preferences
- d. Arrive at mutually acceptable solution
- e. Check patient's willingness and ability to follow the plan.
- f. Identify and enlist resources and supports

End interview

Close
- a. Signal closure
- b. Inquire about any other issues or concerns
- c. Allow opportunity for final disclosures
- d. Summarize and verify assessment and plan
- e. Clarify future expectations
- f. Assure plan for unexpected outcomes and follow up
- g. Thank patient—appropriate parting statement

Fundamental skills to maintain during the entire interview

I. Use relationship building skills
- a. Allow patient to express self
- b. Be attentive and empathic nonverbally
- c. Use appropriate language
- d. Communicate nonjudgmental, respectful, and supportive attitude
- e. Accurately recognize emotion and feelings
- f. Use PEARLS Statements (Partnership, Empathy, Apology, Respect, Legitimization, Support) to respond to emotion instead of redirecting or pursuing clinical detail

II. Manage flow
- a. Be organized and logical
- b. Manage time effectively in the interview

*This model is an expansion of the work of the Kalamazoo Consensus Conference held May 1999 supported by Bayer-Fetzer; in addition other models were consulted directly. These included the Brown Interview Checklist, the Three Function Model, the work of the AAPP Courses Committee-Blue Card, Segue, Calgary-Cambridge Observation Guide, Bayer model, and an extensive review of the literature on communications in medicine completed for the Macy Initiative. This model has been prepared by the Macy Initiative in Health Communication. Please address questions to Regina Janicik (212) 263-2304.

Figure 1-1. The medical interview. (Developed by the Macy Initiative in Health Communication.)

Table 1-4. Self-hypnotic suggestions to enhance interview outcomes.

In this encounter I will:
Focus on the patient and his or her concerns
Not hear outside distractors
Let intrusive thoughts pass through unheeded
Connect meaningfully with this person
Learn something new and surprising about him or her
Have a positive encounter
Leave feeling energized
Help the patient grow, change, and heal
Help the patient leave the interview feeling hopeful and committed

Greeting the Patient

The greeting serves to identify each person, set the social tone, indicate intentions concerning equality or dominance, and to prevent mistaken identity. It also allows the practitioner to establish an immediate connection with patients, presenting oneself as an open, competent, compassionate professional the patient can trust. It enables the physician to learn how patients assert their own identity and how to pronounce their names. Using a standard greeting—saying virtually the same thing each time—provides data based on the uniqueness of a patient's response.

Beginning the Interview

The introductory phase of a medical encounter provides an opportunity for both parties to express their understanding of the purpose and condition of the encounter, to check each other's expectations, and to negotiate differences. For example, the patient may expect to be seen by the head of the clinic, but the physician is only a year out of residency. The patient wants relief from back pain, and the practitioner is worried about the patient's high blood pressure. The cardiologist expects the consultation to lead to cardiac catheterization, whereas the patient thinks the cardiologist's opinions will be sent to his primary care physician for a discussion prior to decision. Perhaps the physician scheduled a 15-minute visit, but the patient feels an hour is needed.

One of the best predictors of the outcome of a dyadic relationship is concordance of expectations; therefore, clarifying and reconciling these is extremely valuable before proceeding to the main part of the interview.

The beginning of the interview, especially with a new patient, sets the interactional tone (although one can always change tone by changing one's behavior). Although many attempt idle social chat, bland social questions may confuse the professional focus or make the patient feel compelled to present a positive tone. It is useful to consider using a fairly stereotyped beginning, such as "what brings you in to see me today?" (As opposed to "… how may I help you," which prejudges the purpose of the interview).

Detecting & Overcoming Barriers to Communication

Many factors that interfere with communication place even more barriers between the doctor and the patient. Sometimes these are tangible barriers: delirium, dementia, deafness, aphasia, intoxication (patient or physician), or ambient noise. Psychological barriers include depression, anxiety, psychosis, paranoia, and distrust. Social barriers often involve language; cultural differences; and fears about immigration status, stigma, cost of the visit, or legal issues. It is valuable to detect barriers early in an encounter. Failure to do so not only wastes time but can seriously and, sometimes, dangerously mislead the physician. For example, residents and students often spend an hour or more trying to extract history from a delirious patient, resulting in an hour lost and highly unreliable historical data. In addition, detecting barriers is the first step toward correction, whether by waiting until delirium or intoxication has cleared, finding a professional interpreter or signer, moving to a quiet place, or deferring difficult issues until trust is established so disclosure is more complete and accurate.

Surveying Problems

Patients come to medical encounters with multiple problems and, for various reasons, may not lead with the most pressing issue. Physicians typically interrupt very quickly (23 seconds on average). It is of vital importance not to jump in at the first important-sounding problem, but instead to elicit all problems. For example, the physician might ask, "What problems are you having?" or "What issues would you like to work on today?" After getting the initial answer or series of answers, the physician can then ask "… what else?" again and again until the list of problems is completed and mutual priorities are established.

Negotiating Priorities

Once the physician and the patient clearly understand the full set of problems, if the physician then asks, "Which of these would you like to work on first?" and the physician believes that something else is more important than the problem the patient selects, a negotiation about this difference can ensue: "Our time is limited today, and I think your shortness of breath is potentially more dangerous than your back pain. Suppose we deal with that first and, if we have time, go on to your back pain. If not, we'll take that up on your next visit."

Appropriate and understandable resentment results when the physician does not ascertain and acknowledge the patient's priorities. This can lead to treatment adherence problems or failure to return to the office.

Developing a Narrative Thread

Once the physician and the patient have decided which problem has priority, exploration of that problem begins. Note the term "exploration." All too often the clinician's approaches are either to jump into a review of systems ("do you have rectal bleeding ... are your gums bleeding ... ?") or to elicit the seven cardinal features of the sign or symptom ("where is it, does it radiate, what makes it better or worse ... ?" and so on). The most efficient method is to explore the problem by asking the patient to tell the story of the problem using an open-ended question, as in "Tell me about your rectal bleeding." Although many will begin at an appropriate point and move toward the present, some patients may need guidance to begin when the patient last felt healthy, when the current episode began, or when the patient thinks the problem started. The patient may not appreciate the necessary level of detail and may be too inclusive or too superficial. It may be necessary to interrupt to indicate a desire to hear more or less about the problem. Clarifying questions shows the patient what is needed, and most patients respond with the appropriate level of detail.

Establishing the Life Context of the Patient

Once the narrative thread is established, the physician can take the opportunity to inquire about specific points. It is important to respond at the patient's first mention of psychosocial matters in order to signal to the patient that such matters are as important as biotechnical ones. Such inquiries help the physician learn in detail about the context of the patient's life—spouse, family, neighborhood, work, and culture. When enough information has been supplied, simply saying, "You were saying ..." or "What happened next?" returns the patient to the narrative. This approach works because almost everyone knows how to tell a story and remembers key points intrinsically organized by what actually happened.

Creating a Safety Net

Once the problems the patient wishes to discuss have been explored, areas or questions may remain. For these, the physician may choose to ask a series of specific review of systems-type questions. Questions may take the form of the seven dimensions of a complaint, delineated as the location, duration, intensity (use a ten-point scale with zero "no pain at all" and ten "the worst possible pain"), quality, association, radiation, exacerbants and ameliorants, or a subset of these dimensions. Such final closed-ended questions tie up loose ends and provide the safety of completeness.

Talking During the Physical Examination & Procedures

During the physical examination, there is a tension between the quiet focusing of the senses needed to observe, hear, and feel findings, and mutually necessary conversation. Practitioners need their senses of smell, sight, touch, and hearing to examine the patient. They need heightened sensory awareness for the encounter. Patients need an explanation of what is being done and what to expect ("this may hurt"), instruction about what to do ("please sit here" ... "bring up your knees" ... "hold your breath"), and a check on how they are doing and responding ("does this hurt?"). The examination often stimulates the memory of relevant experiences and problems the patient may have forgotten to mention. Some physicians like to explain what is happening in detail ("I am looking in the back of your eye because it is the one place in the body where blood vessels can be seen"). Others do their review of systems during the physical examination. In general, it is wise to minimize distractions during the physical examination or a procedure by confining talk to the task and the needs of the patient. Explanation of findings can be reserved and are more efficient at the end of the examination. However, if there is something big, painful, obvious, or worrisome, common sense may suggest dealing with it in the moment.

Presenting Findings & Options

After the history-taking and physical examination have been completed, it is time for the physician and patient to discuss what the problems or probabilities appear to be, related findings, the physician's hypotheses or conclusions, and possible approaches to further diagnostic evaluation and treatment. This should be done in language free of jargon and at the level of abstraction the patient understands and uses.

Bad news includes any information that will change patients from their idealized self-image to a lesser one. While telling someone she has diabetes may seem routine to a jaded practitioner, to a patient who has heard tough stories about diabetes, or has a relative who died of it, or is simply a fearful person, it is certainly life-altering and might seem disastrous. It is valuable to foreshadow any bad or potentially upsetting news (see Chapter 3). This prepares the patient to hear and retain the information. It may be useful to suggest the patient bring along a trusted companion (although this flags the likely news as bad). When bad news is a certainty, it is useful to record the explanation and discussion for the patient. These days, a digital recorder in the room allows the doctor to provide a copy of the encounter when it ends. The patient can review it after shock has cleared and share it with family or friends. It has been documented that listening to such recordings produces better patient understanding and improves outcomes like quality of life. It is essential not to underestimate the potential impact of both positive and negative findings on the patient. After presenting each item, the physician should explore the patient's understanding and reactions. The presentation itself should be problem-oriented and systematic—and as simple and succinct as possible. Although the dictum is "be brief," necessary content and empathy should not be sacrificed for brevity.

Negotiating a Plan

Once patients have been factually informed of the diagnosis and prognosis, it is crucial to involve them actively in making choices and in developing diagnostic and therapeutic plans. Such "activation" of patients has been shown to increase their adherence to plans and improve their medical outcome and quality of life.

When the physician and the patient disagree in emphasis or choice, negotiation is necessary. The principles of negotiation can be summarized as (1) find and emphasize areas of mutual agreement (e.g., live as long as possible, retain dignity, and avoid suffering), and (2) avoid the adoption of inflexible positions that lead only to conflict, wherein one side or the other loses. If physicians take time to understand patients' positions and respect concerns, issues can usually be worked out. For example, it can be agreed upon to do a procedure after a grandchild's graduation or to do noninvasive tests first with hope they will suffice.

Closing the Interview

The closing should include (1) actively reviewing principal findings, plans, and agreements using a talk back or teach back in which the patient is asked to recall what decisions and recommendations have been made; (2) making arrangements for the next visit and giving patient instructions; (3) making sure outstanding issues have been covered; and (4) saying good-bye. As discussed below, both the physician and patient may review the physician's notes together.

THE FUNCTIONS OF THE INTERVIEW

The three functions of the interview are the major purposes of the interview. Each is associated with skills and behaviors that inform the process and outcome. The three functions are as follows:

- Gathering information and monitoring progress.
- Developing, maintaining, and, sometimes, concluding the therapeutic relationship.
- Educating the patient and implementing a treatment plan.

These goals are interdependent. For example, patients cannot be expected to reveal personal or humiliating information until they develop trust in their physician. The physician cannot educate a patient effectively without knowing what level of abstraction, language, literacy, and explanatory models to employ; which concepts to use; how to frame things for clarity; and which formulations will interpose barriers to acceptance. Therefore, the three functions must be integrated and pursued in parallel rather than sequentially.

Function 1: Gathering Information & Monitoring Progress

Many physicians consider information gathering to be the principal focus of the interview. The tasks associated with this function include acquiring knowledge of the patient's current diseases and disorders as well as psychosocial issues and illness behavior, eliciting data relevant to each problem, and generating and testing relevant hypotheses about what is going on that steer physicians' clinical reasoning. Useful skills include use of open-ended questions such as "Tell me about it" and gradually narrowing the queries down to more specific questions, use of minimal encouragers (i.e., "Uh huh" and "Hmmm") to facilitate flow, gentle use of direction to steer without dominating, and use of summarizing and checking ("I think you have said point a, point b, point c; is that right?").

Function 2: Developing & Maintaining the Therapeutic Relationship

The second function of the interview begins with defining the nature of the relationship (short- or long-term, consultation, primary care, and disease–episode-oriented). It requires demonstrating professional expertise; communicating interest, respect, empathy, and support; recognizing and resolving relational barriers to communication; and eliciting the patient's perspective. A relationship that engenders trust and safety is necessary to being able to gather intimate information and actively involve the patient to make lifestyle changes or difficult medical decisions.

The belief that relationships cannot be improved or manipulated has been disproved by empirical psychotherapy literature. It has been shown that the use of appropriate relationship-building skills significantly improves interview outcomes of satisfaction, compliance, data disclosure, quality of life, biological outcomes, and personal growth. These issues are particularly germane in cases involving mental disorders and someone who is experiencing psychosis (see Chapter 31), where skill in managing the patient in a manner compatible with healing is essential.

In general, naming feelings, communicating unconditional positive regard, expressing empathy and understanding, and being emotionally congruent (what you say is actually what you mean and feel) produce the best outcomes. Other skills include reflection, legitimization, partnership, nonverbal skills of touch and eye contact, use of open posture, and avoidance of shame or humiliation (see Chapter 2).

Function 3: Educating the Patient

Patient education and implementation of treatment plans require an awareness of the patient's level of knowledge, understanding, motivation, and cognitive style; a receptive patient who is neither in shock nor disagreement; and the use of plain language that avoids jargon or undue complexity. Cognitive style includes both the patient's conceptual ability and his or her best understood and most fluent ways of thinking. The tasks associated with this function include communicating the diagnostic significance of the problems; negotiating and recommending appropriate diagnostic and treatment options, appropriate prevention, and lifestyle change recommendations; and enhancing the patient's coping ability by understanding and communicating the psychological and social impacts of the illness. Involving the patient in choices, clarifying uncertainties, and eliciting fears and concerns markedly improve outcomes. Having the patient actively review what has been discussed and decided upon (teach-back) is critical to check for understanding and to reinforce memory, thus maximizing the likelihood that the patient can and will do what has been agreed upon (see Chapter 20).

In some cases, the issue is a high-risk health behavior, habit, or addiction such as overeating, smoking, gambling, or medication nonadherence. Two approaches have been demonstrated to be helpful in such situations: (1) the stages of change model and (2) motivational interviewing (see Chapter 19).

The "Stages of Change Model" described by Prochaska and DiClemente involves ascertaining the patient's stage of readiness for change and adapting one's interaction to the patient's stage. Stages assess whether patients have begun to think about changing behavior (precontemplative vs. contemplative). If they have, then it is appropriate to move forward with an action plan by setting key milestones such as a quit date for smokers. A plan includes discussion of barriers and how to respond when relapse occurs. Acceptance of the notion that change may involve several cycles that eventually lead to success unloads the weight and shame of common first failures, reframes them as learning experiences, and may improve the likelihood and stability of eventual success.

Motivational interviewing is a directive, patient-centered counseling approach designed to motivate people for change by helping them clarify goals, explore perceived barriers to behavior change, and commit to such changes. Motivational interviewing has been used widely for health behavior change in areas such as adherence to behavioral weight control programs, dietary and medication adherence, fruit and vegetable intake, and physical activity. Providing objective feedback about behaviors, acknowledging beliefs, minimizing control, and offering behavioral alternatives have been shown to increase patient self-efficacy and intrinsic motivation to adopt recommended health behaviors. Developed initially for use with addictive behaviors, it uses reflective listening to reframe patients' resistance as self-motivational statements by using such devices as a "readiness ruler," which asks the patient to rate on a scale of 1 to 10 (10 highly and 1 very little) how motivated he or she is to modify the target behavior. Even if the patient ranks motivation to lose weight at 2, leverage can be gained by asking, "Why wasn't that a 1?" and building on whatever slim reeds of motivation are there. This approach subtly shifts the physician and patient from confrontation to partnership.

SPECIAL CIRCUMSTANCES & INTERVIEW MODIFICATIONS

Although the preceding principles are applicable to most situations, some circumstances require a modified approach to maximize the usefulness and durability of the interview. Early detection of special situations is crucial, so that appropriate changes in technique can be made. Most special situations require meticulous attention to the particular needs of the patient; for example, with a paranoid patient the clinician may need to tolerate the patient's need for self-protection and distrust of probing questions.

Aids to Diagnosing Mental Disorders

There are a variety of tools to diagnose and monitor mental disorders. The simplest aids have relatively high sensitivity (they detect most cases) but lower specificity (they pick up cases that do not meet diagnostic criteria). Screening devices for depression include the Patient Health Questionnaire-9 (PHQ-9), Beck, Zung, and Hamilton scales. The PHQ-9 is a nine-question quantitative scoring method with an abbreviated two-question (PHQ-2) screen. It is useful for depression in primary care settings (see Chapter 26). Some physicians administer these with the packet of materials to be filled out prior to each initial visit. As with all questionnaires, however, these carry the time-consuming burden to evaluate false positives. The Primary Care Screen for Mental Disorders (PRIME-MD) was developed (with pharmaceutical company support) to screen for common mental disorders. Reasonably sensitive and specific, it is available for telephone use and for computerized administration. However, empathic physicians have two problems with its use: the program asks about feelings but cannot respond, and scoring takes several minutes. The role for such screening adjuncts is still evolving.

When the Patient Uses Another Language or Is From Another Culture: Using Interpreters & Eliciting Explanatory Models

Everywhere in the United States, practitioners frequently encounter patients whose first or only language is not English and who adhere to cultural beliefs different from the practitioner's own. As a result, patients' health-related behaviors are tied more closely to their own health beliefs than to their physician's advice. Kleinman, Leventhal, and others define a patient's health beliefs, or explanatory model, as the conceptual and behavioral framework patients develop to understand the cause of an illness, its likely course, the meaning of specific symptoms, and the implications of these for treatment and recovery. Patient explanatory models tend to be rooted in the experience of their social network, family, ethnicity, and culture, thus reflecting the way people think about their world, themselves, and their health. Physician explanatory models reflect professional ideologies grounded in their medical training (see Chapter 15). Nonconscious bias can affect how physicians communicate critical medical information, as well as how they are perceived by patients. For example, nonminority physicians' implicit bias is associated with Black patients feeling less satisfied and having more negative impressions of the interaction. Lack of trust stemming from nonconscious bias is associated with reduced medication adherence 16 weeks later. When physicians are able to engage in perspective-taking and exhibit empathy, patients may feel more understood and appreciated, which has been linked to increased patient satisfaction and adherence.

For many patients, health beliefs and values intersect with language and acculturation to form a context of experience and expectation discordant from the biomedical model of disease. Patients whose cultural setting is in transition may be confronted with the need to reconcile (or make sense of) the differences between health beliefs that were commonly held in their original culture and the new ones of their care setting. Table 1-5 provides a question set to elicit a patient's health beliefs. Practitioners need to assess patients' salient health beliefs in order to be sure that their teaching, recommendations, and negotiations are not doomed to failure because the patient's cultural beliefs and values suggest that they are contraindicated or irrelevant. Asking about health beliefs enables one to understand them, adjust one's discussion to reflect and respect the patient's cultural concepts and language, and attain mutual agreement consistent with both patient's and physician's belief systems.

Table 1-5. Questions for eliciting patient explanatory models for problems or symptoms.

What do you call your problem?
What causes your problem?
Why do you think it started when it did?
How does it work—what is going on in your body?
What kind of treatment do you think would be best for this problem?
How has this problem affected your life?
What frightens or concerns you most about this problem?

Reprinted with permission from Johnson TM, Hardt E, Kleinman A. Cultural factors in the medical interview. In: Lipkin M, Putnam SM, Lazare A, eds. *The Medical Interview.* New York, NY: Springer-Verlag; 1995.

Explanatory model differences virtually always arise when the patient is using another language (akin to the Sapir–Whorf hypothesis which postulates that language inextricably influences and guides the attitudes, cultural beliefs, and views of the user). They are magnified by interpreter variability and bias. In general, use of interpreters introduces the likelihood of errors and misunderstandings. Tight control of interpreter use standards is essential. Where possible, use a professional interpreter. Use of a friend or family member raises issues of accuracy and privacy. Remote simultaneous interpretation has the advantages of speed and anonymity, but less adventitious relationship building, compared to telephone support or a person in the room. An interpreter in the room should be positioned behind the patient or out of the patient's sight line to keep the focus between the doctor and patient. Interpreters should provide literal translation, not rephrase or become cultural brokers; however, they can be prompted to let you know when they perceive a cultural miscommunication. Principles and standards of interpretation have been defined by the National Council on Interpreting in Health Care (see "Organizations and Websites" at end of chapter).

Electronic Technology: Gateway or Barrier to Effective Communication?

In today's society, electronic technologies are ubiquitous and becoming increasingly central to daily functions including the medical encounter. With more around the corner, three technologies have already achieved significant presence in the medical encounter: the computer and its associated electronic health record (EHR), the telephone, and electronic communication with patients, such as secure messaging by email and text messaging. Secure video chat is now available on smartphones and computers. Technologies such as telemedicine and telesurgery enable physicians to practice remotely. They evoke conflicting sentiments. Promoters and marketers claim that electronic technology provides greater quality, efficiency, cost-effectiveness, and satisfaction. Detractors claim loss of warmth and touch, depersonalization, detraction from patient-centeredness, wasted time, heightened rigidity in practice, and unjustified costs.

The public (i.e., patients) generally likes technology, finds computers easier or safer to "talk" with than practitioners, and accepts technologies as inevitable and related to quality. Physicians may resist most changes and salutatory shifts, such as moving from a paper to an EHR. Consternation is followed by ambivalent acceptance. Practitioners commonly agree that, on the one hand, EHR use enhances legibility, completeness, sharing of records, and data organization. Patients also appreciate the ability to access and review their physician's consultation notes via a patient portal. On the other hand, it slows the encounter and divides the attention between the patient and computer display. Computers magnify the positive and negative attributes of a physician's communication skills. In general, with a computer in the room, practitioners shift away from patients' psychosocial issues and from patient participation and relationship-building in the medical encounter to more physician-dominated biomedical information giving, history-taking, and attention to computerized note-taking. Increased computer use is associated with longer medical visits, less dialogue between the patient and physician, and lower emotional responsiveness by the physician. How much these impacts alter patient outcomes remains to be proven. So, beware of extravagant claims.

Nevertheless, certain computer-related behaviors seem sensible and can enhance the medical encounter, if utilized properly. EHRs can allow physicians to prepare for the visit prior to the patient's entry, saving time during the interview searching for data. With increasing experience (and commitment), physicians can alternate between talking directly to the patient, with good eye contact and open posture, and making explicit breaks to use the EHR for data entry ("I'm sorry, I need to take a minute to ..."). Physicians can use natural breaks in the encounter, such as when the patient is changing or at the end of the visit, for the majority of typing or dictating using voice recognition software. Physicians can choose to share the screen to enhance collaboration by sharing laboratory results, providing patient education, and showing useful images (where the pathology is, what the procedure will do, dietary portions, etc.). Physicians should avoid typing while the patient is talking, since nonverbal cues will be missed and patients will often interpret too great a focus on the computer as a sign of not caring.

An important, ongoing large-scale study (OpenNotes) examines the impact of sharing EHR records with patients. Preliminary findings indicate that such transparency helps patients feel more in charge of their care, promotes increased adherence to treatment plans, reduces content errors, shifts the patient–physician relationship toward greater trust and partnership, and has little adverse impact on the physician's work life. It will take time, however, to understand if and how sharing visit notes affects outcomes and the efficiency of care.

The telephone is not new; it remains a core means of contact between the physician and patient, accounting for as much as 25% of interactions. Use of telephones has extended beyond requests for prescription refills and laboratory results. Phones are now used by practitioners for reminders, monitoring chronic care, delivering manualized treatments, screening, and data transmission from in-home instruments. Phone answering systems are now emblematic of depersonalization, with patients and physicians frustrated by attempts to reach practitioners behind the unbreachable, automated moat of "Please listen to the following options, as they have changed."

Talking with a patient on the phone is rather like looking at a photograph in black and white instead of color. The phone (although it may soon include video) removes the ability to observe nonverbal cues (including lip reading) and forces both parties to listen more, making it possible to hear more. This a-visual quality can be beneficial, especially with patients whose physicality is distracting, but it may be at the expense of nonverbal cues.

Increasingly, physicians are using telephone visits for assessment of acute problems, usefully triaging who should come in urgently, who can wait for the next available appointment, and all options in between. This can save lives, for example, by recognizing an urgent red flag symptom or sign requiring immediate ER intervention or surgery not recognized by the patient. It can prevent ER visits and interventions. A primary care physician who knows her patients well can better interpret the significance of ambiguous complaints than a stranger physician in an emergency room.

Mobile phones extend access and usability further, including texting and image-sharing capabilities. With mobile phone technology, an urgent care visit can be completed virtually through video capabilities, enhancing the ability to provide anytime, anywhere care. Secure text-messaging also offers a means for consistent communication with patients, particularly during times when close monitoring is necessary including when prescribing opioids for pain (see Chapter 25). Mobile technology evidently adds an efficient, safe, private, and cost-effective method for delivery of patient-centered care, but its exact role remains to be evaluated rigorously.

While patient acceptance of and satisfaction with email is high, use of email between physicians and patients remains low. Patient barriers include literacy, computer access, language (if discordant), and comfort with writing skills. Physicians resist email out of fear that it will become intrusive, pose a nonreimbursed time sink, be mistaken for real contact in an emergency, enable patients to avoid reimbursable visits, deny the opportunity for verbal interaction and physical examination, and make the physician accountable 24/7 with a permanent written record. However, many of these perceptions are unfounded. The majority of patients send an average of one email per day and perceive their physician to be more accessible and informed of their individual health care needs when email is used. More importantly, email messages do not totally eradicate the psychosocial and emotional quality of communication. Patients display higher levels of engagement and attentiveness to detail in their email messages than in actual visits. Most physicians tend to exhibit curtness on email, with a majority of the content focused on information giving. As a consequence, it is easier to forget to match language level with the patient when writing in a medium most often used with peers.

Electronic communication such as email and text messaging communication must follow HIPAA (Health Insurance Portability and Accountability Act) guidelines. Patients should be aware of the risks associated with email and text and informed how confidentiality and privacy will be ensured. Each patient should consent to email/text use. Email and text messages should be encrypted and follow authoritative published guidelines.

Screening for & Discussing Social Determinants of Health

There is growing sentiment among some health care providers that addressing patients' medical needs is insufficient to reduce health inequities, which must be addressed to improve patient's health and well-being. To do so requires the practitioner to identify and address social and structural constraints on patients' health behaviors, using methods to screen and address social determinants of health (SDoH) in clinical practice. Less emphasized but equally important is the development of best practices in how to discuss or address unmet social needs with patients. Social needs such as food insecurity, homelessness, and poverty are sensitive and potentially humiliating topics. Once best practices are empirically established, providers will need guidance and training in communication skills to optimize patients' comfort and trust to talk openly about such unmet social needs.

Relationship-centered communication strategies that can be helpful in introducing SDoH screening tools include conveying respect when introducing the topic (e.g., by positioning oneself at the patient's eye level and attending to the patient's privacy), normalizing the topic ("Many people find it hard to talk about…"), asking permission ("Would it be ok if we discussed…"), and expressing appreciation for sharing information about SDoH ("I appreciate your willingness to talk with me about your experiences at home and at work..."). Doing so can decrease shame and increase patient self-disclosure. Asking patients which social needs they want immediate assistance with also demonstrates respect for patients' autonomy and helps patients prioritize while helping the care team focus on needs that are of immediate importance to patients.

SUMMARY

The medical interview is the most commonly used diagnostic and therapeutic procedure in medicine. As such it deserves continued attention and skill enhancement throughout a clinician's professional career. The quality of the clinician–patient encounter, patient satisfaction, the accuracy and completeness of data, patient adherence to treatment regimens, health outcomes, and clinician satisfaction are all influenced by a skillful approach to the medical interview. Attention to both the structure and functions of the interview provides a framework for developing mastery. It also will ensure that the core relationship between the physician and patient remains at the center of all advancements in medicine, including the new technologies of electronic communication and information management.

SUGGESTED READINGS

Delbanco T, Walker J, Bell SK, et al. Inviting patients to read their doctors' notes: a quasi-experimental study and a look ahead. *Ann Intern Med* 2012;157(7):461–470.

Delbanco T, Walker J, Darer J, et al. OpenNotes: doctors and patients signing on. *Ann Intern Med* 2010;153:121–125.

Duffy DF, Gordon GH, Whelan G, et al. Assessing competence in communication and interpersonal skills: the Kalamazoo II report. *Acad Med* 2004;79:495–507.

Frankel R, Altschuler A, George S, et al. Effects of exam-room computing on clinician–patient communication: a longitudinal qualitative study. *JGIM* 2005;20:677–682.

Garg A, Boynton-Jarrett R, Dworkin PH. Avoiding the unintended consequences of screening for social determinants of health. *JAMA* 2016;316:(8)813–814.

Haidet P. Jazz and the art of medicine: improvisation in the medical encounter. *Ann Fam Med* 2007;5:164–169.

Lipkin M, Putnam SM, Lazare A, eds. *The Medical Interview: Clinical Care, Education, and Research*. New York, NY: Springer-Verlag; 1995.

Rao JK, Anderson LA, Inui TS, Frankel RM. Communication interventions make a difference in conversations between physicians and patients. *Med Care* 2007;45:340–349.

Roter DL, Larson S, Sands DZ, et al. Can e-mail messages between patients and physicians be patient-centered? *Health Commun* 2008;23:80–86.

Ventres W, Kooienga S, Marlin R, et al. Clinician style and examination room computers: a video ethnography. *Fam Med* 2005;37:276–281.

Walker J, Leveille S, Ngo L, et al. Inviting patients to read their doctors' notes: patients and doctors look ahead. *Ann Intern Med* 2011;155:891–899.

OTHER RESOURCE

Novack DH, Clark W, Saizow R, et al, eds. *Doc.com: An Interactive Learning Resource for Healthcare Communication*. American Academy on Communication in Healthcare http://www.doccom.org. Accessed September 2018.

ORGANIZATIONS & WEBSITES

American Academy on Communication in Healthcare. www.aachonline.org. Accessed September 2018.

American Medical Association (AMA). Electronic Communication with Patients. https://www.ama-assn.org/delivering-care/electronic-communication-patients. Accessed September 2018.

The Foundation for Medical Excellence. https://tfme.org/. Accessed September 2018.

Motivational Interviewing Network of Trainers. https://motivationalinterviewing.org/. Accessed September 2018.

National Council on Interpreting in Health Care. http://www.ncihc.org. Accessed September 2018.

VIDEOS

Video 1-1. Agenda Setting (2 min, 44 sec)

Video 1-2. Time Efficiency in Clinical Communication (8 min, 40 sec)

Access by scanning the QR code above or visit mhprofessional.com/feldman5evideos.

Empathy

2

Auguste H. Fortin VI, MD, MPH

"I've learned that people will forget what you said, people will forget what you did, but people will never forget how you made them feel."

Maya Angelou

INTRODUCTION

Empathy is a key therapeutic component of clinician–patient interactions and leads to improved patient experience, health outcomes, and decreased clinician burnout. The absence of expressed empathy in clinicians is associated with longer visits and increased risk of malpractice claims. Exactly what empathy is, however, is debated. There are many, sometimes contradictory, definitions in the literature. This may arise from the provenance of this concept, which stems the late nineteenth century, when it described the feeling that a building or artwork can evoke in a person. Only later did the term enter into the field of medicine. More recently, the concept has received renewed attention from a wide spectrum of health practitioners, educators, and the public, which regard empathy as a means to restore compassion and humanism to the clinician–patient relationship (I and Thou), a relationship that has become increasingly impersonal (I and It) because of technology and financial pressures.

While academics debate whether empathy is a cognitive or affective state, an attitude or a behavior, patients increasingly expect it and clinicians increasingly recognize its importance in their interactions. We define empathy as the capacity to understand another person's emotional state, the ability to communicate this understanding, and the desire to be of service to that person. Research suggests that empathy skills can be taught. This chapter will describe how to develop and improve these skills; we will begin by exploring the roots of empathy.

What Is Required to Express Empathy?

Clinical empathy requires certain attitudes, knowledge, and skills. The most important attitude is the recognition that to be a patient is an emotional experience. When clinical work becomes routine or hectic, clinicians can forget this truth and neglect to attend to the patient's emotions, focusing instead on the biomedical tasks at hand. Empathic clinicians try to imagine what it might be like to be the patient; they make it one of their duties to consider the patient's emotional reaction to illness and respond to it. These clinicians care *about* their patients, not just *for* them.

The knowledge domain of empathy includes understanding that many patients offer clues to their emotions, that is, they put their emotion, or at least a hint of it, "on the table"; the clinician merely needs to recognize these clues. Some patients, however, may not express their emotions, but this does not mean that they do not have an emotion to discover and respond to. Because clinicians often have a strong "curative need," that is, the desire to fix problems in their patients (or avoid them if they seem unfixable), it is also important for them to know that patients do not want them to fix everything that they tell them. Many personal and emotional problems cannot be fixed by clinicians, at least in the short term. The tool that clinicians *can* use is empathy—witnessing to the suffering of another human being and, by that witnessing, lighten the burden of it.

In this chapter, we will generally use *emotion* to describe both emotions and feelings. The patient can express *feelings* verbally (e.g., "I was upset"), and/or *emotions* nonverbally (e.g., depressed face and slumped shoulders) or by acting them out (e.g., crying). Paul Ekman identified 15 distinct emotions that can be read from a person's face: amusement, anger, contempt, contentment, disgust, embarrassment, excitement, fear, guilt, pride in achievement, relief, sadness/distress, satisfaction, sensory pleasure, and shame. Feelings, being the conscious, subjective experience of emotion, are much more nuanced and numerous. For example, a patient nonverbally expressing the emotion sadness may say s/he is feeling abandoned, alienated, appalled, bad, betrayed, blamed, blue, etc.

The primary skills of empathy are (1) recognizing when an emotion is being displayed (verbally or nonverbally), (2) helping the patient to express the emotion(s), and (3) seeking to understand the emotion and expressing that understanding by responding with nonverbal and verbal empathy. Many clinicians feel unskilled in assessing and empathically responding to emotion; these skills are addressed below.

BARRIERS TO EMPATHY & OVERCOMING THEM

As mentioned above, empathy involves three components: understanding, communicating the understanding, and an intending to help. The clinician need not have had the same experience to express empathy. Sympathy, on the other hand, is having the same emotional response as the patient or family member, usually emerging from discomfort that is relieved by helping the patient/family member. Both are legitimate forms of affective expression. Empathy is more under conscious control and essentially allows the patient to have and express his/her emotion while the clinician is a witness or nonanxious presence to the patient's suffering. Some clinicians worry that empathy will turn to sympathy and that, in experiencing the patient's emotion, they are being unprofessional. On the contrary, experiencing strong emotions often accompanies working with people in need; these opportunities to bear empathic witness can evoke feelings of gratitude in clinicians and can be an important source of professional meaning and satisfaction.

Eliciting and empathizing with emotions provokes anxiety in some clinicians, for example, raising fears about harming patients or of being intrusive. Patients know how to protect themselves and they usually are forthright when they do not want to engage in a line of conversation. Indeed, most patients feel supported and relieved when they are allowed and encouraged to express emotion. Clinicians must guard against the understandable impulse to shut them down or change the subject and instead draw on the attitudes, knowledge, and skills discussed above.

There are additional barriers that clinicians and patients face to discussing emotions (Table 2-1), from the impersonal office setting to the disinclination of both clinician and patient to address particularly sensitive topics. Nonetheless, appropriate skilled communication can break through these barriers.

Understanding the feelings, attitudes, and experiences of the patient is the first step toward a more effective therapeutic alliance. Many patients, however, may not be skilled in revealing their feelings to their providers. They need to be made aware that their clinician is interested in their feelings and values them, and that feelings are a legitimate topic for discussion in a medical interview.

Table 2-1. Barriers to discussing emotions.

Clinician
1. Takes too much time
2. Too draining
3. Will lose control of interview
4. Cannot fix patient's distress
5. Not my job
Patient
1. Cultural taboo about discussing emotions
2. Preference for interpreting distress in a biomedical model
3. Somatization disorder
4. Desire to meet doctor's expectations
5. Worry about being emotionally overwhelmed
6. Lack of language for emotions

Emotions can be difficult for both clinicians and patients, and clinicians, in particular, may prefer the certainty of science. From the patient's point of view, if difficult emotional issues are manifested as a somatic complaint, denial might be the first reaction to a psychological interpretation of the symptoms. The clinician must appreciate and mirror the terms in which a patient will speak about illness. In many cultures, emotions are simply not discussed. In the United States, where the biomedical model of disease still predominates over the biopsychosocial model in some areas of medicine, patients may feel that it is more acceptable to have physical rather than emotional complaints. Because this expectation is often reinforced by their clinician, it is important to establish a climate conducive to the expression of emotional material and a language useful to that end.

Clinicians often mention the following barriers to discussing emotions with patients.

1. **It takes too much time.** In a busy practice, concerns about time are legitimate. Given an organized framework, however, it takes only a few moments to engage effectively with emotion, and the strategies discussed later in this chapter can prove time efficient. Recent studies suggest that interviews in which physicians respond to emotions may actually be shorter than those in which they do not. An explanation of this finding is that it may be more time consuming to deal with the indirect effects of unaddressed emotions during the rest of the interview. Moreover,

it may be useful to distinguish between "acute efficiency" and "chronic efficiency." "Efficiency" should take into consideration not only the duration of a particular visit but also the total amount of time required to address the patient's concerns. Even if it were to take a few extra minutes to address emotions, that time is more than compensated by fewer phone calls and fewer unscheduled visits.

2. **It is too draining.** It is unrealistic to expect all clinicians to be emotionally available to all of their patients at all times. A clinician who has been awake all night or is emotionally needy may be justified in putting off a discussion of emotions. If the clinician chooses to defer, it would be wise to return to the topic at another time. Clinicians sometimes exert much energy avoiding emotions in the belief that dealing directly with them will be draining. However, it can be far more efficient and satisfying to make an emotional connection than to resist it.

   At times, patients may inadvertently raise issues that are emotionally difficult for the clinician. Sometimes the clinician can discuss the difficulty with friends, family, or colleagues; at other times it may be most fruitfully addressed in the clinician's own therapy. These "difficult" encounters with patients may offer the opportunity for personal growth (see Chapter 4).
3. **The visit will get out of control.** Although many clinicians worry that addressing emotions will cause feelings to escalate, the opposite is usually true. Addressing emotions often helps diffuse them. Learning a language to address emotions creates a comfortable distance from the emotions themselves, so that neither the clinician nor the patient becomes overwhelmed.
4. **I cannot fix it for the patient.** Clinicians are used to "fixing" things. Feelings, however, simply exist, and cannot be "fixed." Patients do not expect their feelings to be eliminated; they just want them to be understood. When a patient keeps returning with the same complaint, unimproved by a clinician's interventions, the patient is trying to communicate a message. Clinicians are often frustrated by these patients; this frustration can be alleviated and the provider's satisfaction improved by the progress that comes with addressing the underlying emotion.

THE ROLE OF EMPATHY IN DIAGNOSIS

Some patients consistently elicit dislike and rejection from their providers. It may seem that the patient is intentionally trying to manipulate the provider into becoming angry or to reject them. When clinicians become aware of these feelings, they should consider the possibility that their own negative feelings may be playing into the patient's self-image as deserving of rejection or punishment. This pattern may be consistent with a personality disorder (see Chapter 30).

The clinician's experience does not invariably reflect the patient's experience. Rather, clinicians should notice their own feelings and ask, "Does the way I feel tell me something about the patient or something about myself?" For example, a clinician who has recently seen a number of drug-seeking patients may begin to feel angry and defensive on noticing that the nurse has recorded "low back pain" as the next patient's chief concern; these negative feelings indicate more about the clinician's recent experiences than they do about the next patient. Feelings are primary data about the person in whom they arise and indirect data about others. The next section clarifies how to test the hypothesis that a patient is feeling a particular emotion and outlines how to respond.

THE THERAPEUTIC LANGUAGE OF EMPATHY

Although empathy is not generally considered a therapeutic tool, discussion of emotional issues can be therapeutic. An empathic relationship is crucial in psychotherapy and enhances the power of all therapeutic relationships. The following sections show how to elicit and talk about emotions using specific skills. A premise of this discussion is that biomedical aspects of disease cannot be effectively addressed without considering their emotional consequences. Emotions, whether related to physiological dysfunction or psychosocial issues, color the discussion in the exam room, and may be so distracting that the patient cannot fully concentrate on other issues until the emotions are addressed.

A clinical scenario helps to illustrate the usefulness of the empathy skills described in this section.

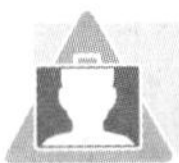

CASE ILLUSTRATION 1

While you are on call, a 45-year-old man is admitted to the hospital because of concern that a 2-week history of chest pain may represent unstable angina. Although the emergency room physician acknowledges that it is a "soft admission," the patient has a history of elevated lipids, a family history of cardiac disease, and his blood pressure in the emergency room is 180/95. The patient describes a sharp substernal chest pain that occurs at rest, when working in the yard, and while trying to fall asleep at night. He does not smoke or have diabetes. On examination, he appears anxious, his blood pressure on the cardiac floor is 160/90, and he is 5% over ideal body weight. The rest of his examination, laboratory tests, electrocardiogram, and chest X-ray are normal, except for his low-density lipoprotein cholesterol, which is 160 mg/dL.

You greet the patient with outstretched hand:

Doctor: *Good morning, Mr. Swenson, my name is Dr. Bergen. I'll be taking care of you while you're in the hospital.*

Patient: *(Anxiously) Well, Doctor, am I having a heart attack?*

Doctor: *You haven't had a heart attack. I can tell from your blood tests and electrocardiograms.*

Patient: *Well is the pain coming from my heart?*

Doctor: *I don't think so.*

Patient: *But you're not sure?*

Doctor: *Well, your age, the character of your pain, and the fact that antacids help reassure me that the problem is most likely acid indigestion or muscular pain.*

Patient: *Don't you think we should do more tests to be sure?*

Doctor: *Although you are at low risk for having heart disease, I would like to do an exercise stress test as an outpatient just to be sure.*

Patient: *What if I have a heart attack in the meantime? I'm still worried.*

Doctor: *You don't need to be. Besides, you were admitted under "observation status" to make sure you didn't have an unstable heartcondition, and we have done that. By standard protocols, you fall into the low-risk category, and your insurance will not allow you to remain an inpatient for further risk stratification. Don't worry, you'll be all right.*

Patient: *Well, okay, if you say so.*

Despite a diagnosis of noncardiac chest pain, providing good information, and attempts to reassure the patient, something goes awry in this interaction. The patient still does not seem satisfied. Let us look at the effect that eliciting the patient's emotion and responding with empathy might have.

Getting Emotion on the Table

Some patients will spontaneously name the emotion they are feeling, but many patients instead express clues to their emotions, as if testing the waters with their clinician, seeing if they can share the impact of their illness on their daily lives and emotions. A study by Levinson, et al., conducted in primary care and in surgical practices showed that this occurred in about half of office visits and in those visits, patients gave about two clues. Unfortunately, physicians responded to a minority of these clues (38% of surgical cases and 21% of primary care cases). Importantly, visits tended to be longer when physicians missed opportunities to express empathy.

Table 2-2. Skills to get emotion "on the table."

Skill	Example
Reading the emotion	"You seem upset."
Direct inquiry	"How is this for you?"
Indirect inquiry	
Impact	"How has this been affecting your day-to-day life?"
Beliefs/attributions	"What do you think might be causing your [symptom]?"
Triggers	"What led you to come in *today* for your [symptom]?"
Intuiting how the patient might be feeling	"I can imagine that this might be worrying for you."

Sometimes patients do not offer clues about the personal or emotional impact of their illness experience but this does not mean that there is no emotion under the surface. The clinician has several options to help get the emotion out in the open. We will present these in general order of our preference for their use (Table 2-2).

Reading the Emotion

The patient's emotion may be easily interpreted from facial expression and other nonverbal cues. It is then appropriate to state the emotion, for example, "You seem sad as you tell me this." The patient will often respond by naming a more nuanced feeling, giving the clinician deeper understanding, which is key to allowing an empathic response.

Direct Inquiry

When it seems clear that the patient could well be expected to have an emotion because what s/he is describing, asking about how the patient is feeling is a highly effective skill. One can ask, for example, "How is this for you?" or "How does this make you feel?" or "How are you doing with this, emotionally?" or "What emotions does this bring up for you?"

Indirect Inquiry

When directly asking about emotions is ineffective, the clinician can often get to the emotion by inquiring in one or more areas:

Impact: One can inquire indirectly about emotion by asking about the impact of the illness on the patient's or the family's life: "How has your back pain affected your day-to-day life?" or "How has your wife's death affected your daughter?"

Beliefs/Attributions: Asking what the patient thinks caused the problem is not only helpful for understanding the patient's medical explanatory model but it may also uncover an underlying feeling or emotion, particularly if the patient believes that a serious condition may be causing the symptom.

Triggers: Determining why the patient is seeking care at this precise time, especially if the problem has been present for more than a few days, can uncover the underlying reason for the visit and provide a window into the patient's feelings and emotions ("What made you decide to see me today for this [symptom]?"). Another common trigger that can lead to emotional expression is personal or interpersonal crisis. When people are in crisis they are worried and distressed, which increases their sensitivity to pain and awareness of bodily symptoms. They often do not make the link between their stress and their symptoms. Asking, "What else is going on in your life?" can uncover the distress and allow for expression of feelings and emotions.

INTUITING HOW THE PATIENT MIGHT BE FEELING

Sharing how the clinician or others might feel in similar circumstances can help the patient identify her or his own emotions and feelings ("I think if that happened to me I would feel upset."). Avoid strong affective terms like "angry" or "depressed" because the patient may not feel comfortable endorsing them; instead use less intense terms like "upset," "unhappy," or "frustrated." If a patient describes a situation that clearly hints at an emotion without clearly naming one, the clinician can express your intuition with a statement like, "I get the sense that this might have been difficult for you." In using this technique, say "might" or "could," rather than "must," in order to encourage the patient to express his/her actual feeling, rather than feeling coerced to validate your inaccurate but strongly presented guess. For example, if one were to say, "You must be very scared about this," the patient may believe that s/he *should* be scared. Better to say, "I can imagine that this might be worrying for you." or "The idea that your neighbor died of the same disease could be worrying." Nevertheless, if the clinician guesses that the patient would have felt worry, but s/he actually felt anger, s/he will likely offer a correction. It is perfectly acceptable (and perhaps preferable) to treat the emotion as having a differential diagnosis and test a hypothesis as one would for any other medical entity: "It seems that you're feeling something strongly, but I'm not sure what it is. Can you help me out?"

Using feelings that arise in the provider during an encounter may be useful in intuiting how the patient might be feeling. For example, a doctor who feels burdened, heavy, or "down" during an interview might consider the possibility that the patient is depressed.

All clinicians have had the experience of trying to help a patient with a behavior change, such as weight loss, only to have each suggestion rejected: "I've already tried that, Doc; it doesn't work." The clinician's own feelings of frustration and powerlessness in trying to motivate the patient are often mirrored by the patient's sense of frustration and powerlessness in attempting to accomplish the change in behavior. The clinician can confirm the hypothesis that the patient is frustrated, as with any other diagnosis, by testing: "I'm feeling frustrated with this problem, and I'm wondering if you're feeling the same way."

Once emotion is "on the table" the clinician should ensure understanding of it by asking for clarification, for example, "Say more about that." or "Tell me more about feeling worried." Avoid asking "why", such as, "Why are you worried?" because the patient may feel the need to defend his/her emotion. The deeper understanding that comes from seeking clarification allows for the communication of precise and effective empathy.

Responding With Empathy

Many if not most clinicians feel an emotional resonance with their patients' suffering, but their response is either an often-futile attempt to "fix" the emotion, or they simply don't know how to respond to the emotion in a helpful way. Empathy skills are behaviors that demonstrate empathy. They are among the clinician's most powerful therapeutic tools. Empathy skills can be nonverbal or verbal and can be expressed by allowing respectful silence, softening the tone of one's voice and moving closer to the patient. Other examples of nonverbal empathy are handing the tearful patient a tissue or respectful touching of the patient. In judging whether touching will be perceived as supportive, invasive, or inappropriate, the clinician should consider such factors as culture, age, gender, sexual orientation, trauma history, and the presence or absence of psychiatric symptoms, such as paranoia. In general, putting a hand on the patient's hand or arm will not be misinterpreted. Many clinicians prefer taking the lead from the patient by matching the patient's nonverbal behavior.

Nonverbal empathy, while important, is often insufficient to make the patient feel understood; verbally expressing understanding of the patient's emotional situation and one's desire to be of service can be powerfully therapeutic. We have all experienced the gratitude of patients, isolated by depression or family loss, for our expression of understanding of their sadness. We recommend the mnemonic "NURS" to help clinicians frame

Table 2-3. The empathy skills.

Skill	Example
Naming	"You're worried."
Understanding	"I can understand your anger with the callous way you were treated."
Respecting	"This has been a difficult time for you" or "You are doing very well handling your grief."
Supporting	"Perhaps we can work together to make you feel better."

empathic responses: *n*aming, *u*nderstanding, *r*especting, and *s*upporting (Table 2-3). Using all four in order is effective in communicating empathy with patients but they can also be used singly or in pairs every time the patient expresses an emotion.

Naming the Feeling/Emotion

To name the feeling or emotion, one simply reflects back the feeling expressed by the patient, "You felt sad" or the emotion one observes, "You look a little teary-eyed."; the result of this reflective naming is that the patient feels heard. For example, when a patient greets a doctor who is 20 minutes late with, "My time is as valuable as yours," the doctor might say, "I'm sorry I'm late. You seem pretty angry with me." The patient might then ventilate about the doctor's lateness or his treatment at the hands of doctors. He might even deny his anger, since many patients might view an expression of anger at their physicians as unacceptable. In any case, the doctor has a chance to deal with the emotion directly and then proceed with the interview, rather than trying to work with a patient who is angry and has not had a chance to express his anger.

After naming an emotion, one should stop talking and see how the patient responds. Although the patient will usually elaborate, if the clinician keeps talking the exploration may be prematurely ended.

Understanding

An "understanding" statement acknowledges that the patient's emotional reaction is comprehended: "Given what you told me it makes sense to me that you'd feel this way" or "I can sure see why." or "I get it; that makes sense to me." These statements legitimize, accept, and validate the patient's expressed emotion, making the patient feel less isolated. For example, to a somatizing patient who has been to several doctors to find a cause for her abdominal pain, the clinician might say, "I can understand how frustrating it's been to be no better after seeking so much help." Some clinicians are reluctant to validate emotions in difficult patients for fear of adding fuel to the fire. If Naming is the empathy skill that opens Pandora's Box, then Understanding is the skill that closes it—it is difficult to remain upset with a person who understands how you feel. Communicating one's understanding of the patient's feelings creates a "shared presence," emphasizing that the patient and clinician are equals in the human condition, although they have different roles in the therapeutic relationship.

One need not have had the same experiences to understand the patient's emotion; understanding usually arises from seeking clarification of the stated feeling: "I've never had that happen, but I can see how that would scare you."

Respecting (praising or appreciating the patient and/or acknowledging their situation)

Respecting may feel like the least natural of the NURS statements. Respect statements show appreciation for the patient's sharing ("Thanks for being so open"), acknowledge the patient's plight ("You've really been through a lot"), or praise the patient's efforts ("I appreciate the way you've hung in there with all of this").

Clinicians may not always know what it would be like to be the patient, but they can respect the patient's experience nonetheless: "I'm not a parent, so I can only imagine what it would be like to lose a child. I can see you're feeling the loss quite deeply."

Supporting

Supporting statements signal to the patient that s/he is not alone and that the clinician is prepared to work with the patient as a partner; for example, "I want you to know that I'm here for you", or "I'm here to help in any way I can."

An advantage of supportive partnership is that it may help motivate patients to take an active role in their own care and may lay the foundation for a contract for behavior change. This is consistent with the notion, especially when illness results from patient behaviors, that clinicians facilitate the patient's healing rather than curing disease in the passive patient. The clinician's use of the pronouns *we* and *us* expresses supportive partnership, as in "Perhaps we can make a plan to help you feel better" or "Let's figure out a way to help you deal with this difficult diagnosis."

Although it is often helpful to use Naming, Understanding, Respecting, and Supporting statements in order when first addressing emotion, these skills can be used throughout the encounter singly and in any order.

Brief Vignette Using NURS Quartet

Patient: (Has just indicated feeling lonely since his dog died)

Clinician: So, this been a pretty lonely time for you. [Naming]

We grieve all our losses—dogs as well as people. It makes sense to me. [Understanding]

This has been a tough time for you. [Respecting]

Sometimes it helps to talk about it. [Supporting]

Patient: It does feel better. I was embarrassed to mention it to anyone else.

This quartet of statements can be powerfully therapeutic. After "NURS"ing the emotion, patients may tear up and say, "No one else knows about this" or "I'm feeling better already." The positive impact on the clinician's sense of professional meaning in these moments can be profound.

Empathy does not equal agreement. Rather, one is expressing one's understanding and appreciation of the patient's point of view and situation. For example, to a patient requesting unwarranted opioids the clinician might say, "I understand why you'd be angry since you came in today expecting that I would prescribe you the oxycodone." Being willing to imagine what it must be like for these more challenging patients can provide us with insights into what motivates them or what might help them. That is diagnostic information. Communicating that insight may encourage patients to change their behavior, and that is therapeutic.

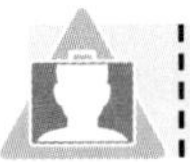

CASE ILLUSTRATION 1 (CONTD.)

Let us return now to the scenario of the 45-year-old man with chest pain to see how that interaction might be improved with a physician who uses empathy skills. The empathy skills used are listed in parentheses.

Doctor: *Good morning, Mr. Swenson, my name is Dr. Bergen. I'll be taking care of you while you're in the hospital.*

Patient: *(Anxiously) Well, Doctor, am I having a heart attack?*

Doctor: *You sound worried. (naming)*

Patient: *Wouldn't you be worried if you thought you were working up to a heart attack?*

Doctor: *I certainly would be. (understanding)*

Patient: *That's what happened to my father. He was raking leaves and just keeled over. I'm the one who found him.*

Doctor: *That must have been so difficult. (respecting)*

Patient: *You can't imagine how awful it was. Every time I think of it, I get upset. Sometimes it even brings on this chest pain. I've been thinking about him more and more lately, especially when I go to sleep at night. It makes me afraid to fall asleep. I'm afraid I'm not going to wake up.*

Doctor: *Say more about feeling afraid. (naming, seeking clarification)*

Patient: *I thought I got over his death. But this is the time of year he died. Just raking leaves, which I do every weekend, makes me think of him. Then I get this chest pain and worry about myself. Heart disease runs in families, I don't have to tell you.*

Doctor: *I can see why you'd be afraid. (understanding) It sounds as though there's a pretty strong connection between thinking about your father and the chest pain.*

Patient: *Yeah. I thought maybe being upset stressed my heart. Do you think maybe this is all in my head?*

Doctor: *I can tell from your lab tests and electrocardiogram that you haven't had a heart attack but I'm sure you really feel the pain, and I suspect your heart still aches for your father-even if only figuratively. It's hard to lose a father. Now, you know there's a pretty strong connection between the body and the mind, and if you've been worrying about your own health, this could be your body's way of making sure you take care of yourself. (respect)*

Patient: *I never thought of it that way. What you say makes a lot of sense, and I think you're probably right. But I still have this nagging worry in the back of my mind.*

Doctor: *That's understandable. (understanding) How about this? Let's work together to reduce whatever risk factors you do have for heart disease to make sure you don't have a problem down the line. (support) Although you are at low risk for having coronary artery disease, I think it would be prudent to do an exercise stress test as an outpatient just to be sure. I'm going to give you my card so that you can call my office to set it up when you get home. Any time in the next few weeks would be fine. And in the meantime, if the pain gets worse or changes in any way, give me a call. Right now, you're having some pretty strong feelings about your father, and if that is the source of your chest pain, it may not go away right away. We'll talk more about it when I see you in the office.*

Patient: *That seems reasonable to me. I appreciate your listening to me.*

Doctor: *Okay, then, I'll see you in a few weeks. And remember, if the pains get worse or you get new symptoms along with them, call me immediately; don't wait till the next day.*

Patient: *Thanks, Doc. See you in a few weeks.*

The patient's experience, as indicated by the patient's responses toward the end of the interview, seems much better than in the first scenario. Although this scenario is longer than the first, using empathic skills added only approximately 1 minute to the interview, and if that additional minute prevents unnecessary visits by allaying the patient's concerns, the time is well spent. Early in the interview the doctor does very little talking, and what he does say primarily addresses the patient's charged emotional state. He initially resists the patient's invitation to confirm conclusively that this is all in his head, and, instead, allows the patient to continue to explore his feeling state. There is uncertainty at the end of the medical interview, but it seems to be an uncertainty that both the doctor and patient can accept comfortably, with a sense of partnership.

IMPLICATIONS FOR PROFESSIONAL DEVELOPMENT

Suppose the content of what the patient reveals is upsetting, distasteful, or even abhorrent to the clinician. In the previous example of the patient with chest pain, suppose that the doctor's mother has just died and his father is scheduled for triplebypass surgery. The mere contemplation of losing his father is so threatening that the physician withdraws into himself. Psychological defense mechanisms may cause the physician to become distracted from the patient's visit and think about his own concerns.

However, suppose that the patient describes a situation that is emotionally charged, but is so alien to the physician's experience that he cannot empathize. If, for example, a patient reveals her sadness that her cat was diagnosed with cancer, the non-pet-owning clinician may pity (feel sorry *for*) the patient but may be unable to relate to the patient's grief and fears. Or suppose the clinician must present certain treatments to a patient that she considers disgusting or repulsive. Her own obvious feeling may prevent the patient from making a truly informed decision.

Finding just the right therapeutic stance is essential; it may be partly intuitive and partly learned, and it may vary from patient to patient—or even with the same patient over time—depending on the patient's needs. Opportunities may be lost when the clinician is unable to empathize with the patient, or when the loss of ego boundaries makes a therapeutic stance impossible. The most effective clinicians are those whose repertoire permits a rapid interplay of objectivity and emotion.

Calibrating responses to patients requires noticing and understanding when clinicians' own emotional issues prevent them from being maximally effective with patients. The first clue may be that a specific patient or type of patient particularly irks a clinician. These "irksome patients" are our "visiting professors." They teach us about ourselves. Personal barriers to effectiveness with patients usually originate in the clinician's own family of origin. Numerous tools are available to help clinicians overcome these barriers: speaking with a trusted colleague, Balint or other support groups, courses that focus specifically on personal awareness, mindfulness practices, and personal psychotherapy.

On Authenticity

When the language of empathy is new, it can feel foreign and, therefore, phony. Some have likened empathy skills to acting. All new skills, whether in sports, cooking, or the performance arts, are awkward and effortful at first. As one gains experience and tailors these concepts to one's own personal style, empathy skills become part of who we are. If a clinician says something he does not believe, with the goal of manipulating the patient, it is likely to be detected and to backfire. We all have had the feeling of being patronized by service workers trained in customer satisfaction. However, if we express what we imagine the patient is feeling with the goal of strengthening a connection, the patient is likely to detect the authentic intent and forgive any awkwardness in the expression. Returning to the "acting" metaphor, there is a distinction in the performance arts between "surface acting" (acting unconnected to emotions) and "deep acting" (grounded in one's own life experiences or imagination of another's experience). There are both ethical and pragmatic arguments against "faking" empathy—only the most skilled actors are likely to possess the capacity to match subconscious nonverbal cues with inauthentic verbal expressions.

Empathy in Medical Training

There is evidence that empathy correlates with the fluctuation of mood state during training (see Chapter 49, "Trainee Well-Being"). It is remarkable how the fresh enthusiasm and caring of new health professions students can quickly devolve into the wry cynicism of senior students. What accounts for this withdrawal? The usual explanation is that insulating oneself in this way is an act of self-preservation in the face of overwhelming demands. It can be torturous to feel another's pain, and if one's self is already stressed because of long hours and the other exigencies of training, it may be more difficult to practice open-heartedly.

The ways in which clinicians withdraw depend on both their personalities and their environment. If the training or practice culture tolerates derogatory labels for patients, it can be easy to see patients as *other*, as not sharing some element of humanity with *us*. Even if such labels are not tolerated and caring for patients is a highly preserved value, dark humor may surface as a means of insulation. To take care of others, one must first take care of oneself. Finding the right balance is a major developmental task of the health-care professional. Perhaps by attending to the well-being of trainees, we will make them better clinicians (see Chapter 44). Since empathy directly correlates with well-being in trainees, it is important that training programs demonstrate that caring for others is valuable. Experienced clinicians can attend to trainees' growth, help them develop effective and healthy working styles, model those styles, and draw attention to the importance of being aware of one's own development. There is a huge contrast between the concept of training as nurturing or mentoring and the concept of it being "trial by fire." And fire, we know, steels metal, making it harder.

Empathy in the Practice of Medicine

What happens after training? For some practitioners, the pressure becomes less, healthy coping styles develop, and the caring clinician reemerges. Far too many, however, are casualties of the training process. Clinicians' compulsive personality styles are susceptible to a pattern of delayed gratification. Constantly nurturing others, clinicians may have no time left for themselves. Relationships with family and friends may atrophy. The most effective clinicians may be those who attend to their own needs as well as those of their patients, who understand their own unique struggles, so that these struggles—by making clinicians aware of their own humanity—can enhance, rather than detract from, their relationships with patients.

Because the culture of an institution strongly influences the practice of medicine within its purview, clinicians who practice together have a unique opportunity to enhance each other's empathic skills. Patient-care conferences can incorporate psychosocial issues into the discussions of difficult cases. Reviewing video-recorded interviews with difficult patients is a powerful tool that allows clinicians to examine their own contributions to the difficulty of such interactions.

Regular video-recorded conferences, in which clinicians take turns presenting cases, allow them to feel at ease in front of the camera, demonstrate collaboration and mutual support, and reinforce the importance and value of empathy to the group. Balint groups or other types of support groups, which may include nonclinician office staff, can help health practitioners cope with collegial interactions or family relationships that have become stressed by practice. Such groups also show that a psychosocial perspective can benefit both clinicians and their patients.

Understanding the interaction between illness and emotion helps us become more effective clinicians. Familiarity and practice with the skills in this chapter can make us more comfortable discussing this interaction with our patients. Becoming aware of our own personal response to patients promotes personal growth as well. The emotional demands of the medical profession can be enriching or impoverishing. Using the skills of empathy, we may become more satisfied and effective clinicians, and at the same time, our patients also may become more satisfied and healthier.

SUGGESTED READINGS

Back AL, Arnold RM. "Isn't there anything more you can do?": when empathic statements work, and when they don't. *J Palliat Med* 2013;16(11):1429–1432.

Back AL, Arnold RM. "Yes it's sad, but what should I do?" Moving from empathy to action in discussing goals of care. *J Palliat Med* 2014;17(2):141–144.

Blatt B, LeLacheur SF, Galinsky AD, Simmens SJ, Greenberg L. Does perspective-taking increase patient satisfaction in medical encounters? *Acad Med* 2010;85(9):1445–1452.

Cripe LD, Frankel RM. Dying From cancer: communication, empathy, and the clinical imagination. *J Patient Exp* 2017;4(2):69–73.

Del Canale S, Louis DZ, Maio V, et al. The relationship between physician empathy and disease complications: an empirical study of primary care physicians and their diabetic patients in Parma, Italy. *Acad Med* 2012;87(9):1243–1249.

Derksen F, Bensing J, Lagro-Janssen A. Effectiveness of empathy in general practice: a systematic review. *Br J Gen Pract* 2013;63(606):e76–84.

Eide H, Frankel R, Haaversen AC, Vaupel KA, Graugaard PK, Finset A. Listening for feelings: identifying and coding empathic and potential empathic opportunities in medical dialogues. *Patient Educ Couns* 2004;54(3):291–297.

Eikeland HL, Ornes K, Finset A, Pedersen R. The physician's role and empathy—a qualitative study of third year medical students. *BMC Med Educ* 2014;14:165.

Finset A, Ornes K. Empathy in the clinician-patient relationship: the role of reciprocal adjustments and processes of synchrony. *J Patient Exp* 2017;4(2):64–68.

Fortin AH VI, Dwamena FC, Lovegrove Lepisto B, Frankel RM, Smith RC. *Smith's Patient-Centered Interviewing: An Evidence-Based Method.* New York, NY: McGraw-Hill; 2019.

Frankel RM. The evolution of empathy research: models, muddles, and mechanisms. *Patient Educ Couns* 2017;100(11):2128–2130.

Hojat M, DeSantis J, Gonnella JS. Patient perceptions of clinician's empathy: measurement and psychometrics. *J Patient Exp* 2017; 4(2):78–83.

Hojat M, Louis DZ, Markham FW, Wender R, Rabinowitz C, Gonnella JS. Physicians'empathy and clinical outcomes for diabetic patients. *Acad Med* 2011;86(3):359–364.

Krasner MS, Epstein RM, Beckman H, et al. Association of an educational program in mindful communication with burnout, empathy, and attitudes among primary care physicians. *JAMA* 2009;302(12):1284–1293.

Lamm C, Decety J, Singer T. Meta-analytic evidence for common and distinct neural networks associated with directly experienced pain and empathy for pain. *Neuroimage* 2011;54(3):2492–2502.

Lown BA. A social neuroscience-informed model for teaching and practising compassion in health care. *Med Educ* 2016;50(3):332–342.

Newton BW, Barber L, Clardy J, et al. Is there hardening of the heart during medical school? *Acad Med* 2008;83(3):244–249.

Novack DH, Suchman AL, Clark W, Epstein RM, Najberg E, Kaplan C. Calibrating the physician: personal awareness and effective patient care. *JAMA* 1997;278:502–509.

Rakel D, Barrett B, Zhang Z, et al. Perception of empathy in the therapeutic encounter: effects on the common cold. *Patient Educ Couns* 2011;85(3):390–397.

Riess H. The science of empathy. *J Patient Exp* 2017;4(2):74–77.

Shanafelt TD, West C, Zhao X, et al. Relationship between increased personal well-being and enhanced empathy among internal medicine residents. *J Gen Intern Med* 2005;20(7):559–564.

Ventres WB, Frankel RM. Shared presence in physician-patient communication: agraphic representation. *Fam Syst Health* 2015;33(3):270–279.

OTHER RESOURCE

Egener B. Responding to strong emotions. Web-based Learning: an Interactive Learning Resource for Healthcare Communication. (doccom.org). Accessed July 2018.

WEBSITE

Academy of Communication in Healthcare Web site. www.achonline.org. Accessed July 2018.

VIDEO

Video 2-1. Empathy Skills (4 min, 49 sec)

Access by scanning the QR code above or visit mhprofessional.com/feldman5evideos.

Delivering Serious News

3

Bethany C. Calkins, MS, MD & Timothy E. Quill, MD, MACP, FAAHPM

INTRODUCTION

With the passage of time, attitudes about how much information is to be divulged to patients about their medical conditions have evolved. In *Decorum*, Hippocrates wrote, "... conceal most things from the patient while you are attending him. Give orders with cheerfulness and serenity, turning attention away from what is being done to him [because] a forecast of what is to come can cause a turn for the worse." In 1847, when the American Medical Association (AMA) published their First Code of Medical Ethics, they agreed, stating that "The life of a sick person can be shortened not only by the acts, but also by the words or manner of a physician. It is, therefore, a sacred duty to guard himself carefully in this respect, and to avoid all things which have a tendency to discourage the patient and depress his spirits."

Over time, there has been a dramatic change in attitudes and practice patterns in this regard among physicians. In 1961, 90% of physicians preferred not to share a cancer diagnosis with their patients. In 1990, the data showed a dramatic upward trend in disclosure with 97% of surveyed physicians disclosing an unfavorable diagnosis to their patients. This could be partly due to the improvement in treatment regimens for chronic diseases, such as cancer and AIDS, over time; with these advances, it has become easier for physicians to deliver serious news to patients while simultaneously offering the hope for effective treatment necessary to sustain them through their illness. However, along with treatments come treatment failures, recurrence of disease and what may be irreversible side effects of those treatments, requiring physicians to also explore these less favorable scenarios with patients. Ninety-five percent of patients prefer to be informed of their diagnoses, though there is some variation in what specifically they want to know. For example, most want to know about their chances for cure and effective treatment options, and fewer want to know about their specific prognosis especially if this news is not positive. Unfortunately, the literature has shown that most doctors receive little or no training in communicating serious news to patients, and even those who do it regularly are unsure of their ability to do it effectively.

COMMUNICATING SERIOUS NEWS

Bad news is defined in the literature as any information likely to alter drastically a patient's view of his or her future. Objectively, serious news can be a life-threatening condition, particularly cancer, but could also include other fatal or serious diagnoses, the death of a loved one, treatment failures, or transitions in care (i.e., to hospice). It is important to remember that serious news is a subjective experience that depends on the patient's expectations and understanding of the situation. For example, patients may be relieved by a diagnosis of a stroke if they had previously believed that they had a brain tumor. Alternatively, the diagnosis of hypertension may be perceived as devastating if it potentially means that they, like their parent, may end up on dialysis. It is hard to know how news will affect a person without this personal knowledge, but effective communication can help patients to better understand and move forward with information tailored to their particular clinical situation.

Prior literature in this area describes these conversations as "breaking bad news." However, in a qualitative study from 2011 on this topic, patients did not like clinicians judging what was considered "bad" news, and valued framing the news as something to work through with the provider, rather than just labeling it as "bad."

Common sense dictates that there are better and worse ways to present serious news to patients. This type of conversation is delicate and challenging and has implications for both the provider and the recipient, yet most physicians are not trained in techniques for carrying out this kind of communication. In one survey, only 5% of oncologists said that they learned to give serious news through a formal teaching program; most had either learned by sitting in on other clinicians giving such information or had no formal teaching at all. Others learn by doing or by relying on their intuition and prior experience in breaking serious news to patients. However, research shows that communication skills do not improve with experience alone (see Chapter 1). Cultural and ethnic variables further complicate the process and will be discussed further toward the end of this chapter.

THE IMPORTANCE OF THE BAD NEWS DISCUSSION

Optimal communication in relaying serious news leads to better outcomes for both the physician and the patient. As providers feel more comfortable with their communication skills, they report less job stress, higher levels of personal accomplishment, higher levels of confidence, and less emotional stress and burnout. Patients will often feel encouraged to participate in difficult decision making when they are connecting with their physician, which can result in higher quality medical decision making. Good, open communication encourages trusting relationships to develop between doctor and patient, and patients report better outcomes, better satisfaction, improved understanding of their condition, and better adherence to treatment plans. Significant decreases in rates of litigation occur when patients feel that they were involved in a conversation that they felt was clear, honest, and empathic.

When communication surrounding the serious news discussion goes poorly, it can negatively affect patients' views of humanity; of the medical field, in general; and of their particular medical-care providers. Patients may see a poorly run conversation as a breach of the patient–physician partnership, which ultimately could affect their compliance with the treatment plan, level of hopefulness, and subsequent psychological adjustment to their disease. When patients' quality of life suffers, so could their health outcomes. There have been many studies to show that the inability of oncologists to deliver serious news effectively leads to short courses of futile, unnecessary chemotherapy being administered at the end of life.

The delivery of serious news is a complex interaction. Providers need to arrange the verbal component of actually giving the news, while simultaneously eliciting and responding to the patient's emotions, dealing with the stress created by patients' expectations for cure, involving patients in decision making, involving as many family members as are present, and all while trying to provide them with hope in the face of a potentially bleak situation. With such an emotionally charged environment, the opportunity for miscommunication is enormous. Given all of the issues surrounding breaking serious news to patients, it quickly becomes evident why learning communication as a skill is important for everyone involved.

Patient-centered communication is an approach in which attention is placed on using verbal and nonverbal behaviors to establish partnerships with patients. Physicians should help create and maintain patient-centered communication by clarifying with patients, in advance, how much information they would like to know before discussing it with them. Using the six-step approach described below—initially created by Dr. Robert Buckman and others—to establish patient-centered goals can smooth the progress in transitions of care.

SPIKES: A PROTOCOL FOR THE DELIVERY OF UNFAVORABLE NEWS

Buckman created a six-step protocol for giving unfavorable information to patients. In a review of the literature on "breaking bad news" published in *JAMA*, most authors agree that following the SPIKES framework reduces stress on the patients receiving the news as well as the physicians charged with delivering the serious news (Table 3-1).

Physicians may have several goals on entering a discussion in which they plan to divulge serious news to a patient: they may wish to gather information from the

Table 3-1. The **SPIKES** protocol for delivering bad news.

Set up the interview	Advanced preparation, pay attention to the physical setting: sit down, make eye contact, avoid interruptions, and invite patient to ask family to stay
Assess patient's **Perception**	"Tell me how you are doing." "What do you understand about what's happened so far?"
Obtain the patient's **Invitation**	"Is it okay to speak freely about the information that I have here?" "Is there anything that you wouldn't want to know?"
Give **Knowledge** and information to the patient	"I'm afraid that I have bad news for you." "The biopsy confirmed cancer."
Address the patient's **Emotions** with empathic responses	"I wish I had better news for you." "I can see that you're upset. Tell me more about what you're feeling."
Set goals	Summarize the conversation and make a plan to go forward

patient in terms of what they know already of their illness as well as how much they want to know; to provide information to the patient that is clear and within the boundaries of what they desire; to support the patient by responding to emotional needs that arise during the conversation; and to develop a treatment strategy with the help of the patient. These are substantial goals, but the SPIKES protocol can assist professionals in realizing them.

Step 1 of the six-step SPIKES protocol (**Set** up the interview) involves advanced preparation for the discussion and choosing an appropriate physical setting in which it will occur. Mentally rehearse what you will tell the patient and family, and anticipate what they may ask or how they may react. Remember that although the conversation that is ahead will be challenging to hear for everyone, it will be important to communicate the information clearly and succinctly to begin preparing patients to plan their future. Consider where the conversation will happen. The space chosen for this purpose should be private, quiet, comfortable, and convenient for everyone involved. Identify the key participants that should be present, including family or friends who the patient identifies as being close supports, as well as practical additions to the team, such as nurses, interpreters, social workers, and consultants who know the patient well. Having a supportive colleague present during the discussion may also potentially bolster the comfort level of the provider when the news is particularly bad. In a hospital, the physical setting adds another level of complexity to an already difficult discussion. Finding a space to have a private conversation where the patient can comfortably attend—while maintaining the peaceful, supportive environment required to openly discuss sensitive information—often proves difficult. Seeking out empty family rooms or offices in advance can be helpful. In the outpatient setting, the physical space may not be as much of a problem as the time constraints. It is recommended in this step of the SPIKES protocol to set aside sufficient time where one does not feel pressured to truncate the conversation in favor of other responsibilities. Many experienced clinicians find that time set aside at the end of a patient-care session is most convenient for this discussion. If possible, providers should hand off their pagers to another colleague and ask staff to hold telephone calls or other interruptions until the conclusion of the bad news discussion.

In addition to the optimal physical setting, physicians should prepare for the conversation by finding out the medical information necessary to answer any anticipated questions. Talking to consultants about specific diagnoses, test results and treatment options in advance will help when formulating a plan with the patient.

Something else to consider before escorting the patient into the conversation is who should be present and who should be delivering the bad news. There is no single right answer, but the health care provider who knows the patient best is the right person in most cases. The use of an interdisciplinary team helps in preventing discrepancies in information presented to the patient, and potentially aids in identification of patient needs. Nurses can also be helpful in acting as a supportive liaison between patients and physicians. Social workers can provide essential services such as talking with patients on how best to communicate with doctors, setting up interpreters, and arranging meetings with key people.

When entering into a discussion, in which sensitive information will be divulged, be mindful of body language and nonverbal cues that could be sending additional information to patients. In addition, be vigilant about identifying what information the patient's body language is providing to you. Sitting down lets the patient know that there is no rush and making eye contact (though sometimes uncomfortable) assists in strengthening rapport between patient and provider.

In **Step 2** of the SPIKES protocol (**Perception**), the goal is to assess the patient's perception of what has thus far occurred to bring everyone together. Introduce yourself and state your role, and invite everyone else in the room to introduce themselves and state their reason for being there. This is a good time to acknowledge any time constraints that you might have. For example, "I have thirty minutes to meet with you before my next meeting." Start then by stating the goals of the meeting, such as, "I asked you here today to discuss Mr. Green's recent test results and how this affects the plan for the future." An excellent rule of thumb at this point of the conversation is "*ask* before you *tell*." Ask what the patient and family know and what they want to know. Some patients may choose less-than-full disclosure in regard to their medical conditions, and you cannot know without asking. Some cultures protect their members from serious news by relaying this information to family instead of the patient; these issues must be explored early in the interview to ensure that this is truly the desire of both the patient and the family. Cultural differences in medical care and in discussing serious news are explored in more detail later in this chapter.

Once it is determined that everyone in the room wants to participate in the ensuing discussion, *ask* the patient to speak freely about their understanding of their experience thus far. Studies have shown that satisfaction in family meetings increases as the proportion of family talk time goes up. Attempt to minimize interruptions and actively listen to what patients and families describe. Invite them to participate freely in the information exchange and to dictate how much information is divulged at this initial meeting. Active listening ensures that nothing is left out of the conversation simply due to over-estimating what the patient and family already know. Step 2 of the SPIKES protocol, when patients are invited to express what they already know, is a great time also to correct any misinformation that the family or the patient may harbor. It is also a good time to assess whether the patient or family are engaging in any sort of denial about their condition. As examples, wishful thinking, unrealistic expectations of treatment or omitting important details of medical care might surface during this time of the interview.

The purpose of **Step 3** of the protocol (**Invitation**) is to obtain the patient's invitation to the clinician to talk further about what he or she knows about the patient's condition. Ideally, one would have previously asked the patient when ordering a test that might result in serious news how they would want to receive the news if the need should arise. Do they want to tell their family on their own? Or would they prefer to let everyone hear together and be able to ask questions of the provider as the news is divulged? When asking the patient for an invitation to speak, ask also if it is okay to speak freely in front of family in the room. Most patients indicate during research studies that they want as much information as possible about their illness, though they may not express their full desire to providers (and they may not retain the details of what has been shared if they have a strong emotional response to the news).

Step 4 (**Knowledge**) is the actual process of giving information to the patient. If the news is bad, clinicians are advised to start with a "warning shot;" this may lessen the shock that follows disclosure and may facilitate processing of the information to follow. The warning shot may be prepared earlier in the process as well. For example, when the office calls a patient to set up an appointment, they might be asked: "Is there anyone that you'd want to bring with you to this appointment? I'm afraid we have some serious things to discuss." The separation in time between the warning shot and the actual disclosure may ease the patient into the coping process.

Once the patient has been told that it is not good news, follow the "Ask, tell, ask" procedure. In Step 3, the patient was asked how much information they wanted to know. Use Step 4 to actually tell them that information in small quantities. Reevaluate the patient's verbal and nonverbal cues throughout the discussion and ask if it is okay to proceed with the conversation. Use nontechnical words, but be sure to use words that will allow the patient to clearly understand what you are telling them when they are ready. For example, instead of telling patients that there is an "invasive mass" in their liver, one might say, "There is a large cancer in your liver" (not a "tumor"). Instead of "metastasized," use "spread." Instead of "dyspnea," say "shortness of breath." Excessive bluntness must be avoided ("There is nothing we can do to treat this cancer") to keep patients feeling engaged in the conversation and to avoid inciting a feeling of isolation and anger—but one should try to gauge what and how much additional information is given by soliciting what additional questions the patient and family may have.

A good rule of thumb along the lines of "ask, tell, ask" is to give at most three pieces of information at a time before checking for understanding. Repeat information as much as is necessary for the patient and their family. Asking patients to summarize periodically what you have shared with them thus far can be helpful in checking to see if information is being received.

Importantly, clinicians should try to help the patient and family find hope. If the hope is no longer in the form of a cure, assist the patient in changing the therapeutic goal or the "hope object." Hope objects will be addressed in more detail later in this chapter. Sometimes patients may have to deal with strong negative emotions (see next section) after hearing serious news before they are able to see hope. But even in circumstances where there is no further effective treatment, one can potentially be hopeful for a good quality of life moving forward or for other important personal or family outcomes.

Step 5 in the SPIKES protocol (**Emotions**) is to respond humanistically to the patient's emotions. Most people find this to be the most difficult part of giving serious news. Although one can hypothesize how a patient might react to life-altering news, the range of potential emotions is wide. Following your disclosure, wait for the patient to react. Begin by acknowledging and if possible naming the emotion ("I see that you're sad, Mr. Green."). It is helpful also to identify the reason for the emotion. "I imagine that you feel this way because you were hopeful that the treatment was going to work." Legitimize the emotions that you have identified ("Most anyone hearing such news would feel [sad, angry ...]"). Rather than trying prematurely to reassure, try exploring the emotion so you fully understand it ("Tell me about the most difficult part ..."). Let patients know that you have connected their emotion to the feeling behind it with a statement to reflect your understanding. "I would probably feel the same way if I were you." It is important to allow patients sufficient time to express their fears and emotions. Listen carefully and do not interrupt. Allowing patients to talk freely about what they are experiencing and express what they are feeling will improve how you both experience the conversation.

An approach to responding to patient emotion.

Acknowledge that emotion is being expressed	"I can see that this is upsetting to you."
Legitimize the normalcy of the emotion	"Anyone receiving this news would be devastated."
Explore more about what is behind the emotion	"Tell me more about that ..."
Empathize with the emotion if you genuinely feel it	"I can imagine that this feels disappointing."
Explore strengths	"In past circumstances, what has helped?"

Empathy is defined as being able to personally imagine what the patient is feeling and experiencing (see Chapter 2). Empathy can be a very powerful tool in building trust and relationships with patients. If done correctly, empathic statements made by the physician are associated with increased family satisfaction. However, if an empathic response is done without sincerity or when a patient is not receptive, it can end up being harmful to a therapeutic relationship. For instance, if a patient is silent at the conclusion of the divulgence of serious news, they are not clearly expressing any emotion to the physician. In this case, it is helpful to explore what the patient is thinking and feeling prior to offering an empathic response. Sometimes the feelings of the provider can provide a clue as to how the patient is feeling, but this is not always accurate. If a physician is feeling anxious while anticipating a response from a patient after having given serious news, this may represent the physician's own response and not necessarily a guide to how the patient is feeling (countertransference).

Addressing a patient's emotions during the conversation may help mitigate anxiety in both provider and patient, prevent depression later in the course of the illness, and improve overall satisfaction with the interaction. Patients report less distress when they feel that their physician detected and addressed their concerns. Although identifying and responding to emotional cues requires focus, experience, and time, clinical interactions may actually take longer when emotional cues are missed.

Physicians often want to respond empathically to a patient's visual cues and feelings, though sometimes physicians may also be experiencing feelings such as hopelessness and perhaps guilt at not having detected the disease earlier. Providers may fear that responding empathically may be construed as evidence of inadequacy, mistakes, or failure. Before expressing empathy, clinicians should try to be sure that they are responding to the patient's feelings and not their own. Clinicians' feelings and reactions are also important, but unless they relate directly to the patient's experience, they should be explored in other settings with trusted colleagues.

When giving serious news to a patient or family, generally avoid apologizing unless you have clearly made a mistake that you are ready to acknowledge. Apologies can be mistaken for admissions of guilt or of error on the part of the clinician. Though we may feel like we need to apologize for being the bearer of serious news, apologies can be problematic to physicians for many reasons. Patients may confuse an apology as an expression of pity or can change the emphasis of the conversation from the feelings of the patient to the feelings of the physician. "I'm sorry" may also limit further exploration of the patient's feelings. A good surrogate expression for "*I'm sorry*" is an "*I wish*" statement. "I wish I had better news for you" allows the physician to walk in the patient's shoes while acknowledging that the news is unlikely to change.

Compassion can take many forms. For instance, empathy can be shown by giving recommendations in light of what the physician knows of the patient's beliefs, goals, fears, and medical situation. For example, "From what I know about your personal values and medical circumstances, Mr. Green, I would recommend switching to a hospice plan of care. This will allow for you to have the best possible quality of life for whatever time you have left."

Factors that improve attentiveness to and empathy for the patient during this difficult discussion include older age, female gender, and personal experience on the part of the physician. One study illustrated that physicians who had personally experienced life-threatening illness were more attentive to the emotional needs of the patient than those who had not. The same study concluded that older physicians give more emotional support to patients than their younger counterparts. Female physicians spend more time giving serious news to patients than male physicians.

Step 6, the final step of the SPIKES protocol (**Set** goals), is to summarize the conversation and to engage with the patient in creating a clear plan for the future. This step is essential in decreasing a patient's anxiety and level of uncertainty. At this point in the conversation, the patient has heard a lot of information that affects them very personally. Ask, first, if the patient and family are ready for a discussion about the plan. If they are not, briefly review the conversation to that point and ask for further questions about what has been said. Most likely at this point patients will be eager to plan for and discuss the next step. Present the possible treatment options in small bits and elicit patients' values and preferences as it relates to the possible treatment options. Clearly state each option and make a recommendation based on your medical expertise and experience as well as your knowledge of the patient's values as to which one you think would work best. Work together to come up with a decision; shared decision making with the patient relieves some pressure for the physician should the treatment not be completely successful. Referring patients to support groups within the community has also shown some benefits in those with terminal illnesses. There has been some evidence to suggest that patients who share experiences with supportive physicians and a group of peers with similar experiences have improved quality of life, experience less pain, and cope more effectively with terminal illnesses than those who do not attend support groups.

Some providers might consider briefly writing down the diagnosis and possible treatment plans for the patient to look up when they feel ready. In some studies, physicians audio-recorded these consultations so that patients could take them home; however, reliving this experience may contribute to poorer mood and increasing rates of depression for patients. Schedule a follow-up appointment with you and other appropriate consultant(s) for the patient before he or she leaves your office. They may not feel up to completing these tasks while they are processing their bad news.

Patients are not likely to ask about prognosis during this initial discussion. In one survey of over 30 patients newly diagnosed with cancer, only 1 patient asked for a specific prognosis. Studies have shown that more patients prefer qualitative estimates of prognosis to quantitative assessments, but there are individual differences. Doctors consistently overestimate survival in terminally ill patients, especially those who have a short life expectancy. Patients may vary in their desire for prognosis disclosure over the course of their illness as well; at their first visit, they may be more interested in information about their disease and possible course of treatment, with curiosity regarding prognosis revealed at later visits. If a patient desires some information at the time of the initial discussion, provide an average range of survival with caveats that they may lie also outside of that range in either direction. *"The average person with your condition will live (3-6) months. Some will live longer, and we will do our best to try to have you be in that group, but also some may live shorter, so you should get prepared just in case."* Clinicians need to be aware if they tend to be optimists or pessimists in their prognostication, but the inclusion of the possibility of being outside the expected range helps compensate for that to some degree.

It has been generally agreed upon by clinicians and researchers in this area that the SPIKES protocol assists both patients and physicians in breaking serious news. Most guidelines are based on expert opinion with little evidence about the best method for breaking serious news. Remember that all guidelines recommend tailoring the interview to the patient, and that each discussion will be different, depending on differences between patients. Not every conversation surrounding unfavorable information will require all six steps, but when it does, the steps of the SPIKES protocol should generally be done in sequence.

STRESS ON THE PROVIDER: BEFORE & AFTER DIFFICULT CONVERSATIONS

Research and anecdotal information remind us that many patients do not often remember most of the initial serious news discussion once the diagnosis is spoken. The divulgence of serious news is a stressful conversation for both providers and patients, but patients still need and want information regarding their disease. Although some stress may be adaptive, stress that is experienced at too high a level or as uncontrollable can have negative effects on the recipient. The emotional response of the patient depends on a number of factors, such as age, familial obligations, and levels of psychosocial support; for example, a 35-year-old father of young children might respond differently to the news of a new lung cancer than would a 96-year-old great-grandfather (but there are exceptions to every rule).

The doctor–patient relationship comes with expectations from both parties. The serious news discussion, when done well, is a good opportunity to strengthen this relationship. Earlier, we discussed shared decision making as a way to mitigate pressure on the physician when deciding on a treatment plan. This model of decision making is the norm in Western culture, but not in all cultures. For this reason, it is important for providers to assess early on how much of a role patients desire in their care. Some patients may want the physician's guidance, while others may only want the medical facts, so that they can then make up their own mind. If a clinician has a recommendation based on her medical knowledge and her knowledge of the patient's values, she should ask if the patient would like to hear what she recommends and why. A multicultural approach to the serious news discussion is addressed in more detail later in this chapter (also see Chapter 15).

The reaction of the provider to the serious news is just as important as the patient's reaction to the difficult discussion. Due to the nature of the relationship between physicians and patients, physicians receive the serious news in advance of the patient. Breaking serious news to patients is stressful and psychologically difficult. There are multiple stressors on those charged with delivering the serious news; challenges include being honest without destroying hope, not knowing what the patient's emotional reaction will be, how to deal with the variety of reactions that might result, and how to deal with one's own feelings and reactions that may be very different from the patient and family. All of these variables create anxiety for the physician, even before the patient knows that anything is wrong. A lack of experience in delivering serious news may also contribute to the stress and anxiety present in the provider before giving the patient the news. This level of stress and anxiety sometimes dissipates quickly after divulging the information to the patient, but other times when the patient and/or family have a strong negative emotional reaction, the clinician's feelings may intensify.

When the physician is stressed, the possibility of avoiding the serious news discussion exists. Also, the physician may convey unwarranted optimism during the actual conversation. Talking with colleagues and getting support from coworkers prior to speaking with the patient can be helpful in difficult cases. Providers must be aware of their personal beliefs about illness, death, and dying prior to sitting down with the patient, to ensure that they are not inadvertently pressuring patients to respond in a certain way. As an example, a provider who recently lost a family member to breast cancer may push harder for her patient with breast cancer to continue with improbably successful treatment. During the conversation, be alert for emotions that you are projecting onto the patient and for emotions that the patient may be projecting onto you. Discussing strong emotional reactions on either side of the relationship with a trusted colleague may help in sorting out these issues and allow clinicians to care for themselves as well as their patients.

Those charged with the task of bearing serious news often experience high levels of stress, anxiety, and fear of negative evaluation. There may be a reluctance to deliver serious news, known as the "mum effect," that may result in the physician holding onto the serious news for a prolonged time prior to contacting the patient. How much stress a physician experiences prior to sharing the news is exacerbated when the physician is inexperienced, when the patient is young, and when there are limited prospects for successful treatment. Physicians may feel uncertain about how the patient will react or how they will manage the patient's emotions. They may fear destroying the patient's hope. Alternatively, physicians may feel embarrassed that they gave too much hope earlier in the process or may feel inadequate in the face of disease that has become uncontrollable. All of these emotions factor into how a physician handles the news prior to getting it to the affected patient and can put up barriers to actually having the serious news discussion. Talking with trusted colleagues and members of multidisciplinary teams can help sort out these complex issues, which is critical to both self-care and patient care.

HOPE AS AN IMPORTANT PART OF THE SERIOUS NEWS DISCUSSION

Hope becomes an important part of the patient's new life after hearing the news of a serious illness. As part of the healing process from the time of diagnosis, hopes will continuously change in the eyes of patients as their disease evolves. Clinicians may at times have to explore and empathize with elements of hopelessness, as when the expectations for a cure or for effective disease-directed treatments are no longer realistic. After exploring and empathizing with the loss of prior aspects of hope, the discussion should eventually refocus, reframe, or find hope again. For the patient with an imminently terminal disease, the hope now is no longer for a cure, but it can be shifted to alternatives, such as hope for a comfortable future or hope for the best-possible quality of life. Exploring hopelessness and potentially reframing hope can be an important role for the physician in a discussion involving the delivery of serious news.

Physicians must walk along a critical path that balances optimism and honesty; patients need enough information to make the decisions that are of value to them, but truthfulness is just as important. However, evidence shows that regardless of the nature of information divulged or the amount of truthfulness as perceived by the patient, patients place more importance on the attitude of the physician and the manner in which the physician gives the news.

In searching for hope, it is helpful to identify that there are two kinds of hope, *specific* and *generalized.* With this knowledge, it becomes possible for providers to help distressed patients find hope even when the chance of a good outcome, in terms of longevity, is small. *Specific hope* is the state of desiring a specific possible event or future state of affairs, called the hope object. For something to qualify as a hope object, it must be possible, though it need not be probable. An example of specific hope is the hope for a cure of a patient's specific disease. Specific hope varies among two dimensions, desire (whose strength varies on a scale between lukewarm and intense) and the perceived likelihood of the event occurring (which varies on a scale between uncertain and nearly certain). The patient's desire for their specific hope and the perceived likelihood of that specific hope occurring are independent of each other.

Generalized hope is a sense that there is some future beneficial, but uncertain, development that is not linked to a particular object, and is broad in scope, in other words, a sense of "open-endedness." Some have argued that the hope that terminal cancer patients experience is not often specific, but generalized; they feel that life still retains the open-endedness that gives people meaning in life. Faith, which is distinct from hope but may play a role in generalized hope, is a belief that life always has meaning, even with its unavoidable loss and suffering. By using two distinct types of hope, physicians can help despairing patients find hope even when the chance of a good outcome is small.

Hope should always be sought with patients, but one must also be truthful. It may sometimes seem hopeless to both patient and physician during a conversation about serious news; in these difficult cases, continuing to honestly explore feelings of hopelessness may eventually help in finding new avenues of hope. Sometimes patients will initially put all their hope in an experimental treatment that is statistically unlikely to be effective. After ensuring informed consent, it is useful to move forward with supporting treatment and "hope for the best," but at the same time, the clinician might offer the patient and family to "prepare for the worst," so that the developmental issues of preparation for death are not necessarily avoided. These two strategies, hoping for the best and preparing for the worst, need not be mutually exclusive. Hoping, while simultaneously preparing, minimizes the weakness of each strategy on its own.

When patients and physicians discuss serious illness only in terms of hope, physicians are potentially missing opportunities to improve upon pain and symptom management, discuss the patient's fears and concerns, and to grow the patient–physician relationship as well as one's relationship with family and friends. By expanding the conversation to include both hoping for the best while preparing for the worst, physicians can now help address needs surrounding symptom management, spiritual, and psychosocial issues. Patients who rely only on hope may not be aware of their limited life expectancy and may go forward with costly, difficult treatments that are unlikely to work. Physicians who focus the relationship on hope alone may feel as if they are being dishonest with the patient and may withdraw from the relationship as the patient becomes sicker.

THE EVOLUTION OF HOPE AND WORKING THROUGH GRIEF

Hope often initially focuses on outcomes that are strongly desired and reflect individuals' varying beliefs, values, and sense of possibility. The main focus of hope can develop and change over time as the disease progresses. At the start of a serious illness, most people will have an implicit hope for cure of their disease and continued life. As the prognosis changes, patients often need to be helped to modify the focus of their hope toward sustaining their quality of life or perhaps having important conversations with family members about "unfinished business." These transitions are initially not only filled with loss and grief but also potentially open up new avenues for hope. Physicians can help patients find hope by offering specific alternate foci that might be adopted when and if they are ready. Near the end of a terminal illness, patients may find hope in the doctor's ability to control symptoms and minimize discomfort. Using "I wish" statements at a time when giving bad news helps to redefine an unrealistic hope as a wish, thereby allowing for empathy without false hope.

Patients normally experience the onset of a life-threatening illness in an evolving state, starting with the idea that something is wrong, then absorbing the diagnosis, adapting to the disease, and, finally, changing their lives to live with the disease. The moment when the clinician is giving the bad news is usually the moment when the reality of the serious news dawns on the patient and stress peaks. After receiving the serious news, patients enter a period of attempted accommodation to changed life circumstances. This may end in denial, acceptance, or anger. Acceptance is usually the optimal outcome for patients. Those who reach acceptance have integrated the illness and the limitations that it imposes by establishing new priorities, shifting the focus of hope, and finding a renewed sense of purpose. This grief work may take a very long time and some patients may never complete it. Often, patients will find a period of "middle knowledge," where they vacillate between continued adjustments and acceptance of life's losses while preparing for death. It is important for clinicians to support over time the evolution of new kinds of hope as well as the preparation for death.

Patients and families are not the only people affected emotionally during the discussion of a serious news. Physicians, too, are often left with feelings of sadness, grief, incompetence, or anger after having to divulge serious news to patients, with whom they may or may not have had a longstanding relationship. These emotions should not be ignored. Allow time for self-reflection and seek out responses from those professionals who experienced it with you, including trainees. Identify the feelings that you have and talk them over with a colleague. Try keeping a journal to elaborate on the experience for the immediate relief of strong feelings and for your future development as a clinician (see Chapter 6).

THE ROLE OF CULTURE IN THE SERIOUS NEWS DISCUSSION

Before giving serious news to patients, physicians must seek out the type of information that the patient and family would like. In some cultures, disclosure of truth is believed to cause bad outcomes, and nondisclosure can be protective and benevolent. Asking the patient and family what their culture dictates in terms of information sharing and decision making prior to giving serious news can strengthen the relationship between provider and patient especially when the patient comes from a culture which is very distinct from the physician's. As an example, pose this question: "If we had to discuss a serious illness, how would you like me to handle this news?" Using open-ended questions to explore cultural differences before the actual disclosure can be helpful in outlining boundaries for clinicians (Table 3-2). Western culture puts a high value on truth-telling and a scientific explanation of disease; however, other cultures may value different degrees of truth-telling and prefer family-centered styles of decision making over patient-centered decision making. Clinicians can ask patients if they would personally want to hear bad news and handle the decision making themselves should something serious arise, or if they would prefer delivering the news to family members. Understanding the patient's reasoning in advance can help circumvent conflict between patient/family and the health care team should they desire serious news information to be withheld from the patient. Having this sort of information about the patient in advance

Table 3-2. **Ways to explore cultural beliefs in discussing bad news.**

What do you think might be going on? What do you call the problem?
What do you think has caused the problem?
What do you think will happen with this illness?
What do you fear most with this illness?
Would you want to handle the information and decision making, or should that be done by someone else in the family?

Source: Back AL, Curtis JR, Communicating bad news. *West J Med* 2002;176:177–180.

will help keep the patient–physician relationship intact when unfavorable news does have to be discussed.

In western culture, patient autonomy and informed consent have created ethical and legal obligations to provide patients with as much information as they want about their illness and treatment. Nondisclosure is unethical unless there is clarity that the patient is deferring decision making, in which case enforcing full disclosure to the patient would be unethical. Hypothetical discussions before the news is actually available can go a long way to avoiding such conflicts. Serious news cannot be unilaterally withheld, but patients can clearly "choose" not to hear it. Communicating serious news must be done sensitively and with high regard given to the patient's readiness to hear and understand the discussion.

If the communication of serious news does not go well, misunderstandings can ensue, causing increased conflict between providers and patients and families, which has been shown to lead to poor quality decision making. Before sitting down with a patient, attempt to identify whatever cultural biases might be present on both sides of the conversation. Recognize also that although some patients may come from a similar cultural background, culture-based preferences vary within groups, and should, therefore, never be assumed. Patients may also have beliefs that vary considerably from their cultural heritage. In terms of decision making, Europeans generally mimic Americans in desire for more information and a stress on patient autonomy. Asians and Eastern Europeans may prefer family to be the decision makers. African Americans tend to prefer family to be heavily involved in the end-of-life decision making. There are wide exceptions to each of these tendencies, so disclosure must always be individualized.

Anytime there is a language barrier in the patient–physician interaction, interpreters should be used to allow the patient to ask questions of the provider and to fully understand the extent of the conversation. The use of family members as interpreters is discouraged, as they frequently misinterpret or omit words either for their own comfort or that of the patient. Children of patients, as an example, frequently leave out words relating to bodily functions. Interpreters who are trained to work in a medical setting are essential in enhancing communication with patients, particularly when the subject matter entails sensitive issues, such as delivery of serious news. Medical interpreters are trained to translate exactly what the provider and patient have said, but also may be used to gain insight into sensitive cultural issues that may help the provider to better understand the patient's context.

SUGGESTED READINGS

Back AL, Arnold RM, Quill TE. Hope for the best, and prepare for the worst. *Ann of Int Med* 2003;138:439–443.

Back AL, Curtis JR. Cultural issues in breaking bad news. *West J Med* 2002:176;177–180.

Back AL, Trinidad SB, Hopley EK, et al. What patients value when oncologists give news of cancer recurrence: commentary on specific moments in audio-recorded conversations. *Oncologist* 2011;16:342.

Baile WF, Buckman R, Lenzi R, Glober G. SPIKES: A six-step protocol for delivering bad news: application to the patient with cancer. *Oncologist* 2000;5:302–311.

Barclay JS, Blackhall LJ, Tulsky JA. Communication strategies and cultural issues in the delivery of bad news. *J Palliat Med* 2007;10:958–977.

Buckman R. Breaking bad news: why is it still so difficult? *Br Med J (Clin Res Ed)* 1984;288:1597.

Casarett DJ, Quill TE. "I'm Not Ready for Hospice": strategies for timely and effective hospice discussions. *Ann Intern Med* 2007;146:443–449.

Fujimori M, Uchitomi Y. Preferences of cancer patients regarding communication of bad news: a systematic literature review. *Jpn J Clin Oncol* 2009;39:201.

Glare P, Virik K, Jones M, et al. A systematic review of physicians' survival predictions in terminally ill cancer patients. *BMJ* 2003;327:195.

Harman SM, Arnold RM. Discussing Serious News. Up-to-Date; Literature review through April 2018; online last accessed May 24, 2018.

Helft PR. Necessary Collusion: prognostic communication with advanced cancer patients. *J Clin Oncol* 2005;23(13):3146–3150.

Ptacek JT, Eberhardt TL. Breaking bad news: a review of the literature. *JAMA* 1996;276:496–502.

Quill TE, Arnold RM, Plass F. "I Wish Things Were Different": expressing wishes in response to loss, futility and unrealistic hopes. *Ann Int Med* 2001;135:551–555.

Quill TE, Holloway RG, Stevens Shaw M, et al. *Primer for Palliative Care*. 5th ed. American Association of Hospice and Palliative Medicine. 2010;1:102–119.

Slevin ML, Stubbs L, Plant HJ, et al: Attitudes to chemotherapy: comparing views of patients with cancer with those of doctors, nurses, and general public. *BMJ* 1990;300:1458–1460.

Whitney JN, McCullough LB, Fruge E, McGuire AL, Volk RJ. Beyond breaking bad news: the roles of hope and hopefulness. *Cancer* 2008;113(2):442–445.

WEBSITES

Ambuel B. Fast Facts and Concepts #29. Responding to Patient Emotion. https://www.mypcnow.org/blank-hecck. Accessed April 2018.

Ambuel B, Weissman D. Fast Facts and Concepts #6. Delivering Bad News part 1. https://www.mypcnow.org/blank-k4ibb. Accessed April 2018.

Weissman DE, Quill TE, Arnold RM. Fast Facts and Concepts #224. Responding to Emotion in Family Meetings. https://www.mypcnow.org/blank-k4ibb. Accessed April 2018.

VIDEOS

Video 3-1. Breaking Bad News Demo (3 min, 31 sec)

Video 3-2. Breaking Bad News (4 min, 29 sec)

Access by scanning the QR code above or visit mhprofessional.com/feldman5evideos.

Difficult Patients/Difficult Situations

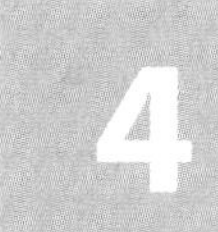

Ryan Laponis, MD, MS & Mitchell D. Feldman, MD, MPhil, FACP

INTRODUCTION

Whenever and wherever health professionals congregate, the topic of difficult situations with patients and families often comes up. Literature suggests clinicians experience up to 20% of their patients as "difficult." These difficult encounters often increase frustration and decrease satisfaction with our work. They may impede our ability to deliver the patient-centered care that is at the heart of high-quality, satisfying, and effective health care.

Fortunately, most difficult situations are both diagnosable and repairable. Most problematic situations are created by unsatisfactory communication between clinicians and patients, or by personal issues the clinician or patient unknowingly bring into the visit. Such issues may mirror similar problems within the clinician or patient's own world and evoke negative reactions to an inherent or overt aspect of the patient's illness, personality, or lifestyle.

Clinicians may view patients as "difficult" based on their similarity to those with whom they have had a close relationship and an interpersonal problem. For example, a clinician whose uncle used anger to control her may now have a strong reaction to an older male patient who responds angrily when she refuses to prescribe an antibiotic for an upper respiratory infection. Another common situation is the clinician who is unusually intolerant of patients who do not engage in behavior change. This clinician may well have had a close relative whom she could not convince to stop smoking and later died from lung cancer. These types of internal reactions are normal, however, allowing them to enter into the encounter often creates discord and unproductive conflict. Developing self-awareness in order to consciously examine one's own internal reaction to a current clinical interaction and then actively choosing a response can ease difficult interactions. The key to success is to carefully examine how visits are progressing while monitoring one's own internal thoughts and emotions in response to the patient and the interaction. Greater self-awareness about our own feelings, experiences, and beliefs can help clinicians approach clinical interactions with less judgment and frustration and hopefully build skill and confidence. The case illustrations that follow focus on some of the more common challenging situations that clinicians encounter, and offer specific approaches. Table 4-1 summarizes some general guidelines. Table 4-2 recommends practical strategies for approaching specific situations.

THE ANGRY PATIENT

CASE ILLUSTRATION 1

Dr. Swanson enters the room to see her fourth of the 10 patients scheduled for her Thursday morning session. Her patient, Ms. B., a 35-year-old social worker, is sitting with arms crossed, refusing to make eye contact. Dr. Swanson greets the patient by asking, "Ms. B., how are you?" She responds, "I've been waiting 35 minutes! This is no way to run an office." The doctor, who is emotionally drained after spending the last 50 minutes talking with a patient about breast cancer, wonders why she's chosen medicine as a career. She follows up by saying, "I apologize for being late. Besides that, are there other things that are upsetting you?"

Ms. B. replies, "You said that when I went to the Emergency Room last week with back pain, you would call and tell them I was coming. When I got there, no one knew why I was there or anything about my medical history. It was very embarrassing."

Diagnosis

It is generally easy to recognize an angry patient. Even without the explicit expression of anger, harsh nonverbal communication, such as rigid posturing, piercing

Table 4-1. General guidelines for working with difficult patients.

- Recognize your own reactions to the encounter
- Seek broader possibilities for the patient's emotions or problems
- Respond directly to the patient's emotions
- Solicit the patient's perspective on why there is a problem
- Seek to discover a common goal for the visit

Table 4-2. Tips for approaching difficult situations or patient behaviors.

Situation	Recommended Techniques
Angry patients	Elicit the patient's reason for being angry: *You seem angry; tell me more about it.* Empathize with the patient's experience: *I can understand why you would be angry.* Solicit the patient's perspective: *What can we do to improve the situation?* If appropriate, apologize: *I'm sorry you had to wait so long.*
Silent patients	Point out the problem: *You are quiet today.* Elicit the patient's reason for silence: *What can you tell me about what is going on?* Explain the need for collaboration: *I'd like to help, In order to, I need you to talk with me more about your problem.* Respond to cues of hearing impairment or language barriers: *Are you having trouble hearing or understanding me?*
Demanding patients	Take a step back from the demand: *It seems the MRI is important to you. Help me understand that?* Acknowledge emotions unexpressed at the time of the demand: *I imagine it is frustrating that your back still hurts.* Solicit the goal of the demand: *Is there something in particular you think the MRI will help us with?* Solicit the patient's perspective: *What do you think is causing your problem? In what way had you hoped I could help you?*

stare, a refusal to shake hands, gritting the teeth, and confrontational or occasionally abusive language, provide unmistakable evidence. More subtle behaviors that may indicate anger include refusing to answer questions; failing to make eye contact; or constructing nonverbal barriers to communication, such as crossed arms, turning away from the clinician, or increasing the physical distance between them.

Table 4-3. Possible causes of patient anger.

- Difficulty in getting to the office
- Problems with the office staff
- Anger toward the illness from which the person suffers
- Anger at the cost of health care
- Problems with consultants to whom the clinician referred the patient
- Unanticipated problems from a procedure or medication recommended by the clinician
- Previous unsupportive or condescending treatment by a clinician
- Absent or miscommunication between members of the health care team
- Other significant news or problems unrelated to health care service, such as work- or family-related conflicts

All too often, clinicians assume that the patient is angry with *them*, and, as a result, feel blamed for something they must have done or forgotten to do. Although that certainly is one possibility, other important reasons must be considered as the cause for a patient's or family member's anger. These include, but are not limited to, those listed in Table 4-3.

Psychological Mechanisms

Many patients come to rely on the special relationship they develop with their clinician. When successful, these relationships are anchored in trust and safety. It is, therefore, quite common for patients to display emotions they would never show to others. Patients want to have their concerns evaluated with compassion and interest. Any perception that their concerns are not taken seriously or are viewed as mundane may be considered a violation of their trust and result in their feeling inappropriately vulnerable, which can lead to anger.

Other violations of expectation may be a trigger for anger. Indeed, patients have lofty expectations of clinicians. They expect timely service, relevant and up-to-date information about diagnostic tests and treatments, and advice on how to cope with their illness. Interactions that fall short, at least from the patient's perspective, may cultivate feelings of shame and rejection. The resulting humiliation can easily turn to anger.

From the clinician's point of view, a patient's expression of anger may trigger feelings as diverse as guilt at having failed the patient, or feeling insulted by the patient's disrespectful behavior. As a result, clinicians may become defensive. This may express itself as a reciprocal anger, a withdrawal from the relationship, or a denial of the clinician's own behavior that may have prompted the anger in the first place. The difficulties are magnified if the expression of anger is or has been problematic in the clinician's own personal life. After recognizing the contributions of one's own experiences, openly exploring a patient's anger can help create a more honest relationship, define the problem more explicitly, and facilitate an accurate and timely response.

Management

In most anger situations, evaluation and understanding should begin the therapeutic process. Responding calmly without judgment or projection with "You seem angry" tests whether the clinician has correctly identified the emotion of the patient. (At times, it may be more effective and less threatening for patients to label the behavior with a less powerful emotion, e.g., "You seem upset"). Failing to acknowledge anger informs the patient that the clinician is impervious to or unsettled by anger, discourages any meaningful sharing of feelings, and ensures eliciting superficial information. However, constructively acknowledging and working with the anger is both efficient and medically appropriate.

Although many patients in this situation respond with, "You bet I'm angry," some deny their anger. Nonetheless, their body language or tone of voice betrays the denial. In this case, the clinician can address the denial: "Maybe 'angry' is too strong a word. You seem upset, I'd like to help. Can you tell me more about it?" This invitation offers patients the opportunity to explicitly express their feelings and conveys a sense of curiosity (as opposed to judgment) while simultaneously cultivating partnership. As a result, the clinician develops a more complete understanding of the patient's point of view; both can reach a deeper agreement on the nature and magnitude of the problem while building their relationship in the process. At this point in the encounter there is usually a reduction in the patient's anger, relief on the part of the clinician, and the restoration of a productive collaborative relationship.

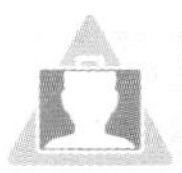

CASE ILLUSTRATION 1 (CONTD.)

The doctor apologizes, saying that the office had gotten busy and that she had simply forgotten to make the call. She explains that to prevent problems like that in the future, the staff decided at a recent meeting to put up a "follow-up" board so that process errors could be reduced. Ms. B. feels better understood, accepts the apology, and ends by saying, "I hope this doesn't happen again; I have enough stress at work as it is." Remembering the same patient's earlier complaint about waiting 35 minutes in the office to be seen, the doctor says, "I should have asked the receptionist to tell you that I was running late—I'm sorry about that. We're really trying hard to make sure that we communicate more effectively with our patients and our consultants." The whole exchange takes 50 seconds—time that is certainly well spent.

Patient Education

It is important for patients to understand that it is not only permissible but also important for them and their families to express their feelings. Encouraging the expression of anger helps to identify unresolved conflicts that can interfere with providing appropriate care. Encouraging patients and their families to express concerns actually offers the clinician an opportunity to become more effective by identifying and then removing significant barriers to effective, honest collaboration. Encouraging the hospital, emergency department, or office staff to use this approach can do the same.

Summary

Too often we assume that angry patients are angry with us. Sometimes this is so, but often there are much more complex reasons for the anger. The patient's reasons must be sought directly before mistakenly projecting our own beliefs onto the patient. By working hard to avoid being defensive, clinicians can acknowledge and then constructively resolve the cause of the anger. Confronted with such a responsive approach, most angry people are satisfied and resume an effective collaborative relationship with their clinician.

THE SILENT PATIENT

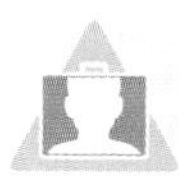

CASE ILLUSTRATION 2

Dr. Cren begins his afternoon office hours with Mr. K., a 47-year-old man who has recently relocated to the area. On entering the room, Mr. K. fails to make eye contact and fiddles with a piece of paper folded over many times. In response to "Good afternoon; I'm Dr. Cren," Mr. K. quietly says, "Good afternoon." When asked what problems he is having, Mr. K. answers, "I've been really tired." After waiting a few seconds, the patient is asked to tell him more. Mr. K. responds, "I don't know what to say."

In response to "You seem quiet," Mr. K. responds, "Today is 3 months since my favorite aunt died." When

Dr. Cren says, "I'm sorry to hear that; would you like to reschedule the visit?" The patient thanks him for the offer, adding that he's concerned about the fatigue and would like to talk about it. With that, the patient becomes more animated and discusses his fatigue. It is subsequently diagnosed as being related to depression.

Diagnosis

Silent patients offer little verbally, but there are a number of important nonverbal cues that deserve attention. The patient may seem withdrawn, as indicated by sitting a greater distance from the clinician than usual, failing to make eye contact, seeming distracted, or not acknowledging the clinician's attempts at interaction. Alternatively, the patient may seem anxious, evidenced by nervous or repetitive habits such as nail-biting, pacing, or folding and refolding papers. Finally, the patient may exhibit signs of sadness like deep sighs, red eyes, or tears. Some of the more common etiologies of silence in patient visits are provided in Table 4-4.

Psychological Mechanisms

In many families, authority figures may demand "silence unless spoken to." This may be transferred to the clinician–patient relationship. This deference may also extend to interactions in which differences in gender, race, sexual orientation, or social class exist. A history of humiliation or perceived mistreatment in previous health care or other hierarchical relationships may also contribute to withdrawn silent behavior.

When patients feel that they have a serious or potentially life-threatening illness, silence may represent denial and serve as a protective function. For example, a woman can avoid confronting her fears about having breast cancer if she does not mention feeling a breast lump while in the shower. Silence may be a sign of a passive personality or, in some cultures, may be consistent with an appropriate way to communicate with clinicians. These individuals want the interviewer to take control and direct the flow. Silence may also indicate a depressed mood, an adverse effect from a medication, or another medical condition that interferes with the patient's ability to communicate. Those struggling with depression or dysthymia may find it difficult to

Table 4-4. Possible causes of silence in patients.

Cause	Discussion
Adverse reaction to prescription medication (e.g., sedation)	Check for overdose or drug interactions
Alcohol or other drug intoxication	Screen with CAGE Questionnaire and elicit history of substance abuse
Alzheimer or other dementia	Age dependent; although some dementias strike as early as the mid-forties, most occur in the 65+ age group. Silence is usually a sign of advanced disease associated with withdrawal from the environment
Anger	The patient is feeling wronged or slighted and is trying to elicit an emotional reaction (see Table 4-3)
Cultural or language barrier	Ask whether the patient can understand; use an interpreter or bilingual staff member, if available
Depression, dysthymia, or adjustment disorder with depressed mood	Name the feelings; request elaboration
Distraction secondary to depression	Associated with drawn features, sad affect, and lack of eye contact
Fear of being told that serious disease is causing the presenting problem	State clearly that, regardless of the outcome, you will be there to help
Fear of clinician authority	Family background, other experience with domineering authority figures may have demanded submissiveness; a gentle demeanor, reassurance, and an explicit request for collaboration can help win the patient's confidence
Hearing impairment	Use the whisper test
Passive or shy personality	Change to a more direct, closed-ended pattern of questions; encourage descriptions and elaboration
Preoccupation with auditory or visual hallucinations	Request additional information from family or attendant
Quiet person	Usually responds to encouragement, offers to elaborate
Stroke, transient ischemic attack (TIA), mass lesion	Conduct thorough neurologic examination for focal findings

express their concerns or even find the energy to initiate conversation.

Management

When confronted with a silent patient, exploring the behavior is usually best begun by reflecting, "You seem quiet today." This offers the p[illegible] acknowledge the behavior an[illegible] Using silence to allow time f[illegible] the space to engender the co[illegible] tive, frightened, or passive p[illegible] When a patient remains passi[illegible] a stance of alliance and mutu[illegible] to earn your trust and help in[illegible] you share with me about wh[illegible] these attempts fail, being mor[illegible] order to help you, I need yo[illegible] experiencing in more detail." [illegible] clues can be useful. For exa[illegible] actively distracted, it is fair [illegible] voices or seeing things you th[illegible] the patient appears angry, co[illegible] be appropriate. If the patient [illegible] "What?" there may be hearin[illegible] nician need only speak loude[illegible]

Patient Education

By explaining that silence may create additional barriers to effective care, clinicians can invite patients to be more involved in evaluation and treatment decisions. Emphasizing the importance of this involvement underscores the value of their taking an active role in decision making. It also discourages the patient from making the clinician solely, and inappropriately, responsible for evaluation or treatment plans.

Summary

There are many reasons for a patient's silence during the visit. Openly acknowledging it and then asking for an explanation offers patients the chance to express a feeling, an extenuating circumstance, fear of an outcome, or fear of the clinician. Further questioning can also result in the diagnosis of an anatomic cause, like sensorineuro hearing loss, or a psychiatric condition. Testing a hypothesis too early runs the risk of insulting patients and worsening the relationship.

Silent patients may be particularly challenging for practitioners who value the social and interpersonal aspects of their work. Learning respectfully to encourage more verbal collaboration is usually beneficial and rewarding. As with anger, the reason for struggling with silent patients may be that they remind us of others from our previous or personal experiences. These reminders can evoke strong negative responses. For example, a clinician easily frustrated by silent patients may be reminded of a parent who died and did not reveal that she was having exertional chest pain. Recognizing the sources of these intense responses can be most helpful in assisting clinicians to focus on the patient and avoid unproductive replays of unsettling past experiences.

[illegible]PATIENT

[illegible]RATION 3

[illegible]ifth patient of the afternoon. [illegible]klayer, who is being seen for [illegible] initial visit, after excluding [illegible]an underlying cancer or spi[illegible] prescribed limited activity, [illegible]steroidal anti-inflammatory [illegible]ting pad. Two weeks later, [illegible]en asked how things have [illegible]responds, "I'm no better. I've [illegible]d back pain chat room and [illegible]have a prescription for some [illegible]ioids." The doctor leans back [illegible]a frustrating encounter.

Diagnosis

Patients often make various requests or demands in the course of their visit for things such as diagnostic tests, referrals to specialists, and for specific treatments. These demands are often tied to dissatisfaction with the recommended evaluation, treatment concern about the accuracy of the diagnosis, or a failure to solicit important aspects of the history. A recommended test or treatment, however, may trigger a memory of a family member or friend's similar and unpleasant experience. The consequence is that the patient projects an undesirable outcome on the recommended plan.

Sometimes the reason for an unexpected demand involves secondary gain, such as workers' compensation, a disability claim or lawsuit, or seeking psychoactive medication. Another possibility is that the patient has found something online, talked to a friend, or read something in the press. The patient may be concerned that the clinician is withholding a more expensive test or treatment to limit cost. Finally, it may be that the patient is frustrated with the lack of relief because additional testing or treatment is actually indicated. By listening carefully to a patient's concerns, the clinician may rethink the diagnosis and/or seek alternatives to the current treatment plan.

Patients who are isolated from family and friends during times of illness may begin to doubt that the clinician is sufficiently interested in their problem to ensure the best possible outcome. If the distrust grows, the patient may feel increasingly responsible and seek alternative sources of care. The patient may become fearful and demanding. If secondary gains are associated with the illness, however, the patient may demand testing to demonstrate greater levels of disability or to prove that the problem is sufficiently severe. This is especially true in chronic pain syndromes for which testing is often unrevealing and treatment not satisfactory.

Clinicians often experience feelings of rejection, distrust, blame, or humiliation in response to demanding patients, leading them to become defensive. By doing so prematurely, the clinician loses the opportunity to explore the patient's subtle reasons for the demands. For example, casual asides; postural shifts in response to a topic; and expressions of fear, agitation, and grief are often ignored and should instead be explored. Possible reasons for demanding additional interventions are listed in Table 4-5.

Management

Rather than responding to the presumed cause, the first step in evaluating or reevaluating the demand is to identify the patient's affect.

Table 4-5. Possible reasons for demanding additional interventions.

Feeling	Discussion
Anger	The patient is feeling wronged or is reexperiencing a previous bad outcome (see Table 4-3)
Fear	The patient may be afraid that the illness is terminal, serious, horrible, disfiguring, and so on, if not attacked quickly
Frustration	The patient may feel that no—or insufficient—progress has been made
Personal responsibility for health outcome	Previous experience may have convinced the patient that physicians are not trustworthy, competent, or interested
Doubt	The patient may wonder if economic reasons are driving decision making or if the practitioner is skilled enough or up-to-date with the current evaluation and treatment technologies

CASE ILLUSTRATION 3 (CONTD.)

Because Mr. G. seems frustrated, the practitioner reflects the feeling: "You seem frustrated." The patient responds, "I am frustrated. My father had a similar condition, and 2 years later they found he had a herniated disk which was successfully treated surgically. I don't want to wait that long to find out what I have."

In response to the clinician's comment about frustration, the patient usually confirms or denies it. If the patient responds affirmatively (e.g., "I am angry, frustrated, sad, nervous"), the clinician would ask, "Why are you ..." This permits the patient to explain and share the experience behind the emotion. Often, this prompts an interaction between clinician and patient that provides important information. In Mr. G.'s case, a better understanding of what prompted the request for more pain medication helps to determine to what extent education, a repeat description of the results of evaluation or treatment, another examination, or questions about possible secondary gain might be most appropriate. As all aspects of a demand are explored, an appropriate response can usually be constructed.

When this approach is less successful, more probing questions may be useful. One is to ask patients what they think is causing their problem; often patients do not offer their opinions without being asked. Given the opportunity, patients frequently say that after an evaluation they were told the test results were all negative, but they believe that the cause of the problem was not addressed. This point cannot be stressed enough: To provide meaningful reassurance, the patient's feelings about what caused the symptom must be elicited and validated.

Another useful question is: "How had you hoped I could help you?" This gives the patient the opportunity to express dissatisfaction with the extent of evaluation, treatment, or perceived commitment by the clinician; it often lightens the clinician's burden, since the patient's request may be significantly less difficult than what the clinician anticipated. A typical example might be the arthritic patient who complains bitterly about the pain in his hip. When the clinician asks, "How had you hoped I could help you?" the patient responds, "I'd like a prescription for a cane." The clinician had anticipated a request for additional imaging (which was not indicated).

Clinicians often find it challenging when patients make requests for opioid pain medication. In response to Mr. G's request for opioids to treat his back pain, the clinician should *acknowledge* the patient's experience of pain and his hope for relief, *reflect* her understanding of the patient's request, and express concern. In addition, the clinician can reframe pain as an "ability." For example, "It's clear that your ability to feel pain is intact. This is important, since pain is an alarm that is wired into us to call our attention to something that may need to be fixed or removed. In your case, unfortunately, there is nothing we can find to fix or remove. Nevertheless the alarm is continuing to go off." It may be helpful to use a metaphor to describe the adaptive nature of pain, for example, "It is like a car alarm designed to signal something to attend to. In the case of chronic pain it is like a car alarm set too sensitively. Rather than removing it, we need to reset the sensitivity of the alarm."

Once validating the patient's experience, only then should the clinician give a rationale for why she is not in favor of using opioids for chronic pain: "It will make the alarm more sensitive." "It can lead to sluggish thinking and interfere with your ability to do your job." "It can lead to addiction." In the common case where patients give a history of previous prescriptions of opioids by other clinicians and that they helped, the clinician may want to comment on how the standard of care in medicine has changed with new knowledge about pain and opioids. "Our understanding of how pain functions and the nature of opioids has changed the standard of care, which is not to use these medications for the kind of chronic pain you are experiencing." It is advisable to avoid personalizing the nonuse of opioids as your preference. Rather refer to it as "the standard of care in this clinic." Finally, suggest that there are a variety of safe pharmacological and nonpharmacological options for managing chronic pain. Instill curiosity, but do not elaborate too soon. "You may not be ready just yet to discuss these with me, but when you are, I'd like you to contact the clinic and set up an appointment so we can discuss the alternatives. I'm confident they can make a difference for you." (This communicates nonabandonment of the patient, even though the patient will not be receiving the desired opioid medication.) (See Chapter 25.)

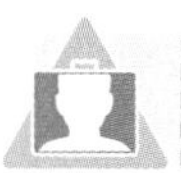

CASE ILLUSTRATION 3 (CONTD.)

Dr. Harwick ends the visit with Mr. G by saying: "What I would like to do is continue our present course of treatment, since in 90% of cases the symptoms you describe resolve within several weeks. If at the end of that time you're still having these symptoms, we can consider further evaluation with imaging studies and a different approach to reducing your pain. I appreciate your suggestions and I will continue to work with you until you feel better."

When clinicians believe that the demand is related to secondary gain (e.g., a desire to remain away from work for an extended period), they can gently confront the patient and offer a plan that provides ample time for recovery.

Patient Education

Patients respond to instruction when they believe it will be helpful in solving their problems. Until there is an agreement on the need for education by clinician and patient, however, the patient might perceive education as the clinician's way to control the visit. The patient's usual response in such an encounter is either to tune out the information or to construct mental barriers to implementing the recommendation. However, once the patient's concerns have been successfully addressed and a partnership formed, the patient often asks for and benefits from information supporting the clinician's point of view.

Summary

Exploring the reasons for a patient's demands in a nonjudgmental manner allows most demands to be understood and addressed. Knowing the cause of the demand, a plan that is mutually agreeable can then be negotiated. If such a negotiation is not possible, the patient should be informed of realistic limits to what the clinician can offer. The patient can then decide whether she is willing to accept the clinician's boundaries or should seek alternative services.

THE "YES, BUT ..." PATIENT

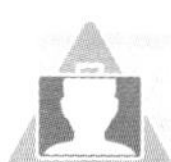

CASE ILLUSTRATION 4

Mrs. M. is a 58-year-old woman being followed for obesity and poorly controlled high blood pressure. Her doctor is frustrated because his continued attempts to get Mrs. M. to lose weight have been unsuccessful. As a result, he is pessimistic about their ability to work together to treat her hypertension, which he feels is a clear risk to her health. When the doctor notes that Mrs. M.'s blood pressure is still elevated, he asks whether she is still taking her medication.

She responds, "Oh, I'm sorry, doctor; I ran out of my medicine 3 days ago and didn't want to bother you for a refill." Later in the visit the doctor asks, "Did you join that exercise program we discussed last visit?" Mrs. M. replies, "I've been so busy. I'll do it next week." The doctor pulls back in his chair, thinking to himself, "This will never go anywhere."

He leans forward and says, "Mrs. M., your actions tell me I'm pushing you to do something you don't want to do. I'm concerned about your weight; what are your thoughts on this?" Mrs. M.'s eyes moisten and she responds, "I want to lose weight, but I can't do it. I've tried for years, and it's so frustrating." The practitioner nods and says, "Let's hold off on the weight control for now. How about taking one thing at a time and focusing on your blood pressure medication?"

Diagnosis

When problems are being discussed, this type of patient's nonverbal behavior is usually engaged and active: leaning forward, bright affect, and dynamic gestures. As recommendations for evaluation and treatment are made, however, the patient typically becomes withdrawn, eye contact diminishes, and language becomes significantly less animated. Verbally, during the discussion of evaluation and treatment, the patient becomes quiet, volunteers little, and characteristically offers no solutions to problems. In fact, as the clinician makes recommendations, the patient often responds with the classic, "I'd like to do that but … ."

The clinician initially feels encouraged to offer the patient suggestions, who then invariably rejects the offer or agrees to the plan but does not carry it out. This may be because the patient is exhibiting "passive/aggressive behavior," but alternatively, perhaps clinician's plan has not taken the patient's perspective into account and is, therefore, unrealistic or economically or logistically impossible. Another consideration is that the patient comes from a highly controlling family and is attempting to follow the recommendations but for psychosocial reasons is unable to. Finally, the patient's previous experiences with clinicians may have been so hierarchical and paternalistic that the thought of disagreeing or negotiating a position does not come to mind, even when the suggested approach is not acceptable.

Psychological Mechanisms

Passive–aggressive behavior may emerge when patients do not feel capable of asserting themselves directly. They may position themselves so that others feel they want to, or must, save them. The clinician's attempt to solve the problem is invariably followed by the patient's frustrating failure to collaborate. The patient successfully transfers responsibly for health problems to the clinician and then rejects each solution offered. Continued failure results in repeated visits, offering the patient continuing attention while increasing the clinician's frustration.

Some patients who are unable to fully collaborate may have been emotionally, verbally, or physically abused or may have had family or other personal experiences that taught unquestioning submission to authority.

Most people who enter the healing professions have a desire to be helpful. Passive–aggressive patients' solicitations for clinicians to save them can be seductive, luring clinicians into believing that these patients will singularly benefit from their expertise. The extent to which clinicians use a patient's recovery to validate their competence or professional value may determine how frustrated and angry they will become when treatment is unsuccessful. Rather than focusing initially on outcomes, the clinician is better served answering the questions "Am I encouraging patients to take a more active role in their care?" and "Am I giving patients the chance to say why they're not using the treatments I thought we agreed on?"

Management

It is important to clearly communicate that to get better the patient must take responsibility for their health. To help differentiate patients who are dependent from those who cannot participate because of a definable medical or personality disorder, the clinician can say, "I'm frustrated with how things are going. Let's start again and see if what I see as a problem is really a problem for you."

The next step is to ask what the patient thinks would be helpful in solving the problem. One can ask, "What barriers do you see in actually doing this?" If the question is asked in a supportive fashion, most patients who initially agreed to fulfill an unrealistic plan (perhaps to please the clinician), respond more honestly. Once this is done, the clinician can encourage collaboration by saying, "Let's explore what realistic options we have to begin to solve this problem together. As we discuss options, it will help if you share what's possible for you and what's not."

If the patient displays passive–aggressive behavior, the clinician can seek agreement on the nature of the problem and then make very specific contracts for what the patient will do. They can be as direct as, "So, until our next visit, you will remain abstinent from alcohol," or "Between now and our next visit, you'll keep a diary and record when, and under what conditions, your headaches occur." The clinician's support and enthusiasm can be directly tied to the degree to which both parties carry out the contract. In this way, the clinician can promote patient autonomy and offer support, without taking full responsibility for the patient's behavior.

Over time, patients learn to respond to the support offered and begin to take a more active role in their care. Of course, there is always the risk that a passive–aggressive individual attempting to control the relationship will choose to seek another clinician who can be more easily manipulated.

Patient Education

Patients who are unfamiliar with a collaborative model can be given specific information about the clinician's understanding and particular style of collaborating. Explicit requests for patients' opinions about collaboration can be extremely useful. Over time, given the opportunity to state opinions and formulate plans, most people find such an approach satisfying, engaging, and motivating. Indeed, there is convincing evidence that patients taught to be more assertive improve their health outcomes, such as lowering blood pressure and controlling diabetes.

Educating patients who exhibit passive–aggressive behavior about such behavior can begin a process of introspection and self-awareness. Encouraging patients to explore the origins of these behaviors and consider a therapeutic relationship that facilitates the process can be rewarding for both patient and clinician. Descriptions of behavior that hit home can provoke emotional responses in patients, but penetrating long-held psychological defenses can spur growth. The clinician might say, for example, "You say your mother was overbearing and controlling and withheld praise. Isn't that what your children are telling you?" In most instances, the benefits outweigh the risks.

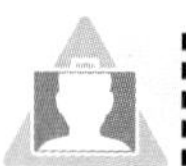

CASE ILLUSTRATION 4 (CONTD.)

Mrs. M. agrees to take her medication and to return for a blood pressure check in 2 weeks. The practitioner gives her a card so that she can record her own blood pressure when she checks it at the drug store or the mall.

Summary

Setting limits and providing explicit feedback can teach patients to collaborate more effectively. Being aware of "yes, but" patterns can help promote a strategy of shared responsibility and prevent the ultimately unhelpful rescuing behaviors that interfere with successful treatment.

Appreciative Inquiry & Difficult Patients

Appreciative inquiry can be applied to our work with difficult patient interactions. It allows us to shift the focus away from the sense of frustration that often accompanies these interactions to recognize and appreciate our successes. One technique is to write a brief narrative of a patient with whom you had initially a difficult interaction, but with whom your relationship became positive over time. As you reflect on the case, keep in mind the following questions to identify the factor or factors that helped transform that initially difficult relationship into one where you felt successful.

- What did you say or do that contributed to moving beyond the difficulty?
- What did the patient contribute to changing your relationship in a positive direction?
- What was it about the environment or circumstances of your encounter that improved the situation or your relationship?
- What changes did you make in your internal appraisal or perception of this patient that made a difference?
- What will you do differently the next time?

INDICATIONS FOR REFERRAL

Indications for referral include inability to make a diagnosis, an objective assessment that the patient is not benefiting from evaluation or treatment, or the clinician's feeling of being threatened or in danger. Outside assistance and advice is always required when an inability to work with a patient impairs the provision of effective care. Since negative feelings often relate to a clinician's previous family and life experiences, a patient who is difficult for one clinician is often not difficult for another.

Once the decision to refer is made, framing the referral in a positive way is particularly valuable. One strategy is to acknowledge the need for assistance in managing difficult situations or problems. The dialogue might take the following form:

Clinician: Mrs. S., for the last 2 months I've been trying to figure out how to help make your headaches better. I think it would help me if you were evaluated by a psychologist; I might be able to get a better handle on what else I could do to assist you in improving the problem.

Mrs. S.: Are you saying that I'm imagining this? Do you think it's all in my head?

Clinician: No, not at all. Nothing we've tried has stopped your headaches and it often helps me to have another person listen to the story and maybe find a new direction to take. Dr. F. has helped me with a number of people in the past, and I'm hopeful she can help us also.

Mrs. S.: What do I have to do? I really do want these headaches to end.

Clinician: I want them to end too. In addition to the referral, let's schedule you for two visits with me over the next 12 weeks to see how things are going and see what else we can do.

Proposing a positive outcome from the referral can be remarkably useful. In addition, scheduling a visit for the person to return after the referral reassures the patient that the referring clinician is truly seeking assistance rather than simply "dumping" the problem on someone else.

Learning to understand the patient's perspective, negotiating for realistic evaluation and treatment plans, and being aware of and responsive to verbal and nonverbal evidence that a recommendation was misunderstood or rejected creates a collaboration that can be satisfying for both participants. Underused skills such as soliciting the patient's attribution for a problem, offering praise and support, listening carefully to the patient's description of a problem, and explicitly confronting problematic or confusing behavior inform the patient that a serious attempt is underway to understand and successfully manage the patient's concerns. To the extent clinicians become more self-aware and address their own feelings, they can become more effective.

Finally, there is increasing recognition of the role the work environment plays in a clinician's effectiveness. As we ask clinicians to be more aware of their emotions, manage the complexities of chronic and life-threatening illnesses, and recognize both verbal and nonverbal clues to overlying psychosocial components of disease, health care systems have a responsibility to create caring, responsive practice settings that nurture clinicians as we ask them to nurture patients.

SUGGESTED READINGS

Beach MC, Inui T. Relationship-centered care: a constructive reframing. *J Gen Intern Med* 2006;21:S3–S8.

Hahn SR, Kroenke K, Spitzer RL, et al. The difficult patient: prevalence, psychopathology, and functional impairment *J Gen Intern Med* 1996;11:1–8.

Hull S, Broquet K. How to manage difficult patient encounters. *Fam Pract Manag* 2007;14(6):30–34.

Lazare A. Shame and humiliation in the medical encounter. *Arch Intern Med* 1987;147:1653–1658.

Quill TE. Partnerships in patient care: a contractual approach. *Ann Intern Med* 1983;98:228–234.

Safran DG, Miller W, Beckman H. Organizational dimensions of relationship-centered care: theory, evidence and practice. *J Gen Intern Med* 2006;21:S9–S15.

Suchman AL, Markakis K, Beckman HB, et al. A model of empathic communication in the medical interview. *JAMA* 1997;277:678–682.

VIDEOS

Video 4-1. Angry Patient Demo (3 min, 25 sec)

Video 4-2. Demanding Patient Demo (4 min, 11 sec)

Video 4-3. Difficult Patients—Difficult Situations (9 min)

Video 4-4. Inappropriate Patient Demo (2 min, 37 sec)

Access by scanning the QR code above or visit mhprofessional.com/feldman5evideos.

Suggestion & Hypnosis

5

John F. Christensen, PhD

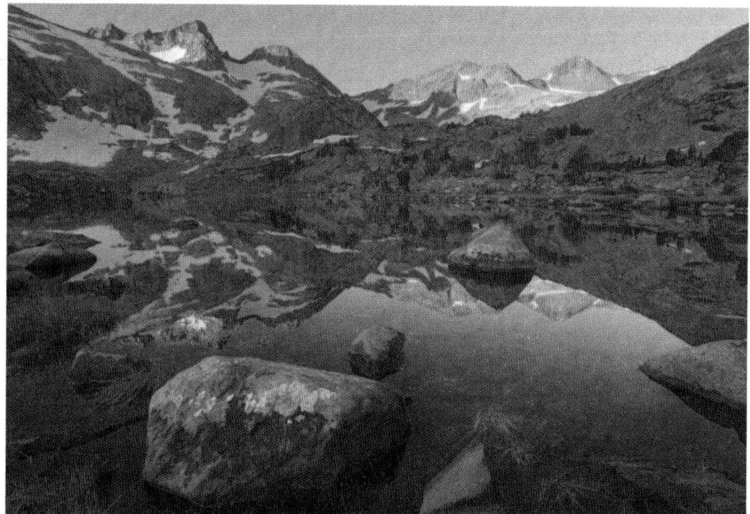

Photo by Hank Christensen (www.hankchristensen.com).

INTRODUCTION

The history of hypnosis as a healing art dates back millennia. Its modern expression as a medical treatment emerged in the eighteenth century, with proponents such as Franz Anton Mesmer, an Austrian physician who practiced in Vienna and Paris in the late 1700s. Mesmer, from whose name the term "mesmerize" was derived, believed that illness was caused by an imbalance of magnetic fluids in the body, which could be corrected by the "personal magnetism" of the hypnotist. Discredited in 1784 by a French royal commission appointed to investigate Mesmer's techniques and chaired by Benjamin Franklin, hypnosis has since regained respectability. Franklin himself wrote an opinion that the patient's beliefs could influence bodily effects. The Scottish surgeon James Braid in 1843 coined the term "hypnosis," from the Greek word for "sleep," and espoused its use as a medical treatment. In the 1930s, Clark Hull and his student Milton Erickson conducted early research on hypnosis. Erickson went on to become a pivotal practitioner, researcher, and teacher of a generation of hypnotherapists. In the 1950s, the British and American Medical Associations recommended incorporating hypnosis into the medical curriculum. The American Psychological Association in 1960 endorsed hypnosis as a branch of psychology. In 1995, the U.S. National Institutes of Health issued a consensus statement with evidence supporting the use of hypnosis for the alleviation of chronic pain.

Hypnosis appears to be a special manifestation of the mind–body system's ability to process information by transforming it from a semantic to a somatic modality. Its therapeutic effectiveness is supported by both research and clinical experience. Today, hypnosis is widely used to treat a variety of conditions—pain, airway restriction, gastrointestinal disorders, skin lesions, burns, and anxiety—as well as to prepare patients for surgical procedures and to facilitate behavior change (such as smoking cessation or weight loss).

Trance and suggestion occur naturally throughout human experience and are a function of how the mind works. Becoming absorbed in a novel and being unaware of surrounding sounds, or daydreaming while driving and not remembering the last few miles, are common experiences that illustrate the ubiquitous nature of trance. Responding to subliminal messages in advertising by purchasing a product represents a familiar reaction to suggestions made in a carefully crafted trance. These common experiences of trance and suggestion also occur with patients in health care.

This chapter will describe the therapeutic use of suggestion within the context of the patient's naturally occurring trance states and in the course of clinician–patient discourse. This application can be used routinely by clinicians in all patient encounters. We will also describe the role of therapeutic hypnosis, usually provided by a specialist trained in this procedure, in treating a variety of medical conditions.

DEFINITIONS

Derived from a Greek word meaning "sleep," hypnosis is, in fact, a therapeutic procedure that requires active cooperation on the part of the patient. The following definitions, used in this chapter, describe the states and processes involved:

Trance: A state of focused attention, in which a person becomes uncritically absorbed in some phenomenon and defocused on other aspects of reality. Trance states can be positive or negative.

Suggestion: A communication that occurs in trance, with special power to elicit a particular attentional, emotional, cognitive, or behavioral sequence of events.

Hypnosis: A communicative interaction that elicits a trance in which other-than-conscious processes effect therapeutic changes in the subject's mind–body system. Hypnosis can be either other- or self-induced.

Induction: The process by which a trance is initiated. This can occur naturally or as the first phase of hypnosis.

Utilization: The therapeutic use of trance to achieve desired outcomes and the phase of hypnosis following induction in which this occurs.

TRANCE & SUGGESTION IN THE MEDICAL ENCOUNTER

Both patient and clinician may undergo a mutual trance induction that, depending on the self-awareness of the participants, can leave either more susceptible to suggestion by the other. This state is neither pathological nor unwarranted, but part of the natural pattern of human awareness in this environment. Generally, because of the power imbalance inherent in help-seeking situations, the patient is more vulnerable to suggestion. Being cognizant of trance and suggestion can give clinicians greater flexibility and influence in leading their patients to more positive outcomes.

Many patients waiting in an examining room are in a trance that has developed through a series of events that started with the onset of the symptom that prompted them to seek help. The patient's awareness of this symptom then leads to an internal search for meaning. Prior beliefs, personal experience, or prompting of family or friends may lead the patient to attribute a particular meaning to the symptom. This attribution constitutes the initial suggestion, perhaps solidifying into a concern, "I wonder if this could be something serious." This preoccupation, in turn, increases awareness of the sensation and further restricts the patient's attentional field. Increased absorption in the symptom and decreased awareness of other sensations are the essence of the trance.

The decision to see a clinician further deepens the trance, and this process continues as the patient, waiting first in the clinician's office and then in the examining room, rehearses how to describe the symptom and discuss it with the clinician. As noted earlier, this process of trance induction around a symptom is not pathological, but is part of the natural unfolding of awareness surrounding a medical visit.

By the time the clinician enters the examining room, the patient is in a trance and consequently susceptible to suggestion. Whatever the clinician says or does not say in the course of the interview can, because of the power generated by the patient's suggestibility, further develop the patient's trance, shift its focus, augment or diminish the patient's somatic awareness, and influence ongoing patient emotions, cognitions, and behaviors surrounding the symptom.

The clinician is also susceptible to trance. Patients can sometimes unwittingly induce a trance in the clinician through a combination of verbal and nonverbal techniques such as the initial verbalization of the problem, hand gestures, grimacing, and changes in voice tone and tempo. All these contribute to focusing the attention of the clinician on the problem or on what hurts. This narrowing of the clinician's focus (even while a differential diagnosis is being developed) may preclude other internal images, such as the future good health of the patient or a positive clinician–patient relationship, which could otherwise give rise to helpful discussions. A too-rapid response by the clinician results in premature closure on the nature of the patient's problem and solidifies the clinician's initial trance. However, attending to and eliciting the whole story from the patient (see Chapters 1 and 2) keeps that focus fluid. Sometimes patients induce a recurrent negative trance in the provider, leading to antagonism or aversion for the patient or to feelings of powerlessness in the face of the patient's problem (see Chapter 4).

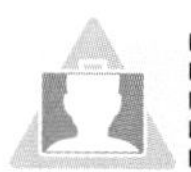

CASE ILLUSTRATION

A 55-year-old single woman was being followed by her primary care physician for chronic chest pain after a thoracotomy. The pain led the patient to withdraw from social activities. Her complaints, which continued for several months, appeared inconsistent with the progress of healing around the surgical wound. Various pain-management strategies that the physician proposed, including physical therapy, acetaminophen, and an antidepressant, had little effect on the complaints. Both patient and doctor became frustrated, with the patient feeling that nothing new was being done for her pain and the physician feeling powerless to alleviate the patient's suffering.

Eventually, seeing this patient's name on the appointment schedule would produce a sinking feeling and tightness in the physician's stomach, and his breathing would become shallow. As he walked into the examining room and observed the patient's slumped posture and grim facial expression, he could predict how the discussion would go:

Doctor: How have you been doing since our last visit?

Patient: (*pointing to her chest and responding with slow speech and long latencies*) This pain really has hold of me, and I can't escape it.

Doctor: (*anticipating a negative answer*) Did you try any of the exercises the physical therapist recommended?

Patient: (*grimacing, shifting position, looking down, and then back at doctor*) I've tried that before, and it only makes the pain worse. (*eyes filling with tears*) Can't you do something for me?

This case illustrates several components of trance in both patient and doctor. The patient's recurring chest pain induces a trance in which her attention becomes narrowly focused on her suffering and disability. Anticipation of a visit to her doctor further restricts her focus, and her rehearsal of how she can convince the doctor of how bad it really is further intensifies the trance. She has learned to associate the image of her doctor's face and the sound of his voice with frustrating discussions about the intractable nature of her pain. Her continued presence at these appointments corresponds with a belief that the power to alleviate her suffering lies outside of herself. If only this doctor knew everything there was to know about her pain, he would be able to help. This expectation keeps her in a suggestible state.

The doctor, too, has shifted into a negative trance by the time he enters the examining room. The induction begins as he anticipates seeing the patient and continues as his accompanying somatic responses shift him from his habitual openness to the field of possibilities to absorption in his own powerlessness to effect change. His trance is deepened by the patient's nonverbal and verbal communications about her continuing pain. The doctor becomes more vulnerable to suggestion, and the patient's plea to do something for her creates the expectation in him that he must do something. This expectation, in the face of the patient's persistent pain, deepens his sense of powerlessness.

Therapeutic Uses of Trance & Suggestion in the Medical Encounter

The clinician can use the patient's trance to make specific suggestions that enhance therapeutic outcomes. The language used in medical encounters can lead to unintended patient beliefs and behaviors that influence both illness and healing. For example, the prediction of continued problems for a patient with a weak knee—"You'll probably always be bothered by some pain in that joint"—in the first postsurgical visit has an enhanced power to influence negatively the patient's future awareness of and belief in the knee's integrity. The warning becomes a self-fulfilling prophecy as the patient unwittingly guards the knee and develops a compensatory gait. A positive suggestion—"Whatever residual discomfort you feel, in time you will notice more freedom of motion and activity"—can create expectations that are more likely to enhance healing and the resumption of activity.

A more subtle strategy is the use of positive images and avoidance of negative modifiers. Consider the following statement to a patient after surgery:

Doctor: Your ankle ought to hurt less in a few weeks.

The unconscious mind tends to delete negative modifiers, in this case "less." The embedded suggestion becomes: "Ankle ... hurt ... in a few weeks." A positive suggestion would be:

Doctor: You will notice much more comfort within a few weeks.

Because the primary words of the sentence are positive, the suggestion might be incorporated as:

Doctor: You will notice ... comfort ... within a few weeks.

In the context of discussing sleep hygiene with an insomniac patient, the well-intended suggestion, "When you go to bed, try not to worry about staying awake," might contain several unintended messages leading to disturbed sleep. The word "try" connotes effort; it becomes associated with "bed"; the negative modifier "not" is deleted by the unconscious mind, leaving the additional message to "worry about staying awake." The suggestion could be positively restated:

> **Doctor:** After you get into bed, you can enjoy a few minutes of deep relaxation before falling soundly asleep.

Clinicians can also use temporal clauses to embed suggestions that lead to positive patient expectations. For example, linking pain with expectations for healing can be accomplished by the following statement:

> **Doctor:** When you first experience postoperative pain, it is important to realize that the healing has already begun.

Predicting positive change that precedes the patient's awareness of it can build positive expectations—even if the discomfort continues. For example, the physician might predict the course of recovery as a patient responds to antidepressant medication:

> **Doctor:** Your spouse and others close to you will notice the changes in you long before you begin to feel better.

The implied suggestion is that you will begin to feel better, and when you do, positive changes will already have occurred.

The clinician can also reframe uncomfortable side effects of some medications as an indicator of their potency, thus enhancing the placebo effect. In prescribing an antidepressant, a physician could disclose the anticipated side effects:

> **Doctor:** If you notice this kind of discomfort as you begin to adjust to the medication, keep in mind that this is a potent drug that has the capability of achieving the results we want.

The message contains two positive associations with the side effects: adjustment to the medication and movement toward the desired outcome.

The clinician who appreciates the trance-like nature of the medical encounter can use the patient's openness to suggestion not only to present positive suggestions and avoid those that are negative but also to promote healing. This is true for both the clinician's own trance and that of the patient.

Shifting From a Negative Trance to a Positive Trance

Clinicians have several options to shift a dysfunctional trance in a more open direction.

CHANGING BODY POSITION

This works directly with the somatic configuration that maintains a trance state. A depressed patient may have a frozen, slumped posture, downcast eyes, and shallow breathing. This frozen posture amplifies negative images and self-statements and inhibits any focus on possibilities for change. The physician can comment on this posture and suggest modifications, such as raising the eyes while walking outside to observe cloud formations, birds, or airplanes, and shifting breathing to the abdomen. The clinician might also suggest that the patient occasionally put on some music and dance—even alone—at home. Clinicians, too, can use a shift of physical position to break an unwanted trance in themselves. A physician who feels ineffectual in the face of an inordinately blaming or demanding patient and reacts physically with chest tightness and throat constriction can stand up, say "Excuse me while I adjust the light," walk to the window, adjust the blinds or shade, move the chair to a slightly different location, and then sit down. During this activity, the physician can shift breathing to the abdomen and prepare to open a new line of discourse with the patient:

> **Doctor:** It's quite obvious how frustrated you are with the way things are going. Let's refocus for a moment on our goals and how things will look for you then.

CONFUSION

Confusion can be helpful in breaking a pattern that locks patient and clinician into repeatedly acting out a script whose negative outcome both can predict. The following caricature illustrates a common script:

> **Patient:** Fix me.
>
> **Doctor:** Try this.
>
> **Patient:** That won't work.
>
> **Doctor:** What do you think will work?
>
> **Patient:** I don't know. You're the doctor.

When the clinician becomes aware of such a circular pattern, it is helpful to ask, "What is the patient anticipating I will say or do next?" If at this point the clinician can do something unpredictable, the result will be temporary confusion, which can be used to shift the patient's trance in a more resourceful direction. The unpredictable action might be the "Columbo technique" (named for the television detective). In this technique, the physician suddenly and dramatically remembers some minor personal problem (e.g., forgetting a spouse's birthday gift), asks the patient's forgiveness for the distraction, and requests the patient's aid (e.g., in suggesting a store to purchase the gift). The momentary confusion that ensues (whether or not the patient is able to offer any help) breaks the previous trance and allows the formation of a new one. This temporary role reversal is only one example of the use of unpredictable behavior to induce confusion and interrupt the pattern, thus allowing greater rapport and more effective communication.

Mining For Gold

This phrase refers to a technique that shifts the focus of discussion away from distress and toward an exploration of the patient's resources. Useful at any time, this strategy is especially helpful when the tone of meetings with the patient is persistently hopeless, when the patient appears to legitimize the visit by focusing exclusively on somatic complaints, or when the patient's continuing complaints make the clinician feel ineffective or frustrated. In "mining for gold," the physician may inquire about things the patient is proud of—past successes, hobbies, travels, relationships, and obstacles overcome. The clinician observes when the patient becomes animated or otherwise shifts out of the negative trance and notes the topic in the chart, returning to this topic briefly in subsequent sessions. Sometimes the change in the patient's state leads to a change in behavior, emotions, or outlook that had been precluded by the "what's wrong with me" trance. Similarly, the clinician's feeling about the patient may change; renewed interest and curiosity about the patient's personal resources may transform a previously difficult relationship.

Eliciting Target States

Here the clinician engages the patient in thinking and talking about a future well-state, asking the patient to describe what things will be like when the medical problem is resolved or no longer interferes with the patient's life. It is important that the patient be able not only to name the target state ("I want to feel good again" or "I want to be free of pain") but also generate visual, auditory, and kinesthetic images of activities associated with that state. This discussion helps physician and patient establish criteria for knowing when the problem is resolved; it also engages the patient in imagining a future well-state unrelated to and incompatible with present suffering. This trance shift may be accompanied by positive physiologic changes and increased animation and hope.

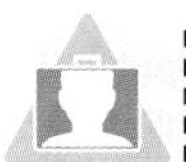

CASE ILLUSTRATION (CONTD.)

In the case of the woman with post-thoracotomy pain, the physician tried using the technique of eliciting a target state to alter the patient's trance.

Patient: (*grimacing*) I feel trapped. I never imagined it would hurt this bad.

Doctor: How do you imagine it will be when you've completely recovered from your surgery?

Patient: Well, I hope I'll feel better.

Doctor: Well, let's think about what that would be like for you. Once you're feeling better, what do you see yourself doing differently?

Patient: Fly fishing.

Doctor: (*smiles; eyebrows raised, voice more animated*) You like to fish? (*the doctor enjoys fly fishing and has shifted automatically into a state of high interest*)

Patient: (*looks at doctor, smiles*) I used to enjoy being out on the river in my waders, fishing for steelhead and Chinook salmon.

The doctor and patient proceeded to discuss various rivers they had fished. The patient had momentarily shifted her mental imagery and her kinesthetic state away from the pain trance toward future health. This created a context in which she could construct a full sensory image of that future well-state that was incompatible with the pain behaviors she had displayed. In addition, her image of the doctor, previously associated exclusively with her pain awareness, became, in subsequent visits, associated with images of recovery and hope. The doctor's impression of the patient also changed so that he looked forward to their meetings instead of dreading them.

MEDICAL APPLICATIONS OF HYPNOSIS

Hypnosis can be an effective therapeutic option for a variety of problems. The neurophysiologic processes by which hypnosis can affect change in such a wide range of complaints are still a subject of exploration. One current theory uses information processing as a heuristic model, with the body, brain, cells, and organs regarded as an information-processing system. In the brain, semantic information (encoded in language) is transduced into molecular information, which uses neurochemical and neurohormonal channels to cause changes in diverse organ systems.

Recent brain imaging studies, employing PET and functional MRI, have shown that the hypnotic state is related to a widespread set of cortical areas involving the occipital, parietal, precentral, premotor, and ventrolateral prefrontal and anterior cingulate cortices. The antinociceptive effects of hypnosis correlated with activity in the mid-cingulate cortex.

In deciding whether to use hypnotic procedures with patients (or to refer them to a hypnotherapist), it is important to consider patients' beliefs about hypnosis, their openness to other therapeutic modalities, and their locus of control. Some religious groups (e.g., Jehovah's Witnesses) forbid use of hypnosis, and some patients may fear that they will surrender control to a powerful "other," who can then control their minds. Brief education by the physician about the nature of hypnosis and its usefulness as a tool to help patients increase control over their symptoms may correct these beliefs. If the patients are not convinced, they are probably not good candidates for hypnosis.

Furthermore, some patients may resist hypnosis because they infer that the physician thinks the problem "is all in their head." For such patients, anything other than a biomedical intervention may be viewed with suspicion. Assuring them that hypnosis is simply part of a comprehensive medical management of their problem may increase their openness.

Locus of control—internal or external—is also a significant factor. Patients with an internal locus of control believe that they can influence many of life's rewards or punishments, and they may be better candidates for hypnosis than those with an external locus of control. This latter group may respond better to biofeedback, which relies on equipment that is external to the patient.

In the following brief descriptions of clinical situations, hypnosis can be considered as an adjunctive or, in some cases, primary treatment.

Relaxation & Stress Management

One of the physiologic effects of therapeutic hypnosis is stimulation of the parasympathetic nervous system (see Chapter 36, "Stress & Disease," Figure 36-2). Several stress-related conditions have been attributed to hyperstimulation of the sympathetic nervous system, which is modulated by the parasympathetic nervous system in a dynamic interrelationship. Sympathetic activation can be part of the fight-or-flight response to perceived threats. Given the plethora of real or perceived threats in today's world, stress-related illnesses may be a common presentation of patients' habitual levels of sympathetic arousal (see Chapter 36). Sympathetic responses include tachycardia, muscle tension, adrenaline release, pupil dilation, inhibited intestinal mobility, shortness of breath, and sweating. This autonomic activation is downregulated during hypnosis, and with parasympathetic stimulation the individual becomes relaxed, leading to energy restoration, conservation, and renewal.

Anxiety

Hypnosis can be quite effective as a primary or adjunctive treatment for anxiety. Patients with an internal locus of control will find self-hypnosis an especially satisfying alternative to anxiolytic medication. When introducing this as an alternative treatment, the physician can say:

> **Doctor:** You have a powerful pharmacy in your brain that can produce significant healing effects. Through hypnosis you can learn to mobilize that pharmacy and let it work cooperatively with the other approaches we use.

The clinician can devote 15–20 minutes to inducing a trance, during which the patient is led to form a full sensory recall of an experience in which he or she felt deeply relaxed. In this process, it is important that clinicians avoid imposing their own images of relaxation, instead facilitating the patient's exploration by means of nonspecific suggestions. These suggestions can lead the patient through each sensory modality (e.g., vision) and submodality (e.g., color, brightness, and quality of reflected light) to allow the patient to become absorbed in a full sensory representation of an actual experience associated with relaxation. If the session is audio recorded, patients can take the recording home for daily practice, thereby learning to self-induce trances and regulate their own levels of autonomic nervous system arousal. The extra time taken for the hypnotic induction can often be compensated by a decrease in time spent on phone calls from anxious patients, since the audio recording allows the patient to access the clinician's voice and suggestions whenever needed.

Pain Management

Because cortical elaboration of nociception is a component of pain, hypnosis can be used to shift the focus of attention away from pain sensations. In some surgical or dental procedures, hypnosis can be used as an adjunct to, or instead of, anesthesia. In addition, patients with chronic pain can be taught to relax the muscles they tense around areas of pain as part of their "guarding" or bracing efforts. This hypnotic relaxation reduces the component of the pain that is due to muscle contraction. Patients with migraine headaches can be taught to dilate blood vessels in their hands and feet through hand- and foot-warming imagery—sitting in front of a campfire, for example. In the early prodromal stage of migraine, this procedure can sometimes reverse the progress of the headache, possibly by increasing peripheral vasodilation and allowing relaxation of blood vessels in the head. Temporomandibular disorders, pain from repetitive strain injuries, and tension headaches have also been treated effectively with hypnosis. In one study, older female patients with osteoarthritis experienced significant increase in their health-related quality of life following a 12-week treatment using guided imagery with relaxation. Brain imaging studies have suggested that in hypnosis-induced analgesia prefrontal and anterior cingulate cortices form important structures in a descending pathway that modulates incoming nociceptive input.

Hospice & Palliative Care

Hypnosis has been used adjunctively with other therapies to help patients with chronic and terminal illnesses. Relaxation, overcoming insomnia, relief from pain and dyspnea, and enhancing relationships with relatives and other support persons are some of the benefits of this modality in the hospice setting.

Cancer

There is evidence that hypnosis is effective in alleviating the chronic pain associated with cancer. In addition, hypnosis can control symptoms such as nausea, anticipatory emesis, and learned food aversion; it is also helpful in managing anxiety and other emotions associated with cancer. Hypnosis may also be effective in reducing hot flashes in breast cancer survivors.

Skin Problems

Certain dermatological conditions, such as warts and alopecia, have been treated successfully with hypnosis. While in trance, patients are given the suggestion to experience tingling or flushing in the affected area. Warts may respond to these suggestions by shrinking in size or—in some cases—disappearing. Burns have also responded to hypnotherapeutic suggestion, both in lessening the degree of the burn and in controlling pain. Other dermatoses for which therapeutic hypnosis may be helpful are acne, atopic dermatitis, herpes simplex, hyperhidrosis, pruritus, psoriasis, and rosacea.

Immune System Function

Hypnosis has been used successfully to treat genital herpes, both in reducing the number of flare-ups and in decreasing the duration of flare-ups. Hypnosis has been shown to decrease blood levels of herpes simplex virus and to increase T-cell effectiveness, NK-cell activity, secretory immunoglobulin A (IgA), and neutrophil adherence. A meta-analysis has shown that hypnosis can reliably alter immune system function. Hypnosis incorporating immune suggestions showed a positive influence on total salivary IgA concentration and neutrophil adherence, along with a modest suppression of intermediate-type hypersensitivity erythema. These effects were mediated through relaxation. Some studies have shown differential delayed skin sensitivity reactions on the right and left arm of subjects depending on which arm was suggested under hypnosis to show no changes.

Respiratory Problems

Patients with asthma have been taught to use self-hypnosis to expand airways and minimize stress-induced attacks, as well as reduce anticipatory anxiety about having an attack. Some patients are able to decrease their bronchodilator use with daily self-hypnosis. Weaning patients off a ventilator in the intensive care unit has been facilitated by the use of hypnosis.

Hypertension

Hypnosis for relaxation can be a useful adjunct to other therapies for hypertension. Individual hypnosis treatments for eight sessions was shown to reduce mild essential hypertension immediately posttreatment and at 1-year follow-up.

Gastrointestinal Problems

Problems such as irritable bowel syndrome (IBS) are amenable to adjunctive treatment with hypnosis. The primary approach is to reduce anxiety, induce relaxation, incorporate abdominal breathing, and suggest warmth in the abdomen and proper functioning in the bowels. Gut-focused hypnotherapy has been shown to have immediate and lasting effects on abdominal pain, bloating, and stool consistency, with significant improvements in somatization and depression. Preoperative suggestions have been used successfully to promote an early return of gastrointestinal motility following intraabdominal surgery, leading to shorter hospital stays.

Sleep Problems

Sleep-onset insomnia—associated with anxiety, obsessive worrying, or sympathetic arousal conditioned to the cue of getting into bed—can be treated with hypnotherapy. By making an audio recording of an induction in which the patient is led into a relaxed state and invited to form positive associations with lying in bed before falling asleep, the clinician can give the patient a new nightly ritual that will enhance relaxation. A relaxing trance can also help the patient return to sleep more quickly after waking up.

Pediatrics

Pediatricians and family physicians skilled in hypnosis find it a useful adjunct in the treatment of children. Children are often amenable to the use of imagination and story-telling as trance induction techniques. Some of the conditions that respond well to primary or adjunctive use of hypnosis include nocturnal enuresis, night terrors, functional abdominal pain, surgical and other office procedures, chronic dyspnea, and symptoms related to cystic fibrosis. Hypnosis was shown to be effective in reducing distress and the duration of an invasive diagnostic test in children with urinary tract abnormalities. In a review of studies on psychological interventions to reduce needle-related procedural pain in children, hypnosis showed the most promise in reducing self-reported pain.

Pregnancy

Hypnosis has been used successfully to reduce symptoms of hyperemesis gravidarum. Habitual aborters have been helped to relieve anticipatory anxiety and lessen the psychogenic risks of spontaneous abortion when organic etiologies have been ruled out.

Childbirth

For pain relief during childbirth, a meta-analysis showed that hypnosis reduces analgesia requirements in labor. In another comprehensive methodological review, hypnosis was consistently shown to be more effective than standard medical care, supportive counseling, and childbirth education classes in reducing pain. Other benefits included better infant Apgar scores and shorter Stage 1 labor.

Preparing for Surgical & Other Difficult Procedures

Patient expectations appear to play a role in the degree of pain and distress felt with surgery and procedures such as colonoscopy. Hypnosis has been used to anesthetize patients who are allergic to anesthetic drugs and to decrease the use of postoperative pain medication. Usually hypnotic anesthesia requires a deep level of trance, which calls for advanced skill on the part of the hypnotherapist along with the patient's ability to be hypnotized. More commonly than for anesthetic uses, hypnotic suggestions can provide a helpful supplement to presurgical communications with patients. Using the naturally occurring trance of patients anticipating surgery, physicians can make simple suggestions to enhance surgical wound healing and reduce postoperative pain. Referring to pain as "discomfort" or an "unusual sensation," the physician can offer the patient a statement such as:

> **Doctor:** No matter what you've been thinking about the time after surgery, you'll be pleasantly surprised at how little discomfort you have.

Presurgical hypnosis can also decrease disorientation and confusion following surgery.

Habit Change

For patients in the preparation/determination or action stage of readiness to stop smoking or to change eating behavior (Chapter 19, "Behavior Change"), hypnosis can be a useful ally. The ritual pattern of patient behavior around smoking can be viewed as a trance phenomenon. There is an automatic, other-than-conscious sequence of kinesthetic (tactile, visceral, emotional, and postural) awareness and behavior usually set in motion by contextual cues (e.g., finishing a meal, drinking coffee or alcohol, and talking on the telephone). Hypnosis can be described to patients in the preparation/determination stage as a useful tool "to help you come out of the smoker's trance and into a more satisfying, health-promoting trance." The clinician can call patients' attention to the automatic behavioral sequence while taking a smoking history (Table 5-1). Asking patients to describe in detail which hand they use to pick up the cigarette pack, take the cigarette out of the pack, hold the lighter or strike the match, and so on, will call their attention to the automatic, trance-like nature of their behavior. After inducing a hypnotic trance, the clinician can suggest that patients visualize in slow motion the entire sequence prior to lighting each cigarette. When the previously automatic behavior is raised to the level of awareness, patients are able to break the previous pattern and approach each episode of smoking with increased deliberation. Once patients are in the action stage of cessation, the parasympathetic effects of self-hypnosis can be used as an alternative stress-reducing activity.

Hypnosis, when combined with cognitive-behavioral therapy, has been shown to be effective in promoting weight loss.

SELF-HYPNOSIS

With proper training, patients who respond well to hypnotic trances can learn to self-induce hypnosis to achieve both relaxation and specific therapeutic effects. A useful transition to confidence in self-hypnosis is the patient's regular use of a recorded hypnotic induction made by the clinician (primary care provider or referral specialist) in the office, thereby extending the clinician's presence into the patient's milieu. As the patient gains experience going into a therapeutic trance by listening to the recording, the clinician can teach the patient one of several self-induction protocols, such as the one shown in Table 5-2 (this can also serve as a handout). Some patients are able to develop their skill at self-hypnosis and retain it as a life-long health resource.

One use of a self-induced trance is to enhance one's inner awareness or state of mind by accessing somatic memories of positive resource states. This can be useful for either patient or clinician when preparing for a stressful encounter. The method (Table 5-3) is based on the observation that various sensory cues (e.g., music or smell) can trigger associated memories of feeling states. By choosing a desired resource state, constructing a

Table 5-1. Hypnotic smoking-cessation interview.

The following questions are designed not only to gather information about the patient's smoking behavior and its parameters but also to raise the patient's awareness about behaviors that are usually automatic and unconscious. The interview presupposes that the patient has already expressed a desire to stop smoking.

- Have you ever quit smoking before? How long were you successful at curtailing your smoking? What allowed you to succeed at not smoking for that long?
- What other habits have you overcome? How have you done that?
- What brand of tobacco have you been using?
- What motivates you to continue smoking?
- Where do you have your first cigarette of the day?
- Where do you have your second cigarette?
- What is the sequence of activities that precede the first cigarette of the day?
- Describe the different situations in which you are likely to smoke.
- Describe the mood or emotional state that usually precedes smoking.
- Describe the urge to smoke in detail.
- Describe how you light a cigarette (if the response is vague, offer the following prompts):
  - Which hand do you use to reach for the pack?
  - Which hand do you use to pull the cigarette out of the pack?
  - Which hand do you use to put it in your mouth?
  - Which hand do you use to light it?
  - Which hand do you use to continue smoking?
- Will you describe in detail all of the reasons that you can think of for not taking a first puff after you have stopped smoking?
- How long will you have to stop before you realize that you are permanently free of smoking?
- How will you tell people that you have stopped smoking?

full sensory memory in which that state was felt, then anchoring that feeling state to a tactile cue, the desired state can be reactivated in the new situation. Clinicians might find this especially helpful in shifting toward a positive trance before a patient encounter.

Table 5-2. Eyeroll technique for self-hypnosis.

1. Find a relaxed, quiet place to sit or lie down.
2. Open yourself to a few minutes of inner renewal and refreshment.
3. Use a one-two-three count:
   One: Roll your eyes up to the top of your head.
   Two: Slowly close your eyelids over raised eyes. Inhale deeply.
   Three: Slowly exhale while you relax your eyes.
4. Continue breathing in a relaxed way from your abdomen.
5. Imagine yourself in some pleasant scene or experience for a few minutes.
6. Imagine the sights, sounds, feelings, and smells.
7. While imagining this scene, focus on the desired outcome of this trance (relaxation, pain reduction, etc.).
8. To alert yourself, use a three-two-one-zero count:
   Three: Tell yourself, "I'm ready to be alert."
   Two: Roll your eyes up under your closed eyelids.
   One: Slowly open your eyes and make a fist.
   Zero: Relax your eyes and your hand. Enjoy reorienting yourself to your surroundings.

REFERRAL FOR TREATMENT WITH HYPNOSIS

The various medical applications of hypnosis described in the above sections require one or more sessions with a trained hypnotherapist. Skilled hypnotherapists spend time with patients prior to hypnosis discussing their understanding and expectations of the hypnotic experience and addressing their anxieties and misconceptions. The aim is to establish rapport and raise positive expectations in the patient's mind. When this preliminary discussion is completed, the clinician proceeds to the induction of a trance, using one of several approaches. (The specifics of these inductions are too numerous and complex to be discussed in detail in this chapter, and special training is required to use them appropriately and with flexibility to the patient's responses.) Once the patient exhibits signs of a trance, the clinician proceeds to the utilization of that trance for the specific benefit desired. This involves offering suggestions for the patient to imagine changes in somatic sensations, emotions, or future behaviors. The clinician then concludes by alerting and reorienting the patient to the external surroundings. After the procedure, the hypnotherapist can discuss the patient's subjective experiences and answer questions.

As noted earlier, some clinicians become trained in hypnosis (see final section) so that they can integrate this treatment into their medical practices. Others may

Table 5-3. Developing resourceful states with self-hypnosis.

This technique is useful when you anticipate a stressful situation where you would like to access a positive internal resource that is already a part of you. It is founded on the reality that you have already experienced all the inner states you need to be effective in the anticipated situation. These inner states are part of the body's kinesthetic memory and the files containing them can be cross-referenced with your mental representation of the new event. This is a reprogramming technique that allows you to rapidly activate the desired kinesthetic state.

1. Allow yourself to become quiet, breathe from your abdomen, close your eyes.
2. Build a full sensory image (visual, auditory, and kinesthetic) of the stressful situation you expect to encounter. Notice your emotional and physical response.
3. Now break your physical state by changing positions. Become quiet again.
4. Think about the kind of internal resource (attitude, feeling state, and level of energy) you would like to have available to you in the stressful situation. Examples would be "confidence," "calmness," or "compassion."
5. Once you have decided on the resource state you want to access, search in your memory for an experience or situation in which you felt that resource to be strong in you. This remembered experience may have nothing to do with the stressful situation you are anticipating and may be from a totally different sphere of your life.
6. Build a full sensory image of the positive experience in which you felt that resource (visual, auditory, and kinesthetic). Allow the resourceful feeling to grow in you as you recall that experience.
7. When the resourceful feeling becomes strong in you, **anchor** it by touching together your right thumb and little finger. (An anchor is any stimulus that can serve as a cue for that resource state—it may be a word you say internally, a melody, a fragrance. The tactile anchor is useful, since it is very portable.)
8. Break your emotional state by changing positions. Now test the anchor you developed by touching your thumb and finger together. Notice what feelings emerge.
9. If you wish to add additional resources to the same anchor to be used in the anticipated situation, repeat steps 4–7 for each additional resource.
10. Now again fantasize the stressful situation. Imagine yourself stepping across a threshold into that scene. As you step across the threshold, activate the anchor (touching right thumb and little finger) and carry the resources you developed with you into the encounter.

choose to refer patients to a specialist (psychiatrist, psychologist, clinical social worker, or psychiatric nurse practitioner) trained in hypnosis and familiar with its medical applications. To maximize the therapeutic outcome, it is essential that the referring practitioner communicate with the specialist—before the visit—about the nature of the medical problem, the desired clinical outcome, and the patient's expectations about treatment. It is also important to prepare the patient by explaining the nature of therapeutic hypnosis and by explaining that its intent is to increase the patient's control over symptoms and their impact.

SUMMARY

Hypnosis has a long tradition as a healing art and as adjunctive treatment for many medical conditions and primary or preferred treatment for some conditions. Clinicians can refer patients for hypnotherapeutic treatment to licensed psychologists, clinical social workers, nurse practitioners, or physicians who have formal training in hypnosis through an accredited organization such as the American Society of Clinical Hypnosis or the Milton Erickson Foundation. Whether or not formally trained in hypnosis, the astute clinician can utilize the naturally occurring trance states frequently found in patients in the medical setting, including the primary care encounter and presurgical consultations, to reduce fear through the reframing of symptoms manifest in common presentations such as chronic nonmalignant pain or anxiety disorders. In these naturalistic trances, careful attention to language is paramount in using suggestion. Avoiding the unwitting use of negative suggestions and maximizing positive expectations for a future experience of healthy functioning can mobilize mind–body healing potentials inherent in the patient.

TRAINING IN HYPNOSIS

Clinicians who are interested in developing their own skills in hypnosis are encouraged to receive formal training from an accredited training program or receive supervision from a licensed health professional with formal training in hypnosis. Several of the organizations listed here provide accredited training:

- The American Society of Clinical Hypnosis (ASCH). http://www.asch.net. Accessed February 2019.
- The Milton H. Erickson Foundation. http://www.erickson-foundation.org. Accessed February 2019.
- Society for Clinical and Experimental Hypnosis. http://www.sceh.us/. Accessed February 2019.

SUGGESTED READINGS

Christensen JF, Levinson W, Grinder M. Applications of neurolinguistic programming to medicine. *J Gen Intern Med* 1990;5:522–527.

Faymonville ME, Boly M, Laureys S. Functional neuroanatomy of the hypnotic state. *J Physiol* 2006;99:463–469.

Hammond CR. Hypnosis in the treatment of anxiety- and stress-related disorders. *Expert Rev Neurother* 2010;10:263–273.

Häuser W, Hagl M, Schmierer A, Hansen E. The efficacy, safety and applications of medical hypnosis—a systematic review of meta-analyses. *Dtsch Arztebl Int* 2016;113:289–296.

Landolt AS, Milling LS. The efficacy of hypnosis as an intervention for labor and delivery pain: a comprehensive methodological review. *Clin Psychol Rev* 2011;31:1022–1031.

Levinson W. Reflections: mining for gold. *J Gen Intern Med* 1993;8:172.

Miller GE, Cohen S. Psychological interventions and the immune system: a meta-analytic review and critique. *Health Psychol* 2001;20:47.

Palsson OS. Hypnosis treatment of gastrointestinal disorders: a comprehensive review of the empirical evidence. *Am J Clin Hypn* 2015;58:134–158.

Pittler MH, Ernst E. Complementary therapies for reducing body weight: a systematic review. *Int J Obes* 2005;29:1030–1038.

Rossi EL. *The Psychobiology of Gene Expression: Neuroscience and Neurogenesis in Hypnosis and the Healing Arts*. Norton, 2002.

Stoelb BL, Molton IR, Jensen MP, Patterson DR. The efficacy of hypnotic analgesia in adults: a review of the literature. *Contemp Hypn* 2009;26:24–39.

Uman LS, Chambers CT, McGrath PJ, Kisely S. Psychological interventions for needle-related procedural pain and distress in children and adolescents. *Cochrane Database Syst Rev* 2006;(4):CD005179.

Practitioner Well-Being 6

Anthony L. Suchman, MD & Gita Ramamurthy, MD

INTRODUCTION

CASE ILLUSTRATION

Don, a 38-year-old primary care physician, sighs as he sees Mrs. D.'s name as a last-minute addition to his patient list. It is mid-afternoon on Friday, and he had blocked out the last hour of the day to attend his son's final softball game of the season. "Of all the days for one of her 'crying headaches,'" Don mutters to himself, "why today?"

Don's skill in handling patients with somatoform problems is respected throughout the health center. Since he assumed responsibility for Mrs. D.'s care, her emergency-department visits have fallen by 90%, and she has even taken a part-time job. Don has almost always been able to help her through these spells by sitting with her, holding her hands, and letting her talk.

When he was growing up, Don was always a leader. In the Boy Scouts, his college newspaper, and student service projects in medical school, he was always the one who could organize everyone and get things done. People came to depend on him for that, and while he never showed it outwardly, his capacity to hold responsibility was a source of pride. "Hey, Don!" The greeting comes from Grace, one of Don's partners, breezing toward the door with briefcase in hand. "What a great afternoon! My last patient just canceled . . . I'm going to go home, pour myself a glass of white wine, sit out on the deck, and catch up on some journals. Hope you have a great weekend!"

The door opens, the door closes, and frustration, sadness, loneliness, and anger come together as Don watches Grace leave.

Primary care practice can be both an enriching source of personal growth and meaning and an unmerciful and depleting taskmaster. It provides us with access to a broad range of human experience—an intimate view of the characters and stories of a thousand novels—and an opportunity to have our very presence matter to others. At the same time, it makes constant demands and surrounds us with perpetual uncertainty; it relentlessly confronts us with our limitations of time, energy, knowledge, and compassion. It is a job that is never done; at best, problems are stabilized until something else goes wrong. And in case the intrinsic challenges of the clinical work were not enough, clinicians now have to contend with unprecedented administrative complexity and burden.

The balance each of us strikes between our own enrichment and depletion is critical to our physical, emotional, and spiritual health and to our ability to care for others. All too often, however, we lose sight of this balance. We become so outwardly focused, attending to clinical problem solving and other workplace demands, that we do not tend to our own renewal. This lack of balance is not surprising; our education has taught us much more about how to care for others than how to care for ourselves. The socialization processes of medical school and residency have cultivated a variety of unrealistic self-expectations and attitudes, especially concerning control, self-sufficiency, and obedience.

Over time, this imbalance can produce a vague but increasing sense of demoralization, exhaustion, and depletion—burnout—in which the joy of work is lost, and patients seem increasingly annoying and adversarial. The prevalence of burnout in the primary care workforce has been estimated to be as high as 50%. When the root causes of this dissatisfaction are invisible to us, we blame external sources such as the government, insurance companies, or lawyers. While there are indeed legitimate complaints about the practice environment and bureaucracy, the most fundamental determinants of satisfaction and well-being are not external but rather are found within.

In this chapter, we will examine important values, attitudes, and skills that affect our well-being. We will also consider the ways in which our work environments and personal practices can keep us healthy.

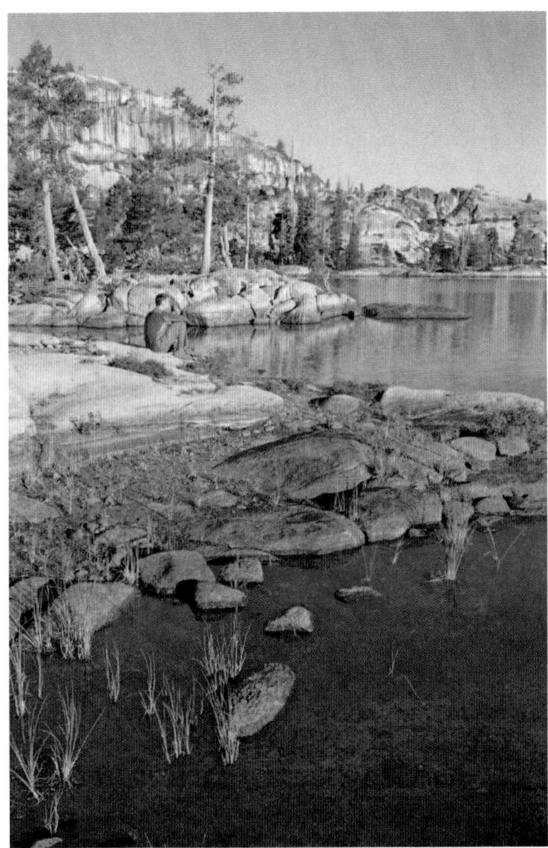

Photo by Hank Christensen (www.hankchristensen.com).

BASIC NEEDS OF PRACTITIONERS

The foundation of our well-being is the acknowledgment that we are human, that we have needs and limits, and that to keep on giving we must know and have reliable access to those things that sustain and revitalize us. Unfortunately, the notion that clinicians have needs has been put off-limits by traditional professional ideals. An excessively narrow interpretation of the scientific model calls on us to be detached and objective observers, leaving no room for our own subjective experience. We are also exposed early, and often, to the ideal of the clinician who is selfless, invulnerable, and omnipotent.

In actuality, each of us has a variety of needs, both universal and neurotic, that cannot fail to assert themselves. Our health and well-being depend on the degree to which we are aware of and attend to them consciously and purposefully.

Among our most fundamental needs are those for human connection, meaning, and self-transcendence—experiencing ourselves as part of something larger than we are. Clinical work is particularly rich with opportunity for human contact and appreciation. Many studies have shown the patient–clinician relationship to be the single most important factor contributing to physician satisfaction (mirroring its central importance to patients). When we are working under excessive pressure or in situations for which we are not adequately prepared, however, clinical work can interfere with the satisfaction of these needs, resulting in depersonalization and alienation from and hostility toward our patients.

Clinical work can also threaten the fulfillment of transpersonal needs by taking too much time and attention from family and community life. Moreover, we sometimes have difficulty shedding the white coat—stepping out of our professional caretaking role to express the spontaneity and vulnerability necessary for intimacy. Alienation in our personal relationships can lead to the breakdown of crucial personal support systems.

In addition to our universal needs for connection and meaning, we also have very individual neurotic needs—born of pain and conflict—that are intimately related to our medical work. These needs influence both our motivation to go into medicine in the first place and the way we practice. Out of a need to feel loved or appreciated, we often find ourselves in the role of overfunctioning caretakers, and our difficulty saying "no" quickly leads to overcommitment. Feelings of impotence engendered by childhood experiences of illness—our own or those of a close friend or relative—may be relieved through our work with patients, but the wishful fantasy of controlling disease is constantly challenged by reality. Voyeuristic desires, fear of death, and the fulfillment of parental expectations are other factors, conscious or unconscious, that can motivate our careers.

These darker, neurotic needs are no less legitimate than those less hidden; they, too, are a normal part of life. When these needs operate outside our awareness, however, they can drive us to work excessively, assume unrealistic degrees of responsibility, and otherwise distort our work lives, thereby causing us to suffer. If we invest ourselves in unrealistic solutions that must inevitably fail, we risk chronic anxiety, substance abuse, and even suicide. Through various processes of self-exploration (such as psychotherapy, peer support groups, or mindfulness workshops) we can become more aware of these needs that underlie our work and find healthier ways to satisfy them. We ignore them at our own peril.

PERSONAL PHILOSOPHY

Another important but under-recognized determinant of our well-being is our personal philosophy—the deeply held beliefs and values that address the most fundamental questions of our lives: the meaning and purpose of life, death, joy, and suffering; why things happen the way they do; the nature of our relationship to other people and to the world; and the nature of our goals and responsibilities as human beings. Our personal philosophies define our expectations of ourselves and other people. They guide the way we perceive and respond to our world and help us identify our place in it. They define the framework by which we imbue things in our lives with meaning, joy, or pain and by which we determine what seems right and what seems wrong.

Developing a personal philosophy tends to be a subliminal process—a gradual internalization of attitudes and values from family, culture, education, and life experience—making it possible for us to be entirely unaware of our core beliefs as an ideology. We may take them so completely for granted that they just seem to be part of the way things are. If we do not understand how these beliefs filter our perceptions and shape our behaviors, then we are unable to subject them to critical reflection and to decide which parts work well for us and which parts need to be changed.

The Control Model

One aspect of personal philosophy with special importance to clinical practice is our attitude toward control. Through the influence of Western culture in general and medical culture in particular, we often perceive being in control (of diseases, patients, and the health care team) to be the ideal state (Table 6-1). We use specific intellectual tools for gathering and applying knowledge: *reductionism*—"Sickle cell anemia is attributable to the substitution of a single nucleotide"; *linear causality*—"*A* causes *B*"; and *generalization*—"Asthma responds to bronchodilators." All have a distinctly controlling, outcome-oriented focus, that is, to manipulate *A* so as to control *B*. Although this approach has led to important technological advances, it also has important adverse consequences.

The control model creates unrealistic expectations that limit our opportunities to feel successful. Consider, for instance, how our expectations of good control in caring for a diabetic patient allow us to feel successful only when the blood sugar is tightly regulated. The patient's blood sugar, however, is influenced by many factors over which we have no control, the patient's own behavior being foremost among them. We become angry at the patient whose "noncompliance" stands in the way of our success. If success for us is defined only in terms of controlling disease, we are precluded from feeling successful in many, if not most, situations. Accepting responsibility for outcomes over which we have little or no control is highly stressful and leads us to feel helpless, anxious, and angry.

Our quest for control also creates distance and detachment in the patient–clinician relationship, which, as we have already seen, is an important factor in professional satisfaction. A strong orientation toward control leads to hierarchic relationships. This, coupled with the reductionism and labeling inherent in medical thinking, turns patients into objects, and we find ourselves working with *things*—organs, diseases, medications, and tests—rather than with people. We, too, become depersonalized in this process, leaving no room for our own subjective experience.

The Relational Model

An alternative philosophy that avoids many of these problems emphasizes relatedness rather than control. This model does not reject the insights of reductionism, but rather builds on them by adding an appreciation of context and relationship. Therefore, although *A* may seem to cause *B*, there are also other mediating factors and bidirectional interactions (*A* and *B* influence each other). For example, the tubercle bacillus causes tuberculosis, but not everyone who is exposed to this bacterium becomes ill; environmental and socioeconomic factors also contribute to the process. The illness, in turn, affects those contextual factors; no portion of the system exists in isolation.

In the relational model, we seek to be with and to understand the patient in a number of dimensions simultaneously—biological, experiential, functional, and spiritual. As we come to understand patients'

Table 6-1. A comparison of control- and relationship-based personal philosophies.

Attribute	Control	Relational (I–Thou)*
Phenomenon of interest	Thing-in-itself	Thing-in-context
Epistemological strategy	Reductionist; linear causality	Emergent; systems model
Clinician's stance	Detached observer	Participant observer
Information deemed relevant	Objective data only	Subjective and objective data
Model for patient–clinician relationship	Hierarchy	Partnership
Focus of attention	Outcome-oriented	Process-oriented

*Terms are from Martin Buber. *I and Thou*. New York, NY: Scribner, 1970.

experiences, we can better identify opportunities to recommend strategies or undertake treatments to ameliorate their suffering. But we also remain mindful that patients are ultimately responsible for their own lives; they may or may not accept our suggestions. In some cases, we may have no suggestions or treatment to offer, but we can still find success in offering, in the words of Arthur Kleinman, "empathic witnessing," honoring the patient's need for connection—a healing intervention in its own right.

This relational model helps us avoid unrealistic expectations of ourselves. It offers us the opportunity to feel successful in situations such as untreatable illness or a patient's refusal to accept our good advice that would seem like failures under the control model. The relational model also leads us to more effective action. In contrast to the control model, which attends exclusively to outcomes, this model calls for explicit attention to process, to the quality of communication, and to the values enacted in the way we work together. Paradoxically, it is by letting go of predetermined outcomes and focusing more on making the process as good as possible that we achieve the best possible outcomes. The relational model also gives us more room to look outside ourselves for guidance and solutions—and to admit our own limitations or powerlessness.

Whereas the control model creates barriers between clinicians and patients, the relational model keeps us closer to the experience of both our patients and ourselves, thereby increasing the opportunities for our work to be meaningful and decreasing the potential for frustration, alienation, and burnout.

SKILLS

There are a number of skills that can make the difference between depletion and thriving in practice.

Time Management

These skills are essential both within the office visit and in arranging work schedules. For example, negotiating an agenda at the start of each visit focuses attention on the issues that are most important to the patient and the clinician, minimizes time spent on unnecessary tasks, and drastically reduces the frequency with which new topics emerge late in the visit ("Oh, by the way, Doc, I've got this chest pain …") that lay waste to office schedules. Informing patients at the outset how long their visits will last and reminding them a few minutes before ending allow them to share responsibility for using time effectively (see Chapter 1). On a more global level, time-management skills can help preserve the balance among work, family, community, and recreation that is so important to life satisfaction. Keeping time logs for several days can help us discover whether we are apportioning our time in accordance with our personal goals and priorities. Time logs can also point out time wasters in daily work habits and help us devise more efficient office procedures.

Communication

Given the important contribution of the patient–clinician relationship as a source of meaning, the communication and relationship skills described elsewhere in this book become critical tools for well-being as well as for good patient care. Learning to *be with* the patient requires broadening the goal of the interview from making a diagnosis to understanding the story of the patient's illness as a lived experience. We need to understand the meaning of the illness to the patient—why this disease in this particular patient at this particular time, how it is affecting the patient's function, and what role it might be playing in the patient's life. Thus, we need skills for eliciting deeper levels of patients' stories, responding to their emotions, and reflecting our understanding back so that they feel heard. As we become better at these relational skills, we will find that there are no longer routine or uninteresting cases—each patient is unique. The patient's personhood enriches our own.

Coaching & Negotiation

Sharing responsibility more effectively and more realistically with patients requires both coaching and negotiation skills. Specifically, we must know how to facilitate patients in articulating their own values, goals, and opinions, including their feedback about their medical care. We must be willing to relinquish our traditional—and burdensome—role of unquestioned authority and adopt instead a more flexible stance, trying to combine synergistically our own knowledge of medicine with patients' knowledge of themselves and the patterns, problems, and balances of their daily lives. We must learn to see patients' increasing capacity for gathering information and making their own decisions as a valuable resource and a sign of our success rather than as a challenge to our competence and authority. Knowing how and when to set firm boundaries without being judgmental and how to discuss communication and relationship problems openly can help resolve impasses with many seemingly difficult patients, making their care less frustrating and more rewarding. We also need to know how to recognize when we are overfunctioning, hooked by unrealistic hopes or expectations of control, and to respectfully, but clearly, give responsibility back to the patient.

Self-Reflection & Self-Care

We need to be able to reflect on our own feelings and actions, to acknowledge our vulnerabilities and needs, to seek and courageously follow our sense of calling, and to act in support of our own health. Rather than judging and shutting out such feelings as anger, attraction, or insecurity that inevitably arise in us, we can learn to accept them with self-compassion, to manage them appropriately, and to harvest from them insights about ourselves and our patients. Through solitary reflection and honest conversation with trusted colleagues (informally or in more organized formats such as Balint groups, workshops, executive coaching, or psychotherapy) we can attend more closely to what our hearts are telling us about the state of our lives. Shedding the mask of omnipotence and invincibility and recognizing our vulnerabilities are essential for working amidst uncertainty and coping with mistakes. And finally, we can thoughtfully examine our lifestyle choices, starting with our work hours. Simplifying our material needs to reduce financial pressures can give us more time for exercise, healthy eating, social interaction, pursuing diverse interests, and whatever else it is that truly gives us joy and meaning.

Collective Self-Care

Over the past 25 years the attention given to clinician well-being has grown enormously. Early pioneers such as the Foundation for Medical Excellence and the Institute for the Study of Health and Illness have been joined by larger mainstream organizations such as the American Medical Association (AMA), Canadian Medical Association (CMA), and American Hospital Association in offering programs and resources. There is now a biennial international conference on physician well-being sponsored by the AMA, CMA, and British Medical Association. Nearly all hospitals and many medical societies in the United States and Canada offer wellness programs of some sort and excellent online resources are available.

These programs may be effective not only by virtue of the education they offer but also because they convene healing communities. Most practitioners experience high levels of isolation, even when they work as part of busy group practices. They seldom talk about their patients in any depth with colleagues and almost never talk about their own responses and struggles. Participants in a program on mindfulness and communication valued the connection and validation that came from honest conversations with peers ("I'm not the only one") as much as the new skills and insights that they gained. The most effective self-care may be that which we pursue in concert with others.

HEALTHY WORK ENVIRONMENTS

Our workplaces have an important effect on our well-being. The local culture of the institutions in which we work—be they hospitals, individual practices, or medical communities—subtly reinforces values through both formal educational processes and everyday policies and practices. The local culture can determine whether we feel able to disclose uncertainty and vulnerability to one another or feel constrained always to maintain an "iron man" façade; whether we see others as collaborators and negotiate collegially or engage in endless "turf" battles with people we perceive as competitors; whether we can discuss mistakes and ask for help or be forced to work in perpetual isolation; and whether we receive encouragement and respect for setting reasonable limits on our workload so that we can be present in our families or feel shamed for being "weak" or "lazy."

Surveys from both industry and academia have identified common characteristics of organizations with greater employee well-being. Organizational cultures characterized by collaborative decision making, ethical behavior toward employees and customers, mutual respect between members, growth and learning toward increasing competence, and a reasonable work–life balance are the most successful in promoting employee trust, engagement, and thriving. In contrast, organizations that ignore employee input, are riddled with political favoritism, and tolerate rudeness appear to breed employee apathy, cynicism, and burnout. Employee trust and engagement—that is, commitment to the organization—correlate positively not only with employee well-being but also with financial and operational success for the organization.

Another dimension of culture that impacts well-being is the degree to which an organization's values are congruent with the personal values of the staff. When clinicians feel that the organizational focus on productivity and financial performance is so intensive and unbalanced that they are forced to provide care that they know to be of substandard quality, they experience a moral injury, resulting in symptoms of burnout. While it's important to eliminate unnecessary variability and inefficiency, clinicians must have adequate time to engage their patients as partners and to think about and manage complex cases. And they need to be confident in the alignment between their personal goals and organizational goals for providing high-quality care.

Creating environments that support relationship-centered care is a large topic; a few general principles must suffice for this discussion:

- As clinicians, we tend to treat patients in the same way that we ourselves are treated within our institutions. Core values such as respect, partnership, honesty, and accountability must not only be articulated but must be consistently embraced and exhibited in institutional policies and procedures. Clinicians and administrators alike may need to learn new communication and relationship skills, and to redesign processes for making decisions and maintaining behavioral accountability.

- The principle of reciprocity governs much of human interaction. Mutually helpful behavior and camaraderie create a virtuous cycle in which employees thrive and succeed. Reciprocity can also tear an organization apart. A few acts of unchecked incivility can spiral into widespread acrimony. Incivility at work has been linked to a lack of job satisfaction, decreased organizational commitment, and impaired job performance. Organizations can foster civility through hiring policies that specifically screen for interpersonal skills, team-development activities, and codes of conduct with meaningful (and respectful) accountability. Respecting values and attending to the quality of process must be embraced as the most effective means to high-quality outcomes at the organizational level, just as at the clinical level. This requires a departure from traditional, hierarchical approaches of top-down decision making and control of the work process.
- Clinicians on the "front lines" of patient care but not in leadership positions may feel helpless to change a dysfunctional organization. The feeling of helplessness reflects the false belief that only the leaders are responsible for organizational culture. In fact, *leaders cocreate an organizational culture with followers*. If leaders are unable or unwilling to promote teamwork, clinicians can take the initiative to reach out across specialties and disciplines to promote a culture of mutual respect and accountability, express appreciation, and begin a virtuous cycle of civility. They can work on "being the change" they seek. Finding like-minded colleagues can create a mutually supportive group that catalyzes creation of a better culture. They can also learn to "manage up," letting their leaders know what they need.
- We can replace the current culture of rugged individualism with a culture of teamwork, accountability, and mutual support. Support groups for all staff, including physicians, may encourage self-awareness, increase sensitivity to patients' concerns, and diminish the isolation and depersonalization that both characterize and accelerate burnout. We can be vigilant to ways in which the local culture reinforces work addiction and inhibits collaboration and work to improve it.
- Recognizing the enormous impact that managers and leaders have on culture and the well-being of employees, organizations can become more skilled and intentional in how they select, orient, train, and evaluate leaders at every level to systematically build relational capacity, self-awareness and emotional maturity.
- As organizations navigate the financial challenges of the current health care landscape, they must maintain their commitment to organizational professionalism with a discipline of ongoing critical reflection on the degree to which their actual behavior remains faithful to their espoused values.

In this time of concern about health care costs and patient safety, clinicians, administrators, patients, and families need to work together in partnership to redesign our medical institutions, making them more respectful and humane, collaborative, accountable, and responsive to the needs of the people they serve and the people who work within them. Clinical outcomes, financial performance, patient satisfaction, and staff satisfaction have all been associated with factors that create healthy work environments for health care providers; thus, institutions have a direct stake in maintaining the well-being of their clinicians and staff.

CONCLUSIONS

Whether the rigors of clinical work become sources of meaning or exhaustion depends on a number of factors. We must be able to know and address mindfully the personal needs that affect our work. Fulfilling our needs for connection and meaning is particularly sustaining. Unrealistic expectations of control interfere with connection and confront us with an ongoing specter of inadequacy and failure. Instead, we need a more mature perspective of balance, acceptance, and relation. We need skills for working with uncertainty, sharing responsibility, and promoting relationship. We need personal disciplines of reflection and self-care, supported by participation in a healing community of peers. We must become more attentive to the values expressed subliminally but powerfully in our work environments and begin to make necessary changes so that these environments call forth the best and healthiest of what we have to offer, both as professionals and as human beings. These approaches can help us to appreciate fully the privilege of caring for patients and to realize our best potential for personal fulfillment and growth.

SUGGESTED READINGS

Egener BE, Mason DJ, McDonald WJ, et al. The charter on professionalism for health care organizations. *Acad Med* 2017;92: 1091–1099.

Friedberg MW, Chen PG, Van Busum KR, et al. Factors affecting physician professional satisfaction and their implications for patient care, health systems, and health policy. *RAND Health Q* 2014;3:1.

Krasner MS, Epstein RM, Quill TE, et al. A continuing education program in mindful communication: effects on primary care physician burnout, empathy and attitudes. *JAMA* 2009;302:1284–1293.

Linzer M, Manwell LB, Williams ES et al. Working conditions in primary care: physician reactions and care quality. *Arch Int Med* 2009;15:28–36.

Shanafelt TD, Noseworthy JH. Executive leadership and physician well-being: nine organizational strategies to promote engagement and reduce burnout. *Mayo Clin Proc* 2017;92: 129–146.

Spreitzer G, Porath C. Creating sustainable performance. *Harvard Bus Rev* 2012;90:92–99.

Suchman AL, Matthews DA. What makes the patient-doctor relationship therapeutic? Exploring the connexional dimension of medical care. *Ann Intern Med* 1988;108:125–130.

Thomas LR, Ripp JA, West CP. Charter on physician well-being. *JAMA* 2018;319:1541–1542.

Vaillant G. Some psychologic vulnerabilities of physicians. *N Engl J Med* 1972;287:372.

WEBSITES

Accreditation Council for Graduate Medical Education Physician Well-Being Initiative. www.acgme.org/What-We-Do/Initiatives/Physician-Well-Being. Accessed February 2019.

Clinician Well-Being Knowledge Hub. nam.edu/clinicianwellbeing/resource-center. Accessed February 2019.

Institute for the Study of Health and Illness: Finding Meaning Discussion Groups. http://www.rishiprograms.org/. Accessed February 2019.

Mindful Practice

7

Ronald Epstein, MD

Excellent patient care requires not only the knowledge and skills to diagnose and treat disease but also the ability to form therapeutic relationships with patients and their families, recognize and respond to emotionally demanding situations, make decisions under uncertainty, and deal with technical failures and errors. These capabilities require that clinicians have self-awareness to distinguish their values and feelings from those of their patients, recognize faulty reasoning early in the diagnostic thinking process, be attentive to when a technical procedure is not going as it should, recognize the need to gather more data, and be able to incorporate disconfirming data into an evolving assessment of the patient. Often, there is no tool or instrument that can help physicians with these situations on a moment-to-moment basis other than their own cognitive and emotional resources.

Mindful practice refers to clinicians' capacity for reflection, self-monitoring, and self-awareness during actual clinical practice in order to practice with clarity, insight, expertise, and compassion. Clinicians generally value the principles of mindful practice—attentive observation, critical curiosity, presence, and the capacity to see a familiar situation with new eyes ("beginner's mind"). Yet, during training and practice, clinicians spend little time "sharpening the saw"—developing, refining, and calibrating their own capacity for self-understanding as they think and feel their way through the complex demands of clinical practice. For psychotherapists, athletes, and musicians, self-calibration and self-awareness are considered fundamental to excellence and are often explicit aspects of training. Yet, for clinicians, there is often the assumption that knowledge and technical expertise are sufficient, when on reflection most clinicians value "adaptive expertise" and cultivating habits of mind that allow the clinician to self-calibrate and reflect continuously during everyday work. This chapter will suggest why mindful practice is important and indicate ways in which it can be cultivated.

Mindful practice is fundamental to excellent patient care. Mindful practice means being attentive, on purpose, to one's own thoughts and feelings during everyday clinical practice and educational activities. Mindfulness implies a stance in which the practitioner can observe not only the patient situation but also his or her own reactions to it. A mindful practitioner can see a situation from several angles at the same time. Mindful practice implies curiosity rather than premature judgment, and presence rather than detachment. Mindfulness is especially helpful when dealing with difficult relationships with patients and families, challenging clinical situations, and in recognizing the need for self-care. Furthermore, recent research among students, residents, and practicing clinicians suggests that mindfulness is associated with better communication, better quality of technical (e.g., fewer errors) and interpersonal (e.g., empathy) care, less implicit racial and gender bias, and greater clinician well-being (e.g., lower burnout).

In contrast, mindless practice involves self-deception, often with the illusion of competence. Blind certainty, ignoring of disconfirming data and arrogance without self-examination or reflection, dooms us to "seeing things not as they are, but as we are." An example of mindlessness is the common practice of reporting findings that were not actually observed, because "they must be true."

Mindfulness is especially important in the diagnosis and treatment of mental disorders, because there are few other anchors than the clinician's own perceptions and judgments to assess the severity or pervasiveness of anxiety, depression, or psychosis in a particular patient. However, mindfulness also applies to other cognitive and technical aspects of health care. For example, hepatobiliary surgeon Carol-Anne Moulton eloquently describes ways in which expert surgeons remain "attentive in automaticity;" they work quickly, yet recognize aberrant and problematic situations and slow down accordingly, switching from automatic to deliberative thinking. This chapter explores several aspects of mindful practice and some ways of recognizing and practicing mindfulness in clinical settings.

MINDFULNESS & CLINICAL CARE

Mindful practice depends on the ability to be aware in the moment. The championship tennis player is being mindful when he or she is not only attentive to the ball but also to his or her state of balance, expectations for what will happen next, physical sensations such as pain or discomfort, and level of anxiety. All of these factors can affect performance and can be modified by specific attention to them. Like tennis players, physicians' lapses in awareness and concentration can have dire consequences. For physicians, these lapses directly affect the patient's welfare and may include avoidance, overreactions, poor decisions, misjudgments, and miscommunications that affect survival and quality of life for the patient. Thus, physicians have a moral obligation to their patients and themselves to be as aware, present, and observant as possible.

CASE ILLUSTRATION 1

Jeffrey Borzak, a patient I knew well, seemed to be recovering from coronary artery bypass surgery. On rounds, I sensed that there was something that was wrong, but I could not put my finger on it. In retrospect, his color was not quite right—he was grayish-pale, his blood pressure was too easily controlled, he was even hypotensive on one occasion, and he seemed more depressed than usual. He reported no chest pain or shortness of breath, and had no pedal edema, elevated jugular venous pressure, or other abnormalities on his physical examination. But still I did not feel comfortable, and although there were no "red flags," I ordered an echocardiogram that showed a new area of ischemia. An angiogram showed that one of the grafts had occluded. After angioplasty, Mr. Borzak looked and felt better, and he again required his usual antihypertensive medications.

By cultivating the ability to be attentive to the unexpected, mindful practice can improve the quality of care and help prevent errors. Case Illustration 1 presents some observations that led to a change in care resulting in an improved outcome. Being aware in the moment and receptive to new information—especially information that is unexpected, unwanted, or upsetting—can help the clinician be more attentive to patients' needs and thus be more likely to meet them. The clinician's job in Case 1 would have seemed easier, at least in the short run, if he had ignored his intuitions.

Mindful practice involves allowing awareness of our own areas of ignorance, as well as our areas of expertise. Yet, many clinicians are not as aware as they should be of the accuracy of their first impressions and tacit judgments. Clinicians, whether beginners or experts, often are aware of things before they are named, categorized, or organized into a coherent diagnosis. For example, the unusual gait of a patient walking toward the chair in the examining room may be the first clue to a neurodegenerative disorder, and such first impressions can often be quite accurate. Educators, psychologists, and cognitive scientists have called these automatic nonconscious mental processes "unconscious competence," the "unthought known," or "preattentive processing."

Conversely, clinicians' capacity for inattentiveness and self-deception can be stunning. Automatic "fast" processing—often helpful in pattern-recognition—can backfire if unexamined biases and preconceived ideas dominate clinical reasoning without some capacity for beginner's mind. Two examples come to mind. Our clinical team suspected adrenal insufficiency in a patient hospitalized with a urinary infection and hypotension. They had noted hyperpigmented skin. Later, they notice that only her forearms and face were hyperpigmented; the rest of the body was pale. Yet, the residents and attending physicians continued to evaluate the possibility of adrenal insufficiency in spite of being aware of their faulty observations and presuppositions. An even more stunning example was reported by Faith Fitzgerald in her classic article on curiosity in clinical education. A patient was presented on rounds as "BKA (below knee amputation) times 2." Fitzgerald, noting that the patient's two warm pink feet were sticking out of the sheets at the end of the bed, asked the resident why he thought that the patient had had amputations. The response was, "It said so in the chart." Apparently, five admissions previously, the patient had been admitted for diabetic ketoacidosis ("DKA"), which the transcriptionist mistranscribed as "BKA", and the error was carried through the subsequent four admission notes. While these examples are dramatic, smaller scale misperceptions are common. For example, patients asking for antidepressant medications tend to receive them regardless of whether they fulfill diagnostic criteria for depression. Patients who are labeled "difficult," "uncooperative," or "demanding," (such as Mrs. Grady, Case Illustration 2), seem to be stuck with such labels for life, and disconfirming data tend to be ignored. Furthermore, clinicians typically attribute the "difficult" to the patient, rather than considering that the physician's expectations and attitudes may also be contributing.

CASE ILLUSTRATION 2

Elizabeth Grady recently came to be a patient in our practice. The practice, despite having long waits for appointments, was recently reopened to new patients to boost productivity. Mrs. Grady left her previous physician's practice because of a disagreement over seeking care in the emergency room rather than in the office for her out-of-control diabetes. Her blood sugar has never been below 400 and often was in excess of 600 mg/dL. Despite claiming to be on a diet, her weight kept increasing, and now she weighed nearly 500 lb. At the first visit, an irate sister accompanied her demanding that the patient be hospitalized immediately. On the second visit, Mrs. Grady was so anxious that she could not sit in the examination room; she was pacing in the waiting room until her appointment and then indicated that she was in a rush to leave even though the appointment was on time. She no-showed for the subsequent appointment and is now returning for her third appointment.

Mindfulness means being simultaneously attentive to external data as well as to internal data—the clinician's own thoughts, feelings, and inner states. Negative thoughts about a patient might promote a pejorative label ("somatizer"); negative feelings might provoke anger or disgust; and negative inner states might induce boredom or hostility. Positive feelings also present difficulties. Sexual attraction toward a patient obviously can be problematic, but so can an unusually keen interest in a patient's illness. As a medical student, I was assigned a patient with hairy-cell leukemia, a disease whose genetic basis was just being uncovered. Although the attending and resident team considered her an "exciting" and "fascinating" case, I was disappointed, when meeting her, that she was a sad, weak, pale woman dying of cancer, hardly "exciting" from her perspective.

Mindfulness of thoughts allows clinicians to follow intuitions while also accommodating for biases and cognitive traps in the process of making clinical decisions. Awareness of feelings is particularly useful in diagnosing mental disorders; clinicians tend to feel "down" when in the presence of a depressed patient, or confused in the presence of patients with subtle delusions and mild dementia. Awareness of their own fatigue can help clinicians recognize when their cognitive, attentional, or technical capacities are not at their best; the fatigued resident in the emergency room late at night might then get corroboration for an important finding on physical examination (such as the degree of nuchal rigidity in a febrile child) from a trusted colleague.

Mindfulness improves learning. Trainees who are more aware of the difference between what they believe and their actual performance can make adjustments and improvements. Key features of mindful learning are the ability to see novelty in familiar situations and to consider facts provisional and contextual. Studies show that mindfulness and self-awareness training can improve reasoning and communication skills. Mindfulness can be a corrective for those who otherwise might believe that they are expert and are surprised when that notion is challenged by an outside observer or objective test. Other types of professionals—not only medical personnel—also can suffer from the illusion of competence. Musicians know the delusion of the "practice-room virtuoso"—an illusion that is often shattered when the performer is put in front of a discerning audience. Clinicians, however, usually practice unobserved, so the opportunities for external validation and learning are much scarcer than for the musician—and the stakes are much higher than a wrong note.

Mindful practice involves cultivating the ability to monitor and modulate one's own emotional reactivity. Faced with emotionally challenging situations, humans often overreact by blaming (oneself, another clinician, or the patient), whereas others underreact by avoiding, minimizing, or distancing. In contrast, a mindful practitioner can observe his or her own reactions and thus have choices about the way she might respond in such a way that enhances quality of care and quality of healing relationships. Clinicians thus respond with empathy based on an understanding of the patient's experience rather than making assumptions about the patient leading to further misunderstandings. Awareness can also clarify the ethical decisions that clinicians make during everyday practice—such as which patient phone call to return first or whether to acquiesce to a patient's slightly unreasonable demand.

Finally, mindfulness involves monitoring the clinician's own needs. Self-awareness can directly enhance clinicians' own sense of well-being by helping them feel more in touch and in tune with themselves. Self-awareness can also motivate the clinician to seek needed help and support. Mindful self-care can lead to greater well-being and job satisfaction; clinicians who report greater job satisfaction and well-being tend to express empathy more readily, report making fewer errors, and have patients who report greater satisfaction. The self-reinforcing process of self-care and well-being can contribute to productivity and reduce burnout and attrition (see Chapter 6).

CULTIVATING MINDFULNESS IN ONESELF & TRAINEES

While it is self-evident that self-awareness is a necessary ingredient in developing and maintaining clinical expertise, achieving a state of moment-to-moment self-awareness in a chaotic and busy health care environment requires effort. For several years, a variety of training venues in medicine, psychology, and other disciplines have offered small group settings for trainees and practitioners to present difficult situations for group discussion, with the intent that the resulting insights then might inform future clinical practice. These sessions have been associated with improvement in communication skills and satisfaction with clinical practice. For example, a year-long course in "mindful communication"—incorporating contemplative practices, narratives about meaningful clinical experiences, appreciative interviews, didactic material, and discussion—led to lower burnout and lower psychological distress, greater empathy, and psychosocial orientation in care and a more attentive and less anxious personality style. Follow-up with participants a year later showed that they preserved a sense of community and continued to value the skills of mindfulness that they learned. Some small group formats are listed in Table 7-1, each with a particular focus but with the common thread of providing both support and insight.

Domains that are amenable to training include the following:

- Clinicians' habits (meditation, body awareness, exercise, interactions with others)
- Clinicians' beliefs and attitudes (health beliefs, beliefs about human behavior and relationships, attitudes toward patient autonomy or psychosocial aspects of care, family, cultural influences)
- Clinicians' feelings and emotions (joy, fulfillment, vigor, attraction, anger, frustration, conflict, setting boundaries)
- Challenging clinical situations (difficult decisions, sharing bad news, facing mistakes, apologizing to patients, dying patients, demanding or "difficult" patients, conflict within the health care team)
- Clinician self-care (impairment, balance between home and work, burnout, healthy approaches to stress, finding meaning in work)

Other educational strategies can enhance the capacity for reflection and mindfulness. Reviewing video recordings of patient sessions can be both sobering and instructive, whether reviewed individually or with a tutor. Learning contracts or agreements can focus learning on areas of deficiency, including becoming more self-aware. Peer evaluations of work habits and interpersonal attributes with medical students can foster greater awareness of how students function on the clinical team and interact with their colleagues and patients. Keeping a journal not only promotes reflection on one's actions but also seems to be therapeutic in itself, offering a venue for self-expression so needed by busy and overwhelmed clinicians.

However, these individual and small group activities may not necessarily translate the insights gained into the moment-to-moment drama of clinical practice. Mindful practice refers not only to reflection on one's actions, but goes one step further by emphasizing habits of mind during actual practice. Mindful practice refers not only to the social and emotional domains of practice but also the cognitive processes of data gathering and making decisions, as well as the technical skills employed during physical examinations, surgery, and procedures. Following are some general suggestions on how to enhance mindfulness in practice, for oneself and for trainees:

- *Priming.* Priming refers to creating the expectation for mindfulness. By observing what they do during clinical practice, clinicians can be more present, curious, and attentive. Sometimes, it is as simple as pausing and taking a breath before entering the patient's room

Table 7-1. Group learning experiences that promote mindful practice.

Type of Group	Description	Qualifications of Facilitator
Mindful practice workshops	Promote attentive awareness through meditation, narrative, appreciative interviews and discussion.	Training in meditation, narrative medicine, communication, and small group facilitation
Support groups	Promote balance between the human and technical aspects of health care by sharing difficult and challenging situations.	Training in psychotherapy and small group facilitation
Balint groups	Recognizing that the clinician is a "drug" (a therapeutic agent), groups aim to improve clinician effectiveness by examining thoughts and feelings that may interfere with care.	Training through the International Balint Society
Family of origin groups	By drawing genograms (family trees), participants learn about influences family and culture have on their values and attitudes.	Family therapy training
Personal awareness groups	Unstructured experience focused on individual needs of participants; these groups examine personal issues that affect a broad array of aspects of being a clinician.	American Academy of Communication in Healthcare offers training courses
Literature in medicine groups	Using published written works or writings of group members, participants explore the human dimensions of health care.	Narrative medicine training
Challenging case conferences	Using videotapes or critical incident reports, participants explore the moment-to-moment actions they took during a clinical encounter.	Facilitation training

or taking time to look at the patient rather than at the chart or screen. Clinicians use these techniques to bring themselves into the present, and then pay attention to how those techniques enhance their capabilities as clinicians. Tutors can set expectations that trainees pay attention not only to the patient but also to their own thoughts and emotions during the clinical encounter. These thoughts and emotions are fodder for discussion following an encounter, whether it occurs in hospital or in outpatient settings. Writing narratives about these experiences can help practitioners recognize their own mental states and learn to be aware of how they contribute to creating a coherent patient story while eliciting what often seems like fragmented information from the patient.

- *Availability.* Just as clinicians should make themselves psychologically and physically available to their patients, teachers should carve out time and space in which they are available to observe and discuss students' progress toward greater self-awareness, whether in a small group setting or individually.
- *Asking reflective questions.* Reflective questions explore the inner landscape; no one can answer them but clinicians themselves. They are designed not to elicit facts or answers but rather to foster reflection in the moment. Teachers can ask reflective questions, but more importantly, clinicians themselves can adopt a habit of self-questioning. Examples of reflective questions are shown in Table 7-2. The internal dialogue that they foster can contribute to mindful practice.
- *Active engagement.* When in learning situations, mindful practice can and should be observed directly. Students' reports of what they said and did during a clinical encounter are biased by their own values, expectations, and anxiety; thus presence of a tutor or observer has no substitute. Imagine if in music instruction or tennis lessons, the student simply reported on his or her progress and difficulties, giving a narrative account of how the piece of music or tennis match went. Ludicrous as it sounds, we often do exactly that in medical education.
- *Thinking out loud.* When facing a challenging clinical situation, it can be useful to describe one's observations, impressions, or clinical reasoning to a colleague or tutor, or to put them down on paper in the form of a written narrative. Similarly, experienced clinicians can think out loud in the presence of learners to demonstrate how recognizing one's own ignorance, biases, and predispositions can lead to more deliberative responses rather than mindless reactions. These methods help clinicians hear the story or rationale as if it were told by a third person, allowing them to examine their own thinking processes and emotional reactions, identify what might be missing in their perception of the situation, and correct faulty logic. These methods can allow for reflection that cannot be accomplished simply by moving forward with problem solving.
- *Practice.* Medicine, like music and tennis, must be practiced; the same is true of mindfulness. There are both formal and informal practices. Formal practices include sitting and walking meditation, yoga, and other self-awareness exercises. Equally important are informal practices that can be incorporated into daily work and may be unobserved by others.

Table 7-2. Reflective questions.

- "What am I assuming about this patient that might not be true?"
- "If there were data that I neglected or ignored, what might it be?"
- "What about my prior experience with this patient (or with other patients) is influencing my thinking and reasoning process?"
- "What surprised me about this patient? How did that surprise affect my clinical actions?"
- "What would a trusted colleague say about the way I am managing this patient?"
- "What outcomes am I expecting from this clinical situation? Are those expectations reasonable?"
- "How do I know when I have gathered enough data?"

Mindfulness practice usually involves stillness. The stillness may happen in frequent brief informal practices—a momentary pause before seeing the next patient or a "huddle" before commencing a surgical operation. Touching the doorknob before going into an examination room, a clinician might develop a habit of stopping momentarily, to a breath; being aware of potentially distracting thoughts, feelings, and preconceptions; and setting aside what has just occurred to be more attentive to the next patient. Formal meditation usually involves longer periods of stillness. Increasingly, workplaces provide space in which employees can engage in meditation during the workday. One powerful means for learning how to be centered, observant, and attentive is a daily meditation practice. Meditation involves watching one's thoughts, feelings, and bodily sensations (such as breathing) without necessarily trying to change them, and thus practicing being attentive and nonjudgmental over and over again, making it easier to evoke similar states of focused calm attentiveness, even briefly, during clinical practice. As a result, the clinician can learn to approach new situations with a lowered reactivity and to tolerate ambiguity. Meditation can be an entirely secular activity and need not have religious or spiritual overtones.

For clinicians and educators, "mantras" for daily practice can be cultivated. Clinicians might use the "it might not be so" mantra when facing a new patient or new diagnosis; the clinician develops a habit of trying to see the situation from another angle that might question an emerging hypothesis. "Unexpecting" is a practice of becoming aware of one's own expectations or eliciting those of a learner, and then actively imagining another outcome (the "it might not happen that way" mantra). The goal of using these techniques is to free one's thinking, recalibrate feelings, and train the mind to consider two or more perspectives at the same time.

- *Praxis.* Clinical skill is not truly learned and known until it is used. Increasing expertise is associated with the development of habits that become second nature. At that point, an expert clinician may not be able to describe easily exactly why he or she is making each decision, because many of the early steps in the decision process may have become automatic or tacit. Just as a habitual approach to history-taking or physical examination becomes second nature, mindfulness training should have as its goal developing habits of reflection, self-questioning, and awareness in the moment during clinical practice.
- *Assessment and confirmation.* As is true for any newly acquired skill, some kind of assessment and confirmation of achievement are important for learning and reinforcement. Facilitated self-assessment, assessment by peers, and feedback from supervising clinicians are important to identify markers of and barriers to practicing mindfully. A supervisor might evaluate, for example, the degree to which the learner was able to articulate his or her reactions to a particular patient. Patients and peers can assess presence and attentiveness.

CONCLUSION

Mindful practice is a process and a goal, not a static state of mind. Even the most accomplished practitioners cannot claim to be mindful all of the time. Efforts toward becoming more attentive, curious, and present, and approaching familiar situations with a "beginner's mind," can lead clinicians to be better listeners and diagnosticians, to recognize biases and assumptions, and to analyze their own technical skills more objectively. Most medical schools and many residency programs now offer training in mindfulness and self-awareness, in recognition that these approaches help in the process of professional development, reduce burnout, and improve communication. Resources for mindfulness and self-awareness training are also available through organizations such as the Mindful Practice Programs at the University of Rochester (www.mindfulpractice.urmc.edu).

SUGGESTED READING

Epstein RM. *Attending: Medicine, Mindfulness and Humanity.* New York, NY: Scribner; 2017.

ADDITIONAL READINGS

Balint E, Norell JS. *Six Minutes for the Patient: Interaction in General Practice Consultation.* London, UK: Tavistock Publications; 1973.

Beach MC, Roter D, Korthuis PT, et al. A multicenter study of physician mindfulness and health care quality. *Ann Fam Med* 2013;11(5):421–428.

Burgess DJ, Beach MC, Saha S. Mindfulness practice: a promising approach to reducing the effects of clinician implicit bias on patients. *Patient Educ Couns* 2017;100(2):372–376.

Dobkin PL, Hutchinson TA. Teaching mindfulness in medical school: where are we now and where are we going? *Med Educ* 2013;47(8):768–779.

Epstein RM. Mindful practice. *JAMA* 1999;282:833–839.

Fitzgerald FT. Curiosity. *Ann Intern Med* 1999;130:70–72.

Krasner MS, Epstein RM, Beckman H, et al. Association of an educational program in mindful communication with burnout, empathy, and attitudes among primary care physicians. *JAMA* 2009;302(12):1284–1293.

Novack DH, Suchman AL, Clark W, et al. Calibrating the physician. Personal awareness and effective patient care. *JAMA* 1997;278:502–509.

Sibinga EMS, Wu AW. Clinician mindfulness and patient safety. *JAMA* 2010;304:2532–2533.

WEB-BASED RESOURCE

Epstein R. Integrating self-reflection and self-awareness. *Web-based Learning Module in Doc.com: An Interactive Learning Resource for Healthcare Communication.* American Academy on Communication in Healthcare Web site. http://www.doccom.org/. Accessed September 2018.

SECTION II
Global Health

Global Health and Behavioral Medicine

8

Patrick T. Lee, MD, DTM&H; Kavitha Kolappa, MD, MPH; & Giuseppe J. Raviola, MD, MPH

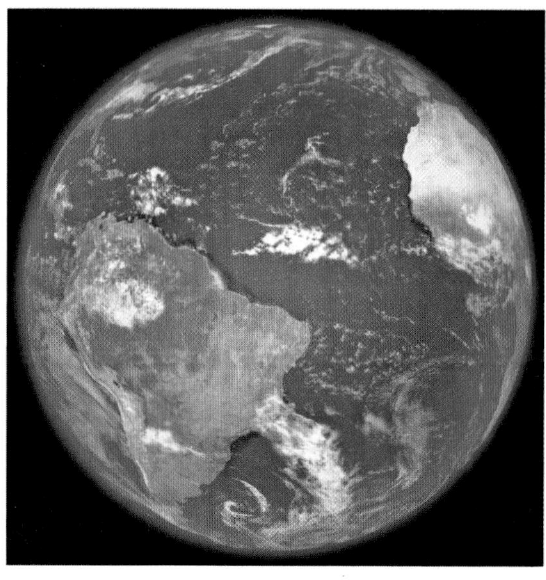

INTRODUCTION

Global health and behavioral medicine intersect in two important ways. First, mental, neurological, and substance use (MNS) disorders affect every community in the world. We relate to MNS disorders at a local level, where they are embedded in our customs, culture, and context. MNS disorders also exert global influence, through their massive burden of disease, the human and economic costs of treated and untreated illness, and their secondary effects on the outcomes of other health conditions.

Second, most MNS disorders are treatable: people get better. Recent advances in behavioral health care delivery have demonstrated that a collaborative (ideally, linked to primary care), nonspecialist, and transdiagnostic approach can deliver evidence-based care with population-level benefits. We understand how to alleviate the suffering of MNS disorders in high, middle, and low-income settings. Given the frequent disenfranchisement of people living with mental illness, an *equity* and human rights-based approach to care is essential.

With the goal of offering students a broad overview of mental health care in the global context, we have organized this chapter into three sections:

1. The global treatment and systems gap.
2. New approaches to addressing behavioral health: collaborative, nonspecialist, and transdiagnostic approaches.
3. The importance of context.

THE GLOBAL TREATMENT & SYSTEMS GAP

The Problem

To appreciate the global treatment and systems gap, we must first understand the level of need. Mental disorders represent the greatest collective cause of disability

BOX 8-1. THE WORLD HEALTH ORGANIZATION (WHO) ON MENTAL HEALTH

The adoption of a mental health programme must be regarded as a truly historic step taken by the Assembly to bring this new field of medicine into the area of inter-governmental action. The programme … will do much for the implementation of one of the W.H.O.'s fundamental principles – namely, that without mental health there can be no true physical health.

–Dr. Brock Chisholm, MD,
psychiatrist and first Director General of the WHO

Since its inception in 1948, the WHO has engaged at the international health policy level in both mental and physical health. Dr. Brock Chisholm, a psychiatrist and the first Director-General of the WHO, helped articulate the WHO's holistic definition of health as "a state of complete physical, mental, and social well-being and not merely the absence of disease or infirmity."* Over half a century later, the 2005 WHO Ministerial Conference in Denmark continued to advocate for an integrated approach, aptly coining the phrase, "No Health Without Mental Health.†

**Outline for a Study Group on World Health and the Survival of the Human Race.*

†WHO Mental health: facing the challenges, building solutions. Report from the WHO European Ministerial Conference. Copenhagen, Denmark: WHO Regional Office for Europe, 2005. Reprinted from Chisholm B. The World Health Organization, *Br Med J* 1950;1:1021 with permission from BMJ Publishing Group Ltd.

globally today. Recent estimates suggest that the disease burden of mental disorders accounts for 32.4% of years lived with disability (YLDs) and 13.0% of disability-adjusted life-years (DALYs). Depression, the most common mental disorder, affects an estimated 350 million people globally. Depression represents the leading cause of disability (as measured by DALYs) around the world-more than ischemic heart disease, road traffic accidents, cerebrovascular disease, and chronic obstructive pulmonary disease. Severe mental disorders, including schizophrenia, affect at least 1 in 100 people globally, across cultures, with significant severity of illness, morbidity, low life expectancy, and economic impact on families. According to a report by the World Economic Forum, the direct and indirect costs of mental illnesses totaled 2.6 trillion dollars in 2010 alone. By 2030, the cumulative costs are expected to exceed 15 trillion dollars.

Although mental disorders significantly impact people in low- and middle-income countries (LMICs) and 80% of the world's population live in these regions, greater than 90% of mental health resources are spent in high-income countries. Resources that do get spent in LMICs are often highly centralized and tend to be funneled toward national-level institutional facilities instead of being "decentralized" to create services at primary care clinics and in communities. Furthermore, the "treatment gap" for people with mental disorders exceeds 50% in all countries worldwide, but approaches rates as high as 90% in the least resourced countries. With regard to child and adolescent mental health, more than 50% of mental disorders start before the age of 14, and 75% before the age of 24. One-quarter of disability-adjusted life years (DALYs) for mental disorders and substance abuse is borne by those 24 years old or younger, the age group that accounts for more than 40% of the world population.

Despite the enormous need, MNS disorders have received insufficient attention globally. Why is this the case? There are numerous reasons for this, not the least important of which has been stigma and discrimination at all levels of society, across high-, middle-, and low-income countries. Stigma leads to the following:

- Underemphasis on MNS prevention, care, and treatment at national and international policy levels, which results in
  - Critical funding gaps for MNS programs, which creates
    - Gaps in the necessary MNS workforce, essential medicines, and access to evidence-based care, as well as
    - Gaps in the reporting of mental health indicators, which obscures the unmet need and perpetuates the underemphasis on MNS disorders at the policy level.

Key findings and selected figures from the 2017 WHO Mental Health Atlas (see Box 8-2 and Figures 8-1 and 8-2) offer a picture of the current state of mental health globally.

In summary, one in four people suffer from MNS disorders in their lifetime, 85% of these are unable to access appropriate care, and trillions of dollars are lost as a result each year. The causes are complex but knowable. Increased investments at all levels of health care systems are needed to close the mental health treatment gap.

EMERGING MODELS OF CARE: SIMPLER, NONSPECIALIST-DELIVERED

The Problem

The delivery of safe, evidence-based, and affordable mental health care to people living with mental disorders is also a major challenge of global health. With the lack of human resources combined with inadequate training, supervision, and professional development, the challenges involved in addressing global mental health delivery in low-resource settings have implications and

BOX 8-2. KEY FINDINGS FROM THE 2017 WORLD HEALTH ORGANIZATION MENTAL HEALTH ATLAS

Key findings

Global reporting on core mental health indicators

- 177 out of WHO's 194 Member States (91%) at least partially completed the Atlas questionnaire; the submission rate was above 85% in all WHO Regions;
- 37% of Member States regularly compile mental health specific data covering at least the public sector. In addition, 29% of WHO Member States compile mental health data as part of general health statistics only;
- 62% of Member States were able to report on a set of five selected indicators that covered mental health policy, mental health law, promotion and prevention programmes, service availability, and mental health workforce.

Mental health system governance

- 72% of Member States have a stand-alone policy or plan for mental health and 57% have a standalone mental health law;
- In the previous five years, 62% of WHO Member States have updated their policy and plan; and 40% their mental health law;
- 94 countries equivalent to 68% of those countries who responded, or 48% of all WHO Member States, have developed or updated their policies or plans for mental health in line with international and regional human rights instruments;
- 76 countries, equivalent to 75% of those countries who responded, or 39% of all WHO Member States, have developed or updated their law for mental health in line with international and regional human rights instruments;
- Human and financial resources allocated for implementation are limited; only 20% of Member States reported that indicators are available and used to monitor implementation of a majority of the components of their action plans.

Financial and human resources for mental health

- Levels of public expenditure on mental health are very meagre in low- and middle-income countries and more than 80% of these funds go to mental hospitals;
- Globally, the median number of mental health workers is 9 per 100,000 population, but there is extreme variation (from below 1 in low-income countries to 72 in high-income countries).

Mental health service availability and uptake

- The median number of mental health beds per 100,000 population ranges below 7 in low- and lower middle-income countries to over 50 in high-income countries;
- Equally large disparities exist for outpatient services, child and adolescent services, and social support; globally, the median number of child and adolescent beds is less than 1 per 100,000 population and ranges from below 0.2 in low- and lower middle-income countries to over 1.5 in high-income countries.

Mental health promotion and prevention

- 123 countries, equivalent to 69% of those countries who responded, or 63% of all WHO Member States, have at least two functioning national, multisectoral mental health promotion and prevention programmes;
- Out of almost 350 reported functioning programmes, 40% were aimed at improving mental health literacy or combating stigma and 12% were aimed at suicide prevention.

importance across all nations, "developing" and "developed." Growing evidence about effective "task sharing" of psychosocial and psychological interventions—care delivered by nonspecialist providers—may be the most important research finding of the field of Global Mental Health (GMH) over the past decade. This was supported by the evolution of the field through a landmark Lancet series in 2007, launching "a new movement for mental health," and subsequently followed with a 2011 Lancet series, a landmark 2011 Nature publication setting out the research priorities for the field, and a 2013 PLOS series on Grand Challenges in Global Mental Health. In 2018 a Lancet Commission report on Mental Health and Sustainable Development highlighted the need for linking the following goals: (1) to increase access to care for mental disorders and (2) to promote mental health as a universal human attribute and an indivisible component of overall health.

The WHO has taken an important role in this process through its Mental Health Gap Programme (mhGAP), which in 2011 published an Intervention Guide (IG) for "mental, neurological and substance use disorders in nonspecialized health settings" based on extensive literature review—an emerging international consensus on best practices that can potentially be adapted to context, and acknowledgment of certain "universal" aspects to the way mental disorders present regardless of cultural context. The WHO mhGAP-IG materials provide guidance for the treatment of disorders in low-resource contexts, including depression, psychosis, and bipolar disorder, suggesting pharmacological as well as psychosocial interventions. A subsequent second edition was

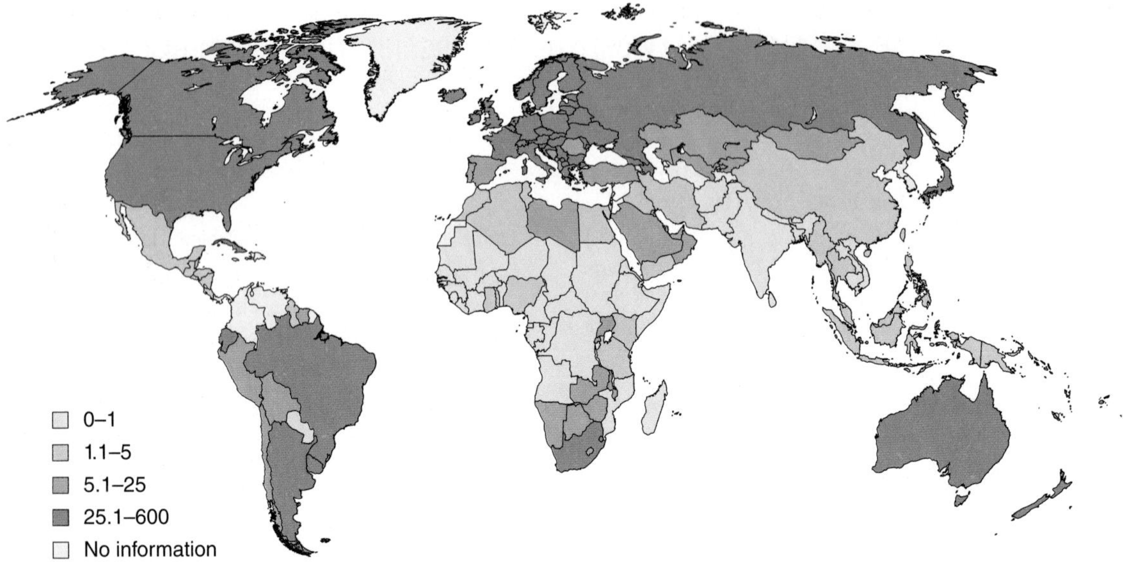

Figure 8-1. Human resources for mental health per 100,000 population. (Data from Mental Health Atlas 2017. © World Health Organization 2018.)

unveiled in 2016, and an additional version developed for use in humanitarian emergencies, and with additional implementation guidance forthcoming.

Best Practices

Several general principles of mental health care transcend context:

- Do no harm.
- Protect confidentiality.
- Respect and protect the autonomy and the safety of the person.
- Maintain therapeutic boundaries with the person, with attention to culture, class, and resource constraints.
- Obtain a good history of the presenting problem.
- Before psychiatric diagnosis, adequate medical evaluation is necessary (i.e., rule out delirium).
- Provide the person and family with clear information about diagnosis, recommended treatments, and treatment alternatives if they exist in context.
- Psychosocial/psychological and psychopharmacologic treatments can each be effective, depending on the problem.

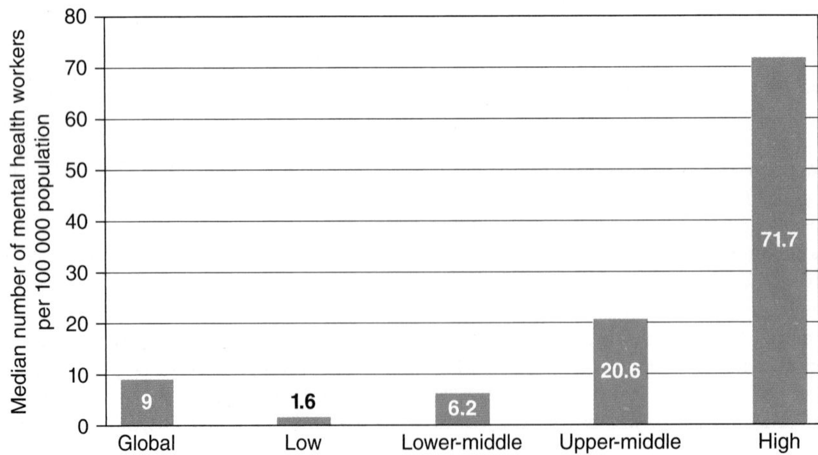

Figure 8-2. Human resources for mental health per 100,000 population. (Reprinted from Mental Health Atlas 2017. © World Health Organization 2018.)

- Mild symptoms can often be treated with social or psychosocial interventions, or psychotherapy alone.
- Moderate and severe symptoms can be treated with a combination of psychosocial support, psychotherapy, and medication.
- A family-based approach to mental health-related problems often can yield the greatest benefits.
- Strength-based and preventive approaches delivered by peers can be highly effective, depending on the problem, whether or not illness is present and/or experienced by the person, and contextual realities (ex: limited health system resources).

Beyond these basic principles, how should mental health services be delivered? Four elements of best practice emerge from the current literature:

1. Collaborative care and primary care integration.
2. Transdiagnostic approaches to psychosocial and psychological care.
3. Use of quality improvement methods.
4. Direct action on adversity and the social determinants of health.

The following sections briefly describe each of these best practice elements.

COLLABORATIVE CARE AND PRIMARY CARE INTEGRATION

Collaborative care is team-based care facilitated by smart systems. Complex care pathways are boiled down to discrete tasks that may be shared across different members of the team. These team members may include community health workers, health coaches, social workers, psychologists, nurse care managers, nurse practitioners, physician assistants, primary care physicians, and/or psychiatrists. Patients, families, and communities are viewed as active team members with specific and outcome-relevant expertise and knowledge.

Protocols provide decision support (i.e., what to do when, when to ask for help, and when to refer), thereby enabling each team member to safely and efficiently perform tasks that might otherwise be outside their usual scope of practice. Smart tools further support this work. These tools range from paper-based population registries (i.e., lists of patients and active issues that facilitate coordination of care) to smartphone-based decision support and data entry applications.

A strong body of evidence indicates that collaborative care models are as or more effective than other ways of delivering mental health care. In addition to demonstrable efficacy, team-based care has the advantages of lower cost, increased coverage, and better resilience in cases of staff turnover.

Principles of collaborative, stepped care for depression and common mental disorders—best practices:

1. Population-based care for specific disorders that prioritizes screening
2. Treatment and tracking of outcomes
3. Self-care support, including family and patient education about illness and treatments, self-monitoring, and adherence support skills
4. Care management and measurement-based care using patient-reported outcomes, focused on adherence, side effects, change in symptoms and course of care following evidence-based guidelines
5. Treatment to target and systematic monitoring of severity, with treatment intensification for patients not improving
6. Case registry to track clinical outcomes (e.g., depression severity scores) and key process steps, to facilitate transparent shared management across nonspecialist workers, primary care providers, and consulting specialists
7. Psychiatric consultation for more complex presentations
8. Use of proven intervention strategies, including brief psychological treatments in addition to medications

There are three compelling reasons for integrating mental health services into primary care. First, such integration locates services closer to people's homes, thereby improving access and reducing costs associated with seeking specialist care in distant locations. Second, it minimizes stigma and discrimination while reducing the risk of human rights violations that may occur in more restrictive settings such as psychiatric hospitals. And third, it generates good health outcomes at reasonable costs. Notably, such integration is not without its pitfalls. Collaborative planning, effective task-sharing among multidisciplinary team members, and adaptation to local context are important adjuncts to care integration. In its 2008 report, *Integrating Mental Health Care into Primary Care: A Global Perspective*, the WHO reviewed the evidence for integration of mental health services into primary care and presented ten best practice case studies from countries around the world. The Case Illustration 1 and Table 8-1 (summary of key messages) are excerpted from the WHO report.

CASE ILLUSTRATION 1

Juan from Chile has suffered from schizophrenia his entire adult life. Before integrated services for mental health in primary care were introduced, his condition was poorly managed and he was shuffled repeatedly in and out of a psychiatric hospital, where he endured and witnessed numerous human rights abuses. This part of his story is unfortunately all too familiar. However, with the advent of primary care services for mental health in his community, Juan's condition became well-managed and he was able to be reintegrated with his family. He hasn't been back to the psychiatric hospital for 4 years now.

Excerpted from: WHO (2008) Integrating mental health into primary care: a global perspective. Geneva: World Health Organization and World Organization of Family Doctors (Wonca).

Table 8-1. Key messages from **WHO** report, "Integrating mental health into primary care: a global perspective."

Key messages of this report
1. Mental disorders affect hundreds of millions of people and, if left untreated, create an enormous toll of suffering, disability, and economic loss.
2. Despite the potential to successfully treat mental disorders, only a small minority of those in need receive even the most basic treatment.
3. Integrating mental health services into primary care is the most viable way of closing the treatment gap and ensuring that people get the mental health care they need.
4. Primary care for mental health is affordable, and investments can bring important benefits.
5. Certain skills and competencies are required to effectively assess, diagnose, treat, support, and refer people with mental disorders; it is essential that primary care workers are adequately prepared and supported in their mental health work.
6. There is no single best practice model that can be followed by all countries. Rather, successes have been achieved through sensible local application of broad principles.
7. Integration is most successful when mental health is incorporated into health policy and legislative frameworks and supported by senior leadership, adequate resources, and ongoing governance.
8. To be fully effective and efficient, primary care for mental health must be coordinated with a network of services at different levels of care and complemented by broader health system development.
9. Numerous low- and middle-income countries have successfully made the transition to integrated primary care for mental health.
10. Mental health is central to the values and principles of the Alma Ata Declaration; holistic care will never be achieved until mental health is integrated into primary care.

Data from Integrating mental health into primary care: A global perspective. Geneva: World Health Organization and World Organization of Family Doctors (Wonca). © World Health Organization 2008.

Transdiagnostic Approaches to Psychosocial and Psychological Care

In settings where the need is great and resources are limited (which is the case for MNS disorders in most of the world), difficult decisions need to be taken regarding what treatments should be provided. Psychosocial and psychological treatments are preferable to medication (although medication can be very helpful) and can be tailored to address both illness and distress that may not meet diagnostic criteria for a disorder. Evidence-based psychotherapies, such as congitive-behavioral therapy and interpersonal therapy for depression, are being increasingly simplified into more basic common elements (i.e., relaxation, behavioral activation, and problem-solving) so that they can be more easily used by nonspecialist providers. These transdiagnostic interventions, delivered by less specialized providers, can be embedded within collaborative health care delivery models that include primary care physicians and more specialized mental health providers. A series of papers published in *PLoS Medicine* reviewed the evidence and proposed a set of evidence-based "packages of care." Table 8-2 is excerpted from one of these papers. It summarizes two evidence-based packages of care for depression, appropriate for low- and high-resourced settings.

Quality Improvement

Quality improvement is the disciplined use of performance data to improve processes, systems, and outcomes. Various approaches exist. All share a focus on clearly defined goals, methods to link actions to outcomes, and steps to translate new lessons into better processes and systems. As distinct from research, which emphasizes methodological rigor at the expense of "real world" relevance, quality improvement takes a more pragmatic approach.

We would suggest all health professional students (and indeed, all health professionals) learn the fundamentals of quality improvement and seek to apply the core principles in their daily practice. One note of

Table 8-2. Packages of care for depression.

Low Resourced Settings	High Resourced Settings
Routine screening for detection	High-risk or routine screening with confirmation of diagnosis by skilled clinician
Psychoeducation	Psychoeducation
Generic antidepressants	Choice of antidepressants
Problem-solving	Choice of brief psychological treatments
	Electroconvulsive therapy

Reprinted from Patel V, et al. Packages of care for depression in low- and middle-income countries. *PLoS Med* 2009;6(10): e1000159.

caution: quality improvement processes, like all tools, are only as useful as the context and skill with which they are applied. Of particular relevance to global health and behavioral medicine, health students and professionals should marry the discipline of performance improvement to a nuanced understanding of local context (see **The Importance of Context** section).

DIRECT ACTION ON ADVERSITY AND THE SOCIAL DETERMINANTS OF HEALTH

"Adversity" refers to traumatic life events and circumstances that place people at greater risk for developing mental health and social problems. In 2016, the WHO published *Problem Management Plus (PM+)*, a pragmatic approach to providing individual psychological help, with integration of transdiagnostic approaches to care, in communities exposed to adversity. In the preface to the PM+ report, Dr. Shekar Saxena, Director of the WHO Department of Mental Health and Substance Abuse, writes:

> There are tens of millions of people in the world who live in extremely difficult circumstances and suffer emotionally. Numerous people live in chronic poverty and live through hardships in urban slums, long-term humanitarian emergencies or in camps for displaced people. They may experience loss of family, friends and livelihoods and may confront extreme stressors such as violent deaths, sexual violence or missing relatives. They often live in communities that lack security, basic services and livelihood opportunities. The term "adversity" is often used to describe such difficult circumstances. People who experience adversity are at greater risk of developing mental health and social problems. They are at greater risk of being impaired by distress. As a result, a range of mental health and psychosocial supports need to be available, including psychological interventions. However, these interventions are rarely accessible to those who need them.

Dr. Saxena presents Problem Management Plus as a simplified, "low-intensity psychological intervention" that "can be quickly learned not only by professionals but also by people who are not mental health professionals."

The PM+ approach suggests four core strategies for managing adversity:

1. Managing stress—Helps patient manage anxiety and stress
2. Managing problems—Helps patient address practical problems
3. Get going keep doing—Aims to improve patient's levels of activity
4. Strengthening social supports—Helps reduce isolation and improve social support

PM+ advocates the following basic helping skills:

- Confidentiality
- Communicating concern
- Nonverbal skills
- Praising openness
- Validating
- Putting aside your personal values
- Giving advice

MNS disorders and social determinants (i.e., the conditions in which people are born, grow, live, work, and age) are closely linked. On the one hand, the incidence of MNS disorders goes up with every step down in the social gradient. For example, the poorest populations in every society have the highest rates of depression and alcoholism. On the other hand, MNS disorders and social determinants actually drive one another in a vicious cycle, as summarized in Figure 8-3.

Traditional models of facility-based care fail to address the root causes of MNS disorders (e.g., poverty, stigma, and local context). Instead, an approach that integrates clinical medicine with public health, community empowerment, and direct action on poverty and stigma is needed. Such an approach tends to reorient the usual workforce pyramid. Instead of the most highly trained providers at the top, it is the team members who are closest to the community that are best able to earn trust, understand the local context, and coordinate care in a patient- and community-centered way.

THE IMPORTANCE OF CONTEXT

The Problem

Context is important for four main reasons. First, the history of global health and behavioral medicine is littered with examples of good (and sometimes not so good) intentions gone awry. A nuanced and locally informed understanding of context can reduce the likelihood of unintended harm.

Second, context influences perception and stigma. The origins and effects of mental health programs can dramatically alter their local acceptability, their cultural meaning, and their eventual impact.

Third, the root causes of mental illness are social as well as biological. Effective action on the social determinants and adversity must necessarily be tailored to local context. Similarly, MNS disorders present and respond differently in different settings. Diagnostic and therapeutic strategies must account for these local variations, while forging past the inaction that sometimes results from such uncertainty.

Fourth, intersecting with all of the above problems is the issue of trust. Given the complex and sometimes troubled history of global health and behavioral medicine, strategies to build and strengthen trust between

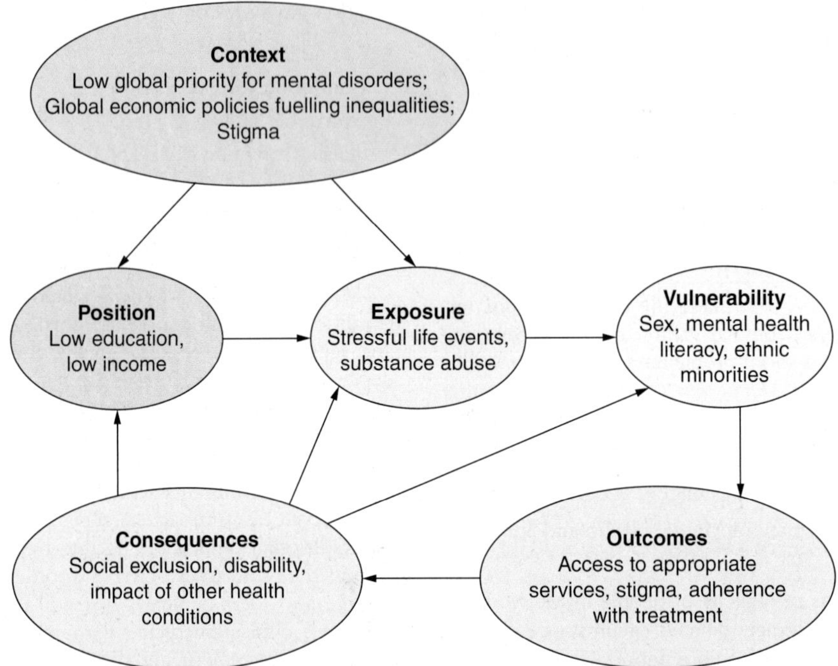

Figure 8-3. Vicious cycle of social determinants and mental disorders. (Reprinted from Patel V, et al. Mental disorders: equity and social determinants. In: Blas E, et al, eds. *Equity, Social Determinants, and Public Health Programmes*. Geneva: World Health Organization; 2010.)

communities and care providers must be grounded in a shared understanding about what truly matters, how best to partner, and how to determine the priorities and metrics for success.

For students interested in reading further about how to consider the issue of context, we recommend Arthur Kleinman's "Four social theories for global health," referenced at the end of the chapter.

Historical Tensions in Global Health & Behavioral Medicine

Behavioral medicine is complicated by a number of historical tensions that persist to the present day. For example, diagnostic systems for MNS disorders (the International Classification of Diseases, developed by the WHO, and the Diagnostic and Statistical Manual of Mental Disorders, produced by the American Psychiatric Association) are not fully supported by scientific evidence, and may to some degree reflect Euro-American concepts of illness. Additional tensions that undermine consensus on how to provide mental health services in different contexts include: spiritual (supernatural or religious) and scientific (natural or biological) approaches to understanding etiology and causation; strength- ("resilience") and illness-based interpretations of human distress in adversity; traditional and biomedical approaches to treatment; and community- and clinic-based approaches to service delivery.

Further controversies arise from the relationship of behavioral medicine to historical precedents. Specifically, psychiatry has at times been used as an instrument of political or government control. This occurred, for example, in Nazi Germany, Communist Russia, apartheid South Africa, and in a number of developing countries during the colonial period. The legacy of these kinds of practices continues to affect the perception of mental health professionals and compounds the already strong cultural predisposition to stigmatize MNS disorders and mental health services.

CASE ILLUSTRATION 2

In January 2010, a major earthquake struck Haiti, crumbling the city of Port-au-Prince and causing massive casualties. Partners In Health (PIH), an international health care organization with 25 years of experience in health care delivery and program implementation in Haiti, was among the first responders to the disaster. At the time of the earthquake, PIH was operating 11 hospitals in partnership with the Haitian Ministry of Health (MOH) and had a staff of approximately 5000 Haitian providers, including 2500 community health workers.

Partners In Health chose to take a long-term view of the problem, recognizing that building mental health systems of care in the context of the disaster would require an integrated, evidence-based, and multisectoral approach. In the weeks following the disaster, immediate linkages were made with the Haitian MOH. Partners In Health also met biweekly with UN and other NGOs interested in post-earthquake mental health services. Initial needs assessments were completed. A proposal was developed for a model of community-based mental health services that could be piloted within the PIH health care system, with the potential to be scaled across the country in partnership with the Haitian MOH.

The empowerment of Haitians to meet locally identified mental health needs was viewed as a critical component for long-term programmatic success. Partners In Health hired additional staff, expanding its team from 3 Haitian psychologists to 17, and from 20 social workers to 50. Approximately 18 months after the earthquake, PIH staff had provided 20,000 individual services for mental health needs. All of these services were linked to a system of social and economic support on the one hand, and advanced medical care on the other. A qualitative study of local beliefs and perceived needs resulted in the creation of locally valid screening tools for use by community health workers. A stepped care model for mental health services—including treatment algorithms, training curricula, and evaluation tools—was developed. Training programs to support the professional development of local implementers were also developed. With increasing experience, the team developed data collection systems and a mental health electronic medical record. The team piloted various models of care, including a mobile team that travels to remote communities. Today the program follows approximately 3000 people in ongoing care, and serves as a point of reference for mental health care in the country.

Informed by decades of collaborative care with local Haitians and the Haitian MOH, PIH was able to respond to a complex humanitarian disaster from a position of trust, resilience, and deep familiarity with local context. This response addressed urgent needs, strengthened local capacity, and positioned mental health services within a continuum of care spanning basic needs, common MNS disorders, and more complex conditions.

BOX 8-3 MENTAL HEALTH CARE DELIVERY: LESSONS AND RECOMMENDATIONS FROM PARTNERS IN HEALTH SITES

- Community-based mental health care, with a focus on both "task sharing" and integration into primary care systems, is feasible.
- Sustained clinical mentorship and supervision are essential and require ongoing commitment, at whatever level you are working within or outside of health systems.
- Work toward multidisciplinary, collaborative, team-based care, and prepare for stigma embedded within and outside of health systems.
- Aim for building local capacity with direct MOH collaboration.
- Seek to adapt evidence-based packages of care (e.g., WHO mhGAP), depending on local priorities, culture, and context.
- Monitoring, evaluation, and continuous quality improvement (MEQ), must be pursued to justify resources and improve quality.
- Be creative in involving specialists, if you can, as mental health care delivery can become complex.
- Seek to directly address social determinants of mental illness (poverty, stigma).
- Research is essential to innovation.

Source: Raviola G. Partners In Health, Boston, MA, USA. 2018.

CONCLUSIONS

This chapter has considered the rationale for integrating the study of global health and behavioral medicine, the magnitude and causes of the global treatment gap for MNS disorders, four elements of best practice for delivering simpler, nonspecialist models of mental health care, and the importance of local context.

We have aimed for breadth, envisioning a concise introduction for a primarily U.S. or European medical student audience. The depth of coverage has necessarily been limited. We hope readers will find the chapter useful, and that those who are interested will be stimulated to read further and perhaps contribute to global health and behavioral medicine in their professional careers.

SUGGESTED READINGS

Becker AE, Kleinman A. Mental health and the global agenda. *N Engl J Med* 2013;369:66–73.

Belkin G, Unützer J, Kessler R, et al. Scaling up for the "Bottom Billion": "5×5" implementation of community mental health care in low-income regions. *Psychiatr Serv* 2011;62:1494–1502.

Bloom DE, Cafiero ET, Jané-Llopis E, et al. The global economic burden of non-communicable diseases. Geneva: World Economic Forum; 2011.

Collins PY, Insel TR, Chockalingam A, et al. Grand challenges in global mental health: integration in research, policy, and practice. *PLoS Med* 2013;10(4):e1001434.

Collins PY, Patel V, Joestl SS, et al. Grand Challenges in global mental health. *Nature* 2011;475:27–30.

Kleinman A. Four social theories for global health. *Lancet* 2010;375(9725):1518–1519.

Kroenke K, Unützer J. Closing the false divide: sustainable approaches to integrating mental health services into primary care. *J Gen Intern Med.* 2016;32(4):404–410.

Mathers CD, Loncar D. Projections of global mortality and burden of disease from 2002 to 2030. *PLoS Med* 2006;3(11):e442.

Patel V, Belkin GS, Chockalingam A, et al. Grand challenges: integrating mental health services into priority health care platforms. *PLoS Med* 2013;10(5):e1001448.

Patel V, Lund C, Heatherill S, et al. Mental disorders: equity and social determinants. In: Blas E, Sivasankara Kurup A, eds. *Equity, Social Determinants, and Public Health Programmes.* Geneva: World Health Organization; 2010.

Patel V, Saxena S, Lund C, et al. The Lancet Commission on global mental health and sustainable development. *Lancet* 2018;392:1553–1598.

Patel V, Saxena S. Transforming lives, enhancing communities–innovations in global mental health. *N Engl J Med* 2014;370:498–501.

Patel V, Thornicroft G. Packages of care for mental, neurological, and substance use disorders in low- and middle-income countries. *PLoS Med* 2009;6(10):e1000160.

Vigo D, Thornicroft G, Atun R. Estimating the true global burden of mental illness. *Lancet Psychiatry* 2016;3(2):171–178.

World Health Organization. Closing the gap in a generation: health equity through action on the social determinants of health. WHO Commission on Social Determinants of Health, 2008.

World Health Organization. Integrating mental health into primary care: a global perspective. Geneva: World Health Organization and World Organization of Family Doctors (Wonca), 2008.

World Health Organization. mhGAP Humanitarian Intervention Guide (mhGAP-HIG): clinical management of mental, neurological and substance use conditions in humanitarian emergencies, 2015.

World Health Organization. mhGAP Intervention Guide for mental, neurological and substance use disorders in non-specialized health settings. Geneva, Switzerland; 2011.

World Health Organization. mhGAP Intervention Guide for mental, neurological and substance use disorders in non-specialized health settings: mental health Gap Action Programme (mhGAP)—version 2.0, 2016.

WEBSITES

Global Burden of Disease Collaborative Network. Global Burden of Disease Study 2016 (GBD 2016) Results. [Internet]. Seattle, United States: Institute for Health Metrics and Evaluation (IHME), 2017 [cited 2017 Dec 19]. http://ghdx.healthdata.org/gbd-results-tool.

World Health Organization: Comprehensive Mental Health Action Plan 2013-2020. Geneva: WHO. http://www.who.int/mental_health/action_plan_2013/en/. Accessed September 2018.

World Health Organization: Mental Health ATLAS 2017. Geneva: WHO. http://www.who.int/mental_health/evidence/atlas/mental_health_atlas_2017/en/. Accessed September 2018.

World Health Organization: mhGAP: intervention guide for mental, neurologic, and substance use disorders for nonspecialists. Geneva: WHO. https://www.who.int/mental_health/mhgap/operations_manual/en/. Accessed February 2019.

World Health Organization: mhGAP-HIG: Clinical Management of Mental, Neurologic, and Substance Use Disorders in Humanitarian Emergencies. Geneva: WHO. https://www.who.int/mental_health/publications/mhgap_hig/en/. Accessed February 2019.

World Health Organization: Problem Management Plus (PM+). Geneva: WHO. http://www.who.int/mental_health/emergencies/problem_management_plus/en/. Accessed September 2018.

Environment, Health, and Behavior

9

John F. Christensen, PhD

If you want to learn about the health of a population, look at the air they breathe, the water they drink, and the places where they live.

Hippocrates, Fifth century BCE

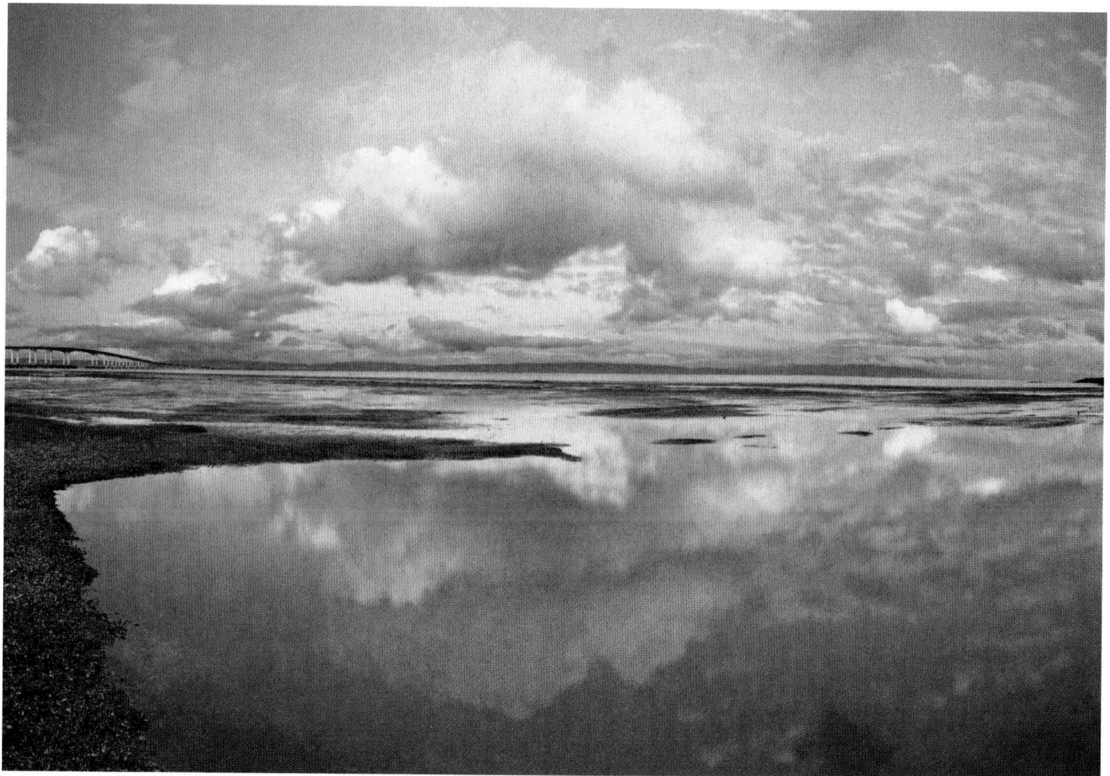

Photo by Hank Christensen (www.hankchristensen.com).

INTRODUCTION

This chapter looks beyond the individual patient and clinician to the behaviors of human populations and their impact on the environment, which itself exerts a profound influence on human health and illness. We will discuss opportunities and strategies for modifying those behaviors—on the individual and societal scale—that affect human health and well-being.

The attention of health professionals to environmental factors is warranted by developments in our scientific understanding of three interrelated domains: (1) the impact of environmental degradation and enhancement on human health, (2) the impact of human behavior on the environment, and (3) the effectiveness of initiatives to modify human behavior on a population scale. This chapter will review each of these domains and conclude with suggestions for clinicians to draw upon this information in the care of patients and to become engaged in the process of societal behavior change for the well-being of the planet.

EFFECTS OF ENVIRONMENTAL DEGRADATION ON HUMAN HEALTH

As Hippocrates observed millennia ago, the quality of the biosphere that supports us has a marked impact on our health. Disease burdens due to environmental degradation include altered fertility rates, challenges to the health of newborns, disorders of human development, malnutrition, vector patterns of infectious diseases, skin cancers due to ultraviolet radiation exposure, respiratory disorders, and obesity. Understanding connections between environmental change and these kinds of health problems has increased as agencies such as the World Health Organization (WHO), U.S. National Institutes of Health (NIH), U.S. Centers for Disease Control and Prevention (CDC), Institute of Medicine (IOM), and others have compiled research on the environment–health connection. A few of these connections are summarized here.

Air Pollution

The WHO estimates that there are 7 million deaths worldwide each year from air pollutants—over five times the number of traffic fatalities. Globally, 9 out of 10 people breathe polluted air. Over an 18-year period, increased death rates from dementias have been linked to a rise in the concentration of pesticides, industrial effluents, car exhaust, and other pollutants in the environment. Sulfur dioxide, produced by combustion of fossil fuels, has been shown to induce acute bronchoconstriction in asthmatics. Particulate air pollution has been implicated in respiratory ailments and in derangement of heart rate variability, a risk factor for cardiac events. Carbon monoxide (CO), primarily emitted from internal combustion engines in motor vehicles, has serious health effects in high concentrations leading to carbon monoxide poisoning. More frequently, however, lower-level exposures to CO may increase platelet activity and coagulation, leading to increased risks of thromboembolism. A global meta-analysis found an association between air pollution and heart failure hospitalization or death, particularly with increases in carbon monoxide, sulfur dioxide, and nitrogen dioxide. In Northern China, where the government's Huai River policy has provided free winter heating with coal, total suspended particulates (TSPs) air pollution has been associated with a lower life expectancy of 5.5 years, compared with populations in the south. A meta-analysis of 17 population cohorts in Europe found a significant association between particulate matter concentrations and lung cancer.

Degraded Water Quality & Availability

The quality of water can be associated with human disease in several ways. Bacterial pathogens, including *Salmonella, Shigella, Escherichia coli,* and *Vibrio cholerae*—all of which cause diarrheal disease, can be spread by water, particularly in developing countries with inadequate water treatment. In Yemen, the cholera outbreak of 2017–2018 led to over 1 million cases, with 2310 associated deaths. Water quality is also compromised by various toxic chemicals that accumulate in ground and surface water from runoff and industrial discharge. Examples are nitrates, pesticides, the gasoline additive methyl *tert*-butyl ether (MTBE), radon, arsenic, lead, and the by-products of disinfectants. These toxins have been associated with a variety of health problems, including various forms of cancer, decreased intelligence quotient (IQ) and behavioral problems in infants and children, adult hypertension, and neurotoxicity.

Water availability per capita is shrinking worldwide. The total amount of freshwater available for human use worldwide is about 0.007 of all the water on earth. Currently, humans use about half of this amount. In many underdeveloped parts of the world, millions of humans live in "hydrological poverty," in which water for direct human consumption through drinking and indirect consumption through grain production is becoming increasingly scarce. In these areas, water for drinking and irrigation is overpumped beyond the recharge rate of underground aquifers. Resource wars, in which arable land is contested in civil wars, such as that occurring in the Darfur region of Sudan, are increasing in frequency due to diminished water availability for irrigation. It is estimated that by 2100 the flow of the Nile into Egypt could be reduced by 75% due to extremes of heat.

Malnourishment

Of the approximately 7.7 billion persons comprising the earth's human population, over 4 billion are prone to some form of malnourishment. Hunger afflicts 1.2 billion; another 2 billion suffer from micronutrient deficiency. Most of these people live in low- or middle-income countries. At the other end of the malnourishment spectrum, 1.2 billion people suffer from overconsumption of food with its associated problems of obesity, cardiovascular disease, and type 2 diabetes.

Climate Change

The earth's climate continues to warm at an alarming rate. Earth's global surface temperature in 2018 was the

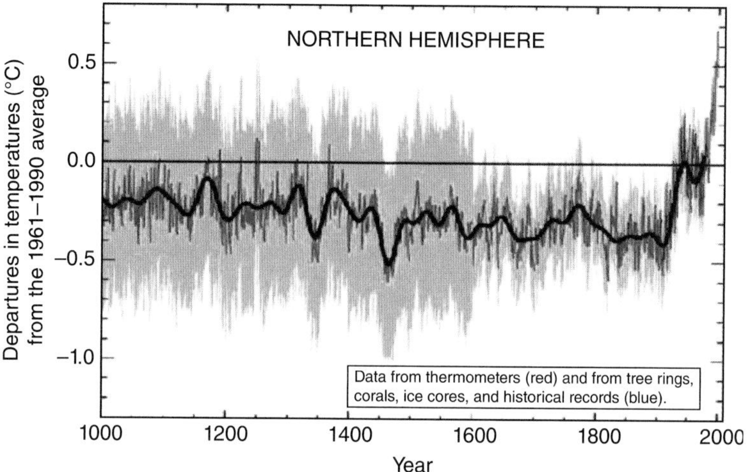

Figure 9-1. Northern Hemisphere temperature changes over last millennium. (The curve of temperature changes takes on a "hockey stick" appearance, with accelerated warming since the Industrial Revolution resembling the blade of the stick.) (Reprinted with permission from the Summary for Policymakers in IPCC 2001: Climate Change 2001: The Scientific Basis. Contribution of Working Group I to the Third Assessment Report of the Intergovernmental Panel on Climate Change [Houghton, J.T, Y. Ding, D.J. Griggs, M. Noguer, P.J. van der Linden, X. Dai, K. Maskell, and C.A. Johnson (eds.)]. Cambridge University Press, Cambridge, United Kingdom and New York, NY, USA.)

fourth warmest since modern recordkeeping began in 1880, according to an analysis by NASA. Global temperatures in 2018 were 1.5°F (0.83°C) warmer than the 1951 to 1980 mean.

Figure 9-1 shows the increase in the Northern Hemisphere temperature over the last thousand years.

Figure 9-2 shows the consensus of five agencies on the earth's warming since record-keeping began in 1880.

The major driver of global warming is the accumulation of "greenhouse" gases—primarily carbon dioxide, methane, and nitrous oxide—which are emitted by industrial pollution and the burning of fossil fuels. These

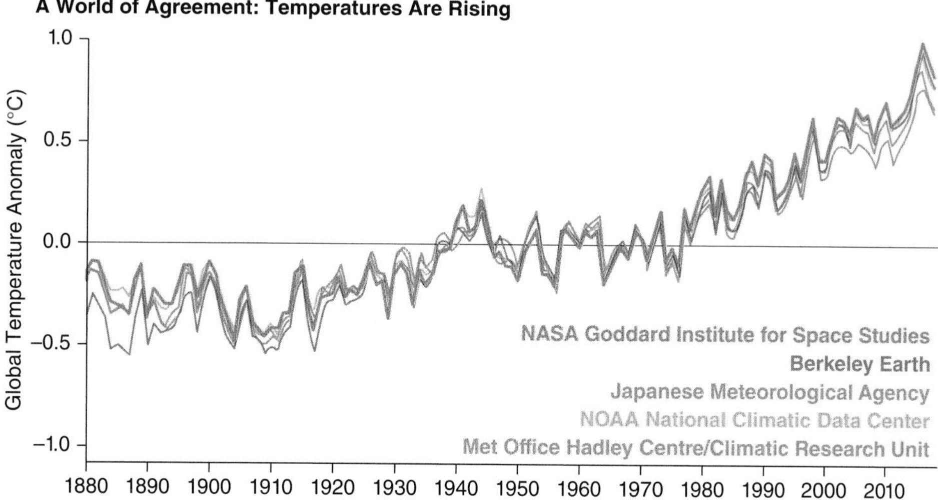

Figure 9-2. Temperature data showing rapid warming in the past few decades, the latest data going up to 2018. According to NASA data, 2016 was the warmest year since 1880, continuing a long-term trend of rising global temperatures. The 10 warmest years in the 139-year record all have occurred since 2005, with the five warmest years being the five most recent years. Credit: NASA's Earth Observatory. (*Source:* Scientific Consensus: Earth's Climate is Warming. NASA's Earth Observatory. Available at: https://climate.nasa.gov/scientific-consensus/)

greenhouse gases allow radiant energy from the sun to be absorbed by water vapor, clouds, and aerosols, and then trap the reflected infrared radiation, absorbing and reemitting it to further warm the lower atmosphere and the earth's surface.

Current estimates are that the earth's warming is accelerating, and climate models predict that the average surface temperature will rise by 2.4 to 6.4°C by the year 2100. Climate scientists have concluded that without significant global efforts to control greenhouse gas emissions, the earth could soon pass a tipping point that would lead to a much higher global average temperature than any interglacial period in the past 1.2 million years and to sea levels significantly higher than at any time in the Holocene epoch. This runaway "Hothouse Earth" effect would result from several self-reinforcing feedbacks. These include permafrost thawing with associated increased releases of carbon dioxide and methane; increased bacterial respiration in the ocean; weakening of land and ocean carbon sinks; Amazon and boreal forest dieback with associated release of carbon dioxide, often through wildfires; decreased "albedo effect" (the reflection of sunlight by ice and snow) due to summer loss of Arctic sea ice, reduction of northern hemisphere spring snow cover, summer loss of Antarctic ice, and loss of the polar ice sheet. All of these feedbacks would amplify and accelerate warming.

The impact of earth's warming on human health is enormous and varied. The *direct effects* of climate change on human health include heat-related illnesses and deaths; increased floods and droughts (often followed by malnutrition due to loss of cropland); the spread of infectious diseases to wider geographical ranges, both in latitude and altitude, as mosquito-borne illnesses such as dengue fever and West Nile virus, tick-borne illnesses such as Lyme disease, and rodent-borne illnesses such as hantavirus follow the warming trends; a longer seasonal duration of biogenic allergens; cardiorespiratory problems due to increased ground-level ozone concentrations and smoke from wildfires; increase in water-related diseases as water scarcity and rising sea levels lead to freshwater contamination; algal blooms with associated cholera outbreaks; increased outbreaks of cryptosporidiosis due to heavy rainfall; and the threat to human health and well-being by the more violent storms associated with warming.

The *indirect health effects* include water scarcity, with the number of people living in water-scarce countries expected to rise to 3 billion by 2025; nutrition deficits driven by a drop in crop yields combined with increased demand due to population growth and higher levels of consumption as affluence promotes shifting to a meat-based diet; undernutrition (indicated by stunting and underweight in children under 5 years) due to lowered crop yields; decreased nutritional content of grains due to increased atmospheric CO_2 concentrations; and finally population displacement—with associated immune system challenges, infectious diseases, housing and sanitation challenges, lack of safe drinking water, malnutrition, violence, and posttraumatic stress disorder (PTSD).

Figure 9-3 shows the various pathways in which a warming climate is having an adverse impact on human health. In addition to the impacts of ocean acidification, elevated temperatures, and increase in air pollutants, the earth's warming also influences social factors such as poverty and population displacement that have a mediating influence on disease. These adverse effects on human health have become more evident and pronounced in recent years. For example, 157 million more people globally were exposed to heatwave events in 2017, compared with 2000. Excessive heat exposure caused more than 7400 deaths in the United States from 1999 to 2010. Across Europe, about 70,000 premature deaths were attributed to the 2003 heat wave. Thirty countries are experiencing downward trends in crop yields, potentially leading to a rise in undernutrition. The global vectorial capacity for the transmission of the dengue fever virus was the highest on record in 2016. Smoke from forest fires and other landscape fires causes about 339,000 premature deaths globally per year primarily due to respiratory and cardiovascular impacts.

Environmental Toxins

The leaching into groundwater of industrial chemicals such as pesticides and herbicides and into the air of substances such as dioxin due to incineration of medical waste has led to an accumulation of persistent organic pollutants (POPs) in the human body. Almost all humans have residues of these chemicals in their tissues, and there is increased concern among public health officials that these levels could reach thresholds harmful to human health. The emerging toxicological field of endocrine disruption focuses on the influence of POPs in imitating or blocking the actions of hormones, possibly leading to a variety of reproductive and neurodevelopmental disorders.

Built Environment

The ways in which cities grow to accommodate increased population may be contributing to worsening human health. The "built environment" refers to the impacts of urban sprawl, traffic congestion, and the associated sedentary lifestyle of the population as people spend more time in cars and in gridlock driving to work or shopping. The U.S. CDC estimates that urban sprawl due to lack of adequate land use planning is associated with increases in obesity, cardiovascular disease, and type 2 diabetes.

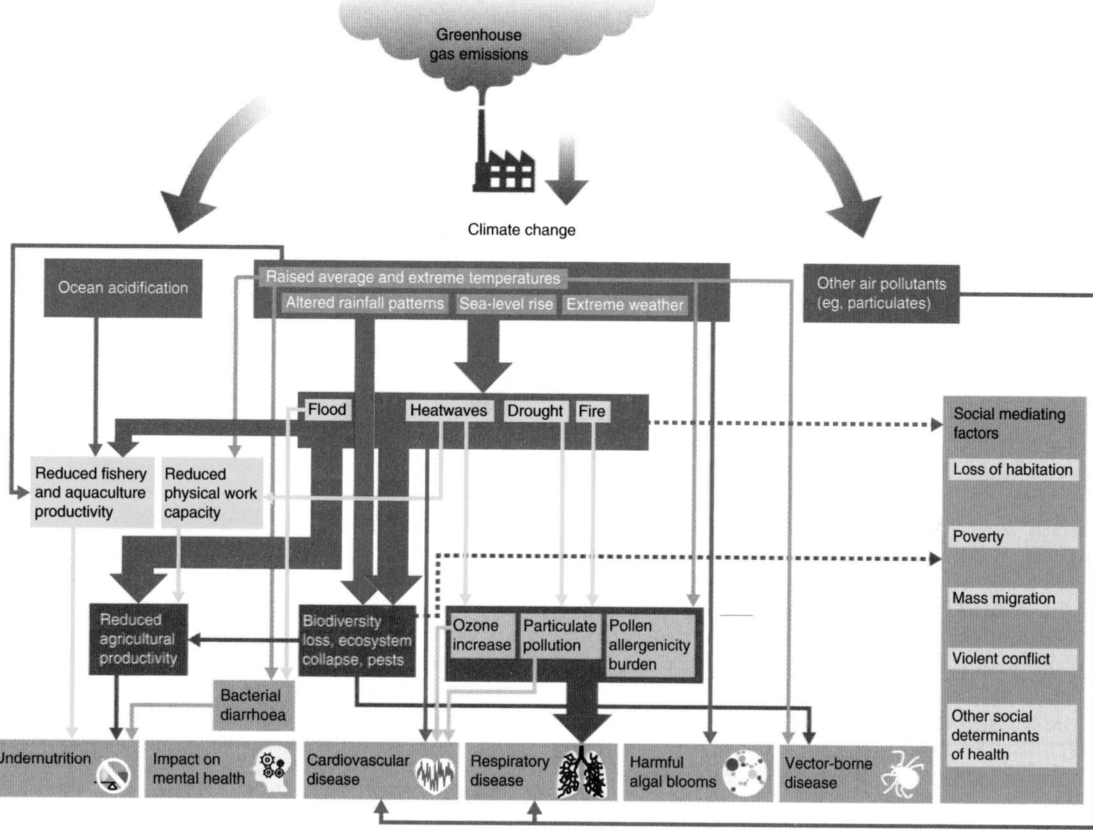

Figure 9-3. Pathways between climate change and human health. (Reprinted from Watts N, et al. The 2018 report of the Lancet Countdown on health and climate change: shaping the health of nations for centuries to come. *The Lancet* 2018; 392:2479–2514.)

POSITIVE HEALTH EFFECTS OF NATURE

A discussion of the connection between the environment and human health would be incomplete without mention of the affinity humans have with the natural world and the positive effect of engagement with nature on human health. The biologist E.O. Wilson proposed in his *biophilia hypothesis* that humans have an innate inclination to affiliate with other forms of life. There is a growing awareness of the restorative benefits of spending time in nature—including physical, mental, and spiritual renewal.

Different theories have been advanced about what constitutes the restorative effects of nature. *Attention restoration theory* suggests that the effort required for focused attention, especially in complex urban environments, requires inhibition of competing demands for attention, often leading to "directed attention fatigue." The restorative benefits of nature involve recovery from this attentional fatigue through the experience of *being away* (having a distance from routine mental tasks), *fascination* (involving interest-driven attention), *extent* (being in a coherently ordered environment of substantial scope), and *compatibility* (the demands and supports posed by the environment match the individual's inclinations).

A theory of *psychological stress recovery* proposes that particular qualities and contents of the natural scene facilitate this recovery—moderate depth, moderate complexity, the presence of a focal point, gross structural qualities, and natural contents (e.g., vegetation and water). These features of the natural scene evoke positive emotions, sustain nonvigilant attention, restrict negative thoughts, and facilitate reduction of sympathetic arousal. From an evolutionary perspective, humans are biologically prepared to respond positively to environmental features that signal possibilities of survival.

There is growing evidence supporting the restorative and health-promoting influence of nature. Several studies have shown that children who have access to green environments with trees and other vegetation have an increased ability to focus and concentrate. Children with attention-deficit/hyperactivity disorder (ADHD) have shown improvement in symptoms when they are in contact with nature. A study of childhood asthma and the number of street trees in neighborhoods in New York City found that an increase of tree density of one standard deviation was associated with a lower prevalence of asthma. Neighborhood greenery has also been associated with lower body mass index (BMI) in children, indicating the value of urban planning for greenspaces as a means of addressing childhood obesity.

A number of studies have shown positive impacts of natural environments on cognitive performance and attentional enhancement in adults. Recovering breast cancer patients who participated in nature-based restorative activities showed better coping ability and attentional performance than those who did not. College students whose dormitory windows had views of nature functioned more effectively on daily tasks requiring directed attention than those with views of buildings. These studies lend support to the attention restoration theory of how nature influences human performance.

There is also evidence supporting the role of engagement with nature in psychological stress recovery. Hospital inpatients recovering from cholecystectomy whose rooms had views of trees had a shorter length of hospitalization and lower need for pain medication than patients with views of buildings. Bronchoscopy patients exposed to images and sounds of nature had significantly better pain control than those who did not.

The influence of natural environments on physiologic parameters related to stress and illness suggests some of the pathways mediating the positive impacts of nature on human health. Studies in Japan on *shinrin-yoku*, or "forest bathing trips," have shown significant effects of time spent walking in forest settings on enhanced immune function, including increase in natural killer cell activity, decreased levels of adrenalin and noradrenalin, and increased activation of the parasympathetic nervous system.

IMPACT OF HUMAN BEHAVIOR ON THE ENVIRONMENT

Figure 9-4 shows the growth over the last two millennia of the earth's human population, which has doubled since 1950 to 7.7 billion as of 2019. Population growth, coupled with increased human extraction of resources from the earth (the "ecological footprint") has led to a cumulative and negative impact of human alteration of the environment.

The consensus of the scientific community is that the earth is warming due to human activity. The dramatic rise in atmospheric concentrations of carbon dioxide since the Industrial Revolution—especially due to carbon emissions from automobiles, coal power plants, and other industrial sources—coupled with a destruction of natural carbon sinks due to deforestation, especially the loss of tropical rainforest, is correlated with the increased warming trend noted over the same period (Figure 9-5). For the first time in geological history, the behavior of a single species is now altering on a global scale the sustaining fabric of all life. Earth scientists have proposed a new term, "the Anthropocene," for the geological age that is now emerging. It is based on the observation that human impacts on planetary processes have become so profound that they have driven the Earth out of the Holocene epoch in which agriculture, sedentary communities, and eventually, socially and technologically complex human societies developed.

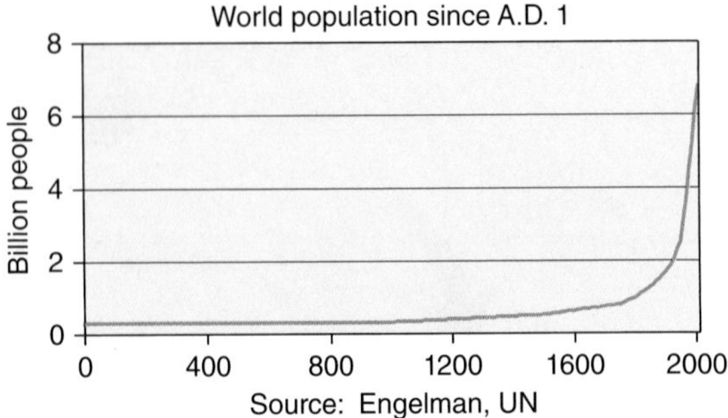

Figure 9-4. Growth in the earth's human population over the last two millennia. (The acceleration of population growth over the last century assumes a "hockeystick" curve, similar to Figure 9-1 for northern hemisphere warming.)

The "ecological footprint" of humans on the earth is unequally distributed among nations. China's total CO_2 emissions are the highest (27% of the world's total), compared to the United States (18%), the European Union (13%), and India (5%). To make a fair comparison of CO_2 emissions, however, it is important to compare emissions in terms of CO_2 emitted per person. The United States, with one of the highest rates of carbon emissions per capita, released 15.7 tons per person in 2017, compared to China (7.7 tons), the European Union (7.0 tons), and India (1.8 tons) (Figure 9-6).

Human behavior is implicated in all of the environmental threats to human behavior mentioned above. Poor or absent land use planning; waste of water and the overpumping of underground aquifers below their recharge rate; deforestation; overfishing of the seas; indiscriminate discharge of pollutants into air, ground, and water; overcultivating and mismanaging the soil; and overconsumption of material goods whose manufacture and disposal further degrades the environment—all are behaviors that in the aggregate alter the fabric that sustains life and supports human health.

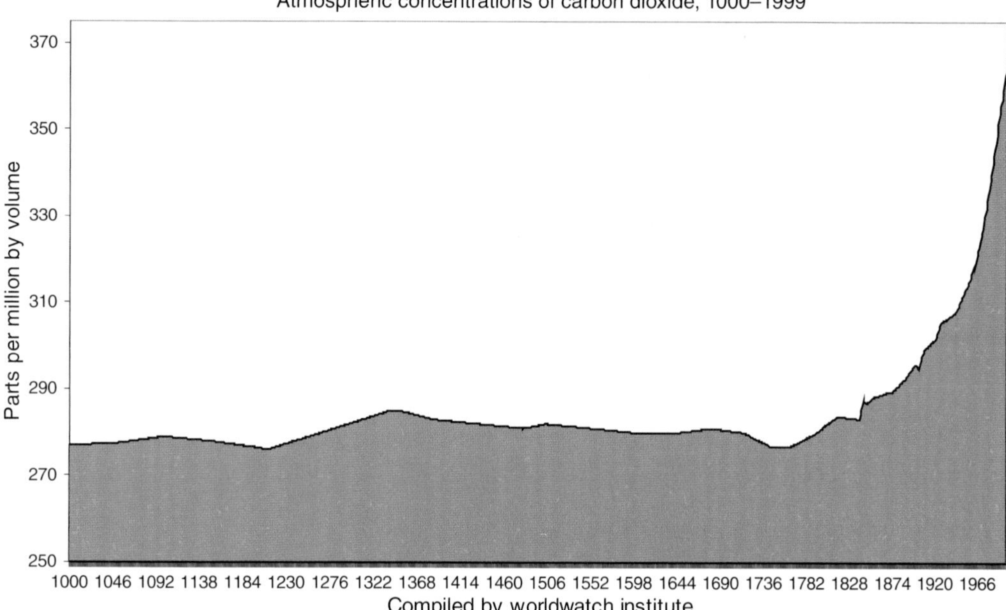

Figure 9-5. Increase in atmospheric concentrations of carbon dioxide over the last millennium. (The accelerated increase in CO_2 since the Industrial Revolution assumes the familiar "hockey stick" curve, as in Figures 9-1 and 9-4.) (Compiled by Worldwatch Institute.)

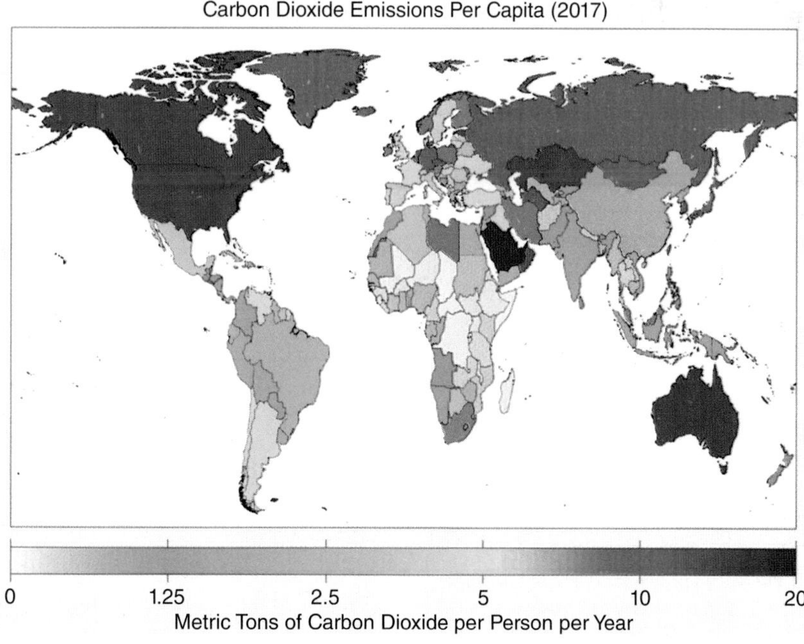

Figure 9-6. Carbon dioxide emissions per capita among nations. (Twitter posting by Robert Rohde, PhD. Lead scientist at Berkeley Earth @RARohde.)

Behavioral medicine, especially as practiced in the individual clinician–patient encounter, traditionally targets the behaviors, emotions, and relationships of patients and clinicians in the amelioration of disease in the individual patient. *In the context of the environment–health connection, however, behavioral medicine focuses more broadly on the behavior of populations, while maintaining the individual patient encounter at its core.*

CHANGING POPULATION BEHAVIOR IN RELATION TO THE ENVIRONMENT

There is consensus among climate scientists that future rise in global average temperatures must be held to well below 2°C above preindustrial levels. The safer target should be 1.5°C. Meeting these targets will require a major restructuring of human behavior globally, including the following: a complete decarbonization of power generation away from fossil fuels, reversing a trend that began with the industrial revolution; a reorientation toward sustainable global food and agricultural systems; a rethinking of the structure and function of spatial infrastructure and cities, and methods of transport within and between them; the reversal of deforestation and land-use change trends; and profound changes in the methods of delivery of health care.

In 2016 the American College of Physicians (ACP) adopted the following policy recommendations to guide physicians and the public in efforts to mitigate climate change:

1. *A global effort is required to reduce anthropogenic greenhouse emissions and address the health impact of climate change. The United States must commit to taking both a leadership and collaborative role in developing, implementing, and ensuring the success of such a global effort and in reducing its own contributions to greenhouse emissions. Climate change adaptation strategies must be established, and mitigation measures must be adopted.*
2. *The health care sector, within the United States and globally, must implement environmentally sustainable and energy-efficient practices and prepare for the impacts of climate change to ensure continued operations during periods of elevated patient demand.*
3. *Physicians, both individually and collectively, are encouraged to advocate for climate change adaptation and mitigation policies and communicate about the health cobenefits of addressing climate change in objective, simple language to their community and policymakers. For its part, the American College of Physicians is committed to working with its international chapters and with other professional membership and public health organizations within the United States and globally to pursue the policies recommended in this paper.*
4. *Physicians are encouraged to become educated about climate change, its effect on human health, and how to respond to future challenges. Medical schools and continuing medical education providers should incorporate climate change-related coursework into curricula.*
5. *Governments should commit to providing substantial and sufficient climate change research funding to understand, adapt to, and mitigate the human health effects of climate change.*

Although the actions of world governments are necessary to create the public policy framework for restructuring human society as a carbon-free economy, the involvement of health professionals is critical in changing societal behavior to protect and promote human health. How can health care clinicians influence behavior change at the population level? There is a growing awareness that several approaches have either demonstrated effectiveness or hold promise for exerting a meaningful influence, if professionals organize to take action.

Leading by Example

Individual clinicians can adopt environmentally friendly practices by the way their offices and clinics are furnished. The use of low-watt fluorescent or LED lighting and low flow toilets, and the purchase of products from vendors known to use environmentally sensitive practices demonstrate to patients that their clinician is committed to sustainability. In their personal lives as well, health professionals can lead the way in the choices they make by using mass transportation and lower-carbon-emission vehicles, owning energy-efficient homes and appliances, using renewable sources of energy, being mindful of consumer patterns that favor eco-friendly products, and dealing responsibly with waste.

Patient Education

Mentioning the link, where appropriate, between patients' illnesses and environmental factors that are the result of human behavior can plant the seed for behavior change. For example, mentioning the link between exposure to diesel exhaust and asthma, or between pesticide overuse and endocrine disruption, can in the aggregate begin to educate a community, using teachable moments related to individual health care. The Pediatric Environmental Health Toolkit developed by Physicians for Social Responsibility (PSR) and endorsed by the American Academy of Pediatrics (https://peht.ucsf.edu/index.php) to assist pediatricians in educating parents about POPs is one example. Another resource is *Healthy Aging and the Environment: A Pocket Guide*, developed by the Collaborative on Health and the Environment (https://www.healthandenvironment.org/docs/healthy-aging.pdf). Having literature available in the waiting room linking environmental factors with human health may provide a context for further clinician–patient dialogue on this issue.

Community Education

Health professionals can offer community education lectures through their hospital systems, civic clubs, community associations, schools, and churches. Resources such as the Worldwatch Institute, Collaborative on Health and the Environment, CDC, PSR, and others have websites and databases from which presentations can be easily assembled. One helpful resource for health professionals in preparing presentations to educate the public about climate change is "Conveying the Human Implications of Climate Change: A Climate Change Communication Primer for Public Health Professionals" (see link in list of websites at end of chapter). Letters to the editor and op-ed submissions to local newspapers are other ways of informing communities about the link between the environment and health, as well as about behaviors that can mitigate deleterious health impacts.

Land Use Planning

Decisions made at the neighborhood, municipality, state, and national levels about the built environment and the protection and promotion of natural areas have relevance for human health and well-being. Health professionals can play an informative role with land use planning bodies, providing testimony about the importance of wilderness areas, parks, and open spaces in promoting human health.

Public Policy Advocacy

Professional associations at the local, state, and national level are potent vehicles for public policy advocacy. Clinicians who are interested and informed about environmental issues and their health effects can organize interest groups and public policy advocacy teams within their organizations. They can also work with the governance structure of their organizations to endorse policy positions both to influence public opinion and to lobby local, state, and federal government for legislation and regulations to promote eco-friendly practices. Several U.S. states have enacted legislation to cap greenhouse gas emissions, and health professionals have played important roles in these efforts.

The Clean Air Act of 1970 is an example of a public policy success involving regulation of industrial pollution in the United States. With support from the medical community, the Clean Air Act provided a broad regulatory framework for air pollution standards. It set ambient air emission standards, including acceptable levels for particulate matter, ozone, carbon monoxide, nitrogen dioxide, sulfur dioxide, and lead. The law required the U.S. Environmental Protection Agency to use scientific evidence relating air quality to public health in setting standards. Over the last 40 years this has led to a progressive national reduction of these air pollutants. Even in the first year after the law went into effect, there was a sharp reduction in total suspended particulates of air pollution and infant mortality, with a 1% decline in TSPs resulting in a 0.5% decline in the infant mortality rate.

The Precautionary Principle

Many professional associations have adopted versions of this principle, which states: "When an activity raises threats of harm to the environment or human health, precautionary measures should be taken even if some cause and effect relationships are not fully established scientifically." When applied to a phenomenon such as global warming, this principle states that the probable connection between human behavior and planetary warming, coupled with the probable and irreversible health consequences to humanity and other species if preventive action is not taken, creates a moral imperative for governments and human society to act now to reduce greenhouse gases, even before all the scientific causality is established. Health professional associations have played a role in getting this principle adopted by municipal and local governments.

Changing the Corporate Behavior of Health Care Organizations

The U.S. health care sector is second only to the food industry in overall energy use. Health professionals affiliated with medical centers and other health care organizations can influence these organizations to alter practices that have an impact on the environment. Examples are the use of "green" building design to make new facilities more energy efficient and utilize materials that leave a lower environmental footprint, environmentally preferable purchasing of supplies, healthy food options for patients and staff, safe disposal of medical waste, and recycling of materials produced by the health care enterprise.

CONCLUSIONS

These are but some of the ways in which clinicians and health professionals can influence the behavior of populations, corporations, and governments. The principles of behavior change (see Chapter 19) may be applicable not only to individuals but also to whole societies, as they move through stages of readiness to alter lifestyles that strain the earth's carrying capacity. In the aggregate these behavior changes can reduce the human footprint on the earth.

Finally, the health and well-being of our personal lives and of the organizations within which we work is embedded within the health of our planet. Being mindful of the factors that promote environmental and planetary health can give us insights into the sustainability of our lives and careers in medicine. Land use planners, when determining where human population growth in a region should be allowed to occur, employ the following equation: **C – L = M** (*Capacity – Load = Margin*). Here, *capacity* refers to the carrying capacity of the land, which includes available water, natural resources, transportation corridors, and the ability of the land to absorb the wastes of human activity. *Load* refers to the impact or "ecological footprint" of that human activity upon the land. When the carrying capacity of the natural environment is greater than the additional load of human activity, then there will be a *positive margin* and population growth is *sustainable*. Conversely, when the load exceeds the capacity of the land, then there is a *negative margin* and growth is *unsustainable*.

This same equation, **C – L = M**, can be applied to our own lives and the organizations within which we work. When our capacity as persons is chronically overloaded by work, family, and other commitments, then we are in a negative margin state, which is a way of defining *burnout*. At this point our lives as human beings are unsustainable. It is as if we are drawing off the principal of our resources rather than living off the interest. Conversely, when our capacity routinely exceeds the load we assume, then we are in a positive margin state, and our lives are sustainable.

We must awaken to the full context of our lives on this planet. Restoring the proper relationship of humans with the earth in a way that promotes sustainability in the whole system is what Thomas Berry has called "the great work" of our generation. Physicians and other health professionals have a vital role to play in this work, for our own health will only be as good as the health of the planet.

SUGGESTED READINGS

Amel E, Manniing C, Scott B, Koger S. Beyond the roots of human inaction: fostering collective effort toward ecosystem conservation. *Science* 2017;356:275–279.

Berry T. *The Great Work.* New York, NY: Bell Tower; 1999.

Chen Y, Ebenstein A, Greenstone M, Li H. Evidence on the impact of sustained exposure to air pollution on life expectancy from China's Huai River policy. *PNAS* 2013;110:12936–12941.

Clayton S, Devine-Wright P, Stern PC, et al. Psychological research and global climate change. *Nat Clim Chang* 2015;5:640–646.

Crowley RA. Climate change and health: a position paper of the American College of Physicians. *Ann Intern Med* 2016;164:608–610.

Epstein PR, Ferber D. *Changing Planet, Changing Health.* University of California Press; 2011.

Hansen J, Sato M, Ruedy R. Perception of climate change. *PNAS* 2012;109:E2415–E2423.

McCally M, ed. *Life Support: The Environment and Human Health.* MIT Press; 2002.

Raaschou-Nielsen O, Andersen ZJ, Beelen R, et al. Air pollution and lung cancer incidence in 17 European cohorts: prospective analyses from the European Study of Cohorts for Air Pollution Effects (ESCAPE). *Lancet Oncol* 2013;14:813–822.

Samet JM. The Clean Air Act and health—a clearer view from 2011. *N Engl J Med* 2011;365:198–201.

Shah ASV, Langrish JP, Nair H, et al. Global association of air pollution and heart failure: a systematic review and meta-analysis. *Lancet* 2013;382:1039–1048.

Steffen W, Rockstrom J, Richardson K, et al. Trajectories of the earth system in the Anthropocene. *PNAS* 2018;115:8252–8259.

Watts N, Amann M, Arness N, et al. The 2018 report of the Lancet Countdown on health and climate change: shaping the health of nations for centuries to come. *Lancet* 2018; 392: 2479–2514.

Weart SR. *The Discovery of Global Warming.* Harvard University Press; 2003.

WEBSITES

350.org (an online grassroots movement dedicated to reducing CO_2 concentrations in the atmosphere from its current 411 parts per million to below 350 ppm). www.350.org. Accessed March 2019.

Centers for Disease Control articles on the built environment and health. https://www.cdc.gov/healthyplaces/. Accessed March 2019.

The Collaborative on Health and the Environment (CHE). http://www.healthandenvironment.org/. Accessed March 2019.

Healthy Aging and the Environment: A Pocket Guide available for download. https://peht.ucsf.edu/index.php. Accessed March 2019.

Intergovernmental Panel on Climate Change (IPCC). http://www.ipcc.ch/. Accessed March 2019.

Maibach E, Nisbet M, Weathers M. (2011) Conveying the Human Implications of Climate Change: A Climate Change Communication Primer for Public Health Professionals. Fairfax, VA: George Mason University Center for Climate Change Communication. https://publichealth.yale.edu/alumni/benefits/events/4C%20Communication%20Primer%20-%20

Conveying%20the%20Human%20Implications%20of%20Climate%20Change_86971_1095_31769_v1.pdf. Accessed March 2019.

Myers N, Stein J, Schettler T, et al. *Environmental threats to healthy aging.* Greater Boston Physicians for Social Responsibility and Science and Environmental Health Network, 2008. http://www.agehealthy.org/pdf/GBPSRSEHN_HealthyAging1017.pdf. Accessed March 2019.

Physicians for Social Responsibility. http://www.psr.org/. Accessed March 2019.

PSR Environmental Health Toolkit for pediatricians. https://peht.ucsf.edu/index.php. Accessed March 2019.

The Worldwatch Institute. http://www.worldwatch.org/. Accessed March 2019.

Training of International Medical Graduates

10

H. Russell Searight, PhD, MPH; Jennifer Gafford, PhD; & Vishnu Mohan, MD, MBI, FACP, FAMIA

INTRODUCTION

This chapter will review issues involved in the training and education of international medical graduates (IMGs), including differing views of psychiatric conditions and treatment, differences in educational experiences, clinical issues involving interactions with patients and nonphysician staff, technology and documentation, psychosocial issues, and medical ethics. General suggestions are offered regarding possible modifications to residency education to address the special needs of these trainees. As in any discussion of cross-cultural differences, the tremendous variability in the backgrounds of IMGs must be acknowledged. Generalizations will always be qualified and may not reflect the experience of all IMGs.

BACKGROUND

CASE ILLUSTRATION 1

The primarily U.S.-trained family medicine residency faculty meets one last time to review candidates before submitting their final rank order list to the National Resident Matching Program (NRMP). With few exceptions, the rank order begins with the U.S. medical graduates (USMGs) and ends with IMGs, who comprise two-thirds of the total list. Visa issues further complicate the selection process. "She is a strong applicant, but her visa status is likely to cause some administrative difficulties." Thoughtful, sensitive discussions sort out which applicants, particularly among the IMGs, appear genuinely interested in family medicine; which applicants are more familiar with the U.S. medical system; which applicants might effectively relate to and communicate with this residency's low-income, urban population; and which applicants might appreciate and attend to psychosocial issues in patient care. One faculty member comments, "The ranking process was more straightforward when we considered only USMGs." Another adds, "So was residency education!" A third retorts, "Don't forget, some of our strongest residents have been IMGs!"

Since our original research paper on the topic published in 2006, the past decade has seen a growing number of studies—primarily qualitative—focusing on the experience of international medical graduates. Recently, there has been a growing educational and evidence-based literature on the topic including systematic reviews. Many of the issues that we reported—lack of experience in the biopsychosocial model, a narrow biomedical orientation, collaborative versus hierarchical physician–patient relationship, hierarchical versus more egalitarian interaction with faculty, disclosure of medical bad news, the individualist focus on patient autonomy supported by law in the United States versus a collectivist or family-centered communication style—have been reported in studies conducted in the United States, Canada, the United Kingdom, and Germany.

GROWING NUMBER OF IMGS

International medical graduates provide a good deal of primary care in the United States; about 30% of practicing physicians in primary care specialties are IMGs. A similar pattern exists for Canada, Britain, and Australia. For example, in Britain, one-third of all practicing physicians are IMGs. The top three specialties for non-U.S. citizens who were graduates of international medical schools were internal medicine, family medicine, and pediatrics. It is estimated that IMGs will soon represent 35% of the U.S. primary care physician workforce. In Germany, IMGs comprise about 10% of the medical workforce. In the United States and Great Britain, the majority of IMGs are from East Asian and Middle Eastern countries. In the United States, the most common countries in which currently licensed IMGs received medical education are, in order: India, the Caribbean, the Philippines, Pakistan, and Mexico. Over half of the Caribbean graduates are U.S. citizens. In the United States, International Medical Graduates currently provide a disproportionate share of health care in medically underserved areas.

IMGs & Residency Education

In 2019, non-U.S. citizen IMGs comprised 18% of MATCH candidates—the second largest group after U.S. allopathic medical school graduates. From 2014 to 2019, the MATCH rates of foreign trained physicians (excluding U.S. citizen IMGs) have averaged slightly above 50%. This is in contrast to the 98–99% acceptance rates of seniors from U.S. allopathic medical schools.

For non-U.S. citizen IMGs, the 2019 match rate was 58.6%. While the number of non-U.S. citizen IMG applicants has declined slightly over the past four years, the 2019 rate is the highest in 25 years.

As noted by geographic data, a high proportion of U.S. and Canadian noncitizen physicians come from less developed countries with diminished in resources. In addition to the differences in educational content and pedagogy, many IMGs come from cultures in which norms differ from the United States regarding communication style, physician–patient and teacher–student interaction, male–female relationships, and views of children and the elderly. Given this increased internationalization of medical residents, assumptions about prior medical training, based on U.S.-educated physicians, are likely to be inaccurate.

PRIOR TRAINING IN THE BIOPSYCHOSOCIAL MODEL

In the United States, the biopsychosocial model has strongly influenced primary care and community medicine. While the diverse backgrounds of IMGs are valuable in caring for a multiethnic and increasingly diverse U.S. population, the extent to which IMGs have been trained in the biopsychosocial model differs tremendously depending on the country in which the resident was trained. For instance, with a few exceptions, such as Canada, England, Australia, South Africa, and the Netherlands, applied behavioral science and psychology is much better developed in the United States than elsewhere in the world. A study examining IMGs' recognition of late-life depression through standardized vignettes found significant differences between U.S.-trained and IMG physicians. Among 178 primary care physicians and 321 psychiatrists, IMGs were significantly less likely than the U.S. medical graduates (USMGs) to make the correct diagnosis of depression or recommend treatment with a first-line antidepressant.

A biopsychosocial framework also implicitly underlies sexual medicine and pain management, topics also largely absent in non-Western medical school curricula. In the case of sexual medicine, cultural factors associated with prohibitions regarding premarital sex, sexual orientation, and sexual activity in later life may make it less likely that IMGs will broach these topics with patients. For example, in a large sample of Turkish University students, 6% of females and 40% of males reported having had sexual intercourse with comparable rates of 0.6 % of females and 16% of males in Iran. This reluctance is likely to extend to assessing and treating medication-induced sexual dysfunction. With respect to pain management, a recent report found that only 5 out of 300 medical schools in India included pain management and/or palliative care in their curricula. Recently trained physicians in India tended to view pain associated with cancer as inevitable and unmanageable.

Our experiences in family medicine residency training are consistent with these observations. As our programs matched greater numbers of IMGs, physician faculty increasingly commented that many of these residents did not appear to appreciate the psychological and social components of primary care. For example, without prompting and even with direct modeling, an IMG resident might interview a 17-year-old pregnant patient without inquiring about the patient's feelings about the pregnancy; the father of the child; parental/family support; whether and how she plans to continue her education; and the availability of other social supports.

Moreover, comments by the IMGs with whom we worked suggested that many of the common mental health conditions seen in the United States were not commonly diagnosed or treated in their home countries. These comments are supported by cross-cultural research. For example, in Japan major depressive disorder, as defined in the *Diagnostic and Statistical Manual of Mental Disorders, 5th Edition* (DSM-5), has only recently gained acceptance. Historically, *Utsobyo* was the term for clinically significant depression; however, this condition is severe and involved debilitating psychotic symptoms requiring inpatient care. A related condition, *Yuutsu*, a melancholic state having moral connotations, was often prized in Japanese culture. *Kokoro no kaze*, the Western construct of depression, is beginning to gain acceptance as a "cold of the soul."

Many IMGs that we trained viewed attention-deficit hyperactivity disorder (ADHD) as misbehavior rather than a medical condition requiring medication. These differences in practice appeared to stem both from differences in previous training (i.e., limited education in behavioral medicine) as well as acculturation factors (i.e., the way mental health was conceptualized in the resident's home country).

DIFFERENCES IN EDUCATIONAL EXPERIENCES PRIOR TO U.S. RESIDENCY TRAINING

While medical schools vary widely internationally, residents from non-Western countries describe vastly different educational experiences than the typical U.S. graduate. First, in many Asian countries, entrance into medical school occurs directly after completion of high school. While there are some 6-year medical school programs in the United States that take students at a similar point in their educational career, most students in the United States earn a bachelor's degree before applying to medical school. While meeting medical school requirements in the sciences, many U.S. medical school applicants major in fields such as English literature, history, psychology, foreign language, or even art history. A growing number of U.S. medical schools actually encourage potential applicants to have a broad-based liberal arts undergraduate education. In contrast, in those countries in which students enter medical school at 17 years of age, a direct career trajectory heavily loaded with education in the biological sciences precludes broadening the student's scope of knowledge and intellectual exploration in the humanities.

At the post-graduate level with the emphasis on standards of professionalism in the United States, there has been increased attention to behavioral science in most specialties. Indeed, some medical schools now require that applicants have at least two courses in psychology or social science. In many IMGs' home countries, education is certainly valued but the educational focus is on "hard" science alone.

Approaches to teaching and evaluation of students' knowledge also frequently differ by country. In many international schools, rote memorization of information from textbooks and lectures is the principal learning style. In the United States, there is more emphasis on the application of medical knowledge and on small group learning experiences such as "problem-based learning" (PBL), rather than pure memorization of information. The current U.S. medical school emphasis on evidence-based medicine (EBM), combined with PBL, encourages critical analysis of knowledge and its applicability to a given context rather than retention of facts alone. In addition, PBL stands in contrast to the view that esteemed faculty ("eminence-based medicine") are absolute authorities on medical knowledge regardless of research reported in journals, a view still common in many developing countries.

The interactional style of many U.S. educators, often including games requiring learner participation (e.g., "Pharmacotherapy Jeopardy"), is a new experience for many IMGs. Ironically, however, the United States relies heavily on multiple-choice exams to evaluate medical students, residents (in training exams), and practicing physicians (board exams)—thereby reinforcing the memorization of facts. Outside of the United States, essay and oral exams are more commonly used to assess medical students' knowledge. In addition, Objective Structured Clinical Examinations (OSCEs), featuring role playing by standardized patients, are not as widely used outside of the United States, Canada, and Western Europe. In many developing countries, rather than being observed by faculty, it is assumed that directly observing faculty mentors' interactions with patients will provide adequate training to medical students. In these societies, the physician-patient relationship component of the clinical encounter is often minimized.

International medical graduates frequently come from societies in which there is a rigid hierarchy between students and teachers. International graduates often demonstrate much greater deference toward faculty than their U.S.-trained counterparts. A Canadian study concluded that an IMG's medical school experience is characterized by ". . . an authoritarian didactic professor in large group settings." In these countries, two-way exchanges of ideas are also very rare—a learner openly questioning a faculty member would be considered impolite, if not disrespectful. These differences are particularly evident when learners are asked to evaluate their teachers. The U.S.-trained residents and students have considerable experience evaluating faculty; student evaluations are commonly used for promotion and tenure decisions in undergraduate colleges and universities. International Medical Graduates often indicate that they are very uncomfortable evaluating their U.S. faculty and consider it inappropriate. Additionally, in residency programs, IMGs may be particularly motivated to establish a positive relationship with program directors since their title suggests that they have substantial authority.

This reticence to speak up in the presence of authority often extends to rounds and precepting interactions, frequently leading the U.S.-trained faculty member to conclude erroneously that the IMG has a deficient knowledge base. Moreover, the IMG's knowledge may not be evident in precepting encounters. Rather than providing to preceptors the presenting problem, evaluation results, diagnosis, and plan as USMGs are trained to do, some IMGs may provide only the patient evaluation findings, and not offer problem lists, diagnoses, or treatment recommendations. This reticence is often mistaken for a deficient knowledge base by the U.S.-trained faculty. IMGs from some cultures may perceive that offering this concluding information without specific prompting from the supervising physician is "showing off" and a sign of disrespect for a faculty member. In many Asian countries, teachers are held in very high esteem and a learner who "knows too much" would be seen as offending a supervising clinician. Even when presenting diagnoses and treatment recommendations, this information may be tentatively communicated out of respect. Similarly, when desiring assistance with a patient, the IMG resident may not make a direct request but expect that the omniscient faculty member will recognize their difficulties and spontaneously provide the necessary help.

CLINICAL ISSUES

Patient Care & Physician–Patient Interaction

Many IMGs come from developing countries and have a wealth of experience with diseases that their U.S. counterparts rarely see. For example, early childhood death due to diarrhea and parasitic diseases are relatively uncommon in the United States compared with the developing world. The physician–patient relationship also differs across cultures. Many IMGs come from countries in which a paternalistic style of medical practice still predominates. The concept of patient-centered care and shared decision-making between physician and patient is a radical departure from the style of medical practice in many IMGs' home countries. As an IMG in Germany observed, "*When the doctor says something, one has to listen. [. . .] people listened, there was no need to have hour long discussions with them.*"

Under the basic tenets of informed consent, patients have a right to know what is wrong with them, what treatments are being recommended, the risks and benefits of the treatment(s), and alternatives—including no treatment. The ultimate decision maker is the patient with the physician acting more as an expert facilitator. This model is in stark contrast to the approach in India described by a family medicine resident from that country:

> *In India, the doctor is God-like. "The doctor cured me, saved my life, my God." Whatever the doctor says, that's enough . . . . Patients don't ask questions, they don't doubt. That wouldn't be taken very nicely. "I am the physician. If you are coming to me, my rule goes."*

The hierarchical differences between residents and faculty parallel relationships between physicians and patients. The idea of shared decision-making with patients is unusual. In their home countries, physicians make the decisions and patients follow advice. IMGs are often accustomed to respectful, deferential patients. Coming from this background, IMGs are likely to be disoriented and perhaps insulted by American patients coming to them requesting specific tests or medications that they have seen on television or on the Internet, or that have been recommended by friends.

Because much of primary care in the United States emphasizes chronic disease management rather than treatment of acute illness, patient adherence has become a particularly relevant issue. Some IMGs were brought up in systems that have little respect for patients who do not take their antihypertensive medications or follow their diabetic regimen. The concept of having a repertoire of communication skills for enhancing patient adherence is new to IMGs trained in a country where physician authority, power, and control are unquestioned. The idea of a difficult patient, requiring specialized interpersonal management skills, may not be viewed as part of the physician's responsibility. Models such as the transtheoretical approach in which patient adherence is conceptualized by stages of change (e.g., precontemplation, contemplation, preparation, and action) are unlikely to be part of the IMG's knowledge base. Health behavior change requires active listening, negotiation, setting initially small goals, and providing social support for the patient (see Chapter 19). These skills are unlikely to be taught in developing countries nor are health behavior models that provide a conceptual framework for counseling these patients. Because of these cultural and educational differences, IMGs may not know how to address issues of nonadherence. As an illustration, Verma and colleagues present this exchange between an IMG physician in the United Kingdom and a patient recently hospitalized for an asthma attack:

> *[Physician]: "So we need to make sure that, you know, couple of things like ensuring compliance with the medication, you need to go strictly on your asthma inhalers, and you need to take these regularly as well and so these are the views of . . ."*
>
> *[Patient]: "But if I don't feel like that's helping, why would I take it?"*
>
> *[Physician]: "Umm, one thing is that, you know, all the medications that we have given you should be taken in regular dosages and there's a protocol for these. I mean, obviously, we can escalate the thing as well for you, the dosages wise. And you, we always start the people on low dosages of the medication."*

Verma and colleagues found that physicians from countries with less tolerance for medical uncertainty often did not answer direct questions from patients. Unfortunately, this lack of response or indirect style often increased patients' anxiety. Qualitatively, investigators noted that IMGs often appeared uncomfortable when patients posed direct questions.

Even if the IMG begins practice with an appreciation of the American patient as a consumer, there are still concrete challenges, such as language barriers. Often IMGs who have spoken English much of their lives still find conversations with U.S. patients challenging:

> *My first day in clinic in the United States, I couldn't understand most of my patients. My entire education has been in English but these patients could have been from Mars.*

Particularly for those IMGs who have learned English as a second language, they may find it confusing that their patients do not speak "proper" English. American English is strongly impacted by regional and ethnic factors influencing word choice, idioms, intonation, and emphasis. Similarly, U.S. patients may be unfamiliar with the accent and terminology (some of which includes British words) of IMGs who acquired much of their English outside the United States. Finally, social psychologists suggest that 90% of communication is nonverbal. As anthropologists and international businessmen have noted, gestures and other physical styles of communication are culture bound. For example, the shaking of the head from side-to-side, while meaning "no" to most Westerners is often an expression of agreement among persons from India.

The unexpected directness of many patients in Western countries may be unnerving for the IMG resulting in poorer communication in their second language. The patient-centered perspective emphasizes that patients must understand relevant medical information so that they can collaborate with the physician in their care. Because of a lack of experience with patient-centered care, IMGs may have difficulty presenting relevant findings and treatment implications in ways that patients can readily comprehend. In this example from the Verma study, when the patient asks the physician a direct question, they receive a technical, jargon-filled response:

[Patient]: What do, do you think this is what it is?

[Physician]: No, actually from the history I have taken and then received these blood tests. I'm thinking of some blood-related problem.

[Patient]: "What, what do you think it is?"

[Physician]: "Um, probably related to the blood. Your hemoglobin is quite low. And, your ESR, that's a marker of some inflammation in baseline, some disease activity, some certain disease activities, is quite high, as well. And your symptoms—like weight loss."

Interactions With the Nonphysician Staff

U.S. medical care is multidisciplinary. International medical graduates need to learn to work with and respect social workers, pharmacists, nurses, care managers, nurse practitioners, physicians' assistants, physical therapists, and other professions who are all involved in the care of patients. These teams often have a horizontal rather than hierarchical power configuration. Physicians frequently manage patients as a member of a complex team, and though in many cases they coordinate care, in other instances (e.g., hospice care), nonphysician providers take the lead in many aspects of patient care. As one IMG said: *"I can't believe the number of people who tell me how to do things their way—and I'm the one who went to medical school."*

In many countries, the interdisciplinary nature of health care is not as well developed, if recognized at all. Physicians are the lead decision makers, and their orders are obeyed unquestioningly. Additionally, in countries with social and economic distinctions, ancillary workers are typically from different social strata than physicians. In U.S. outpatient settings, the easy familiarity existing between staff, including calling physicians by their first names, is often seen as disrespectful and overly familiar by those trained in a more formal, hierarchical system.

Medical Ethics

Many IMGs come from societies where physician paternalism is still the rule. In countries in which physician paternalism predominates, ethical principles such as autonomous informed consent are often not culturally normative. Ethical dilemmas can be evaluated from the perspective of four principles: autonomy, benevolence, nonmaleficence (do no harm), and justice. Over the past 50 years, U.S. health care has deemphasized beneficence and increasingly valued autonomy as a preeminent principle. Changes in disclosing a cancer diagnosis to patients clearly illustrate this historical shift. In 1961, 90% of American oncologists indicated that they would not disclose a cancer diagnosis to a patient. Twenty years later, this pattern had been reversed, in that oncologists routinely informed patients of their condition. The U.S. emphasis on autonomy, which takes the form of giving patients choices about how to treat their condition (e.g., "You could take any of these three medicines; which one would you like to try?"), is likely to be disorienting to IMGs from countries where the physician remains an unchallenged authority.

While not typically labeled as such, a communitarian model of ethical reasoning, which recognizes the role of cultural values, often prevails in non-Western countries. This ethical theory stands in contrast to *principlism*, the dominant framework in U.S. medical ethics. For a number of years, the first author often polled groups of internal medicine residents (comprised of approximately 75% IMGs) about whether physicians in their home countries routinely disclosed serious or terminal conditions to patients. Many, if not most, residents from India, Pakistan, and Eastern Europe responded "no."

The individualistic focus of American medicine supported by policies such as HIPPA was also found to be unusual. In IMGs' home countries, patients' relatives had routinely been involved in receiving information about family members and making treatment decisions with the patient not being directly informed. Cross-cultural research suggests that beneficence typically guides nondisclosure. In these societies, it is seen as cruel to inflict emotional distress on an already ill person through such a disclosure. In Jain and Krieger's study of IMGs' communication strategies, a third-year resident expressed distress about American medicine's standard of honesty:

The one thing I don't like about the American system is that you are telling the patient face-to-face that he is going to die . . . You are telling a dying patient that he only has a few weeks or months left . . . . [if I was the patient] I wouldn't want to know that.

East Asian IMGs, practicing in Western countries, may use language that obscures the diagnosis and instead use euphemisms such as "growth" or "mass" or "lesion" to describe cancer.

In societies in which patients are not informed of their diagnosis, the locus of decision-making is likely to differ from the U.S. norm. Family members, often within a network that includes the physician, make medical decisions for the patient. In Pakistan, where family decision-making is common, the physician may become adopted into the family and addressed as "parent," "aunt," "uncle," or "sibling."

This collectivist value may conflict with U.S. laws and ethics emphasizing individual autonomy. International Medical Graduates from traditional societies, particularly when treating a patient in the United States from their own ethnic background, may feel caught between the legal requirements for disclosure and their own culture's ethics about proper physician conduct.

Technology

Many IMGs are from countries with far less access to sophisticated laboratory and radiologic testing or choices for pharmacotherapy. As a result, they are often particularly skilled in obtaining maximum information from the history and physical examination, since other data sources are limited. The educational system in many international medical schools rewards acumen in physical exam skills, which is heavily emphasized in evaluating the competence of medical students and residents. The routine of ordering multiple tests is initially surprising to many IMGs: *"When I first started my training in the US, I was stunned by the number of tests that we ordered. I wish I had the luxury of ordering an echocardiogram for every heart murmur or a CT scan for every head injury back home!"*

The influence of technology has spread to commonly used pharmaceutical reference sources and treatment guidelines—all of which are increasingly digitized in the United States. Electronic medical records further challenge physicians trained in systems with significantly less technology.

Meghani and Vijay noted that many IMGs had rarely or never prescribed opioid analgesics. This lack of experience often reflects the limited availability of these drugs in their home countries. For example, the amount of fentanyl available to one person in the United States is the same quantity available to 2323 individuals in the Philippines.

Documentation & Litigation

Depending on their training, IMGs have varying degrees of exposure to medical documentation formats common in the United States. While some are aware of the Subjective, Objective, Assessment, and Plan (SOAP) format, others, once exposed to this approach, cannot understand its significance. The vast majority indicate that the amount of detail required in patient notes far exceeds customary practice in their home countries. Additionally, the presence of third parties "looking over the physician's shoulder" at the chart notes creates some anxiety. One IMG resident observed: *"Documentation is a huge issue here. Not just documenting in a professional way, but in a legal way. Every word is important."*

Malpractice litigation is a relatively new concept in many developing countries. Concerns such as patient abandonment, negligence, and the dictum "if it isn't written in the chart, it didn't happen," are new to many IMGs. Some report frequently being worried that they have "missed something" in a patient's care that could lead to a lawsuit.

In addition, in the United States, HIPAA regulations tightly regulate the release of medical information—even to family members. In describing IMGs from collectivist cultures in Germany, Klinger and Marckmann note that they may inadvertently violate medicolegal policies:

If a relative calls the ward and wants to talk to a doctor. In [country of origin] you talk to them. It's family. Here the patient needs to first sign a release from confidentiality and then you can talk to them. I did not know that at the beginning. I did talk to the partner. God bless, [. . .] They did not want to sue me.

PSYCHOSOCIAL & MENTAL HEALTH ISSUES

IMGs' Views of Psychiatric Conditions

International medical graduates often have different views of psychiatric conditions compared to U.S.-trained residents and faculty. In a qualitative study investigating the behavioral science training of IMG residents prior to coming to the United States, the majority of respondents commented that rates of mental disorders appeared to be higher in the United States than in their home countries. IMG residents will sometimes attribute higher rates of depression in the United States to differences in the U.S. social structure—such as the widespread use of nursing homes, elders without visitors in the hospital, and mothers raising several children alone. These residents perceive family support to be stronger in their home countries, buffering against mental illness. The well-established finding by the World Health Organization of better outcomes for persons diagnosed with schizophrenia in less-developed versus more-westernized countries provides some indirect support for these observations.

IMGs also tend to perceive strong religious faith as a valuable coping skill. These residents suggest that Americans often become "depressed" in response to chronic or daily struggles, in contrast with their international counterparts who may be more likely to accept their fate and avoid converting emotional distress into a medical condition:

> *It is a religious society (India), so if there is a difficult life event, people accept it and move on... The strong belief in God means that if something bad happens, that's because of God.*

Other cultures share with the United States the belief that psychiatric disorders are a form of illness, but the perceived causes of mental illness may differ. For example, in Karachi, Pakistan, Qidwai and Azam found that 30% of primary care patients believed that psychiatric illness was caused by supernatural powers and spirits. These patients commonly sought treatment from a Hakim (12%), spiritual healer (12%), and family support (2.5%).

The stigma of mental illness also affects how these issues are addressed by IMG residents in primary care. In many cultures, mental health issues are viewed as shameful and taboo: "You practically never do this . . . [in my country] . . . psychiatry is for the mad man." Due to their own culturally based misgivings about mental health issues, many residents fear they will offend patients and therefore avoid such questioning.

Views of Mental Health Treatment

Not surprisingly, many IMGs report minimal exposure to behavioral medicine prior to residency education in the United States. Many cultures view anxiety and milder mood disorders as variations on normal functioning rather than as illnesses. In these societies, the prototype of a psychiatric condition is a severe illness such as psychotic depression, bipolar I disorder, or schizophrenia. Clinical training often involves observerships or walking rounds in institutions for patients manifesting debilitating psychiatric conditions. One resident from India reported:

> *I had minimal training or no training in anxiety and depression. I was in a mental hospital and I had one month. It was in my fourth year. We had lectures for 2 weeks and 2 weeks in an institution. We looked at locked-up people all the time. We did not interview patients; we just walked through. It was like looking at specimens.*

Even in countries in which primary care physicians inquire about and treat psychiatric symptoms, there may be little diagnostic specificity. For example, one IMG from Bosnia stated:

> *Mental health does not look the same there as it does here. In my country, our people are simply "nervous." All psychiatric problems, depression, posttraumatic stress disorder, everything, it is just "nervous."... People in my country, they come to the office and say they are nervous, so we just give them some benzodiazepines.*

The sociopolitical history in IMGs' home countries may influence how they approach mental disorders. Family physicians in Russia revealed a reluctance to refer for mental health care, in part due to a history in which psychology and psychiatry were used by the State to control political dissidents. In the Stalinist era it was said, "No person, no problem." Diagnoses such as schizophrenia meant that there was "no person," and the "patient" could be locked up indefinitely in a mental hospital, which was little different than a prison. (This practice has recently been resurrected in Russia by the Putin government.) People became afraid of psychiatrists. As one of the interviewees said, "The fear of that kind of specialist is probably somewhere in the genetic code."

Family Life

International medical graduates, particularly from East Asian countries and the Philippines, may be startled by many aspects of U.S. family life, including single-parent families, cohabiting relationships, and serial monogamy. In discussing IMG psychiatric residents, Pumareiga and colleagues note that common U.S. childhood experiences such as living in two households with divorced parents, being part of the stepfamily, or dating during high school would be considered highly unusual in many developing countries—particularly those with strong religious influences. The common recommendation for infants to sleep in their own crib may often conflict with cultures in which co-sleeping—often until the child reaches school age—is the norm. Before beginning residency, IMGs obtain their knowledge about U.S. families from several sources, including television "talk" shows, as well as from listening to the discussions of the personal lives of office staff in settings where they were completing observerships.

IMGs are often stunned by the permissive parenting practices in the United States and the childhood behavior problems that they believe result from this approach. Many find it odd that conditions like childhood ADHD, not commonly diagnosed in their home countries, are so common in the United States. As one resident from Eastern Europe said:

> *Parents in this country, they let the kids do whatever they want... ADHD is not diagnosed in my country—it's simply a matter of discipline. Here it seems to calm down parents and teachers when you give the kids medicine.*

International medical graduates tend to view parental discipline, even when physically harsh, as important for preventing oppositional and disrespectful behavior among children. The notion of child physical abuse is new to many IMGs. They are surprised that the state becomes involved when parents physically discipline their children. Child protective services' power to remove children from their parents' custody is very troubling to many of these residents. What is considered abusive in the United States may be seen as responsible parenting that builds character in their home countries. A resident from India noted that the children of strict parents do very well in school and college. In addition to influencing the clinical context, many IMGs have children of their own that they are raising in a new country with different parenting practices. They may themselves be experiencing conflicts regarding appropriate discipline.

Nonmarital cohabitation is also a unique experience for many IMGs. In one instance, a resident from the Asia-Pacific region was seeing a hospitalized patient with injuries reportedly sustained through an assault by her boyfriend. The supervising physician had urged the resident to address the issue with the patient and provide her with resources for victims of domestic violence. The IMG was confused and didn't follow through at first. When asked about her reluctance, she responded: "It's not domestic violence. They are just boyfriend and girlfriend; they're dating. Each of them has their own house." The resident was surprised to learn that adult "boyfriends" and "girlfriends" often live together, and domestic violence can indeed occur in these situations.

The increased nuclearization and isolation of generations among U.S. kinship networks is troubling for IMGs from non-Western cultures, where extended families are common. To those from East Asia, for example, domestic violence in their home country was not a dyadic event with a perpetrator and a victim, but a situation in which the wife's family members would rightfully intrude into the marriage to protect her. The family should handle this problem rather than the medical–legal system:

> *Back home, if I hit my wife, they would not take that to the doctor. There is family support. Women are abused here, and they often do not want to do anything about it. Back home, women are hit and their dad says: "Come home." Here, women get put out on the street.*

Caring for geriatric patients in institutional settings contributes to a view of American families as isolated and cut-off from their extended kinship network. Residents from societies that care for aging family members at home have difficulty comprehending the practice of placing senior family members in impersonal nursing homes: "*Nursing homes do not exist in India*—because no son or daughter would ever lose the honor of caring for his or her elders, especially a parent." Similarly, hospitalized patients receiving no visitors—even when family members live nearby—are troubling to IMGs. One resident commented that he could now understand why he saw so many depressed patients here in the United States compared with his home country: *"Back home families are crucial. Here, people are left alone. You have a chance to get depressed much more here."*

Sexual Behavior

Early sexual experiences are particularly troubling to IMGs raised in traditional societies governed by strong religious and collectivist values. Sciolla and colleagues suggest that IMGs raised in many non-Western cultures may view sexuality as intensely private or even shameful. Premarital sex, while occurring, is a taboo subject.

Our observations of IMG residents suggest two common patient management styles. One approach is to avoid discussing sexuality with adolescents seen in the office. Preceptors often need to remind residents repeatedly to raise these issues. Even then, residents often appear uncomfortable with the topic—speaking awkwardly while looking at the floor rather than the patient. The other approach is to accept that the West is a sexually permissive society. The resident may address sexuality in a matter-of-fact, almost business-like manner. For example, an IMG seeing a 14-year-old girl who recently had her first sexual intercourse approached the patient in much the same way as an adult. A PAP smear and pelvic examinations were conducted, and customary guidance about pregnancy, contraception, and safe sex provided. There was no discussion about the circumstances under which the girl had intercourse (e.g., was it coerced?), the age of the partner, or the patient's perspective on the experience. Despite research evidence that early sexual activity is associated with sexual abuse history, smoking cigarettes, and using marijuana, the resident raised none of these issues until some of them were suggested by the behavioral scientist observing the encounter.

Challenges in Learning Behavioral Science

At a fundamental level, many IMGs are challenged by the inclusion of psychiatry and psychosocial aspects of the patient's life as a significant component of Western medical practice. Coming from societies where diagnosis of mental health problems was often less common and those syndromes that were diagnosed were typically severe, many resident IMGs initially feel inadequate to diagnose and treat these conditions. Early in residency, some IMGs respond by referring nearly all depressed and anxious patients to psychiatrists. It is important that preceptors establish early in training that diagnosis and treatment of common mood and anxiety disorders, dementias, childhood behavior and adjustment problems, as well as sexual dysfunction, are expected competencies for primary care physicians. Unless the case is complicated and beyond the scope of a nonspecialist (e.g., schizophrenia), the resident should learn to manage the patient.

Diagnostic interviewing for mental health conditions is particularly challenging for IMGs. After taking the United States Medical Licensing Exam (USMLE), most IMGs are familiar with the Diagnostic and Statistical Manual of Mental Disorders (DSM) system and the use of explicit criteria for diagnosis. It may be difficult for them, however, to convert these dimensions to conversational questions. Often the questions tend to be verbatim recitations of the DSM criteria and have a stilted quality that confuses the patient (e.g., "Are you having feelings of worthlessness or inappropriate guilt?" Or "Are you experiencing pervasive anhedonia?"). IMGs often recognize that they do not know how to ask about these types of symptoms and consequently omit them. This reluctance may be particularly pronounced for questions about self-harm, suicide, abuse, and illegal acts. One IMG resident describes his experience of learning how to ask sensitive questions:

First, you are very uncomfortable, then you feel better and better... how to ask questions, how to ask about suicide. For me, that was very embarrassing. I was surprised people responded normally to these questions. "How will this influence her relationship with me?"

Another IMG said:

In my country, if I asked a woman with a child if she was married, she'd get mad at me.

During their behavioral science training, we have noticed unspoken discomfort when IMG residents are asked to interview, for example, a 14-year-old unwed mother, a lesbian couple, or divorced parents—each present with their new spouse. The resident who has done quite well interviewing other patients with psychosocial issues often seems at a loss about how to proceed with these family configurations. After sensing that they are uncomfortable asking the patient(s) further questions, the behavioral science faculty member will take over the interview for a while. Later in the interview, we typically try to turn it back over to the resident who often at this point appears less confused and can follow the faculty member's lead. After the encounter, when asked about their reaction and reason for not continuing the interview, a common response is something like:

I know these relationships exist in America, but I have never seen them face-to-face. I don't know what to say to these people.

RECOMMENDATIONS FOR IMPROVING THE EDUCATION & TRAINING OF INTERNATIONAL MEDICAL GRADUATES

General Suggestions

While we have pointed out areas of concern for IMGs receiving training in U.S. residencies, the few comparative studies on clinical outcomes suggest that non-U.S. citizen IMGs perform well in caring for patients. Tsugawa and colleagues found lower mortality rates for hospitalized Medicare patients treated by IMGs compared with U.S. graduates. When U.S. citizens who attended international medical schools were removed from the comparison, the distinction between U.S.-trained and IMG physicians remained. A similar pattern was found for a large sample of hospitalized patients with congestive heart failure and/or myocardial infarction. In a later study, Norcini and colleagues examined the association between IMGs' performance on Step 2 of the U.S. Medical Licensing Examination (Clinical Knowledge) and patient mortality. It was found that each additional point earned on Step 2 was associated with a 0.2% decrease in mortality.

A consistent theme arising in recent research on IMGs is their experience of being "second class citizens." Having been educationally and often professionally successful in their home countries, proving oneself in a new country and health care system is frustrating and onerous. This issue is particularly sensitive for those IMGs who had practiced independently in their home countries and now are having to undergo retraining. Alienation, loneliness, and anger are common emotional reactions to these challenges. Some residents have shared their fear that they may be unsuccessful in the long sought-after U.S. residency program and be required to return to their home countries. Fears of revealing any knowledge deficiencies may prevent IMGs from directly asking for appropriate faculty assistance. When providing clinical supervision to IMGs, educators should maintain awareness of these underlying dynamics.

International medical graduates would benefit from early acclimatization. Instead of the typical July 1 start date, it would be helpful if some preparatory experiences could begin at least 8–12 weeks before the formal residency year begins. English immersion, and when possible including information on common U.S. medical abbreviations as well as idiomatic English expressions, would be helpful for IMGs with uneven abilities in written and/or spoken English. For those residents who learned English late in life and whose accent is a barrier to understanding, there are specialists in accent reduction who can be quite helpful. There are CD-ROMs and other resources for learning specialized medical terminology.

Other areas that could become part of a preresidency curriculum include medical documentation, the mechanics of ordering lab work and radiographic studies, writing prescriptions, and use of the electronic medical record. An overview of the U.S. health care system including legal, ethical, and insurance issues would also be valuable. Basic medical interviewing skills can be taught through use of videotapes, simulated patients, and role-plays. One resource that may be helpful is the *Doc.com* interactive web-based curriculum on clinician–patient communication, produced by the American Academy on Communication in Healthcare (see "Other Resources" at the end of chapter). The general "style" that a primary care physician uses when relating to patients, however, is difficult to reduce to a set of skills. IMGs might benefit from shadowing faculty or seasoned primary care physicians as they see patients.

The individualist–collectivist distinction that plays a significant role in ethics and determining moral responsibilities should be discussed explicitly in the context of ethical decision-making, end-of-life care, and other relevant areas in medicine. In addition, for both U.S.-trained physicians and IMGs, an open exploration of these issues, including their cultural and religious background, would allow all physicians to be more sensitive with a broader cultural array of patients. With skillful leadership, Balint groups and other opportunities for reflective practice may provide IMGs an opportunity to understand and manage the emotional impact of these cultural differences on their conceptualization of and response to the patient's illness and healing experience as well as the physician–patient relationship. Left unaddressed or unexamined, strong emotional reactions to patients can trigger a cascade of clinical and behavioral responses that stifle or even interrupt development as a physician; but when explored with curiosity and within the context of a safe, nonjudgmental format such as Balint, the IMG as well as U.S.-trained resident has the potential to develop more fully with openness and meaningful engagement.

When IMG residents are having apparent difficulty meeting performance criteria, faculty should consider both cultural and language issues. As anyone who has learned a second language knows, people can appear to understand even if they are only picking up bits and pieces of what is being said. The deference that IMGs show toward faculty may be misinterpreted as a lack of assertiveness, an absence of independent thinking, inadequate knowledge base, or poor motivation. Before drawing conclusions, it would be helpful to have several supportive, noncritical conversations with these residents to better understand their background. During observation of clinical interactions with patients, we noted that an IMG from Pakistan never sat down during any of four to five encounters. In our discussion afterward, the resident indicated that she knew that sitting was the correct thing to do in terms of carrying out an effective interview, but thought it would be disrespectful to sit while the supervisor was present. If we had not clarified this point, we would have "graded" her interview skills as less than optimal.

Suggestions for Teaching Psychiatry & Psychosocial Medicine

Psychosocial content should be introduced early in the first year of residency. To address educational and training needs in behavioral science, a formal block rotation can be scheduled during the resident's first year. At our program, we added a first-year rotation in addition to the second-year rotation that had been in place for many years. The first-year behavioral science rotation focused more on effective interview skills and several common psychiatric conditions, while the second-year block focuses exclusively on diagnosing and treating mental disorders.

To help residents with wording questions about psychiatric symptoms, we heeded their advice and developed a series of "cheat sheets." Specifically, we made up a series of laminated cards (they easily fit into a lab coat) with helpful questions to elicit symptoms for many common psychiatric disorders. These became very popular among residents.

Faculty should be aware that patients with diverse backgrounds, customs, and family configurations are likely to be somewhat disconcerting to the IMG resident. In an individual discussion with a resident, the faculty member may want to begin by asking questions such as, "How often have you had the experience of . . . interviewing an openly gay male, a teenager being raised by foster parents, or a patient who requests a specific test that you don't think is indicated? Would physicians see patients or situations like these in your home country? Why do you think it's different here?" The faculty member should demonstrate genuine interest in the resident's experiences, respect, and intellectual curiosity during this exchange. These conversations can be useful learning experiences for both parties. Next, the clinical instructor should provide some focused information on the topic (e.g., "In the inner city, up to 50% of children are being raised by grandparents. Research shows that raising grandchildren has a negative effect on the grandparents' health compared to grandparents not raising grandchildren." Or, "About a third of the U.S. children are born to unmarried women. What is your reaction to that norm?")

We typically do joint patient interviews with residents as part of their behavioral science training. This allows observational learning of the faculty's unspoken acceptance of patients and a way of responding to them "like anyone else." In discussing these issues with IMGs, faculty should appreciate the extent to which patterns of family organization, views of the physician role, and so forth, are culturally relative. For example, many Westerners who automatically accept the norm of "companionate marriage"—a product of an extended friendship, dating relationship, and often a period of cohabitation—may be disturbed by the East Asian custom of arranged marriage. However, the teacher's genuine, noncritical interest in the background of arranged marriages often creates a climate in which the IMG is receptive to learning about the U.S. relationship variations.

As many seasoned clinical faculty members know, patients can be great teachers. IMGs who have been successful in understanding U.S. patients in a cultural context approach these patients with respect, intellectual curiosity, concern, and a genuine desire to learn. While obtaining pertinent historical and symptomatic information, these physicians can also encourage patients to "tell their story," and in so doing provide meaning and satisfaction for both doctor and patient.

SUGGESTED READINGS

Huijskens EGW, Hooshiaran A, Scherpbier A, et al. Barriers and facilitating factors in the professional careers of international medical graduates. *Med Ed* 2010;44:795–804.

Jain P, Krieger JL. Moving beyond the language barrier: the communication strategies used by international medical graduates in intercultural medical encounters. *Patient Educ Couns* 2011;84:98–104.

Kales HC, DiNardo AR, Blow FC, et al. International medical graduates and the diagnosis and treatment of late-life depression. *Acad Med* 2006;81(2):171–175.

Kitanaka J. *Depression in Japan: Psychiatric Cures for a Society in Distress. Princeton*, NJ: Princeton University Press; 2011.

Klingler C, Ismail F, Marckmann G, Kuehlmeyer K. Medical professionalism of foreign-born and foreign-trained physicians under close scrutiny: a qualitative study with stakeholders in Germany. *PLoS One* 2018;13(2):e0193010.

Klingler C, Marckmann G. Difficulties experienced by migrant physicians working in German hospitals: a qualitative interview study. *Hum Resour Health* 2016;14(1):57.

LeBaron V, Beck SL, Maurer M, et al. An ethnographic study of barriers to cancer pain management and opioid availability in India. *Oncologist* 2014;19(5):515–522.

Meghani SH, Rajput V. The need for practice socialization of international medical graduates—an exemplar from pain medicine. *Acad Med* 2011;86:571–574.

Norcini JJ, Boulet JR, Dauphinee WD, et al. Evaluating the quality of care provided by graduates of international medical schools. *Health Aff (Millwood)* 2010;29:1461–1468.

Norcini JJ, Boulet JR, Opalek A, Dauphinee WD. The relationship between licensing examination performance and the outcomes of care by international medical school graduates. *Acad Med* 2014;89(8):1157–1162.

Pettigrew LM. The NHS and international medical graduates. *Educ Prim Care* 2014;25(2):71–75.

Rao NR, Roberts LW (eds). *International Medical Graduate Physicians: A Guide to Training*. New York: Springer; 2015.

Sciolla A, Ziajko LA, Salguero ML. Sexual health competence of international medical graduate psychiatric residents in the United States. *AcadPsychiatry* 2010;34:351–368.

Searight HR. *Cross Cultural Issues at the End of Life*. New York: Springer; 2019.

Searight HR, Gafford J. Behavioral science education and the international medical graduate. *AcadMed* 2006;81:164–170.

Searight HR. *Health and Behavior: A Multidisciplinary Perspective*. Rowman and Littlefield; 2019.

Sternlieb JL. A guide to introducing and integrating reflective practices in medical education. *Int J Psychiatry Med* 2015;49(1):95–105.

Tsugawa Y, Jena AB, Orav EJ, Jha AK. Quality of care delivered by general internists in US hospitals who graduated from foreign versus US medical schools: observational study. *BMJ* 2017;356:j273.

Verma A, Griffin A, Dacre J, Elder A. Exploring cultural and linguistic influences on clinical communication skills: a qualitative study of International Medical Graduates. BMC medical education. 2016 Dec;16(1):162.

WEBSITES

American Academy of Communication in Health Care. http://www.doccom.org/. Accessed February 2019.

American Balint Society. https://s3.amazonaws.com/ClubExpressClubFiles/445043/documents/Helping_Doctors_Develop_1946604484.pdf?AWSAccessKeyId=AKIAIB6I23VLJX7E4J7Q&Expires=1551198404&response-content-disposition=inline%3B%20filename%3DHelping_Doctors_Develop.pdf&Signature=1t80vTfezY46quuzlphraxnzXas%3D. Accessed February 2019.

American Medical Association. International Medical Graduates Section. https://www.ama-assn.org/about/international-medical-graduates-section-imgs. Accessed July 2019.

Educational Commission for Foreign Medical Graduates. https://www.ecfmg.org/news/category/2018-match/ /. Accessed July 2019.

National Resident Matching program. The MATCH. http://www.nrmp.org/main-residency-match-data/. Accessed July 2019.

SECTION III
Working With Specific Populations

Families

11

Mitchell D. Feldman, MD, MPhil, FACP & Steven R. Hahn, MD

INTRODUCTION

The Family Is the Social Context of Health and Illness

Our experience of health, illness, and health care, as patients and as practitioners, occurs in a social context. The "family" is at the heart of that context. Practicing "family-centered care," that is, making the patient's social context an explicit part of medical care, will affect every step of the clinical process, from basic assumptions about who the patient is to the conceptual framework for the database, theories of causality of symptoms, and the implementation of treatment. Our patients with chronic diseases survive by virtue of the help their families provide and suffer from the burdens their families impose; often both occur at the same time. Consider the following vignettes:

1. Despite wondering whether she could have done something more for Joe, the doctor is gratified and reassured by the family's overwhelming thanks for the "wonderful care" she provided for the past 10 years, and in particular during the time preceding the patient's death. The family is grateful for her help in family discussions about end-of-life care.
2. Eric is a 40-year-old man with diabetes who has extraordinary difficulty following a reasonable diet. His partner has been unwilling to change his expectations about their meal plans and he has been unable to negotiate a change with him.
3. Mary, 50 years old and previously without complaints, presents with headaches that have been ongoing for 2 months. She is afraid she has a tumor or "something bad." A brief discussion about her family reveals that her 60-year-old husband has been depressed and forgetful for at least 6 months. Two months ago he got lost on his way home from the hardware store. After her doctor listens to her story, she agrees that she too is depressed and very concerned about her husband. She is upset that he has refused to see a doctor. She accepts her doctor's offer to help her get him evaluated, but she is still worried that her headache is something bad.
4. Eva, who is 27 years old, has multiple somatic complaints and panic disorder. She was raised by her grandmother after her mother died, and when her grandmother died 4 years later, by an aunt 20 years her elder. She and her aunt became very close, "almost like sisters, we did everything together." After completing college she returned to live with her aunt, who had recently begun the first serious relationship of her life. Eva does not understand why her aunt needs a boyfriend, and reports that her panic attacks often interrupt her aunt's plans to spend time alone with her fiancé.

In every case, the family context is critical to understanding the situation. In the case of Joe, the doctor has attended to both patient and family and the family is a partner in care and grief. Eric's partner's unwillingness to adapt their diet to Eric's diabetes has become a significant barrier to critical self-care. Mary is having a psycho-physiologic reaction to family stress. Eva is a vulnerable young woman whose panic attacks are not only a response to her aunt's perceived abandonment but also a high-cost and inadequate "solution" that temporarily is keeping her aunt more attentive and attached.

All health care providers have an intuitive understanding about "the family" and how families work and develop. However, lack of clinically useful tools for making the family an explicit part of care may prevent successful application of this knowledge. On the one hand, caring for the patient in the context of the family goes beyond involving family members in some of the tasks of chronic disease self-management. On the other hand, family-centered care is also a matter of perspective and is often conducted with only the patient in the room and without direct contact with other family members.

A Family-Centered Perspective Provides the Structure for Office Counseling

Our patients come to us with the full spectrum of medical, psychiatric, social, and interpersonal problems. As primary care clinicians, internists, and family physicians, we have always understood that assessing our patients' psychosocial problems, and offering some form of "counseling" is part of our mandate. However, the nature of "office counseling" as a practical procedure and the boundaries between an internist's counseling and a behavioral health clinician's therapy is less clear. It is also common for medical clinicians to be reluctant to explore their patient's psychosocial problems because they confidently anticipate that they are likely to be overwhelming and seemingly unsolvable, leaving them wondering whether the exploration left the patient better off or worse for the experience. Although competence in applying psychopharmacology to the frequently accompanying axis I psychiatric disorders has grown substantially in contemporary practice, addressing interpersonal, psychosocial problems still seems a daunting task, and physicians often feel reluctant to in because of the mistaken belief that they are expected to fix the problems they find.

There are two remedies to this uncomfortable situation. *The first* is to understand that the principal goal for the medical clinician is not to fix the problems that they encounter when they explore the patient's psychosocial context. Rather, the goal should be to reframe the patient's attention to those problems and help the patient understand that, in addition to any medications they may be offering for concomitant axis I disorders, counseling or therapy from a mental health professional will help them address the problems they face. *The second* remedy is to understand that a semistructured four-step family-systems-based assessment described in this chapter, can be an effective strategy that can be applied in the context of primary care clinical practice.

THE FAMILY AS THE CONTEXT OF ILLNESS

The family is the primary social context of experience, including that of health and illness. The individual's awareness and perception of health and disease are shaped by the family, as are decisions about whether, how, and from whom to seek help. Use of health care services and acceptance of and adherence to medical treatments are all influenced by the family.

Reciprocal Relationships

There is a reciprocal relationship between healthy family systems and the physical and mental health of its members. Physical symptoms and illness can significantly influence the family's emotional state and behavior, often causing dysfunction in family relationships; and dysfunction in the family system can generate stress and lead to physical illness. Dysfunctional family systems can incorporate a physical illness and symptoms into the family's behavioral patterns, thereby reinforcing the sick role for one or more members and sustaining or exacerbating illness and symptoms. In these "somatizing" families, the presence and persistence of the symptom or illness cannot be understood without examining its meaning in the context of the family.

What Is a Family?

Our understanding of family is based on our experience with our own family and experiences with the families of others. The variety of groups that make up a family is enormous: two-parent nuclear families, single-parent families, foster parents with children from different biological families, families of divorcees blended through remarriage, families with transgender, gay and lesbian couples as parents, and married or cohabiting couples without any children. In some cultures, the "family" may be other members of the clan who are not related by blood or marriage. Isolated elderly individuals may think of their home health attendants as family, and for other solitary individuals the only family they may know is their pets.

All of these groups can be experienced as families. They share similarities in the structure of the relationships between their members and the role that the family group plays for the individuals and for the society in which the group exists. So, rather than define the family in terms of its members, we describe it as a *system having certain functional roles.*

The Role of the Family

Family relationships are described more by their roles than by the labels traditionally applied to individuals. For example, in one family an elderly woman may obtain companionship and emotional support from a home health attendant, a friend at the local senior citizen's center, and a daughter, whereas a woman in another family may find these needs met by her marital partner. In one society, the primary education and socialization of children may be accomplished in the household of the child's parent(s) and in community schools.

Table 11-1. The role of the family: a partial list.

- Reproduction
- Supervision of children
- Food, shelter, and clothing
- Emotional support
- Education: technical, social, and moral
- Religious training
- Health care—nursing
- Financial support
- Entertainment and recreation

In another, parent collectives or unrelated individuals may accomplish these educational tasks, and play a more prominent, family-like role in children's lives. Hence, for health care practitioners, the patient's family context must be understood as the individuals in the social system, who are involved in the roles and tasks that are of central importance to the patient (Table 11-1).

The Family as a System

Families as systems are characterized by the following:

1. External and internal boundaries
2. An internal hierarchy
3. Self-regulation through feedback
4. Change with time, specifically family life cycle changes

The qualities of these four system characteristics in a particular family help shape the family's internal milieu and functioning.

Boundaries

The family is partially separated from the outside world by a set of behaviors and norms that are embedded in specific cultural systems. Family boundaries are created by norms that determine who interacts with whom, in what way, and around what activities. For example, teaching children "not to talk to strangers" creates a boundary around the family. Different parts of the family system (i.e., subsystems), such as "the parents" and "the children," or each "individual," are separated from one another by boundaries. Internal boundaries work in the same way: children who speak back to a parent may be told that they "don't know their place"; they have crossed a boundary that defines their role. Healthy boundaries balance the individual identity of family subsystems with the openness required for interaction and communication across boundaries.

Internal Hierarchy

Subsystems of the family relate to one another hierarchically: parents have authority over the children, the older children over the younger children, and so on. A healthy hierarchy is clear and flexible enough to evolve with the needs of the family, and localizes power and control in those who are the most competent. Hierarchies may become dysfunctional for a number of reasons; for example, when they are unable to adapt to change, when the allocation of power or authority is not consistent with the location of expertise or competence in the family, or when the lines of authority are blurred and effective decisions cannot be made.

Norms for hierarchies vary dramatically across cultures. Clinicians should be aware that their assumptions about who has the authority to make decisions for and about others may be incorrect. For example, the adult sons of a patient from Africa who lacked decisional capacity were offended when physician spoke to the patient's wife about medical decisions when they believed that it should have been obvious that the eldest son would be the decision-maker.

Self-Regulation Through Feedback

Relationships within the boundaries of the family system and its subsystems are regulated by "feedback." All behaviors in the family set actions in motion that in turn influence the original actor.

Feedback maintains the integrity of the family system as a unit, establishes and maintains hierarchies, and regulates the function of boundaries in accordance with the individual family's norms and style. This tendency toward maintaining "homeostasis" is critical. All family systems must learn to balance the desire for stability with the inevitable need to evolve and change.

Change and the Family Life Cycle

The family must continually adapt as its members evolve both biologically and socially (Table 11-2). For example, the family with young children must protect them within the boundaries of the family (or that of specific delegates, such as the schools). Adolescents need to achieve a degree of independence and the ability to function without immediate adult supervision. To facilitate this, the family must develop new norms of behavior and relax the boundary between the child and the world and redraw the boundaries between parent and child (e.g., provide more areas of autonomy and privacy). Each stage of the family life cycle presents new challenges, and healthy families are able to modify their hierarchic relationships and boundaries. Families whose boundaries, hierarchies, and self-regulatory feedback are dysfunctional have difficulties at each transition.

Cultural norms have a dramatic impact on the family life cycle. For example, the stage of "single adult living alone" may not exist, particularly for women, in many cultural milieus. The independence granted to adolescents that differentiates the life cycle stage of "families with adolescents" from the preceding "family with young children" varies enormously across cultures.

Table 11-2. The family life cycle.

Life Cycle Stage	Dominant Theme	Transitional Task
The single young adult	Separating from family of origin	Differentiation from family of origin Developing intimate relationships with peers Establishing career and financial independence
Forming a committed relationship	Commitment to a new family	Formation of a committed relationship Forming and changing relationships with both families of origin
The family with young children	Adjusting to new family members	Adjusting the relationship to make time and space for children Negotiating parenting responsibilities Adjusting relationships with extended families to incorporate parenting and grandparenting
The family with adolescents	Increasing flexibility of boundaries to allow for children's independence	Adjusting boundaries to allow children to move in and out of the family more freely Attending to midlife relationship and career issues Adjusting to aging parent's needs and role
Launching children	Accepting exits and entries into the system	Adjusting committed relationship to absence of children in the household Adjusting relationships with children to their independence and adult status Including new in-laws and becoming grandparents Adjusting to aging or dying parents' needs and role
The family later in life	Adjusting to age and new roles	Maintaining functional status, developing new social and familial roles Supporting central role of middle generation Integrating the elderly into family life Dealing with loss of parents, spouse, peers; life review and integration

Data from Carter CA, McGoldrick M, eds. *The Family Life Cycle: A Framework for Family Therapy.* New York, NY: Gardner Press; 1980.

HEALTH AND ILLNESS IN FAMILIES: THE "SICK ROLE"

Behavior in social settings can be understood in terms of "roles" that are shaped by shared expectations, rules, and beliefs. All roles have prerequisites, obligations, and benefits or dispensations. One such role is the "sick role," which is temporarily and conditionally granted to individuals when they have an illness perceived to be beyond their control, seek professional help and adhere to treatment, and accept the social stigma associated with being sick. Individuals in the sick role are exempt from many of their usual obligations and entitled to special attention and resources. The sick role therefore has a profound effect on relationships within the family.

The exemption from obligations that is part of the sick role is critical to recovery from illness and adaptation to disability. The obligations and stigmatization of the sick role serve to insure that the benefits of the sick role are not abused. Physicians play a critical role in establishing the legitimacy of the sick role by certifying the prerequisite illness or disability, and attesting to adequate adherence to treatment. Because the sick role has such a profound effect on the family of the sick individual, physicians' obligate role in establishing the sick role makes them a powerful actor in the patient's family system, and makes the family system an intrinsic part of the doctor–patient relationship, whether the physician is aware of these ramifications or not.

The Doctor–Patient–Family Relationship & the Compensatory Alliance

A positive relationship with an active and concerned family can be one of the physician's most powerful tools and rewarding clinical experiences. In these circumstances, working with the family seems quite natural and the complexities of the doctor–patient–family relationship are not apparent. On the other hand, when significant family problems exist, the doctor–patient relationship can become entangled in the family system's dysfunction.

When one or more members have assumed the sick role in response to family problems, the task of providing appropriate care for the patient may be subverted and subsumed by family dysfunction. Some families can achieve internal stability and meet the needs of their members only when one member is perceived as being sick.

The physician's role in determining that the patient is entitled to the special prerogatives and dispensations of the "sick role" makes the physician a central and powerful member of these family systems. The authority to prescribe changes in role function for the patient further involves the physician in the life of the entire family. In effect, the physician and patient develop an alliance that compensates for the dysfunction and deficit at home. Hahn, Feiner, and Bellin have termed this a *compensatory alliance.*

When the physician is unaware of underlying family dysfunction, the compensatory alliance can become dysfunctional and contribute to somatization and noncompliance, and support the ultimately inadequate coping mechanism afforded by the sick role.

PATIENT CARE IN THE CONTEXT OF THE FAMILY: FAMILY ASSESMENT & INTERVENTION FOR PRIMARY CARE

General Considerations

Treating the patient in the context of their family requires a practical method that can be learned and used by health care providers in real-world practice and training. The large number of tasks that occupy the provider places limits on the complexity of and time available for family assessment and intervention. A family assessment and intervention method must be focused, time efficient, and consistent with the general scope of care.

All patients should receive a "basic" family assessment that allows the doctor to understand how the family milieu will influence the basic tasks of care, and that identifies family problems requiring intervention (Table 11-3). Basic family assessment consists of two processes: (1) conducting a genogram-based interview and identifying the relevant family life cycle stages, and (2) screening for family problems that are associated with family life cycle stage tasks, or the patient's medical problems. A subset of patients with problems rooted in more serious family dysfunction requires the four-step family-systems-based counseling intervention described below.

Table 11-3. Goals of basic family assessment and intervention.

- Understand the pattern of family involvement with the patient's medical problems
- Communicate with other family members about the management of the patient's medical problems
- Recognize the presence of problem behaviors (e.g., alcohol or drug abuse, somatization, domestic violence, physician experience of the patient as "difficult") and family dysfunction affecting the patient's medical problems or functional status, which require further assessment and intervention
- Assess the family's behavioral and emotional response to the patient's medical and behavioral problems, and provide emotional support to the patient and family
- Provide counseling to enhance the family's emotional and functional adaptation to the patient's medical problems
- Understand the doctor–patient–family relationship and recognize a "dysfunctional compensatory alliance" when present or developing
- Refer the patient or family for further behavioral assessment and intervention
- Understand the triangular relationships and repetitive patterns of interaction among members of the family system, including the development those affecting the doctor–patient–family triangular relationship(s).

Treating the patient in the context of the family does not necessarily mean bringing the family into the examining room and in adult medicine usually does not. Family assessment and intervention can be accomplished by meeting exclusively with the patient, though meeting with other family members is very often desirable, sometimes necessary, and almost always enhances care. Using a family systems orientation without meeting directly with other family members requires the ability to explore the life of the family and bring the family into the room through the patient's narrative.

The genogram-based interview, described below, is a powerful technique for accomplishing this goal. However, the task of understanding the patient's family system in this way can be complicated by the fact that patients often give a distorted and incomplete presentation of family life. Such distortion may be conscious, unknowing, or some of both. Therefore, clinicians need to learn to infer what is going on at home—to "see the family over the patient's shoulder"—by imagining how members of the patient's family might be reacting or behaving in ways that the patient does not understand or will not report.

BASIC FAMILY ASSESSMENT: CONDUCTING A GENOGRAM-BASED INTERVIEW, IDENTIFYING FAMILY LIFE CYCLE STAGE ISSUES, & SCREENING FOR PROBLEMS

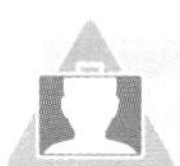

CASE ILLUSTRATION 1

Ariana is a 40-year-old Italian-American woman with multiple somatic complaints. She has complained of chronic diarrhea, dyspepsia, and "asthma" but has had a thorough normal gastrointestinal and pulmonary evaluation. She has made multiple visits to her primary provider and to an urgent care clinic, has been hospitalized two times, and has been seen in several subspecialty clinics. She has made an average of 15 visits per year for the past several years.

Constructing a Genogram

The first step to treating the patient in the context of the family is to create a picture of the family by conducting a "genogram-based interview." A

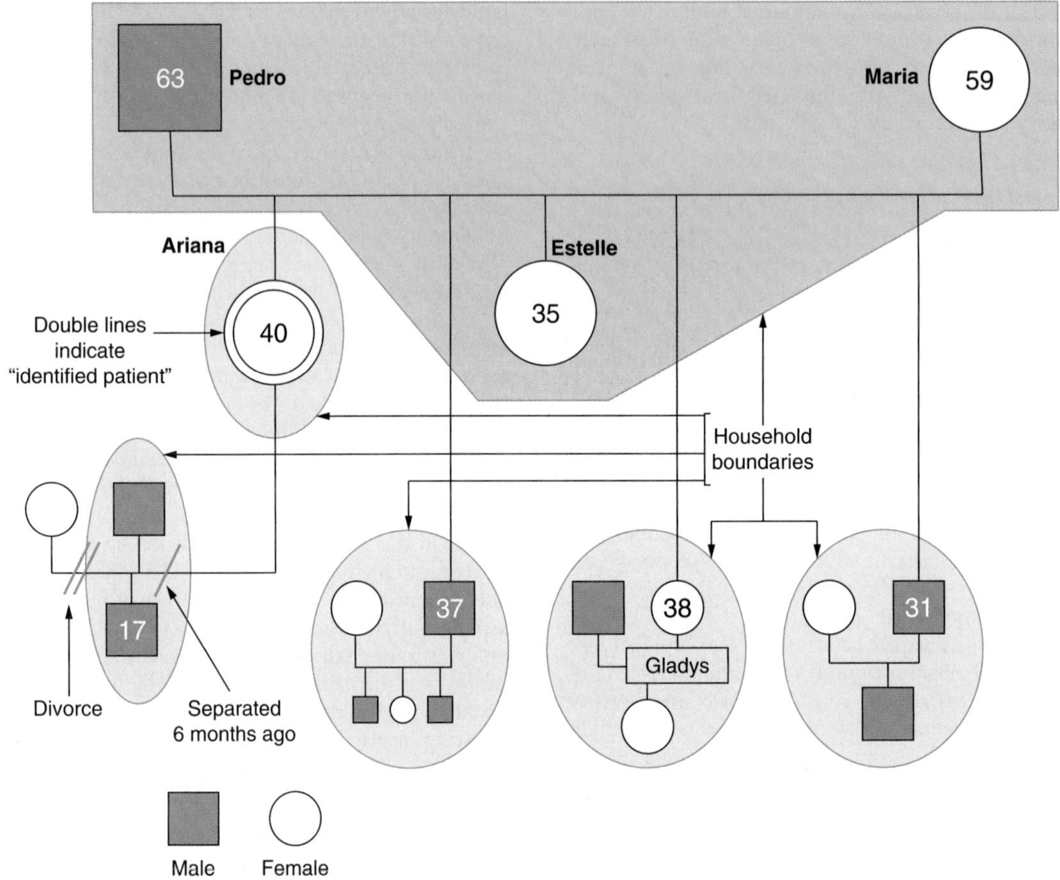

Figure 11-1. Genogram showing household composition and key family members in Ariana's family (Case Illustration 1).

genogram is a graphic representation of the members of a family. It uses the iconography of the genetic pedigree (Figures 11-1 and 11-2) and can be used to record data ranging from family medical history to life events and employment, as well as family issues. The overall objective of the genogram interview is to help the patient tell their story, framed in the life of their family.

Conducting a Genogram Interview

Begin with a blank page, placed where the patient can see it, and draw a family tree with the patient's help. Note important dates such as marriages, divorces, and deaths, and the general location of individuals in other households. Family systems data can be recorded using lines to enclose household boundaries, double lines between individuals to indicate strong relationships or coalitions, jagged lines to indicate conflict, and triple lines to indicate dysfunctional overinvolvement. At subsequent visits a brief look at the genogram helps to recall the patient's family context, and the genogram can be expanded or altered as the family changes or new issues arise.

Focusing the Genogram

The type of information explored, the number of generations, and the level of detail included in the genogram depend on an initial sense of the importance of family issues. A detailed, comprehensive genogram interview going back more than one generation can be a powerful clinical tool but is too complex for everyday practice. The genogram should be focused on the most clinically useful information while providing the foundation for treating the patient in the context of the family. As with most clinical databases, it is harder to know what can safely be excluded than it is to include the entire range of family-oriented data. However, skillful parsimony is acquired with experience, and efficiency is produced by following three principles:

1. Engage patients and encourage active participation—they will take you to the heart of the story.
2. Focus the interview on family life cycle tasks and issues—they are almost always the focal point of stress and dysfunction.

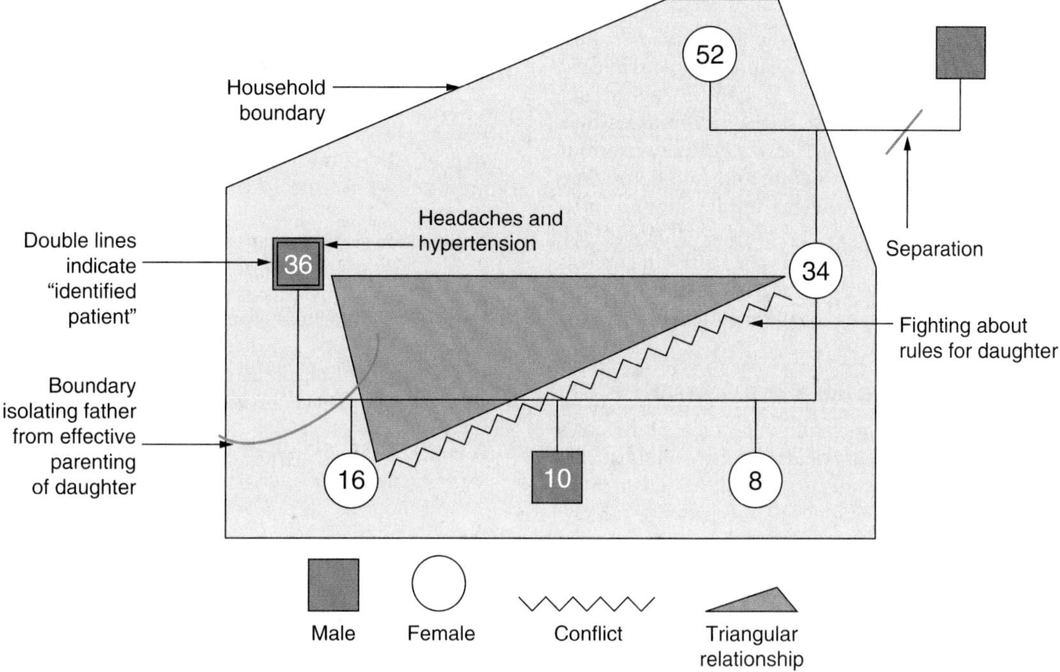

Figure 11-2. Genogram of the family in Case Illustration 2.

3. Draw and examine the genogram—a picture is worth thousand words (e.g., picture a single mother, six children, parents, and siblings in another country; three different fathers in various places; and a new boyfriend).

Begin with the core members of the family, that is, household members, parents, children, and past and present partners and spouses. Identify the family life cycle stage of the patient's family from the ages, relationships, and household composition of the nucleus of the patient's family. As described below, the family life cycle stage will almost always predict the locus of stress, challenge, or conflict in the patient's family system.

Inquire about the family's responses to any known or presenting problems, and to issues identified using the family life cycle screening questions described later. If no significant major problems or dysfunctions are identified, stop the focused genogram interview when you understand the family well enough to take the family into consideration in addressing the patient's medical and other problems. If significant family problems are discovered, continue with the four-step family-systems-based counseling intervention described later.

Figure 11-1 shows the skeleton of the genogram for Case Illustration 1. The amount of information you gather about each individual and the family should be guided by the evolution of your hypotheses about family function as you go along. When major family issues emerge from the shape of the genogram or the patient's narrative, exploration of family relationships and history can be very focused. If the nature of family issues is initially obscure, but you suspect something important is going on, expand the genogram to include more peripheral family members and examine individual relationships more completely.

In general, it is useful to obtain brief descriptions of family members and important relationships, the history of major life events, immigrations, and comings and goings from the household(s). Record important information on the genogram as the interview progresses to create a picture of the family. Remember, the greatest efficiency in the genogram interview comes from the patient's active participation.

Identifying the Family Life Cycle Stage & Predicting Stress & Conflict

Family Life Cycle Stage Assessment

Determining the life cycle stage of the family is a helpful first step in conducting a genogram-based assessment. The stages of the life cycle are a road map for exploring the important issues in the life of a patient and family.

The family life cycle consists of six stages (see Table 11-2). Each stage is grounded in biologically driven and socially and culturally shaped patterns of individual development. The cycle usually "begins" with the separation of the individual from the family of origin (stage 1), followed by the formation of a new family (stage 2), the raising and "launching" of children into the world (stages 3, 4, and 5), and the family later in life (stage 6). Each of these stages is dominated by a theme and principal task. Each task requires two to four major changes in family structure and function. More often than not, family problems revolve around difficulty with one or more of the developmental tasks of the family's life cycle stage. Of course, the family life cycle is grounded in a specific sociopolitical and cultural context that helps to determine and shape the themes and tasks of each stage.

The Family Life Cycle: Roles and Generations

With each stage of the family life cycle individuals acquire new roles: for example, from single adult to husband or wife and simultaneously to son or daughter-in-law. Note these roles as you and the patient scan the genogram. A directed open-ended question to screen for problems in each role is an efficient way of exploring the patient's relationships: "What's it like being a grandmother of six? Joe's wife? The daughter of a 95-year old?" If the patient is suitably activated, the whole story may come out after the first inquiry: "Being a grandmother is great, it's being a mother-in-law that I can't stand!"

The Life Cycle and Patterns of Parenting

In probing for life cycle problems, be sensitive to the influence of culture, ethnicity, and social class on norms and expected patterns. Pay particular attention to the structure of the parental subsystem: the adaptational strategies of families with one parent, one "working" and one "child care" parent, two working parents, families with extended-family parenting, blended families, and so on have differences that can be anticipated.

Case Illustration 1: Discussion

Ariana (see Figure 11-1) is in the first stage of the family life cycle, an unattached young adult, in her case, "between" families. Her divorce from her husband suggests difficulty forming a new family and establishing the second, "couple without children," stage of the family life cycle. It is noteworthy that the patient's sister Estelle is still at home and having difficulty with the first phase of the life cycle.

Screening for Family Function

After drawing the genogram and determining the life cycle stage of the family, the next step is to screen for family problems (Table 11-4). An activated patient will do the work of screening for you and immediately describe the "real problems." If the patient is reticent or the problem more obscure, the following strategies should aid the exploration.

Table 11-4. Presentations and problems associated with family dysfunction that should trigger screening for family dysfunction.

- Noncompliance with self-care regimens
- Alcohol or substance abuse
- Mental disorders, especially psychotic, mood, and anxiety disorders
- Unexplained medical symptoms and somatization
- Physician-experienced difficulty in the doctor–patient relationship (i.e., the "difficult patient")
- Health-related habitual behaviors—smoking, eating disorders
- Newly diagnosed, rapidly deteriorating, or frightening illnesses (e.g., HIV infection, cancer, end-stage renal disease, and myocardial infarction)
- Disruptions and change in the family system—divorce, separation, death, immigration, or emigration
- Natural and social disaster or trauma—fires, floods, earthquakes, crimes
- Sexually transmitted illness
- Anniversary dates and important holidays
- Domestic violence
- Reproductive health—pregnancy, termination of pregnancy, family planning

Global Family Function

Begin screening for family problems with open-ended questions about global family function (Table 11-5). The tone and content of the questions should be nonjudgmental, and even normalize the presence of problems, for example, "All families have their ups and downs, how's yours doing these days with all that is going on in your life?" An effective initial inquiry directs the patient's attention to family issues in general, leaving the patient free rein to respond.

Screening for Family Life Cycle Problems

If a question about global function does not provide the necessary information, ask a few screening questions about the life cycle tasks that confront the patient's family. For example, the genogram in Figure 11-2 indicates that this family will be dealing with the tasks of "the family with young children" and "the family with adolescents" (see Table 11-2). Six questions, one for each of the three tasks in these two different life cycle stages, can screen for life cycle problems (Table 11-6). However, it is likely that not all of these six questions will have to be asked to identify sources of difficulty, especially if the unique features of any particular family are used to select the initial questions.

Screening for Family Difficulty With the Patient's Medical Problems and Symptoms

The presence of somatization is one of the most important indications for exploring the patient's

Table 11-5. Family assessment screening questions.

Category	Example
Open-ended assessment of family problems	"How are things going with your family? How is everyone getting along?" "Are you having any problems with (name the key individuals in the genogram)?"
Family problems with the patient's medical problems	"How is your family dealing with your medical problems?" "How is (name the key individuals in the genogram) dealing with it. What is their reaction?"
Problems associated with family dysfunction (see Table 11-4)	"I know you have been feeling quite depressed lately, how has your family reacted to that?" "What has (name the key individuals) said or done about your depression?"
Family life cycle problems	"I see you have a houseful of adolescents. I know that can be quite difficult. How have you been bearing up?"
Problems in the doctor–patient–family relationship: the compensatory alliance	"What does your family think and feel about the suggestions I have made?" "What were you hoping I might say to or do about your family?"

Table 11-6. Family life cycle screening questions for families with young children and adolescents.

Stage 3—The family with young children
How are you doing with making time and space in your lives for three children?
How are you and your wife managing with child care responsibilities?
How are you getting along with the children's grandparents, *particularly your mother-in-law,** and your other in-laws?
Stage 4—The family with adolescents
How are you doing with a teenager, *your daughter*, in the house, and setting rules and expectations?
How are you and your wife doing with your work or careers?
Your youngest is going to go to school all day now. Will that change your or your wife's responsibilities or activities?
What concerns do you have about the health or functioning of your parents or in-laws, *particularly your mother-in-law?*

*Generic questions for this stage of the family life cycle are shown in regular type, questions or elements in italic are modifications *specific for the family of the father* (see Figure 11-2).

family, because it is usually driven by the patient's and/or family's need to have the patient occupy the sick role. An effective strategy for exploring the role of symptoms and medical problems in families is to follow the sequence: *symptom—function—family response. Symptom*—"Tell me about your symptom." *Function*—"How does your symptom affect your functioning, your normal activities, and ability to do what is expected?" *Family response*—"If you can't do these things, who does? What does your family do and say?"

Screening With Red Flag Problems

Whenever a problem associated with family dysfunction is present, the physician should screen for the family's reaction and response (see Tables 11-4 and 11-5). Many of these problems are emotionally charged and stigmatizing. Nonjudgmental, normalizing, and directive questions are therefore critical. These issues often have immediate clinical and legal implications and raise issues of confidentiality that need to be addressed.

Screening for Problems in the Doctor–Patient–Family Relationship

Throughout the family assessment, consider what role you may be playing in the family system and be alert to the development of dysfunctional alliances with the patient or other family members. Ask the patient or other family members what reactions the family has had to health care providers' suggestions or interventions. It is also useful to determine what the patient wants you to say to other family members. Often these hopes and expectations are implied by patients' words or behavior rather than stated, because patients may not be fully aware of what they want, are too embarrassed to ask for it, or do not feel they have permission to make the request explicit.

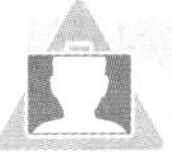

CASE ILLUSTRATION 1 (CONTD.)

In response to an open-ended question about how things are going at home, Ariana immediately identifies the major problem as the stress that Estelle's illness places on her mother and the pressure her mother then puts on her (Ariana) to help out. Regarding her family's reaction to her own medical problems, Ariana says her mom has difficulty understanding why she's always so sick. Ariana reports that her sister Gladys has come right out and said that she doesn't think Ariana's problems should be taken seriously. Ariana feels that the pressure of Estelle's problems and her mother's demands makes it difficult to think about getting involved with anyone. She blames her divorce on her ex-stepson's wildness and her ex-husband's inability to control him. Ariana thinks her mother is depressed about Estelle's illness, and suspects that she is burdened by and resents Estelle's continued

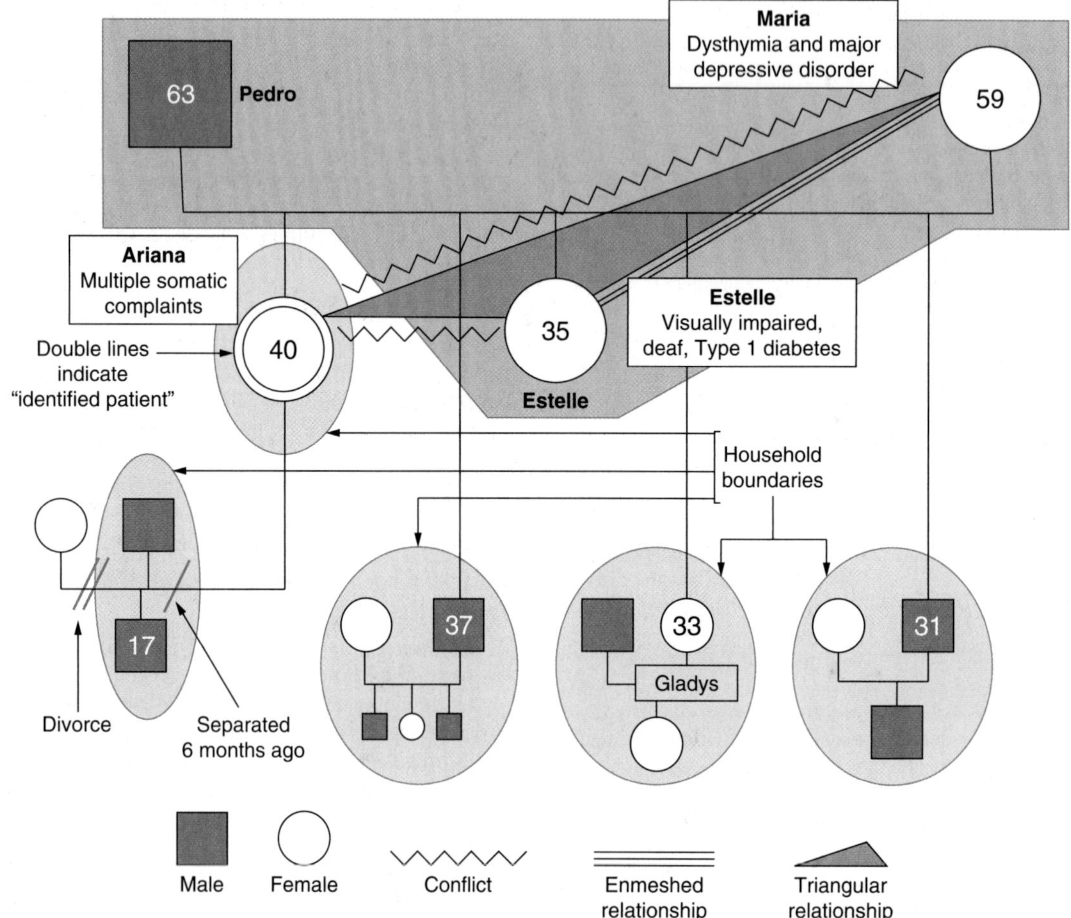

Figure 11-3. Annotated genogram for Ariana in Case Illustration 1.

dependence but can't admit it to herself or anyone else. Asked what she would like her physician to do in terms of her problems at home, Ariana says that she would like the physician to make her family understand that she really is sick. (Figure 11-3 shows the genogram at this stage of the family assessment.)

Treating the Patient in the Context of the Family: Communicating About & Caring for the Patient's Medical Problems

After completing the basic genogram, assessing the family life cycle stage, and screening for problems in family function, the practitioner should be able to provide basic medical care for the patient in the context of the family (Table 11-7). With the majority of families, the interventions described in this step accomplish the basic goals of family assessment and no further intervention is needed (see Table 11-3). A basic family assessment will, by itself, facilitate the following goals.

Enhancing the Therapeutic Alliance

Perhaps the most important consequence of conducting a family systems assessment is to enhance the therapeutic alliance between the patient and provider, and other family members. Patients' perception that their physician cares for them is probably the single most important variable in the formation of a successful doctor–patient relationship. Few things accomplish this better than talking to patients about the most important people in their lives (see Chapter 2).

Communicating With the Family

Family assessment enhances communication with the family about the patient's medical problems. This may involve educating them about the patient's condition, discussing self-care regimens and monitoring family

Table 11-7. Basic family interventions.

- Enhancing the therapeutic alliance by demonstrating interest and concern about the patient's family and life situation
- Communicating with the family about the patient's medical condition
- Providing information about the patient's problems: discussing prognosis and answering family members' questions about medical problems
- Discussing self-care and enlisting family assistance with medical management
- Facilitating the family's participation in decision making about therapeutic options
- Discussing and mediating the effect of the patient's loss of function on the roles of other family members
- Providing emotional support to the patient and the family
- Counseling the family about simple family system problems
- Identifying problems requiring attention from the family
- Preparing for further family assessment, intervention, and referral for further family interventions
- Working in collaboration with family therapists or other mental health specialists

involvement with the medical regimen, facilitating the family's role in decision making and advance directives, and helping the family adjust to changes in the patient's functional capacity.

Assessment and Support

Assessing the family's emotional response to the patient's problems and providing needed support are challenging and rewarding family-oriented tasks. Addressing caregiver burden in the adult children of elderly patients with dementia is a classic example. However, it is often difficult for the physician to witness the emotional distress experienced by patients and their family in the face of serious medical problems. The temptation to "stick to the facts" and restrict attention to biomedical issues is both strong and understandable, especially in light of the physician's perception that he or she "can do nothing" about the emotional pain caused by complex and seemingly overwhelming family and/or social problems. It is important to understand that empathically listening to the family and the patient is a powerful therapeutic intervention in itself—even if it appears to "fix" nothing (see Chapter 2).

CASE ILLUSTRATION 2

A 36-year-old man with hypertension presents to a walk-in clinic with tension headaches that have been going on for 2 weeks. The genogram interview (see Figure 11-2 and Table 11-6) reveals that he is distressed by ongoing conflict between his wife and teenage daughter about rules governing her behavior with peers outside the home. At home, the father remains silent until the fights between mother and daughter become intolerable. Their fights stop only when he complains about the headaches the fights have given him. He has never discussed his own ideas about rules for his daughter's behavior—or of family arguments—or negotiated a common position with his wife.

An appropriate intervention would be to suggest that the patient and his wife discuss the situation before the fights begin and try to develop a plan on which they both agree. If the family has the flexibility to respond to this suggestion, it may help them with the developmental life cycle challenge. If this intervention fails to help sufficiently, it may be a sign that further family assessment and interventions are required. It is important that suggestions be based on at least as thorough an evaluation as that produced by the preceding steps of this method; premature suggestions based on incomplete assessment are likely to fail.

Caregiver Collaboration

If the patient or family is receiving treatment from mental health specialists, the physician should actively collaborate, and they should consult with one another when issues come up that are relevant to the other's expertise. Patients may attempt to play one health care provider against the other; for example, they may present somatic symptoms to the mental health specialist and attempt to engage the medical provider in issues being examined in therapy. Patients or family members may complain about the therapist, especially when the family or patient is being challenged to change. Active communication between treating providers is critical if this "splitting" behavior occurs.

Focusing on the Dysfunction

Some problems have a clear and potentially devastating effect on the family. Focusing the family's attention on the problems associated with family dysfunction is a crucial clinical task. For example, if a patient or a member of the patient's family has a problem with alcohol abuse, it is important to assess the family's response, help the family accept the reality of the problem, and support their need to address it. Many families are waiting for just the kind of professional, extra-familiar attention that the physician can provide. Validating their feelings, and providing information about resources such as Alcoholics Anonymous (AA), may be all that it takes to precipitate action.

However, the patient's and family's resistance to change may be so strong that basic family assessment is not enough to help them take action. In these cases, it is appropriate and sometimes effective to refer the patient to a mental health specialist without further family intervention. However, it is often necessary to proceed to the next level of family intervention in order to make the referral a success.

FOUR-STEP FAMILY ASSESSMENT & INTERVENTION

If serious family dysfunction is interfering with medical management, the doctor–patient relationship, or the patient's functional status and quality of life, a four-step family systems based evaluation and intervention is required (Table 11-8). The goals of family assessment and intervention as described go beyond those of routine medical practice but also differ from the structural systems changes that are employed in family therapy.

Step 1: Assessing the Family: "Bringing the Pain Into the Room"

The previously described basic family assessment is the core and foundation of the first of the four steps of intervention with dysfunctional families (see Table 11-8). The difference lies in the need to achieve two goals that go beyond a basic understanding of family functioning. The physician must: (1) develop a substantial understanding of the major conflicts or issues in the family and conduct the interview so that the patient can bring the full intensity of their feelings about the family problems out, that is, "bring the pain into the room"; (2) understand how the sick role, if present (and it usually is), is functioning as a coping strategy for the patient and the family.

The goals of the first step of family assessment and intervention are achieved when the clinician is confident that the patient will agree with the statement that is used to conclude Step 1 and transition to Step 2, "It seems to me that the family problems we are discussing are extremely painful, and worthy of our attention." Bringing the pain of the patient's life into the room during the interview is a critical goal because the shared emotional experience will drive the remaining three steps of the process. The following interviewing techniques will help accomplish this task.

EMOTION ELICITING AND SUPPORTIVE TECHNIQUES

Patient-centered emotion-supporting interviewing techniques are instrumental in "bringing the pain into the room." Simply asking about the patient's feelings when they are recounting a distressing situation is a powerful technique, "That must have been very distressing. How did it make you feel?" A three-step "normalizing" sequence that couples a normalizing or universalizing statement giving permission to express feelings,

Table 11-8. Family intervention.

Step	Objective	Statement
Analyze, and "bring the pain into the room"	1. Understand the major conflicts in the family system. 2. Understand how the sick role functions in the family system. 3. "Bring the pain into the room," that is, help the patient (and family if present) experience the pain of their problems during the interview.	"Tell me about [anything you see in the genogram that is often difficult], e.g., . . . having your mother-in-law living with you or, raising teenagers."
Reframe	1. Direct the patient's (and family's) attention to the underlying family problems and away from the sick role establishing somatization, excessive functional impairment, or dysfunctional self-management behavior. 2. Endorse the patient's objectives while separating them from the use of the sick role to obtain them.	For 1. "*In addition to* your [symptom/problem] these family problems are equally worthy of attention." For 2. "*Even if you were in perfect health* I could understand why you would want your [family problem] resolved in a way that meets your needs."
Empathically witness	1. Provide emotional support and empowerment to the patient. 2. Enhance the therapeutic alliance.	"I am so impressed with how well you are doing despite all your problems. You're really determined to be a good wife . . . father . . . daughter."
Refer	1. Restate the problem from Step 1 as a question the patient needs to answer with help from an expert. 2. Address resistance to psychotherapeutic treatments.	"You have important questions to answer about how to change your communication . . . relationship . . . you're your mother . . . husband. You need the help of a counselor to answering those difficult questions."

followed by a closed-ended screening question, and then an open-ended follow-up question to a positive response is particularly effective in asking about embarrassing or socially undesirable situations. For example, you might say to a new grandmother whose single-parent daughter Marianne is hoping for child care for her new baby, "Setting limits with Marianne so that you can be a grandma rather than a nanny can be difficult and "even cause a lot of guilt," [the normalizing statement]. Has that been a problem for you?" [Closed-ended screen]. Followed by the open-ended invitation, "Please tell me about it" if the answer to the screen is "yes."

Getting the patient to talk about their feelings often requires gentle persistence. This is a good situation to use the request, "Tell me more about feeling sad . . . angry . . . disgusted." Patients often use vague descriptors of negative emotion such as "upset" or "it got to me." It can be helpful to ask the patient to clarify their own understanding and to elaborate with questions like, "What kind of 'upset?' " or " 'Got to you' in what way?"

Asking About Triangles and Looking for Circles

It is helpful to be aware of two characteristics of dysfunctional families that can help guide the interview: first, although patients often experience and describe their problems as a conflict or problem with one person, for example, "my wife," "my kid," "my mom," these conflicts between two people inevitably draw others in and "triangulate." Second, families that are having difficulty, are stuck in circular patterns of behavior (as reflected in the family therapists' saying, "What do families in trouble do? The same, thing but harder"). These repetitive sequences are the best that the patient and family can do to cope with their problems. An example of repetitive, triangulated behavior is described by Salvador Minuchin and colleagues in their seminal study of the "psychosomatic families" of adolescents with brittle diabetes, poorly controlled asthma, and anorexia. They observed the following pattern: unresolved marital conflict erupts into an argument between the adolescent's parents; the adolescent, in response to the stress of the fight and sometimes volitionally, becomes acutely ill (skips a dose or two of insulin and develops DKA or skips their asthma medicine, or intensifies their refusal to eat); the parents temporarily stop fighting to focus on caring for their child but are distracted from finishing their fight or resolving their problem; the exacerbation of the child's illness resolves; the unresolved marital conflict erupts into another fight, and the process is repeated. It is clear that the outcome of the seemingly dyadic parental conflict cannot be understood without knowing how the parents and child are triangulated and the adolescent's seemingly spontaneous episodes of illness cannot be understood without knowing about the role they play in the repetitive triangulated behaviors. It is important to note that in families stuck in this pattern of triangulation, the child's episodic illness serves the unconscious needs of all three members. The parents in these families were not able to resolve their problems and conflicts on their own and were relived to be interrupted by the illness episodes.

These aspects of family dynamics can guide interviewing strategy: ask about triangles and look for circles. The best way to understand what is happening between two people in conflict is to find out what the proximal third parties think, do or say. For example, in talking to a mother about her problems with her estranged adult daughter Stephanie, if you ask (or observe) what her husband, or other children or own mother say or do about the conflict you will probably learn more than you will by asking what happens between her and Stephanie.

Exploring Sick Role Coping Behavior With Psycho-Physiologically Reactive Symptoms

Patients who present with psycho-physiologically reactive symptoms[1] whose presence or associated functional impairment cannot be explained on the basis of organic pathology alone are common in medical practice. Kurt Kroenke and colleagues demonstrated that overall, only 15% of the most common physical symptoms presenting in primary care are determined to be caused by a physical illness that would normally be associated with the symptom. In the PRIME-MD 1000 study, "somatoform" disorders were present in 14% of primary care patients (varying from 9% to 29% across four clinical sites and associated with lower socio-economic status) and present in half of "patients experienced as difficult" by their physicians. Medical specialization offers no safe haven from this phenomenon; every specialty has its iconic psycho-physiologically reactive presentation: atypical chest pain in cardiology, irritable bowel syndrome, and fibromyalgia are a few examples. Invariably it is the need to be in the "sick role" as a coping strategy that drives and sustains this somatoform presentation. The exacerbations of asthma, diabetes, and anorexia described by Minuchin et al. are classic examples and demonstrate both the power of the sick role and the fact that the whole family system is invested in the sick role coping strategy. Although Minuchin's adolescents' parents were genuinely dismayed by their child's episodes of illness, at the same time they were relieved to be "rescued" from their marital strife by the need to attend to their child's acute problem. Often, the child's illness episode was the only way that the parents acute conflicts could stop. Unfortunately, while providing temporary respite

[1]The term psycho-physiologically reactive is preferable to psychosomatic because the latter implies an absence of "organic" or physiological causality when in most instances these symptoms have "real" physical etiologies that are dramatically influenced by psychological states.

from marital discord, the underlying marital problems remained unresolved. The price of the sick role as a "solution" to interpersonal and family problems is high for all involved, and will fail in the long run. But when patients present with psycho-physiologically reactive symptoms that are generated and sustained by sick role coping strategies it needs to be respected as the best that the patient and family can do to cope with the their problems.

CONDUCTING A FAMILY MEETING

Typically, physicians need to understand the patient's story and family situation by talking to the patient alone. But often, at least one other family member will be present and this offers a powerful opportunity to rapidly understand the patient's situation and bring the pain into the room more quickly. Ideally, the key members of the family, especially those that the patient is having a problem with should be present, but much can be learned by simply having one other knowledgeable person in the room. The objective of the family meeting is to have the family discuss the family's interactions and have other members directly report their responses to the patient's behavior and sick role symptoms. The most effective family interview will result in the family enacting their drama in the room with the patient and the physician.

Although clinicians may be afraid that such an enactment will get out of hand, it is actually relatively easy to keep the process under control by using the statement that concludes Step 1 and begins the process of executing Step 2 when the conflict has come out into the open and the pain is in the room. Even in the midst of raised voices, the physician will be able to say:

- "Ok, timeout." That will stop the discussion. Use a hand signal if necessary.
- "I have feeling this is not the first time you all have had this fight." The family will appreciate that you are bearing witness and that you are insightful.
- "It seems to me that what has just happened here and the problems you've been talking about are extremely painful for everyone involved and definitely worthy of attention, and that you have been unable to resolve them on your own." This is the Step 2 statement.

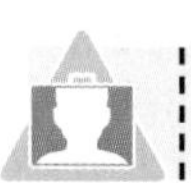

CASE ILLUSTRATION 1 (CONTD.)

Ariana greatly appreciated the opportunity to describe the situation at home, especially when the physician expressed sympathy for the burden that Estelle's illness placed on everyone and for the disappointment resulting from Ariana's failed marriage. The physician now had a general feel for Ariana's family. It was clear that Ariana needed to be labeled as "sick" and that every diagnostic test, referral to a specialist, and symptomatic treatment helped to establish the sick role. Ariana, clearly feeling that the physician was on her side after the genogram interview, readily agreed to a family meeting.

During the family interview, the tremendous burden placed on the family by Estelle's visual impairment, deafness, and diabetes care became painfully clear as the physician struggled to communicate with her; a process that required writing notes in letters 6 inches high, or having Ariana or her mother slowly and carefully speak so that Estelle could read their lips (Estelle was unable to read anyone else's lips, and the family had tried but failed to learn sign language). When asked what her most important question or request was, Estelle, an insulin-requiring diabetic said, "Can I stop the insulin?" It also became clear how much the family depended on Ariana and how she stepped ambivalently into the fray whenever Estelle needed attention.

When the subject turned to Ariana's failed marriage and social life, the mother (Maria) expressed some hope, immediately labeled as ridiculous by Ariana, that she (Ariana) would get back together with her ex-husband. Ariana said, "with all this," gesturing around the room and referring to the just demonstrated problems with Estelle, "how can I find time to get involved with anyone?"

Further discussion revealed that Maria was a "worrier" and was determinately preoccupied with whichever of her children was having difficulties, especially medical problems, at any given time. Ariana's medical problems elicited sympathy from her mother, who suggested that since Ariana was no longer married, she should move back into the family house.

Ariana immediately rejected that idea and said that her medical problems were the primary reason she could ***not*** *move back into the house; she didn't want her mother to see her when she was sick because her mother would worry too much. Ariana added that when she was feeling sick, she needed to stay home by herself, and at these times she didn't even answer the phone (these were pre-cellphone events) or know what was going on in her parents' house.*

The physician concluded that Ariana's somatization was embedded in the repetitive pattern of events dominated by her triangular relationship with Estelle and their mother. Ariana's physical symptoms allowed her to remain connected to and receive attention and emotional support from her mother, and simultaneously allowed her to control the family's expectations that she would always be there to help with Estelle. In order to be effective and acceptable to everyone in the family, Ariana's reason for remaining away from her mother and Estelle needed to be an illness; that is, something beyond her control. Ariana's desire to achieve some separation from her mother and Estelle and devote more of her life to herself was not something she could readily acknowledge to herself let alone explicitly ask for.

Step 2: Reframing Attention to the Underlying Family Problems

The goal of Step 2 of family intervention, "reframing," is twofold (see Table 11-8): The first and most important goal is to focus the patient's (and family's) attention on the underlying family problems, and away from physical symptoms and sick role-justifying problems. The second goal of reframing is to help the patient understand that the goal of their sick role behavior can be justified and might eventually be achieved without using the sick role as a strategy. That is, the patient would be entitled to what they want or need even if they were not sick. In Ariana's case, she would be entitled to set some boundaries around her involvement with her mother and Estelle even if she were "the picture of perfect health."

Reframing, "In Addition to Your Pain . . ."

The transition from Step 1 to Step 2 occurs when the interview has "brought the pain into the room," and patients are in touch with their distress, that is, when they agree with the first critical reframing statement, "It seems to me that the family situation you have just described is extremely painful, and that *in addition to* your [problematic symptom or behavior], this [family problem] is also worthy of attention."

A critical component of the first reframing statement is "*in addition to*" in contrast to either "instead of" or "because of." Even if your understanding, based on a psycho-physiological or "psychosomatic" hypothesis, is that family stress is "causing" the somatoform presentation, you must resist saying so. The legitimacy of the sick role and coping strategies that the patient and family currently need to function depends on there being a "disease beyond one's control" to justify the sick role. If the family intervention begins to have effect, and healthier coping strategies are adopted, then the family will be able to relinquish sick role–based coping. Until that time they must be allowed to retain the sick role strategy. Therefore, the goal of reframing is to establish a *parallel* concern directed at the underlying family problems. Occasionally, a patient or family member will be able to make the connection themselves: "Doctor, do you think that maybe my headache is being caused by all these problems?" In such cases, the patient's hypothesis can be endorsed. The mistake is to make the connection before the patient and family are ready. This will result in the all too familiar, "Doctor, you think it's just all in my head. It's not in my head, my pain is real!"

Reframing, "Even If You Were the Picture of Perfect Health You, Would Be Entitled to . . ."

Unless your patient's objectives in occupying the sick role are antisocial, you should be able to identify an essential core of their objective that you can endorse—a new grandmother who does not want to be treated as a nanny, a father who wants peace in his home and rules for his teenage daughter, a young woman who does not want to become her sister's home health aide and unpaid medical concierge, and so on.

The second objective of reframing is to separate the objective from the strategy of occupying the sick role and to empower the patient and family to adopt other, healthier strategies. This can be done by telling the patient, "*even if you were the picture of perfect health, you would be entitled to*—be a grandmother not a nanny, have your daughter follow some agreed-upon rules, set limits on your role in taking care of your sister," and so on. This part of the reframing addresses the fundamental function of the sick role, which is to establish entitlement, and uses the authority of the physician to legitimate the desired entitlement on other, healthier grounds.

Case Illustration 1: Discussion (Contd.)

It was relatively easy to reframe the burden of caring for Estelle as a problem worthy of attention after the painful demonstration of just how difficult it was to just have a conversation with her. It was also easy to reframe Ariana's desire to have some time and space for herself—a need she was unwilling to claim on her own—as something that would be important for "a woman in her situation" *even if she was not ill.* Ariana was willing to accept the suggestion that her failure to develop the kind of intimate relationship she desired was also a problem worthy of consideration.

Step 3: Empathic Witnessing: "I Am So Impressed With How Well You Are Doing Despite . . ."

The most immediate way to ensure that the four-step counseling process has a positive and therapeutic effect is to "empathically witness" the patient's (and family's) problems and their efforts to cope (see Table 11-8). If the interview has succeeded in exposing the patient's distress and their best attempts to deal with their problems, the patient will recognize that the physician knows them (and their family, especially if they have been directly engaged) in a very intimate way. If the physician acknowledges the special nature of this awareness, and responds empathically to the patient, the effect can be very therapeutic. The general format for empathic witnessing is to mitigate the sense of failure by acknowledging how difficult their situation is and complementing them on their intent. "*I am very impressed with how well you are doing despite all your problems and difficulties, you are really determined to . . . help your daughter take care of your grandchild, . . . be a good father for your daughter and partner to your wife . . . help your sister and mother.*" It is helpful to remember that even if the patient is failing in their efforts, seeing them and praising them for who they are trying to be is powerfully therapeutic, and is appropriate as long as their intentions are not antisocial or abusive.

CASE ILLUSTRATION 1 (CONTD.)

The family admitted that the current situation was very distressing and that they had not been able to solve their problems despite their best efforts. The physician was able to tell Ariana and her mother: "I am so impressed with how well you are both doing despite the tremendous problems you have had to deal with." The physician also remarked on the magnitude of the sacrifice Ariana had made, neglecting her own social life to be available to the family. The physician also commented that it was easy to understand how this area of Ariana's life might be difficult for her to deal with because of her past problems.

Step 4: Referral for Family & Psychotherapy

FEAR OF LOSING THE SICK ROLE

Referral for therapy is not always indicated. Sometimes the first three steps of this family-based counseling intervention can empower patients and their families to address their difficulties with new energy, insight, and courage to change. However, it is not the physician's job to "fix" the problems they discover when they bring the pain into the room, and behavioral health intervention is often needed to help patients develop the new coping and interpersonal behaviors they need to address their problems. When patients are referred for counseling or therapy as soon as their clinicians realize that it is indicated, patients and their families are often not ready to accept it (see Table 11-8). One of the goals of the first three steps of the counseling process is to prepare the patient for a discussion of how and why counseling will be helpful in addressing the problems that have been uncovered and validated.

It is very important at this stage to frame the patient's interpersonal problems as being "in addition to" to their physical symptoms and presenting complaints. This will help patients feel comfortable that therapy does not threaten their use of the sick role before they are ready to give it up.

FEAR OF ADDRESSING PAINFUL EMOTIONS AND PROBLEMS

Resistance to therapy may be due to fear of dealing directly with painful and powerful emotions. Empathic witnessing and reframing can make this challenge seem more surmountable by demonstrating that the problems can be talked about and that the patient can feel better about themselves after doing so. Introducing the therapy by saying "What do you think about the idea of continuing *a conversation like this one* with a counselor who has special expertise in helping with this kind of problem. . . ." The message is, "If therapy is like this conversation, it can't be that bad."

TURNING THE PROBLEM THE PATIENT HAS INTO A QUESTION FOR THE PATIENT TO ANSWER: HELPING PATIENTS UNDERSTAND HOW THERAPY CAN HELP

Finally, patients may accept the reality of family problems yet not accept the fact that therapy will help: "What's talking going to accomplish?" The process of therapy may indeed seem obscure to patients. Therefore, the key to making the referral is to restate problems as questions and describe therapy as the process of looking for answers. For example, "You have a serious question to answer. You have to determine how much child care you actually want to provide, and then how to talk to your daughter about it. Therapy can help you find answers to these questions."

It may take a long time for patients to accept the need for therapy; and some may never go despite our best efforts. However, when a discussion of how therapy can help is based on the shared emotional experience created during the first three steps of the family assessment process, the discussion about therapy will have a positive and therapeutic effect. *After* bringing the pain into the room, reframing attention to the interpersonal problems and empathic witnessing, even if that experience occurred many visits previously, the physician may say the words recorded in our conclusion to Case Illustration 2, below, to the patient who has not followed through with referral for therapy and who returns with persistent or recurrent symptoms (as did the father in this case):

CASE ILLUSTRATION 2 (CONCLUSION)

"I am sorry that your headache is still bothering you. Your wife and daughter are still fighting, aren't they? It's too bad that you haven't gotten to the therapist yet. I truly wish that there was more that I could do for

you, but why don't you go ahead and schedule that appointment. Now, why don't we check your blood pressure."

The patient—aware that the physician has witnessed the family conflict—knows that the clinician understands the importance of the conflict at home and that this understanding is empathic. Although it may be helpful to hear a periodic update of the original story, the physician does not have to perform the first three steps with every encounter. It is sufficient to merely recall it for the patient. The physician is in a position to respect the meaning of the patient's symptoms and reorient the patient to a potentially fruitful pathway for addressing their problems, without allowing those problems to divert the process of care into unnecessary testing, medication, or referrals for more evaluation.

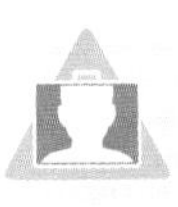

CASE ILLUSTRATION 1 (CONCLUSION)

The physician (1) referred the family for family therapy to explore better approaches to coping with Estelle's medical problems; (2) suggested that Ariana would benefit from individual counseling to explore her difficulties in forming a satisfying intimate relationship; (3) asked the mother's (Maria's) physician to consider the diagnoses of dysthymia and major depression; and (4) recommended that the family try to obtain a home health aide for Estelle to give Maria a break. The family agreed to all four of these suggestions. When Ariana returned for her next visit, she still had numerous symptoms but spoke of them only briefly, allowing the physician to turn the discussion to what was going on at home. Ariana reported that the family had taken no steps toward family therapy and that she was still considering whether to go to individual therapy. She did report feeling more comfortable setting limits on her mother's expectations of assistance in dealing with Estelle, and reported success in obtaining a home health aide for Estelle. Maria had been placed on an antidepressant, made a few visits to a community mental health center, and was much less symptomatic.

Eight months later, Ariana entered individual therapy and her somatization decreased dramatically and her limit-setting improved. Eventually, she started dating and entered a steady relationship but has not remarried.

It is not unusual for patients to predict that other family members will be unwilling to participate in family therapy, and often they are right, especially initially. This is no barrier to the family systems approach because, as family systems therapists commonly point out, if one member of a family changes, the rest of the family will have to change to. When patient's raise their family members unwillingness the physician should help them understand that they may have to start the work of answering the important questions that have been framed in the fourth step by themselves, but that one of the things that they will have to learn and get help with in therapy is how to engage those other family members by changing the things that they do. Help them understand that if they change, the others will have to change too.

SUGGESTED READINGS

Carter CA, McGoldrick M, eds. *The Family Life Cycle: A Framework for Family Therapy.* New York, NY: Gardner Press; 1980.

Doherty WJ, Baird MA. *Family-Centered Medical Care: A Clinical Case Book.* New York, NY: Guilford Press; 1987.

Doherty WJ, Campbell TL. *Families and Health.* New York, NY: Sage Publications; 1988.

Haley J. *Problem Solving Therapy.* San Francisco, CA: Jossey-Bass; 1976.

McGoldrick M, Gerson R. *Genograms in Family Assessment.* New York, NY: Norton; 1985.

Minuchin S. *Families and Family Therapy.* Cambridge, MA: Harvard University Press; 1974.

Parsons T. *The Social System.* Glencoe, IL: The Free Press; 1951.

Children

12

Adam L. Braddock, MD, MPhil & Howard L. Taras, MD

INTRODUCTION

This chapter reviews some important concepts in child behavior and the primary care provider's role in assessing and providing guidance on common behavioral challenges. Pediatric behavioral medicine is closely linked to child development because many problematic childhood behaviors are developmentally normal. Clinicians who work with children need to identify parents' behavioral concerns, even if parents do not initially volunteer this information at the visit. Clinicians also need to become comfortable with principles to address behavioral challenges in order to help parents learn skills to manage these behaviors. The second half of this chapter includes case illustrations of some common behavioral concerns in pediatric primary care such as aggression, oppositional behaviors, and infant sleep patterns.

UNDESIRABLE BEHAVIOR: PART OF NORMAL CHILDHOOD DEVELOPMENT

A child's ability to understand and interact with the environment is constantly evolving. To learn more about the world, a child experiments with ways of interacting with it. Most often, children test the reactions of the people, such as parents, to whom they are closest. Colloquial phrases such as *"the terrible twos"* and *"she's going through a stage"* indicate that some undesirable childhood behaviors are commonly accepted as "normal." But when a child is demonstrating an undesirable behavior, parents can have a hard time accepting the behavior, and many parents need guidance. The clinician's goal in these cases is to educate parents about normal child development, provide reassurance and advice, and emphasize the positive aspects of a child's behavior and development in order to maintain a warm and supportive relationship between parent and child.

BEHAVIORAL DISORDERS

Behavioral challenges associated with normal childhood development must be distinguished from behavioral disorders, such as attention deficit hyperactivity disorder (ADHD), which are not the focus of this chapter. Disorders are diagnosed in children when problems are not related to normal development, symptoms meet the threshold set out by the *Diagnostic and Statistical Manual of Mental Disorders* or related criteria, and the behaviors cause distress or impairment for the child. The diagnostic requirement for distress or impairment is critical because behaviors or mental states such as anxiety, sadness, and inattention occur in healthy children and do not necessarily reflect pathology.

ENVIRONMENT AND BEHAVIOR

Aberrant childhood behaviors can be secondary to life stresses. This applies to children who witness violence, are members of communities that have experienced a natural disaster or catastrophic event, are exposed to continuous marital discord, have a frequently absent parent (such as military deployment), have a chronic illness or a chronically ill sibling, or who do not feel wanted. Children living under any condition that seriously threatens healthy and successful transition through a developmental stage are at risk for behavioral problems.

Children, like adults, may appear to be the dysfunctional member of an otherwise healthy family unit even though the problem actually stems from family issues. This is particularly the case with childhood behaviors, because children are dependent on adults in almost every way. Take, for instance, the child who refuses to attend school. This behavior can occur when one or both parents send subliminal messages to the child to remain home. Although the primary problem is parental anxiety about separation, it is the child who exhibits the apparent symptoms.

Stresses causing unwanted childhood behavior may be different than those described above. For example, children of immigrants often successfully acculturate to the prevalent culture. But when these children's attitudes and behaviors are not culturally acceptable or understood by their parents, children can be perceived as having behavioral problems, or they may develop behavioral disorders at least in part due to the stresses of this culture clash.

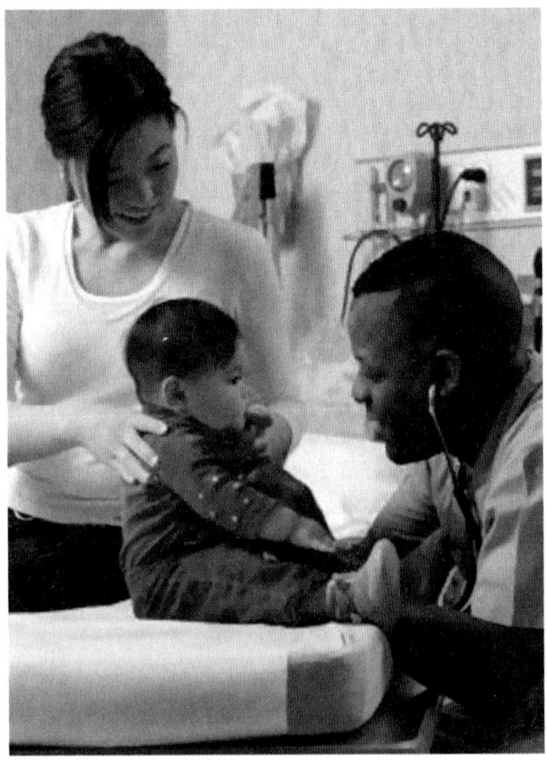

ADVERSE CHILDHOOD EXPERIENCES

Childhood exposure to violence, abuse, neglect, and other forms of "toxic stress" does not only increase the probability of behavioral problems in children. Accumulating evidence demonstrates that these adverse childhood experiences increase the risk for diseases in adulthood such as cardiovascular disease, cancers, asthma, depression, and obesity. A "dose-response" relationship has been demonstrated in which higher exposures to adverse childhood experiences are associated with worse health. These associations are likely due to the impact of toxic stress on the neuroendocrine–immune network (see Chapter 36). Dysregulation of the hypothalamic–pituitary–adrenal (HPA) axis and proinflammatory immune responses can impact both brain development and other organ systems. Epigenetic changes (regulation of genes) due to toxic stress can cause exaggerated HPA response. Adverse childhood experiences also increase the risk for smoking and substance abuse (illicit drugs, alcohol), which can mediate the increased risk for chronic disease in adulthood. Providing interventions to reduce toxic stress could improve both physical and mental health for children and adults.

SCREENING FAMILIES FOR DIFFICULTIES WITH CHILDHOOD BEHAVIORS

Pediatric primary care providers must screen families for difficulties with childhood behaviors, consider possible causes for the behaviors, recognize when a mental health referral is appropriate, and manage those problems that are likely to respond to simple environmental changes or behavioral management techniques.

Practitioner concern versus time constraints. Many parents do not know where to seek help for behavioral problems such as their baby's night awakenings, their toddler's tantrums, or their fourth grader's class clown behavior. They do not realize that their child's primary care clinician can assist them. To overcome these barriers, health care providers should take every opportunity to talk about behavioral issues, although time constraints may limit the practitioner's ability to listen to extensive histories. Therefore, clinicians need to screen for behavioral information in ways that are efficient and that leave time to reflect on issues that can be discussed more fully at another time.

Trigger questions and questionnaires. One way to elicit behavioral information from parents is to ask a list of screening questions specific to each age group. Use of a screening questionnaire that is mailed home in advance or that parents can answer electronically is a reliable way to elicit history. Numerous such questionnaires have been available since the 1990s. While primary care clinicians commonly use developmental questionnaires such as the Modified Checklist for Autism in Toddlers, Revised with Follow-Up (M-CHAT-R/F) and Ages and Stages Questionnaires (ASQ) to screen for autism and developmental delays, behavior-focused questionnaires are not as prevalent. Some feel these questionnaires merely confirm what a clinician would suspect once the patient and family are in the office for a clinical evaluation. Nevertheless, clinicians should consider using brief behavioral screening tools such as the 17-item Pediatric Symptom Checklist. The American Academy of Pediatrics recommends universal screening for depression in children 12 years of age and older using a formal self-report screening tool such as the PHQ-9. These tools can help clinicians identify children at risk for behavioral disorders and trigger a follow-up interview to determine if further evaluation and intervention are necessary.

To effectively identify childhood behavioral problems, practitioners need to develop their skills of observation and follow their intuitions. Parent–child interaction in the office can be an excellent indicator of problems occurring at home. It is a warning sign when reported childhood behavior problems are combined with a clinician's suspicion that there is an aberrant pattern of attachment between parent and child. Incidents in the office that induce parents to discipline their child are opportunities for clinicians to better understand the parent–child relationship and to model behavior management techniques for parents. Experienced clinicians have learned to become aware of subtle signs in the office that are indicative of a family's dynamics. A mother who seems uncomfortable feeding her baby, a pattern of nonadherence to provider recommendations, or parents who are disengaged from their child should register concern with the clinician. Involvement of grandparents and other extended family, comments parents make about their own upbringing, and other family characteristics are also worth noting. Positive impressions that clinicians form about families also provide clinically useful information.

Asking parents about their children's screen time on electronic devices can be a window into family habits and childhood behavior. Video games, texting, smartphones, computers, and social media have assumed central roles in children's daily lives, but there is increasing awareness of the potential risks of excessive or inappropriate screen time for children. For example, early media exposure may put children at risk for later attentional problems, and screen time late in the day can disrupt sleep. The blue light emitted from television, computer, smartphone, and tablet screens delays the release of melatonin and damages the quality and duration of sleep. Children with insomnia or other sleep disturbances should be asked about screen time and should receive counseling about sleep hygiene, including elimination of evening screen exposure. Screen time should also be a concern if it is associated with the emergence of behavior problems, and it is worthwhile to ask about screen time if a child has a history of problem behaviors.

Interviewing young children. Primary care providers can find themselves in a quandary when they try to elicit information directly from children. Most children by age 2½ to 3 years are capable of communicating certain thoughts and feelings to an inquiring health provider. But children do not typically divulge such information to clinicians when questioned directly. Children freely offer their honest opinions on just about any topic, sensitive or banal, but they often do so when it is unsolicited. Parents are often surprised when their children first reveal their feelings about a delicate personal issue to an adult with whom they are not ostensibly very close (a preschool teacher, a friend's mother in their car pool, and so on).

Therefore, primary care providers should use tools that help children more freely and predictably disclose their thoughts and feelings. One way is to ask children old enough to understand and comply to draw a picture, for example, to draw "anything you want," "something scary," "your family," or "the worst day at school." The position of the characters in the drawings, facial expressions, and choice of colors can yield important information about what children are thinking, may be indicative of how they are feeling, and can be used as a starting point for discussion. Children often find it easier to speak about themselves when the conversation is in the third person, such as "Why would that little girl in the picture want to hit her mommy?"

Other oblique ways of eliciting information from children are to ask open-ended questions that children like to respond to: "Pretend a magical genie in a bottle wanted to grant you three wishes; what would they be?" And "If you could magically turn into any animal you wanted, what would it be?" To the child's response to the last question, then say, "Well that's wonderful! And why would you be happy as that animal?"

Sentence completion games are also useful. The clinician begins the first few words of a sentence and asks the child to complete the sentence by making something up. Examples of some are given in Table 12-1. These (and clinicians can improvise on others like them) can be typed onto colorful cards so that children can choose one at a time and perceive it as a game, not a real interview. Allow the child to be imaginative with responses, and indicate that their responses can be truthful but do not have to be.

Toddlers and school-age children are often aware of the clinician's intent when these interviewing techniques are used. Despite this, children seem to enjoy going along with this form of questioning and appreciate having an easy way to express themselves. Children respond best when they are comfortable with the clinician. Arranging a number of office visits can help to establish that relationship.

When using drawings, questions in the third person, or questions evoking the child's imagination, it is

Table 12-1. **Samples of "sentence completion" items for interviewing young children.**

- I really like it when . . .
- I am ashamed . . .
- I worry a lot about . . .
- My mother . . .
- I hate . . .
- It makes me sad to . . .
- It makes me happy to . . .
- People think that I . . .
- I really hope one day that I . . .

important not to read too deeply into children's responses. Children have active imaginations: they play around with frightening ideas and wishful thinking. Sometimes they are merely obsessed with speaking about what they have recently seen on television. Responses of young children that fit into a general pattern of concerns that the clinician has derived from the parent interview and the child's symptoms should be taken more seriously.

Beyond the physician–child–parent triad. Many toddlers are placed in the care of a day care provider, babysitter, or relative. Most children older than 5 years of age spend a large portion of their waking hours in school. Yet despite this, clinicians traditionally rely almost exclusively on parents (and the children themselves) to gather a behavioral history. Some clinicians send questionnaires to school staff to elicit information, or they ask parents about their children's progress at school or day care. It is rare, however, for clinicians to routinely engage in direct telephone contact with child care providers and teachers. Yet these people occupy many, and occasionally most, of children's waking hours. The value of attaining parental permission to speak directly with education professionals in a child's life cannot be overstated. Teachers and child care providers can provide valuable insight. Many have years of experience with all types of children, and their observations rarely include the emotional biases that sometimes confound a parent's interpretation and recollection of details. Once a behavior plan has been recommended, a relationship with daytime caregivers may extend the plan's implementation to that setting and render it more effective.

NORMAL CHILDHOOD DEVELOPMENT

Knowledge about stages of normal childhood development can assist a clinician in understanding the etiology of a problematic behavior. It allows the clinician, and in turn the parent, to attribute an undesirable behavior to a developmental stage of childhood. An understanding of child development can guide parents to respond to a problem behavior using a strategy that is consistent with that child's stage of development. For example, it is often appropriate to give a firm "no" to a child's behavior when they are very young, but that response would be insufficient for an older child who has developed skills of reasoning.

There are several thinkers who have attempted to systematize stages of childhood development. Sigmund Freud's psychoanalytic theories emphasized unconscious and conscious mental processes that reflect different stages of development. Each stage, which is several years long, is a turning point where a child can become vulnerable or strong in relation to a certain characteristic. For example, according to this theory, in the anal stage at 1½ to 3 years of age, children are personally focused on elimination. Interpersonally, they are focused on "rebellion versus compliance" with parental demands and may fear loss of parental love.

Erik Erickson's stages are an expanded version of psychoanalytic theory. According to his theory, infants develop trust or mistrust through their experiences up to about age 18 months. In the next stage (ending around age 3 years), children develop autonomy or self-doubt, and in preschool (up to age 6 years) children learn to either take initiative or feel inhibited to do so. School age children can acquire the psychological skills to feel competent in work or experience repeated frustration and feelings of inferiority. No stage is ever completely resolved, but the experience of those critical years is present in some way as the person moves throughout life.

Jean Piaget described stages of cognitive development. Though his theories have since been proven to underestimate children's abilities, they are still useful guides. For example, until around age 7 years children are what Piaget termed "preoperational." They engage in make believe, which parents should not misconstrue as lying. Complex concepts such as cause and effect are not yet well developed, and parents should be wary of trying to rationalize with them. Once well into elementary school, they are at the "concrete operational" stage, meaning they are less egocentric and understand how events outside of their own actions can lead to concrete changes. Hence, parental explanations for behavior are important for children at this age. Adolescence is marked by the increasing ability to work with abstract concepts. Adolescents may test out these new skills by how they interact with their peers. They can begin to moralize about their own and others' behaviors.

Another important aspect of normal childhood development is temperament. Healthy children demonstrate a wide range of behaviors and dispositions in mood, adaptability, intensity, and other dimensions. A child's temperament is the stable response to the environment across these various dimensions. Temperamental variation is normal and does not imply pathology. Sometimes parental expectation regarding a child's behavior can be unrealistic given the child's temperament. Unrealistic expectations can occur if there is a mismatch between parental and child temperament. In these cases the clinician should aim to educate the parents about this difference and how to manage the most problematic behaviors while accepting that many behaviors may simply reflect the child's temperamental profile.

ATTACHMENT THEORY

Newborns are dependent on caregivers for all their needs and are vulnerable to environmental threats. Attachment theory explains how infants respond to this vulnerability by developing a strong emotional relationship with a primary caregiver in the first year of life. The primary caregiver becomes a source of comfort, security, and encouragement during the first year as the infant's ability to act independently grows. Different patterns of attachment have been examined in a study named Ainsworth's Strange Situation. In this experiment, infant-caregiver dyads are separated, reunited, and a stranger is introduced to test the infant's attachment to the caregiver. In secure attachment, the infant seeks the caregiver for reassurance and uses the caregiver as a "home base" for exploration. The infant's distress is resolved by contact with the caregiver. In anxious-avoidant attachment, the infant shows reduced affect and interest toward the caregiver and treats the stranger and caregiver in a similar manner. In anxious-resistant attachment, infants are unable to be consoled by the caregiver. Finally, disorganized attachment occurs when the infant demonstrates inconsistent behavior that reflects fear of the caregiver.

Insecure attachment patterns (anxious-avoidant, anxious-resistant, and disorganized) are associated with caregiving that is not responsive to infant needs, including maltreatment and abuse. Insecure attachment has been linked to mental health problems later in life, including anxiety, depression, antisocial behavior, and dissociative symptoms. Maladaptive responses to stress and loss may be related to early life insecure attachment. The lack of a responsive primary caregiver in infancy can have lifelong effects on social and emotional functioning.

BEHAVIORAL MANAGEMENT IN PRIMARY CARE

Primary care providers can and should evaluate and manage common child behavior problems in their own offices. Mental health referrals may be unnecessary since so many problematic child behaviors are manifestations of normal child development. There are occasions when the need for psychiatric assessment, medication, or psychotherapy is apparent from the start. But for many problems that present to primary care practitioners, children respond well to brief, solution-focused strategies. Although no single behavioral management technique works well for all children, clinicians can quickly learn to tailor their management plans to suit the individual needs of each family. These plans should be based on families' cultural characteristics, size, work schedules, and other factors. A management failure should first be considered a problem with the behavioral management technique prescribed, not with the child or family.

It is useful for primary care clinicians to have some understanding of psychotherapeutic interventions and concepts. Expertise in these therapies takes years of specialized training, which is not feasible for most primary care providers. Providing psychotherapy in the clinical setting takes many sessions, and for some, many years. However, just knowing the premise behind these psychotherapeutic techniques may guide a clinician on how best to frame a conversation with a child and family when they face relatively minor behavioral problems.

Family therapy is based on the premise that every family is a system (see Chapter 11). When a child has a problem behavior, it can be analyzed in terms of being one outcome of the relationships among all members of the family. By first understanding and then intervening with the nature and dynamics of the family as a system, family therapy can help parents understand the complex etiology of their child's behavior. In the primary care setting, this concept can help underpin the etiology and management of relatively minor behavior problems. For example, a clinician working with a child who refuses to eat meals can consider inviting the entire family to the office when the problem hinges on a doting live-in grandmother who slips cookies to her granddaughter between meals.

Cognitive behavioral therapy (CBT) comprises a series of techniques based on the notion that there is a close relationship between a person's thoughts, feelings, and behavior. It involves interrogating these thoughts and revealing the cognitive distortions that can lead to unhelpful emotional reactions and behaviors. Dysfunctional behaviors can also be targeted. CBT is the most evidence-based psychotherapy for anxiety and depression in children and adults. The concepts of CBT can be useful for a primary care provider who is trying to coax parents to recognize that their child's obstinate "no" to every directive need not raise their parental ire. The clinician can help the parents recognize that their emotional reaction to their child's misbehavior may be rooted in their own unrealistic thoughts about acceptable behavior (e.g., "my child should always do what I say"), and may actually promote such behaviors by providing further attention to the child.

Motivational interviewing was designed as a technique to improve treatment outcomes for people with substance abuse disorders (see Chapter 19). However, many clinicians have recognized that the philosophy and techniques of motivational interviewing can be helpful when trying to change other patient behaviors. Many people come to a health professional stating that they would like to stop smoking or lose weight, but they may be less than ready to do so. Motivational interviewing recognizes the client's stage of readiness to make a change. These stages include precontemplation, contemplation, preparation, action, and maintenance. Behavioral experts in this technique learn to determine the client's readiness to change and help the client push him or herself to the next stage. Helping patients recognize the discrepancy between their stated desire and their current predicament is an important part of the process. In addition to engaging children and adolescents around behaviors such as healthy eating and physical activity, motivational interviewing can be used to engage parents. For example, parents might state that they dislike their child sleeping in the parental bed each night but do not seem motivated to change this behavior. The clinician can show sympathy for the parents and point out how it is common to be ambivalent about changing the status quo. The clinician can then encourage the parents to think about what would motivate them to act and what they perceive as barriers to behavior change.

Promoting *emotional intelligence* can be a useful part of the treatment plan for behavioral problems in children. Emotional intelligence is defined as the ability to identify one's own feelings, to identify the feelings of others, and to solve problems that involve emotional issues. Emotional intelligence is associated with, for example, having a lower risk for smoking during one's youth. Parents who provide their child with "tools" to handle emotional challenges may be able to increase the emotional ability of their child. By learning a vocabulary of words that describes emotions, such as "frustrated," "anxious," and "envious," children may become more likely to use them *in lieu* of acting out behaviors. Clinicians can also encourage parents to foster an environment in which children will want to describe their feelings. Naturally, this is more easily accepted by parents in your office than at home. Clinicians can ask about specific and recent situations at home that demonstrate the child's personality and stage of emotional maturation. By understanding these details, a clinician can offer step-by-step suggestions that are pertinent to the child's emotional development.

Fostering *resilience* in children is another strategy to improve behavioral outcomes. Resilience reflects a child's ability to recover from negative or traumatic experiences. There are significant individual differences in sensitivity to negative and positive experiences, and a child's resilience is probably based on neurobiological and epigenetic processes. There is growing evidence that one can promote childhood resilience through intervention during critical stages of development. Positive relationships with caring adults and effective parenting promote attachment. Problem-solving skills, self-regulation, and self-efficacy are associated with resilience. Societal factors such as close friends, faith (i.e., hope, spirituality, and belief that life has meaning), and effective teachers and schools appear to be correlated with resilience. High-quality schools, child care settings, and other developmental programs are critical in the effort to promote resilience and improve mental health for children. The resilience of a child's family and community also influences outcomes. This point reinforces the importance of eliciting a history that takes into account family and community strengths and vulnerabilities.

Advocacy is a tool that clinicians can use to modify the environments that affect child health and behavior outside the walls of the clinic or hospital. Such environments include schools, playgrounds, parks and recreational centers, and child care centers. Advocacy is most powerful when clinicians use their own experiences with patients and families to educate legislators and the public about the needs of children. School-based behavioral interventions are one example of programs that clinicians can support through advocacy. In these programs, children are taught in the classroom that anger is an emotion that can be recognized before it is acted upon. School-based programs have helped students discuss and act out situations that trigger anger, learn how to temper these emotions, and develop the skills to de-escalate a situation. Clinicians can play an important role in advocating for these and other behavioral programs at the local, state, and national levels.

EXAMPLES OF COMMON BEHAVIORAL ISSUES

Infancy: Night Waking

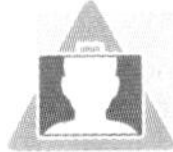

CASE ILLUSTRATION 1

Parents of a 12-week-old girl complain that their daughter rarely sleeps more than a total of 4–5 hours between 8 P.M. and 6 A.M. She may fall asleep at 8 P.M., only to awaken an hour later. She seems to fall asleep during or after short feeds and then remains awake for hours later on. Each night is a struggle of long periods awake between short spells of sleep. Her parents note that she cries when left alone. She seems content at night when parents walk around with her.

Child development in early infancy is characterized by large fluctuations in temperament and schedules. In the first few weeks of life, infants often sleep as much during the day as at night. In the first 2 months of life, two night awakenings are common, but by 3 months of life most infants are sleeping for 5–6 hours uninterrupted. In this case, the child did not naturally "learn" the difference between night and day, and parents did not train her to do so.

CASE ILLUSTRATION 1 (CONTD.)

On further questioning in this case, the parents reported that their baby falls asleep immediately after daytime feeds and sleeps for 3–5 consecutive hours thereafter. Since this baby did not adapt to an acceptable day/night schedule, the doctor recommended waking the baby up after no more than 2–3 hours of daytime sleep. Parents were to occupy their infant's daytime hours by walking around, talking, playing music, and other activities. It was recommended that nighttime feeds be made minimally stimulating: soften the lights, produce minimal noise, and avoid "fun" interactions at night. Although sleeping and feeding "on demand" does not need to be discouraged if parents find it acceptable, in this case the infant's pattern was distressing to the parents. After 5–6 days of compliance with this schedule, it became easier for the parents to keep their daughter awake during the day, and they settled for a nighttime feed before they went to bed at 11 P.M. and another feed at 4 A.M.

It is important to note that the likely causes for night awakenings change with developmental stages. This same sleep history told by parents of a 9-month-old child would be more likely related to the child's ability to recognize that parents still "exist" after they leave the room. At that age, if there were no other likely cause, other recommendations would be in order. A nightlight or a transitional object could be helpful. The clinician could devise a careful behavioral intervention schedule that includes parental reassurance for the child but may also include an allowance for the child to "cry it out" for a couple of nights.

Toddler: Aggression

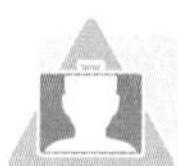

CASE ILLUSTRATION 2

The parent of a 3-year-old boy reports that her son throws himself on the floor, throws objects, and screams . . . usually when he does not get his own way. This seems to happen daily. At his child care center, he has begun to bite other children when he is angry, and other parents have begun to complain about him.

Angry outbursts are common at 3 years of age, when children often begin to direct their anger at others. Parental response to a given level of aggression differs widely from family to family. Parental expectations of children's behavior, not solely the magnitude of the child's behavior, help define whether a behavior is a problem. A child who explores the environment very actively may be described as "curious" in one family but as "always climbing the walls" in another. A "difficult and stubborn" child in one family is "persistent—just like his successful grandpa" in another.

Assessment of this behavior begins with elucidating the extent and nature of the child's aggression, the circumstances surrounding the aggression, and the antecedents and consequences for the behavior. Detailed examples of what instigated the last one or two aggressive behaviors are more revealing than letting the parent say, "Oh it happens for just about anything." Always ask parents how they feel when their child acts out. Also ask what parents have done in response to misbehavior and whether this reaction helped.

Certain questions may help clinicians assess the etiology of aggressive behavior: Is the child generally unhappy or irritable? Is the child exposed to frequent violent (physical or verbal) outbursts from others at home? Did the aggression start with a specific change in environment or family stressor? Is the child delayed in some aspects of development? Positive responses to these questions may point to a specific etiology and treatment plan.

Children with well-developed cognitive abilities, but with comparatively delayed language abilities, often become frustrated with their inability to communicate and may act out in an aggressive manner. In addition, children at this stage often strive for adult attention and have found aggressive behaviors to be a guaranteed way of getting it. Parents who report feeling "I just don't have time for this" may indicate that the child is trying to get attention. Children at this stage also need to express their independence and may become aggressive if caregivers are unable to find ways to allow for independent behavior. If the caregiver's first reaction is to feel that it is a power struggle, then the child's wish for independence may be his or her primary incentive.

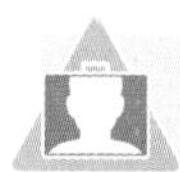

CASE ILLUSTRATION 2 (CONTD.)

In this case, the child's tantrums began as a result of typical frustrations experienced by children his age. Over a period of months, as his parent became busier with other family needs, however, he discovered that expressing anger was an excellent way to get adult attention, and the frequency of these behaviors increased. As part of the management plan, his parent was instructed to ignore his anger and put him in his room for three minutes when he became physically violent toward others. She was also advised to increase time spent doing positive things with him, like playing games, going on walks, and having him help around the house. At day care he was given increased attention during times he was behaving well. Child care providers were asked to ignore him when he was aggressive toward other children and to shower a noticeable amount of attention on the other child.

Within a couple of weeks he stopped biting and seemed happier. Although he still had tantrums, these strategies gave his mother the feeling that she had some control over the situation.

Toddler: Oppositional Behavior

CASE ILLUSTRATION 3

A 32-month-old boy refuses to go to bed on time. He prolongs bedtime rituals by making numerous requests (e.g., for water, use of bathroom, and adjusting the door). He repeatedly leaves his bed. On many nights he finally falls asleep in the living room or his parents' bedroom while spending time with his parents.

CASE ILLUSTRATION 4

A father solicits your opinion on vitamin supplements to counterbalance his 28-month-old daughter's picky eating habits. She drinks apple juice and eats hot dogs and Honey-Nut Cheerios and little else. When these foods are not offered, she protests violently and eats nothing.

The behaviors described in these cases are typical for this age group. Toddlers commonly oppose parents for many sorts of issues, including the eating and bedtime cases illustrated here (e.g., getting dressed, putting toys away, and wearing a seat belt). A tendency to challenge parents' instructions subsides naturally as children grow older. When parents interpret a child's behavior as a personal offense, they react to the behavior in a way that creates additional conflict and heightens oppositional behavior. Therefore, it is important for clinicians to emphasize what is developmentally normative behavior. Sometimes oppositional behaviors can safely be ignored if they do not pose a serious threat to a child's health or safety. Ignoring the behavior can also help extinguish it by removing the reinforcing attention children receive when caregivers react emotionally. Coupling positive reinforcement (praising and rewarding good behavior) with ignoring undesirable behavior can be a powerful tool to reduce oppositional behavior. In the first case, praising and rewarding the child when he does eventually sleep in his own bed and avoiding punishment or criticism when he does not might be enough to change the undesired behavior.

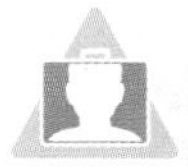

CASE ILLUSTRATION 4 (CONTD.)

In the second case, the child was offered three wholesome meals and one snack at preset times of the day. After telling their daughter once about the meal, parents were not to engage in any discussion with their child about the volume eaten. No other foods in the house were made available to her during this behavioral management period. Between meals this girl was allowed an unlimited quantity of water, but nothing else. After a difficult period of $1^1/_2$ days (thrown silverware, persistent crying, etc.), she began to nibble at new foods and to enjoy the positive attention for doing so. Although the child still enjoyed only a limited range of foods, parents were able to expand her repertoire to include broccoli, milk, and pasta.

Parents often worry about harming their child by restricting access to food after a missed meal, so they need to be reassured that this is not harmful and will ultimately improve nutrition. It is common for a well-meaning grandparent who resides in the home to "save" the child by sneaking her a cookie between meals (Case Illustration 4) or lying down with the child after a designated bedtime (Case Illustration 3). Such well-intentioned behaviors prolong the child's maladaptive behavior, extending the period of inadequate nutrition and sleep. It is imperative that clinicians invite all adult household members to their offices when prescribing a management plan to ensure that all involved endorse both the intent and methods. It is useful to write behavioral management "rules" down on a prescription pad to be taped to the refrigerator door. This helps prevent conflict among adult household members that may arise later. Clinicians should also routinely recommend follow-up visits to monitor progress once the management plan has been implemented.

Toddler: Toilet Training

Children should be developmentally ready before parents initiate toilet training. First, physiologic sphincter control is necessary. This usually develops between ages 1 and 2 years, and parents often know when their child is beginning to sense a bowel movement because of a characteristic grimace or stance. The ability to follow sequential instructions, the motivation to imitate parents, and the patience to sit on a potty should also be present. It is reasonable to try toilet training at age 2 years if these milestones have been achieved. But disinterest or undue difficulty should alert parents to terminate their attempt and wait 2–3 months before trying again. Some children may not be ready until age 3 while others are ready at 18 months.

Although a number of effective toilet training methods exist, only one method is described here. Place the potty in the bathroom the child typically uses and explain what it is for by associating it with the toilet that parents use. The child should be encouraged with praise to sit on the potty for a couple of minutes a day, initially with diaper and pants on and after a few days without them. The child should accompany the parent to empty soiled diapers into the potty. Parents should avoid commenting on the foul odor of the stool, as some children identify what they have produced as extensions of themselves. Gradually, the child should be asked to sit on the potty more frequently during the day, particularly if there is a time when bowel movements are likely to occur. Encourage the child to let the potty "catch" the stool. Parents should never scold a child for an inability to use the potty or for any "accidents." Night training, standing at urination, and using a larger toilet are secondary skills that should be introduced only after the child has mastered the basics.

Preschooler: Sexual Behaviors

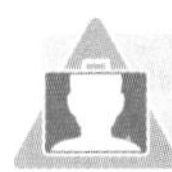

CASE ILLUSTRATION 5

A 3-year-old girl has shown her genitals to a peer and has commented on her father's genitals. One week prior to their visit to your office, the little girl began masturbating at home and occasionally in public. Not knowing how to react, her parents have been begging their daughter to stop. They are concerned that her sexualized behavior indicates something is wrong.

The clinician was initially concerned by these behaviors. Sexualized behavior in young children can be a sign of sexual abuse and should prompt a thorough evaluation. The nature of the sexualized behavior, frequency, persistence, and response to redirection by caregivers are among the factors that determine if the behavior is normal curiosity or a possible sign of abuse. After taking a careful history and completing a physical examination looking for signs of abuse, the clinician found no suspicions of sexual abuse, physical abuse or neglect, or recent emotional trauma. The clinician then instructed the parents to simply ignore or redirect the behaviors. On follow up, the clinician learned that these behaviors self-resolved within a week when they were no longer reinforced with parental attention.

School Age: Primary Nocturnal Enuresis

One definition for nocturnal enuresis is at least one bedwetting incident weekly for a boy older than 6 years of age or a girl older than 5 years of age. It is considered secondary enuresis if a child had been dry previously for a period greater than 6 months. This is one of the most commonly asked questions of pediatric primary care providers. Other urinary tract problems (infection, neurogenic bladder, etc.) can be ruled out with a basic history, physical examination, and if needed, urinalysis or other testing. Constipation is a common and underappreciated cause of enuresis. It is important to recognize that primary nocturnal enuresis is a self-limiting condition that resolves spontaneously. If a child and his or her parents are not bothered by it, then no treatment is necessary. This is worth pointing out to families whenever the option for intervention is offered.

Both children and parents must be motivated to treat this condition. When a child is not genuinely motivated to try something new in order to be dry, clinical attention should be directed toward the parents. Reducing parental anxiety around enuresis may limit unnecessary stress for the child. Children should never be punished for enuresis. Even if parents insist that their child help to change wet bed sheets, this task should be carried out with the same attitude as other household responsibilities that are expected of the child.

Commercially available enuresis alarms assist clinicians and parents in instituting "conditioning therapy." This method is clinically proven to be effective in reducing or eliminating bedwetting. The alarm awakens the child with the first few drops of urine, and eventually this teaches the child to awaken with the sensation of a full bladder. The child is still responsible for getting to the bathroom. The alarm is usually effective when used nightly for a couple of months. Setbacks might occur after removing the alarm, but these are often corrected by another trial with the device.

Desmopressin (DDAVP) tablets, an analog of antidiuretic hormone, is the pharmacologic therapy of choice for enuresis but is rarely necessary. Children who respond to this medication usually do so within 2 weeks. Relapses after withdrawal are not uncommon, however, and this therapy is best offered when the enuresis alarm has failed and for temporary relief (e.g., summer camp). Imipramine has also been shown to be useful in certain circumstances. Sphincter control exercises, fluid restrictions in the evening hours, and urine retention training may be tried, but these methods have shown only limited success.

School Age: Bullying

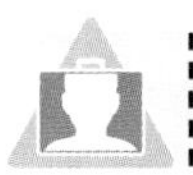

CASE ILLUSTRATION 6

During a routine health supervision visit of a 12-year-old girl, your customary questioning of social development reveals that this seventh grade student has been having problems with peers at school. She dislikes school and many of her classmates. Problems began about 3 months ago when another girl knocked an apple out of her hand and onto the cafeteria floor. Your patient tried to swat at the girl (but missed) and was reprimanded by the lunch monitor. Your patient broke into tears at that time and has since been the butt of jokes among a group of girls. False rumors about her have been spread at school and through social media.

Victims of bullying are likely to internalize bad situations, and it is likely that this child did not reveal much of her distress to her parents at the onset of her problems. Signs that a child might be a victim of bullying include an increasingly apparent dread of going to school, depressive signs, psychosomatic symptoms of anxiety (e.g., headaches and stomachaches), or worsening academic performance. Many children who internalize threats and fears of bullying may believe they are somehow to blame for the behavior of others. Some parents and school staff members view bullying among school-age children as a normal part of growing up and need to be educated about the serious harms of bullying.

Although some victims of bullying respond with aggression, many more are passive. Sometimes, certain personality characteristics or maladaptive behaviors have made children prone to becoming a victim of bullying. Problems such as having poor social skills, difficulty making friends, or even just being quiet, withdrawn, or shy can be sufficient. Victims are often those who easily become upset or have difficulty defending themselves in public. Some feel more comfortable socializing with adults than with age-appropriate peers.

Primary care providers need to assess the severity and persistence of bullying and the factors that might make a child vulnerable to bullies. Are there signs that this occurs in more than one environment, including the home? Have basic interventions such as making teachers aware of the bullying failed? Are there too few positive social interactions with one's own age group? For some, victimization is a sign that the child needs evaluation by a mental health specialist.

CASE ILLUSTRATION 6 (CONTD.)

The primary care physician made an agreement with the girl and her parents that they would work together on the problem until the bullying was over. The girl would share her experiences with her parents, despite embarrassment, and her parents would take these events seriously and keep her from facing them alone. The parents would speak with the school administration and suggest a plan. Further history taking revealed that she was an excellent artist. The parents were encouraged to praise her for her artistic accomplishments as well as other achievements, and they encouraged school staff to do the same. They also sought new opportunities for their daughter to exhibit these strengths to herself and to others.

The youngster's parents kept a record of bullying episodes and communicated these with the school principal. Eventually, enrollment in an after-school art class helped this girl develop new friendships, which improved her self-esteem and made her less vulnerable to being bullied.

Interventions initiated by primary care physicians may be inadequate to resolve bullying, and schools need to play a prominent role in detecting and managing bullying behavior. An experience with a bullied patient presents an excellent opportunity for a primary care provider to advocate for bullying prevention programs in local schools. Successful bullying prevention programs require more than just a single school counselor with a plan or policy. The Olweus Bullying Prevention Program has been relatively well researched and demonstrates encouraging results. Interventions should occur at several levels: school-wide interventions (e.g., staff training and development of school rules against bullying), classroom interventions (e.g., regular classroom meetings and class parent meetings), and individual interventions (interacting one-on-one with bullies and victims). School administrators and school staff must be committed, and each site needs a coordinator responsible for assuring that the plan is carried out.

It is equally important for primary care providers to help parents take note of signs that their children might be bullies. Bullies and victims often share problems with friendships, but they manifest these problems in different ways. Parents and clinicians need to be alert to children who are often in trouble at school (but are great at talking themselves out of blame) and who need to control their friends and peers. Often the only intervention for these bullies is to punish them, but punishment is typically ineffective because it does not address the underlying psychological factors associated with bullying. Close supervision and communication with the school are important interventions for parents, and assessment and treatment by a mental health specialist may be appropriate for persistent bullying behavior. When bullies have unaddressed psychological problems that lead to poor conduct, poor peer relationships, and emotional upheaval, they have a significantly higher chance of engaging in criminal activity later in life.

CONCLUSION

Pediatric primary care clinicians need to be comfortable evaluating and managing a wide variety of common behavioral challenges in children. Understanding normal development, family dynamics, and principles of behavior management can assist the provider in generating practical solutions for problematic behaviors. Educating parents about normal development and healthy differences in child temperament can reassure parents that an undesirable behavior is not pathologic. Assisting families with childhood behavioral challenges is an important part of primary care practice and builds a trusting relationship between providers and families.

SUGGESTED READINGS

American Academy of Pediatrics; Policy Statement. The future of pediatrics: mental health competencies for pediatric primary care. *Pediatrics* 2009;124(1):410–421.

Anda RF, Felitti VJ, Bremner JD, et al. The enduring effects of abuse and related adverse experiences in childhood. *Eur Arch Psychiatry Clin Neurosci* 2006;(256):174–186.

Brown ML, Pope AW, Brown EJ. Treatment of primary nocturnal enuresis in children: a review. *Child Care Health Dev* 2011;37(2):153–160.

Carlson EA, Sampson MC, Sroufe LA. Implications of attachment theory and research for developmental-behavioral pediatrics. *J Dev Behav Pediatr* 2003;24(5):364–379.

Dixon SD, Stein MT. *Encounters with Children: Pediatric Behavior and Development.* Philadelphia, PA: Mosby Elsevier; 2006.

Hagan JF, Shaw JS, Duncan PM, eds. *Bright Futures: Guidelines for Health Supervision of Infants, Children, and Adolescents.* 4th ed. Elk Grove Village, IL: American Academy of Pediatrics; 2017.

Hayutin LG, Reed-Knight B, Blount RL, Lewis J, McCormick ML. Increasing parent-pediatrician communication about children's psychosocial problems. *J Pediatr Psychol* 2009;34(10): 1155–1164.

Johnson SB, Riley AW, Granger DA, et al. The science of early life toxic stress for pediatric practice and advocacy. *Pediatrics* 2013;131(2):319–327.

Njoroge WF, Bernhart KP. Assessment of behavioral disorders in preschool-aged children. *Curr Psychiatry Rep* 2011;13(2):84–92.

Olweus D. School bullying: development and some important challenges. *Annu Rev Clin Psychol* 2013;9:751–780.

Sanci L, Lewis D, Patton G. Detecting emotional disorders in young people in primary care. *Curr Opin Psychiatry* 2010;23:318–323.

Sapienza JK, Masten AS. Understanding and promoting resilience in children and youth. *Curr Opin Psychiatry* 2011;24(4):267–273.

Schonhaut L, Armijo I, Schönstedt M, et al. Validity of the ages and stages questionnaires in term and preterm infants. *Pediatrics* 2013;131(5):e1468–e1474.

Zimmerman FJ, Christakis DA. Associations between content type of early media exposure and subsequent attentional problems. *Pediatrics* 2007;120(5):986–992.

Zuckerbrot RA, Cheung A, Jensen PS, et al. Guidelines for adolescent depression in primary care (GLAD-PC): part I. *Pediatrics* 2018;141(3):e20174081, 1–21.

WEBSITES

American Academy of Pediatrics Web site for parents. http://www.healthychildren.org. Accessed July 2018.

Cambridge Center for Behavioral Studies. http://www.behavior.org/. Accessed July 2018.

"Kids Health for Parents." http://kidshealth.org/. Accessed July 2018.

Olweus School Interventions for Bullying. http://www.clemson.edu/olweus. Accessed July 2018.

Pediatric Symptom Checklist. https://www.massgeneral.org/psychiatry/services/treatmentprograms.aspx?id=2088&display=forms. Accessed August 2019.

Search Institute. http://www.search-institute.org. Accessed July 2018.

Adolescents

13

Lawrence S. Friedman, MD

INTRODUCTION

This chapter offers a practical behavioral framework to assist those who provide health care to teenagers. Stages of adolescent development along with behavioral correlates are discussed, as are suggestions for effective patient–doctor communication, interviewing, and provision of health services. From a physiologic perspective, adolescence is the interval between the onset of puberty and the cessation of body growth. In psychosocial and behavioral terms, it is the time during which adult body image and sexual identity emerge; independent moral standards, intimate interpersonal relationships, vocational goals, and health behaviors develop; and the separation from parents takes place. Although some of these tasks may begin prior to puberty and evolve into adulthood, they provide the foundation for understanding adolescent behavior.

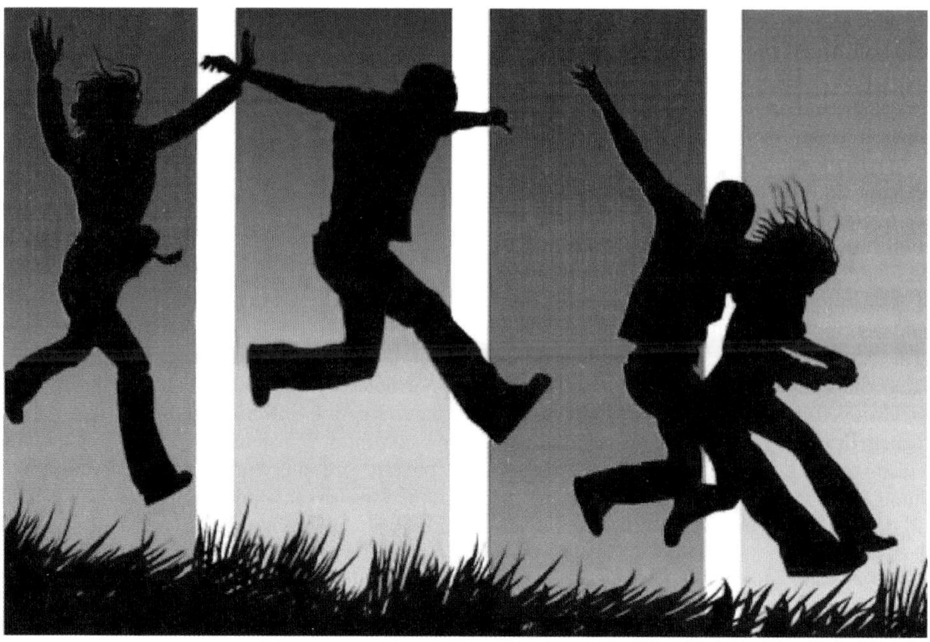

Health Status & Trends

Most teenagers are healthy. Compared with other age groups, mortality rates for teenagers are low. The majority of health problems in teenagers are behavior related and include unwanted pregnancy; sexually transmitted infections (STIs); weapon carrying; interpersonal violence; suicidal ideation; alcohol, cigarette, and illicit drug use including inappropriate use of prescription medications and various forms of opiates; and dietary and exercise patterns. Nationally, accidents are the leading cause of death for most populations of teenagers, although homicide (often gang related) leads in some geographic locations. Socioeconomic status and population density, rather than ethnic or racial grouping, define the neighborhoods most at risk for interpersonal violence-related death. The most common reasons for acute medical office visits for teenagers are routine or sports physicals, upper respiratory infections, and acne. One of the major challenges to a provider caring for teenagers is eliciting a history that reveals health-risk behaviors. Because most adolescent mortality and morbidity are preventable and because many behaviors such as sexual practices, diet, exercise, and substance use that result in adult disease begin in adolescence, ignoring this age group means missing a major public health opportunity.

In 1992, the American Medical Association published Guidelines for Adolescent Preventive Services (GAPS), the first set of developmentally and behaviorally appropriate comprehensive health care guidelines for adolescents. These guidelines remain the gold standard to this day. They emphasize anticipatory, preventive, and patient-centered services. Guidelines for Adolescent Preventive Services suggest that promotion of adolescent health and prevention of disease involve a partnership encompassing patients, parents, schools, communities, and health care providers. Although these guidelines have existed for several decades, and have been shown to be valuable as care standards and as quality measures, there is little evidence that they are being widely implemented.

Adolescent health outcomes—perhaps more than for any other population—are closely linked to cultural, educational, political, and economic policies at the local and national level. Guns and bullying are both relevant examples. For example, the availability of guns is not a problem that the health practitioner can resolve during an office visit, yet making them less available would substantially benefit the health of many teenagers. There would very likely be less depression and suicidal ideation if more schools instituted zero tolerance programs for bullying and developed programs that promoted diversity and tolerance.

The Internet and all forms of related electronic communication, including social media, texting, and instant messaging, have profoundly changed the way we all interrelate socially and how we receive and disseminate health-related and behavioral information. Adolescents and young adults are, and will likely continue to be, at the forefront of this communication transformation. It is essential that those providing care to adolescents understand how these communication developments might have beneficial and detrimental influences on this population. Social media are a good example. Social media and electronic interaction for adolescents with chronic diseases might serve as a positive influence to improve medication compliance and decrease the sense of isolation. Conversely, bullying through social media has been the cause of depression and suicide. It is especially important to understand these influences because there is compelling evidence that teens who feel connected to parents, school, and community are less likely to participate in health-compromising behavior than teens who feel isolated or disconnected. It should be expected that the evolution of new forms of electronic communication will continue to play a role in how teenagers connect to all facets of their environment including those that relate to health and well-being. We have also entered an age of virtual medical visits through various forms of telemedicine that theoretically makes medical care more accessible to teenagers but simultaneously raises issues of confidentiality, parental consent, and privacy.

STAGES OF DEVELOPMENT

Medical services for teenagers need to be appropriate for each developmental stage. Each of the three recognized developmental stages in adolescence is distinguished by physical, cognitive, and behavioral hallmarks. Not all adolescents fit perfectly into each phase, and they often progress at different rates from one phase to the next. Moreover, rates of physical, cognitive, and behavioral development may not be congruent. For example, a 14-year-old girl who is physically mature may be emotionally and cognitively unable to decide about sexual intimacy and the potential consequences.

Early Adolescence (Ages 11–14)

PHYSICAL

Rapid growth causes physical and body image changes. Many teenagers question whether their growth is "normal," and commonly there is a good deal of somatic preoccupation and anxiety. Gynecomastia, for example (a common transient problem for boys), may cause concern and prevent participation in physical education class. Because the topic may be too embarrassing for an already self-conscious teenager, clinician-initiated reassurance is essential when the condition is identified during a physical examination. Early or later onset of puberty has widely variable effects. Early puberty may be associated with the increased likelihood of weight concern and excessive dieting and other eating disorders in girls, but it may result in greater self-esteem and athletic prowess in boys. Because self-esteem is linked closely with physical development and peer group attractiveness, teens who develop later than their peers may have self-esteem problems. Among early adolescents, questions and concerns about menstruation, masturbation, wet dreams, and the size of their breasts (too large or too small) and genitals are common. These questions need to be anticipated and specifically and carefully addressed. Endocrine disorders related to sexual maturation are likely to emerge; early diagnosis and treatment can improve health and self-esteem.

Social

In adolescence, peer group involvement increases and family involvement decreases. Friendships are idealized and are mostly same gender. Close peer relationships coupled with curiosity about body development may result in homosexual and other sexual experimentation, anxiety, and fear. Although some heterosexual relationships are initiated, contact with the opposite sex frequently occurs in groups. Often by this age adolescents have access to the Internet, participate in social media, and use cell phones. How they are used and potentially monitored should become an important topic of family discussion.

Cognitive

The transition from concrete to abstract thinking begins. Because experience and emotion play important roles in decision making, improved cognition alone is not enough to prevent many teenagers from making impulsive decisions with little regard for consequences. Increased cognitive ability linked with the search for identity often leads teenagers to test limits both at home and at school. Daydreaming is common.

Middle Adolescence (Ages 15–17)

Physical

The issues of early adolescence may continue, although most physical development is complete by the end of this phase.

Social

Independence, identity, and autonomy struggles intensify. Peer groups may become more important than family to some teenagers and result in increasing teen–parent conflict. Experimentation with alcohol, drugs, and sex is common. A sense of invincibility coupled with impulsiveness leads to relatively high rates of automobile accidents and interpersonal violence. Suicide, impulsively linked to failed love relationships, or poor self-esteem because of difficulty finding peer group acceptance may also occur during this phase. Despite adhering to peer group norms regarding music, dress, and appearance (including body piercing, tattoos, clothes, hair color, and makeup), the expression of individuality is common. Many teenagers find identity and support in school, sports, community, or church activities. For teenagers whose support systems or community resources are inadequate, gangs may supplement personal strength and provide a sense of identity. Teenagers from alienated and disenfranchised ethnic groups are at particular risk for gang activity. In spite of improving cultural acceptance, gay, lesbian, and transgendered teenagers may feel increased isolation, alienation, and bullying (see Chapter 17). This may lead to depression, sexual promiscuity, or suicide. The Internet provides easy linkage to social media for minority youth, such as those with chronic diseases, who in the past might have felt isolated and now can gain access to social and psychological support. Those same media, however, also make it much easier for sexual encounters and resulting exposure to STIs or unintended pregnancy.

Cognitive

Improved reasoning and abstraction allow for closer interpersonal relationships and empathy in this group. Evaluation of future academic and vocational plans becomes important. Poor school performance may heighten anxiety and concern about vocational choices and lead to "escape" in drugs and alcohol. Practical guidance that identifies strengths and builds self-esteem can help avoid frustration and failure.

Late Adolescence (Ages 18–24)

Physical

Body growth is usually no longer a concern. The quest to become comfortable with one's physical appearance often continues throughout adulthood.

Social

If the adolescent's development has occurred within the context of a supportive family, community, school, and peer environment, individual identity formation and separation will be complete. In reality, however, at least some developmental issues usually remain unresolved into adulthood. Late adolescents typically spend more time developing monogamous interpersonal relationships and less time seeking peer group support. Ideally, decision making, based on an individualized value system, is modulated by limit setting and compromise.

Cognitive

Vocational goals should now be set in practical terms, and there should be realistic expectations about education and work.

ADOLESCENTS & THE MEDICAL INTERVIEW

A general health assessment should include a review of systems and an evaluation of health-related behavior. This should include risk factors for accidents, STIs, including human immunodeficiency virus (HIV), pregnancy, interpersonal violence (including past physical or sexual abuse), nutrition, substance use including prescription medication abuse, exercise, sleep, learning, and mental health problems. Guidance about promoting healthful behaviors and preventing disease should be integrated into the discussion. Inclusion of these factors is considered community standard of care for adolescents. Documentation of health encounters should be done electronically; it is therefore recommended that a standard protocol be developed with discrete searchable fields, so that all elements described above can be documented and searched for quality assessment. From the patient's perspective, the clinician's inquiries and assessment of some behaviors may be viewed as embarrassing, intrusive, or trivial. It is therefore helpful to explain, prior to questioning, that (1) the same questions are asked of all patients and that (2) the encounter goal is patient self-awareness and health education. During the interview it is important to reinforce and praise healthy decisions, such as sexual abstinence.

Confidentiality

Certain ground rules are important. Ensure the adolescent that, unless homicide or suicide is threatened or abuse is reported, all conversations are confidential, and the information will not be shared with parents, teachers, or other authorities without permission. Discussions about sex and drugs should always occur in private unless otherwise requested by the patient. If the patient is accompanied by a parent, solicit parental concerns, and then ask the adult to leave the room and conduct the interview in private. It is also helpful to let the parent know (if present) about the confidential nature of the patient–clinician conversation.

Although most teenagers want to receive health information and discuss personal behavior, these discussions must generally be initiated by the physician. Many teenagers are not accustomed to interacting in such participatory, nonjudgmental conversations with adults. The willingness of a teenager to share personal or intimate information depends on the perceived receptiveness of the provider. Teenagers need to feel that they have permission to share personal, behavior-related information. For example, it is usually not difficult for patients and clinicians to discuss routine chronic medical conditions such as diabetes or asthma. Control of these conditions in some teenagers, however, may be related more to dietary indiscretions and cigarette use, than to insulin or inhaler use. Such health-compromising behaviors must be identified before they can be dealt with; comments, facial expressions, or body language indicating disapproval can undermine the patient's willingness to disclose confidential behavior (Table 13-1).

Most electronic medical record systems now include patient web-portals that allow secure communication between patient and provider. This type of system potentially makes communication easier and faster for all involved. Issues around confidentially and parental access make independent use by minors problematic, although it is often supported by many parents. See Table 13-2 for Quality and Safety suggestions.

Table 13-1. Interview suggestions.

1. Ensure doctor–patient confidentiality. Do not inquire about health-related behaviors in front of parents.
2. Use the HEADSS format to organize the interview.
3. Assess the patient's cognitive and developmental level through interactive dialogue.
4. Initiate discussions about behavior and offer anticipatory guidance that is culturally and developmentally appropriate.
5. Listen actively to patients' opinions and perspective.
6. Be familiar with and refer to local resources for cases of domestic violence, runaways, and substance abuse.
7. Include patients in discussing and making all diagnostic and therapeutic decisions.
8. Review the behavioral stages of development with parents. Emphasize the importance of instilling confidence and building self-esteem in their children.
9. Reinforce good behavior. Congratulate teenagers who do not use drugs and who are not sexually active.
10. Address all teenagers with respect, and be nonjudgmental about their behaviors and traits.

Legal Issues

Many practitioners worry about the legality of evaluating and treating teenagers without parental consent. Because laws vary by state, it is essential to become familiar with the applicable local statutes. Many states permit the diagnosis and treatment of teenagers with sex-, drug-, and alcohol-related problems without

Table 13-2. Recommendations for care quality.

1. Written documentation (electronic documentation ideal for audits) of behavior-related health risk factors
   a. Alcohol and drugs
   b. Tobacco
   c. Violence/gang involvement
   d. Seat belt use
   e. Helmet use
   f. Firearms and storage
   g. Sexual behavior
   h. Nutrition/diet/exercise
2. *Chlamydia* screening in patients who are sexually involved
3. Vaccines (assuming up-to-date with childhood vaccination)
   a. HPV males and females
   b. Meningococcal booster
   c. Tdap
   d. Influenza

parental notification or consent. States do vary at the age about which teens can receive such services without parental permission. Likewise, most states permit medical care if a condition is potentially life threatening. Documentation of the rationale leading to the decision to proceed without parental permission, in a potential "life-threatening" situation, is essential.

Interview Organization

A comprehensive health-risk assessment should cover issues dealing with home, education, activities, drug use, sexual practices, and suicidal ideation (HEADSS). Using the HEADSS format helps with organization and standardization. Assessing cognitive ability using interactive dialogue needs to be done in the first few minutes of the interview. The following interview goals and questions facilitate communication.

Home

1. **Goal**—Determine household structure, family structure and function, conflict-resolution skills, the possibility of domestic violence, and presence of chronic illness in the family (see Chapter 11).
2. **Questions**—"Who lives where you live?" If only one parent is at home, the interviewer should inquire about the other parent's whereabouts, visitation pattern, reasons for leaving (especially domestic violence and substance abuse), and whether the teen moves back and forth between parents. Teenagers caught between divorced parents or those who feel neglected may "act out" and get into trouble to gain parental attention, sometimes in the hope that their problems will reunite separated parents. For single-parent families, the patient can be asked, "Does your mom or dad date? How do you get along with the people he or she dates?" Questions about domestic violence should include "What happens when people argue in your house?" and "Does anyone get hurt during arguments? How about you?" and "What if someone has been drinking or using drugs and they argue?" and "Have you ever seen your mother hit by anyone?" "Are there guns in your house?" If there are, ask if they are always locked and who has a key. Educate parents and patients about accidental gunshots. Ask about siblings, including their health and whereabouts. Somatization may be learned by observing a family member who receives attention for a chronic medical condition. Learning about extended family members living in the household is also important and will likely be revealed with the first question above.

Education

1. **Goal**—Identify attention deficit hyperactivity disorder (ADHD) and other learning disabilities, school performance, cognitive ability, and vocational potential.
2. **Questions**—"What grade are you in?" "What type of grades do you get?" "How do they compare with your grades last year?" Falling grades may indicate family, mental health, or substance-abuse problems. "Have you ever been told you had a learning problem?" "Can you see the blackboard?" Most teenagers respond that everything in school is okay. Specific questions about courses and content need to be asked, including the student's favorite and worst subjects and his or her career aspirations. Generally, teenagers who perform well in school are less likely to participate in multiple health-risk behaviors. The teen should be asked about attendance and truancy or other school troubles. Teenagers with drug problems may enjoy going to school because, although they may rarely attend class, school is where they visit friends and purchase or sell drugs. Students who get all "A's" should be asked about school-related stress and what would happen if they did not receive high grades. Depression and even suicide can be related to unrealistic grade expectations by teenagers and their parents.

Activities

1. **Goal**—Evaluate the patient's social interactions, Internet use and purposes of use, interests, and self-esteem.
2. **Questions**—"What do you do for fun?" "Are you involved in school, community, or religious activities, such as youth groups, clubs, or sports?" Self-esteem is often related to successful participation in these activities. Teenagers actively involved in "productive" activities are less likely to participate in delinquent behavior. The clinician should ask about gang or fraternity/sorority membership, either of which can be a source of inappropriate peer pressure. Gangs may provide the strongest sense of family or community available to some teenagers.

Questions should be asked about dietary habits, including the frequency and amount of "junk" food, who cooks, and dieting or self-induced vomiting (see Chapter 23). It is also important to inquire about patients' physical activities, and to educate and to make recommendations about regular exercise, protective headgear, and seatbelts. Internet assessment should include types of sites visited, amount of time daily, and purpose of use.

Drugs

1. **Goal**—Evaluate the patient's current habits, patterns of use, and the genetic or environmental risk factors (Table 13-3). Distinguish between those who drink because of social, cultural, and peer pressure; those who are genetically predisposed; and those who

Table 13-3. Substance abuse risk factors for adolescents.

1. Family history of use
2. Low self-esteem and body image
3. Depression or thought disorder
4. Antisocial personality traits
5. Peer and cultural pressures

drink or use illicit drugs because of comorbid mental health problems.

2. **Questions**—It is less threatening to begin by asking, "Are you aware of alcohol or drug use at your school?" and "Do any of your friends drink or use drugs?" followed by "Have you ever tried alcohol or drugs?" The clinician should inquire specifically about cigarettes, alcohol, marijuana, recreational "pills" (e.g., ecstasy and ketamine), cocaine, lysergic acid diethylamide (LSD), crystal methamphetamine, anabolic steroids, heroin, and prescription pills for problems such as ADHD or pain that are used inappropriately. The quantity, frequency, circumstances, and family patterns of use are important. To learn about family drinking, ask specific questions about each parent and both maternal and paternal grandparents, including whether anyone in the family attends Alcoholics Anonymous (AA) or other self-help groups. When parents do not recognize or admit to a problem, a child may not identify them as alcoholics. The teenager should be asked to describe the parent's pattern of alcohol use. "Have you ever seen your mother or father drunk?" If the answer is yes, then ask "When and how frequently?" The CRAFFT questions have been validated as a useful brief screening test for teenagers suspected of substance abuse (Table 13-4). Two or more YES answers on the CRAFFT indicate a significant problem.

Table 13-4. CRAFFT* questions.

1. Have you ever ridden in a **C**AR driven by someone (including yourself) who was "high" or had been using alcohol or drugs?
2. Do you ever use alcohol/drugs to **R**ELAX, feel better about yourself, or fit in?
3. Do you ever use alcohol/drugs while you are by yourself, **A**LONE?
4. Do your family or **F**RIENDS ever tell you that you should cut down on drinking or drug use?
5. Do you ever **F**ORGET things you did while using alcohol or drugs?
6. Have you gotten into **T**ROUBLE while you were using alcohol or drugs?

*Two or more YES answers indicate a significant problem.

Recognition of a parental problem is also essential. Even the best treatment program will fail if a teenager is discharged back into the home of an actively using parent. The willingness of parents to change either their own drinking or family behavior patterns is one of the best predictors of adolescent treatment success.

Among many teenagers, the use of drugs and alcohol is often not considered abnormal or dangerous. Only about 5–10% of teenage drinkers or drug users develop substance-abuse problems as adults. Because serious physical consequences, other than accidents, usually do not occur until later in life, there is little negative association with alcohol or drug use. Abused, neglected, disabled, or chronically ill teenagers may consider drugs or alcohol one of the few things that, at least temporarily, make them feel good and accepted by peers. If legal involvement, school problems, or family conflict are present, it is important to assess the role of alcohol and drugs. Even if use seems minimal, it should be pointed out that problems are best solved sober.

Referral to a substance-abuse expert is indicated when use significantly interferes with school, family, or social functioning. Anticipatory guidance should address age-appropriate concerns. Advising teenagers to stop smoking cigarettes because of the possibility of future lung cancer and heart disease is usually meaningless. Talking about wrinkled skin, bad breath, and yellow teeth is much more relevant to body image concerns and far more likely to prevent or stop cigarette use. Similarly, the association between alcohol and date rape is more important to teenage girls than are other future consequences.

SEX

1. **Goal**—Determine the level of the patient's sexual involvement and sexuality, use of birth control, protection against STIs, and any history of abuse.
2. **Questions**—An opening question such as "Have you ever been sexually involved with anyone?" is preferable to "Are you sexually active?" The word *active* is notoriously misinterpreted. Questions need to be open ended and should not assume heterosexual orientation. Assumptions about boyfriends or girlfriends inhibit discussion or questions about homosexual partners or feelings. Because teenagers frequently practice serial monogamy, the sequential number of different partners and their ages should be determined. Ask whether they have ever met anyone on the Internet for sexual reasons and the circumstances related to that encounter. A 15-year-old teenager with a peer group partner is at less risk for STIs, especially HIV, than is one with a substantially older partner. For the sexually involved, discuss birth control techniques and condoms. One of the most

common reasons for not using a condom is the belief that birth control pills provide adequate protection against STIs. When appropriate, physicians should reinforce sexual abstinence with congratulations and support.

Sexual abuse is unfortunately common. A history of such incidents should be sought by asking, "Have you ever been touched sexually when you did not want to be?" Obtaining this history may be pivotal in helping a teenager who has developed abuse-related behavioral problems, such as sexual promiscuity, depression, substance abuse, delinquency, or an eating or somatization disorder.

Unwanted pregnancy among teenagers is still unfortunately common. Risk factors are complex but include ignorance, lack of access to family planning services, cultural acceptance, and poor self-esteem.

SUICIDE

1. **Goal**—Identify serious mental health problems and distinguish them from normal adolescent affect and moodiness. Primary risk factors are listed in Table 13-5.

   Distinguishing significant psychiatric illness from normal fluctuations in a teenager's affect is challenging. In spite of the general perception to the contrary, most teenagers are not maladjusted, and the rates of mental health problems are no higher than in adults. Few teenagers announce that they are feeling depressed or are in emotional turmoil. Depression may be reflected in sexual promiscuity, drug and alcohol abuse, or in the commission of violent and delinquent acts. Chronic somatic complaints such as headache, abdominal pain, or chest pain without an identifiable biological explanation may also indicate depression secondary to abuse.
2. **Questions**—Practitioners should identify vegetative signs of depression, such as sleep disturbance, decreased appetite, hopelessness, lethargy, continuous thoughts about suicide, hallucinations, or illogical thoughts. It should also be noted that many of these symptoms may also be caused by substance abuse. Evaluation of lethargy should be done from the patient's perspective. Energy may be low relative to the parents' desires or expectations—but sufficient for the teenager. There may be insufficient energy to clean, help with household chores, or complete homework but plenty of energy available to play sports, go on a date, party with friends, travel miles, and wait for hours to obtain concert tickets.

Table 13-5. Risk factors for major depression and suicide.

1. Prior episode of serious depression or suicide
2. Family history of suicide or mental health problems
3. History of victimization
4. Substance abuse or dependency
5. Gay or lesbian sexual identity
6. Availability of handguns (increases rate of success)
7. Recent loss of significant friends or family
8. Extreme family, school, or social stress

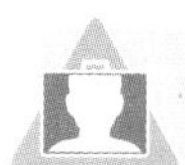

CASE ILLUSTRATION 1

Lauren is a 15-year-old girl admitted to the hospital with an arm fracture requiring surgical repair. The fracture occurred during cheerleading practice while climbing a pyramid of other cheerleaders. She reported being distracted while climbing, lost concentration, and fell to the ground. During the admission history the patient was talkative and easily distracted. Although she did not report taking any medications to the admitting nurse, when asked "are you supposed to be taking" any medications, Lauren reported that she should be taking medication for ADHD (see Chapter *28). She had not taken medication for the last several days because she was staying with a friend and did not want her friend to know that she took medication.*

This case illustrates several important adolescent issues. First, teenagers may concretely interpret questions. When Lauren was asked by the nurse if she was taking any medication, she answered honestly. A combination of clinical judgment at the time of interview related to Lauren's inattentiveness, knowledge that teenagers may interpret concretely, and that they may not make the connection between behavior and health consequences are all important to this case. Second, teenagers seek peer conformance. Medication compliance problems may relate to avoiding peer awareness of medications and, therefore, being labeled as different. Taking medication at school, camp, or at the house of a friend may all make a teenager feel different. Lastly, instructions about medications should be given in terms of what is important to the patient. Lauren may have known that medication was beneficial for school performance, but may not have realized that it would improve concentration with other tasks that required focus and attention.

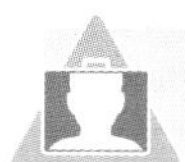

CASE ILLUSTRATION 2

Two days after sustaining minor injuries in a traffic accident, Jeff, a 17-year-old teenager, comes to the physician's office complaining of left shoulder pain.

He is accompanied by his mother, who is concerned because Jeff was also recently arrested for driving under the influence of alcohol. There is no history of medical or behavioral problems, although, on questioning, his mother describes a 12-month history of moodiness and falling school grades. Using the HEADSS format assessment, the physician assesses Jeff's health risks:

Home: Jeff lives at home with his biological mother and father. The parents are first-generation immigrants who both work full time. There are few arguments at home, and Jeff describes both parents as stoic, religious, and unemotional.

Education: Although he was an above-average student until last year, Jeff's education is now being adversely affected by his truancy and lack of interest.

Activity: Although Jeff previously played several sports at school, watching television is now his favorite activity.

Drugs: Jeff admits to using drugs frequently. He drinks alcohol at least twice a week and smokes marijuana daily. Since this use is no more frequent than that of his friends, he does not consider it excessive.

Sex: Jeff has no steady sexual partners, but has had several short-term relationships.

Suicide: Jeff denies being suicidal or depressed. When asked about significant losses, however, he becomes tearful and talks hesitantly about his older brother, a construction worker, who died accidentally 2 years ago. Since the burial, his brother was never talked about at home.

The connection between increased substance use, declining grades, and the brother's death seems obvious. Because the substance use began insidiously, and significant trouble did not occur until more than a year after his brother's death, neither Jeff nor his parents associated the events. Furthermore, this is a family that seemingly does not share emotions, and Jeff never learned how to discuss his feelings. In this case, simply learning about his drug use, home situation, school performance, and activities was not enough. The facts all confirmed his substance abuse but did not explain it. With a teenager who previously has been without significant behavioral problems, it is crucial to search for personal or family events, including losses, which underlie and precipitate behavior change.

Both Jeff and his parents must be made aware of the connection between the substance use and the brother's death. It is imperative that Jeff acknowledge his drug problem and be referred to a practitioner experienced in treating adolescents with substance-abuse problems (see Chapter 24). Although Jeff should respond to psychotherapy that addresses his grief and loss, psychotherapy may not be effective if mind-altering substances are being used concomitantly.

SPECIFIC AT-RISK POPULATIONS

Homeless & Runaway Teenagers

There is a heterogeneous group of between 500,000 and 2 million homeless teenagers in the United States. Some are homeless because their families are, some live on the streets for brief periods of time, and others find shelter with friends or relatives. Those who leave home, do not return, and no longer depend on parents for financial support or shelter constitute a significant proportion and may be more precisely called *throwaways.* Before they leave home, these teenagers have usually had repeated contacts with social service agencies and have histories of severe parental conflict and high rates of physical and sexual abuse. Family abandonment because of sexual orientation is sometimes a factor. The social network designed to protect them has failed, and their experience of neglect, abuse, and abandonment results in a distrust of adults and institutions.

Leaving home and living on the streets may initially be a liberating experience. Once on the street, multiple substance use is common, often becoming a short-term pleasant escape from an otherwise dismal existence. Survival often depends on trading sex for drugs, food, or shelter. Other survival techniques, such as selling drugs and theft, create risks for interpersonal violence and victimization. Poor self-esteem, depression, and suicidal ideation are common in this group. Usually—within weeks or months—the liberating experience of independence becomes one of desperation and hopelessness.

The initial medical evaluation may seem overwhelming. Many of these patients qualify for emancipated minor legal status and may be eligible for Medicaid or other entitlements. Distrust of adults, the inability to navigate a complicated health system, and reluctance to disclose personal information may, however, keep them from receiving benefits and proper health care. It is important for the clinician to prioritize such a patient's health issues and be familiar with community referral sources. Shelter, food, safety, social support, substance abuse and mental health counseling, and medical evaluation are all usually necessary. Developing a trusting working relationship is essential and may require several visits. Keeping medical appointments and complying with referrals may be complicated by a reversed sleep–wake cycle. In some cases, it may be that texting can be used beneficially for appointment and medication reminders. As with other teenagers, questions about sex and drugs are best kept in a medical context; it should be made clear that they are asked only because of their health implications. Rather than asking whether a teenager has been a "prostitute," asking, "Have you ever had sex in order to obtain drugs, food, or a place to sleep?" is nonjudgmental and will be readily understood. Questions about sexual orientation may be confusing to a teenager with a history of sexual abuse and survival sex and may provoke anxiety and shame. These issues are best raised after a stable living situation and support system have been established.

Chronic Disease & Disability

At least 2 million teenagers in the United States have chronic disabilities or diseases. Although this is a diverse group, its members share some similar behavioral issues. Unlike other teenagers whose identity and self-esteem are molded by the acceptance of a peer group, chronically ill or disabled teenagers have limited ability to conform and often have poor self-esteem. Too frequently this leads to depression, family conflict, and social isolation.

Like those of other teenagers—issues usually revolve around physical, social, and sexual development. Frank discussions, including realistic assessments of their hopes and expectations, need to be initiated by the physician. It is crucial to identify and encourage the interests and skills that may realistically be expected to strengthen self-esteem. Predictors of successful coping include friendships with healthy as well as ill or disabled peers, parents who are not overly protective, involvement with family activities, and appropriate household responsibilities.

Chronically ill teenagers are often "noncompliant" with medical regimens. Adolescence is no less a time of experimentation, self-discovery, and testing of limits for the chronically ill teen than for other teens, and chronically ill teenagers—like others—are often noncompliant. Issues about compliance are often issues about control and of testing of limits. The struggle for independence conflicts with the limitations of the disability itself as well the relationship with parents and health care providers. Supportive social media for teens with similar disorders might greatly decrease the sense of social isolation, and texting reminders has the potential for improving medication compliance. Table 13-6 lists some suggestions for ways of improving compliance.

Table 13-6. Strategies for improving compliance.

1. Have patients participate in all therapeutic and diagnostic decisions.
2. Discuss developmentally appropriate consequences of noncompliance. For instance, the renal or neurologic complications of poor diabetes control will not seem very important to a 14-year-old teenager. Emphasize the positive instead—such as how proper glucose control will allow continued participation in sports and other peer activities.
3. Parents need guidance on how to balance protectiveness with their teenager's need to make independent decisions. Role-playing in specific scenarios may be helpful.
4. When possible, communicate directly with the patient without using the parent as a conduit. Let patients know that their opinions and questions are important.
5. Refer patients and parents to local peer support groups such as diabetes, asthma, and epilepsy societies. Support groups exist for almost all chronic illnesses and can usually be found through local telephone directories or agencies such as United Way.

Gay, Lesbian, & Transgender Youth

Gay, lesbian, and transgender teenagers are at risk for social isolation, depression, STIs, substance abuse, and interpersonal violence. The relationships they develop with a health care provider may help them cope with the negative stereotyping they receive from other parts of society. A nonjudgmental and supportive attitude by the clinician helps lessen the weight of such cultural negativity.

Although some teenagers may volunteer information about their sexuality concerns or ideation, many do not unless they are specifically asked or given permission to do so. Some teens may have feelings of anxiety, shame, and guilt about same-sex experiences. Such experiences are common, especially among young adolescents who may not yet have firm sexual identity. Such experiences do not necessarily reflect future sexual orientation. The risk of HIV infection increases when gay teenage boys have older partners, who themselves may have had multiple partners. Inquiry about Internet use and actual sexual encounters is essential to get a sense of potential health-risk behaviors and exposure to STIs. Table 13-7

Table 13-7. Recommendations for addressing needs of gay or lesbian youth.

1. Assess the patient's level of comfort and self-acceptance.
2. Evaluate and discuss external stressors, such as parents, school, and the patient's social and religious environment. Refer the patient (and parents, if necessary) to mental health experts if the stressors are severe and interfere with daily activities.
3. Reassure the patient that from a medical perspective, homosexuality is a normal variant like left-handedness.
4. Refer patients to local gay youth groups for peer support; most cities and colleges provide resources for lesbian and gay youth, and telephone directories usually list local resources. Refer parents to local parent support groups, especially the local chapter of Parents and Friends of Lesbian and Gay Youth (P-FLAG).

lists some suggestions for working with gay and lesbian youth.

SUGGESTED READINGS

Committee on Adolescence. Policy statement: achieving quality health care services for adolescents. *Pediatrics* 2016;138(2).

Committee on Substance Abuse. Policy statement: alcohol use by youth and adolescents: a pediatric concern. *Pediatrics* 2010;5:1078–1087.

Confidentiality Protections for Adolescents and Young Adults in the Health Care Billing and Insurance Claims Process. Position Paper of the Society for Adolescent Medicine. *J Adolesc Health* 2016;58:374–377.

Elster AB, Kuznets NJ, eds. *AMA Guidelines for Adolescent Preventive Services (GAPS).* Philadelphia, PA: Williams & Wilkins; 1994.

Kann L, McManus T, Harris W, et al. Youth Risk Behavior Surveillance—United States 2017. *MMWR Surveill Summ* 2018;67(8):1–114.

Media Use in School-Aged Children and Adolescents, Policy Statement. *Pediatrics* 2016;138(5).

WEBSITES

A Consensus Statement on Health Care Transitions for Young Adults With Special Health Care Needs. American Academy of Pediatrics, American Academy of Family Physicians and American College of Physicians-American Society of Internal Medicine. *Pediatrics* 2002;110:1304. http://pediatrics.aappublications.org/content/110/Supplement_3/1304.full.pdf. Accessed February 2019.

Official Position Papers on Multiple Relevant Topics. Society for Adolescent Medicine Web site. https://www.adolescenthealth.org/Advocacy/Position-Papers-Statements.aspx. Accessed February 2019.

Older Patients

14

Elizabeth Eckstrom, MD, MPH; Leah Kalin, MD; & Nicholas Kinder, MSN, APN, AGNP-C

INTRODUCTION

We are an aging society. In 2014, 14.5% (46.3 million) of the U.S. population was 65 and over. This will increase to 23.5% (98 million) by 2060. During this same time period, the share of the older population that is non-Hispanic white is projected to drop from 78.3% to 54.6%. Those living with Alzheimer's disease and other dementias could nearly triple from 5 million in 2013 to 14 million in 2050. The oldest of the old, those over 85, are expected to reach 19 million by 2050, and present special challenges to health care providers. Good clinical care of older adults relies on knowledge of normal aging and the common diseases of older age. This chapter focuses on these aspects of mental health and illness.

At a population level, older adults are staying in the workforce longer, having "encore" careers, contributing to our economy in a myriad of ways, and pushing the boundaries of social engagement. Eighty-seven percent of people 65+ want to stay in their own homes and communities as they age ("aging in place"). Health care and aging services providers will need to adapt to changing demographics and perceptions of aging. For example, an increased sensitivity to terminology about aging is critical. "Elderly" and "senior" can have negative implications, whereas "elder" and "older adult" are more respectful. Rather than using the term "dementia facility," "memory care home" speaks to the fact that this setting truly is an elder's home. Frameworks Institute, with support from AARP, the American Geriatrics Society, and others developed a model called "Reframing Aging" that offers tools and thought pieces to improve public understanding of older adults' needs and societal contributions and is valuable for all older adult health and community providers.

NORMAL PSYCHOLOGICAL AGING

Many older adults are active, engaged, pleasure seeking, and remain curious and continue to learn throughout their lives. Temperament (i.e., energy, intensity, and reactivity) remains stable through adult life, whereas personality (learned behavior patterns) undergoes refinement and change over time in most healthy adults. Predictable changes in intellect occur in most people as they age. Changes that are normal with aging include problems with multitasking; slowed speech, word retrieval, and naming; decline in episodic memory (a conscious recollection of a person's experienced events); and decline in motor coordination, motor response time, and balance and gait. Impairments that are not normal with aging and are associated with dementia include decline in visual-motor tasks (hand eye coordination), semantic memory (facts, meanings, concepts, and rote knowledge), physical memory (ability to knit or play the guitar), sensory perception, and written/spoken language comprehension.

Successful adaptation to growing old is difficult to define and variably expressed. Signs of successful aging include acceptance of change, affectionate relationships with family and friends, and a positive view of one's life story. Another indicator is the ability to find new sources of self-esteem independent of raising children, career, physical strength, or beauty. Factors that promote successful adaptation are luck (good genes, avoiding injury) and healthy behaviors, including proper diet, adequate sleep, plenty of physical activity, social engagement, and good stress management. Having enough money for basic needs as well as strong kinship and extended family bonds add extra protection from disease and despair; as do spirituality, having friends and confidants, and feeling valued by society. Opportunities to be productive and assist younger generations can provide a sense of connection to one's community and a feeling of completeness.

Patients and families will often ask for advice on staying engaged and active. Many communities have senior centers, agencies, or programs that organize discussion groups, lectures, hobby groups, travel groups, book groups, adult education classes, and volunteer activities. Similar programs or groups can be created, even in the smallest communities, by forming book or knitting groups, foster grandparent services, or peer support programs. The local Area Agency on Aging may have information for specific resources and volunteer opportunities in your community. The Blue Zones Project is the dissemination of strategies gathered from studying the five places in the world where people live the longest (the Blue Zones of Okinawa, Japan; Sardinia, Italy; Nicoya, Costa Rica; Icaria, Greece, and among the Seventh-day Adventists in Loma Linda, California).

Social conditions that contribute to demoralization in old age include highly mobile and rapidly changing communities, youth-oriented aesthetics, the deaths of friends and family members, and forced retirement. Physical conditions that limit function and increase isolation, such as urinary incontinence, chronic pain, gait and mobility problems, and hearing and vision loss also contribute to demoralization. Declining hygiene, poor nutrition, falls, alcohol abuse, social withdrawal, difficulties managing finances, and denial of severe health problems are clues that an older person is failing at home because of diminishing physical, emotional, or intellectual function. Recognizing these problems can be difficult. Health care practitioners may not detect problems if older patients are reclusive, try to look their best in the office, or avoid discussion of problems they face functioning at home. Often it is family members, friends, neighbors, and others who first recognize a person's functional decline. Their impressions can be very helpful to clinicians, but sometimes family need to be specifically asked about the well-being of the patient. In extreme cases, Adult Protective Services or a local Council on Aging may be asked to investigate patients' safety in their own environment. The challenge is to obtain the needed information while abiding by HIPAA (Health Insurance Portability and Accountability Act) regulations and retaining the confidence of the patient. If time permits, a home visit by the physician, nurse, or other clinician may be especially revealing.

Older adults experience obstacles to obtaining medical care. In the United States, financial barriers to mental health care are compounded by lower coverage for mental illness compared to physical illness under Medicare. Health care reform has attempted to reduce these disparities, but much remains to be done. Older patients may also deliberately avoid seeking help, particularly for emotional and cognitive problems. Some older adults do not view emotional distress as something to discuss with primary care providers. They suffer silently or disguise their distress with physical symptoms or irritability and withdrawal from family, friends, or caregivers. Health practitioners need to watch for subtle signs of cognitive or emotional decline, and respond sensitively and respectfully to maintain a good patient-provider relationship.

Providing medical care to older patients requires an understanding of normal changes in mental and emotional functioning in old age, and skill in determining when intervention is needed. Addressing the concerns of family and caregivers, accessing community services, and advising patients about end-of-life and long-term care options all require sensitivity and skill. Diagnosing mental disorders in older people is challenging as multiple clinical syndromes often overlap. In the following sections we will review an approach to geriatric conditions and highlight cases that illustrate how clinicians can effectively treat this population.

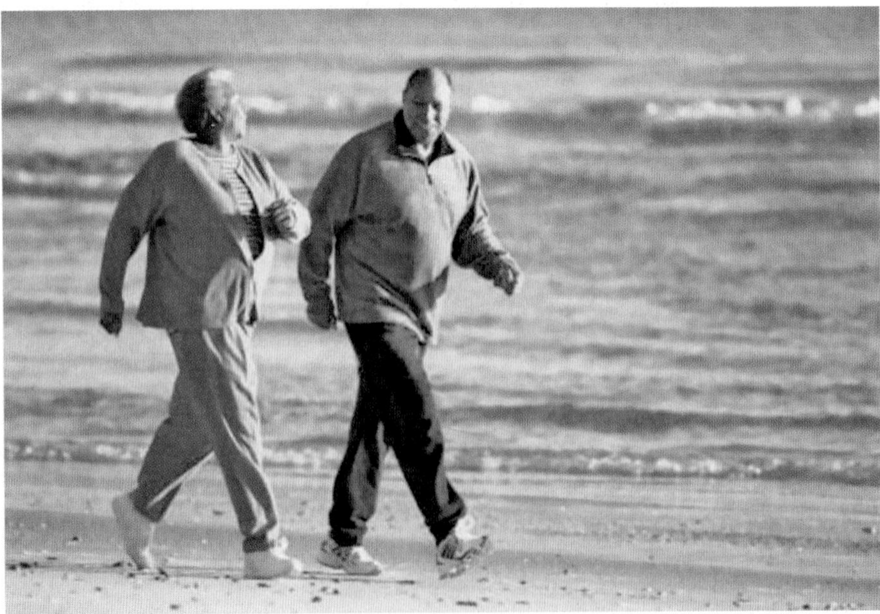

Source: The McGraw-Hill Image Library.

THE CLINICAL ENCOUNTER

Considerations for Communicating With Older Patients

THE CLINICAL SETTING

Seeing older adults in a primary care practice can be challenging due to the unique needs of this population. Adaptations to the clinic space, such as wheelchair-accessible doorways and rooms, can make it easier for patients to mobilize. Loud noises from the waiting room or adjoining rooms can be distracting and can limit the provider's ability to obtain a focused history. If possible, appointments should be made later in the day to allow older adults to arrange transportation. Adopting a more liberal "no-show" policy may be necessary as rescheduling and cancellations in this age group are not uncommon. Forms and educational materials in larger, clear fonts should be made available to accommodate older adults with vision deficits.

PATIENT INTERVIEW

Clinicians should inquire early in the interview whether they are being heard and understood. Projecting one's voice and speaking distinctly are helpful for many older persons, but clinicians should not assume this is necessary and shout at patients just because they are older. Speaking slower facilitates communication much better than speaking louder. Assistive devices, like a Pocket Talker® portable amplifier, can be invaluable in obtaining useful information. Active listening methods, such as maintaining eye contact, nodding, and paraphrasing the patient's questions and statements should be used (see Chapter 1). Attention to the light source is important, being careful not to sit or stand with your back to the window or light fixture, so patients can see your face. Shorter, more frequent visits for patients with many symptoms or greater need to talk may reduce the provider's frustration, improve communication, and better meet the patient's emotional needs for interpersonal contact with a clinician. One of the true pleasures of caring for older patients is hearing their life stories, but time constraints may mandate that this occur over several visits.

FAMILY AND CAREGIVER INTERVIEW

Most frail older patients should be accompanied by a family member or caregiver so that the clinician can obtain a complete view of the issues to be addressed during the visit. If this is not possible, a phone conversation with family or caregivers, once permission from the patient is obtained, can be just as illuminating. Patients with dementia may not be aware of their memory impairment and can actively deny they have any problem. They may also have limited insight into functional decline in their own activities of daily living (ADLs), depressive symptoms, or paranoid thinking. Delusional thoughts may seem perfectly logical until the family or caregiver is consulted (sometimes, of course, the patient is correct—reports of abuse and exploitation should be thoroughly considered and investigated). Family consultation must be pursued with sensitivity to the patient's feelings; discussions may need to occur outside the examination room (with permission from the patient) to avoid alienating the patient. It is during these separate interviews that clinicians can obtain more candid reports of impaired ADLs, psychiatric symptoms, and memory problems.

TRANSCULTURAL AWARENESS

Beliefs, values, and practices associated with culture or ethnicity often impact behavioral health (see Chapter 15). These effects can present in many ways, including relationships with clinicians and health care systems, perceptions and expectations regarding wellness and disease, and integration of new knowledge or prescribed interventions. Although it is impossible for any clinician to know all cultural and ethnic preferences, it is imperative to develop an awareness rooted in patient-centered care. This approach is particularly meaningful considering the increasing diversity of the U.S. population and significant disparities in disease burden and health care quality that have historically affected persons of color, immigrants, sexual minorities, and other individuals who are part of a nondominant community. It is also important to remember that older adults may not always fully embrace every belief, value and practice that is commonly associated with a specific culture or ethnicity. In most cases, respectfully asking questions about individual preferences and deferring to the patient and family will aid in establishing a trustful rapport.

Assessment

HISTORY

When assessing older adults, clinicians should pay particular attention to recent changes in function and a review of the most common geriatric syndromes. These include cognitive impairment, falls, urinary incontinence, hearing and vision loss, malnutrition, frailty, and mood disorders. A meticulous medication reconciliation is one of the hallmarks of a geriatric assessment. Polypharmacy, the prescription or dispensation of unnecessarily numerous or complex medicines, use of potentially inappropriate medications, and medication interactions are quite common. Scores of medications can result in behavioral side effects, and many medications for mental health conditions can cause serious medical adverse events. Further complicating the picture, vitamins, homeopathic medications, and over-the-counter therapies are increasingly being used but not often regarded as medications. A careful assessment of alcohol intake is essential. Though misuse and abuse are not uncommon, everyday alcohol use is commonly overlooked in this population, and the results can be devastating. Additionally, clinicians often mistakenly omit assessment for recreational and illicit substance use due to preconceived notions about their use in older adults. A useful acronym we have developed for a geriatric review of systems (MOMS AND DADS) is given in Table 14-1.

PHYSICAL ASSESSMENT

Though a complete physical exam is always informative, there are certain elements that are especially important in older adults. General appearance and hygiene can help determine whether the patient is well cared for or able to adequately provide self-care. Tracking weight is useful for assessing nutritional status. Many medications used to treat mental health problems come with potential side effects that may affect blood pressure, gait, and balance. Checking orthostatic blood pressure, the hemodynamic response to changes in body positioning, can help determine a patient's risk for dizziness and falls. Gait and balance, which can be evaluated with tools like the Timed Up and Go or the Tinetti Gait and Balance tests, should also be used to determine fall risk. The oral exam can be critical in this population, as poor dentition or ill-fitting dentures can contribute to weight loss, malnourishment, and frailty and may in fact point to self-neglect. A careful neurologic exam can reveal conditions such as Parkinson's disease and Lewy body dementia. Evidence of physical abuse, such as suspicious bruises or injuries, and neglect should prompt an adult protective services referral through the local Area Agency on Aging or as directed by the regulations applying to your jurisdiction.

Table 14-1. The acronym MOMS AND DADS is a helpful tool in assessing new neuropsychiatric symptoms in older adults, especially those with dementia.

M	mobility	Recent change in gait or balance
O	output	Urine output, retention, incontinence, fecal impaction
M	memory	Change in orientation, recall, awareness of situation
S	sleep	Increased lethargy, daytime sleepiness, insomnia, abnormal sleep behaviors, sleep breathing disorders
A	aches	Evidence of pain-associated behaviors
N	neurologic	Weakness, aphasia, seizures, acute lethargy
D	depression	Mood and anxiety symptoms
D	delusions	Paranoia, suspiciousness, hallucinations
A	appetite	Change in PO intake of food and fluid
D	dermis	Skin integrity, pruritis, cellulitis, dental or periodontal pain
S	sensory	Hearing and vision problems that may be contributing to misperceptions, isolation, confusion

MENTAL AND COGNITIVE STATUS EXAMINATIONS

When there is concern for cognitive changes or mood disorders, the clinician should keep in mind that dementia and depression share some prominent symptoms and can occur simultaneously. Although there are subtle differences in presentation, difficulty concentrating and making decisions, slowed psychomotor response, sleep pattern disturbances, decreased appetite, and loss of interest in activities previously enjoyed may be apparent in both disorders. Because of the similitudes, adequate screening for and treatment of depression generally should take place prior to making a diagnosis of cognitive impairment or dementia. Validated screening tests used to examine orientation, memory, insight, judgment, executive function, mood, and affect are therefore invaluable components of a thorough cognitive assessment.

The U.S. Preventive Services Task Force (USPSTF) updated its guidelines in 2016 to recommend depression screening for all adults, provided systems are in place to treat and follow up. The Geriatric Depression Scale is a standardized mood rating scale that can be administered by the clinician or the patient. The yes-no answers allow for use in an ill or cognitively impaired population. The original is a 30-question version, but a shorter 15-question version has been validated and can be a more efficient tool. Obtaining reliable reports of depressive symptoms from older adults with dementia may be difficult. The Cornell Scale for Depression in Dementia is a useful, validated tool intended for persons with moderate to severe dementia. It incorporates interviews from both the patient and an informant (e.g., a caregiver and family member) along with the clinician's impressions.

Although the USPSTF found insufficient evidence to recommend cognitive impairment screening for all older adults, it is required in patients' Medicare Annual Wellness Visits. There is consensus among many professional societies and governmental bodies that screening is indicated if: (1) the patient, family members, or others express concern about cognitive changes; (2) the clinician directly observes changes in memory or thinking; and (3) the patient is age 80 or over. Other risk factors that may trigger screening for cognitive impairment include cardiovascular disease, diabetes, stroke, depression, low educational status, and difficulty managing finances or medications.

Providers might choose a preliminary screening with the simple and time-efficient Mini-Cog™ wherein 3-word recall and clock-drawing differentiate between a positive or negative screen for dementia. If any of the words or clock are incorrect or missing elements, the patient requires further evaluation with a broader test of cognitive function. The St. Louis University Mental Status Exam (SLUMS) is sensitive for detecting dementia in its earlier stages. It consists of an 11-item assessment of orientation, memory, attention, calculation, naming, visuospatial relationships, and executive function. The Montreal Cognitive Assessment (MoCA) is another instrument that is sensitive for detection of mild cognitive impairment and dementia. In addition to the domains tested in the SLUMS, the MoCA also assesses conceptual thinking. Additionally, the MoCA is offered in two different forms to minimize test learning that may artificially influence scores. It is also available in 37 languages, with instructions for administration and scoring, as well as normative data for the examination. Both the SLUMS and MoCA have been validated across numerous settings and comorbidities, have scoring systems that can be adjusted for educational level, are available in multiple languages, and can be downloaded for free (see list of "Web sites" at end of this chapter). The Folstein Mini-Mental State Exam (MMSE) is another widely used tool to assess cognition, and it is perhaps most practical for serial assessment of dementia severity and treatment response; however, because the MMSE is copyrighted and copies must be ordered through the company that holds the intellectual property, it may not be readily accessible in some clinics. The 100-point Modified Mini-Mental State Exam (3MS) includes verbal fluency assessment and more extensive testing of memory while offering increased sensitivity and specificity over the 30-point MMSE.

Functional Assessment

Another element that sets the evaluation of older adults apart from that of younger patients is the importance of performing a functional assessment. The ability to perform basic ADLs, including bathing, dressing, grooming, eating, transferring, and toileting, can be affected by both medical illness and mental disorders. Instrumental activities of daily living (IADLs), such as telephone and computer use, money and medication management, shopping, cooking, driving, and transportation, are impacted by even mild dementia. Commonly used assessment tools are the Katz Index for ADLs and the Lawton Scale for IADLs. ADL and IADL functional capacity can inform the clinician about a person's safety at home. Treatment of mental health issues may result in functional status improvement with the goal of allowing patients to remain at home and independent for as long as possible.

Social System Assessment

When frail older adults are dependent on others, the caregiver's capacity and coping also become the clinician's concern as caregiving is often associated with depression and physical health problems. The clinician should tactfully probe for indicators of stress, feelings of burden, and breakdown in the caregiver's ability to provide care. There are a number of tools available to assess caregiver burden, such as the *Caregiver Self-Assessment Questionnaire*. The potential for abuse and mistreatment of vulnerable older adults should also be assessed, keeping in mind that hostile remarks and impatience are risk factors for physical aggression and neglect. Many states require health care providers to report suspected abuse, and all communities are required by federal law to have Area Agencies on Aging that provide adult protective services.

Environmental Assessment

Community nursing and senior care agencies can assist health care providers by making home assessments and evaluating patients' safety in their own environment. These services are often covered as a Medicare benefit, especially if the patient is homebound. Fall risk, fire safety, medication management, and hygiene concerns are among the many things that can be assessed. Removing loose throw rugs, keeping the path to the bathroom free of clutter and lit at night, adding bars next to the toilet, and other simple interventions can markedly increase safety and prolong independent living.

MAJOR MENTAL DISORDERS

Depression

Major depression is common in community dwelling older adults (2–4%), and more common in residents of long-term care homes. Depressive symptoms are even more prevalent, affecting up to 20% of older adults. Chronic medical conditions increase the risk of developing depression. Major depression in geriatric patients can manifest in all the usual ways seen in younger adults, but nonspecific and atypical symptoms are common and may dominate the clinical presentation (see Chapter 26). Although depressed mood and hopelessness have diagnostic value, anhedonia—or loss of interest in previously pleasurable behaviors-anxiety, fearfulness, irritability, cognitive impairment, apathy, dependency, and numerous somatic complaints should prompt the consideration of depression even when the patient denies feeling depressed.

The most efficient tool for assessing mood is the 2 questions screen: "In the past month, have you felt depressed or down?" and "In the past month have you had little interest or pleasure in activities and/or hobbies?" If either question is answered in the affirmative, further testing is indicated. The Geriatric Depression Scale is a more complete screening tool and can be followed over time to monitor progression or response to therapy (see section "Mental and Cognitive Status Examinations").

The prognosis for acute symptoms of depression in old age is fairly good, and patients need to be told this to counter the hopelessness they might feel. However, partial remissions and relapses are common, especially in patients with previous episodes of depression. Other predictors of recurrence include persistent health problems that compromise function or comfort, poor social support, and ongoing psychosocial stressors.

The pillars of treatment for depression are psychotherapy, antidepressant medications, mood stabilizers, and electro-convulsive therapy (ECT). Informal "psychotherapy" for depressed older adults can be provided by primary care clinicians through frequent brief visits, and often is the most acceptable approach for older adults who may have negative attitudes toward seeing mental health providers. Disease education, cognitive reframing of hopelessness, simple problem-solving, and—most important of all—compassionate listening can all make a big difference. In complex cases, referral to a mental health professional is warranted. Outcome data for brief, structured psychotherapy for depression in older adults are quite good, especially for mild to moderate depression. Antidepressant medications have been shown to improve outcomes and reduce the risk of relapse in older adults, though they must be started in low doses and increased gradually (e.g., start Sertraline 25 mg daily, increase by 25 mg every 2–4 weeks until an adequate response is achieved, with a maximum dose of 200 mg daily). Sustained clinical responses are seen only about half the time for the first medication trial. Appetite, sleep, and energy often improve before mood itself, and patients often need to be seen frequently to encourage them to continue treatment. Residual symptoms such as anxiety are very common even in those with good initial responses. Fortunately about half of patients will respond to a second trial of a different medication. Those who don't may need psychiatric referral or a trial of an added medication for augmentation. Augmentation strategies include adding a nighttime dose of a complementary antidepressant such as mirtazapine or, in rare situations, addition of a mood stabilizing antipsychotic medication (the most supportive data are for the atypical antipsychotics: olanzapine, aripiprazole, risperidone, or quetiapine). Patients with prominent fatigue or apathy may respond to bupropion. Patients who are restless, agitated, and have intense, labile affects in response to medication may actually carry a diagnosis of bipolar disorder and may benefit from a mood stabilizer as the primary treatment.

ECT has high efficacy rates and can be used for drug resistant depression, as well as for patients with psychotic features. Randomized trials show ECT to be more effective than placebo in geriatric depression, and observational data show ECT works better than antidepressants for psychotic depression in older adults. In patients hospitalized with depression, ECT improved mortality over the subsequent 5 years compared to medications alone. There are no absolute contraindications, but many patients experience short-term memory loss after this treatment.

Cognitive impairment associated with depression may improve with remission of the mood disorder, but it is predictive of an underlying dementia. These patients should be followed closely to determine if cognitive changes are related to their depression or a sign of a separate cognitive disorder.

Anxiety Disorders

Many older adults who suffer from anxiety have an underlying depression, and should be treated as such. Apart from depression, the differential diagnosis of anxiety in older adults includes transient apprehension and fear, adjustments to life changes, phobic avoidant behaviors, obsessive-compulsive disorder, panic disorder, post-traumatic stress, and generalized anxiety disorder (see Chapter 27). Secondary anxiety disorders are also very common; medications, chronic obstructive pulmonary disease, and endocrinopathies such as thyroid disease are often implicated.

The mainstay of therapy for anxiety in all adults is SSRIs. Benzodiazepines have impaired drug excretion as well as changes to the benzodiazepine receptors making older adults exquisitely sensitive to this class of medications. Increased somnolence, unsteadiness, falls, memory loss, and disinhibition are common and dangerous reactions. Long-term use of benzodiazepines has also been associated with an increased risk of developing dementia, and these drugs should be avoided in older adults. If an older adult has been on a long-term benzodiazepine, a slow taper will be required, and patient buy-in is important to successfully complete the taper.

Delusional Disorders

Delusional thinking arises from a number of disturbances in old age. Hallucinations can be seen in both dementia and delirium. Dementia with Lewy Bodies is the dementia most frequently associated with visual hallucinations, although they may occur in Alzheimer

Dementia (AD) as well (see below). Charles Bonnet Syndrome is a condition that causes patients with vision loss to have complex visual hallucinations. These hallucinations are often not bothersome, and the patient frequently has insight that the visions are not real. While there is no specific treatment for Charles Bonnet Syndrome, education about the nature of the hallucinations can be very reassuring to patients who think they are going "crazy." If hallucinations are distressing to the patient, antipsychotic medications may be helpful. Musical hallucinosis is an auditory variant of hallucinosis associated with acquired deafness, in many ways analogous to Charles Bonnet Syndrome. Hearing aid upgrades or masking sounds may be helpful. Delusional disorder, a primary disorder of unknown etiology, previously known as paranoia, is sometimes seen in older people who live alone. Classic delusions include people "living in the attic" or coming in the house or apartment to steal things. Although these patients describe persecutory delusions of an intense nature, highly suggestive of schizophrenia, they do not have other manifestations of this disease, such as hallucinations, loose associations, disorganized behavior, and functional decline. Elders who do exhibit these cardinal symptoms of schizophrenia have usually had the disease for many years. Paranoia and delusions can also be the presenting symptoms of dementia, depression, mania, and alcohol abuse.

Dementia

Dementia is an acquired, persistent, and usually progressive impairment in multiple cognitive domains, usually including memory. There must also be a significant decline in function that is severe enough to interfere with work or social life. Dementia is a common disorder with a prevalence that doubles every 5 years after the age of 60 years, affecting up to 45% of those aged 85 years and older. Today, over 5 million Americans are living with Alzheimer disease and related dementias. By 2050, up to 16 million will have dementia. Dementia is the 6th leading cause of death in the United States. Dementia is covered in much greater detail in Chapter 34.

OTHER PROBLEMS

Polypharmacy

Because of their greater number of chronic medical conditions, older patients generally take more prescription medications than younger patients. Polypharmacy is defined as the use of multiple medications by a patient, including both prescriptions and over-the-counter medications. Though the exact number of medications varies, polypharmacy generally involves between 5 and 10 medications according to some studies. Unfortunately, this is a common problem—in a sample of Medicare beneficiaries discharged from the hospital to a skilled nursing home, patients were prescribed an average of 14 medications. Polypharmacy increases the risk of adverse drug events (ADEs), which can lead to serious consequences. Confusion, falls, depression, functional decline, or any other new symptom should be considered to be drug-related until proven otherwise. Polypharmacy can also lead to "prescribing cascades," whereby a new symptom is misinterpreted as a new medical condition and an additional drug is then prescribed to treat it.

Many medications must be used with caution due to age-related changes in drug metabolism and decreased drug clearance, often due to naturally reduced renal clearance in older adults. Therefore, dosing must often be reduced. In addition, the volume of distribution for benzodiazepines and opioids is increased in older adults, and thus older adults often have increased sensitivity to these medications due to increased plasma concentrations.

Frequent medication review and reduction should be part of the care of every older adult. Deprescribing, whereby medications are either removed or tapered over time, is an essential component of the physician visit with older persons who are taking multiple, often unnecessary medications. The decision to discontinue a medication is not only influenced by the possibility of ADEs, but also by the goals of care for a particular patient. When deprescribing, it is necessary to consider safer alternative medicines, using the lowest possible dose, to remove one medication at a time, and to consider nonpharmacological treatments such as cognitive behavioral therapy for depression and anxiety, stress reduction activities for anxiety, cognitive rehabilitation for mild cognitive impairment, and a change in environment for dementia.

Specific criteria have been developed regarding high-risk and inappropriate medications for use in older adults. The Beers Criteria, which was most recently updated in 2019, is the most widely used and includes many psychotropic medications. It is available on the American Geriatric Society website. The new updates include stricter use of antipsychotics for behavioral issues when other options such as behavioral modification have failed or there is a threat of harm to the patient or others. Of note, atypical antipsychotics are among the most frequent causes of ADEs in long-term care homes, and the U.S. Food and Drug Administration (FDA) issued a warning regarding increased risk of fatal adverse events in patients with dementia being treated with atypical antipsychotics.

Table 14-2 shows the preferred antidepressant and antipsychotic medications for use with older patients.

Grief

During their lifetime many older adults experience the loss of a loved one. The loss of a spouse can be one of

Table 14-2. Antidepressants/antipsychotics and better alternatives for older patients.

Antidepressants	
Instead of:	Use:
Amitriptyline	Sertraline
Doxepin	Escitalopram
Imipramine	Mirtazapine
Paroxetine	Citalopram* FDA guidelines suggest a max of 20 mg/d patients >60
	Bupropion
	Trazodone
Antipsychotics	
Instead of:	Use:
Haldol	Risperidone (avoid in dementia with Lewy bodies)
Thioridazine	Quetiapine
	Acetylcholinesterase inhibitors and memantine may reduce psychotic symptoms in dementia

the most devastating life experiences. Grief is defined as the reaction to bereavement, which is the situation when a loved one has died. Though often very distressing, grief is a natural response to the loss of a loved one and should not be diagnosed as a mental disorder. However, it should be noted that bereavement may worsen underlying mental diagnoses or lead to new mental disorders such as major depressive disorder. Rather, bereavement is regarded as a stressor that can trigger a depressive episode. This represents a change from the previous edition of the Diagnostic and Statistical Manual, Fourth Edition, Text Revision (DSM-IV-TR), which did not permit clinicians to diagnose major depression within two months of bereavement (commonly referred to as the "bereavement exclusion").

Grief comes in many different forms, and the patterns and course of grieving are influenced by many factors, including religion, culture, and social norms. The stages of grief vary by individual and do not necessarily occur in a standard order. Though often intensely distressing, acute grief is typically integrated such that the distressing emotions gradually diminish over time.

When grief becomes prolonged, debilitating, or leads to dysfunctional thoughts or maladaptive behaviors, it is defined as "complicated grief." Complicated grief should be recognized as a mental disorder and treated appropriately.

Substance Use

Definitions and Diagnosis

Although often overlooked, substance use is very common in older adults and has become a significant public health concern in this population. The prevalence of alcoholism is greater for older men than for older women. Alcoholism is the third most common mental health disorder in older men. This is typically an exacerbation or relapse of life-long alcoholism in men. Late-life onset of alcohol dependence is more common in older women.

Any substance greater than the recommended level is considered *at-risk use*. For adults >65 alcohol use should not exceed more than 7 standard drinks per week or more than 1-2 drinks per day. For other substances, there are no specific, agreed-upon standards for overuse. *Problem substance use* is defined as consumption of a substance that results in at least one problem, for example, falls related to alcohol consumption.

Of note, the Diagnostic and Statistical Manual of Mental Disorders, 5th Edition (DSM-5) no longer includes the terms substance abuse and dependence. Rather, "substance use disorder" is the recommend diagnostic term. According to the DSM-5, substance use disorder is defined as a problematic pattern of substance use leading to clinically significant impairment or distress, with at least two of the following occurring within a one-year period:

- The substance is often taken in larger amounts or over a longer period than was intended.
- There is a persistent desire or unsuccessful efforts to cut down or control use of the substance.
- A great deal of time is spent in activities necessary to obtain the substance, use the substance, or recover from its effects.
- Craving, or a strong desire or urge to use the substance.
- Recurrent use resulting in a failure to fulfill major role obligations at work, school, or home.
- Continued use despite having persistent or recurrent social or interpersonal problems caused by or exacerbated by its effects.
- Important social, occupational, or recreational activities are given up or reduced because of use.
- Recurrent use in situations in which it is physically hazardous.
- Use is continued despite knowledge of having a persistent or recurrent physical or psychological problem that is likely to have been caused or exacerbated by the substance.

Tolerance and withdrawal are also included in these criteria and are discussed in more detail in Chapter 24.

Signs and Symptoms

Older adults are particularly sensitive to the physical and cognitive effects of alcohol, nicotine, and psychoactive medications. Harmful consequences include, but are not limited to, kidney and liver disease, peptic ulcer disease, cognitive impairment, unsteady gait, falls, sleep disturbance, impaired driving, worsening of mood disorders, and increased risk for suicide. Older adults with alcohol use disorder are nearly three times more likely to have a lifetime diagnosis of another mental disorder. There are also harmful interactions between alcohol and certain prescription medications such as Warfarin that are common in older adults. Unexplained falls, ataxia, confusion, malnutrition, burns, head trauma, and depression should prompt questions about surreptitious alcohol use.

Prescription pain medication, sedative-hypnotic medications, over-the-counter remedies for constipation, and numerous vitamins and supplements are also overused. Seeing multiple physicians and practitioners and patronizing several pharmacies are clues to the clinician that prescription drug use disorder is likely.

Screening and Treatment

There is a growing body of effective treatment for substance use disorders, which has led to a reduction in substance use among older adults. Therefore, it is vital for primary care providers to identify such disorders so that they may be treated appropriately. The USPSTF recommends that all adults be screened to identify unhealthy alcohol use. There are several well-validated screening tools for use in primary care. The AUDIT-C tool is well-validated in older adults and is used to screen for unhealthy alcohol use. We recommend the AUDIT-C over its counterpart, the AUDIT screening tool, since it is easier to administer. It is comprised of three questions: "How often do you have a drink containing alcohol?" "How many drinks containing alcohol do you have on a typical day when you are drinking?" "How often do you have six or more drinks on one occasion?" Positive scores indicating unhealthy alcohol use are greater than or equal to 3 points for women, with 73% sensitivity and 91% specificity, and 4 points or more in men, with 86% and 89% sensitivity and specificity, respectively.

Specific to older adults, the Comorbidity Alcohol Risk Evaluation Tool (CARET) is also used to screen older adults at risk for alcohol overuse. This tool incorporates medication use and comorbidities and may also be useful in the primary care setting.

The primary care provider should also monitor prescription medications closely, as these are often abused by older adults (in particular, benzodiazepines, opioids, and sedative-hypnotics). The primary care provider should avoid prescribing these medications if possible. Otherwise, re-evaluation of the necessity of these medications should occur at least every 3–6 months. If benzodiazepines are required, such as in treating anxiety, it is best to use shorter-acting formulations to help prevent adverse reactions and withdrawal symptoms.

Treatment for substance use disorders varies by the substance used and the severity of the disease. Common interventions include simple education and advice, psychotherapy and/or counseling, peer groups, and more formal treatment such as rehabilitation and pharmacologic agents if necessary. Withdrawal from alcohol and benzodiazepines can be fatal, and inpatient detoxification may be necessary. Benzodiazepine dependence may be managed by replacing the medication with a 24-hour equivalent dose and then tapering the dosage by 10% every three half-lives.

The outpatient treatment of substance use disorder is typically relegated to specialized clinics. However, given the increasing public health concern, it is becoming necessary to recognize and treat substance use disorders in the primary care setting. This is of particular importance in older adults, who are often reluctant to utilize specialty addiction services.

SPECIAL CONSIDERATIONS

Maintaining Functional Independence

The focus of treatment planning with frail older patients always includes provision of comfort and maintenance of independence. To achieve this in the face of aging and progressive disease, treatment planning must include utilization of community resources, skillful medical management, and rehabilitation therapies. If there is doubt about a senior's driving safety, many driving schools and outpatient occupational rehabilitation programs offer driving safety evaluations for older adults.

Community Care Options for Frail Elders

Clinicians should familiarize themselves with services available in their community that provide care management, in-home assistance, and emotional support to older patients and caregivers. Local and county agencies providing services for seniors, private case management firms, local chapters of the Alzheimer's Association, and home health care agencies will be resources to you and your patients in arranging the services necessary to keep your patients at home longer than would otherwise be safe. In rural areas without these resources, family, neighbors, and lay networks of helpers can sometimes fill in the gaps and keep frail elders in their home. Patients with round-the-clock care needs will eventually exhaust many family caregivers. Caregivers, family, and paid professionals all face depression and health risks beyond their peers. There comes a time when placement in a long-term care facility may become necessary for both the patient's and family's well-being. Physicians, nurses, and other practitioners play important roles in assisting patients and families through this transition. Clinicians can help them anticipate the need to leave home for supervised living settings, familiarize them with different long-term care options in the community, and address families' feelings of guilt when they have to make the decision on the patient's behalf. This role requires clinicians to know what the patient's care needs are and what type of facility can safely meet those needs. People who need assistance only with housekeeping and cooking will do fine in retirement homes and residential care facilities. Residential care facilities may be able to administer medications and provide assistance with ADLs for additional cost. Adult foster homes provide a home-like alternative to residential care facilities for up to five older adults per home. Additional care needs may be met by an independent or assisted living facility. Assisted living or independent living facilities may provide some nursing supervision and occasionally may even have a medical director. However, the amount of nursing and medical involvement varies greatly based on state regulations and the management philosophy of the owners. These facilities are very popular with patients and families and are increasingly seen as alternatives to skilled nursing facilities, because they are less expensive and have less of an institutional feel than nursing homes. Many assisted living facilities allow patients to age in place and allow them to receive hospice-level care at the end of life without having to move to a nursing facility.

MEDICAL TREATMENT PLANNING

The motto of the British Geriatrics Society, "Adding Life to Years," is useful to keep in mind when treating older patients. Comfort, meaningful engagement, and increased activity become the goals of treatment. Providing adequate pain relief, physical therapy, and treatment of depression are all integrated into comprehensive treatment plans.

Immunizations, smoking cessation, weight loss, exercise, and proper nutrition should continue to be a focus of preventive care in older adults. It is also important to explore the expectations of both the patient and the caregiver and to discuss end-of-life treatment decisions. If possible, this discussion should take place before an acute medical condition leads to interventions that may be invasive, futile, or unwanted. These "advance directives" should extend beyond cardiopulmonary resuscitation and include the patient's goals of care. If the decision is to forego these interventions, the clinician should provide assurances that the comfort of the patient will be maintained (see Chapter 42).

CASE DISCUSSIONS

CASE ILLUSTRATION 1

Mr. J is a 78-year-old man with hypertension and hypothyroidism who is brought in by his daughter, who has noticed a decline in his ability to care for himself. She noticed the decline after her mother, his wife of over 50 years, died 6 months ago. Since that time, he has lost 20 pounds and has not been going to his weekly bridge games. He has been forgetful, initially losing his keys or missing appointments, but progressing to the point where he became lost driving in his own neighborhood. He has become increasingly disheveled.

When approached with his daughter's concerns, Mr. J reports that he thinks he is doing just fine and simply hasn't felt like playing bridge recently. As to getting lost in his neighborhood, he says he just wasn't paying attention. He answers questions in short phrases. His biggest concern during the visit is low back pain, which has been acting up recently. On exam, he is poorly groomed. He scores a 23/30 on the SLUMS test, missing all the orientation questions and several of the recall questions. He scores 10/15 on the GDS.

This case highlights the difficulty in distinguishing dementia from depression. Cognitive deficits can be associated with depression. While Mr. J may have some cognitive impairment as well, he will have to be re-evaluated after his depression resolves or remits. The abrupt onset, timed with the passing of his wife, is more consistent with depression than dementia, which usually has a more insidious onset. Then again, his wife may have been covering for pre-existing deficits that became evident after her death. Medical causes such as drug side effects and hypothyroidism should be ruled out. Some depressed mood is normal after the death of a loved one, but his symptoms are starting to affect his ability to take care of himself. Treatment should be initiated with counseling and/or anti-depressant therapy, with up-titration if needed or a switch to another medication if the first has no effect. ECT is an option for drug resistant depression. If his symptoms do respond to therapy, his cognition should be re-evaluated as he may also have an underlying dementia.

CASE ILLUSTRATION 2

Mrs. R is an 84-year-old woman with a history of hypertension and bilateral cataracts who is brought in by a neighbor out of concern for hallucinations. Her neighbor brings her groceries once a week and notes that lately the patient has been making comments about children and animals that are not there. The patient admits that she does sometimes see one young boy and two small cats in her home. She knows they aren't really there, but she isn't bothered by them. In fact, she somewhat enjoys their company. On further questioning you find that she drinks one martini each night before bed and occasionally takes diphenhydramine to help her sleep. On presentation, she is well groomed, and aside from her vision the exam is unrevealing. She scores 24/30 on the SLUMS test but misses only the questions that require intact vision. Her attention is normal, as she is able to participate in activities such as spelling "world" backwards and naming days of the week backwards. A laboratory workup is also unrevealing, showing no signs of infection or electrolyte abnormality.

This case highlights the differential diagnosis of a patient presenting with visual hallucinations. Dementia, delirium, psychosis, intoxication, and medication effects should all be considered in this patient. Though she had an abnormal score on the SLUMS test, her memory was intact. In delirium, inattention is a hallmark of the disease, accompanied with fluctuations in consciousness. Her alcohol intake and diphenhydramine use may be implicated, and these should be stopped. This patient may be suffering from Charles Bonnet syndrome if workup of the other diagnoses is negative. If medically stable, the patient should undergo surgical removal of her cataracts, as this may cure her of her hallucinations.

ACKNOWLEDGMENTS

Clifford M. Singer, MD, Jay Luxenberg, MD, and Robin Telerant, MD, were authors of prior editions of this chapter.

SUGGESTED READINGS

2019 American Geriatrics Society Beers Criteria® Update Expert Panel. American Geriatrics Society 2019 Updated AGS Beers Criteria® for Potentially Inappropriate Medication Use in Older Adults. *J Am Geriatr Soc* 2019;67(4):674–694.

Kok RM, Reynolds CF. Management of depression in older adults: a review. *JAMA* 2017;317(20):2114–2122.

WEBSITES

AARP Livable Communities. https://www.aarp.org/livable-communities/info-2014/livable-communities-facts-and-figures.html. Accessed August 2019.

Alzheimer's Association. http://www.alz.org. Accesssed August 2019.

American Association of Geriatric Psychiatry. www.aagponline.org. Accessed August 2019.

American Geriatrics Society. www.americangeriatrics.org. Accessed August 2019.

Family Caregiver Alliance. www.caregiver.org. Accessed August 2019.

Geriatric Depression Scale. https://geriatrictoolkit.missouri.edu/cog/GDS_SHORT_FORM.PDF. Accessed August 2019.

Geriatrics and Palliative Care Blog. www.geripal.org. Accessed August 2019.

The Hartford Institute for Geriatric Nursing "Try This" Series. https://consultgeri.org/tools/try-this-series. Accessed August 2019.

Katz Index for ADLs. https://consultgeri.org/try-this/general-assessment/issue-2.pdf. Accessed August 2019.

Lawton Scale for IADLs. https://consultgeri.org/try-this/general-assessment/issue-23.pdf. Accessed August 2019.

Mini Cog: http://mini-cog.com/wp-content/uploads/2018/03/Standardized-English-Mini-Cog-1-19-16-EN_v1-low-1.pdf. Accessed August 2019.

Montreal Cognitive Assessment (MoCA). https://www.mocatest.org/. Accessed August 2019.

National Institute of Aging. www.nia.nih.gov. Accessed August 2019.

National Council on Aging. https://www.ncoa.org/centerforbenefits/mippa/. Accessed August 2019.

Reframing Aging. http://frameworksinstitute.org/reframing-aging.html. Accessed August 2019.

St. Louis University Mental Status Exam (SLUMS). https://www.slu.edu/medicine/internal-medicine/geriatric-medicine/aging-successfully/pdfs/slums_form.pdf. Accessed August 2019.

Timed Up and Go Test. https://www.cdc.gov/steadi/pdf/TUG_Test-print.pdf. Accessed August 2019.

Tinetti Gait and Balance Tests. http://hdcs.fullerton.edu/csa/research/documents/TinettiPOMA.pdf. Accessed August 2019.

Cross-Cultural Communication 15

Thomas Denberg, MD, PhD & Mitchell D. Feldman, MD, MPhil, FACP

INTRODUCTION

Effective clinician–patient communication involves verbal and nonverbal sharing of information across cultural and linguistic boundaries. In the medical arena, these boundaries are populated on the one side by clinicians who represent the esoteric world of biomedicine, and on the other side by patients and families who often lack familiarity with biomedical concepts and procedures and may have their own strongly held beliefs about illness—what it means, how it should be diagnosed, and how it should be treated. The goals of effective cross-cultural communication (or "cultural competency," as it is sometimes called) are threefold: (1) to understand illness from the perspective of the *patient*; (2) to assist patients in understanding diseases and treatments from the perspective of *biomedicine*; and (3) to help patients and their families navigate, express themselves, and feel comfortable within large, complex, and often impersonal health care organizations. These activities require some awareness of the wider context of patients' lives, and of how the worlds of biomedicine and the lay public interact and, at times, conflict and misunderstand each other.

Cross-cultural communication skills are best developed through practice, reflection, and reading about and interacting with diverse patient populations. Knowing a few facts about the illness beliefs of an immigrant group or ethnic minority is not enough. It is important to develop ways of perceiving and interpreting what *individual* patients say and do in the context of their previous experiences with illness, structural positions within society, and membership within particular ethnic and religious communities. True cultural awareness also involves understanding how biomedicine is itself a cultural system, and how it is likely to be perceived and (mis) understood by patients.

As the dominant form of health care in the United States, biomedicine is practiced by highly specialized professionals and relies on detailed, scientific information about the human body and the use of pharmaceutical and surgical interventions to prevent or treat anatomic and physiologic disorders and their associated symptoms. It has a definite body of knowledge, set of practices, strengths and weaknesses, nonevidence-based biases, and inherent limitations. Each of its many specialties and subspecialties has unique conventions, systems of knowledge, and ways of making sense of people and events. To patients of all backgrounds, much about biomedicine is obscure; difficulties agreeing with and accepting medical explanations and recommendations are commonplace. Therefore, the perspective that orients the discussion in this chapter is that although cross-cultural communication is especially important and challenging for immigrant and minority patients, it has relevance to *all* patients.

CULTURE & SOCIAL LOCATION

Culture

Culture refers to beliefs, values, rituals, customs, institutions, social roles, and relationships that are shared among identifiable groups of people. Typically, one's own culture is taken for granted; it feels entirely natural, consisting of those assumptions and routines that make the world what it is "supposed" to be. Unconscious learning and modeling play important roles in the acquisition of cultural assumptions and routines. Within the family, one of the most influential cultural systems, there is generally a clear-cut division of labor, regular routines such as meal and work times, explanations (or myths) about family origins, and strategies for fulfilling common goals and passing down shared values. It is also within the family that beliefs are first developed about the causes of illness, acceptable ways of expressing symptoms, and strategies for diagnosing illness and restoring health. Individuals, of course, are also shaped by, and participate in, cultures related to work, school, worship, political affiliation, social clubs, and so on, each of which may also have important—and sometimes contradictory or inconsistent—influences on beliefs about and responses to illness.

Cultures are neither pure nor static, but constantly intermix and evolve. Particularly in the United States—a highly mobile, diverse, and media-saturated society—millions of people move in and out of multiple domains, borrowing and adapting ideas and customs from other groups. Because cultural change over time and across generations is considerable, it should not be *assumed* that particular patients have certain beliefs or engage in certain behaviors solely on the basis of their last name, physical appearance, or national origin. Inferences—always open to revision—should be based on detailed knowledge of patient attributes that go beyond race and ethnicity alone.

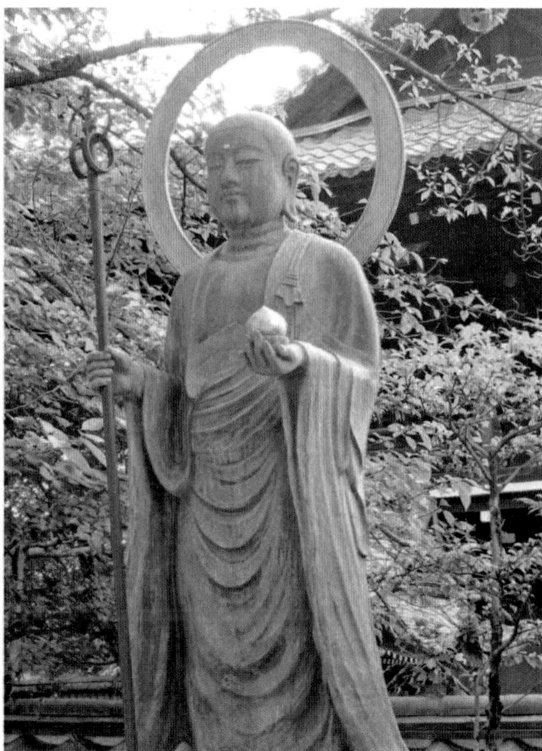

(Photo courtesy of Mitchell D. Feldman, MD, MPhil, FACP.)

THE RELATIONSHIP OF CULTURE TO RACE, ETHNICITY, AND NATIONAL ORIGIN

Some cultural competency training takes the approach that various racial, ethnic, and national groups possess distinctive cultural traits with which the clinician should become familiar to render more effective care. Commonly cited examples include beliefs in "fallen fontanelle" and "evil eye" among Latinos and "high blood/low blood" among African Americans, as well as values such as "individualism" among North Americans, and "family centeredness" among Asians. Although these generalizations (or stereotypes) may illustrate a wide spectrum of cultural influences on illness and healing, this approach is too simplistic. It implies that race, ethnicity, and national origin are the most important determinants of an individual's understanding of and response to illness and ignores the tremendous heterogeneity among individuals *within* these groups and among individuals who may inhabit multiple groups simultaneously. Common notions of cultural competency assume that culture can be reduced to a technical skill that clinicians can develop without necessarily engaging with people in their local worlds and understanding the ambiguity and ambivalence that many people feel as a result of living within these multiple worlds.

Take the case of the United States, in which the primary racial/ethnic categories include African American, white, Asian, American Indian, Pacific Islander, and Latino. Some people may self-identify using these terms, and the labels are often important politically, but there are significant differences among people within each of these categories in terms of age, place of birth, religion, social class, sexual orientation, level of education, and so on. Conceptualizing differences in health beliefs and behaviors on the overarching levels of race and ethnicity promotes stereotyping and does little to advance more effective medical care. In general, assumptions about cultural beliefs and practices should be based on more specific identification of group membership, such as recent immigrants; particular U.S. subpopulations such as the homeless, southern rural African Americans, or inhabitants of particular city neighborhoods.

Social Location

As we move beyond ideas of culture determined solely by race and ethnicity, knowledge of patients will be enhanced by awareness of their *social location*. Social location specifies one's position in society relative to others and is based on an amalgam of characteristics that include not only race and ethnicity but also gender, age, immigration status, language(s) spoken, neighborhood of residence, length of time and number of generations in the United States, educational attainment, income, occupation, religion, sexual orientation, and prior experiences with racism. Gender and age are two fundamental variables that influence how patients give meaning to illness and express themselves in relation to it. Men and women, and people over the age of 50 years and under the age of 20 years, although from the same city or region, will generally belong to distinctive subcultures: they may share certain core beliefs, values, and customs, but not others. Another fundamental influence on disease risk, health behaviors, and familiarity with biomedicine is degree of acculturation. One's neighborhood of residence, with its quality of housing and schools, population density, associated level of crime, and access to public transportation, also dramatically shapes one's understanding of the world and strategies for dealing with adversity. Religion, spirituality, and membership in a community of like-minded believers also have significant bearings on attitudes toward health and illness. Historical experiences of racism can engender feelings of helplessness, anger, and distrust that may, in turn, significantly affect attitudes toward medical providers as well as interpretations of illness. Finally, the elements of social class—education, income, and occupation—have a profound influence on beliefs about illness and opportunities and strategies for restoring health.

The attributes of social location are more complete, specific, and clinically relevant than race and ethnicity alone. In this way, a clinician will not simply note that a patient is Latino, or even Mexican American, and then attempt to remember "typical" cultural traits that apply to members of this group. Instead, they will observe that the U.S.-born patient is 20 years old, unemployed, has completed high school, speaks little Spanish, and lives with her Mexican-born, primarily Spanish-speaking, rural-origin parents in a mixed race, working-class neighborhood. Each of these characteristics, alone and in combination, provides important clues about *this* patient—clues that help in interpreting the patient's statements and symptoms and that facilitate patient education and tailored treatment.

Of course, the more experience that practitioners have with patients from a specific, narrowly defined population or community, and the greater the language concordance between practitioner and patient, the more they are likely to become aware of the health problems and themes important to that group as a whole. The ability to communicate effectively with patients from such groups can be enhanced by spending time in the local community—in senior citizen centers, at cultural and sporting events, churches, and schools—as well as by reading relevant neighborhood newsletters, ethnographies, social histories, census reports, novels, and biographies. Although such activities and materials do not constitute the normal corpus of medical duties or references, they can sensitize the clinician to the issues that are important to patients—in their own terms and from their own points of view. Detailed knowledge of a specific population as well as the ability to communicate in the patient's native language can also help the clinician understand not only the literal sense of a patient's words, but also other kinds of meanings contained in what the patient says (or chooses not to say), and in what the patient does (or chooses not to do), such as adhere to prescribed treatments.

IMMIGRANTS & ETHNIC MINORITIES

Recent immigrants bring a number of unique issues and challenges to medical cross-cultural communication. Relocating to a new country often results in dramatic alterations in social status, occupation, and daily routines; isolation from previous friendships and networks of social support; and the upending of traditional roles as older individuals rely on those who are younger to support the family, locate housing, and interpret local events. Anomie (a sense of purposelessness) and alienation (lack of feelings of belonging) can contribute to anxiety, depression, and a decreased ability to cope with the new stresses of daily life. Refugee experiences of war and natural catastrophe exacerbate these problems. The astute clinician will be aware that many individuals somatize this distress.

Recent immigrants are more likely to hold beliefs and practices that to "Western" trained physicians may seem colorful or strange. These illness beliefs and behaviors are often cited in discussions of cultural competence but are generally most applicable to elderly and/or recently arrived immigrants. Processes of globalization, including the growth of tourism, the opening of commercial markets, and the spread of popular culture from the United States and Europe, have familiarized large numbers of third-world immigrants with life in industrially advanced, capitalist societies. In addition, a substantial proportion of first- and second-generation residents quickly assimilate into U.S. society, often because of a keen desire to "fit in" or "become American." Even among individuals who speak English poorly, are poorly assimilated, or actively resist assimilation, many will have had a significant amount of experience with biomedicine in their countries of origin. Although they may not have previously encountered the technological and organizational complexity that characterize biomedicine in the United States, they may be familiar with its reductionistic, scientific foundation, status as a profession, and its conventions for diagnosing and treating illness. It is difficult, if not impossible, to accurately gauge a patient's level of sophistication about biomedicine and "Western" disease categories through visual inspection or knowledge of the patient's race and ethnicity alone; the clinician should avoid assumptions and instead learn by observing and asking questions of the patient.

BIOMEDICINE AS A CULTURAL SYSTEM

Developing cross-cultural communication skills may involve a transition from having no insight about the role of patient culture on medical care; to accepting that a patient's culturally informed beliefs, values, and behaviors have an important influence on health, disease, and treatment effectiveness; and, finally, to unconsciously integrating attention to patient culture into all areas of clinical practice. Equally important, however, is that clinicians develop an awareness of their *own* cultures and the unquestioned assumptions that are informed by their personal histories, the nonprofessional aspects of their daily lives, and the socialization imparted by their significant, lengthy engagement in biomedical training and practice.

Focusing on "culture" primarily in relation to immigrant or minority patients may convey the notion that biomedicine is itself without culture. In fact, although biomedicine is informed by scientific knowledge (a "culture" with its own values and beliefs), it is also shaped by the politics of government funding, insurance reimbursement, rivalries among specialties, as well as by competing ideologies of profit versus altruism, changing fashions and trends, best guesses, and regional biases. Biomedicine comprises many cultural worlds and languages—primary care, cardiology, surgery; the hospital, the clinic; nursing, physicians, pharmacists; and so on—that for many patients are strange, potentially threatening, and difficult to understand. Awareness of how different kinds of patients are likely to experience and interpret biomedicine is essential to enhancing cross-cultural communication. It is equally important for clinicians to be aware of their own roles in perpetuating the culture of biomedicine, and to realize the extent to which they are both the products and practitioners of this cultural system.

Table 15-1 lists several characteristics that have been associated with biomedicine and its practitioners. Tensions and misunderstandings between practitioner and patient are often strongly rooted in many of the attributes listed under (A) in Table 15-1. Often most problematic from the perspective of patients is biomedicine's tendency to sharply differentiate body from mind and to emphasize organic pathophysiology over the psychosocial ramifications and origins of illness. Nonetheless, many of biomedicine's major successes have been achieved despite—or often because of—such tendencies. These are the characteristics that set biomedicine apart from other systems of healing. They are also quite resistant to change. The clinician's goal should be to act as a cultural broker, making these features of biomedicine more accessible and understandable to the patient while at the same time exploring and attending to the psychosocial dimensions of illness from the patient's perspective.

Individual practitioners vary greatly in the degree to which they conform to the attributes of professionalism listed under (B) in Table 15-1 (see Chapter 47). Although common, none is a *predictable* feature of biomedicine in the same way as those listed under (A). A central problem, however, is that many patients have difficulty understanding or sympathizing with the

Table 15-1. Characteristics of biomedicine and its practitioners.

(A) ***Biomedicine as a system of healing rests upon and esteems the following:***

- Empiric science
- Written knowledge as opposed to oral tradition
- Rigorous and lengthy training
- Technological sophistication and innovation
- Action orientation and interventionism ("doing something rather than nothing")
- Materialism (disease in the individual, physical body rather than in the family, social group, mind, or spirit)
- Differentiating among acute illness, chronic illness, and prevention
- Reductionism (pathophysiology is molecular and anatomic; symptoms are expressions of underlying disease rather than diseases themselves)
- High levels of bureaucratic organization; complexity and subspecialization
- Team-based care
- Efficiency
- Cost containment
- "Defensiveness" or avoiding malpractice
- The prolongation of life

(B) ***Many*** **clinicians** ***value these traits:***

- Hard work
- Self-sacrifice
- Self-reliance and autonomy
- Strong career orientation
- Status consciousness
- Respect for authority and hierarchy
- Hygiene
- Punctuality
- The physician as the expert
- Deliberateness
- Articulateness
- A clear separation between personal and work lives
- Conservatism in dress and expressions of emotion
- Quality judged by one's colleagues

(C) ***Common attributions that*** **patients** ***have about biomedicine and its practitioners:***

Negative	Positive
Arrogant	Highly competent
Elite	Honest
Judgmental	Careful
Remote and inaccessible	Thorough
Narrow minded	Methodical
Difficult to comprehend	Caring
Money hungry	Accurate
Rushed	Reliable
Dogmatic	Responsible
Rigid	Impartial
Entitled	Hardworking
Uninterested in the patient as a person	Putting the patient's welfare first and foremost

attributes in either category, compounding communication difficulties, and leading some to hold many of the negative impressions listed under (C) in Table 15-1. This is especially true when patients desire a more personal and less professional relationship with their physicians, or when social distance compounds the patient's feelings of powerlessness. The culturally competent clinician will understand these common features and negative patient perceptions of biomedicine, recognizing when they contribute to misunderstandings and impair a patient's ability to feel at ease, communicate, and benefit from a biomedical approach.

COMMUNICATION

Communication involves the exchange, processing, and interpretation of messages—both verbal and nonverbal. In this complex process, there are myriad opportunities for miscommunication: messages can be incomplete, confusing, and contradictory; language barriers as well as emotional and physical distractions can interfere with the receipt and relaying of information; and unspoken assumptions can influence the meaning one person attributes to another's statements or actions. Much of this takes place outside of conscious awareness. With this in mind, this section reviews three fundamental aspects of communication to which the clinician should direct particular attention: (1) attempting to understand the illness from the *patient's* perspective; (2) ensuring that the patient understands, as much as possible and at an appropriate level, *biomedical* explanations of the illness and its treatment; and (3) guiding patients through the *ritualized* clinical encounter and the health care bureaucracy in ways that increase their familiarity and comfort with it.

The Patient

Barriers to health care affecting both immigrants and disadvantaged minority groups—such as lack of insurance and other financial resources, physical distance, and low literacy—often make biomedical treatment an option of last resort. Clinical consultations for such patients will frequently be more time consuming and require increased patience by the clinician. Extra effort may sometimes be needed to teach such patients to be assertive, ask questions, and raise concerns. Clinicians who treat large numbers of such patients will benefit the most from reading about and becoming personally familiar with them outside of medical settings.

EXPLANATORY MODELS

Explanatory models refer to theories of disease causation, prognosis, typical symptoms, and appropriate treatment. Eliciting patients' explanatory models of disease offers unparalleled insight into their sense of self and relationships with significant others while yielding clues about how they are likely to interpret, resist, or accept biomedical explanations and treatments. Knowledge of the patient's perspective also facilitates the ability to ease patient fear and anxiety. Understanding the patient's *explanatory model* of illness is especially important when treating potentially debilitating chronic conditions, where nonadherence is a common concern and where the psychosocial dimensions of illness loom large.

Table 15-2. Questions to elicit a patient's explanatory model of illness.

- What do you think caused your problem?
- What do you think you have?
- What is the name you give to this condition?
- Why do some people get this illness but not others?
- What do you think needs to be done to relieve this problem?

Typically, the most important component of a patient's explanatory model is the idea of illness *causation* (Table 15-2). To elicit this belief the clinician can ask, "What do you think caused your problem?" and then listen carefully to the answer as it is likely to reveal crucial feelings related to moral failings, discord with significant others, financial and practical challenges in daily life, and whether there is a sense of hope for the future. The clinician should not expect patients to answer questions about causation with simple and mechanistic explanations. Additional probing may also be required. For example, the clinician could follow up with questions, such as "What do you think you have? What is the name you give to this condition?" "Why do some people get this illness and not others?" "Who or what is responsible (or to blame) for this problem?" and "Do you ever think that you did (or didn't do) something to bring this on yourself, or that someone else did (or didn't do) something?" Additional questions can allow patients to elaborate on their explanatory model: "What do you think should be done to treat you?" "Do you think a complete cure is possible?" "How long will the problem last?" "What do you think needs to be done to relieve this problem?" The advantage of such questions is that they are open ended, are applicable to every patient, and can help to correct or refine initial clinical assumptions or preconceptions. They are also powerful in their ability to provide clues about what the patient may find difficult to understand or accept when it comes to explaining the illness in *biomedical* terms.

Some patients, especially recent immigrants, may be reticent about sharing their explanatory models of illness out of concern that their beliefs will be viewed as ignorant or superstitious. Alternatively, such patients may feel that they have come to hear the doctor's expert opinion, and that their own perspective is of little consequence.

It is sometimes prudent to allow patients' explanatory models to emerge slowly, through gentle probing, over the course of several visits. Inference combined with direct questioning (e.g., "other patients believe X, what do you think about this?") and background knowledge of the patient's social location will often be necessary to form a coherent picture.

Shared Decision Making

Patient centeredness and involving patients in complex decisions about their health care are important goals in medical care; however, it is still the case that most medical decisions are made by physicians with little input from patients or families. In shared decision making, a patient and clinician work together to evaluate tradeoffs based on the patient's values and preferences in light of the risks and benefits of various treatment options. Shared decision making is most important for preference-sensitive conditions in which there are at least two legitimate treatment options available, but each has different levels of risk or types of side effects.

Imparting accurate information about the nature and course of the disease, framing numerical risks, and eliciting a patient's outcome preferences are all important for shared decision making. Successfully sharing decisions, however, also requires a consideration of cultural influences. For example, certain patients (e.g., some older patients or patients who grew up in authoritarian societies) may not wish to participate in making a final treatment decision but instead wish to be involved only in articulating preferences and in selecting the most desirable outcome. Thus, the process of promoting patient centeredness should involve directly asking patients how involved they would like to be in decision making.

In emphasizing the importance of rational decision making, traditional shared decision-making approaches implicitly stress how patients "should" behave while often overlooking how they, in fact, do behave. To address these challenges, clinicians should strive to meet patients closer to where they actually begin the decision-making process. Eliciting patient explanatory models may allow patients and clinicians to consciously recognize and correct misconceptions. Sources of patient fear can be elucidated and, where possible, reassurance can be offered. Patients can also be asked to recount stories about other people who faced similar illnesses so that their attitudes and perceptions can be clarified, and they can be helped to understand key differences between these stories and their own circumstances.

Sometimes there is medical uncertainty about the value of a medical test or intervention (e.g., prostate-specific antigen [PSA] screening), or there may be more than one treatment option, none of which is clearly superior in terms of prevention, cure, or control of symptoms, but each of which differs significantly in terms of cost or in the likelihood of various adverse effects on quality of life. In these instances, before taking action the clinician should attempt to gauge both the patient's desire for information as well as preferences for decision making. Studies have shown that most patients wish to be "maximally" informed about their diseases as well as medical treatments and evaluations, but there is variability in their desire to assume or share responsibility for making actual treatment decisions. Only through probing is it possible to determine how much information patients want and how much they want to share in the decision-making process. Providing too much information or attempting to make the patient accept responsibility for a medical decision can be counterproductive, but so can an approach that is overly paternalistic. One strategy is for the provider to state that there is a choice and perhaps some medical controversy or uncertainty; briefly mention the pros and cons of each option; elicit patient outcome preferences; and then wait for the patient to ask for more details, voice concerns, or express a preference.

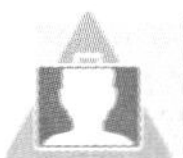

CASE ILLUSTRATION 1

A 72-year-old World War II veteran was diagnosed with localized prostate cancer. The patient is adamant about his desire to undergo curative treatment with radical surgery after the urologist explains that the likelihood of cure is the same with radiation therapy, after he reviews the specific and significant numerical likelihood of serious side effects associated with surgery and radiation, and after he proposes that watchful waiting and active surveillance are also reasonable options. After carefully eliciting the patient's understanding of the disease and its treatment, the urologist learns, from the patient's perspective, that: "cancer is a death sentence," "the only way to cure cancer is by cutting it out," and "radiation is dangerous." By taking the time to understand the patient's explanatory model of illness, the urologist is in a position to more effectively address his misconceptions and fears, thus allowing the patient to make a more genuine, high-quality decision about his care.

Fatalism

Members of some groups, including many immigrants, may seem to be fatalistic in their attitudes toward illness. They may be passive about seeking treatment, persist in unhealthful behaviors, or accept misfortune because they believe it is preordained. It is important not to assume that this style of explaining and dealing with illness is indelibly rooted in the culture or religion of the patient's racial or ethnic group. In fact, fatalism is widespread and is common among people who have little control over the circumstances of their lives. It also emerges out of a kind of valid logic that observes that serious illness can befall even those who have no bad habits and live a "clean" or "virtuous" life. Fatalism does not usually imply a lack of interest in preventing or treating disease. Rather, it can be viewed as an idiom for describing a person's perceived powerlessness in the world, lack of hope, and even distrust. The doctor can approach this problem by acknowledging the real challenges the patient faces, and by clearly articulating the practical steps the patient can take to resolve or manage the illness.

CASE ILLUSTRATION 2

A 56-year-old woman who completed a grade-school education declines colon cancer screening. On questioning, she believes that cancer is not preventable and cannot be cured. Cancer terrifies her and she therefore sees no point in learning she might have it. The clinician explains that from a medical perspective cancer takes many years to develop, and that in people aged over 50 years it can happen in a few individuals out of a hundred. She then tells the patient that the purpose of colon cancer screening—a relatively safe procedure performed thousands of times every year—is not to find a big cancer (which would be extremely unusual) but to save lives by finding a few areas (polyps) where cancer could develop and then snip them out. She provides the patient with an illustrated brochure to look over and consider.

In addition to the patient's beliefs about cancer, the clinician suspects that she distrusts the idea of doctors doing something to her that she, herself, has not requested or previously thought about. Over the course of several appointments, the clinician gently revisits the issue. A year later, the patient agrees. Trust—developed through a continuing relationship, manifest concern on the part of the clinician, and openness in explaining the purpose of medical tests—was a key factor in the patient's decision. Had the patient continued to decline screening, however, the clinician appropriately would have respected her decision, without overt negative judgment.

The Passive Patient

Some immigrants and older patients may be exceptionally reserved or deferential in clinical interactions, often preferring to avoid direct eye contact. The clinician should not assume that such patients are shy, uninterested, unintelligent, or uneducated simply because they avoid eye contact, agree with everything the doctor says, express a great deal of uncertainty about instructions, or are not forthcoming with information. In these circumstances, the clinician should speak clearly without reverting to an overly simplistic, commanding, frustrated, or patronizing tone of voice. Further clinic visits and gentle elicitation of questions and concerns may be necessary before the patient begins to interact more openly. The patient's behavior may reflect not only cultural norms toward those in authority, but uncertainty, fear, the expression of trust through passivity, or a desire to attain a better impression of the clinician before revealing intimate details.

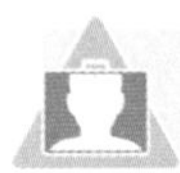

CASE ILLUSTRATION 3

An older patient, originally a schoolteacher from the Philippines, is hospitalized for community-acquired pneumonia. The hospitalization is uneventful and on the day of discharge, the medical team enters his room to review his discharge instructions. When asked for his input about preferred follow-up or his understanding of the ongoing treatment, he averts his eyes, speaks quietly, and seems unable to comprehend the discharge plan. He repeatedly asks for instructions about the various forms. The team leaves the room uncertain of his understanding. Later that morning, the pharmacist on the team returns to review his discharge medications with him. She sits down and speaks softly and respectfully. Eventually, he opens up and it becomes apparent that he understood the prior conversation completely and speaks articulately about his concerns, although he continues to avoid eye contact.

Interpreters

Trained medical interpreters can greatly facilitate patient–clinician communication and improve quality of care. Unfortunately, perhaps because of economic constraints and clinicians' beliefs in their own ability to simply "get by," well-trained interpreters are underused in many medical settings, with negative consequences for patient care. For example, although clinicians with some ability in conversational Spanish may assume they understand a Puerto Rican patient's use of the term "ataque de nervios" (literally a "nervous attack"), the patient is actually referring to a culturally specific syndrome with identifiable precipitants and clear symptoms that has little to do with a "nervous breakdown."

Although family members often act as de facto interpreters, this can also introduce problems. For example, a relative who "already knows" what is wrong with the patient may not wish to bother the physician with the full details of the patient's complaints, thereby omitting important symptoms. Children and adolescents are inappropriate interpreters for many reasons, including an often incomplete mastery of English, insufficient knowledge of the subtleties of translation, and issues of relationship and status.

Trained medical interpreters can provide more than literal paraphrasing: they can serve as "cultural interpreters" by explaining patient's illness labels and idioms for the practitioner and translating biomedical concepts and instructions into the patient's vernacular. Interpreters should be treated as full members of the health care team. Prior to the interaction, the clinician may want to meet briefly with the interpreter to review the goals for that discussion (e.g., addressing the patient's understanding of and compliance with a particular medication). In addition, the clinician should periodically stop the interview to seek clarification from the interpreter: "The patient has mentioned 'nerves' a few times. I was assuming that she felt nervous, but now I'm not so sure. Could you explain to me what she means?"

When using an interpreter, it is important to consider the physical arrangement of the participants. The clinician should always face and speak to the patient directly. The interpreter can sit next to the physician (though some patients may find this arrangement threatening), or the patient and interpreter can sit side by side. Some clinicians prefer the traditional triangular arrangement so that all parties have equal space and symbolic power, but the easy flow of conversation may be compromised as patient and provider often cannot resist the impulse to direct their attention toward the interpreter instead of toward each other.

The Clinician

Understanding illness from the patient's perspective—traditionally regarded as the essence of cultural competence—must be balanced by the equally important task of knowing how to communicate *biomedical* explanations about the disease and its treatment to the patient (i.e., serving as interpreter of biomedical culture for patients). The desire for such information is usually one of the patient's primary motivations for visiting a doctor. The clinician should offer explanations in terms the patient can understand and then gently test this understanding.

Naming and Explaining the Disease in Neutral Terms

Naming a disease helps to transform a patient's inchoate fears into something that can be perceived and addressed directly. Speaking about disease in neutral and mechanistic ways can also dispel feelings of shame and ideas about etiology that are rooted in personal weakness and social failure. Patients will often seize upon, and benefit from, explanations that appropriately relieve them of personal responsibility for their misfortune. Giving a specific name to a disease and explaining it in neutral terms should be regarded as one of the primary goals of communication. Reaching this point, of course, may depend upon an initial period of testing and observation.

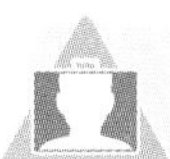

CASE ILLUSTRATION 4

A 65-year-old immigrant and former physician is diagnosed with cancer. The clinician is able to elicit the patient's belief that cancer often occurs in people with "repressed personalities." Believing that he brought his disease upon himself because of such a character flaw, he feels a lack of hope and is less inclined to treat the disease. He benefits from an impersonal biomedical interpretation of cancer that focuses on damaged cellular DNA leading to unchecked cellular proliferation, and treatment aimed at destroying aberrant cells.

Medicalization

Although reductionistic disease labels and explanations are often helpful, they may contribute to the medicalization of conditions whose etiologies reside in adverse environmental (e.g., polluted air and water) or social circumstances (e.g., racism, intimate partner violence, sexual abuse, and work-related stress). In other words, defining illness entirely in terms of how it adversely affects the body can direct attention away from other, more fundamental causes. It is important to remain mindful of, and at times acknowledge, the broader context that gives rise to the illness. This is often very difficult for physicians to do, in part because they are not trained to recognize these links and are limited in their ability to resolve problems such as poverty, unemployment, poor housing, or lack of education and opportunity. For example, declaring that a patient's asthma is made worse by living near a factory from which, for economic reasons, the patient cannot easily move away may imply that nothing can be done about the problem. Nonetheless, awareness of such constraints can help the clinician to better understand and sympathize with the patient and tailor therapies that are realistic and appropriate. In addition, it is extremely common for patients of all backgrounds to believe that illness is caused by breaches in the moral order, social discord, and the failure of one's self or significant others to fulfill expected roles. Purely mechanistic biomedical explanations cannot simply replace these types of beliefs, which tend to be deeply rooted and resistant to change. Educating the patient about disease terms and pathophysiology should complement but not supersede the importance of understanding and acknowledging these other aspects of the patient's explanatory model.

"Blaming the Victim"

When it is possible to trace the etiology of disease to potentially destructive personal behaviors, such as "risky" sex, smoking, alcoholism, and drug abuse, or the worsening of disease to medical nonadherence, two pitfalls should be avoided. One is emphasizing personal culpability at the expense of helping the patient to understand the nature of the disease itself. Without adequate education, patients may have a difficult time perceiving the relationship between their behavior and the outcomes these generate, and will therefore see less reason to make changes. Although it is important to stress that certain habits are harmful and should be altered or discontinued, this should be done in a straightforward and nonjudgmental manner. The second pitfall is failing to acknowledge the personal situations and social contexts that contribute to or sustain these behaviors. Low self-esteem, depression, chronic pain, social isolation, lack of "legitimate" employment, and a strong desire to experience a sense of social belonging can contribute to many varieties of harmful and risky practices. To the extent possible, clinicians should attempt to determine the factors that perpetuate or encourage harmful behaviors and discuss these with their patients in an open and frank manner. Doing so will demonstrate empathy and concern, and help patients understand how their behavior (arising as it might for understandable reasons) should nonetheless be modified, and how this might be achieved.

Communicating Bad News

Naming the disease is a cornerstone of communication in the biomedical model. However, a more flexible approach to informing patients of their diagnosis is often appropriate, particularly when the diagnosis is cancer or a terminal illness. Knowledge of a patient's social location and explanatory models of illness (including cancer), as well as in-depth questioning of the patient and family, will provide the best understanding of cultural differences and preferences. Chapter 3 offers a more complete discussion of this topic.

Evidence-Based Medicine and Minimizing the Overuse and Misuse of Clinical Services

Promoting clinician stewardship over limited health care resources and ensuring the delivery of cost-conscious, evidence-based care have become increasingly important as health care expenditures have risen to unsustainable levels in the United States. Influences that promote the overuse and misuse of clinical services include financial gain for clinicians as well as defensive medicine (ordering tests, procedures, or visits primarily in order to reduce perceived exposure to malpractice liability). Patient expectations—shaped by clinicians themselves, the popular media, direct-to-consumer advertising, and anecdotes of friends and family—are also important drivers of medical overuse. It can be a significant challenge convincing patients that more care, more expensive care, or even the latest technology do not necessarily mean better care, especially because unmet expectations for care can be associated with less patient satisfaction and reduced intentions to adhere to prescribed therapy. Nonetheless, evidence-based practice often depends on a clinician's ability to elucidate patient expectations that are unrealistic or not medically valid, the beliefs and worries that underlie these, and then on an ability to engage patients in conversations that educate and, where possible, reassure. Helping patients to feel like they have been understood is a key way of earning their trust and realigning their expectations.

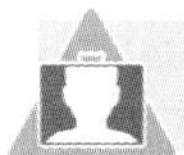

CASE ILLUSTRATION 5

A 32-year-old woman, the daughter of a prominent local philanthropist, complains of chest pain and demands that her physician obtain a stress test to make sure she is not at risk of having a heart attack. The patient, an avid runner, does not experience exertional chest pain and otherwise has no cardiac risk factors. On questioning, the physician learns that the patient recently broke up with her boyfriend and that her parents are contemplating a divorce. The physician obtains an EKG and informs the patient that it is normal. She explains to the patient that chest pain is not unusual among patients living through significant stress, that these symptoms almost always resolve with time, and that she has no risk factors for cardiac disease. She further explains that stress testing in her situation has a real likelihood of leading to false positive results, prolonged anxiety, more clinic visits, and perhaps even additional, invasive testing. Ultimately, the physician is able to help the patient understand that a stress test is unnecessary. The patient agrees to return in a week to reassess how she's feeling and consider whether referral to a therapist might be helpful.

Psychiatric Diagnoses

For patients of many backgrounds, profound stigma is often attached to behavioral and psychiatric diagnoses. Labels such as "depression," referrals to psychiatrists, or prescriptions for "mind-altering" medications may be strongly resisted, interpreted as insulting by some, and may severely compromise the practitioner–patient relationship. For such patients, somatization is often the most "legitimate" way of expressing distress. If there is any doubt regarding the patient's perception of psychiatric labels and referrals, the clinician should carefully explore the meanings that patients and their families attribute to them.

CASE ILLUSTRATION 6

An immigrant, working-class mother is taken aback by the pediatrician's diagnosis of "attention deficit disorder" in her child and concomitant referral to a child psychiatrist and prescription for stimulant medication. She believes these recommendations imply that her child is "crazy" and, by extension, that she, first and foremost, as well as the family as a whole, have somehow failed. Her anguish is compounded by the extreme importance she attributes to her role as a mother and homemaker. Furthermore, she holds that psychiatric medicines are "too powerful" for her child who, like all children, is "sensitive and vulnerable." She would have benefited from a discussion that elicited these beliefs in advance, followed by an approach that acknowledged her fears, reaffirmed her maternal skills and concern, and attempted gently to address her beliefs and values.

Patient Interpretations of Acute Illness, Chronic Illness, and Preventive Medicine

Many patients do not clearly differentiate acute from chronic illness, nor do they make distinctions among curing, managing, and preventing disease. Commonly, they assume that symptoms or diseases are self-limiting or curable with a single course of therapy. This can frustrate the clinician's ability to provide education and can contribute to poor adherence. If in doubt, the clinician should determine whether patients believe a cure is possible (*not* generally the case with chronic illness) or whether patients believe the absence of current symptoms implies the absence of future disease (suggesting poor understanding of preventive medicine). Gently correcting patients' misconceptions should be viewed as an ongoing process that takes time and bears repetition.

Patients with Poor English Literacy

It is estimated that up to 21% of American adults are functionally illiterate and many more are only marginally literate, limiting their ability to understand medical information and engage in meaningful discussions with their providers. Feelings of embarrassment may lead patients to conceal this problem. Strategies for managing such patients include speaking slowly, using simple terms, targeting written materials to at most a fifth-grade reading level, and using clear pictures and diagrams whenever possible. Instruments such as the Test of Functional Health Literacy in Adults (TOFHLA) can provide rapid estimates of the ability to read and comprehend common medical and lay terms. Such tools can assist clinicians in tailoring both written and spoken information, and are probably more accurate at assessing the patient's reading and numerical skills and ability to function effectively in health care settings than subjective clinician impression alone.

Reviewing Medications

Failure to discuss medications is one of the most frequent lacunae in practitioner–patient communication. Misunderstandings and fears about medications are extremely common and are major contributors to nonadherence. Pharmaceuticals, however, are generally the most tangible and therapeutically important products that result from the clinical encounter. Special care should therefore be given to explaining their purpose, mechanism of action, and common side effects. Eliciting patient concerns and questions to uncover erroneous beliefs is also important. This is particularly likely to benefit patients who are reticent or unable to express these concerns on their own.

Sometimes it may be helpful for clinicians to personalize information by acknowledging common challenges they face in educating and treating patients.

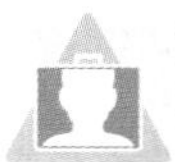

CASE ILLUSTRATION 7

A patient has been diagnosed with hypertension. After explaining the benefits and risks of treating hypertension with medication, the physician tries to help the patient see the clinical challenge from her perspective. She explains, "As doctors, we often have difficulty helping patients understand why they should take medicines even when they have no unpleasant symptoms. Understandably, patients often hate to take medicines, especially if they feel perfectly fine. Yet medicines are important for preventing very serious problems down the road."

This kind of approach may help some patients to understand and sympathize with the challenges faced by the clinician, promoting a sense that the two are allies in achieving a common objective.

Assessing Patient Understanding

To ensure that biomedical explanations are correctly understood, the clinician should ask patients close- and open-ended questions about their disease process and ask them to repeat instructions. For example, "Tell me what you understand about the cause of your diabetes and what you think will happen if we cannot adequately control your blood sugar. How often should you check your blood sugar? What should you do if you feel lightheaded and sweaty?" Such checks will help to reinforce knowledge and understanding and identify areas that benefit from further counseling.

The Clinician as Cultural Broker & Institutional Guide

As described above, cross-cultural communication is enhanced by attention to patients' social location because it allows provisional inferences to be made about how patients, as *individuals*, are likely to interpret and respond to their illness. Initial clinical impressions are then modified by eliciting patients' explanatory models of illness. This information helps to tailor communication regarding the *biomedical* perspective. Finally, communication is further enhanced by understanding how patients perceive key features of the clinical process and by guiding them through its ritual and bureaucratic aspects.

Clinical Rituals

Repetitive and predictable patterns and rules circumscribe patient–clinician interactions. In the ambulatory setting, for example, the nurse measures the patient's blood pressure and then brings the patient to see the physician, who directs the proceedings according to a predefined format of greeting the patient, asking questions in a certain order, examining the patient, and offering explanations and recommendations. The patient is given a specific place to sit and generally knows that the consultation will last a fixed amount of time. In the hospital, the medical team rounds in the morning and obtains a standard template of subjective and objective information. The basic format of these rituals is fairly simple and can be readily learned by patients and by the new initiates into the profession.

Such ritual aspects of medicine can both facilitate and impede effective communication. For example, consistency minimizes confusion about what is acceptable and unacceptable and about what will happen. Ritual offers a sense of security when patients are undressed or are sharing personal information. The ground rules and scripts of ritual are translatable from one setting to another and operate even if practitioner and patient have never met. They allow the involved actors to focus greater attention on the *content* of their exchanges and, in themselves, these rituals can be comforting and even therapeutic.

On the other hand, rituals can impair communication if patients and practitioners differ in their expectations about how they are supposed to work, or if rituals become inflexible, blind routines that leave little room for digression, variation, and opportunities for patients to express themselves freely and in fully emotional ways. This frequently happens when the clinician is pressed for time and wants the patient to provide the "facts" as tersely as possible, or when the patient yields all spontaneity of self-expression to the perceived all-knowingness and authority of the doctor. Ritual should not become so fixed that its participants become inflexible. Awareness of these pitfalls and the ability to make spontaneous adjustments to unspoken aspects of ritual can do much to enhance communication with the patient. Brief, unexpected, or even surprising disruptions to ritual—such as a joke, a doctor's personal reflection, allowing the patient to shed a tear or relate a piece of medical history during the physical examination, or briefly and politely answering a patient's personal question about the doctor or his family—can, when judiciously applied and without breaking the overall structure of the encounter, foster more effective communication and enhance the therapeutic relationship.

For almost all patients, illness is not simply an individual malady, but a social disruption that both affects and requires the involvement of significant others. The paradigmatic private, dyadic nature of biomedicine's doctor–patient relationship can also impair communication when working with patients for whom the involvement of family members is very important. When desired by the patient, and to the extent possible, allowances and arrangements should be made to incorporate the family into diagnostic and treatment plans (see Chapter 11).

Institutional Guide

Health care is often highly fragmented. The increasingly sharp separation between hospital and ambulatory medicine, a large variety of subspecialists, and the growing importance of health care "teams" means that patients often interact with a bewildering variety of individuals whom they have never previously met and whose roles are not always apparent. Carefully guiding patients—anticipating their possible confusion, explaining the function of different health care workers, and encouraging patients to ask questions at any point during their trajectory through an illness episode—can go a long way toward alleviating their fear, misunderstanding, and distrust. Providers should be especially sensitive to immigrants and other vulnerable patients who may have a particularly poor understanding of how the health care system works. Providing education about where to report for laboratory work and procedures, when results will be returned and what will be done with these, the roles of various office staff, the hours of operation, rules pertaining to the presence of children, and so on will increase efficiency, improve patient use of resources, and also increase patient trust and adherence by demystifying what seems to be a complex and threatening bureaucracy. Of note, some patients may not wish to fill out forms because of fears of deportation; it is important to be explicit about the purpose and confidentiality of medical information.

"COMPLEMENTARY" & "ALTERNATIVE" HEALERS

Despite its depth of knowledge and undeniable efficacy in many areas, biomedicine is for many patients simply *one* healing option among many others, some of which are employed simultaneously and without apparent contradiction. If the patient wishes to discuss or solicit the provider's opinion about other healing modalities, the clinician—unless there are concrete reasons to the contrary—should be willing to acknowledge the beneficial role that nonbiomedical approaches may have for the patient. If there are potential adverse interactions or side effects of "alternative" therapies, or if there is concern that potentially beneficial biomedical therapies might be thwarted by other types of healers, the clinician should express these concerns but should always respect the fact that patients are the ultimate arbiters regarding the healing modalities for which they are best suited (see Chapter 33).

RACE/ETHNICITY & GENETICS

By virtue of their race or ethnicity, patients are sometimes said to be "at risk" for certain diseases. Examples include diabetes mellitus among Native Americans, breast cancer among Ashkenazi Jews, and prostate cancer among African Americans. Particular forms of treatment are also believed to be more (or less) effective among certain racial/ethnic groups compared with others. For example, among African Americans compared with whites, it is said that the combination of isosorbide dinitrate and hydralazine is more effective for treating heart failure, angiotensin-converting enzyme (ACE) inhibitors are less effective for essential hypertension, and a therapeutic response to selective serotonin reuptake inhibitor (SSRI) antidepressants takes place at lower doses. Each of these examples is highly controversial, reflecting long-standing, often heated disputes about whether race and ethnicity are primarily social constructs or, instead, meaningful and valid surrogates for biological difference. It is beyond the scope of this chapter to summarize the elements of this debate. We believe, however, that in communicating with patients it is important for clinicians to avoid oversimplifying the relationship between race/ethnicity and genetics. Although knowledge of race or ethnicity might prompt genetic testing or detailed family history taking in particular instances, the issues are simply too complex and the evidence too uncertain in a relatively small number of conditions for clinicians to make unqualified assertions to patients that they are "at risk" for a particular illness or unlikely to respond to therapies solely on the basis of their racial/ethnic background. In very real ways, believing that one is "at risk" can unnecessarily increase stress, fear, and feelings of stigma, uncertainty, and worthlessness. When discussing with patients the possible relevance of race and ethnicity, clinicians should openly acknowledge that experts do not always agree, and they should quantify and convey individual risk through a consideration of as many relevant variables as possible.

CONCLUSIONS

Cross-cultural communication can be learned and enhanced through reflection and practice with a variety of patients from different cultures. Biomedicine has its own distinct culture and practices that may be difficult for many patients to comprehend and access. Cultural stereotypes are rarely useful in clinical encounters; instead, clinicians should attempt to understand the social location of their patients as reflected in their race and ethnicity, gender, age, immigration status, literacy level, occupation, sexual orientation, and other characteristics. As their skills develop, clinicians will find enormous gratification in caring for patients who are very different from them.

SUGGESTED READINGS

Denberg, TD, Melhado, TV, Steiner, JS. Patient treatment preferences in localized prostate carcinoma: the influence of emotion, misconception, and anecdote. *Cancer* 2006;107(3):620–630.

Fadiman A. *The Spirit Catches You and You Fall Down.* New York, NY: Farrar, Strauss & Giroux; 1998.

Helman C. *Culture, Health, and Illness*, 2nd ed. Oxford: Butterworth-Heinemann; 1992.

Kaiser Permanente National Diversity Council. *A Provider's Handbook on Culturally Competent Care.* (Available for Latino, African American, Asian/Pacific-Islander, and Eastern European populations.)

Kleinman A. *Patients and Healers in the Context of Culture.* Berkeley, CA: University of California Press; 1980.

Kleinman A, Benson P. Anthropology in the clinic: the problem of cultural competency and how to fix it. *PLoS Med* 2006; 3(10):e294.

WEBSITES

Centers for Medicare and Medicaid Services, Office of Minority Health. A Practical Guide to Implementing the National CLAS Standards: For Racial, Ethnic and Linguistic Minorities, People with Disabilities and Sexual and Gender Minorities. December, 2016. https://www.cms.gov/About-CMS/Agency-Information/OMH/Downloads/CLAS-Toolkit-12-7-16.pdf. Accessed July 2019.

Industry Collaborative Effort (ICE) Cultural and Linguistic Workgroup. Resources to Assist Communication with a Diverse Patient Population Base. http://www.iceforhealth.org/library/documents/ICE_C&L_Provider_Toolkit_7.10.pdf. Accessed July 2019.

National Institute on Minority Health and Health Disparities. Health Information in Multiple Languages for Priority Health Conditions. https://www.nimhd.nih.gov/programs/edu-training/language-access/health-information/index.html. Accessed July 2019.

U.S. Department of Health and Social Services, Office of Minority Health. Think Cultural Health: A Physician's Practical Guide to Culturally Competent Care. https://cccm.thinkculturalhealth.hhs.gov/. Accessed July 2019.

Women

16

Diane S. Morse, MD; Misa Perron-Burdick, MD, MAS; & Judith Walsh, MD, MPH

INTRODUCTION

This chapter describes the broad array of behavioral issues for women using a developmental framework. We discuss expected behavioral issues occurring as part of the normal life cycle, as well as problematic ones requiring medical surveillance or intervention.

ADOLESCENCE: A TIME OF POWER IN THE MIDST OF INSECURITY

The task of adolescence is to find one's own beliefs, moving from childhood to adulthood physically and in relationships (see Chapter 13). Several events can occur during this time that will require the sensitive attention of the primary care provider, but numerous studies have demonstrated that confidentiality must be maintained for the provider to be trusted and helpful to an adolescent.

Approach to the Gynecologic Examination

Some women fear a pelvic examination, especially when they are undergoing it for the first time. Little research has been done on what strategies are best in performing a pelvic examination, but several techniques have been found to be helpful in clinical practice.

Before performing the examination, clinicians should make the patient as comfortable as possible when taking a history by asking open-ended questions, demonstrating empathetic communication skills such as eye contact and nonjudgmental reactions, and not making assumptions about sexual activity and orientation. In addition, they should ask if the patient has had a previous pelvic examination. When taking a complete sexual or gender identity history, they should inquire about prior sexual abuse or challenges with past examinations, inviting the patient to suggest techniques for making the exam more comfortable. The exam may need to be done at a separate visit after the clinician has built rapport with the patient.

It is useful for the clinician to describe exactly what is being done before and during the examination. Both female and male clinicians should consider offering to have a chaperone or support person present to reassure the patient about the professional content of the examination. Clinicians may also use chaperones at their discretion, such as in the case of adolescents or patients with development delay, psychiatric illness, or a history of physical or sexual abuse. Other techniques include draping all areas of the body not being examined; using a warm, lubricated speculum; using the narrowest speculum that will allow adequate visualization of the cervix; being as gentle as possible; and encouraging the patient to use relaxation techniques including abdominal breathing and mental imagery, techniques which are especially useful for young women and those who have experienced sexual abuse. In addition, elevating the head will facilitate communication and may help the patient feel less vulnerable. In situations where a patient has significant anxiety, an anxiolytic medication prior to the examination may be useful. Specific recommendations for examining patients with a history of trauma can be found at https://www.reproductiveaccess.org/resource/trauma-informed-pelvic-exams/.

Research has shown that the experience of the first pelvic examination influences attitudes about subsequent examinations; therefore, it is important to make the first pelvic examination as positive an experience as possible. In a study describing women's experiences of the first pelvic examination, a negative evaluation of the examination was associated with pain, embarrassment, having insufficient knowledge about the examination and what the clinician was doing, and not knowing that they could stop at any time. Taking time to provide knowledge, encourage realistic expectations of the examination, and reminding patients that they may stop the exam at any time may help shape attitudes about subsequent examinations.

If a gynecologic examination is being carried out on an adolescent in the context of reproductive health care or to screen for sexually transmitted infections, it is important to be aware of the legal requirements of confidentiality in the United States, which vary by state and are listed on the Guttmacher Institute website (http://www.guttmacher.org). Adolescents should be encouraged to involve their parents or guardians in medical decisions, and providers should be aware of mandatory reporting laws in the case of nonconsensual sexual activity, sex with an older adult, or other abuse.

Chronic Pelvic Pain & Vulvodynia

A condition that can affect women starting in teen or early adult years is chronic pelvic pain (CPP), which is commonly defined as pain of at least 6 months duration that occurs in the pelvis, abdominal wall, lower back, or buttocks, and is serious enough to cause disability or require medical care. CPP affects up to 15% of women and accounts for 20% of the hysterectomies performed in the United States. Up to 40% of women with CPP have other diagnoses, which may be the cause and/or effects of the CPP, such as depression, anxiety, sexual dysfunction, substance use disorders, and other pain syndromes, requiring in-depth investigation into all contributing factors. A history of sexual or physical abuse, including intimate partner violence, has been identified in over 50% of CPP patients, and therefore must be included in the history (see Chapter 40). This evaluation often requires many visits, as well as providing patient education such as that provided by the International Pelvic Pain Society (http://www.pelvicpain.org).

CPP is usually multifactorial and a definitive diagnosis is not made for the majority of CPP patients, but for those with diagnoses, they are more commonly of urologic or gastrointestinal than gynecologic origin. Common nongynecologic and gynecologic causes include irritable bowel syndrome (IBS), painful bladder syndrome (PBS), endometriosis, myofascial disorders, and neuralgias. The treatment of CPP requires a multidisciplinary approach of physical therapy, behavioral therapy, and pharmacotherapy. Physical therapy is the most effective treatment for CPP regardless of etiology. Cognitive behavioral therapy can teach patients to identify pain triggers and develop responses to ameliorate the pain experience. First-line pharmacologic treatments when a gynecologic cause is suspected include analgesics such as non-steroidal anti-inflammatories and hormonal contraceptives (including the levonorgestral intrauterine device). Anticonvulsants and antidepressants, specifically norepinephrine reuptake inhibitors (SNRIs), are helpful in other chronic pain conditions although studies on CPP are limited. Amytriptyline is recommended for patients with PBS but may only have a mild effect. A strong therapeutic relationship with a trusted provider and lifestyle modifications to improve overall health and reduce stress (exercise, diet, or meditation) have also been shown to improve CPP.

Vulvodynia is vulvar discomfort with no identifiable cause, usually described as burning–diffuse, constant, and unprovoked, and less commonly, localized and provoked. Comorbidities associated with vulvar pain are low back pain, PBS, migraine, and fibromyalgia. Approaches to the patient with vulvar pain may include a variety of nonpharmacological modalities: education about vulvar care, addressing sexual and psychological issues, and pelvic floor physical therapy. Topical anesthetic ointments such as lidocaine have been shown to improve pain. Tricyclic antidepressants and gabapentin have been used, although there have been few controlled trials. Topical estrogen may be helpful in women who also have low estrogen such as in breastfeeding or menopause. For the primary care provider, recommendations include counseling the patient about the disorder, giving emotional support, and facilitating appropriate subspecialist involvement.

SCREENING & DETECTION OF EATING DISORDERS

Issues Around Food & Eating Disorders

Eating disorders are common and challenging in young women, and the primary care provider plays an important role in their detection (see Chapter 23). The primary care provider also manages the medical complications, determines the need for hospitalization, and coordinates care. In addition, for patients with milder forms of disordered eating who may not be seeing a mental health specialist regularly, the primary care provider may have responsibility for ongoing care, including exacerbations that may mandate coordination with mental health and/or nutritional support. Although the diagnostic criteria for anorexia nervosa and bulimia nervosa are clearly defined, women may also have disordered eating that does not meet the criteria for anorexia nervosa or bulimia nervosa, but is nonetheless abnormal. In addition, two groups at particularly high risk for eating disorders include female athletes and women with diabetes.

Female athletes who participate in sports and activities valuing thinness are at increased risk for developing the female athlete triad disorder. The definition of the triad includes disordered eating (a spectrum of abnormal patterns of eating, including bingeing; purging; food restriction; prolonged fasting; and the use of diet pills, diuretics, or laxatives), menstrual disorders, and low bone mineral density. Half of all athletes with amenorrhea have bone density at least 1.0 standard deviation below the mean. The bone density is decreased even in those areas subjected to stress during exercise. The diagnosis is made when the female athlete meets the three criteria of the triad.

Eating disturbances have been estimated to be present in up to one-third of young women with diabetes mellitus. Eating disorders are more common in female adolescents with diabetes than in their nondiabetic peers, and in women with type 1 diabetes. Mortality is particularly high in individuals with both diabetes and eating disorders.

For diabetes, the dietary regimen emphasizes intense meal timing and consistency. In addition, the hunger associated with hypoglycemia encourages binge eating. Diabetic patients with disordered eating have been shown to have an increased risk of retinopathy. Given the emphasis that young women often place on body weight, maintaining optimal diabetes control is a particular challenge. The diagnosis is typically made in a diabetic patient who has worsening diabetic control, when other causes of worsening control have been ruled out.

Binge eating disorder, more common than anorexia nervosa or bulimia nervosa, is recognized as a diagnosable eating disorder in the *Diagnostic and Statistical Manual of Mental Disorders,* 5th Edition (DSM-5). Binge eating disorder is much more common in women and is associated with obesity, although not all individuals with binge eating disorder are obese. Obesity-related complications are likely to occur, and the disorder may be more common in weight cycling patients. Psychiatric comorbidities are common.

Binge eating consists of episodes of eating a large amount of food in a discreet period of time with a sense of lack of control. The binges must have at least three of the following criteria: (1) eating much more rapidly than normal; (2) eating until uncomfortably full; (3) eating large amounts of food when not feeling physically hungry; (4) eating alone because of embarrassment; and (5) feeling disgusted, depressed, or very guilty after overeating. The episodes must occur at least once a week for 3 months, and must not be associated with any compensatory behaviors (e.g., purging or fasting). The estimated population prevalence is 3.5% in women. Binge eating has been strongly associated with obesity; in weight control programs, an estimated 15–50% of individuals have binge eating disorder.

Treatment goals focus on decreasing the patient's binge eating episodes and may include weight loss and treatment of other psychiatric comorbidities. As in bulimia nervosa, cognitive behavioral therapy is the mainstay of treatment. Interpersonal therapy has also been shown to be effective. Pharmacotherapy with selective serotonin reuptake inhibitors (SSRI) is also helpful, but does not appear to be better than cognitive behavioral therapy. If the woman does not respond to an SSRI, then topiramate and lisdexamfetamine (a medication typically used for attention deficit hyperactivity disorder) have also shown some efficacy. Whether cessation of binge eating disorder has an impact on subsequent weight loss or other obesity-related complications is not clear.

Screening for Eating Disorders

Because many women will not seek care for an eating disorder, the clinician must remain alert for clues, such as amenorrhea, concern about weight loss by a family member, abdominal bloating, and cold intolerance. Questions that are useful in ascertaining eating habits include: "Are you trying to lose weight?" "What did you eat yesterday?" and "Do you ever binge eat (eat more than you want) or use laxatives, diuretics, purging, or diet pills?" One screening tool, the SCOFF questionnaire, may prove to be useful in screening for eating disorders. The questions included the following: (1) Do you make yourself **S**ick because you feel uncomfortably full? (2) Do you worry you have lost **C**ontrol over how much you eat? (3) Have you recently lost more than **O**ne stone (fourteen pounds) in a 3-months period? (4) Do you believe yourself to be **F**at when others say you are too thin? (5) Would you say **F**ood dominates your life? A "yes" answer to any question is worth 1 point and a score of 2 is highly predictive of anorexia nervosa or bulimia nervosa. The Eating Disorder Screen for Primary Care (ESP) has also been proposed as a screening tool. The questions include: (1) Are you satisfied with your eating patterns? (no is abnormal); (2) Do you ever eat in secret? (yes is abnormal); (3) Does your weight affect the way you feel about yourself? (yes is abnormal); (4) Have any members of your family suffered with an eating disorder? (yes is abnormal); (5) Do you currently suffer with or have you ever suffered in the past with an eating disorder? (yes is abnormal). Both of these scales need to be evaluated in broader populations.

Clinicians should remain alert for the possibility of binge eating disorder in obese patients. Questions such as, "Do you ever binge eat?" "Do you often eat alone?" and "Do you ever feel guilty or depressed after overeating?" may be useful in detecting this disorder.

Treatment of Eating Disorders: A Framework

The first step is assessment of patients' safety, knowledge, and attitudes toward their condition by a primary care provider. They may then agree to work with one member of the treatment team, for example, a nutritionist. Similarly, counseling for developmental or family issues, or treatment for depression, may be acceptable to patients. Family counseling may be helpful in limiting pressure from the family, as pressure may be less likely to result in changed behavior than to generate resistance from patients. A counselor trained in treating adolescents may be able to help patients navigate peer issues involved in the behavior. Whether or not referral to a nutritionist or psychologist is accepted, periodic medical visits to follow the presenting symptom(s)–for example, amenorrhea, low heart rate, or gain or loss of weight–allow the primary care clinician to monitor the severity of symptoms (particularly cardiac status or other indications for hospitalization) while gently informing patients of the medical risks of their condition. Evidence of associated medical risks, such as osteopenia, dental erosion in the case of bulimia, or concerns about fertility (particularly when patients have low weight, are estrogen-deficient, or have polycystic ovary syndrome) may encourage patients to acknowledge their diagnosis and begin full treatment. Danger signs such as bradycardia and electrolyte disturbances may mandate involuntary hospitalization.

In summary, the primary care practitioner should be equipped to detect an eating disorder, and then must work as a nonjudgmental member of a multidisciplinary team, including a mental health professional and a nutritionist, to support weight gain as appropriate, modification of eating habits, and appropriate psychological and/or medical therapies.

YOUNG ADULTHOOD: LEAVING HOME & PUTTING IT ALL TOGETHER

In this phase of life, individuals begin to accept financial and emotional self-responsibility, to differentiate from the family of origin, and to develop intimate relationships with peers.

Healthy Behaviors & Health Care Maintenance

Safety in relation to sexuality, substance use, contraception, motor vehicles, and preventive care are ultimately the patients' responsibility, but the primary care provider can play an important role in establishing lifelong healthy habits and collaboration in this realm. The provider who uses gender-neutral and nonjudgmental styles of history-taking and is alert to patient cues will be more likely to be told about challenges for the patient that may have long-term modifiable consequences such as gender-identity issues, substance use disorders, condomless sex, intimate partner violence, eating disorders, and depression. Engaging with patients in partnership works best, allowing them to identify pros and cons of their choices, and supporting their ability to make changes if needed. Autonomous motivation to change and patient belief in ability to make a change are positively associated with successful changes in behavior and maintenance of those changes.

Role of Culture

Identity also includes patients' self-definition of cultural role within the context of their families of origin, and this can impact health and illness behavior (see Chapter 15). If, for example, she feels great pressure to succeed as an engineer, but prefers to be an artist, this dissonance can cause stress-related symptoms that bring her to the health care system. Somatoform behavior and medically unexplained symptoms (MUS) are common across all cultures and may be reinforced in preference to the expression of emotions in some families, masking a mental health disorder (see Chapter 29).

For women, unique issues regarding culture can relate to appearance and behavior as well. Some may feel pressure from the dominant culture regarding slender body weight, but conflict may arise if their internal or family value system and/or sex partner is concordant with a larger body habitus. Other women could be encouraged verbally and through their cultural customs to be subservient to men, though this can be manifested to varying degrees, and may or may not result in conflict. Social support may be lacking as immigrant women become more acculturated in the United States. Also, immigrants engaged in a cultural transition process may experience criticism from older relatives as they assimilate to the prevailing culture and from younger relatives or friends if they maintain connection with the culture of origin. Traditional cultures may promote respect for elders and traditional gender roles, often a family-strengthening behavior, but reinforce secrecy around family violence and abuse. Family violence may also be kept secret if immigrant, black, or Latina women mistrust authorities such as police or social workers whether or not they have an illegal immigration status. It is important for providers to remember that family violence may include intimate partner violence, violence from extended family, and honor crimes (violence toward an individual whose behavior is interpreted as shaming the family). These issues may affect women of all ages uniquely, in their traditional role in the family, and providers should be on alert for clues that problems are occurring and when warranted use direct inquiry or screening.

Reproductive Life Planning: Psychosocial Issues

Reproductive life planning is defined as a set of personal goals regarding whether, when, and how to have children based on individual priorities, resources, and values. A woman's reproductive life plan may also be influenced by the preferences of a partner or the beliefs of her family and community. Given these many considerations, women may feel ambivalent or uncertain about the desire for or timing of pregnancy. Clinicians should strive to create a supportive environment by asking open-ended questions to help patients clarify their own wishes and offering resources for preconception heath counseling or contraception if appropriate.

UNINTENDED PREGNANCY

Almost half of the 6.7 million pregnancies in the United States each year (3.2 million) are unintended, and more than half of these unintended pregnancies are continued. Given these statistics and the risks of neural tube defects, it is appropriate for providers to advise all women of childbearing age who are not using effective contraception to take a daily multivitamin containing folic acid. Unintended birth is more common in women aged 18–24 years and in lower income women, and is associated with worse maternal and neonatal outcomes than intended birth. These include late presentation to prenatal care; smoking, drug use, and drinking during pregnancy; premature birth; negative pediatric mental health effects; and not breast-feeding. Nearly 40% of unintended pregnancies end in abortion; at current rates, 30% of women will have an abortion in their lifetime.

Several factors contribute to unintended pregnancy, most importantly not using effective contraception at all or consistently. Fifty-four percent of women undergoing abortion report that they had used a contraceptive, most commonly the pill or condoms, during the month they became pregnant. Forty-six percent had not used contraception, and of these women many reported concerns about contraceptives, a quarter had had unexpected sex, and 1% had had forced sex. Contraceptive nonuse was more common among black, Latina, poor, and less educated women.

It is important to anticipate potentially sensitive issues in communicating with women who have unintended pregnancies. For example, among black and Latina women in the United States, there is a history of unethical medical experimentation and eugenics in the development of contraception that have left many mistrustful of both abortion and long acting contraception. Women with well-managed substance use disorders, including prescribing methadone or subutex, can have healthy babies, yet often face judgment from health care professionals. Incarcerated pregnant women face difficult and varied policies from state to state such as shackling during delivery and enforced separation after delivery. Women who are trafficked sex workers may have little control over their reproductive health. Providers should be prepared to address these concerns either themselves, with trained staff, or knowledgeable colleagues.

Preventing unintended pregnancy and associated poor outcomes is an important goal of reproductive health counseling. Patients interested in contraception should be asked about prior contraceptive experience and current contraceptive values, which may include efficacy, side effects, convenience, confidentiality, and time to reversal. Low-income women and women of color are more likely to report coercion during contraceptive counseling and thus a shared decision-making model prioritizing patient preference should be used to preserve reproductive autonomy. Providers should also be aware of their own biases when counseling women about pregnancy and contraceptive options.

To help women prevent unintended pregnancy it is imperative that clinicians counsel reproductive-aged, women who have sex with men who are not trying to become pregnant about contraception. They should include the highest efficacy reversible methods such as intrauterine contraception and implants in the discussion, address patient's concerns about methods, and help women choose the best method for them. Although oral contraceptives are the most commonly prescribed reversible contraceptives, they have a high failure rate of up to 8%, and require women to fill a regular prescription and take it daily. One recent study found that women, on average, do not take five pills each month, which likely contributes to its high failure rate. In contrast, the long-acting reversible methods have much lower failure rates of less than 1%.

PREGNANCY OPTIONS, COUNSELING, AND REFERRAL: PROFESSIONAL RESPONSIBILITY

Clinicians should provide objective, nonjudgmental pregnancy options counseling to women with newly diagnosed pregnancies. This includes asking whether the pregnancy was intended or is desired; educating them about the options of pregnancy continuation, including parenting, adoption, and pregnancy termination; offering supportive counseling if they are undecided; and providing appropriate referrals. At times this can be challenging for individual clinicians who have strong feelings about the woman's preference. For some, they may feel morally opposed to and uncomfortable referring a woman for abortion. For others, they may feel that her desire to continue the pregnancy is not wise due to factors such as her age, resources, relationship status, or potential interference with her educational or career goals. These feelings may interfere with one's ability to provide unbiased counseling and referral for patients. This raises the issue of conscientious refusal and whether clinicians can opt out of such counseling.

The vast majority of U.S. states allow health care providers to decline direct participation in abortion services; nine states permit clinicians to refuse to provide contraception for patients, and six permit pharmacists to refuse to dispense contraceptives. States offering varied access to abortion, with potential for difficulties to increase, have placed the United States on the international abortion rights watch list. However, ethicists and medical organizations, such as the American Congress of Obstetricians and Gynecologists (ACOG), argue that it is the clinician's responsibility to provide a timely referral when they do not, due to conscience, provide the services the patient requests. Studies show that in practice most provider support these guidelines. To provide adequate counseling and referral, it may be helpful for clinicians and office staff to clarify their values about pregnancy options through facilitated discussion of different scenarios, decide on a policy about counseling and referral, and learn about the closest sites to obtain counseling and abortion services as well as financial and transportation assistance if needed.

Abortion

Many well-designed studies have demonstrated that abortion is not associated with poor mental health outcomes. However, unintended pregnancy can be stressful for patients and requires significant psychosocial support, regardless of decision about pregnancy outcome. Women with unintended pregnancies are more likely to have a history of depression than women with intended pregnancy, and these women are at higher risk of a depressive episode at the time of or after an abortion. Thus, it is important to screen women with unintended pregnancy, regardless of their plans for the pregnancy, for depression. Also, whereas most women experience great relief after abortion, a few seek support as they grieve the loss of the pregnancy and may be referred to counseling services (https://all-options.org/).

When a woman seeks an abortion it is important to refer her as early as possible, because although abortion is extremely safe, its morbidity increases as women enter and proceed through the second trimester (although it is still lower than term birth). Women who have had an abortion are at increased risk of having a repeat, unintended pregnancy, and therefore require extra support for choosing and using contraception effectively. Also, studies have found that two modifiable factors, intimate partner violence and substance use, increase a woman's risk of abortion and therefore warrant screening and subsequent referral.

Infertility

Psychosocial stress is common in individuals struggling with infertility, increases as treatment becomes more complex and expensive, and makes discontinuation of treatment more likely. Although studies of baseline stress and conception rates with fertility treatments are mixed, a recent large meta-analysis found no relationship between baseline stress and pregnancy rates. The prevalence of psychiatric disorders also appears to be higher in infertility. Risk factors include past psychiatric illness, particularly discontinuation of medication due to anticipated pregnancy; longer duration of infertility; and history of pregnancy loss. Therefore, it is important to screen these patients for psychiatric illness, especially for anxiety and depression, as well as for the effects of infertility on various aspects of their lives such as partner relationships, sexual health, and financial health. A recent systematic review also found that women with infertility from low- and middle-income countries may be at increased risk for IPV and therefore screening is recommended in some populations. Prior cancer treatment of a female or male can also be a risk factor in infertility and it is worth discussing with patients prior to treatment whether eggs or sperm can be frozen.

Many studies have been conducted on the effect of psychosocial support—including counseling, support groups, and training in relaxation techniques and stress management—on pregnancy rates. Some studies have shown increased birth rates in patients participating in these services. A meta-analysis found an increased relative risk of pregnancy in patients participating in support groups compared with controls. Thus, it is appropriate to screen patients seeking to become fertile for psychiatric illness and treat appropriately, and to recommend participation in a support group or similar social intervention.

Premenstrual Syndrome & Premenstrual Dysphoric Disorder

Premenstrual syndrome (PMS) is characterized by cyclic occurrences of a variety of symptoms prior to and resolving within a few days of the onset of menses. As many as 150 symptoms have been attributed to PMS, but the most common are fatigue, irritability, bloating, anxiety or tension, breast tenderness, mood lability, depression, and food cravings. Whereas up to 80% of women describe at least one PMS symptom, the more severe form, premenstrual dysphoric disorder (PMDD), occurs in only 3–8% of women and impairs daily living. Five symptoms characterize PMDD: (1) sadness, hopelessness, or being self-critical; (2) tension or anxiety; (3) labile mood interspersed with frequent tearfulness; (4) persistent irritability or anger; and (5) increased relational conflicts. Additional emotional and physical symptoms may also be present, and other psychiatric illnesses must be ruled out.

Because of varied symptoms and overlap with other conditions, a prospective daily symptom scale—demonstrating onset of symptoms around the time of ovulation and cessation of symptoms after the menses—is critical for diagnosis. Several calendars have been validated, including the Calendar of Premenstrual Experiences (COPE), in which women document symptoms daily on a 4-point Likert scale for 10 physical and 12 behavioral symptoms. A total score of less than 40 during days 3–9 of the cycle combined with a score greater than 42 during the last 7 days of the cycle is an effective screening tool for PMDD.

Treatment for PMS is approached in a stepwise fashion, first with behavioral changes and progressing to pharmacotherapy. Encouraging patients to exercise regularly, limit salt and caffeine intake, and keep a regular sleep schedule may be beneficial. Calcium and vitamin D supplementation are associated with a lower incidence of PMS symptoms. The prospective daily symptom scale may be therapeutic as well as diagnostic by allowing the patient to be proactive in anticipating, managing, and avoiding symptoms. Since stress has been shown to increase symptoms, relaxation exercises and counseling may be effective.

Most patients with PMDD require pharmacological therapy for significant improvement. The SSRIs are considered first-line therapy and have been proven to be effective in multiple studies, for both behavioral and physical symptoms. Fluoxetine is FDA-approved for this indication at doses between 20 mg and 60 mg, with lower doses equally effective and better tolerated. Other effective SSRIs are sertraline, paroxetine, and citalopram, and all can be administered continuously throughout the month, intermittently from ovulation to the onset of menstruation, or semi-intermittently with increased doses in the late luteal phase. The benzodiazepine alprazolam can be used in the luteal phase to reduce symptoms, but with less effect than SSRIs. Patients who do not respond to SSRIs or anxiolytics can try agents to suppress ovulation; options include continuous oral contraception or contraceptive rings (the patch cannot be used continuously due to increasing weekly levels of ethinyl estradiol). One pill formulation with drospirenone improves PMS when prescribed traditionally, with a hormone-free interval, but only in comparison with placebo and only in the short term compared with other pill formulations (by 2 years symptoms are equivalent to the effects of other pills). Also, GnRH analogues, which require add-back estrogen therapy if used for more than 6 months, can treat symptoms. Other treatments showing some benefit are vitamin B6 supplementation and spironolactone. Although studies on the impact of hormonal contraception on mood are conflicting, some women with underlying mood disorders may experience worsening symptoms and should be made aware of this possibility and screened for mood changes in subsequent visits.

Depression in Pregnancy

Pregnancy is often thought to be a joyous and positive experience, however it is also a time of significant stress and transition. Many women experience depression for the first time during pregnancy and up to 50% are undiagnosed and untreated. Women with a history of major depression are at highest risk of depression in pregnancy. Other risk factors include discontinuing or decreasing antidepressant medications, life stressors, and trauma. Psychotherapy for depression has been shown to be equally effective when compared to antidepressant medications in the general population (see Chapter 26). For those without premorbid depression, the focus of psychotherapy in this setting is often on the transition to motherhood and the acquisition of the requisite skills.

The decision about prescription of psychotropic medications is complex: the risk of medication exposure to the fetus must be balanced against the risk of untreated depression for the mother, other children in the home and, ultimately, the infant. Medication risks to fetus are based on low-quality evidence but may include cardiac defects and abnormal neonatal neurodevelopment. The risks of untreated maternal depression are significant and include miscarriage, preterm birth, and abnormal emotional and cognitive development in offspring. Decisions about medication include factors such as the severity of the depression, the number of prior depressive episodes, and a woman's history of response to medications. All the evidence comes from observational studies.

Selective serotonin reuptake inhibitors are typically prescribed for patients who are naïve to pharmacotherapy, with sertraline being the most studied. Patients successfully treated with other antidepressants should consider restarting or continuing that medication in consultation with a psychiatrist experienced in pregnancy and postpartum. Pregnant women taking medications for depression are recommended to engage in psychotherapy.

Postpartum Depression

During the postpartum period, women can experience mood changes, including postpartum blues, postpartum depression, panic disorder, and postpartum psychosis. Transient postpartum blues are common, occur within a few days of delivery in 40–80% of women, include mood swings, irritability, sadness and crying spells, and resolve within 2 weeks. Postpartum depression has been estimated to occur in 5–9% of women. The clinical diagnostic criteria are feeling depressed or hopeless most of the day almost daily for at least two consecutive weeks, with onset usually within 1 month but up to within a year of birth. The biggest risk factor for postpartum depression is a personal history of depression. Other risk factors include lack of social support, history of miscarriage or other pregnancy loss, not breast-feeding, pregestational or gestational diabetes, and family psychiatric history. Some of the symptoms of postpartum depression such as fatigue, sleeping problems, and decreased sexual drive are common symptoms of the immediate postpartum period, making the disorder more difficult to detect. Feeling overwhelmed or guilty, being unable to care for or bond with the baby, or not sleeping even when the baby is sleeping, should all alert the clinician to the possibility of the diagnosis.

The Edinburgh Postnatal Depression Scale has been validated and used in multiple settings to screen for postpartum depression. Clinicians should ask about mood, appetite, sleep, and being overwhelmed during postpartum visits. A woman who expresses thoughts about harming herself or the baby should receive immediate evaluation by a mental health professional. When evaluating a woman for possible postpartum depression, thyroid disorders should be ruled out, as both hypothyroidism and hyperthyroidism are more common in the postpartum period. Women with mild to moderate symptoms should be initially treated with nonpharmacological measures, including sleep hygiene, education, psychotherapy, CBT, or family therapy.

There are no randomized controlled trials of pharmacotherapy for postpartum depression, so recommendations are based upon observational studies and extrapolation from the general population. Antidepressant drugs are generally initiated in the same fashion as in the usual treatment of major depression, using a medication previously effective whenever possible. The SSRIs are the drug of first choice, given their safety profile and relative low risk of side effects, with the evidence slightly favoring sertraline and paroxetine. Although there is limited evidence about antidepressant use in breast-feeding women, there are only few reports of adverse effects. The benefits of depression treatment and of breast-feeding are generally felt to outweigh the risks of the medications.

Irritable Bowel Syndrome

Young adult women may present to their providers with IBS, as it is the most common gastrointestinal disorder seen in primary care. It is characterized by chronic abdominal pain and altered bowel habits in the absence of an organic cause. IBS is estimated to occur in 1–20% of the population with a female predominance of 1.5:1. Only about 15% seek medical care for their condition, yet the volume of patients is large and the burden to society in health care costs and missed work is significant.

The pathophysiology of IBS remains unknown. It is thought to be a disorder of gastrointestinal motility, dysregulation of the nervous system, increased visceral sensitivity, and possibly bacterial overgrowth. Psychosocial stressors have been shown to precipitate and exacerbate symptoms but are not thought to be a cause of the underlying condition. Women who have a history of physical or sexual abuse are more likely than controls to suffer from IBS and other functional bowel disease. Patients with a history of abuse have poorer health outcomes as manifested by an increase in pain, provider visits, and surgical procedures than patients without an abuse history. Although women seeking treatment for IBS are more likely to suffer from depression, anxiety, panic disorder, somatization, or other mental illness, those who do not seek treatment have the same incidence of these problems as the general population. Hence, it is unclear whether psychiatric stressors exacerbate the disease or contribute to the underlying etiology, perhaps varying in different individuals. Other conditions related to IBS include sleep disturbance, depression, and fibromyalgia. Interestingly, health-related quality of life appears to be more related to extraintestinal symptoms rather than traditionally elicited gastrointestinal symptoms in patients with IBS.

Effective treatment for IBS involves an integrated behavioral and pharmacological stepwise approach individualized to the patient's main symptom. Treatment for mild disease can involve only education, bulking laxatives, and antispasmodics. Both the SSRIs and the tricyclic antidepressants (TCAs) are effective for symptom relief in some patients but the TCAs can exacerbate constipation. Loperamide is helpful for treatment of diarrhea, but does not relieve other symptoms. Rifamaxin, a nonabsorbable antibiotic given for a short course, has been shown to relieve some symptoms of IBS. Newer treatments include alosetron, a 5-hydroxytryptamine-4 (5-HT-4) antagonist, which was removed from the market because of serious complications, but is now again available for limited use. Cognitive behavioral therapy (CBT) has been shown to be helpful in several studies. Dynamic psychotherapy and hypnotherapy have also been shown to be useful in reducing IBS symptoms, although results are somewhat mixed and effects were of short term in some studies. In the largest trial testing CBT in women, CBT was significantly more effective than education alone. Certain subgroups of IBS sufferers may be especially responsive to CBT. Simple educational interventions designed to help patients learn more about their bodies and IBS can be helpful in reducing anxiety and improving health-related quality of life. However, similar to other disorders overlapping with a history of childhood or adult abuse, sexual trauma, psychiatric comorbidities, or somatization disorder—sensitive communication strategies and avoidance of unneeded interventions are crucial.

Criminal Justice Involvement & Substance Use

While the United States accounts for only 4% of the world's female population, the nation accounts for over 30% of the world's incarcerated women and those numbers are increasing for women at faster rates than for men. The increasing rate of arrests for women is attributed to many causes, including mandatory minimum sentences for drug convictions and harsher sentences for women. Many of the women will recidivate in and out of county jails for short periods of time such as days to months with smaller but growing numbers committing violent crimes incarcerated in federal settings for years. When a woman commits a violent crime is not unusual for it to be self-defense for IPV perpetration, in contrast to men who are often not arrested since women have more safety concerns about pressing charges and testifying. Women re-entering the community from incarceration face comorbid health conditions on top of barriers to care on multiple levels ranging from intrapsychic through systemic. This is related to increased rates of substance use, mental health, and medical disorders compared with incarcerated men and the general population; abuse histories; poverty; lack of safe housing and childcare; inadequate care for these problems during incarceration including a lack of medically assisted treatment for opioid use disorders; appointments being repeatedly missed; social instability engendered by recidivism; release without medication; unplanned pregnancies with 75% being active parents of young children; sexually transmitted infections; and routine interruption of Medicaid which then must be reactivated. Women need help in addressing these problems to prevent cycles of sex work to support themselves, substance use, and reincarceration. Primary care providers can be helpful by using nonstigmatizing clinical approaches and having an infrastructure to address medical, psychiatric, substance, and social risks. These risks should be addressed using gender and trauma-informed strategies such as peer navigators, social workers, and linkages with community programs.

THE MIDDLE YEARS: FAMILY AND TRANSITIONS

Women with children negotiate a myriad of changes in themselves, their children, their families of origin, and their committed relationships. In the childbearing years, depending on their own relationship situation, women need to integrate the child into a diversity of potential relationship environments: same- or opposite-sex partner, marriage, cohabition, monogamous, or nonmonogamous. Relationships are mapped upon changes in the emotional and physical self, career, and the rest of the family on all sides. This often requires profound multitasking. As children age, the parent(s) must accommodate varying tasks in the children's lives, helping them with their transitions, even as the parents, sometimes paradoxically, make their own transitions. Women, with and without children, are the most likely ones to care for aging parents, parents-in-law, and other older relatives. Expected physiologic changes or unexpected illness further impact women in these years. It is imperative that primary care providers anticipate these developmental processes and incorporate them into their approach to these patients.

Menopause: Managing Symptoms

Personal, cultural, and family attitudes can have a large effect on the emotional and functional impact of menopausal symptoms. A biopsychosocial approach, which includes inquiring about the impact of these developmental processes and ascertaining whether symptoms can be managed without medication, is crucial. Since publication of the results of the Women's Health Initiative, which showed increased risk of breast cancer and cardiovascular disease associated with use of estrogen/progestin, many women and their providers are reluctant to use hormone therapy (HT) for treatment of menopausal symptoms. However, estrogen can be extremely helpful for the treatment of hot flashes and vaginal dryness. Use of systemic estrogen, with progesterone if the woman has a uterus, is an option that some women may choose if symptoms are severe or if other therapies are not successful. The primary care provider can help female patients sort through the multitude of options, including assessing the risks and benefits of HT, and make their own best decisions. Comorbidities such as family history of breast cancer, use of cigarettes, and personal or family history of thromboembolic disease may impact this decision.

The average age of menopause in the United States is 51 years. More than 50% of postmenopausal women experience "hot flashes," a manifestation of vasomotor instability associated with the abrupt withdrawal of estrogen. Hot flashes, also known as hot flushes, are sensations of feeling warm, frequently associated with perspiration, palpitations, and anxiety. When they occur at night, they can be manifested by night sweats, frequent awakening, and consequently, sleep disturbance and chronic insomnia. In the SWAN study, a multiethnic, multiracial observational study of over 3000 women at seven sites, among those women who reported frequent vasomotor symptoms, the symptoms lasted an average of 7 years. Potential treatment options must be considered within the context of this symptom duration.

Another troubling menopausal symptom is urogenital atrophy. The loss of estrogen causes thinning of the vaginal epithelium and may lead to vaginal irritation, dyspareunia, and increased risk of vaginal infections. When the urethra is affected, urinary frequency, incontinence, and bladder irritation or infection can also occur.

Treatment of Vasomotor Instability

Symptoms such as hot flashes and changes in sexual function can have a profound effect on a woman's mood and quality of life. Many women with mild vasomotor symptoms will try nonpharmacological interventions, such as lifestyle changes, relaxation, and exercise, but the evidence for these therapies is limited. Obesity, however, is a risk factor for hot flashes, therefore it is possible that weight loss will help to reduce hot flash severity.

Determining the efficacy of pharmacological treatments for vasomotor instability is challenging, as many women will respond to placebo. However, although most therapies have not been compared head to head, estrogen seems to be the most effective in reducing the frequency of hot flashes, associated with an 80% reduction in hot flash frequency.

Nonestrogen therapies that have been used for vasomotor symptoms include SSRIs, SNRIs, high-dose progestins, clonidine, gabapentin, and several complementary therapies. Several trials have evaluated antidepressants (SSRIs and SNRIs) in the treatment of postmenopausal hot flashes. Drugs that have been found to be effective include venlafaxine and desvenlafaxine (SNRIs) and paroxetine and escitalopram (SSRIs), and are generally associated with about a 60% reduction in hot flash frequency. A formulation of the SSRI paroxitene (Brisdelle) is the only nonestrogen therapy that is FDA approved for hot flashes. In addition a combination of bazedoxifene and estrogen is available for menopausal symptom treatment. Bazedoxifene is a selective estrogen receptor modulator that can be considered for women in whom progestins are not appropriate. High-dose progestins (megestrol acetate or Megace) have been associated with about a 50–60% reduction in hot flashes, although prolonged therapy can be associated with weight gain. Clonidine has been associated with about a 40% reduction in hot flashes. Gabapentin has also been associated with a reduction in hot flash frequency of about 30–45% and may be particularly useful when taken at bedtime for symptoms that awaken women from sleep at night.

Several complementary and alternative therapies have been used for treating hot flashes, although the trials are often small, short in duration, lack a placebo arm, and use variable doses. The North American Menopause Society recently conducted a systematic review of nonhormonal menopause treatments. The treatments were divided into three categories based on the available evidence: (1) recommend, (2) recommend with caution, and (3) do not recommend at this time. Recommended treatments included cognitive behavioral therapy and stellate ganglion block. Although paroxitene is the only nonhormonal treatment that is FDA approved, the authors acknowledged that other SSRIs, SNRIS, gabapentin, and clonidine also have proven efficacy. "Recommended with caution" are weight loss, mindfulness based stress reduction, S-equol derivatives of soy isoflavones, and stellate ganglion block. Strategies not currently recommended include cooling techniques, avoidance of triggers, exercise, yoga, paced respiration, relaxation, OTC supplements and herbal remedies, acupuncture, chiropractic, and calibration of neural oscillations.

When recommending nonhormonal treatments for menopause, clinicians should be aware of the limited evidence supporting them. Although many proposed menopause treatments may not have been proven to be beneficial for vasomotor symptom treatment, some may be relatively benign (e.g., cooling techniques) or have other benefits (e.g., yoga and exercise).

Many women go through menopause without medications, using behavioral strategies and taking short daytime naps to compensate for hot flash-interrupted sleep. It is important for primary care providers to establish a collaborative relationship with patients, allowing them to discuss issues that may compound menopausal symptoms. Normalizing these sometimes stressful transitions may help a woman to accept a trial of watchful waiting or even psychotherapy to address the stress of these changes. Discussion of menopausal symptoms may not necessarily be a request for medications, but should trigger discussions about the variety of available management strategies.

Treatment of Urogenital Atrophy

The mainstays of treatment for urogenital atrophy are currently vaginal moisturizers, lubricants and topical vaginal estrogen in tablet, cream, or ring form. Vaginal therapy can be safely used in most women, although there is some controversy about use in women with estrogen-dependent tumors. Regular use of vaginal moisturizers and use of lubricants during intercourse can be beneficial to relieve symptoms but do not treat the underlying genital atrophy. Topical estrogens can also reduce the symptoms of recurrent urinary tract infections and symptoms of overactive bladder. Typically vaginal estrogen is given daily for the first 2 weeks or two and then can be given at a lower maintenance dose two to three times a week. In addition, there is a new medication, ospemifine, a novel selective estrogen receptor modulator for treating dyspareunia associated with postmenopausal vulvar and vaginal atrophy. It may be useful for women who cannot (due to obesity or arthritis) or prefer not to use a vaginal product.

Maintaining Sexual Function

It is important for providers to inquire about sexual function; a national study of 1749 women and 1410 men aged 18–59 years found a prevalence of sexual dysfunction of 43% for women (see Chapter 33). Sexual function in women is both emotional and physical. As some women age, they experience a liberation from the responsibilities of young children, relationship struggles, and financial concerns that allows them to enjoy sex more than they ever have. This may also be due, in part, to a relative rise in testosterone, as estrogen levels decrease, which improves sexual function in some women. Others experience physiologic changes described above that diminish sexual function, such as urogenital atrophy or sleeplessness from hot flashes. Expectations may be different between male and female partners, especially if the male is able to treat erectile dysfunction medically. Besides lubrication, women can be advised to try a slower pace of sexual activity, as it is normal for reaction time to diminish with age in both genders. If estrogen is used to treat vasomotor symptoms of menopause, the relative drop in testosterone can diminish sexual drive or function in some women, and that subgroup of patients may benefit from the addition of small amounts of testosterone. A primary care provider may defer prescription of medications and behavioral treatment to specialists in gynecology, endocrinology, or sexual medicine, but should be familiar with the physiology and be able to make recommendations accordingly.

LATER LIFE: SHIFTING ROLES & OPPORTUNITIES

Women in their later years are achieving the tasks of shifting generational roles and changes in couple and family functioning. Challenges may include loss of spouse, family members, and friends, along with physiologic aging and financial concerns. Opportunities exist, however, for life review and integration, along with time for new friendships and activities. Additionally, a woman may enjoy being appreciated for her wisdom, without many of the burdensome responsibilities of younger years. A primary care provider should be prepared to assist in these challenges and supportive of the opportunities (see Chapter 14).

Osteoporosis & Falls

Both osteoporosis and falls are more common in older women than in men. More than half of all women will develop osteoporosis by the age of 80 years. Fractures are 2.2 times higher in women over the age of 65 years than they are in men. Women appear to recover more slowly from these injuries, which may contribute to increased medical costs. Hence, prevention of falls is an important issue for older women and has several behavioral components. Interventions shown to reduce falls include muscle strengthening and balance retraining, multidisciplinary health and environmental risk factor screening and intervention programs, group exercise with tai chi, home hazard assessment, and withdrawal of psychotropic medications.

Screening for osteoporosis with a DEXA scan is recommended for all women aged 65 and older. Osteoporosis is defined as a T-score 2.5 standard deviations or more below that of a healthy 30-year-old female. Osteopenia is defined as a T-score between 1 and 2.5 standard deviations below that of a healthy young adult woman. Regular weight bearing exercise can slow the progression of bone loss. The USPSTF recommends against daily supplementation with 400 IU or less of vitamin D and 1000 mg or less of calcium for the primary prevention of fractures in community-dwelling, postmenopausal women. They give a grade I (insufficient) recommendation to supplementation above these amounts. For women with osteoporosis, medication such as a bisphosphonate is recommended.

Fear of falling can significantly impact an older woman's life by inhibiting activities, leading to a loss of independence. In one survey, 80% of women answered that they would rather be dead than experience the loss of independence and quality of life that results from a bad hip fracture and subsequent admission to a nursing home. Clinicians caring for older women should address this fear and consider interventions not only to reduce osteoporosis risk but also to reduce risk and fear of falling. Some of the same activities that reduce incidence of falls can reduce fear of falling; these include tai chi and strength training.

Urinary Incontinence

Up to 50% of elderly women report some urinary incontinence. Daily incontinence occurs in about one-fifth of community-dwelling women aged 85 years or older. More than half of the women with urinary incontinence do not tell their health care provider about their situation and just try to live with it. The psychological morbidity from this "hidden" problem can be high. Problems may include social withdrawal, depression, and sexual dysfunction. The clinician can uncover these problems with a thorough history and physical examination to assess for volume overload, constipation, musculoskeletal limitations, bladder integrity, and vaginal atrophy. Specialist referral should be considered in those with abdominal or pelvic pain, hematuria, fistula, pelvic mass or prolapse, complex neurologic conditions, and those who fail conservative management.

Several behavioral treatments are helpful in urinary incontinence. For stress, urge, and mixed incontinence, avoiding overfilling of the bladder and regular muscle contraction (Kegel) exercises are beneficial. In urge and mixed incontinence, bladder retraining in cognitively intact women along with biofeedback is effective. In cognitively impaired women, prompted voiding by a caregiver can further reduce incontinent episodes. Smoking, caffeine, alcohol cessation, and weight loss are of benefit. Anticholinergics, antispasmodics, or combinations are the most commonly used and effective pharmacological options in conjunction with behavioral treatments for urge and mixed incontinence. Topical estrogen is another potentially helpful option. If these conservative measures are not effective, timely referral to a specialist for evaluation for pessary placement, electrical stimulation, pelvic floor physical therapy, or surgery is recommended. Surgical options for urinary incontinence include low-risk procedures that are safe for older patients with comorbid conditions and are shown to significantly improve quality of life.

Cognitive Dysfunction

Cognitive dysfunction, including mild cognitive impairment and dementia, are major issues facing older women, with an estimated annual incidence for Alzheimer dementia of 0.6% for people over the age of 65 years and 8.4% of those over the age of 85 years. Women appear to be at higher risk of developing dementia and, because of women's longer life span, there are many more older women suffering from dementia than men. Prevention of dementia would be optimal in reducing the burden of this disease, and many of the prevention strategies involve behavioral approaches (see Chapter 34). Risk factors for dementia include hyperlipidemia, diabetes, hypertension, smoking, low levels of physical activity, low levels of mental activity, and poor social network. Women are often encouraged to adopt a "brain-healthy" diet, which includes a decrease in overall fat and an increase in foods high in monounsaturated fats and antioxidants (fruits, vegetables, nuts, and cold-water fish) and engage in regular physical and mental activities. However, while there is unproven benefit for this approach for dementia prevention, there may be other health benefits.

It has been hypothesized that HT after menopause would help decrease the risk of cognitive dysfunction and dementia. Several prospective population cohort studies found fewer declines in cognitive function in women taking HT. Earlier small clinical trials have shown some cognitive improvement in women taking HT, but the Women's Health Initiative actually showed an increase in cognitive decline in some groups taking HT, both estrogen-alone and estrogen–progestin groups. As this study started several years after menopause for most of the participants, no conclusions regarding early postmenopausal therapy can be made. Using current evidence, HT should not be prescribed for the sole purpose of preserving cognition. Since many cardiovascular risk factors can be associated with an increase in cerebrovascular disease, modification of these risk factors may be helpful in dementia prevention.

SUMMARY

There are a number of behavioral issues in the primary care of the woman patient, and these should be integrated into preventive care and management of medical issues from a biopsychosocial perspective. Although the developmental stages women experience include challenges, there are also opportunities for fulfillment both for the patients and those who care for them.

SUGGESTED READINGS

Boivin J, Griffiths E, Venetis CA. Emotional distress in infertile women and failure of assisted reproductive technologies: meta-analysis of prospective psychosocial studies. *BMJ* 2011; 342:d223.

Brownley KA, Berkman ND, Peat CM, et al. Binge-eating disorder in adults: a systematic review and meta-analysis. *Ann Intern Med* 2016;165(6):409–420.

Goldstein I, Kim NN, Clayton AH, et al. Hypoactive sexual desire disorder: International Society for the Study of Women's Sexual Health (ISSWSH) expert consensus panel review. *Mayo Clin Proc* 2017;92(1): 114–128.

Hammerli K, Znoj H, Barth J. The efficacy of psychological interventions for infertile patients: a meta-analysis examining mental health and pregnancy rate. *Hum Reprod Update* 2009;15(3):279–295.

Hay P, Touyz S. Treatment of patients with severe and enduring eating disorders. *Curr Opin Psychiatry* 2015;28(6):473–477.

Jones RK, Kooistra K. Abortion incidence and access to services in the United States, 2008. *Perspect Sex Reprod Health* 2011;43(1):41–50.

Joy E, De Souza MJ, Nattiv A, et al. 2014 female athlete triad coalition consensus statement on treatment and return to play of the female athlete triad. *Curr Sports Med Rep* 2014;13(4): 219–232.

Murray L, Carothers AD. The validation of the Edinburgh Postnatal Depression Scale on a community sample. *Br J Psychiatry* 1990;157:288–290.

The North American Menopause Society. Nonhormonal management of menopause-associated vasomotor symptoms: 2015 position statement. *Menopause* 2015;22(11):1155–1172; quiz 1173–1174.

Stellar C, Garcia-Moreno C, Temmerman M, van der Poel S. A systematic review and narrative report of the relationship between infertility, subfertility, and intimate partner violence. *Int J Gynaecol Obstet* 2016;133(1):3–8.

USPSTF Fall Prevention in Community Dwelling Older Adults. April 2018. https://www.uspreventiveservicestaskforce.org/Page/Document/RecommendationStatementFinal/falls-prevention-in-older-adults-interventions1. Accessed October 3, 2018.

Vall E, Wade TD. Predictors of treatment outcome in individuals with eating disorders: a systematic review and meta-analysis. *Int J Eat Disord* 2015;48(7):946–971.

Wisner KL, Parry BL, Piontek CM. Clinical practice: postpartum depression. *N Engl J Med* 2002;347(3):194–199.

WEBSITES

All-Options Pregnancy Support. http://all-options.org/. Accessed October 2018.

Guttmacher Institute. http://www.guttmacher.org. Accessed October 2018.

The International Pelvic Pain Society. http://www.pelvicpain.org. Accessed October 2018.

Reproductive Health Access Project. https://www.reproductiveaccess.org/resource/trauma-informed-pelvic-exams/. Accessed October 2018.

Lesbian, Gay, Bisexual, Transgender, & Queer Patients

17

Richard E. Greene, MD, MHPE, FACP; Jason Schneider, MD, FACP; & Tiffany E. Cook, BGS

INTRODUCTION

Lesbian, gay, bisexual, transgender, and queer (LGBTQ) people face many challenges when approaching the health care system. Among the most important is finding access to effective, informed, and affirming care. The medical literature has expanded its discussion of the health needs of LGBTQ people, though often addressing the issues from a strictly sexual behavior perspective (e.g., "men who have sex with men"). Specific knowledge and skills are essential for the health care provider to ascertain the sexual orientation and gender identity of patients; communicate acceptance and understanding of LGBTQ health needs; screen for conditions amenable to behavioral and biomedical interventions; and provide information and resources specific to the lives of LGBTQ patients. Only by employing these skills can providers ensure competent medical care for the LGBTQ community.

DEFINITIONS & CONCEPTS

LGBQ people make up anywhere from 1% to 10% of the general population—depending on the source quoted and the sampling method used in the study. Recent estimates suggest that transgender and gender nonbinary (TGNB) people make up 1.4% of the population in the United States. Whatever the exact percentage, LGBTQ persons constitute a significant group of patients with unique medical, psychological, and social needs. Sexual orientation and gender identity are largely invisible. Consequently, many health care providers caring for LGBTQ patients do not recognize or acknowledge their identities and unique needs.

Sexual Orientation, Sexual Behavior, & Identity

Sexual orientation refers to attraction to another person, including fantasies and the desire for sex, affection, and/or love. Sexual orientation is distinct from and not necessarily predictive of *sexual behavior* or activities. Identifying as gay, lesbian, bisexual, and/or queer assumes awareness of this sexual attraction to people of the same gender or other genders, respectively, and the development of one's identity based on this awareness. Emotions, psychological responses, societal expectations, individual choices, and cultural influences are all factors that form this identity. Compared to the term homosexual, often interpreted as more clinical and sometimes pejorative, gay, lesbian, bisexual, and queer are more accepted terms.

Sexual orientation, sexual behavior, and identity are interrelated but function independently. Most self-identified lesbians and gay men are sexually active with a partner of their own gender. However, despite this identity, some lesbians and gay men are celibate (not having sex with other people) or have sexual partners of other genders. Because of the variable relationship between orientation, behavior, and identity, clinicians must remain sensitive, open-minded, and nonjudgmental (see section "Provider–Patient Interactions").

Many LGBTQ people hold intersectional identities, including gender, race, ethnicity, religion, and ability. Individuals from racial and ethnic minority communities may be less likely to identify as LGBTQ due to the complex interactions of homophobia (see section "Homophobia & Transphobia"), religious influences, and cultural norms. Cultural factors, such as race and ethnicity, do not seem to hamper the formation of identity but may delay the integration of identity with behavior. When sexual behavior is in conflict with sexual or other identities held by individuals, the overt or subtle discrimination they face by the health care and other systems can make seeking care more difficult. For example, a US-born, English-speaking, white lesbian may have an easier and time accessing care than a lesbian who is born in Mexico who speaks Spanish as her first language. This decreased access can lead to increased social stress, known as "minority stress," which has been linked to increased risk-taking behaviors (see section "Clinical Issues").

Gender Identity & Gender Expression

Gender identity refers to one's internal sense of self, of being either a man or woman, a combination of the two, neither, or a different gender altogether. Transgender individuals have a gender identity that is different than their sex assigned at birth. The term *cisgender* is used when referring to a person whose gender correlates with their sex assigned at birth. A person with a gender identity that falls outside of the *gender binary* of female or male may identify as *gender nonbinary* or *gender nonconforming*. *Gender expression*, how one portrays their gender identity to the world via fashion, hair, accessories, etc., is the behavioral manifestation of gender identity.

Transgender people also have widely varying gender expression, influenced by personal preference and access to health care resources. Some transgender people may only desire an outward physical appearance (e.g., hair style, cosmetics, clothing) consistent with their identity. Not all transgender individuals experience gender dysphoria; however, those who do may seek gender affirming medical treatment, including access to hormone therapy and/or gender affirming surgeries. Gender identity is distinct from sexual orientation and behavior. As such, providers must discuss both a patient's gender identity and the sexual behaviors they engage in, including determining the patient and partner's body parts to have a more complete understanding of a patients' risk of pregnancy or sexually transmitted infections.

Homophobia & Transphobia

Homophobia is defined as an irrational fear of or prejudice against gay men, lesbians, bisexuals, and queer people. *Transphobia* reflects a similar fear or prejudice against transgender and gender nonconforming individuals. In daily life, LGBTQ individuals experience homophobia and transphobia as interpersonal, workplace, societal, or political bias. In other words, homophobia and transphobia reflect prejudice or hatred based solely on perceptions of sexual orientation and gender identity. LGBTQ people often find it difficult to act in accordance with their identity for fear of bias, discrimination, or violence.

The stigma that accompanies attitudes of homophobia and transphobia contributes to chronic stress, also known as minority stress, and negative health outcomes for LGBTQ persons. Societal discrimination both creates a disparity in social support and resources and limits access to appropriate health care resources. Internalized homophobia and transphobia (i.e., self-hatred) and self-concealment can create adverse mental health outcomes. Conversely, disclosure of LGBTQ identity often leads to better psychological adjustment. However, lack of support of self-disclosure by an LGBTQ individual can lead to stress and risky behaviors, including higher rates of smoking, drug and alcohol use and increased sexual risk-taking (see section "Coming Out").

Provider Bias

LGBTQ patients frequently report detrimental experiences with health care providers. Recent studies document implicit bias against sexual minorities among heterosexual health care providers. Even in urban communities with presumed acceptance of LGBTQ people surveys of patients describe behaviors of providers indicating inadequate knowledge or training and disrespect. Each negative experience with a health care provider decreases the likelihood that LGBTQ patients will continue to seek health care. This can have long-lasting impact and can affect health-seeking behaviors into senior age. Providers must work to overcome judgmental attitudes and biases toward LGBTQ patients. The Code of Ethics of the American Medical Association states that professional obligation limits a physician's prerogative to choose whether to enter into a relationship with a patient, in that "physicians cannot refuse to care for patients based on race, gender, [or] sexual orientation . . . ." Health care providers must recognize that they will likely encounter patients of all orientations and identities in the daily practice of medicine (see section "Provider–Patient Interactions").

PROVIDER–PATIENT INTERACTIONS

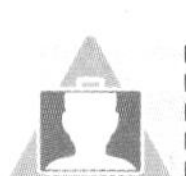

CASE ILLUSTRATION 1

Jessica, a young law student, comes to the doctor's office. Her last doctor left the practice and this is her first visit with the doctor who will be taking over her care. The doctor notes the name David on her chart and sees a notation that she identifies as a transgender woman. Jessica is visibly anxious when entering the room.

The doctor starts the introductions:

Doctor: *Hello, nice to meet you. What name would you like me to call you?*

Jessica: *Thanks for asking, I'm Jessica.*

Doctor: *And, Jessica, what pronouns do you use?*

Jessica: *I use she, her, and hers. (Jessica seems noticeably less anxious.)*

Doctor: *Thanks for sharing that information with me, I'll be sure to make note of it. So, what brings you in today?*

Further questioning reveals that Jessica has been on hormones since the age of 18, spironolactone to block testosterone, and estrogen for feminization. On surgical history, the doctor learns that she has had breast augmentation surgery, and a tracheal shave, but she has not had "bottom surgery" and has testicles, a penis, and a prostate. She is considering having "bottom surgery" to have an orchiectomy and to create a neovagina, but the surgery is quite expensive and she has not been able to afford it. She notes this makes dating difficult as she identifies as straight and dates mostly cisgender men. She reports a history of depression and one suicide attempt in the past, prior to beginning gender affirming hormone therapy, and reports her mood is much better now, despite significant stress in her life.

A robust provider–patient relationship is key to providing competent and respectful care to LGBTQ patients. Providers who are uncomfortable working with LGBTQ patients, or who fail to recognize the sexual orientation and gender identity of a patient, cannot provide quality care. Without a trusting provider–patient relationship, patients may avoid medical care and miss out on competent primary care services, including screening and health risk and psychosocial counseling. They are likely to have a lower health status than their heterosexual or cisgender counterparts. Inclusive and nonjudgmental history-building skills are the cornerstone of providing affirming and effective LGBTQ health care.

Overcoming Barriers to Communication

Many LGBTQ individuals are reluctant to share their sexual orientation with health care providers for fear of negative judgment and homophobic or transphobic responses. Some fail to share this information even when asked directly. Unpleasant experiences with health care providers have led to LGBTQ people being more likely to avoid health care and routine screening, and even the most sympathetic health care providers are often uncomfortable with the interaction. For example, LGBTQ identified providers are not necessarily experts in caring for LGBTQ identified patients and may not recognize their own biases or lack of knowledge. They may lack experience with LGBTQ health issues, despite their own identity, or feel unsure as to what language to use to elicit information respectfully from these patients. When the patient and/or provider are uncomfortable, important information may not be shared or missed.

The Affirming Social and Sexual History

LGBTQ identities are important to a patient's social history, outside of the sexual history. The social history may be a more comfortable part of the interview to bring up gender and sexuality. By asking questions that do not make assumptions about a patient's identities, the provider can increase the opportunities for, and comfort level in, discussing these issues. Providers learn about the patient's relationships, family structure, stressors the patient may have, and personal and community resources on which patients would be likely to draw.

Gathering information about a patient's sexual orientation, gender identity, and/or sexual behaviors, however, is often a challenge for health care providers. Many people with same-gender partners do not identify as LGBQ and sexual orientation is a complex, multifaceted concept. Asking about orientation only while taking a sexual history and not at other times can limit the opportunity to learn important details about the patient.

The focus of the sexual history may then be on sexual behavior, not identity. During the sexual history, the provider should avoid questions that presume behavior or identity. For example, "What form of birth control do you use?" may not be relevant, and the patient must either provide false information or awkwardly stop and explain. Forcing a patient to "out" themself or a partner, by not asking appropriate questions can make obtaining a sexual history even more difficult for both parties. To avoid this awkwardness, patients may play along with the assumption about their gender or sexuality, which may negatively impact their health care.

Because LGBTQ people may not be identified by their outward appearance, providers need to use questions that avoid bias with all people, not just those they suspect of being LGBTQ. Sensitive questions make no assumptions about sexual orientation and are easily phrased (Table 17-1). Many sexual health history questions taught in medical school, such as "Do you have sex with men, women, or both?" presume the identities and bodies of sexual partners. Reframing questions to be more inclusive and open-ended, such as "Who are your current sexual partners, if any?" and following up with more specific questions, like "What types of sex do you have? How do you engage in sex with your partner(s)? Do you use sex toys?" can provide space for LGBTQ individuals to out themselves and/or share more information that is relevant to their medical care. Simply identifying the gender of one's sexual partners may miss important information about sexual risk.

Some electronic health records are now collecting information about a patient's sexual orientation or gender identity. While this can be extremely helpful for providers, LGBTQ patients may not want this information in the record and may choose not to disclose this information. Youth may not be ready to be "out" to parents and many adult LGBTQ persons keep their sexual orientation hidden for legal, employment, or child custody reasons. In the initial visit with the patient, it is important to discuss explicitly the documentation of sexual orientation and gender identity in the chart. A direct question, such as, "How do you feel about my

Table 17-1. Suggested questions.

- To begin the visit:
  - "What name do you prefer?"
  - "What pronouns do you use? For example, I use [he/she/they]?"
- During the medical history:
  - "What body parts do you currently have?"
  - "What words do you use to describe your anatomy?"
- During the social history:
  - "Are you in a relationship?"
  - "Who forms your support system?"
  - "If you become ill, is there someone important whom I should involve in your care?"
- During the sexual history:
  - "Over your lifetime, who have your sexual partners been?"
  - "What types of sex are you having?"
  - "Can you tell me more what sex looks like between you and your partner(s)?"
  - "What choices do you make to reduce your risk of contracting HIV or other sexually transmitted infections?"

documenting your sexual orientation and gender identity in the chart?" may be asked. When an LGBTQ patient does not want sexual orientation documented, providers can use a coded entry. The code serves to remind providers of the patient's sexual orientation for medical purposes but will prevent inadvertent breaches of confidentiality.

Enhancing the Relationship

As a relationship develops between the patient and the provider, it is appropriate to inquire more deeply about how a patient's gender identity or sexual practices may impact their health. For example, a provider may use one of the following questions: "If you become ill, is there someone important whom I should involve in your care?" or "What choices do you make to reduce your risk of contracting HIV or other sexually transmitted infections?" It is important to note that transgender individuals, especially those early in a transition to another gender, may have an appearance that is discordant from their gender identity. Additionally, they may have not yet changed their assigned sex or name on legal documents or the medical record. Providers should inquire about the patient's personal pronouns: "What name do you prefer? What pronouns do you use? For example, I use [he/she/they]?"

Consider the health system or practice environment in a comprehensive, holistic way. Ensure each member of the health care team with whom a patient may interact has training at regular intervals to provide inclusive care to LGBTQ populations. Examine relevant policies and practices (e.g., nondiscrimination and visitation policies, patient registration processes) to ensure they are inclusive of the full spectrum of sexual orientation, gender identity, and expression. Be cognizant of visual imagery represented on the walls and in the hallways of the physical space in which you practice and include pictures and symbols indicating to patients that they are welcome. Examples include the rainbow pride flag, the transgender pride flag, and pictures of diverse couples and families.

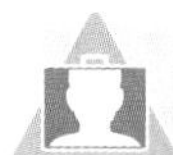

CASE ILLUSTRATION 2

Robert, a middle-aged high school teacher, comes to the doctor's office. This is his first visit, and he has not completed the intake history form. After the introductions, the physician looks at the form and prepares to take a social history.

The doctor starts the social history:

Doctor: *Are you single, partnered, married, widowed, or divorced?*

Robert: *I'm divorced, with a 20-year-old son, and I'm partnered now. His name is Tim.*

Doctor: *How long have you been together? How's the relationship?*

Robert: *Six years, and going well.*

Further questioning reveals that Tim is younger than Robert—and openly gay. Although openly gay with his friends and family, Robert is uncomfortable being that open at work; he is afraid of a scandal at school and the loss of his job. As the history taking continues, the physician asks how Robert feels about having the fact that he is gay documented in the chart. After some discussion, the two decide on a coded entry of the information. At the end of the visit, Robert thanks the doctor for being so understanding; he especially appreciates the advice to establish a durable power of attorney for health care, something that he and Tim have not discussed yet. The doctor is also happy with the visit because he has been able to screen the patient appropriately and provide him with his first physical examination in 6 years.

COMING OUT

The process of discovering one's sexual orientation and/or gender identity and revealing it to others is known as coming out and can occur at any age. Stage theories for coming out have been well described and have been summarized as a four-step process:

1. Awareness of same-gender attraction and/or transgender feelings

2. Testing and exploration
3. Identity acceptance
4. Identity integration and self-disclosure

Recent research suggests that there may be different sequences of coming out for younger and older individuals, with individuals who come out in adolescence often identifying and disclosing LGBTQ identities prior to any consensual sexual experiences. The process of coming out involves a shift in core identity that can be associated with significant emotional distress, especially if family and peers respond negatively. Prevailing social attitudes also influence the experience. Individuals may come out to other people in person, or choose to come out through virtual arenas, a process with its own potentially complicating factors, including issues of privacy or unintended disclosure to other individuals. Societal and internalized homophobia and transphobia often cause LGBTQ individuals to perform a fatiguing "cost–benefit" analysis for each situation in which they consider coming out. This process can be even more taxing for transgender individuals as each situation may involve outing their orientation and gender identity. If the costs of self-disclosure are repeatedly high, an individual may ultimately become socially isolated or revert to denying their LGBTQ identity. On the other hand, disclosing at work and working for more LGBTQ-supportive organizations correlate with higher job satisfaction and lower anxiety at work.

Adolescents

LGBTQ adolescents are particularly vulnerable to the emotional distress of coming out, and this distress can make adolescent development even more difficult (see Chapter 13). Adolescents who self-identify as LGBTQ prior to consensual sexual experiences may have a more rapid progression through the coming out stages, have fewer or no heterosexual encounters, and may engage in less risky sexual experiences. Parental acceptance of the adolescent during the coming out process may be the primary determinant of healthy self-esteem. Research by Ryan et al (see Suggested Readings) demonstrated that teens who have been rejected by their families are more than eight times more likely to have attempted suicide than those who have not been rejected. They were also more likely to suffer from depression, anxiety, and low self-esteem, to perform worse in school, and more likely to engage in risk-taking behaviors such as high-risk sexual behavior or substance abuse. Teens who come out in school may be more likely to be teased or bullied and even threatened with a weapon. In many instances, these teens feel unsupported by teachers or parents. Indeed, teens may feel fearful of or bullied by their parents or siblings and feel unsafe at home. This can lead to increased feelings of isolation, hopelessness, and suicidality.

Primary care providers need to screen for signs that adolescents are questioning their sexual orientation and/or gender identity. These signs may include depression, diminished school performance, alcohol and substance abuse, acting out, and suicidal ideation. Providers noting these signs need to consider distress regarding sexual orientation and gender identity in the differential diagnosis, along with depression and substance abuse. Providers should also ask their adolescent patients directly about feelings of same gender attraction, and gender distress or dysphoria, as this may allow the patient to feel comfortable disclosing these feelings for the first time. If providers respond to a patient's disclosure with reticence, dismay, or contempt, the adolescent may be less likely to share their feelings with others and either revert to denial or engage in more covert, risky behaviors.

Older Adults

Later adulthood is a period of continued growth but also, for many, the onset of disease. During this period, LGBT people may become dependent on health care providers and feel uncomfortable disclosing their LGBTQ identities. Because there are varying degrees of disclosure, older individuals may be "out" to themselves and a partner or close friends but no one else beyond that trusted circle. Older LGBTQ individuals are vulnerable to social isolation, and primary care providers are often among the primary support resources for older individuals. Older individuals are more likely to engage in heteronormative sexual experiences prior to self-identifying as LGBTQ than adolescents and thus may be at greater risk for adverse health consequences because of risky sexual behavior. In exploring the social support network for their older patients, primary care providers need to be alert to the possibility of LGBTQ identities and the needs they engender.

LGBTQ seniors are more likely to be single and without children compared to heterosexual counterparts and, thus, have inadequate social supports as they age. When transitioning to assisted living or skilled nursing facilities becomes necessary, LGBTQ seniors can face types of bias and discrimination not previously faced when they were living independently. Various media outlets regularly report such occurrences. Providers caring for LGBTQ seniors must be proactive in discussing social supports for their patients and work to identify inclusive resources and facilities in their communities.

RELATIONSHIPS, SOCIAL SUPPORT, & COMMUNITY

Community

Many LGBTQ individuals experience support and nurturing from their biological families after coming out to them. For others, the support network of LGBTQ individuals may not include their biological family, as many families do not accept the sexual orientation or gender identity of the individual. In either situation, partners, friends, and community organizations can serve as an extended family, sometimes colloquially referred to as "chosen family." Primary care providers should be aware of resources to which they can direct patients (some are listed at the end of this chapter). LGBTQ people in rural or suburban areas may have difficulty in accessing community-based support networks more readily available in urban environments. In a study focused on men who have sex with men (MSM), those outside concentrated urban areas were less likely to identify as gay, be in a long-term relationship, be involved in a gay community, and were more likely to be out to a smaller number of people. In rural areas, a caring, open-minded clinician may be an especially important source of support for LGBTQ patients.

Social Media

In the past, LGBTQ individuals have sought out others in the community by finding bars, social clubs, or community spaces frequented by other LGBTQ people. This is difficult in more rural areas or where the population of LGBTQ people is sparse or where many people are not out. The Internet, and more specifically social media along with dating and hook-up apps, allows LGBTQ individuals to find each other worldwide. An adolescent is no longer isolated to their geographic location but can find a social support network on the Internet, including anonymously through Tumblr or more visibly through Instagram. For adults looking to date, there are many options for both long-term partnerships (OKCupid, HER, LGBTQutie, etc.) and short-term hook-ups (Grindr, SCRUFF, etc.).

Partners

Many LGBTQ people express a desire to find partners and develop long-lasting relationships. LGBTQ individuals get married, own homes together, share finances, and raise children. Clinicians should be aware of local, state, and federal laws that affect LGBTQ individuals in family-building, establishing health insurance and access, retirement benefits, documenting advance directives, and securing inheritance rights.

Because of potential isolation from family, coworkers, and religious organizations, the relationship with a partner, or partners, can be particularly important to an LGBTQ individual's well-being. As a result, discord in relationships may be even more stressful and an individual may have limited resources for help in coping. Primary care providers should screen for such stressors and be able to provide appropriate referrals for LGBTQ-affirming individual, couple, and family therapy.

Parenthood

Family building is an important part of the lives of many LGBTQ people, and the decision to become parents is often deliberate and carefully made. LGBTQ individuals may have children from previous relationships, through adoption, via artificial insemination, in vitro fertilization and surrogacy, vaginal sex with a partner or surrogate, or service as foster parents. LGBTQ families are built in many different ways and are becoming increasingly common.

Current evidence indicates that children of LGBTQ people develop normally and fare better in relationships where parents share responsibilities equally and have a low level of interpersonal conflict. Though they may face additional stigma in school or the community, children of LGBTQ parents, like all children, are resilient and cope well with this challenge. Many professional medical associations, including the American Academy of Pediatrics and American Medical Association, have policies supporting LGBTQ families.

Loss & Grief

Grieving the loss of a partner may be more difficult for an LGBTQ-identified person if they do not have an adequate support system. The family of the deceased partner may exclude the survivor or will not allow them to take part as a spouse in the funeral. Occasionally, parents and family of deceased LGBTQ people are shocked and embarrassed to learn of the individual's sexual orientation or gender identity. In such cases, the family may feel intense guilt or the need to hide their grief, unable to share it with their support network because of embarrassment.

Transgender people may hold deep concerns that their families will not respect their gender identities and attempt to bury them in a way that emphasizes their sex assigned at birth over their true gender identity. Family members of LGBTQ individuals can find information and support for this and other issues by contacting Parents and Friends of Lesbians and Gays (PFLAG), a national organization with local chapters (see the list of resources at the end of this chapter).

Primary care providers can assist patients in advanced planning by encouraging them to complete advanced directives indicating their wishes. Providers can assist the surviving spouses or close friends in talking about the loss and expressing their feelings, identifying and interpreting normal grieving behavior and timelines, providing ongoing support throughout the grief process, encouraging the survivor to develop new relationships and support structures, and helping the survivor adapt to new roles and patterns of living. In some cases, the health care provider may be the only individual in whom the survivor can confide.

CLINICAL ISSUES

Historically, medicine has marginalized LGBTQ patients by pathologizing their identities. It was not until 1973 that the American Psychiatric Association removed homosexuality from its list of mental disorders. Just recently, in 2013, the diagnosis of "Gender Identity *Disorder*" was finally removed from the *Diagnostic and Statistical Manual of Mental Disorders*, Fifth Edition (DSM-5) and replaced with "gender dysphoria," which focuses on the symptoms experienced by TGNB people. Psychiatric and behavioral interventions like conversion therapy, also known as reparative therapy, used to "cure" patients of homosexuality or transgenderism, have proven ineffective and harmful, yet only 14 states have made it illegal to subject minors to conversion therapy. Nonetheless, primary care providers must be aware of the unique psychosocial issues that face many LGBTQ people and the specters of pathologizing treatments that still impact the psyches of many LGBTQ patients.

Depression & Suicide

Multiple studies indicate a higher prevalence of depression among LGBTQ people. Higher rates of suicidal behavior are also evident compared with the general population. Lesbians are four times more likely to report suicidal ideation than heterosexual women, and gay men are six times more likely to attempt suicide than heterosexual men. Multiple studies document rates of suicidality among transgender individuals as much as eight times the rate in the general population.

Adolescents are particularly vulnerable to depression and suicide. One report suggests that approximately one-third of LGBTQ adolescents will attempt suicide. Much of the literature on this topic, however, comes from surveys of self-reported behavior subject to report bias. Whatever the exact prevalence of suicidality, LGBTQ youth face additional risk of suicide related to coming out early, rejection by family members, rejection by religious institutions, interpersonal violence, and additional levels of marginalization (e.g., homelessness, racial and ethnic minority status, etc.).

Smoking

Data from the National Health Interview Study documents 20.5% of LGBQ people smoke compared to 15.3% of their heterosexual counterparts. The Women's Health Initiative survey data documented a 10–14.4% smoking prevalence among lesbian respondents, compared with 7.2% among heterosexual counterparts. The Urban Men's Health Study data indicate a 31.4% prevalence of smoking among MSM. While data from transgender populations are more limited, evidence indicates rates of smoking higher compared to the general population. Theories supporting the increased rates of smoking among these groups include higher levels of stress secondary to homophobia and discrimination, bars as a frequent social focus, potentially higher rates of associated drug and alcohol use, and targeted advertising by cigarette manufacturers.

Substance Abuse

The National Survey on Drug Use and Health in 2015 documented use of illicit drugs in the past year among LGBQ respondents at rates more than two times that of heterosexual respondents (39.1% vs. 17.1%). For the first time in 2013, the National Health Interview Survey (NHIS) asked participants about sexual orientation. The NHIS was one of the first population-based surveys to document increased rates of binge drinking (more than five drinks in one day) among an LGBQ population. Inquiring about drug and alcohol use is also important for LGBTQ patients (see Chapter 24). A provider should specifically explore the type, frequency, and quantity of substances, and whether patients use them during or preceding sexual activity. Many substances have a disinhibiting effect on the user and may make individuals more likely to engage in unsafe sex practices. In a multivariate analysis of drug use among MSM, amyl nitrate ("poppers"), crystal methamphetamine ("crystal meth"), cocaine, and heavy alcohol use were all associated with condomless anal intercourse, independent of partner-specific variables. Similar to many other populations, crystal meth, with its highly addictive potential, has had a profound impact on many gay men. There is a strong association between crystal meth use and prolonged, condomless sexual activity.

Sexual Risk & HIV Prevention

In 2012, the Food and Drug Organization (FDA) approved the use of the antiretroviral medications emtricitabine/tenofovir disoproxil fumarate for daily use to prevent transmission of HIV to individuals at increased risk. Until this time, the primary messaging from health care providers had been exclusively to use condoms for all sexual activity in individuals at high risk. Often, this message was delivered heavy-handedly, reinforcing and connecting fear with sexual activity. With preexposure prophylaxis (PrEP), the conversation about HIV prevention has become more nuanced.

While condoms are still an important tool in preventing many sexually transmitted infections, the importance of a thorough conversation about the types of sex LGBTQ patients are engaging in has become more important than ever. Among MSM, regular discussion of risk to guide testing and screening is important. PrEP has been shown to increase engagement in primary care and may provide an opportunity to provide prevention to people who might not otherwise have engaged.

Data for PrEP in transgender women are also promising for preventing HIV infection, but data in transgender men are still lacking. While women who have sex with women are at lower risk for HIV, more information is needed to ascertain their risk, and they may be at risk for other sexually transmitted infections depending on the kinds of sexual activities in which they engage. In all patients, assumptions should not be made about with whom patients are having sex and what body parts may be inserted where, which is at the root of sexual risk.

Intimate Partner Violence

Contrary to some popular beliefs, battery of LGBTQ persons by their partners exists. LBQ women are disproportionately affected by intimate partner and domestic violence (IPV) as nearly 44% of lesbian women, and 61% of bisexual women have experienced rape, physical violence, and/or stalking in their lifetime. Bisexual men, similar to bisexual women, experience higher rates of violence as well, with nearly 38% experiencing IPV compared to 26% of gay men. Gay men's IPV prevalence appears to be similar to that of heterosexual men. Transgender individuals also experience high rates of IPV, with some studies indicating prevalence as high as 50%. It should be noted that this violence can be perpetrated by both heterosexual and LGBTQ individuals. Unfortunately, gender-role stereotyping both in the likelihood of the perpetrator inducing injury and the seriousness of the violence exists and likely influences the recognition of IPV, the consequences to the perpetrator, and empathy for the victim when they are LGBTQ. Due to the lack of awareness about violence faced by LGBTQ individuals, many community resources are not responsive to their specific needs. For example, women's shelters may not know how to offer support and safety to LBQ women, and very few services know how to work with gay and bisexual men related to battery. Many providers of sexual assault forensic examinations have not been trained in how to appropriately gather evidence for LGBTQ survivors of violence or how to modify their examinations for transgender individuals who have undergone surgery and/or utilize prosthetics.

Minority stress negatively influences IPV perpetration and victimization among LGBTQ persons. Health care providers should screen their LGBTQ patients—and all patients—for the possibility of IPV and be able to give referrals to LGBTQ-inclusive resources, including hotlines, shelters, and counselors (see Chapter 40).

Hate Crimes

Also known as *bias crimes*, hate crimes are words or actions directed at an individual because of membership in a minority group. The U.S. Department of Justice reports that LGBTQ individuals may be the most victimized group in the nation and that the incidence of hate crimes against LGBTQ persons is rising. 2016 data reported by the Department of Justice indicated a 2% increase in crimes motivated by sexual orientation bias and a 9% increase based on gender identity. Many studies report crimes ranging from verbal abuse and threats of violence to property damage, physical violence, and murder. The number of hate crimes reported by LGBTQ persons is increasing every year. Lesbians at universities, for example, report being victims of sexual assault twice as often as heterosexual women. Youths who report same-sex or both-sex romantic attractions are more likely to be both victims and witnesses of violence.

Perpetrators of hate crimes often include family members and community authorities. Many LGBTQ adolescents leave home because of an abusive family member, and homeless LGBTQ youths are of increasing social concern. LGBTQ survivors of hate crimes display more symptoms of depression, anger, anxiety, and post-traumatic stress than other recent crime victims. When patients present with symptoms of depression or anxiety, providers should consider violence, including hate crimes, as a possible correlate.

EDUCATION, REFERRALS, & RESOURCES

Patient education is a cornerstone of primary care. Providers who care for LGBTQ patients must know how to advise patients on health issues, refer them to appropriate educational and community resources, and provide appropriate reference materials during visits.

Referrals should include other providers and community-based resources sensitive to the needs of LGBTQ people. Specialists of particular importance to delivering appropriate, multidisciplinary care include gynecologists, urologists, general or colorectal surgeons, plastic surgeons, and endocrinologists. Health care providers can obtain additional information about specific health issues and communicating with LGBTQ patients through published and online resources and workshops at both national and regional medical conferences. See next for details on individual resources.

RESOURCES & WEBSITES

1. General Resources

GLMA: Health Professionals Advancing LGBTQ Equality. www.glma.org. Accessed August 2018.

- Resources for providers and patients
- Provider referral network

National LGBT Health Education Center. www.lgbthealtheducation.org. Accessed August 2018.

- Resources for providers and patients

National Association of Gay and Lesbian Community Centers (Centerlink: The Community of LGBT Centers). www.lgbt-centers.org. Accessed August 2018.

- Directory for centers throughout the United States

GLBT National Help Center. www.glnh.org. Accessed August 2018.

- National nonprofit organization offering toll-free peer counseling, information, and local resources, including local switchboard numbers and gay-related links: 888-THE-GNLH (843-4564)

2. Lesbian & Bisexual Women's Health

The CDC Lesbian and Bisexual Health Fact Sheet. https://www.cdc.gov/lgbthealth/women.htm. Accessed August 2018.

ACOG Health Care for Lesbians and Bisexual Women. www.acog.org/Clinical-Guidance-and-Publications/Committee-Opinions/Committee-on-Health-Care-for-Underserved-Women/Health-Care-for-Lesbians-and-Bisexual-Women. Accessed August 2018.

3. Gay & Bisexual Men's Health

The CDC Gay and Bisexual Men's Health Page. www.cdc.gov/msmhealth/. Accessed August 2018.

Gay Men's Health Crisis. www.gmhc.org. Accessed August 2018.

4. Bisexual Health

Bisexual Resource Center. www.biresource.net. Accessed August 2018.

5. Transgender Health

World Professional Association of Transgender Health. www.wpath.org. Accessed August 2018.

UCSF Center of Excellence for Transgender Health. http://transhealth.ucsf.edu/. Accessed August 2018.

National Center for Transgender Equality. transequality.org. Accessed August 2018.

6. Youth

The Trevor Project. www.thetrevorproject.org. Accessed August 2018. 1-866-4-U-TREVOR (1-866-488-7386).

- A national organization providing crisis intervention and suicide prevention services to lesbian, gay, bisexual, transgender, and questioning (LGBTQ) youth. Services are available by phone or online chat.

National Youth Advocacy Coalition: Youth Guide. www.nyacyouth.org. Accessed August 2018.

7. Elders

SAGE: Services and Advocacy for Gay, Lesbian, Bisexual, and Transgender Elders. www.sageusa.org. Accessed August 2018.

8. Support & Resources for Family & Friends of LGBT People

PFLAG (Parents, Families, and Friends of Lesbians and Gays). www.pflag.org. Accessed August 2018.

- Promotes the health and well-being of gay, lesbian, bisexual, and transgender persons, their families and friends

The Gender and Family Project. www.ackerman.org/gfp/. Accessed August 2018.

- Promotes the health and well-being of transgender and gender non-binary youth and their families.

9. Intimate Partner Violence

National domestic violence hotline 1-800-799-SAFE (7233) (24 hours in English and Spanish), TTY: 1-800-787-3224 (www.thehotline.org). Accessed August 2018.

- Local referrals, including LGBT-sensitive

The Anti-violence Project. www.avp.org. National Hotline 212-714-1141. Accessed August 2018.

- Provides support for LGBTQ and HIV+ survivors of violence.

FORGE. www.forge-forward.org/. Accessed August 2018.

- Provides support for transgender and non-binary survivors of violence; resources include gender-neutral body map for sexual assault forensic examinations.

10. General Information: National LGBT Rights & Advocacy

Human Rights Campaign. www.hrc.org. Accessed August 2018.

- National organization working for LGBT equal rights on federal government level

Lambda Legal. www.lambdalegal.org. Accessed August 2018; Legal helpdesk: 1-866-542-8336

- National LGBT legal and policy organization protecting civil rights of LGBT and people living with HIV

National Center for Lesbian Rights. www.nclrights.org. Accessed August 2018; Hotline: 1-415-392-6257

National Gay and Lesbian Task Force. www.thetaskforce.org. Accessed August 2018.

- National organization supporting LGBT advocacy efforts at state and federal levels

11. Media/Brochures (for Waiting Room)

American Cancer Society. http://www.cancer.org. Accessed August 2018.

- Breaking Down Health Care Barriers for LGBT Community
- Cancer facts for gay and bisexual men
- Cancer facts for lesbians and bisexual women
- Tobacco and the LGBT community
- Place order for free brochures by phone: 1-800-ACS-2345

American College Health Association. www.acha.org/ACHA/Resources/Brochures.aspx. Accessed August 2018.

- Man to man: three steps to health for gay, bisexual, or any men who have sex with men
- Woman to woman: three steps to health for lesbian, bisexual, or any women who have sex with women

SUGGESTED READINGS

Daniel H, Butkus R; Health and Public Policy Committee of American College of Physicians. Lesbian, gay, bisexual, and transgender health disparities: executive summary of a policy position paper from the American College of Physicians. *Ann Intern Med* 2015;163(2):135–137.

Floyd FJ, Bakeman R. Coming-out across the life course: implications of age and historical context. *Arch Sex Behav* 2006;35(3):287–296.

Hembree WC, Cohen-Kettenis PT, Gooren L, et al. Endocrine treatment of gender-dysphoric/gender-incongruent persons: an Endocrine Society Clinical Practice Guideline. *J Clin Endocrinol Metab* 2017;102(11):3869–3903.

Institute of Medicine Committee on Lesbian, Gay, Bisexual, and Transgender Health Issues and Research Gaps and Opportunities. The National Academies Collection: reports funded by National Institutes of Health. In: *The Health of Lesbian, Gay, Bisexual, and Transgender People: Building a Foundation for Better Understanding*. Washington, DC; National Academies Press (US) National Academy of Sciences; 2011.

The Joint Commission. *Advancing Effective Communication, Cultural Competence, and Patient- and Family Centered Care for the Lesbian, Gay, Bisexual, and Transgender (LGBT) Community: A Field Guide*. Oak Brook, IL; October 2011. LGBTField-Guide.pdf.

Katz-Wise SL, Rosario M, Tsappis M. LGBT youth and family acceptance. *Pediatr Clin North Am* 2016;63(6):1011–1025.

King M, Semlyen J, Tai SS, et al. A systematic review of mental disorder, suicide, and deliberate self harm in lesbian, gay and bisexual people. *BMC Psychiatry* 2008;8:70.

Marcus JL, Levine K, Grasso C, et al. HIV Preexposure prophylaxis as a gateway to primary care. *Am J Public Health* 2018;108(10):1418–1420.

O'Hanlan K, Cabaj RP, Schotz B, et al. A review of the medical consequences of homophobia with suggestions for resolution. *J Gay Lesbian Med Assoc* 1997;1:25–39.

Ryan C, Huebner D, Diaz RM, Sanchez J. Family rejection as a predictor of negative health outcomes in white and Latino lesbian, gay, and bisexual young adults. *Pediatrics.* 2009 Jan;123(1):346-52. doi: 10.1542/peds.2007-3524. PubMed PMID: 19117902.

Sabin JA, Riskind RG, Nosek BA. Health care providers' implicit and explicit attitudes toward lesbian women and gay men. *Am J Public Health* 2015;105(9):1831–1841.

Stall R, Mills TC, Williamson J, et al. Association of co-occurring psychosocial health problems and increased vulnerability to HIV/AIDS among urban men who have sex with men. *Am J Public Health* 2003;93(6):939–942.

Vulnerable Patients

18

George W. Saba, PhD; Neda Ratanawongsa, MD, MPH; Teresa Villela, MD; & Dean Schillinger, MD

OBJECTIVES

In this chapter, we will cover the following key learning objectives:

- Describe the elements of building a therapeutic alliance, eliciting the patient's narrative and assessing the patient's vulnerabilities and strengths.
- Explore critical components of the therapeutic alliance: building trust, conveying empathy, and collaboration.
- Describe the relevance of the therapeutic alliance to the effective care of vulnerable patients.
- List the benefits of eliciting the patient's narrative.
- Review common psychosocial vulnerabilities and points of resilience and illustrate how identifying them can help create a patient-centered clinical encounter.
- Describe strategies for clinician sustainability in working with vulnerable populations.

INTRODUCTION

CASE ILLUSTRATION 1

Ms. Sviridov is a 67-year-old woman with chronic arthritis pain, hypertension, prior stroke, diastolic dysfunction, and diabetes. Despite a sizable, guideline-based medication regimen and frequent visits to both a primary care physician and a cardiologist, she has recalcitrant heart failure, requiring multiple hospital admissions. An extensive cardiac workup has been unrevealing.

Ms. Sviridov's new primary care physician asks about her life. She describes an active singing career and a rich family life in the past, and the importance of her church. She acknowledges that profound depression and concern over the welfare of her drug-abusing son, however, now interfere with caring for herself.

Ms. Sviridov's physician suggests he make a home visit. Exploring her initial refusal, he learns that her son deals drugs from her apartment. Eventually, with the support of her physician and adult protective services, she is able to demand that her son leave. She receives support and assistance from home-health services and her church group. Her conditions stabilize, and she is not rehospitalized.

Social characteristics—living in poverty, having a low level of education and limited literacy skills, being from a community that has experienced racism and discrimination, having no health insurance, speaking little English, among other factors—make individuals vulnerable to contracting illness and to facing overwhelming obstacles in the care of that illness. Vulnerable populations tend to experience these health risks in clusters, making both individuals and communities more susceptible to declines in health. For example, it is not uncommon for an individual living in poverty to have limited literacy skills and no health insurance; to simultaneously have diabetes, heart disease, or depression; and to smoke or to live in a community with limited access to high-quality grocers and safe outdoor space for physical activity.

Clinicians must learn to successfully engage those most at risk by virtue of this clustering. Unfortunately, vulnerable patients experience a triple jeopardy when it comes to health care: they are more likely to be ill; more likely to have difficulty accessing care, and when they do, the care they receive is more likely to be suboptimal. This reflects the mismatch between the psychosocial vulnerabilities that they bring to the clinical encounter and the knowledge, attitudes, skills, and beliefs of the clinicians caring for them, as well as the priorities and policies of the health systems in which they receive care. Patients who are vulnerable often come from communities that have been historically under-resourced and have faced structural racism and discrimination. Further they have experienced racism and discrimination in the

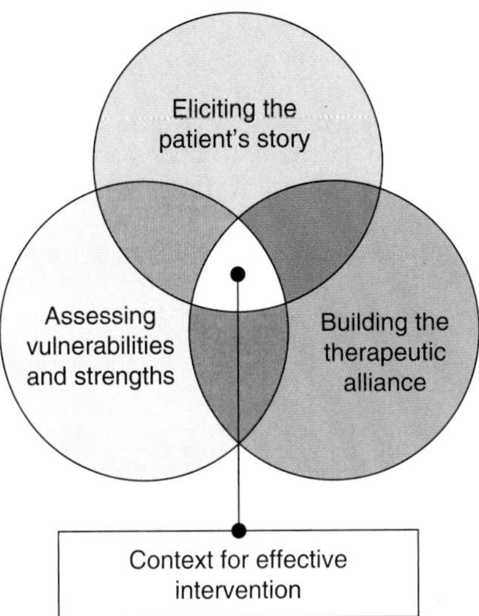

Figure 18-1. Creating a context for effective intervention in the clinical care of vulnerable patients.

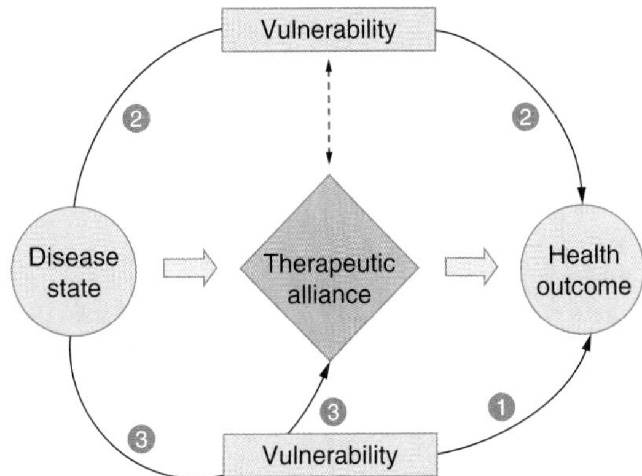

Figure 18-2. Pathways by which psychosocial vulnerabilities affect health and health care in the clinical encounter (see text for details).

interpersonal interactions with health care clinicians who have fostered mistrust and contributed to avoidance of the health care system and inequities in their health and health care. While there are many avenues into addressing these problems, in this chapter, we focus on the centrality of strong provider–patient relationships to all efforts to improve the health of vulnerable patients. Three essential strategies are recommended to promote a context for effective care for vulnerable patients: building a therapeutic alliance, eliciting the patient's story or "narrative," and assessing for the patient's psychosocial vulnerabilities and strengths. Clinicians can use a combination of these approaches to create more productive and effective interactions and relationships with vulnerable patients (Figure 18-1).

VULNERABILITY & THERAPEUTIC ALLIANCE

Psychosocial vulnerabilities can affect health and health care, either alone or in concert (Figure 18-2). The first path is a direct one, a situation in which the vulnerability in and of itself leads to poor health. Concrete examples of this mechanism might be intravenous drug abuse and skin abscesses or intimate partner violence and head trauma. A second path is an indirect one, where the vulnerability attenuates the benefits of medical treatment on coexisting medical conditions; that is, the vulnerability presents a barrier to optimal acute, chronic, and/or preventive care, thereby accelerating disease course. Examples of this include the effects of depression on nonadherence to medications among patients with heart disease, or inability to pay for medications and poor diabetes control. The third mechanism, also an indirect one, is mediated entirely through the therapeutic alliance. In this path, the vulnerability affects components of the relationship or therapeutic alliance with the provider (such as open disclosure, mutual trust, caring, and engagement), thereby limiting the benefits of a collaborative relationship on care. Examples of this include a patient with an undisclosed illness that is inconsistent with a prescribed treatment plan; a physician whose belief systems regarding addiction impedes true engagement with a patient with a substance use disorder; a physician whose implicit bias about the race of the patient may doubt their motivation for self-care; a patient with depression that impedes follow-through with a prescribed treatment plan, thereby leading to mutual frustration and blame; a patient who is transgender experiences discrimination from the physician and does not return to the clinic resulting in adverse health outcomes.

What Is the Therapeutic Alliance?

In the field of medicine, a therapeutic alliance exists when the patient and provider develop mutual trusting, caring, and respectful bonds that allow collaboration in care and treatment. "Patient-centered" and "relationship-centered" care models build on the notion of the therapeutic alliance, and research reveals that patients reporting greater trust, increased satisfaction, and more collaborative relationships with clinicians have increased adherence to medication and treatment regimens and better health outcomes.

Key dimensions of the therapeutic alliance include:

- **Mutual trust**—Patients need to trust in their clinicians' integrity and competence, and clinicians need to trust that patients enter the relationship trying to do their best.

- **Empathy**—Demonstrating empathy, or recognizing and understanding the beliefs and emotions of another without injecting one's own, allows the clinician to connect emotionally with the patient without pity or overidentification.
- **Respect**—Expressing respect for patients and treating them with dignity are important and require creating a context in which communication can occur as equals.
- **Collaboration**—Collaboration requires a meaningful partnership in which the clinician and patient perceive that they are working together toward a common goal and committed to resolving conflicts that inevitably emerge about treatment goals.

The therapeutic alliance must be broadened beyond the one-to-one relationship between the clinician and patient to include other important people (e.g., family, patient navigators/health coaches, consulting clinicians). Health systems can foster or erode the therapeutic alliance based on the policies they promote.

Therapeutic Alliance & Vulnerable Patients

CASE ILLUSTRATION 2

Mr. Jackson is a 52-year-old man with type 2 diabetes, hypertension, and end-stage renal disease. He receives care intermittently at a public clinic. He was recently referred for dialysis but missed his appointment for evaluation. He was a construction worker and now is unemployed; he lives alone and is episodically homeless. He is African American and has two sons living in the area.

He was admitted to the Family Medicine Service of a county hospital and found to be in diabetic ketoacidosis. During the admission, the inpatient team rediscusses his need for dialysis. His initial meeting with the Renal Team ends with him becoming angry and refusing dialysis. The resident assigned to his care urges him to reconsider, and he becomes withdrawn. She attempts to arrange dialysis again, and the Renal Team, citing his history of alcohol use, his intermittent homelessness, and his lack of follow-through, declares him a "poor candidate" for dialysis.

The resident meets with Mr. Jackson to better understand his thinking. Initially he remains distant; as she expresses her concern for helping him receive the best care, he is able to express his anger at the medical system over the years. He feels he has not been given information about his illness in a manner that he understands; he is unable to implement the many self-care suggestions, given his living situation; and feels that doctors have only been interested in him if they can "learn medicine" by experimenting on him. The resident expresses her concern and regret for how he has been previously treated and offers to do her best to help him now. He is able to talk about his experience with diabetes, his fear about dying, and his desire to change. She expresses her appreciation for his willingness to be forthright and offers to become his primary care physician. She also offers to advocate for him with the Renal Team to initiate dialysis both in and out of the hospital.

A growing body of evidence suggests that it is precisely with vulnerable patients that the therapeutic alliance can have its most profound benefits. Through a therapeutic alliance, clinicians offer a professional relationship aimed at helping patients feel comfortable to be as open and honest as is necessary to receive the best care. Clinicians are permitted access to the interior of patients' lives that few other people are allowed. Using this privileged position, they can help build an alliance that empowers patients and reduces barriers to their care.

Empowerment—Vulnerable patients often experience human relationships as broken or disrupted (e.g., due to violence, immigration, mental illness, homelessness, and illness). Through the therapeutic alliance, clinicians can offer a reliable, dependable, and continuous presence that is supportive, accepting, and nonjudgmental. They can provide safety, thus allowing patients to tell the stories of their lives and illness and disclose their vulnerabilities. By examining the patients' strengths and resources, clinicians can provide a sense of dignity and hope. Through validating their experiences, clinicians can help patients feel less marginalized. In supporting patients as competent and strong, clinicians can help empower them to become actively involved in their care.

Access to care and related resources—Vulnerable patients often face limited access to health care and social services. In part, they may be unaware of what is available and may not have the facility to negotiate complex, bureaucratic systems. Clinicians are in a position to remedy both of these barriers. Through the therapeutic alliance, clinicians can help patients feel safe enough to reveal concerns or problems beyond the presenting problem, which they might not otherwise have done. For example, a patient seeking care for her diabetes may disclose that she lives with an abusive partner, drinks alcohol regularly, or is only sporadically housed. The clinician has the ability to collaborate on treatment plans and to facilitate entry into the various health and social systems that can help address vulnerabilities. The therapeutic alliance can help patients feel assured that clinicians will not abuse the disclosure of information (e.g., leading to rejection or legal action) but will help them access resources critical for their health.

What Can Happen When the Therapeutic Alliance Is Absent?

The absence of a therapeutic alliance can result in serious consequences for the health of vulnerable patients.

Trust—Clinicians often enter into relationships with patients assuming they share the same goals and will trust each other to do their best to attain them. However, many patients enter into the relationship with a degree of mistrust. This may result from personal experiences with institutions in which they have felt betrayed or unwelcome or may be rooted in broader, historical experiences of their community. Clinicians should not automatically assume that they have patients' immediate, total trust; rather, they should earn it by demonstrating trustworthiness.

Clinicians can indicate their trustworthiness by:

- *Being transparent*: Vulnerable patients often experience external intrusions into their lives and little privacy; they may not understand why clinicians ask about personal information. Explaining the context of questions that may not seem immediately pertinent to the patient's concern may dispel patients' concerns about hidden agendas (e.g., "I am asking about who you live with, not to pry, but to see who might be available to care for you following your operation."). Similarly, vulnerable patients may believe clinicians are interested in ordering particular laboratory tests, imaging studies, or procedures to learn at the expense of the patient or to increase financial resources. On the other hand, patients may fear that they are being denied particular treatments to save the health care system money. Explaining why one is recommending a particular diagnostic course or treatment regimen can build trust (e.g., "I want you to get the treadmill test, because I think it is the best way we have to know how best to help you and to decide the best treatments.").
- *Following through*: Vulnerable patients are accustomed to hearing that something will occur (e.g., appointment scheduled; prescription ordered; referral to social service made) and then learning, for whatever reason, that it did not happen. By taking the extra time to follow-through on promises, clinicians can show patients that they can be counted on to ensure the best care ("I told you I would call when I found out how to help you find housing; here's what I've learned." "My homework after your last appointment was to find out about Spanish-speaking support groups for patients with diabetes; there is one not too far from your home.").
- *Addressing concerns*: Vulnerable patients may experience clinicians as rushed, interested in their own agendas, and nonresponsive to those of the patient. By taking the time to ask and answer questions and focus on what the patient needs, clinicians can indicate that they are interested in helping the patient and can be trusted to care ("While there are many things that I want to talk to you about, what are you most concerned about?"; "I know that I am more worried about your high blood pressure than you are. I also know you are more concerned that you cannot work because your elbow is so painful. Let's work on both today.").

Caring—Patients who are poor and/or have historically faced racism and discrimination frequently receive care in teaching hospitals and community health centers with high provider turnover. Patients may question providers' motivation and commitment, fearing that they are educational fodder for trainees who will go on to care for the privileged. When clinicians do not offer certain treatments, patients may be suspicious about the clinicians' willingness to expend resources for them. When clinicians persuasively argue for unwanted treatments, they may fear being used as experimental "guinea pigs." Rather than risk raising concerns or disagreements with a clinician whose motives they question, patients may choose not to follow-through on recommended treatment or simply not return for care.

Respect—Disrespect and discrimination due to race or socioeconomic status has been associated with lower satisfaction with the health care system and worse health outcomes among patients with chronic illness. Significant proportions of people from African American, LatinX, and Asian communities and those with lower educational attainment have reported that they were treated with disrespect, were treated unfairly, or received worse care because of their position in society. These perceptions influence whether patients follow recommended advice or delay needed care for chronic illness. Communicating respect is essential to convincing vulnerable patients that clinicians are willing to enter into a relationship based on equality and dignity.

Mutual agreement and collaboration—In the absence of a trusting relationship, true collaboration may be difficult to achieve. Fear of being punished or treated unfairly for speaking truthfully can lead patients to withhold their beliefs and values about a suggested treatment or to refuse to follow through on a recommendation. Clinicians, in turn, feel frustrated and mistrustful when they wonder if they are being misled or if patients really care about their health.

Shared decision making is often promoted as a model for mutual agreement and collaboration. However, research with diverse populations suggests that clinicians and patients, seemingly engaged in the cardinal behaviors of shared decision making, may still not perceive that a collaborative partnership exists between them. Indeed, being treated with respect and dignity may be more important than engaging in shared decision making and may itself lead to positive outcomes (i.e., higher satisfaction, adherence, and receipt of optimal preventive care).

BUILDING A THERAPEUTIC ALLIANCE WITH VULNERABLE PATIENTS

There are no simple, protocol-like statements or behaviors that we can employ to make another human being feel cared about or respected. However, if clinicians consciously strive to transmit a sense of trust, caring, and respect, along with a desire to enter into true partnership, they increase the likelihood of forming productive relationships with patients. Some guidelines to consider in this process include the following:

- **Demonstrate commitment to the relationship**. Clearly state your desire to be available to your patients within the scope of your practice (e.g., "I will be your regular doctor. Here is my telephone number with a voice mail; I check it daily and will get back to you as soon as possible."); be clear about what you will do for the patient between visits (e.g., "I will check into support groups and tell you at our next appointment."; "I know how your inability to walk keeps you isolated in your apartment, I will make sure you receive the wheelchair you were supposed to have."); and follow-through as promised.
- **Allow for the humanity of the patient and the clinician to emerge**. The humanity of the health care worker and the patient should be expressed and elicited. This may include the sharing of beliefs, values, and feelings as they relate to the clinical issues facing them (e.g., express concern about suffering, "I am sorry you have to deal with this pain;" offer self-disclosure to identify a shared history or common interests with the patient, "As a parent, I can't imagine how incredibly strong you had to be to escape with your children.").
- **Elicit patients' stories or health "narratives."** This interviewing approach can provide critical insights into a patient's illness model, allow for expression of the patient's humanity, and uncover important psychosocial vulnerabilities (see section "Eliciting the Patient's Story or 'Narrative'").
- **Search actively for patients' strengths and resources**. We commonly focus on what is wrong or dysfunctional in the patient's life. Just as vital as the search for deficits is the identification and validation of the strengths and *resilience* each patient has (e.g., "You have been through a lot of suffering in your life; how have you been able to survive?" "Who gives you the strength to deal with difficult things?"). Reflecting on how the patient has used these resources in previously difficult times can provide a positive starting point for healing (e.g., "You have talked about turning to God when dealing with other major crises in your life; have you thought of doing that now?"). The power for healing does not rest solely with the clinician, but must involve an empowered patient and family (e.g., "Your sister gave you strength to leave an abusive relationship; can she help now in dealing with your diabetes?").
- **Express caring overtly**. When patients describe difficult or painful experiences, clinicians can acknowledge the patient's perspective (e.g., "I can't imagine how difficult your life has been;" "What you have lived through sounds so frightening;" "I know you're afraid of going through these tests and treatments; is there anything I can do to make it less scary?"). A number of nonverbal behaviors and verbal statements can also express that we care: (1) body language (e.g., *sitting in proximity; a focused, unhurried posture)*; (2) active listening and reframing (e.g., "It sounds to me that you felt betrayed by the people you trusted most; am I right about that?"); (3) support (e.g., "I know you are trying very hard to live on your own now; I think you are doing great, and I want to do whatever I can to support you."); and (4) validation (e.g., "You are right to feel that you do not deserve to be abused."). Caring can also be communicated in a number of indirect ways, such as making an unexpected phone call to follow-up with a patient in crisis (e.g., "I know you had your colonoscopy yesterday, and I wanted to see how you are doing."). Not all patients (nor all clinicians) are comfortable with touch. Some patients may even believe clinicians are afraid to touch them. Respectful physical contact during painful or uplifting moments can help cement a mutual human connection.
- **Create a context for conflict to emerge and get addressed**. We need to convince patients that when they have beliefs, opinions, or ideas different from ours, we will welcome discussing them. We must allay any fears patients have that voicing disagreement will incur displeasure or even punishment from the provider. A corollary to this is that patients need to understand that they can change their minds about treatment plans and decisions at any time. Patients need repeated reassurance and reminders that disagreement will not cost them the provider's regard and care (e.g., "I will not be angry or upset if you disagree; it would be very helpful to know how you really feel, because together we can figure out the best thing to do."; "I want you to let me know if I do or say anything that is disrespectful or discriminating. You deserve the best care, and I want to make sure I give that to you."). Building a therapeutic alliance does not require clinicians to deny their viewpoint but to adopt nonthreatening ways of communicating differences with their patients.
- **Clarify boundaries**. Vulnerable patients may often experience considerable intrusion into their personal lives by government institutions or social service agencies. They may be required to disclose more information than others and then find it shared across agencies without their knowledge or permission. We should clarify why we are inquiring about certain information

(e.g., "I want to ask more specifically about your family because they seem important in your care, and I want to understand how they help you.") and what is confidential or required to be shared (e.g., "I will keep whatever you tell me confidential unless I think you may harm yourself or someone else; then I must tell others to protect you from any harm.").

We should also clarify our own boundaries; it is not uncommon for a relationship between a clinician and a patient to evolve into one of unhealthy dependence or unrealistic expectations. For example, as we learn more about the hardships our patients face and their difficulty navigating the system, we may feel tempted to reach out to them differently than we would for nonvulnerable patients. We may be inclined to give them a pager number or even our home phone because we want to improve access; we might lend them money or give them a ride. While these behaviors might not, in and of themselves, prove problematic, they do represent a crossing of boundaries that are commonly set with patients and signal us to reflect upon and to consider potential consequences. We can avoid creating problematic relationships by remaining mindful of the role we play in the therapeutic relationship and by regularly reflecting on our interactions. Communicating with colleagues about our patient challenges (including boundaries) can provide a critical and supportive perspective as we strive to make appropriate decisions in building the therapeutic relationship.

- **Address the therapeutic alliance directly**. When caring for a patient who is doing poorly clinically but receiving optimal "medical" management, we should consider if the therapeutic alliance needs attention. We can directly state our desire to have a strong relationship and a real sense of partnership. We can ask if the patient would want any changes in the relationship, reassuring them that speaking honestly is not only acceptable, but essential to working together.

ELICITING THE PATIENT'S STORY OR "NARRATIVE"

What Is the Patient's Perspective?

Many factors—individual, familial, societal, spiritual, and cultural—shape a person's concepts and experiences of health and illness. These inform an individual's sense of responsibility as a patient, expectations of health care providers and family members, and the meaning of healing and recovery. Personal concepts of health determine what preventive and self-care behaviors are considered appropriate, which symptoms seem worrisome, and when to seek help from health care professionals. These explanatory models encompass the meaning of the illness, the presumed cause, its proposed trajectory, the degree of hope of cure, and how treatment should be conducted (see Chapter 15).

The same factors that influence how people think about health and illness also impact other aspects of their lives, and eliciting information about these influences can uncover perspectives important to health care. For example, how individuals make decisions about health care may resemble how they make decisions about parenting or work; the process for how a family decided to immigrate to the United States may be very similar to how they will approach a difficult treatment decision; one's explanation of life difficulties and the narrative of how one has prevailed over them may illustrate how one will face challenging health problems as well. Illness may be framed hopefully or pessimistically; patients may identify themselves as efficacious or as victims; they may prefer being independent or isolated or they may find strength in support from others.

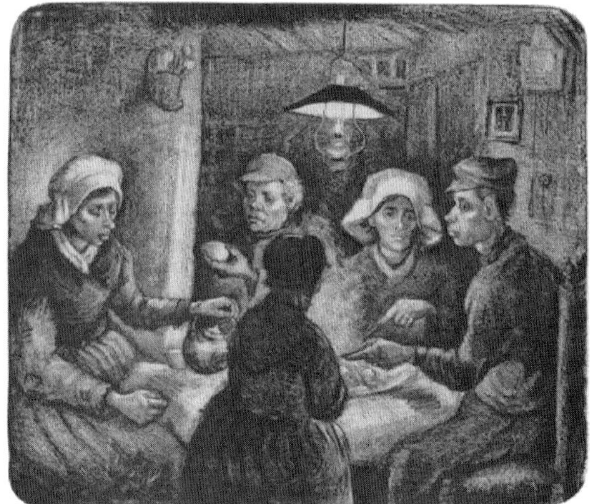

Potato Eaters, by Vincent van Gogh, 1885. National Gallery of Art. Located at: https://images.nga.gov/en/search/do_quick_search.html? q=potato+eaters. Accessed July 4, 2013.

Importance of Eliciting the Patient's Perspective

Patient's perspectives—a complex mixture of very personal beliefs, values, and assumptions reflecting multiple influences—can determine how they develop a relationship with their clinician, and whether they feel understood and respected or misunderstood and discounted. Clinicians, in turn, have their own individual perspectives on health and illness, and ascribe specific meaning to their role as healers (see Chapter 15). Assuming a shared understanding and not exploring the differences may in fact lead to greater distance and misunderstanding. Eliciting patients' perspectives allows for accurate empathy and can uncover interests or experiences common to both patient and clinician, thereby reducing the social distance that often impedes the development of a therapeutic alliance. Eliciting the patient's story can also improve patient trust, satisfaction, and adherence. It enriches and brings meaning to interactions and allows providers to be more effective and engaged.

Furthermore, sometimes the way people frame their illnesses can cause suffering. Within the context of a strong therapeutic alliance it is possible, as part of the healing process, to recast some narratives. A patient who feels incompetent, for example, might grow, through learning to control his illness, to feel capable and empowered in realms beyond the medical.

ASSESSING & ACKNOWLEDGING PSYCHOSOCIAL VULNERABILITIES

Much of clinical training and guideline development focuses on pathophysiology, disease, diagnosis, and treatment. Seasoned clinicians, however, are acutely aware of the gap between the outcomes that are expected (e.g., from reading textbooks or following guidelines) and the outcomes that are actually achieved in practice. While there are many reasons for the observed variation in quality and health outcomes, one of the most important and frequently least appreciated factors is the patient's social context. A wide range of psychosocial vulnerabilities can impinge on a patient's ability to carry out the treatment plan and interfere with the therapeutic alliance (Table 18-1).

When faced with a patient who is doing poorly from a clinical standpoint, many clinicians do not reflect on the psychosocial factors that may be influencing the patient's course. They may simply throw up their arms and attribute a patient's clinical decline to his or her social milieu in a global or at times derogatory fashion, referring to such a patient as "nonadherent," a "difficult patient," or a "social nightmare," without digging deeper. Such clinicians often believe that addressing psychosocial problems is "not my job," stating, "I can't fix his social problems." Still others may not have the communication skills to uncover underlying psychosocial problems, or to address them and integrate this knowledge into treatment plans to forge a more genuine, engaged therapeutic alliance.

Screening for psychosocial vulnerabilities is central to caring for patients in any setting and at many points during the process of care, particularly when treatments appear to be failing. Some vulnerabilities will be apparent from the first encounter, whereas others may be hidden. For some problems, it is not until a collaborative relationship has been established that a patient might feel comfortable enough to disclose sensitive information. Similarly, patients may perceive a problem to be irrelevant to their health and neglect to discuss it. When assessing for areas of vulnerability, the clinician should be nonjudgmental, allowing the patient to respond at his or her own pace. Using open-ended questions and responding to patient cues may enable a patient to reveal the important nonclinical factors that may be impeding progress (Table 18-2).

It is important to raise four important *caveats* about assessing for psychosocial vulnerability. The first is that in the pursuit of identifying vulnerability, the clinician should be reminded of the importance of simultaneously identifying and acknowledging an individual's *strengths*, *resilience*, and range of *resources*, such as one's belief in a higher power or support from a religious community; or the love and support provided by a spouse, friend, or pet. Reviewing and reflecting patients' past experiences of overcoming difficulty and helping them identify patterns of success is critical to building self-efficacy and developing a therapeutic alliance in the face of vulnerability. We have created a framework of resilience domains to use to help clinicians listen for and/or elicit patients' resilience factors (Table 18-3).

Table 18-1. Generating a differential diagnosis of psychosocial vulnerabilities.

Violence
Uninsured
Literacy and/or language barriers
Neglect
Economic hardship
Race/ethnic discordance, discrimination
Addiction
Brain disorders (e.g., depression, dementia, personality disorder)
Immigrant
Legal status
Isolation/informal caregiving burden
Transportation problems
Illness model
Eyes and ears (vision and hearing problems)
Shelter

Table 18-2. Common pitfalls in assessing for vulnerability.

- Failing to recognize the contribution of psychosocial vulnerabilities to the patient's illness.
- Failing to acknowledge vulnerability and to explore how vulnerability may be affecting care.
- Failing to address specific vulnerabilities.
- Failing to integrate knowledge of vulnerability into treatment plans.
- Failing to recognize the shame and stigma associated with vulnerabilities.
- Neglecting to identify and acknowledge strengths, resilience, and range of resources.

Table 18-3. Resilience factors.

RESILIENCE Factors	Sample Questions
Religion/spirituality/philosophy	"Do you have a spirituality, a religion, or a philosophy of life? If so, how has it helped you deal with life's challenges."
Expertise/employment	"What do you feel expert at doing?"; "What work have you done in your life?"; "What have you learned from those experiences."
Social support and network	"Who would you say are people or communities you feel support you?"
Intimates	"Who are the people you feel the closest to?"; "Who do you trust?"
Laughter	"What makes you laugh?"; "When was the last time you had a really good laugh?"
Institutions	"Are there any institutions or organizations that support you?"
Energy and enthusiasm	"What helps you feel energetic?"; "What do you get really enthusiastic about?"
Navigation of life's difficulties	"How have you made it through the challenging times in your life?"; "Who has helped you during those times?"
Cultural assets	"What strengths do you get from your culture"; "How have your cultural beliefs and values helped you deal with challenges?"
Entertainment/enjoyment	"What do you enjoy doing?"; "What do you do for fun?"

Second, vulnerability is *context dependent*. For example, in countries with universal health care coverage, lack of insurance simply does not contribute to vulnerability. Conversely, absence of interpretation services may exacerbate the effects of limited English proficiency when compared to settings with medical interpretation; presence of a methadone treatment program or a mobile treatment van in one's clinic may mitigate the untoward health effects of heroin addiction and housing instability, respectively. As such, the effects of vulnerability on health care can be influenced by altering the context in which caregiving takes place, which most frequently means adapting the clinical encounter. This suggests that when caring for vulnerable populations, clinicians and systems should also perform *self-assessments*, and carefully explore the ways in which the caregiving context can be adapted to best attenuate (or even eliminate) the health effects of vulnerability.

Third, in the process of assessment, the clinician should be sensitive to the concerns of patients with respect to shame and stigma. It is clear that a number of factors listed in Table 18-1 may elicit feelings of shame, such as having limited literacy, being marginally housed, having mental illness, or being addicted.

Fourth, after identifying vulnerability, the clinician should not forget the important step of exploring with the patient, in a supportive and nonjudgmental manner, how the vulnerability may be affecting health and care and how to mitigate these effects. Only by doing so can the clinicians develop a more effective treatment plan while simultaneously enhancing the therapeutic alliance.

SUSTAINABILITY IN BUILDING THE THERAPEUTIC ALLIANCE WITH VULNERABLE PATIENTS

There are several additional strategies that may be useful especially in developing and sustaining a therapeutic alliance with socially vulnerable patients. These include *showing* patients in concrete ways that you care (i.e., "going the extra mile"); *advocating* for patients with the myriad bureaucracies with which they struggle; *connecting* them to appropriate community resources (e.g., immigration lawyer, domestic violence counselor, exercise groups); *networking* with others, including family, friends, public health, and community resources, so as to encourage them to support the patient's efforts to achieve health; and *engaging* in *self-disclosure* to narrow social distance and encourage the sharing of personal stories.

Building a therapeutic alliance with vulnerable patients comes with both special rewards and challenges. Working with the underserved allows a clinician to apply his or her skills to assist those who are most in need, fulfilling one of the basic humanitarian ideals in medicine. Developing a therapeutic bond with patients that do not represent the "typical patient," or that many consider too difficult to manage, can be rewarding in and of itself, often involving a process of shared discovery and reflection.

It is not uncommon, however, for even seasoned clinicians to be overwhelmed by the many challenges inherent to caring for vulnerable patients. Developing patterns of codependency, such as repeatedly "rescuing" patients from the decisions that are in their control, may be a prelude to clinician "burnout." In addition, the work environment plays an important role. Although clinicians in underserved clinical settings report serving higher proportions of medically and psychosocially complex patients, they are more likely to report a chaotic work environment and less likely to feel in control. In these contexts, clinicians who perceive high proportions of challenging patient encounter have higher odds of burnout and reduced job satisfaction. Finally, with the widespread implementation of electronic health record systems, clinicians increasingly report dissatisfaction with both the high burdens of documentation and the barriers computer use creates in their communication and relationships with patients.

Clinicians should be aware of signs of "burnout," such as exhibiting their anger and frustration at patients or staff, or developing an overly passive style of patient engagement. To minimize burnout and maximize sustainability, clinicians caring for vulnerable populations may draw on personal, interpersonal, and environmental supports. In a qualitative study exploring why clinicians work in underserved clinics, clinicians cited the importance of personal motivators (such as opportunity for personal growth and concordance of service with self-identity and mission-based values); career motivators (such as work–life balance and loan repayment assistance); and environmental factors, primarily supportive interprofessional colleagues and teams.

Clinicians who have been able to sustain therapeutic relationships with vulnerable patients and maintain fulfilling careers in the care of vulnerable populations tend to (1) elicit patients' agendas so as to establish an understanding of patient expectations, (2) set realistic goals for what they can accomplish and share these goals with their patients, (3) limit what they aim to accomplish in any given encounter and see their work with patients as evolving over a long period of time, (4) continually clarify boundaries, (5) maintain a sense of curiosity and discovery about the patients' clinical and personal profile, (6) acknowledge that many of the problems experienced by vulnerable patients are structural/societal in nature, and not always a result of patient choice, (7) engage in public health-related or social advocacy efforts to affect structural determinants of health, (8) seek the advice and support of colleagues who share common ideals and practices, and (9) engage with interprofessional colleagues to draw on their expertise as part of an integrated team. Health care systems wishing to recruit and retain clinicians caring for vulnerable populations should provide opportunities for clinicians to develop these intrapersonal and interpersonal skills and enhance the clinical resources that allow clinicians to feel successful in this work.

CONCLUSION

A strong therapeutic alliance creates a trusting context for patient care, contributes to a higher quality of care, and can improve patient safety. Building a therapeutic alliance, eliciting the patient's narrative and assessing for vulnerabilities and strengths are critical to creating this context. Fostering the therapeutic alliance requires developing trust, conveying empathy, and collaborating about treatment goals. Depending on the skills, attitudes, and orientation of clinicians and the systems in which they work, the clinical encounter can increase social distance and exacerbate the effects of vulnerability on health, or it can lead to productive engagement with patients to mitigate or even eliminate the effects of vulnerability on health. Though it may be especially challenging to develop and sustain a therapeutic alliance with those who are socially vulnerable, the benefits to patient and clinician can be profound.

KEY CONCEPTS

- Vulnerable patients often experience fragmentation and disconnection in their lives and in their health care.
- The therapeutic alliance is an important means to reduce the effects of vulnerability on health outcomes.
- Eliciting the patient's story or perspective is an effective means to uncover health beliefs, develop shared meaning, enable empathy, and enhance the therapeutic alliance. It also serves to uncover patient vulnerabilities and reveal patients' resilience.
- By identifying vulnerabilities and acknowledging these to the patient and to other clinicians involved in the patient's care, clinicians will be better equipped to develop effective treatment plans.
- Though it may be especially challenging to develop and sustain a therapeutic alliance with those who are socially vulnerable, the benefits to the patient and clinician can be profound.

DISCUSSION QUESTIONS

1. Discuss clinical experiences you have had with vulnerable patients in which the presence or absence of strategies such as building a therapeutic alliance, eliciting patients' narratives, and assessing for vulnerabilities and strengths influenced the process and perhaps the outcome of their health care.
2. Consider what structural and health policy changes would need to be made to better incorporate the strategies of building a therapeutic alliance, eliciting patients' narratives, and assessing for vulnerabilities and strengths into the day-to-day clinical care of vulnerable patients.
3. What are some of the most surprising or fascinating non-medical pieces of information you learned about the last patient you cared for, and how did it influence either the treatment plan or your relationship with the patient and his or her family?
4. Discuss how personal beliefs, values, and assumptions about vulnerable patients affect your ability to create a context for effective care, using strategies such as building a therapeutic alliance, eliciting patients' narratives, and assessing for vulnerabilities and strengths.
5. What special rewards and challenges have you encountered in caring for vulnerable populations, and what strategies would help you sustain therapeutic alliances with your patients and families?

SUGGESTED READINGS

Beach MC, Branyon E, Saha S. Diverse patient perspectives on respect in healthcare: a qualitative study. *Patient Educ Couns* 2017;100(11):2076–2080.

Beach MC, Sugarman J, Johnson RL, et al. Do patients treated with dignity report higher satisfaction, adherence, and receipt of preventive care? *Ann Fam Med* 2005;3:331–338.

Blanchard J, Lurie N. R-E-S-P-E-C-T: patient reports of disrespect in the health care setting and its impact on care. *J Fam Pract* 2004;53:721–730.

Copper LA, Roter DL, Carson KA, et al. A randomized trial to improve patient-centered care and hypertension control in underserved primary care patients. *J Gen Intern Med* 2011;26:1297–1304.

Gottlieb L, Sandel M, Adler NE. Collecting and applying data on social determinants of health in health care settings. *JAMA Intern Med* 2013;173(11):1017–1020.

Hayashi AS, Selia E, McDonnell K. Stress and provider retention in underserved communities. *J Health Care Poor Underserved* 2009; 20(3):597–604.

Lyles CR, Karter AJ, Young BA, et al. Provider factors and patient-reported healthcare discrimination in the Diabetes Study of California (DISTANCE). *Patient Educ Couns* 2011;85(3): e216–e224.

Moskowitz D, Lyles CR, Karter AJ, et al. Patient reported interpersonal processes of care and perceived social position: the Diabetes Study of Northern California (DISTANCE). *Patient Educ Couns* 2013;90(3):392–398.

Odom Walker K, Ryan G, Ramey R, et al. Recruiting and retaining primary care physicians in urban underserved communities: the importance of having a mission to serve. *Am J Public Health* 2010;100(11):2168–2175.

Paradies Y, Ben J, Denson N, et al. Racism as a determinant of health: a systematic review and meta-analysis. *PLoS One* 2015;10(9):e0138511.

Piette JD, Bibbins-Domingo K, Schillinger D. Health care discrimination, processes of care, and diabetes patients' health status. *Patient Educ Couns* 2006;60:41–48.

Saba GW, Wong S, Schillinger D, et al. Shared decision-making and perceived collaboration in primary care. *Ann Fam Med* 2006;4:54–62.

Schillinger D. Improving chronic disease care for populations with limited health literacy. In: Nielsen-Bohlman LEA, ed. *Health Literacy: A Prescription to End Confusion.* Washington, DC: Institute of Medicine, National Academy Press; 2004:267–284.

Varkey AB, Manwell LB, Williams ES, et al. Separate and unequal: clinics where minority and nonminority patients receive primary care. *Arch Intern Med* 2009;169(3):243–250.

SECTION IV
Health-Related Behavior

Behavior Change

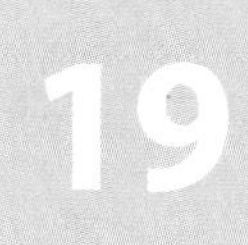

Daniel O'Connell, PhD

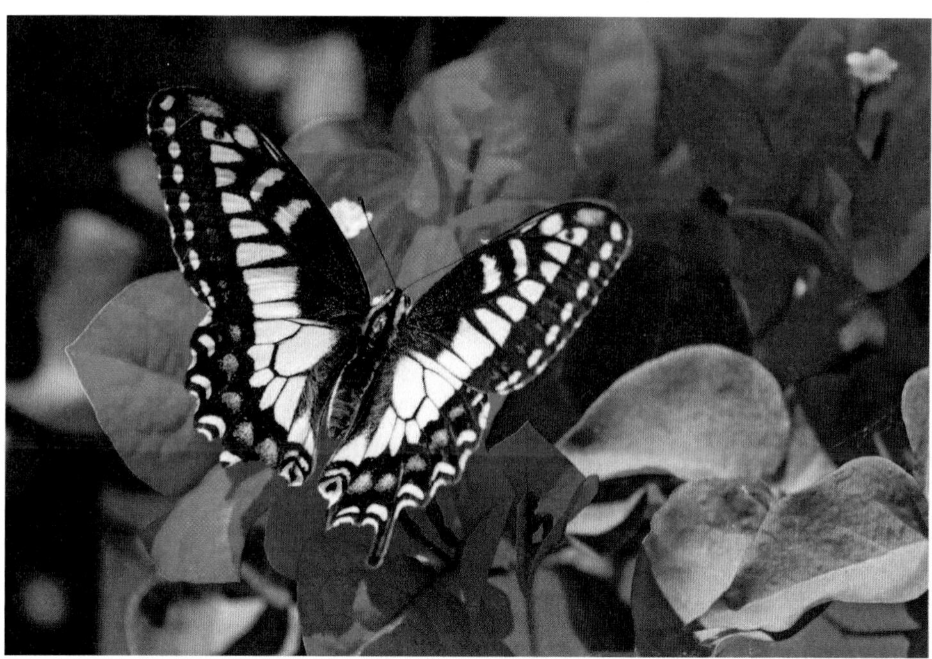

Photo by Hank Christensen (www.hankchristensen.com).

INTRODUCTION

It is clear that many contemporary health problems, such as diabetes, heart disease, and cancer, are related to patients' lifestyles and specific behaviors. As a result, the clinician must cultivate the skills to influence patient lifestyles, including the reduction or elimination of destructive behaviors (e.g., smoking and alcohol dependence), promotion of healthier behaviors (e.g., weight control, regular exercise, stress management, and safer sex), and increasing adherence to medical regimens intended to treat acute or chronic illness (e.g., taking medications, dietary restrictions, and checking blood glucose). Yet not everyone's vision of the good life involves careful attention and effort toward the healthiest behavior. Many patients prefer either to live with a risk (e.g., smoking or obesity) or prefer a medication or procedure over behavior change to ameliorate a problem. Much of clinical practice, particularly with limited visit time, conforms to a "find it and fix it" approach. The clinician assesses and identifies the problem and tells the patient what needs to be done about it. Sometimes this works. Often however, the "fix" requires patients to be convinced of the necessity of burdensome behavior changes which they must commit to, carry out, and maintain for years to come. How to best promote this kind of change is the objective of this chapter.

Fortunately, work done in the field of psychology and behavioral medicine in the past 40 years has clarified the most effective approaches to successful behavior change. In this chapter, we will incorporate the contributions from the most evidence based approaches: the *Stages of Change Model, Motivational Interviewing, Self-Efficacy, Harm Reduction, Communication Theory, Social Support/Influence, Willpower, Goal Setting, and Behavior Therapies.*

Table 19-1. Stages of change and patient characteristics.

Stage	Patient Characteristics
Precontemplation	The problem exists, but the patient minimizes or denies it.
Contemplation	The patient is thinking about the problem and the costs and benefits of continuing with the problem or trying to change.
Preparation	The patient commits to a time and plan for resolving the problem.
Action	The patient makes daily efforts to overcome the problem.
Maintenance	The patient has overcome the problem and remains vigilant to prevent backsliding.
Relapse	The patient has gone back to the problem behavior on a regular basis after a period of successful resolution.

BEHAVIOR CHANGE MODELS

The **Transtheoretical Model** (TTM) (see Prochaska and DiClemente) is perhaps the most researched and applied of all comprehensive approaches to behavior change. It describes the stages through which change progresses as well as the change processes (e.g., insight development, self-reevaluation, behavior modification strategies like changing settings and stimuli and using rewards to encourage constructive behavior) that prove effective at each stage. The **Stages of Change** (SOC) aspect of TTM describes how people move in a spiral manner through a succession of five relatively distinguishable stages in intentional behavior change. The succession is "spiral" because patients rarely move in a linear path through the stages but instead linger and often relapse into prior stages before eventually achieving maintenance of healthier behaviors. Some critics have found this forward and backward aspect of patients' time courses to undermine the validity of the SOC approach. For most clinicians, however, the value of being able to assess the patient's stage of readiness for changing a specific behavior lies in focusing discussion or assistance where it is most efficient and effective. Many of the other behavior change models and strategies we will discuss work best when integrated into this framework, matching the clinician's approach to the patient's current stage of change. The stages are outlined in Table 19-1.

The following descriptions and examples illustrate each of the stages of behavior change:

Precontemplation: The patient gives little thought to the problem and how best to solve it (e.g., adolescent drinks heavily but is apparently oblivious to consequences or resentful when discussed).

Contemplation: The patient thinks about the pros and cons of the problem and the potential methods, costs, and benefits involved in trying to address it but makes only inconsistent attempts at changing behavior (e.g., promised dietary changes that last intermittently or only for a few days/weeks).

Preparation/Commitment: The patient commits to a specific course of action and timetable within the next 30 days (e.g., patient decides to join Weight Watchers this month with a girlfriend from work, or hires a personal trainer for four sessions to initiate an exercise program). Note that this activates *social support* to assist change both practically and emotionally. The *preparation* stage can also entail *behavior therapy* strategies such as *stimulus control* (positive cues, reminders, removing tempting stimuli such as high calorie snacks or alcohol to reduce the burden of *limited willpower*), *goal setting* (using specific goal targets and self-monitoring for guiding and encouraging change), and *reinforcement*, perhaps by using large or small intermediate rewards along the way to long-term health improvement (e.g., a patient agrees not to buy a new car until he has 6 months abstinence from cigarettes so he does not foul the car with stale smoke).

Action: A plan is being carried out on a regular basis with relatively clear goals, strategies, and reinforcers (e.g., walking at least 30 minutes in the morning or evening 5 days a week and using a chart or diary to mark accomplishment and perhaps link to a previously determined reward).

Maintenance: Successful changers incorporate *Action* stage behaviors into a "new normal" way of living.

For example, an alcoholic with 5 years of sobriety still attends AA meetings on occasion and *has* altered his social network and leisure activities to maintain sobriety (e.g., joining a hiking group or deepening involvement with yoga practice that provides and expands a constructive network of social support antithetical to drug/alcohol abuse).

Relapse: While not a stage itself, relapse describes the retreat from a more advanced stage to an earlier stage of change (e.g., a patient who has quit smoking relapses back into regular smoking; a person who has committed to checking blood sugars daily fails to follow through, saying "I got too busy").

Fewer than 20% of patients report willingness to take a specific action on a health behavior change in the next 30 days (e.g., quit smoking or start a weight loss program). Therefore, in 80% of patient encounters the clinician's immediate objective is to increase patients' readiness to contemplate the pros and cons of the problem and the paths to change. The long-range objective is that patients eventually will commit to, initiate and stick with specific actions until the improved behavior has become the new normal. Moving from contemplation to maintenance in smoking cessation, for example, has been shown to take years and involve multiple periods of progression and relapse before long-term success. More than half of all the people in the United States who have ever smoked have now quit (i.e., progressed to *maintenance)*, and more than 70% of current smokers report the desire to quit at some future point (i.e., *contemplation on the way to commitment)*. The goal of each clinician–patient conversation is to encourage movement through the stages. Most of patients' work is done outside the visit, as they think about, plan, commit, and then carry out the new behaviors. The clinician is attempting to link up with all the other forces and resources that promote healthier behaviors, including laws, restrictions on smoking in many settings, employee drug testing, taxes on tobacco and alcohol, and media reports of harms such as the opioid epidemic and obesity crisis.

The TTM provides a useful framework for clinicians to tailor their approach in any given patient encounter to the patient's stage of change in modifying health-risk behaviors. Appropriate clinician strategies for each of the stages are summarized in Table 19-2.

Motivational Interviewing, with its recognition of the power of *intrinsic motivation*, is particularly valuable in showing how best to talk with patients about health-risk behaviors in a way that increases their own motivation to change. *Reactance theory* emphasizes that people are inclined to resist coercion and so have trouble making behavior changes that do not meet their own internalized values and goals (*intrinsic motivation*). *Communication theory* differentiates influence styles as either *Pushing or Pulling*. *Pushing* entails statements directed from the influencer toward the one being influenced that include advice-giving, teaching, directing, ordering, pleading, threatening, cajoling, lecturing, and criticizing. Pushing communications are overused by clinicians who naturally assume the expert role and feel it is most time efficient to simply tell the patients what they need to know and do. Research has found little support for the sustained effectiveness of lecturing, threatening, or otherwise trying to inspire behavior change in patients. *Pulling*, in contrast, is communication intended to encourage others to self-reflect and re-evaluate their own ideas and feelings about an issue. *Pulling* is used when we recognize that the necessary answers are within the other person and need to be explored if understanding and motivation for change is to be identified and encouraged. *Reactance theory* suggests that people, who might otherwise have admitted and explored a problem, may instead feel compelled to defend their behavior when criticized, pressured, or coerced. *Motivational interviewing* utilizes *Pulling* by eliciting the patient's own ideas, values, motivations, concerns, feelings about the problem, and potential solutions. The clinician's role is to help patients gather and reflect on the relevant data, weigh the pros and cons of change, determine the importance and urgency of change for themselves, and then commit to a course of action when they feel ready.

Motivational Interviewing is accomplished through a conversational style that encourages expressions of empathy, acknowledgment of ambivalence about change, curiosity about feelings and ideas, and respect for the patient's ownership of the problem and autonomy in deciding when and what to do next. Listening for and highlighting "*change talk*", in which patients themselves are providing the arguments for change and exploring how it might be accomplished, can be very effective. *Clinician: "I can hear that you don't want to risk another heart attack. Your plan for joining a health club makes sense and there is nothing in your exam today that would restrict you from exercising."* Expressing concern instead of control, and curiosity rather than advice, are the hallmarks of this approach.

The clinician is often the one providing the worrisome information that precipitates the behavior change conversation, thus stimulating *precontemplators* to engage in contemplation of the problem and explore their own motivation for change. *Clinician: "Your hemoglobin A1c has gone from 8-9 this year. What do you understand that means in terms of potential harm to you?"*

Communication theory and *motivational interviewing* encourage a conversational sequence of *provide–elicit–provide*. The clinician *provides* a piece of information ("Your elevated liver enzymes indicate that your liver is having trouble with what it is being asked to detoxify.") and immediately *elicits* the patient's thoughts, ("What do you know about the burden that drugs and alcohol put on your liver?"). This style makes for a more active

Table 19-2. Stages of change and clinician strategies.

Stage of Change	Patient Characteristics	Clinician Strategies
Precontemplation	Denies problem and its importance. Is reluctant to discuss problem. Problem is identified by others. Shows reactance when pressured. High risk of argument.	Ask permission to discuss problem. Inquire about patient's thoughts. Gently point out discrepancies. Express concern. Ask patient to think, talk, or read about situation between visits.
Contemplation	Shows openness to talk, read, and think about problem. Weighs pros and cons. Dabbles in action. Can be obsessive about problem and can prolong stage.	Elicit patient's perspective first. Help identify pros and cons of change. Ask what would promote commitment. Suggest trials.
Preparation/ Determination	Understands that change is needed. Begins to form commitment to specific goals, methods, and timetables. Can picture overcoming obstacles. May procrastinate about setting start date for change.	Summarize patient's reasons for change. Negotiate a start date to begin some or all change activities. Encourage patient to announce change publicly. Arrange a follow-up contact at or shortly after start date.
Action	Follows a plan of regular activity to change problem. Can describe plan in detail (unlike dabbling in action of contemplator). Shows commitment in facing obstacles. Resists slips. Is particularly vulnerable to abandoning effort impulsively.	Show interest in specifics of plan. Discuss difference between slip and relapse. Help anticipate how to handle a slip. Support and reemphasize pros of changing. Help to modify action plan if aspects are not working well. Arrange follow-up contact for support.
Maintenance	Has accomplished change or improvement through focused action. Has varying levels of awareness regarding importance of long-term vigilance. May already be losing ground through slips or wavering commitment. Has feelings about how much the change has actually improved life. May be developing lifestyle that precludes relapse into former problem.	Show support and admiration. Inquire about feelings and expectations and how well they were met. Ask about slips, any signs of wavering commitment. Help create plan for intensifying activity should slips occur. Support lifestyle and personal redefinition that reduce risk of relapse. Reflect on the long-term—and possibly permanent—nature of this stage as opposed to the more immediate gratification of initial success.

and involved patient, who is encouraged to self-reflect rather than deflect and defend or passively nod and smile while quietly waiting for the subject to change.

Self-efficacy theory predicts that for individuals to become more *committed* to change they must become sufficiently *convinced* both that the change is needed and also that the specific change being considered would be *effective* in meeting their objective (e.g., "Is losing weight really necessary for me? *And* If I were able to follow a Mediterranean or a programmed diet, would I really lose significant amounts of weight?"). *Self-efficacy* research also reminds us that people must feel sufficiently *confident* that they can reliably perform the changed behavior before they will commit themselves to action. The clinician thus tries to help the patient create manageable and achievable steps that can be embraced with more confidence. *Clinician: "Where do you think it would be easiest for you to reduce the calories you are taking in—by cutting out sweets or by reducing portion sizes at meals?"* "Ultimately, the change must strike patients as sufficiently *important* that it feels worth all the effort in light of all the other demands on their energy and time. *Harm reduction* research teaches us that benefits can accrue with less than comprehensive behavior changes. Examples of harm reduction include drinking and using drugs less often or in lower doses, switching from cigarettes to nicotine vapor, prescribing controlled opioid partial agonists to replace uncontrolled street opioids or prescription drug abuse, or losing 5% of body weight. All or nothing thinking about behavior change can leave people stuck in the *Contemplation stage* (weighing pros and cons without resolution) or *Commitment stage* (making unrealistic promises that have little chance of being enacted and maintained). *Conviction, confidence, and importance* are continuous variables (more/less) rather than dichotomous all or none thinking. Increased conviction that the change is important and necessary, combined with increasing confidence that the specific steps are doable, ultimately results in the tipping point being reached where the patient is willing to commit to a course of action that can reduce harm.

Tying in Stage of Change With Motivational Interviewing & Self-Efficacy Theory

Depending on the patient's stage of change, the clinician could promote further contemplation of the problem and potential solutions, encourage commitment to a specific course of action already contemplated, help tailor the patient's current actions to accelerate desired outcomes, or assist incorporation of successful actions into the patient's ongoing lifestyle. For example, in the contemplation stage assessing and building conviction is usually the place to start, since a patient who is not sufficiently convinced that the problem is important and the proposed behavior change would lead to success is unlikely to think much about how to solve it or what the challenges might be. Research shows that unless the balance of *pros vs. cons* of change shifts in the change direction, changed behavior is unlikely to be initiated and maintained. *Patient: "I see that I over-relied on benzos to relax me, where I needed to get my work and home life in better balance to really become less stressed."*

Clinician: (Provides information) *"I am concerned that your hemoglobin A1c has gone up further. What do you think might have contributed to that rise?"* (Encouraging self-reflection on the problem) (Pause for a response) *Clinician: "What do you understand that increased hemoglobin A1c means for you?"* (Encourage *contemplation of the harms of current behavior*). *Clinician: "What do you think may be needed to turn that around?"* Many patients already have a good idea of possible needs (e.g., watch diet more closely, get more exercise, and check blood sugars more regularly). If not, the clinician can *provide* information (e.g., teach/suggest). After discussing ways to get blood sugars under control, the clinician can ask how ready the patient is to *commit* to one of those behaviors by asking about *conviction* and *confidence*. *Clinician: "How convinced are you that reducing sweets and deserts could get your blood sugars back in a safer range?"* (Pause for patient to genuinely self-reflect and respond.) If the patient is reasonably convinced, then the clinician can ask: *"How confident are you that you could start to make those changes today?"* (Pause for an answer). *"Is that something you are willing to commit yourself to start?"* If patient agrees, it can help to anchor that commitment by making a note in the electronic health record (EHR) right then and including that commitment in the after-visit summary for the patient to take home. *Clinician: "So you are committing yourself to eliminate desserts after meals for 3 months, and we will keep the rest of your plan the same and recheck your hemoglobin A1c in 3 months."*

As we have learned through research on *motivational interviewing*, the clinician will be tempted to fall back into the "find it and fix it" process, particularly if the problem is serious and the clinician is feeling pressed for time and feels the responsibility to be directive with the ambivalent or resistant patient. Yet research suggests that this is a trap to be avoided. Instead clinicians are more effective if they can continue to show respect for patient autonomy while also empathizing with the patient's ambivalence. *Clinician: "Sounds like you would like to lose weight but feel discouraged about how hard you have found it to eat less. I might have some ideas for how to make best use of the willpower you do have if you think that might be helpful."* (The patient owns the problem, and clinician is a helper; rather than the clinician owns the problem, and the patient says "yes, but . . . ")

Exploring the patient's *self-efficacy* entails accessing how able and confident the patient feels to succeed at a specific behavior change. Ask the patient how *convinced* he is that quitting smoking would be helpful right now. If the patient is barely *convinced* that the change is valuable at this time (e.g., *"I don't see how that would really help."*), then focusing on the impact of smoking on his chronic obstructive pulmonary disease (COPD) will be the place to start. *Clinician: "What do you know about the connection between smoking and the increasing shortness of breath you have been experiencing?"* If the patient is already sufficiently *convinced* that the change would be very valuable (*Patient: "I know that smoking is killing me, but I have never been able to quit for more than a few days."*), then the clinician's time is best spent talking about ways to enhance *confidence* that the patient can accomplish quitting. *Clinician: "What aspect of quitting smoking has been the most difficult for you?* (Pause for answer) *Let's see what we might have to offer to help with that by way of strategies or medications that other patients have found helpful."*

These same open-ended and scaling questions about *conviction, confidence, and importance* can be used with almost any health behavior. Here are more examples of questions.

Clinician: "How surprised were you to learn that you reported the key symptoms of depression on that questionnaire that my MA asked you to complete?" (Pause for a response) *"How convinced are you now that depression is a part of your feeling so tired and discouraged these last few months?"* (Pause and elicit a response) If the patient now agrees that depression is contributing to the chronic fatigue for which they sought treatment, then there is a natural opening to talk about treatment options. Conversely, if the patient continues in the view that the fatigue is unrelated to a mood disorder, then the clinician can encourage the patient to simply *contemplate* the possibility further with reading material, websites, or suggesting the patient talk with family members and friends about whether they have seen signs of depression. The clinician can also suggest that the patient might consider sitting down with a behavioral health provider for a single visit to explore the issue of how psychological/neurobiological factors could be contributing to the fatigue. The key point is that the clinician should not be most motivated person in the room for long. It is the patient who needs to become more concerned that psychological distress, lifestyle, or behavior may be contributing to their medical concerns. The clinician should not argue or criticize as that tends to build resistance (*reactance theory)* but can and should express concern. *Clinician: "I am concerned that you may not have the outcome we are both wanting for you without understanding and addressing all the behaviors that could be contributing to the problem."*

CONCLUSION

Although clinicians are convinced that behavior change would be helpful in many patient conditions, they often lack confidence in their ability to influence patients' behavior in brief medical interviews. The goal of this chapter has been to map out pragmatic approaches that can be utilized in even the briefest encounters to have a positive influence on the patient's behavior. Assessing a patient's *stage of change* promotes a more focused conversation by pointing up where the patient's next efforts might be most productive. *Motivational interviewing* teaches the demeanor of empathic and respectful curiosity that acknowledges patients' autonomy while exploring the ambivalence that marks all difficult choices. The clinician learns to *Pull* from the patient self-motivational thoughts and feelings rather than *Push* at the patient with lectures, threats, and inspiration. *Reactance theory* reminds the clinician of the natural urge of patients to resist coercion, and research on *intrinsic motivation* makes clear that for change to be initiated and sustained individuals must relate the effort and outcome to their own goals and values, ultimately deciding if the effort is sufficiently important. Research on *goal setting* emphasizes that the most effective actions are ones in which the patient has clearly identified goals and monitors both behavior and outcomes on a regular basis. *Willpower* is a necessary but limited commodity in the patient's life. Techniques from *behavior therapy* can reduce the burden on willpower by making healthy behavior and choices more accessible and unhealthy behavior less easily triggered. For example, *stimulus control* addresses cues that tempt problem behavior (having cigarettes in the house; having liquor, high calorie, or high glycemic index foods easily accessible) and replacing them with cues and alternatives that make healthy behavior an easier default. *Reinforcement management* refers to how a patient can build in intermediate rewards to encourage movement on the way to longer term health improvements. *Social network* and influence strategies enable the patient to build activities and interpersonal connections that promote healthier behavior and replace social networks that have been associated with problem behaviors (e.g., less time with heavy drinkers and drug users and more involvement in leisure time activities such as yoga classes where the problem behavior is antithetical).

Intentional behavior change is built on the underpinning of careful contemplation of the problem and ways to overcome it, a clear commitment to goal setting with a specific course of action, anticipation of temptations to slip and relapse, and modification of the environment to make the right choices easier and the wrong choices harder until healthier behavior has become the new normal. *Social learning theory* teaches that behavior changes when both *conviction* and *confidence* build to a level of self-efficacy that supports the ability to act. At each stage of change the clinician must understand what is influencing patients' conviction that the problem requires attention as well as their confidence that success is possible. The principle and reality of *patient autonomy* reminds us to respectfully inquire about, thoughtfully attempt to influence, and ultimately accept patients' decisions about how important a change is for them. We must accept that patients' behavior is affected by many forces and influences, only one of which is us. The more clinicians can link up with and build upon the broader array of motivators and resources for healthier behavior and lifestyle, the more they will enjoy this fundamental aspect of effective patient care.

SUGGESTED READINGS

Baumeister R, Tierney J. *Willpower.* New York, NY: Penguin Press; 2011.

Miller WR, Rollnick S. *Motivational Interviewing: Helping People Change,* 3rd ed. New York, NY: The Guilford Press; 2012.

Prochaska JO, Norcross JC, DiClemente CC. *Changing for Good.* New York, NY: The Guilford Press; 1994.

Rollnick S. Readiness, importance and confidence: critical conditions of change in treatment. In: Miller WR, Heather N, eds. *Treating Addictive Behavior,* 2nd ed. New York, NY: Springer US; 1998.

Rollnick S, Mason P, Butler C. *Health Behavior Change: A Guide for Clinicians.* New York, NY: Churchill Livingstone; 1999.

WEBSITES

The Motivational Interviewing Page. http://www.motivationalinterview.org/. Accessed August 2018.

Positive Psychology Program. What is Self-Efficacy Theory in Psychology? Definition and Examples. May 28, 2018. www.postive psychologyprogram.com. Accessed August 2018.

Transtheoretical Model Cancer Prevention Resource Center, University of Rhode Island. http://www.uri.edu Search: Cancer Prevention Research Center. Accessed August 2018.

Patient Adherence

20

Veronica J. Sanchez, PhD & M. Robin DiMatteo, PhD

INTRODUCTION

In the context of medical treatment, the term adherence refers to a patient's success in following the recommendations of a health care provider for disease prevention and treatment. Nonadherence (also called noncompliance) refers to a patient's failure to follow these recommendations, such as by not filling a medication prescription or by stopping the medication before being instructed to do so, improperly using a medical device, carrying out prescribed behaviors (e.g., specific exercises) incorrectly, or entirely ignoring medical advice (such as to avoid certain foods, or to engage in disease screening). Nonadherence can be purposeful or not. The term "unintentional nonadherence" is used to describe cases in which patients believe (mistakenly) that they are adhering to what has been prescribed, whereas "intentional nonadherence" is used for cases in which patients choose to disregard treatment recommendations completely or to modify their prescribed regimens.

Across a variety of disease conditions, 25% of patients (on average) do not adhere to prevention and disease management activities (including taking medications, going to medical appointments, obtaining screening, exercising, and/or dieting); for some medical conditions, adherence can be as poor as 50% or less. Even in the context of well-controlled clinical trials for treating chronic conditions, medication adherence has been as low as 43%. Adherence is a behavior that is strongly connected to health outcomes. On average, the odds of a good health outcome for patients who are adherent are 2.88 times higher than for nonadherent patients. Nonadherence can take a significant toll not only on patient health outcomes but also on providers and the health care system. At the interpersonal level, the inability to achieve health care goals due to nonadherence can be frustrating for both patients and their providers and may result in an estimated 125,000 avoidable deaths per year. From a societal standpoint, nonadherence produces a significant economic burden (calculated at $100 billion dollars annually in preventable health care costs alone).

According to the World Health Organization, adherence is affected by many factors such as: (1) the health care system, including the provider–patient relationship, (2) the patient's disease type and severity, (3) the type of treatment regimen and its complexity, (4) patient characteristics, and (5) socioeconomic factors. This chapter will focus on the interplay of these factors in the provider–patient relationship and communication quality in promoting adherence among all, including the most vulnerable, patients. These include patients of ethnic minority status, low socioeconomic standing, low education level, and/or low health literacy. Emphasis will be placed on targeting individual patients' needs to promote adherence through the use of a recently devised heuristic model offered by DiMatteo and colleagues, called the Information–Motivation–Strategy Model©.

OVERVIEW OF THE INFORMATION–MOTIVATION–STRATEGY MODEL©

Although the elements of the Information–Motivation–Strategy Model© (IMS Model) were first introduced in the early 1980s, there was insufficient empirical research on which to build support; now, many large-scale empirical trials and meta-analytic reviews provide evidence for the framework of the model. The primary purpose of the IMS Model is to offer health care providers a valid and practical rubric for remembering and using three broad elements of care that are essential for improving patient adherence. The three components of the IMS Model are Information, Motivation, and Strategy. They reflect the fact that patients can only follow treatments about which they have been informed and which they understand; patients will only adhere to treatments to which they are motivated; and patients only do what they are able to within their resource limitations and available strategies.

Information

The information component emphasizes the importance of the knowledge held by patients about their condition and its treatment, and it suggests that this knowledge depends most upon effective provider–patient communication. Patients are unlikely to follow a treatment unless its importance is clear to them and they fully comprehend the care instructions. Unintentional nonadherence commonly stems from failure at this stage in the process of care. Research from hundreds of studies indicates that many patients' health literacy is low and their ability to understand the health information they receive is inadequate. Therefore, health care providers have a responsibility to communicate effectively with their patients and to inform them thoroughly, as well as to check on how well patients understand the information that they are given. A meta-analysis found that in more than a hundred empirical studies, good physician communication skills were associated with increased patient adherence. To encourage patient adherence, health care providers should focus considerable attention on communicating information effectively and on determining patients' degree of understanding of the treatment regimen. When interacting with vulnerable patients, adequate communication is especially challenging because low health literacy, language barriers, and low levels of education can hinder patients' full and accurate understanding of what they must do to care for themselves. Health professionals need to identify any specific barriers to communication and attempt to build patient trust in the therapeutic relationship, promote shared decision making, listen to patients, and allow patients to offer essential information on how they plan to follow through with their medical recommendations (see Chapter 18) (Figure 20-1).

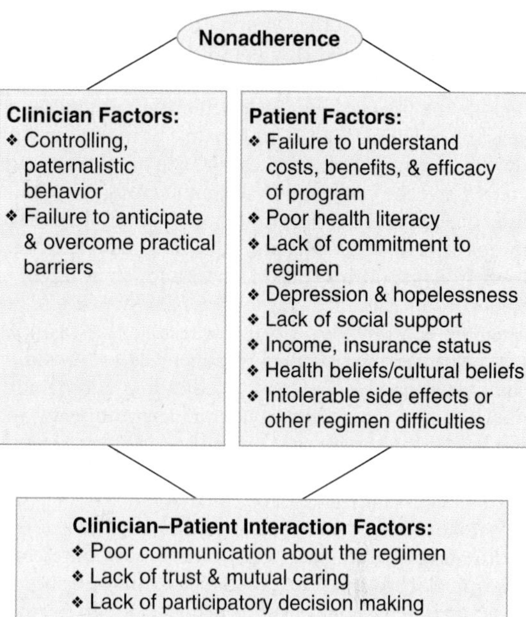

Figure 20-1. Clinician–patient barriers to adherence.

Motivation

The motivation component of the model highlights the notion that patients will only follow treatments that they believe in and are motivated to pursue. Therefore, a major goal of health care providers should be to work with each patient to develop a treatment plan to which the patient can be fully committed. Health care providers should keep in mind that patients' beliefs about the value of a treatment (such as about the risks, benefits, and efficacy of treatment) and their sense of confidence that barriers to adherence can be overcome are crucial to influencing their motivation to adhere. In addition, patients' beliefs in the consequences of nonadherence are important; if nonadherence is perceived as likely to produce problematic health outcomes, patient adherence will be higher than if consequences are not believed or fully understood. Cultural factors, including social group norms, may also impact adherence; providers need to be aware of and sensitive to their patients' cultural beliefs and practices so that treatment recommendations do not conflict with cultural norms. Furthermore, it is important to note that motivation to adhere may be especially compromised in disadvantaged patients who experience cultural barriers between them and their physicians. If patients and their physicians are not of a similar cultural background, for example, physicians should learn about their patients' culture to find the best way to help motivate them to adhere; providers should be careful to avoid introducing cultural impediments to adherence (see Chapter 15). Lastly, patients often desire to participate in the process of caring for their health; thus, it is beneficial to promote shared decision making between physicians and patients within the context of a strong therapeutic relationship. Doing so would allow providers to openly discuss patients' beliefs, concerns, confusions, and apprehensions about treatment regimens. Furthermore, meta-analytic research has indicated that patient motivation to adhere may be augmented through the use of cognitive-based behavioral strategies such as motivational interviewing. Such approaches can help patients express their concerns regarding adherence-related behaviors and allow clinicians to encourage intrinsic motivation in patients by tailoring individual adherence plans (see Chapter 19).

Strategy

Finally, the strategy component of the model underscores the fact that patients must be capable of adhering and have the resources necessary to follow the prescribed treatment. Patients need the tools and strategies necessary for effectively following their treatment, as well as the capacity to overcome any barriers to adherence that may arise. Thus, another important task for health care providers is to help patients identify and surpass obstacles to adherence. The concrete barriers patients face might include the financial cost of a medication, difficulties in remembering the medication schedule or in dealing with the treatment complexity, coping with unpleasant side effects, and the challenge of accommodating changes in lifestyle such as diet and exercise. Social support from family and friends is instrumental in helping patients adhere to treatments. In this context, social support is useful in terms of the assistance that individuals who are close to a patient can provide. A patient's relative, for example, can help overcome barriers to adherence by providing transportation, helping with medication affordability, offering child care to attend medical appointments, and reminding the patient to take medications. Past research has found that family cohesiveness can positively influence patient adherence, and that family conflict can threaten it severely. Providers should know their patients well enough to evaluate whether and how the people who are close to a patient can assist in promoting adherence; providers should also help their patients identify other formal systems of aid, including workplace-based interventions and community-based resources. Obtaining aid is particularly valuable for patients of low socioeconomic status. Disadvantaged patients may need help from their health care providers in building a social support network (e.g., if they are recent immigrants) and acquiring financial resources for covering medical care expenses (such as the costs of medications and medical devices if no insurance coverage is available).

Understanding how the three components of the IMS Model can be applied to promote patient adherence may be facilitated by the use of a case illustration.

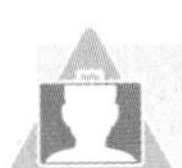

CASE ILLUSTRATION

Lucy is a 62-year-old married Hispanic woman with hypertension, adult-onset diabetes mellitus, and obesity. She lives with her husband who is ill and has two loving and supportive adult children who live nearby. She has not been feeling well for the last couple of weeks and decided to see her physician, Dr. Ruiz, at the nearby publicly funded clinic. Lucy has seen Dr. Ruiz twice before and she likes her and feels that they are developing a good relationship. Dr. Ruiz sees Lucy as a friendly and generally optimistic person.

During their second medical visit, Dr. Ruiz determined that Lucy has not been adhering to the treatment regimen prescribed by her previous physician. Dr. Ruiz prescribed two medications to control her diabetes and hypertension, offered Lucy a detailed explanation of how to take the medications, and described any serious side effects that Lucy should report. Next, Dr. Ruiz discussed the behavioral changes that Lucy would need to engage in—to check her blood sugar levels daily (before and after each meal), improve her diet (e.g., consume less sugar and salt and more vegetables), and incorporate light exercise into her daily routine (e.g., 30-minute walks). As Dr. Ruiz explained these changes to Lucy, she realized that Lucy had trouble understanding how to take her medications and how to interpret her blood sugar levels. Lucy did not believe that she needed to take medications when she felt well. Furthermore, Lucy was concerned about how she would be able to cook healthier meals and go out for walks; her time and attention were consumed by concerns for her husband's health.

APPLICATION OF THE INFORMATION–MOTIVATION–STRATEGY MODEL©

Stage One: Achieving Patient Understanding of Treatment

One of the primary reasons for nonadherence is that patients do not understand what they are supposed to do when a physician provides them with a treatment regimen. Lucy speaks Spanish fluently but is limited in her understanding of English and in her ability to speak it. Medical terminology and treatment descriptions are difficult to understand, even in her native language (i.e., she has low health literacy). Dr. Ruiz tries to speak to Lucy in terms that she can grasp, and employs a communication feedback loop (or teach-back method). She carefully explains to Lucy what having diabetes and hypertension means for her health and the importance of taking her medications, eating healthy foods, and exercising regularly. Subsequently, Dr. Ruiz can ask Lucy to state in her own words what she has understood. Then, Dr. Ruiz can try to make clear anything that Lucy has not comprehended. This process may continue until Lucy has achieved an adequate level of understanding. These techniques can be used with a medical translator as well. Good communication can help compensate for factors that inhibit proper patient understanding of medical information and can increase the likelihood that a patient adheres to treatment. Furthermore, patients who, like Lucy, tend to be disadvantaged feel empowered by understanding the medical dialogue and would be more capable of making decisions jointly with their physician and implementing their treatment regimen.

Stage Two: Motivating Patients to Adhere

A second reason why patients may not adhere to their treatment is that they may lack the motivation to do so. If Lucy did not understand the information provided by Dr. Ruiz (if stage one of the IMS Model is not effectively employed), she would likely not believe that untreated diabetes and hypertension are serious threats to her health. She may also not believe that she must take her medications and change her diet and physical activity level to remain healthy. Dr. Ruiz would need to motivate Lucy to adhere by helping her accept the seriousness of her conditions and recognize the efficacy of treatment. She can do so through motivational interviewing techniques by prompting Lucy to discuss her cognition-based challenges including her beliefs, negative attitudes that she may have about her treatment, and behavior-related obstacles for adherence. Once Lucy believes that the benefits of adhering outweigh her concerns, Dr. Ruiz can work with Lucy to state a firm commitment to focus her efforts on adhering to the treatment, and Dr. Ruiz can provide encouragement to build Lucy's sense of her own capability and efficacy in caring for herself.

Stage Three: Creating a Feasible Strategy for Attaining Patient Adherence

A third key obstacle for achieving patient adherence is that patients sometimes lack a workable strategy for following their prescribed treatments. Lucy is preoccupied with worrying about her husband's illness and needs. She does not know how she will incorporate into a manageable daily routine the many tasks—including taking her medications on schedule, checking her blood sugar level before and after each meal, buying fresh vegetables, and cooking healthy meals instead of those that are typical for her Hispanic culture. She worries that she cannot go out for walks, tend to her housekeeping, and care for her husband. In addition, she has a very limited financial budget and is not sure that she can afford three expensive elements of her treatment: the device for checking her blood sugar level, her medications, and healthy food options. Lucy is also uncertain about her ability to remember to test her blood sugar throughout the day and to take the correct medication at the accurate time.

Dr. Ruiz can try to help Lucy address all of her concerns by first assessing all of the resources that are available to Lucy. Upon asking Lucy about close relatives, Dr. Ruiz would learn that Lucy has two adult children who live fairly nearby. She could then ask about Lucy's willingness to ask her children for assistance with bringing her groceries or helping her care for her husband, and Dr. Ruiz would realize that Lucy can potentially obtain considerable social support from her children. With regard to taking her medications, Dr. Ruiz, or her nurse, could write out a simple schedule in Spanish for when to take which medications, and Lucy could place it on her refrigerator. Dr. Ruiz could also suggest that Lucy keep the device for measuring her blood sugar levels in the kitchen where she typically eats her meals. Moreover, she could inform Lucy of financial assistance programs or discount programs where she can sign up to obtain medications and medical equipment at either no cost or at reduced prices. Dr. Ruiz or members of her team could also provide Lucy with ideas for how to adjust her current cooking style to one that slowly introduces healthier options to her traditional cuisine. Lastly, Dr. Ruiz or the team could assist Lucy with finding the best times throughout the week when she can go out for a walk and achieve the goal of increased physical activity. A general summary of the suggested care for vulnerable patients using the IMS Model is provided in Table 20-1.

Table 20-1. Adherence challenges for vulnerable patients and potential solutions using the IMS Model©.

Model Component	Challenges	Suggested Care
Information: Patients need to *know what to do* to adhere.	Low health literacy, low education level, and language barriers can severely challenge adherence. Patients may have limited understanding of the treatment regimen but remain reluctant to ask questions.	Physicians should thoroughly explain the treatment in terms the patient can understand, utilizing medical team members to work with the patient. Providers should use a communication feedback loop, having patients express their understanding while physicians clarify any confusion. Medical translators should always be present when needed.
Motivation: Patients need to *want to adhere.*	Ethnic minority patients may experience culture-based obstacles to adherence. They may have difficulty believing in the importance of adhering and reconciling their cultural beliefs with the treatment plan.	Physicians should allow patients to express their concerns and negative attitudes about the treatment. Physicians should listen, be culturally sensitive, and help patients to understand the reality of their conditions, the efficacy of the treatment, and their capability to adhere.
Strategy: Patients need help to *be able to adhere.*	Patients of low socioeconomic status may lack necessary resources and have difficulty affording their medications and medical devices. They may have many competing demands on their time, and many practical limitations that stand in the way of adhering.	Physicians should offer patients information about sources of financial assistance for their medication, as well as help them determine how to draw on the social support resources available to them. Physicians should address all patient barriers for implementing their treatment regimen.

CONCLUSION

The IMS Model asserts that patient knowledge, belief in and commitment to a treatment, and capability to adhere are essential for maximizing adherence. Nonadherence is a multifaceted problem and addressing it requires the involvement of health care providers, patients, and the other individuals who are a part of a patient's social support network. The implementation of the three components of the IMS Model can have a positive influence on the process of care for all patients, particularly those who are most vulnerable, and can improve the physician–patient relationship, communication quality, and favorable health outcomes.

SUGGESTED READINGS

Bussel JK, Cha ES, Grant YE, Schwartz DD, Young LA. Ways health care providers can promote better medication adherence. *Clin Diabetes* 2017;35(3):171–177.

Cutler DM, Everett W. Thinking outside the pillbox—medication adherence as a priority for health care reform. *N Engl J Med* 2010;362(17):1553–1555.

DiMatteo MR, Haskard-Zolnierek K, Martin LR. Improving patient adherence: a three-factor model to guide practice. *Health Psychol Rev* 2012;6(1):74–91.

DiMatteo MR, Haskard-Zolnierek K, Williams SL. Health beliefs, disease severity, and patient adherence: a meta-analysis. *Med Care* 2007;45(6):521–528.

Haskard-Zolnierek KB, DiMatteo MR. Physician communication and patient adherence to treatment. *Med Care* 2009;47(8):826–834.

Kleinsinger F. The unmet challenge of medication nonadherence. *Perm J* 2018;22:18–033.

Oung AB, Kosirog E, Chavez B, Brunner J, Saseen JJ. Evaluation of medication adherence in chronic disease at a federally qualified health center. *Ther Adv Chronic Dis* 2017;8(8-9):113–120.

Palacio A, Garay D, Langer B, Taylor J, Wood BA, Tamariz L. Motivational interviewing improves medication adherence: a systematic review and meta-analysis. *J Gen Intern Med* 2016;31(8):929–940.

WEBSITES

Agency for Healthcare Research and Quality: Medication Adherence. https://healthit.ahrq.gov/ahrq-funded-projects/emerging-lessons/medication-adherence. Accessed August 2019.

Centers for Disease Control and Prevention: Overcoming Barriers to Medication Adherence for Chronic Diseases. https://www.cdc.gov/grand-rounds/pp/2017/20170221-medication-adherence.html. Accessed August 2019.

World Health Organization: Adherence to Long-Term Therapies Evidence for Action. http://www.who.int/chp/knowledge/publications/adherence_full_report.pdf. Accessed August 2019.

ACKNOWLEDGMENTS

Supported by a Robert Wood Johnson Foundation Investigator Award in Health Policy Research (PI: M. Robin DiMatteo) and by the Committee on Research of the U.C. Riverside Academic Senate.

VIDEO

Video 20-1. Patient Adherence (6 min, 44 sec)

Access by scanning the QR code above or visit mhprofessional.com/feldman5evideos.

Tobacco Use

21

Nancy A. Rigotti, MD & Sara Kalkhoran, MD, MAS

INTRODUCTION

Cigarette smoking is the leading preventable cause of death in the United States, responsible for an estimated 480,000 deaths per year, or one in every five deaths. Physicians care for the health consequences of their patients' tobacco use, and it is equally important for them to prevent smoking-related disease. There is no safe level of tobacco use. Smoking as few as one cigarette per day increases the risk of myocardial infarction and stroke. Smoking cessation extends life and treating tobacco use is one of the most cost-effective preventive actions available to clinicians.

The prevalence of cigarette smoking in the United States rose rapidly in the first half of the twentieth century and peaked in 1965, when 40% of adult Americans smoked cigarettes. Since then, smoking prevalence has decreased to 15.5% of adults in 2016. This dramatic decline reflects growing public awareness of the health risks of tobacco and decades of public health efforts to discourage tobacco use. More recently, smoking prevalence has stabilized but the pattern of tobacco use has changed. Nearly a quarter of current smokers do not smoke every day, and the average smoker smokes only 14 cigarettes daily. In addition, an increasing number of cigarette smokers also use other tobacco products such as smokeless tobacco, small cigars, or even newer alternative tobacco products.

Over the past decade, newer products that aim to reduce a smoker's exposure to the toxins in cigarette smoke have appeared. These so-called alternative tobacco products are expected to reduce the health risks of cigarette smoking because most of the risk is attributable to inhaling the toxins other than nicotine. Electronic cigarettes (e-cigarettes) are the most widespread of the alternative tobacco products. Despite their name, electronic cigarettes (e-cigarettes) are fundamentally different from conventional cigarettes that burn tobacco to generate smoke. E-cigarettes are battery-powered nicotine-delivery devices that heat a solution usually containing nicotine, solvents, and flavors, to create an aerosol that users inhale. E-cigarettes reduce exposure to the many other toxins in cigarette smoke and are therefore likely to have less health risk than smoking cigarettes, but the long-term health effects of e-cigarette use remain unknown.

Cigarette smoking starts during childhood and adolescence. Nearly 90% of smokers begin to smoke before the age of 18 years and 98% start by the age of 26 years. The behavior is sustained due to the addictiveness of nicotine and as a deeply ingrained habitual response to multiple cues. Eventually, most smokes seek to stop smoking, but often struggle to sustain abstinence long term, giving smoking the characteristics of a chronic disease, but one for which sustained remission is possible. In the United States, smoking is concentrated among individuals with lower socioeconomic status, comorbid psychiatric disorders, and other substance use disorders.

HEALTH CONSEQUENCES OF TOBACCO USE

Cigarette smoking increases overall mortality and morbidity rates and is a cause of cardiovascular disease (including myocardial infarction and sudden death); cerebrovascular disease; peripheral vascular disease; chronic obstructive pulmonary disease; and cancers at many sites, including the lung, larynx, oral cavity, esophagus, stomach, bladder, kidney, pancreas, and uterine cervix. Approximately 30% of tobacco-related deaths are due to cardiovascular disease. Lung cancer, once a rare disease, increased dramatically during the twentieth century, becoming the leading cause of deaths due to cancer among men in 1955 and among women in 1986. Lung cancer incidence is now declining among both men and women, reflecting the decline in smoking prevalence by U.S. adults that occurred decades earlier.

Smoking is associated with many pregnancy complications, especially low birth weight (<2500 g). This is primarily attributable to intrauterine growth retardation (IUGR), although smoking in pregnancy also increases the risk of preterm delivery. Other adverse pregnancy outcomes linked to smoking are miscarriage (spontaneous abortion) and stillbirth. Smoking during pregnancy affects children even after birth. Sudden infant death syndrome is two to four times more common in infants born to mothers who smoked during pregnancy. Cognitive deficits and developmental problems in childhood are also linked to maternal smoking during pregnancy.

Cigarette smoking also increases a woman's risk of postmenopausal osteoporosis and fracture. Smokers have higher rates of upper and lower respiratory infections, diabetes, peptic ulcer disease, cataracts, macular degeneration, and sensorineural hearing loss than nonsmokers. Smokers have more prominent skin wrinkling than nonsmokers, independent of sun exposure. Smoking causes the majority of residential fire deaths.

The health hazards of smoking are not limited to those who smoke. Nonsmokers are harmed by exposure to the smoke produced by nearby smokers, a phenomenon called secondhand smoke (SHS). According to the 2006 U.S. Surgeon General's Report, there is no safe level of exposure to SHS. The children of parents who smoke have more serious respiratory infections during infancy and childhood, more respiratory symptoms, and a higher rate of chronic otitis media and asthma than the children of nonsmokers. Among adults, chronic SHS exposure increases a nonsmoker's risk of lung cancer and coronary heart disease. An estimated 7300 lung cancer deaths and 34,000 heart disease deaths in U.S. nonsmokers are attributable to SHS exposure. Even after tobacco smoke has dissipated, it leaves a residual of chemicals on clothing and surfaces in the area where tobacco was smoked. This phenomenon, called thirdhand smoke, produces an even more prolonged exposure to tobacco toxins.

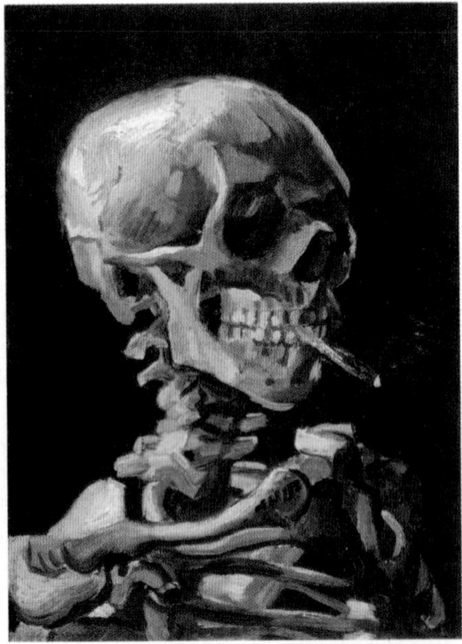

Source: **Van Gogh Skull with a Burning Cigarette.** WikimediaCommons. https://commons.wikimedia.org/wiki/File:Vincent_van_Gogh_-_Head_of_a_skeleton_with_a_burning_cigarette_-_Google_Art_Project.jpg.

HEALTH BENEFITS OF SMOKING CESSATION

Smoking cessation has health benefits for men and women of all ages, even for those who stop smoking after the age of 65 years or who quit after the development of a smoking-related disease. Smoking cessation decreases the risk of lung and other cancers, heart attack, stroke, chronic lung disease, and peptic ulcer disease. After 10–15 years of abstinence, overall mortality rates for smokers approach rates of those who never smoked. The risk reduction for cardiovascular disease occurs more rapidly than the risk reduction for lung cancer or overall mortality. Half of the excess risk of cardiovascular mortality is eliminated in the first year of quitting, whereas for lung cancer, 30–50% of the excess risk is still evident 10 years after quitting and some excess risk remains after 15 years.

The benefits of stopping smoking translate into a longer life expectancy for former smokers compared with continuing smokers. Smokers who benefit the most are those who quit when they are younger, have fewer pack-years of tobacco exposure, and are free of smoking-related disease. The health benefits of smoking cessation far exceed any risks from the small weight gain that may occur with cessation.

SMOKING BEHAVIOR

Cigarettes and other tobacco products are addictive because they contain nicotine, a drug that creates tolerance and physical dependence in habitual users with symptoms of nicotine withdrawal when smoking stops. Nicotine withdrawal symptoms include: (1) cravings for a cigarette, (2) irritability, (3) restlessness, (4) anger and impatience, (5) difficulty concentrating, (6) anxiety, (7) depressed mood, (8) excessive hunger, and (9) sleep disturbance. These symptoms begin within a few hours of the last cigarette, are strongest during the first 2–3 days after quitting, and gradually diminish over a month or more. Other than craving for a cigarette, the symptoms are nonspecific, and many smokers fail to recognize them as nicotine withdrawal. The severity of nicotine withdrawal is variable across smokers and is related to the level of prior nicotine intake. Smokers who smoke more than 20 cigarettes daily or smoke their first cigarette within 30 minutes of awakening are likely to suffer from more nicotine withdrawal symptoms when they quit.

The discomfort of nicotine withdrawal is one reason smokers fail in their efforts to stop. However, the attractiveness of smoking is attributable to more than nicotine dependence. Smoking is also a habit, a behavior that has become an integral part of a daily routine. Smokers come to associate cigarettes with enjoyable activities, such as finishing a meal or having a cup of coffee. These actions trigger the desire for a cigarette in smokers who are trying to quit. Smokers also use cigarettes to cope with stress and negative emotions, such as anger, anxiety, loneliness, or frustration. Quitting smoking represents the loss of a valuable coping tool for many smokers.

SMOKING CESSATION

Over half of the living Americans who have ever smoked have now quit smoking. According to surveys, 70% of the remaining smokers would like to stop smoking and over half of them tried to do so in the past year. However, most quit attempts fail, in part because only one in three smokers trying to quit use any assistance when quitting, despite the existence of effective treatments that improve the success rate of a quit attempt.

Approximately 25–30% of smokers who use state-of-the-art treatment are not smoking 1 year after their quit attempt, though many more smokers quit for a short time and then relapse. Most relapse occurs in the first week of a quit attempt. Only 6% of smokers who try to quit without assistance succeed for 1 year. Behavioral scientists regard smoking cessation to be a learning process rather than an action requiring a discrete episode of will power. Smokers learn from mistakes made during a prior attempt at quitting, thereby increasing the likelihood that the next attempt will succeed. Psychologists have identified a series of cognitive stages through which smokers pass as they move toward nonsmoking: (1) initial disinterest in quitting, (2) thinking about health risks and contemplating quitting, (3) preparing to quit in the near future, (4) currently taking action to stop smoking, and (5) maintained nonsmoking (see Chapter 19).

Surveys of former smokers reveal how and why they stop smoking. Fear of illness is the reason most often cited. However, awareness of health risks alone is not sufficient to motivate smoking cessation. Over 90% of current smokers know that smoking is harmful to their health, though they may not know the full extent of tobacco's health risks. Many smokers rationalize that they are immune to the health risks of smoking until these risks become personally salient. Current symptoms (e.g., cough, breathlessness, and chest pain), even if they represent minor illness rather than the onset of a smoking-related disease, stimulate change in smoking behavior more powerfully than does fear of future disease. Illness in a family member may also motivate smoking cessation. The price of cigarettes and the social unacceptability of smoking are other frequently cited reasons.

SMOKING CESSATION METHODS

Evidence-based clinical guidelines for smoking cessation were released by the U.S. Public Health Service in 2000 and updated in 2008 (https://www.ahrq.gov/professionals/clinicians-providers/guidelines-recommendations/tobacco/index.html). These guidelines identify two methods, psychosocial counseling and pharmacotherapy, as having strong evidence of efficacy. Each is effective individually, but combining the two produces higher cessation rates. The U.S. Preventive Services Task Force's 2015 update agreed with this finding and it categorized treating tobacco use as a high priority (Category A) preventive service. There is no strong evidence to support the efficacy of hypnosis or acupuncture for smoking cessation.

Psychosocial Support

Effective psychosocial support provides smokers with both practical behavior change strategies and also support and encouragement as part of treatment. Cognitive behavioral treatment methods address the barriers to quitting smoking that are rooted in habit. These methods are effective in aiding smoking cessation. In a typical program, smokers monitor their cigarette intake to identify the things that trigger the smoking, change their habits to break the link between the trigger and smoking, and learn to anticipate and handle the urges to smoke when they occur. The counselor also provides social support to bolster the smoker's confidence in the ability to stop smoking.

Psychosocial support was originally developed for in-person delivery. To broaden the reach of behavioral treatment, in-person methods were adapted for delivery by telephone and found to be effective. These techniques have also been adapted for delivery using newer communication tools, including websites, text messaging, mobile phone applications, and social media.

Pharmacological Treatment

Seven products have been approved by the U.S. Food and Drug Administration (FDA) as smoking cessation aids and rated as first-line drugs by the U.S. Public Health Service tobacco treatment guidelines (Table 21-1). These include five nicotine replacement products, bupropion (an atypical antidepressant), and varenicline, a nicotine receptor partial agonist. Cytisine is another nicotine receptor partial agonist that has shown efficacy for smoking cessation in recent randomized clinical trials. It has been used in Eastern Europe for many years but is not currently available as a smoking cessation aid in the United States. Nortriptyline and clonidine have also shown efficacy for smoking cessation in clinical trials but have not been submitted for approval by the FDA for this indication and are considered second-line drugs by the U.S. Public Health Service guideline panel.

Nicotine Replacement Therapy

The rationale for nicotine replacement therapy (NRT) is to supply nicotine in a form other than a cigarette to block the symptoms of nicotine withdrawal. Nicotine

Table 21-1. Pharmacotherapy for smoking cessation.*

Name	Dosage per Day	Recommended Duration of Use
Nicotine Replacement Products		
Transdermal nicotine patch	1 patch/24 h 21 mg (smoke ≥10 cig/d) 14 mg (smoke <10 cig/d)	8–12 weeks
Nicotine gum	9–12 pieces/d[†] 2 mg (smoke 1st cig >30 min after waking) 4 mg (smoke 1st cig >30 min after waking)	3–6 months
Nicotine lozenge	9 pieces/d (max 20) 2 mg (smoke 1st cig >30 min after waking) 4 mg (smoke 1st cig <30 min after waking)	3–6 months
Nicotine nasal spray	1–2 doses/h (min 8/d, max 40/d)	3–6 months
Nicotine inhaler	6–16 cartridges/d	3–6 months
Bupropion SR	150–300 mg/d[‡]	3–6 months
Varenicline	1mg BID[#]	3–6 months

*Products approved by the U.S. FDA as smoking cessation aids.
†Chew as needed or one piece every 1–2 h while awake.
‡Start 1–2 weeks before quit day. Use 150 mg/d for 3–5 days then 150 mg twice a day.
#Start 1–3 weeks before quit date. Uptitration of dose: 0.5 mg/d for 3 days, 0.5 mg twice daily for 4 days, then 1 mg twice daily.

replacement permits the smoker to break the smoking habit first and subsequently taper off nicotine. Five forms of nicotine replacement are approved for use in the United States. Nicotine in the form of a gum, a transdermal skin patch, and an oral lozenge are sold without prescription. A nicotine nasal spray and an oral inhaler are prescription-only products. Of all these products, the nicotine patch produces the most constant blood level of nicotine, a substantially different pattern from the fluctuating nicotine levels produced by cigarette smoking. The gum, lozenge, inhaler, and nasal spray produce nicotine levels that vary more than the patch, but less than smoking a cigarette. They provide more control over nicotine level. The nicotine supplied by the gum, patch, or nasal spray is sufficient to reduce nicotine withdrawal symptoms, but does not reproduce the rapid rise in nicotine blood levels that results from smoking a cigarette.

Randomized, placebo-controlled trials demonstrate that nicotine gum, patch, lozenge, inhaler, and nasal spray all reduce symptoms of nicotine withdrawal and approximately double the rates of smoking cessation compared with placebo. Combining the patch with another NRT product is safe and more effective than using a single NRT product. The effectiveness of all products depends on the instruction and counseling that accompany them. This is particularly true for the gum, nasal spray, and inhaler, which require careful instruction for proper use. Adherence is less of a problem with the nicotine patch. Any NRT product is more effective if used with some behavioral smoking cessation support. Clinicians should refer smokers to these resources when they recommend or prescribe NRT products.

Nicotine replacement is safe to use in smokers with stable coronary artery disease and evidence indicates that it is not harmful even when used in hospitalized smokers with acute coronary syndromes. Nicotine does increase heart rate and blood pressure and causes vasoconstriction, but is not thrombogenic and a smoker who substitutes NRT for cigarettes also avoids exposure to carbon monoxide and oxidant gases generated by burning tobacco.

TRANSDERMAL NICOTINE PATCH

The nonprescription nicotine patch contains a reservoir of nicotine that is released at a fixed dose and is absorbed through the skin. The patch can be started before or on a smoker's quit day. To use, the smoker applies a patch and removes it 24 hours later. A new patch is applied to rotating skin sites each morning afterward for 2–3 months, although there is evidence that prolonging use beyond 3 months produces better long-term results. Smokers who smoke 10 or more cigarettes (half of a pack) daily start with the 21-mg patch; lighter smokers start with the 14-mg patch. After 6 weeks, the smokers progressively switch to a lower dose patch. The most common side effect is local skin irritation, which rarely requires discontinuation of treatment and can often be managed with topical steroids. Vivid dreams or insomnia can be managed by removing the patch at bedtime. Long-term dependence on the nicotine patch rarely occurs.

NICOTINE GUM

Nicotine gum is available without prescription in 2-mg and 4-mg strengths and in several flavors. Smokers who smoke their first cigarette within 30 minutes of waking use the 4-mg gum; all others use the 2-mg gum. Proper chewing technique is essential for the nicotine released by chewing to be absorbed through the oral mucosa as intended, rather than being swallowed. The gum should not be chewed like regular gum. Initially, it should be chewed only long enough to release the nicotine, producing a peppery taste, and then placed between the gums and buccal mucosa to allow for nicotine absorption. When the taste disappears, the gum is chewed again until the taste reappears, then "parked" again. After 30 minutes, it is discarded. The smoker should not eat or drink while the gum is in the mouth, and should avoid beverages, especially acidic beverages (e.g., coffee) for 30 minutes before gum use. Common side effects include those related to nicotine (nausea, dyspepsia, hiccups, dizziness) and to chewing (sore jaw, mouth ulcers). The product is approved for use as needed to handle urges to smoke, but its onset of action is slower than smoking. Most patients chew fewer than the recommended 9–12 pieces daily. Consequently, many experts use fixed-dose schedules (e.g., chewing one piece for the first 30 minutes of every hour) to achieve blood nicotine levels adequate to prevent withdrawal. It is used for 3 months. Long-term dependence on the gum is uncommon.

Nicotine Lozenge

A nicotine lozenge whose pattern of nicotine delivery resembles the gum is sold without prescription in 2-mg and 4-mg doses. Smokers whose first cigarette of the day is smoked within 30 minutes of awakening should use the 4-mg dose; others use the 2-mg dose. In randomized controlled trials, it doubles cessation rates compared with a placebo lozenge. It is placed in the mouth between cheek and gum. Nicotine in the lozenge is gradually absorbed through the oral mucosa over 30–40 minutes. The user should not eat or drink when the tablet is in the mouth. The lozenge differs from the gum in that no chewing is required, making it easier to use properly. People with dentures or poor dentition who generally cannot use the gum can use the lozenge. A smoker uses a lozenge as needed to control cravings, usually every hour or two, and uses it for 3–6 months. A mini-lozenge formulation that is smaller and dissolves more rapidly than the original nicotine lozenge is also available.

Nicotine Inhaler

The nicotine inhaler, sold only by prescription in the United States, is a handheld device containing nicotine in a plug that is vaporized when the smoker inhales. The nicotine is absorbed through the oral mucosa rather than in the lungs. Therefore, the inhaler delivers nicotine in a pattern similar to the gum or lozenge with peak nicotine levels reached 20 minutes after the start of use. The inhaler mimics the hand-to-mouth behavior of cigarette smoking, a feature that appeals to some smokers. The inhaler doubles the cessation rate compared to placebo in randomized trials. Side effects are minimal; throat irritation and cough are the most common.

Nicotine Nasal Spray

Nicotine nasal spray is sold only by prescription. Nicotine is more rapidly absorbed from the nasal mucosa than it is through the oral mucosa, but less rapidly absorbed than through the lungs when a cigarette is smoked. The nicotine nasal spray doubles cessation rates compared with a placebo spray in randomized controlled trials, but has a high incidence of side effects (nose and throat irritation, watery eyes, sneezing, and cough). Careful instruction is required for its proper use. The dose is one spray in each nostril as needed; this delivers a dose of 1 mg of nicotine. It is used for 3–6 months.

Bupropion

Bupropion is an antidepressant with dopaminergic and noradrenergic activity. In its sustained-release form (Zyban, Wellbutrin SR), bupropion doubles smoking cessation rates compared with a placebo and is FDA approved for smoking cessation. The most serious side effect is a reduction in the threshold for seizure. The risk of seizure is 1 in 1000 patients or less, but the drug is contraindicated in patients with a seizure disorder or predisposition. Common side effects are insomnia, agitation, headache, and dry mouth. Doses of 150–300 mg/d for 12 weeks are effective for smoking cessation. The drug is started 1 week before the smoker's quit date to allow for blood levels to stabilize before quitting occurs. Bupropion reduces but does not eliminate weight gain after smoking cessation (see section "Weight & Smoking Cessation"), but the effect disappears when the medication is stopped. Nonetheless, this effect may appeal to smokers who are concerned about postcessation weight gain.

Varenicline

Varenicline is a selective partial agonist at the $\alpha4\beta2$ nicotinic receptor, the subtype of nicotine receptor in the brain that appears to mediate nicotine dependence. It is thought to have a dual mechanism of action. As a partial agonist, it partly relieves nicotine withdrawal symptoms. In addition, if a smoker using varenicline smokes a cigarette, the drug blocks the nicotine in cigarette smoke from binding to the nicotine receptor, thereby making smoking less rewarding. In randomized controlled trials comparing the drug with placebo and with bupropion, varenicline produced a higher long-term cessation rate than both and nearly tripled the cessation rate compared with placebo. Nausea is the most common side effect, occurring in nearly 30% of subjects in clinical trials. In practice, it can often be managed successfully by taking the pill with food and a full glass of water. Varenicline is used for 12 weeks at a dose of 1-mg bid, starting with a 1-week gradual uptitration in dose to minimize nausea. The quit date should be set at least 1 week after starting the drug to allow blood levels to stabilize before quitting occurs, but delaying the quit date until 4 weeks after starting the drug is also an effective strategy.

Previous concerns about varenicline's and bupropion's safety in terms of changes in behavior, depressed mood, and suicidal thoughts and actions led to the FDA requiring both medications to add boxed warnings about this to their labels. This was removed in December 2016 after results of a large trial comparing nicotine patch, bupropion, varenicline, and placebo found no significant differences in rates of psychiatric side effects among smokers with or without mild to moderate psychiatric disorders. All three drugs in that study produced higher cessation rates than placebo, but varenicline generated higher cessation rates than either bupropion or nicotine patch. Combination NRT is an alternative for individuals who are reluctant to use varenicline.

Nortriptyline & Clonidine

Nortriptyline, a tricyclic antidepressant, has demonstrated efficacy for smoking cessation in randomized controlled trials. A meta-analysis found that its efficacy resembled that of the atypical antidepressant bupropion. Nortriptyline is not FDA approved as a smoking cessation aid. Hypotension and dry mouth are the most common side effects. There is no evidence to support the use of any other antidepressants or any antianxiety agents for smoking cessation.

Clonidine, a centrally acting α-adrenergic agonist, is used to treat craving for psychoactive drugs other than nicotine. In randomized, placebo-controlled trials, both oral and transdermal clonidine reduced nicotine withdrawal symptoms and increased rates of smoking cessation. Clonidine is not FDA approved for smoking cessation, and side effects (sedation, dizziness, and dry mouth) generally limit its use in practice.

Electronic Cigarettes & Other Alternative Tobacco Products

Newer products that aim to reduce the health harms of smoking by reducing a smoker's exposure to the toxins in cigarette smoke have appeared on the market in the past decade. These so-called alternative tobacco products are expected to reduce the health risks of cigarette smoking for individuals who are unable or unwilling to quit. Electronic cigarettes (e-cigarettes), the most widespread of these products, are battery-powered nicotine-delivery devices that heat a solution usually containing nicotine, solvents, and flavors, creating an aerosol that users inhale. Unlike conventional cigarettes that burn tobacco to generate smoke, e-cigarettes reduce an individual's exposure to the many other toxins in cigarette smoke and are therefore expected to have a lower health risk than smoking cigarettes, but the long-term health effects of e-cigarettes are currently unknown.

In 2016, 15.4% of U.S. adults reported ever using an e-cigarette and 3.2% reported currently using them. E-cigarette use is most common among current and former smokers who quit within the past year. Most adults report using e-cigarettes either to quit or reduce their cigarette smoking, or to reduce their health risks. Few randomized controlled trials have assessed whether e-cigarettes are an effective tool for smoking cessation, and e-cigarettes have not been approved for this purpose by the FDA. Smokers seeking to quit should be encouraged to first use one of the FDA-approved smoking cessation medications. If smokers choose to use e-cigarettes for smoking cessation, they should be advised to switch completely to e-cigarettes. Approximately 70% of e-cigarette users continue to smoke cigarettes, and dual use results in much less reduction in exposure to toxicants in tobacco smoke than exclusive e-cigarette use. Because the long-term health effects of e-cigarette use remain uncertain, smokers who quit smoking using e-cigarettes should be encouraged to eventually set a quit date for the e-cigarettes as well.

Heat-not-burn tobacco products are newer devices developed by the tobacco industry as a way to reduce the health risks of smoking. They heat tobacco to create an aerosol rather than burning it as cigarettes do. Little is yet known about their health effects. These products are marketed in many countries, but not yet available in the United States, but the FDA is currently reviewing applications to market the product in the United States as reduced-risk tobacco products.

BARRIERS TO SMOKING CESSATION

Weight & Smoking Cessation

Smokers weigh 5–10 lb less than nonsmokers of comparable age and height. When smokers quit, 80% of them gain weight. The average weight gain is 10–15 lb (4.6–6.8 kg). Women and heavier smokers (>25 cigarettes per day) gain more than men and lighter smokers. The mechanism is incompletely understood, but a nicotine-related decrease in metabolic rate and possibly increases in food intake appear to be largely responsible. Postcessation weight gain does not counteract the overall health benefits of smoking cessation but it can discourage weight-conscious smokers from making a quit attempt. A good strategy is to help smokers accept a small weight gain and reassure them that the expected amount is less than they may fear. A vigorous exercise program reduces postcessation weight gain and promotes cessation and even moderate exercise will reduce postcessation weight gain. Smokers who use nicotine gum or bupropion gain less weight than those who quit with a placebo, and this may help weight-concerned smokers to make a quit attempt.

Social Support

Smokers with nonsmoking spouses are more likely to quit than smokers whose partners smoke. Smokers whose efforts to stop are supported by partners, family, and friends are more likely to succeed than smokers without this support. Those who live with smokers can ask them to restrict smoking to outdoor areas to provide a smoke-free home. Formal cessation programs provide an additional source of social support that can be valuable when a smoker's own environment is not supportive of quitting.

Psychiatric Disorders

There is a strong association between smoking and psychiatric disorders. Smokers have more depressive symptoms than nonsmokers and are more likely to have a history of major depression. Smoking prevalence among smokers with bipolar disorder and schizophrenia is over twice as high as smoking prevalence in the general population. Smokers with psychiatric disorders have similar interests in quitting smoking as smokers without psychiatric disorders but are less likely to receive treatment. The medications that are effective for smoking cessation in the general population, including varenicline and bupropion, are effective and safe in adults with psychiatric disorders, but the cessation rates achieved by smokers with psychiatric comorbidity is generally lower than the rates achieved by smokers without comorbid psychiatric illness. Evidence indicates that symptoms of mental illness do not worsen after smoking cessation and may actually improve. Nevertheless, smokers with a history of psychiatric disorders should be monitored for the reemergence of symptoms during a quit attempt.

Substance Use Disorders

There is a high rate of smoking among individuals with other substance use disorders. Substance use should be considered as a potential comorbid disorder in smokers who repeatedly try and fail to quit. Even among smokers who do not abuse alcohol, drinking is frequently an ingredient in relapse situations. Smokers attempting to quit are commonly advised to avoid alcohol temporarily after quitting. Behavioral and pharmacologic smoking cessation treatments are effective in individuals with other substance use disorders and they do not worsen other substance use outcomes. Some studies have suggested improved substance use outcomes after smoking cessation treatment. However, smokers with other substance use disorders have lower quit rates when compared to smokers without substance use disorders.

TREATING TOBACCO DEPENDENCE IN THE HEALTH CARE SYSTEM

The Physician's Role

Because tobacco use begins early in life, preventing young people from starting to smoke is a task for physicians who care for children and adolescents. The challenge for physicians caring for adults is smoking cessation. Physicians have the opportunity to intervene with smokers because each year they see an estimated 70% of the smokers in the United States. They also see smokers at times when their symptoms have caused them to be concerned about their health and therefore be more willing to consider changing their smoking behavior. For example, one-third of smokers stop smoking after a myocardial infarction; this can be increased further with a cessation intervention at that time. Approximately 30% of female smokers stop smoking while pregnant, although many resume smoking after delivery. Other smoking-related conditions also provide "teachable moments" when smokers are more receptive to advice to stop smoking.

Providing brief advice to stop smoking to all patients in office practice increases patients' rates of smoking cessation. Although advice alone is effective, randomized controlled trials in general medicine and family practices have demonstrated that supplementing advice with brief counseling in office practice is more effective. Brief interventions prompt smokers to attempt to quit, but the clinician's responsibility should not stop there. The clinician should also ensure that smokers are linked to effective treatment to maximize the success of a quit attempt. Providing tobacco cessation treatment in office practice is as or more cost-effective as other preventive health care services.

A System-Level Approach to Treatment

Because tobacco dependence is a chronic health condition characterized by periods of remission and relapse when cessation is attempted, tobacco cessation treatment in outpatient practice should resemble the management of other chronic conditions, such as hypertension or diabetes, in health care systems. Treatment should not be viewed as exclusively a physician's responsibility. Instead, it should be a system-level effort in which each member of the clinical team has a specific role. Delivering treatment should be done collaboratively by individuals who are provided adequate training, institutional support, and reimbursement from health insurers. In this model, a physician's role is to give strong advice to quit, offer tobacco cessation treatment to every smoker, and help the smoker to access evidence-based resources such as medication and behavioral support. Other office staff can assist the physician by identifying a patient's smoking status, making specific referrals to resources, and providing in-office counseling and medication management.

SMOKING CESSATION COUNSELING STRATEGY FOR OFFICE PRACTICE

Evidence-based clinical guidelines for smoking cessation treatment from the U.S. Public Health Service recommend a five-step protocol, called the 5A's, for use in the outpatient care of adults. The steps include **A**sking all patients about tobacco use, providing strong **A**dvice to all smokers to quit, **A**ssessment of a smoker's readiness to quit, offering **A**ssistance for those smokers who are ready to stop, and **A**rranging follow-up for all smokers. This model has been adapted by several professional organizations to better integrate tobacco treatment into busy clinical settings. The newer models have abbreviated the 5A's, usually to 3-steps that are designed to be delivered collaboratively by the care team and to require less time of the physician member of the team. Examples of these abbreviated models include "Ask/Advise/Assist" and "Ask/Assist/Refer." Here, we describe the full 5-step model (**Table 21-2**).

1. **ASK:** The initial step is to identify every patient's tobacco use status at every visit and document it in the health record. A staff member in the office who has the initial patient contact can be responsible for this task. Some individuals who smoke only occasionally do not consider themselves to be smokers. Therefore, patients should be asked if they ever smoke cigarettes or use other tobacco products, including electronic cigarettes. Those who do not use tobacco should be advised to be sure to avoid secondhand smoke exposure by adopting a smoke-free policy for the home and car and avoiding it in other venues.
2. **ADVISE:** The physician's responsibility is to deliver to every smoker clear advice to stop smoking. The message should be strong and unequivocal; for example, "Quitting smoking now is the most important action you can take to stay healthy." Advice is more

Table 21-2. Smoking cessation counseling protocol for physicians.

1. **ASK**—about smoking and secondhand smoke exposure at every visit: "Do you ever smoke cigarettes or use tobacco?" "Do you live with any smokers?"
2. **ADVISE**—every smoker to stop and nonsmokers to avoid secondhand smoke exposure.
   a. Make advice clear: "Stopping smoking now is the most important action you can take to stay healthy."
   b. Tailor advice to the patient's clinical situation and focus on benefits of quitting.
   c. Advise nonsmokers to adopt a smoke-free policy for home and car and avoid smoke in other venues.
3. **ASSESS**—Offer treatment: "Stopping tobacco use can be challenging, but there are proven treatments to help smokers quit and I can help you use them. Would you like to try?"
4. **ASSIST**—the smoker to stop smoking.
   a. For smokers willing to accept treatment
      (1) Ask smoker to set a quit date within 4 weeks.
      (2) Prescribe pharmacotherapy.
      (3) Refer for psychosocial support to free telephone quitline (800-QUIT-NOW), text messaging (www.smokefree.gov) or in-person counseling program in the health system or community.
   b. For smokers not willing to accept treatment
      (1) Discuss advantages and barriers to cessation, from smoker's viewpoint.
      (2) Advise smoker to avoid exposing family members to secondhand smoke.
      (3) Indicate willingness to help when the smoker is ready.
      (4) Ask again about smoking at the next visit.
5. **ARRANGE**—follow-up visits.
   a. Make follow-up contact to assess progress 1–2 weeks after visit via phone, patient portal, or in person
   b. For smokers who have quit:
      (1) Congratulate!
      (2) Ask smoker to identify future high-risk situations.
      (3) Rehearse coping strategies for future high-risk situations.
   c. For smokers who have not quit:
      (1) Ask: "What were you doing when you had that first cigarette?"
      (2) Ask: "What did you learn from the experience?"
      (3) Ask smoker to set a new quit date.

Data from Clinical Practice Guideline. Treating Tobacco Use and Dependence: 2008 update (Located at: https://www.ahrq.gov/sites/default/files/wysiwyg/professionals/clinicians-providers/guidelines-recommendations/tobacco/clinicians/update/treating_tobacco_use08.pdf).

effective when phrased positively, emphasizing the benefits to be gained from quitting rather than the harms of continuing to smoke. If possible, advice should be tailored to the clinical situation that led to the office visit, especially to any current symptoms attributable to or worsened by tobacco use. Electronic health records can use information collected at the Ask step to prompt the physician to deliver this advice during an encounter.

3. **ASSESS:** The third step is to assess a smoker's interest in quitting smoking. Categorizing smokers in this way is a clinically useful approach that helps the physician to determine which counseling strategy is appropriate and to set achievable goals. However, this step is de-emphasized in newer treatment models that characterize smoking as a chronic disease for which treatment should be offered proactively at every opportunity, rather than first asking about readiness to accept treatment. In this newer model, the clinician offers treatment with a statement such as, "Stopping tobacco use can be challenging, but there are proven treatments to help smokers quit and I can help you use them. Would you like to try?"

4. **ASSIST:** The physician's approach to assisting smokers will depend on the smoker's readiness to accept treatment.
   - *For smokers willing to accept treatment*, the physician should ask whether they are ready to set a "quit date," a date within the next 4 weeks when they will stop smoking. If so, the date should be recorded in the chart and on take-home material given to the smoker. The physician and patient should discuss which approach is most likely to be successful considering the smoker's level of nicotine dependence, past efforts to quit, and barriers to cessation. Both behavioral treatment and pharmacotherapy should be offered, because combinations of pharmacotherapy and behavioral counseling are more effective than either one alone. Behavioral smoking cessation programs teach practical behavior change skills and social support. More intensive treatment is indicated for smokers who have been unsuccessful in previous attempts. Decision support can be built into electronic health records to facilitate clinicians' prescription of smoking cessation medications and referral of smokers to behavioral support resources. Behavioral support resources include in-person or telephone counseling, text messaging programs and web-based programs. Free telephone counseling for smoking cessation is accessible nationwide by calling a central number (800-QUIT-NOW). Text messaging programs and other resources can be accessed through the website www.smokefree.gov.
   - *For smokers not willing to accept treatment*, the physician should elicit the smoker's views about the benefits and harms of smoking to the individual smoker. With this perspective, the physician can provide missing information about health risks and correct misconceptions about the process of smoking cessation. The discussion should focus on short-term benefits rather than distant risks, and the physician should be prepared to discuss common barriers to smoking cessation. The clinician should advise the smoker to avoid exposing family members to secondhand smoke by adopting a no-smoking policy for their homes and cars. Finally, the physician can make it clear that he or she is available to help is when they are ready to make a quit attempt.

5. **ARRANGE:** Randomized trials have demonstrated that arranging follow-up visits to discuss smoking increases the success of physician counseling. Sustaining contact with smokers who are attempting to quit is especially important for smokers using pharmacotherapy to monitor for side effects and dosing changes needed based the level of nicotine withdrawal symptoms. While follow-up can be accomplished at an office visit, practice staff can also monitor smokers' progress using phone calls, patient portals, or other means of contact not requiring an in-person visit.
   - *A smoker who is not smoking at the follow-up contact* deserves hearty congratulations paired with a warning that continued vigilance is necessary to maintain abstinence. The level of nicotine withdrawal symptoms and any side effects should be assessed to determine whether a change in medication dosage is indicated. To help prevent relapse, patients should be asked to identify future situations in which they anticipate difficulty remaining abstinent. The physician can help to plan and rehearse coping strategies for these times.
   - *For a smoker who has not been able to remain abstinent*, the physician's role is to redefine a failure into a partial success. The patient can be told that even one day without cigarettes is the first step toward quitting and be reminded that it takes time to learn to quit, just as it took time to learn to smoke. To help the patient learn from the experience, the physician should ask about the circumstances that preceded the first cigarette smoked after the quit date, what was learned from the experience that could be used for the next attempt to quit, and whether a new quit date should be set.

SUGGESTED READINGS

Anthenelli RM, Benowitz NL, West R, et al. Neuropsychiatric safety and efficacy of varenicline, bupropion, and nicotine patch in smokers with and without psychiatric disorders (EAGLES): a double-blind, randomised, placebo-controlled clinical trial. *Lancet* 2016;387:2507–2520.

Babb S, Malarcher A, Schauer G, et al. Center for Disease Control and Prevention. Quitting smoking among adults—United States, 2000–2015. *MMWR Morb Mortal Wkly Rep* 2017;65:1457–1464.

Benowitz NL, Pipe A, West R, et al. Cardiovascular safety of varenicline, bupropion, and nicotine patch in smokers: a randomized clinical trial. *JAMA Intern Med* 2018;178(5):622–631.

Cahill K, Lindson-Hawley N, Thomas KH, Fanshawe TR, Lancaster T. Nicotine receptor partial agonists for smoking cessation. *Cochrane Database Syst Rev* 2016;(5):CD006103.

Cochrane Tobacco Addiction Group. https://tobacco.cochrane.org/our-reviews (*Regularly updated systematic reviews with meta-analyses of smoking cessation interventions, both pharmacologic and non-pharmacologic.*)

Fiore MC, Baker TB. Treating smokers in the health care setting. *N Engl J Med* 2011;365:1222–1231.

Fiore MC, Jaen CR, Baker TB, et al. *Treating Tobacco Use and Dependence: 2008 Update.* Clinical Practice Guideline. Rockville, MD: U.S. Department of Health and Human Services. Public Health Service, 2008.

Hartmann-Boyce J, Chepkin SC, Ye W, Bullen C, Lancaster T. Nicotine replacement therapy versus control for smoking cessation. *Cochrane Database Syst Rev* 2018;5:CD000146.

Hughes JR, Stead LF, Hartmann-Boyce J, Cahill K, Lancaster T. Antidepressants for smoking cessation. *Cochrane Database Syst Rev* 2014;(1):CD000031.

Prochaska JJ, Hilton JF. Risk of cardiovascular serious adverse events associated with varenicline use for tobacco cessation: systematic review and meta-analysis. *BMJ* 2012;344(e2856):1–11.

Rigotti NA. Balancing the benefits and harms of e-cigarettes: a National Academies of Science, Engineering, and Medicine Report. *Ann Intern Med* 2018;168(9):666–667.

Rigotti NA. Strategies to help a smoker struggling to quit. *JAMA* 2012;308(15):1573–1580.

Rigotti NA, Clair C, Munafò MR, Stead LF. Interventions for smoking cessation in hospitalized patients. *Cochrane Database Syst Rev* 2012;(5):CD001837.

Siu AL for the U.S. Preventive Services Task Force. Behavioral and pharmacotherapy interventions for tobacco smoking cessation in adults, including pregnant women: U.S. Preventive Services Task Force Recommendation Statement. *Ann Intern Med* 2015;163(8):622–634.

Stead LF, Koilpillai P, Fanshawe TR, Lancaster T. Combined pharmacotherapy and behavioural interventions for smoking cessation. *Cochrane Database Syst Rev* 2016;3:CD008286.

WEBSITES

BecomeanEx website (Mayo Clinic). https://www.becomeanex.org/# (tips for preparation, quitting, and staying quit). Accessed August 2018.

Centers for Disease Control Web site. http://www.cdc.gov/tobacco (comprehensive web site of information about tobacco use, prevention, and cessation). Accessed August 2018.

U.S. National Cancer Institute Web site. http://www.smokefree.gov (tips for preparation, quitting, and staying quit, links to access telephone counseling (quitline) and text messaging programs). Accessed August 2018.

U.S. Preventive Services Task Force Web site. https://www.uspreventiveservicestaskforce.org/Page/Document/RecommendationStatementFinal/tobacco-use-in-adults-and-pregnant-women-counseling-and-interventions. Accessed August 2018.

Obesity

22

Robert B. Baron, MD, MS

INTRODUCTION

Obesity is one of the most common problems in clinical practice. Defined as a body mass index (BMI) of greater than 30 kg/m^2, over 39% of adult Americans are obese. An additional 35% are overweight, with BMIs between 25 and 30 kg/m^2. 18.5% of children are obese and over one-third of children are overweight or obese. Because obesity is at the center of chronic disease risk and psychosocial disability for millions of Americans, its prevention and treatment offer unique patient care and public health opportunities. If all Americans were to achieve a normal body weight, it has been estimated that the prevalence of diabetes would decrease by half, whereas hypertension, coronary artery disease, and various cancers would decrease by 10–20%.

Obesity is often one of the most difficult and frustrating problems in primary care for both patients and physicians. Considerable effort is expended by primary care providers and patients, often with little benefit. Weight-loss diets, for example, even in the best treatment centers, result in an average 5–10% reduction in body weight. This modest clinical success has created a never-ending demand for new weight-loss treatments. Approximately, half of women and one-quarter of men are "dieting" at any one time, spending billions of dollars each year on diet books, diet meals, weight-loss classes, diet drugs, exercise programs, and other weight-loss aids. The challenge for health care providers is to identify those patients with obesity who are most likely to benefit medically from treatment and most likely to maintain weight loss, and to provide them with sound advice, skills for long-term lifestyle change, and support. For patients not motivated to attempt a weight-loss program, health providers must continue to be respectful and empathic and focus on other health concerns. Whenever possible, providers should emphasize prevention of obesity and further weight gain and the importance of physical fitness independent of body size.

DEFINITIONS

Obesity is defined as an excess of body fat. Body fat can be measured by several methods, including isotope-labeled water, underwater weighing, bioelectric impedance, dual-energy X-ray absorptiometry, computerized tomography, and magnetic resonance imaging. In clinical practice, however, obesity is best defined by the BMI—body weight divided by height squared (kilograms per square meter). The BMI correlates closely with measures of body fat and with obesity-related disease outcomes. According to the National Institutes of Health (NIH), an individual with a BMI lesser than 18.5 kg/m^2 is classified as underweight, 18.5–24.9 kg/m^2 as normal, 25.0–29.9 kg/m^2 as overweight, and greater than or equal to 30.0 kg/m^2 as obese. Obesity is further classified as class I (BMI 30–34.9 kg/m^2), class II (BMI 35–39.9 kg/m^2), and class III or extreme obesity (BMI ≥40 kg/m^2). The term "morbid obesity" is best avoided for those with class III obesity, since obesity-related morbidity can occur at any obesity level. Measurements of waist circumference, waist-to-hip ratio, and skinfold thickness can also be performed in clinical practice.

PREVALENCE OF OBESITY

Globally the prevalence of obesity has nearly tripled since 1975. According to the World Health Organization, in 2016 39% of adults were overweight and 13% were obese. Although previously considered a problem of high-income nations, overweight and obesity are increasing in low-and middle-income nations as well. For example, almost half of the world's overweight or obese young children live in Asia.

While overall the prevalence of obesity in the United States has increased dramatically over the last four decades in both adults and children, differences between demographic groups are common. In women, for example, obesity is substantially more common in non-Hispanic black and Hispanic women (55% and 51%, respectively) than in white women (38%). Similarly, in youth age 2–19 years, non-Hispanic blacks and Hispanics (22% and 26%, respectively) have higher rates of obesity than whites (14%). Other subpopulations have dramatically increased rates of overweight and obesity. Eighty three percent of patients with mental illness, for example, are obese or overweight. Geographic differences in prevalence are also prominent in the United States. Obesity is more common in the southeastern United States than in other regions.

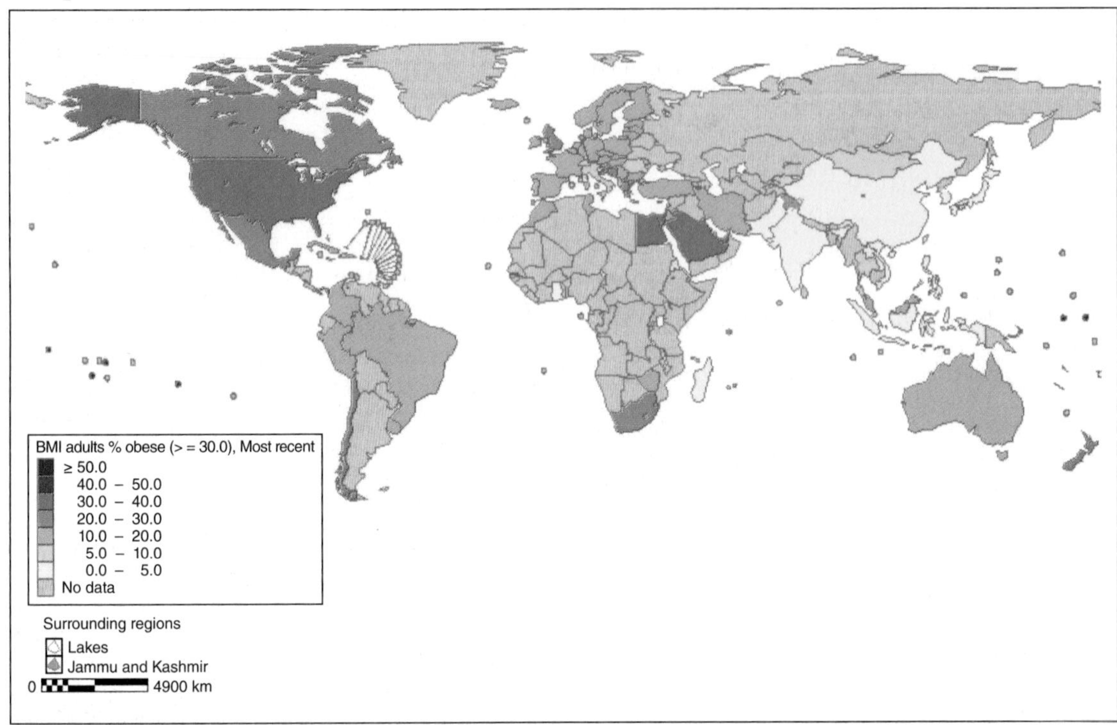

Figure 22-1. Reprinted with permission from World Health Organization (WHO), Worldwide BMI adults % obese world map (≥30.0). (http://apps.who.int/bmi/index.jsp). Accessed 8/28/19.

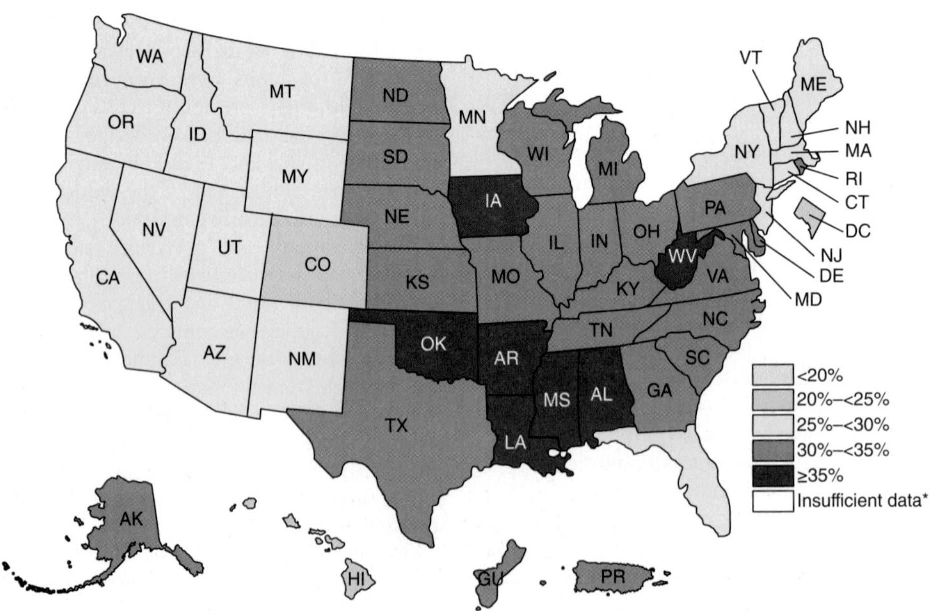

Figure 22-2. Self-Reported Obesity Among U.S. Adults by State and Territory, BRFSS, 2017 (https://www.cdc.gov/obesity/data/prevalence-maps.html). Accessed 8/28/19.

HEALTH CONSEQUENCES OF OBESITY

The relationship between body weight and mortality is curvilinear, similar to other cardiovascular risk factors. Most studies have demonstrated a J-shaped relationship, suggesting that the thinnest portion of the population also has an excess mortality. This is primarily due to the higher rate of cigarette smoking in the thinnest group except in the elderly, in whom being underweight is predictive of excess mortality independent of cigarette use. Recent analysis of the National Health and Nutrition Examination Study (NHANES) has suggested that overweight individuals may not have as much excess mortality as previously described and that the impact of obesity on mortality overall may be decreasing over time. Racial and ethnic factors may also impact the relationship of weight and mortality. In African Americans, the weight associated with the point of lowest mortality is greater than in whites, whereas in Asian Americans it is lower. Guidelines of the American Diabetes Association, for example, suggest screening for diabetes in people of Asian descent at a BMI of 23 kg/m^2 rather than 25 kg/m^2.

The increase in total mortality related to obesity results predominantly from coronary heart disease (CHD). Although it is not fully established that obesity is an "independent" risk factor for CHD, obesity is clearly an important risk factor for the development of many other CHD risk factors. Obese individuals aged 20–44 years, for example, have a three- to fourfold greater risk for type II diabetes, a five- to sixfold greater risk for hypertension, and twice the risk for hypercholesterolemia. The obese also have an increased risk for some cancers, including those of the colon, ovary, and breast.

As a result of these conditions, mortality from all causes for persons with class I obesity (BMI 30–34.9 kg/m^2) is 20% greater than for those with a normal BMI. Individuals with class II obesity, BMI 35–39.9 kg/m^2, have an 80% increase in mortality from all causes. Mortality for extreme obesity, although less well studied, is estimated to be at least double that of normal weight individuals.

Obesity is also associated with a variety of other medical disorders, including degenerative joint disease of weight bearing joints, diseases of the digestive tract (gallbladder disease, gastroesophageal reflux disease), thromboembolic disorders, cerebrovascular disease, heart failure (both systolic and diastolic), respiratory impairment including sleep apnea, and skin disorders. Obese patients also have a greater incidence of surgical and obstetric complications, are more prone to accidents, and are at increased risk of social discrimination. Several studies have also shown a rate of depression higher in the obese than in normal weight subjects and a higher rate of binge eating disorder.

In addition to the total amount of excess body fat, the location of the excess body fat (regional fat distribution) is a major determinant of the degree of excess morbidity and mortality due to obesity. Increased upper body fat (abdomen and flank) is independently associated with increased cardiovascular and total mortality. Body fat distribution can be assessed by a number of techniques. Measurements of skin folds (subscapular and triceps) reflect subcutaneous fat. Measurement of circumferences (waist and hip) reflects both abdominal and visceral fat. Computed tomography (CT) and magnetic resonance imaging (MRI) scans measure subcutaneous and visceral fat. Clinically, measurement of the waist and hip circumference is most useful, especially in individuals with BMI 25–35 kg/m^2. A circumference in men greater than 102 cm (>40 in.) and in women greater than 88 cm (>35 in.) can be used to identify individuals at increased risk of developing obesity-related health problems.

ETIOLOGY OF OBESITY

Numerous lines of evidence, including both epidemiologic studies of adoptees and twins and animal studies, suggest strong genetic influences on the development of obesity. In a study of 800 Danish adoptees, for example, there was no relationship between the body weight of adoptees and their adopting parents but a close correlation with the body weights of their biological parents. In a study of approximately 4000 twins, a much closer correlation between body weights was found in monozygotic than in dizygotic twins. In this study, genetic factors accounted for approximately two-thirds of the variation in weights. Studies of twins reared apart and the response of twins to overfeeding showed similar results. Studies of regional fat distribution in twins have also shown a significant (but not complete) genetic influence.

Genetic studies have confirmed a clear relationship between genetics and obesity in both animals and humans. In humans, at least eleven rare monogenic forms of obesity have been identified and over 300 loci have been identified in genome association studies. Studies suggest that genetic influences may impact both energy intake (control of appetite and eating behavior) and energy expenditure.

Differences in the resting metabolic expenditure (RME), for example, could easily result in considerable differences in body weight as RME accounts for approximately 60–75% of total energy expenditure. The RME can vary by as much as 20% between individuals of the same age, sex, and body build; such differences could account for approximately 400 kcal of energy expenditure per day. Evidence suggests that the metabolic rate is similar in family members, and, as expected, individuals with lower metabolic rates are more likely to gain weight. Differences in the thermic effect of food, the amount of energy expended following a meal, may also contribute to obesity. Although some investigators have shown a decreased thermic effect of food in the obese, others have not.

Environmental factors are also clearly important in the development of obesity. The U.S. Centers for Disease Control and Prevention (CDC) estimates that urban sprawl due to lack of adequate land use planning is associated with increases in obesity, cardiovascular disease, and type 2 diabetes (see Chapter 9). Decreased physical activity at work and during leisure activities and food availability and choices that result in increased energy intake also clearly contribute to the development of obesity. Medical illness can also result in obesity, but such instances account for less than 1% of the cases. Hypothyroidism and Cushing syndrome are the most common. Diseases of the hypothalamus can also result in obesity, but these are rare. Major depression, which more typically results in weight loss, can also present with weight gain. Consideration of these causes is particularly important when evaluating unexplained, recent weight gain. Numerous medications can also result in weight gain, including antipsychotics such as clozapine, olanzapine, and risperidone; antidepressants such as amitriptyline and cyproheptadine; anticonvulsants such as valproate, carbamazepine, and gabapentin; and diabetic medications such as insulin and thiazolidinediones. Of note, each of these categories of medications includes drugs that do not cause weight gain. Weight gain is also common following smoking cessation. On average, patients gain 4–5 kg within 6 months of quitting smoking but some patients may gain much more.

PATIENT SELECTION FOR WEIGHT LOSS

The BMI should be measured and recorded at each clinical encounter. As with other clinical abnormalities, patients should be nonjudgmentally informed of their BMI and how it conforms to definitions of overweight and obesity. Patients who are told that they are overweight or obese by their clinician are more likely to classify weight as a health concern and have greater desire and more attempts to lose weight. Using language such as "your weight is unhealthy" or "your weight may be damaging your health" may be preferred by patients than medical terms such as overweight and obesity.

Weight loss is indicated to assist in the management of obesity-related conditions, particularly hypertension, type 2 diabetes mellitus and prediabetes, hyperlipidemia, and metabolic syndrome in any patient who is obese (BMI >30 kg/m^2). Many patients with BMI 25–30 kg/m^2 who have one of these conditions also often benefit from weight reduction.

Weight loss to prevent complications of obesity in patients without current medical, metabolic, or behavioral consequences of obesity is more controversial. In young and middle-aged individuals, particularly those with a family history of obesity-related disorders, treatment should be based on the degree of obesity and body fat distribution. Such individuals with upper body obesity (increased waist circumference) should be considered for treatment; those individuals with lower body obesity and no significant consequences of obesity can be reassured and monitored. Many such patients, however, desire weight loss for psychological, social, and cosmetic reasons. A careful discussion of the risks and benefits of weight loss in such instances helps patients make informed decisions about various weight-loss strategies.

A medical or psychosocial indication for weight loss is necessary but not sufficient to begin treatment. Treatment must be designed in the context of the patient's readiness to change. The Transtheoretical Model of Change, also commonly known as the Stages of Change Model, is a useful framework for helping patients to modify their behavior. Developed and applied initially in smoking cessation, the model has also been used to modify eating and exercise behavior. It defines behavior change as a process of identifiable stages, including precontemplation, contemplation, preparation, action, maintenance, and relapse. By understanding the patient's stage of readiness to change, the clinician can work specifically with each patient to move him or her to the next stage (see Chapter 19).

Clinical assessment should also focus on how the current attempt compares with previous attempts; a realistic assessment of the patient's goals for the amount and rate of weight loss; the extent to which outside stressors, mood disorders, or substance abuse might impair the attempt; and the degree to which others can provide support. Patient readiness to change can be further assessed by requiring the patient to complete specific pretreatment assignments. For example, patients can be asked to complete a 3-day diet record and to submit an exercise plan that includes both the type of aerobic exercise the patient plans to begin and how the patient plans to fit it into his or her schedule. When obesity coexists with other significant psychiatric disorders, particularly depression, binge eating disorder, and substance abuse, treatment should initially be directed at the concurrent disorder.

DIET THERAPY

The goal of diet therapy for weight loss is to achieve a daily energy deficit whereby energy intake is less than energy expenditure. Daily energy expenditure can be estimated based on age, gender, and activity level. Two thousand calories (kcals) per day is often used as a reference level, but different individuals' requirements may vary by hundreds of calories per day. The goal of most weight-loss diets is to achieve an energy deficit of approximately 500 kcal/d. Since a pound of fat equals approximately 3500 kcal, this will result in approximately 1 lb of weight loss per week.

Meta-analyses of randomized studies of dietary therapy to achieve weight loss have demonstrated an average weight loss of 5–10% of the starting weight in patients followed for 3 months to 1 year. Follow-up for up to 5 years suggests average long-term weight loss of 2–4% of initial weight. Of note, all studies have a substantial variation of response. Some patients, approximately 20%, are able to lose substantially more weight and keep it off for longer periods of time. Studies of commercial weight-loss programs also demonstrate modest amounts of weight loss but with wide variations. Weight Watchers, for example, reports 3.2% weight reduction at 2 years.

The optimal composition for weight-loss diets has been the subject of numerous clinical trials and, of course, thousands of popular weight-loss books. Most nutrition guidelines such as the Dietary Guidelines for Americans, recommend a low-fat, high-fiber, "balanced" diet. This approach emphasizes consumption of a wide variety of foods to achieve a balanced mix of macronutrients, that is, 20–35% of total calories from fats, 45–65% of total calories from carbohydrates, and 10–35% of total calories from protein. These ranges are substantially wider than earlier federal guidelines and allow for flexibility in diet design. The DASH (Dietary Approaches to Stop Hypertension) eating plan, originally developed for treatment of hypertension, is an example of a balanced diet that meets these macronutrient ranges and is supported by federal guidelines. A Mediterranean-style diet and most types of vegetarian diets can also be used to achieve an energy deficit for weight loss and remain within these ranges.

Numerous clinical trials have compared this balanced approach with low carbohydrate diets such as the Atkins and South Beach Diets. These studies have consistently shown equivalent amount of weight loss independent of the macronutrient composition of the diet. Rather than nutrient composition, weight loss was predicted by adherence to the diet. Satiety, hunger, lipid levels, insulin levels, and other metabolic factors were also found to be equivalent despite large differences in macronutrient composition. Similar findings have been published with comparisons of the very low-fat Ornish diet, the Zone diet, and other diets with various combinations of macronutrients. Thus, patients can be reassured that almost any whole food diet can result in safe weight loss as long as the patient consistently follows the diet.

An important alternative in the dietary treatment of obesity is the use of safe and effective very-low-calorie diets (VLCDs). Previously known as protein-sparing modified fasts and protein-formula liquid diets, these diets restrict calorie intake to less than or equal to 800 kcal/d. Patients ingest only prepackaged, often liquid, food that provides adequate protein, vitamins, and minerals. Additional intake is limited to 2–3 quarts of calorie-free beverages per day. The major advantage of these diets is the removal of patients from the food environment to facilitate short-term adherence. In addition, the significant energy deficit results in rapid weight loss, usually 2 lb/week, encouraging the patient to continue. Ongoing concerns about these diets include their cost, side effects, and long-term results. Clinical trials suggest that the use of 800-kcal VLCDs can lower cost and prevent most of the significant side effects associated with the lower-calorie (400–600) VLCDs, including gallstones and fluid and electrolyte disorders, with equal long-term efficacy.

As with standard diet therapy of obesity, VLCDs require adherence during the diet, and long-term nutritional and behavioral changes to maintain weight loss. Well-planned programs that combine VLCDs with nutrition education, behavior therapy, exercise, and social support report improved long-term results. For example, an average weight loss of 55 lb with 75% and 52% of the loss maintained at 1- and 2 1/2-year follow-up, respectively, and maintenance of an average of 24 lb after 2- to 3-year follow-up have been reported. Meta-analyses of published VLCD trials suggest that while initial weight loss is greater with VLCDs than standard diets, both approaches have equal long-term results. As with other approaches, however, there is a wide variation of response with VLCDs, and some patients can achieve long-term weight loss. Because of the quicker and greater amounts of weight loss, VLCDs may be particularly useful in situations in which rapid weight loss is clinically indicated such as preoperative treatment (joint replacement, transplant surgery, bariatric surgery) or for initial management of severe medical conditions (severe sleep apnea, poorly controlled diabetes, heart failure, or coronary artery disease).

Recent studies have helped elucidate predictors of long-term weight maintenance after diet therapy for weight loss. Most important has been information from the National Weight Control Registry. This cohort of individuals who have lost an average of 33 kg and maintained the loss for 5 years report consumption of low-calorie diets averaging approximately 1400 cal/d; high levels of physical activity averaging 60 min/d; regular self-monitoring of body weight; eating breakfast daily; and maintaining consistent dietary patterns on weekdays and weekends.

HEALTH CONSEQUENCES OF DIETING & WEIGHT LOSS

Few studies have examined the effects of weight loss on mortality. Studies examining the effect of weight loss on cardiovascular risk factors generally show beneficial changes with weight loss but no impact on cardiovascular mortality. Descriptive studies on mortality show inconsistent results. Such descriptive studies are unable to clarify if changes in mortality are caused by the weight change, if disease or other factors that contribute to disease, such as cigarette smoking, cause weight loss, or if both are related to a third factor.

Because so many Americans are dieting at any one time, and having so little long-term success, considerable interest has focused on the potential adverse effects of weight cycling ("yo-yo" dieting). Numerous adverse effects of weight cycling have been hypothesized, primarily from animal studies. These include making further weight loss more difficult, increasing total body fat and central obesity, increasing subsequent calorie intake, increasing food efficiency, decreasing energy expenditure, increasing levels of adipose tissue lipolytic enzymes and liver lipogenic enzymes, increasing insulin resistance, increasing blood pressure, and increasing blood cholesterol and triglyceride levels. Most experts currently feel that these phenomena occur inconsistently, if at all. Descriptive studies that have addressed this question by looking at the impact of weight fluctuations on CHD incidence, CHD mortality, and total mortality have shown mixed results.

There is also debate over whether weight-loss diets cause eating disorders or binge eating. Although a history of dieting often precedes the development of eating disorders, there is no evidence proving a causal link. In addition, approximately 50% of individuals with binge eating disorder report that binging preceded dieting. There is also some evidence to suggest that successful weight loss may reduce binge eating in the obese (see Chapter 23).

Thus, there is only indirect evidence suggesting that dieting has negative health effects. This remains an important question, however, and reinforces the idea that casual attempts at quick weight loss should be avoided. At present, however, committed attempts at long-term weight loss should not be discouraged because of adverse health effects or the potential of regaining weight.

Dieting also has a significant effect on energy balance both during and after weight loss. As every successful dieter has observed, the rate of weight loss slows during the course of dieting. Because this can be quite discouraging to the unwary patient (or uninformed health care provider), it is important to inform the patient prior to initiating a weight-loss diet that this is likely to occur. Weight loss is most rapid during the initial days of hypocaloric feeding due to changes in sodium and water balance caused by early loss of glycogen and protein (both contain water) and, depending on the degree of calorie deficit and type of diet, loss of sodium associated with ketonuria. Following this initial phase, weight loss depends on the extent of energy deficit. With time, however, the rate of weight loss slows again as the body's metabolic rate decreases and the energy deficit becomes smaller. This change in metabolic rate can be two to three times greater than that predicted from changes in body weight. The lower the energy content of the diet, the lower the metabolic rate. Although it was initially suggested that exercise occurring during a period of hypocaloric feeding could prevent this decrease in metabolic rate, recent studies have suggested that it has no direct effect during hypocaloric feeding.

Following the period of hypocaloric feeding (resumption of normal energy intakes), the resting metabolic rate increases, but to a level below that observed before beginning the diet. This reduction is in part a reflection of the loss of lean body mass and in part due to additional, poorly understood effects on energy metabolism. Overall energy expenditure is further reduced due to a decrease in the thermic effect of food (the individual eats less) and in differences in physical activity (it takes less energy to perform the same amount of activity for a smaller person). Thus, to maintain weight loss, individuals need to consume less energy than before dieting and increase energy expenditure by increasing the amount of physical activity.

EXERCISE

Exercise offers a number of significant advantages to patients attempting to achieve long-term weight loss. First and foremost, exercise increases energy expenditure, helping to create the energy deficit necessary for weight loss. Unfortunately, the amount of energy expended during most aerobic exercises (e.g., walking, jogging, and swimming) for the typical periods performed (30 minutes four to five times per week) is modest, approximately 1000–1500 kcal/week. Thus, exercise can be predicted to have little effect on short-term weight loss. Clinical trials reflect this modest effect: some studies demonstrate weight loss with exercise alone or extra weight loss when exercise plus diet is compared with diet alone, but other studies do not show such an effect. In a meta-analysis of 43 studies, exercise combined with diet lead to 1.1 kg greater weight loss than diet alone. Studies comparing high-intensity exercise to low-intensity exercise demonstrated a 1.5 kg greater weight loss.

The importance of exercise for successful maintenance of weight loss is more clearly established. As discussed above, an hour per day of exercise was one of the predictors of long-term weight maintenance in the National Weight Control Registry. In addition to the cumulative effect of increased energy expenditure, exercise affects the composition of the body substance lost during weight loss. When exercise is directly compared with diet, or when exercise plus diet is compared with diet alone, exercise results in greater preservation of lean body mass. That is, for each pound of weight lost, less fat and more muscle are lost during weight-loss programs without exercise.

The observation that much of the long-term effect of exercise is through preservation of lean body mass has resulted in an increased interest in the potential role of resistance training (e.g., weight lifting and circuit training). Preliminary results suggest that resistance training during dieting does result in maintenance of lean body mass compared with the result from dieting alone. Thus, highly motivated patients can be instructed to add resistance training to their aerobic exercise program.

Regular aerobic exercise results in a number of other benefits to the obese patient, including improved cardiovascular training effect (increased exercise tolerance), decreased appetite (per calorie expended), a general sense of well-being, decreased blood pressure (in hypertensives), improved glucose metabolism and insulin action (in diabetics), improved blood lipids (in lipid disorders), and based on descriptive studies, decreased mortality from cardiovascular disease and all other causes.

Young patients with mild-to-moderate obesity can be started directly on a regular aerobic exercise program. Patients are commonly instructed to select two exercises and to perform either one of them six times per week for 30–60 min/d. Patients are taught to take their pulse and to generate a sustained tachycardia at 70–80% of their maximum predicted heart rate. Sedentary patients, older patients, and patients with severe obesity are instructed to begin walking programs without initial concern about meeting target heart rates. In these patients, the focus is on frequency and duration, rather than intensity. As weight loss proceeds and patients become used to exercising regularly, they can be advanced to formal aerobic programs.

BEHAVIOR THERAPY & SOCIAL SUPPORT

Sustained weight loss requires long-term changes in eating and exercise behavior. Patients must learn specific skills to facilitate decreased calorie intake and increased energy expenditure. Behavior therapy, combined with diet and exercise, forms the core of the most standard "lifestyle modification" approaches to weight management. Behavior therapy can be implemented in groups or in individual therapy. Trained psychologists and dieticians commonly lead such efforts, but office-based clinicians can often learn to use many of the same techniques. Intensity of interaction appears to be one of the predictors of success. In the highly successful Diabetes Prevention Project, for example, lifestyle modification was taught in 16 individual sessions over 24 weeks.

Meta-analysis of 36 studies of behavior therapy for weight loss showed that behavior therapy alone resulted in significantly greater weight loss, a decrease of 2.5 kg, than placebo. When behavior therapy was combined with diet and exercise and compared to diet and exercise alone, the combined treatment also resulted in greater weight loss in five of six studies. Two studies compared cognitive behavioral therapy (CBT) plus diet and exercise with diet and exercise alone. In these studies, the combined treatment lost 4.9 kg more.

Standard behavior therapy relies on specific techniques to teach the skills needed to change problematic behaviors.

1. **Goal-setting:** Patients are taught to set specific quantifiable, realistic goals at the outset of behavior therapy and during each week of therapy. Succeeding at meeting realistic goals creates a sense of self-efficacy and can reinforce further change.
2. **Self-monitoring:** Patients are taught to monitor both food and beverage intake and physical activity. Specific attention must be directed at teaching patients how to estimate portion sizes since patients may underestimate intake by 50%. The context, degree of hunger, and emotional state of each time of eating are also recorded. This may allow eating-related factors to be targets for modification. Patients are also instructed to record all programmed physical activity. Additional tracking of physical activity can be done with activity monitors.
3. **Stimulus control:** Patients are instructed to identify stimuli that increase the likelihood of both desired and undesired behaviors. Particular emphasis is placed on attempting to modify nonfood cues that are associated with eating. Similarly, simple techniques such as keeping certain problem food out of the house may be useful.
4. **Cognitive skills:** Patients are taught skills for problem solving and cognitive restructuring. Patients are asked to identify problems, consider potential solutions, list the advantages and disadvantages of each, select a feasible solution, and evaluate the results. Cognitive restructuring involves identification of dysfunctional thoughts that interfere with goals and replacing such thoughts with more rational ones. Formal CBT can also be used as part of weight management. CBT places more emphasis on cognitive change, rather than behavioral change, as the primary focus of treatment.

Social support is an additional essential component for any successful weight-loss program. Most successful programs use peer group support. Diet partnerships and financial incentives are effective for some patients. Involvement of family members is also important. A comprehensive review of published results of weight-loss programs strongly suggests that close provider–patient contact is a better predictor of success than the particular weight-loss intervention.

MEDICATIONS FOR TREATMENT OF OBESITY

Six medications have been approved by the U.S. Food and Drug Administration to treat obesity. The oldest of these, phentermine, was approved in 1959 for short-term weight loss (≤ 3 months) and is the most widely prescribed. It has not been evaluated as a single agent in long-term studies. Five newer medications include three single agents and two combination drugs. Each has been studied in trials of 1 year or longer and has shown either 5% or more weight loss than placebo or that at least 35% of patients lost 5% of their starting weight. Weight loss associated with these medications is associated with improvements in metabolic risk factors. Long-term studies of cardiovascular outcomes are in progress. Of note, one additional medication, sibutramine, was withdrawn from the market in the United States in 2010 due to a large randomized controlled study that showed a 16% increase in cardiovascular events in patients in the medication group.

The three single agents are lorcaserin, orlistat, and liraglutide. Lorcaserin is a selective serotonin receptor agonist that increases satiety. Common adverse events include headache, dizziness, fatigue, dry mouth, and nausea. Other concerns include attention and memory disturbances, depression, priapism, and serotonin syndrome. No increase in valvulopathy (as seen previously with other serotonin receptor agonists) has been reported. The medication is contraindicated in pregnancy. Orlistat inhibits pancreatic lipase causing fat malabsorption and reduced energy intake. Side effects include flatulence, fecal urgency, oily stool, and fecal incontinence. Liraglutide is a glucagon-like peptide-1 (GLP-1) agonist. It is thought to work by slowing gastric emptying to increase satiety. Side effects include nausea, vomiting, constipation and diarrhea, headache, fatigue, abdominal pain, and dizziness.

The two combination medications are phentermine–topiramate and naltrexone–bupropion. Topiramate is a gamma-aminobutyric acid (GABA) receptor modulator. The combination of phentermine and topiramate reduces appetite. Side effects include insomnia, dry mouth, constipation, tingling, dizziness, and changes in taste. Mood disorders, increased suicidal thoughts, impaired concentration, and cognitive dysfunction have also been described. Naltrexone is an opioid antagonist, and bupropion is a norepinephrine and dopamine reuptake inhibitor. The combination reduces appetite. Side effects include nausea, vomiting, constipation and diarrhea, headache, and dry mouth. All of these medications are contraindicated in pregnancy.

Considerable controversy exists about the use of these medications in clinical practice and their overall use is less than might be expected. Weight loss is modest and commonly regained with discontinuation of the medication. Side effects are common and costs to patients are high. The lack of long-term outcome studies remains a concern.

The NIH guidelines state that the FDA-approved weight-loss drugs may be useful as an adjunct to diet and physical activity for patients with BMI greater than or equal to 27 kg/m^2 and obesity-related risk factors or diseases, and for any patient with BMI greater than or equal to 30 kg/m^2. Based on the modest efficacy noted above, however, these guidelines have not been widely implemented by clinicians. Prescriptions for weight-loss drugs should be limited to patients adhering to weight-loss diets and physical activity. In addition, weight loss early in treatment use correlates highly with weight loss at 12 months. Thus, for patients in whom no weight loss is achieved within the first several months of use, weight-loss medications should be discontinued.

SURGERY FOR WEIGHT LOSS

Several surgical options can also be considered for patients with severe obesity. The NIH guidelines state that weight-loss surgery may be an option for selected patients with BMI greater than or equal to 40 or greater than or equal to 35 kg/m^2 with comorbid conditions. Such patients must be at high risk for obesity-related morbidity and mortality, must have failed medical therapy, must have stable psychiatric status, and must be fully committed to lifetime lifestyle changes.

In recent years, the use of surgery to treat obesity has grown substantially. With implementation of new techniques and the use of less invasive approaches, obesity surgery is now one of the fastest growing operations in the United States. A majority of procedures are now done laparoscopically.

The two most common procedures in the United States are the roux-en-Y gastric bypass and the vertical sleeve gastrectomy. Adjustable gastric banding is less commonly performed due to a lack of efficacy and a high rate of reoperation. Malabsortive procedures, such as duodenal switch and biliopancreatic diversion, are also infrequently performed due to concerns of metabolic and nutritional sequelae analogous to those observed with jejunoileal bypass procedures in the past.

The roux-en-Y bypass remains the gold standard bariatric procedure in the United States. Weight loss, approximately one-third of initial weight, is greater than with other procedures and the durability of weight loss is better established. Serious perioperative complications including bleeding and gastrojejunostomy leaks can occur. Approximately 4% of patients will have early complications including deep venous thrombosis, surgical reintervention, or spend greater than 30 days in the hospital. Perioperative mortality is low and reported to be equivalent to cholecystectomy or hysterectomy. Intentional weight loss of 5–10% of initial weight before weight-loss surgery is associated with reduced perioperative complications. Longer term complications include nutritional deficiencies of fat-soluble vitamins, especially vitamin D, iron, B_{12}, folate, and calcium.

Beneficial effects of weight-loss surgery include marked improvement in diabetes, hyperlipidemia, hypertension, sleep apnea, and other obesity-related symptoms. Overall mortality over 11 years is improved by 24%, but the number needed to treat to prevent one death per year is approximately 850 patients.

SUMMARY

Obesity and obesity-related illnesses are major public health concerns. Currently available treatments with diets, exercise, and behavior therapy provide limited efficacy for most patients. Some patients, however, can achieve long-term weight loss. Currently approved medications demonstrate limited efficacy. Surgical treatment of obesity is the most effective treatment but must be balanced against risk of complications. Given the lack of effective therapy, preventive measures are essential. Broad and ambitious public health approaches are required to impact the obesity epidemic. For most individual patients, dietary changes that emphasize calorie reduction by consuming smaller portions, more plant foods, fewer high-calorie beverages and other foods with added sugar, and less fast food are necessary even to maintain current weight. Similarly, striking increases in daily physical activity are needed to maintain body weight and achieve fitness.

SUGGESTED READINGS

Dietz WH. Obesity and excessive weight gain in young adults: new targets for prevention. *JAMA* 2017;318(3):241–242.

Fothergill E, Guo J, Howard L, et al. Persistent metabolic adaptation 6 years after "The Biggest Loser" competition. *Obesity (Silver Spring)* 2016;24(8):1612–1619.

Haire-Joshu D, Hill-Briggs F. Treating obesity-moving from recommendation to implementation. *JAMA Intern Med* 2018; 178(11):1447–1449.

Hales CM, Carroll MD, Fryar CD, Ogden CL. Prevalence of obesity among adults and youth: United States, 2015–2016. NCHS Data Brief, No. 288, October 2017.

Heymsfield SB, Wadden TA. Mechanisms, pathophysiology, and management of obesity. *N Engl J Med* 2017;376(3):254–266.

Igel LI, Kumar RB, Saunders KH, Aronne LJ. Practical use of pharmacotherapy for obesity. *Gastroenterology* 2017;152(7): 1765–1779.

Ma C, Avenell A, Bolland M, et al. Effects of weight loss interventions for adults who are obese on mortality, cardiovascular disease, and cancer: systematic review and meta-analysis. *BMJ* 2017;359:j4849.

O'Connor EA, Evans CV, Burda BU, Walsh ES, Eder M, Lozano P. Screening for obesity and intervention for weight management in children and adolescents: evidence report and systematic review for the US Preventive Services Task Force. *JAMA* 2017;317(23):2427–2444.

Piercy KL, Troiano, RP, Ballard, RM, et al. The physical activity guidelines for Americans. *JAMA* 2018;320(19):2020–2028.

Thom G, Lean M. Is there an optimal diet for weight management and metabolic health? *Gastroenterology* 2017;152(7):1739–1751.

Vidal J, Corcelles R, Jiménez A, Flores L, Lacy AM. Metabolic and bariatric surgery for obesity. *Gastroenterology* 2017; 152(7):1780–1790.

Webb VL, Wadden TA. Intensive lifestyle intervention for obesity: principles, practices, and results. *Gastroenterology* 2017;152(7): 1752–1764.

Eating Disorders 23

Erin C. Accurso, PhD & Sarah Forsberg, PsyD

INTRODUCTION

Eating disorders are complex psychiatric illnesses characterized by pathological eating and related behaviors, and disturbances in body image that cause significant distress and/or impairment. In the United States, approximately 30 million individuals are affected by an eating disorder in their lifetime, with prevalence rates of about 1% for anorexia nervosa (AN), 1.5% for bulimia nervosa (BN), and 3% for binge eating disorder (BED). Eating disorders that have more recently been included in Diagnostic and Statistical Manual of Mental Disorders, Fifth Edition (DSM-5) include avoidant/restrictive food intake disorder (ARFID) and other specified feeding and eating disorders, including atypical AN, BN, and BED of insufficient frequency and/or duration, and purging disorder. Preliminary estimates suggest that prevalence rates are approximately 5% for ARFID, 3% for atypical AN, 4% for BN or BED of insufficient frequency and/or duration, and 3% for purging disorder. Eating disorders are more common in women than men. Among women in the United States, the prevalence of AN, BN, and BED is similar across major racial/ethnic groups (non-Latina Whites, Latinas, Asians, and African Americans). However, prevalence is higher in gay men and transgender individuals, with some research suggesting that prevalence is lower in lesbian women than heterosexual women.

Eating disorders can have severe medical complications and carry the highest mortality rate of any psychiatric disorder due to high suicide rates, particularly in AN, and serious medical concerns, including cardiovascular, pulmonary, gastrointestinal, and electrolyte complications requiring medical intervention. Prevention and early identification are critical as these disorders can become chronic and have serious psychiatric, psychosocial, and medical consequences. Unfortunately, only about one-third of those with an eating disorder ever receive treatment. Primary care providers are often well-poised to identify potential risky behaviors and to recognize the onset of an eating disorder early on where medical management (sometimes including medical stabilization on an inpatient unit) is critical. Indeed, about one in five individuals with an eating disorder require medical hospitalization, and two in five of those require rehospitalization within 1 year. Despite knowledge about eating disorders, most medical and psychiatric practitioners lack competence in the treatment of eating disorders. Because of the complexity and breadth of clinical presentations, extent of co-occurring psychopathology, general lack of familiarity and training in the assessment and treatment of eating disorders, and the importance of a multidisciplinary treatment approach, referral to a specialist is typically required. Comprehensive treatment includes evidence-based psychotherapy in the context of medical management, in which nutrition counseling can also play a complementary role. Pharmacological interventions have less empirical support as direct targets of eating disorder behavior, though may enhance effects of psychotherapy, particularly among individuals with BN or BED. Psychotropic medications are often used in those with eating disorders to address common comorbid anxiety and mood disorders.

DIFFERENTIAL DIAGNOSIS

Anorexia Nervosa

AN is characterized by persistent dietary restriction leading to a significantly low body weight (in context of what is minimally expected for age, sex, developmental trajectory, and physical health) and an intense fear of gaining weight or becoming fat. Given that AN is usually egosyntonic and some individuals may deny fear of weight gain, this diagnosis can be made if there is persistent behavior that interferes with weight gain. Finally, individuals with AN have a significantly distorted view of their body (often see themselves as fat) or their weight/shape has an undue influence on their self-evaluation; in the absence of these two criteria, the diagnosis can be made if there is a persistent lack of recognition of the seriousness of the current low body weight. Individuals who meet the above criteria but who have a BMI within the average or above average range despite significant weight loss are classified as having atypical AN. Atypical AN is not as readily identified in primary care, although its psychological and medical presentation is comparable if not more severe than typical AN.

Individuals with AN and atypical AN typically develop a large number of food rules related to quantity (e.g., set calorie limits and counting food items), and food type (e.g., avoid certain foods or macronutrients, such as fats or carbohydrates). They develop an obsessive preoccupation with food, eating, dieting, weight, and body shape, and frequently exhibit ritualistic behaviors involving choosing, preparing, and ingesting meals (e.g., cutting food into very small pieces or chewing each bite a specific number of times). This rigidity makes it very difficult to eat in settings that are not highly controlled (e.g., food prepared by others or in restaurants). Individuals with AN frequently engage in exercise that is driven and compulsive. Binge eating and/or purging (including self-induced vomiting, or laxative or diuretic misuse) can be present in the binge/purge subtype of AN.

Lack of appetite or decreased intake, with or without subsequent weight loss, is encountered in a number of psychiatric disorders. These include depression, anxiety, conversion, other psychosomatic disorders, schizophrenia, and certain delusional disorders, but each of these is associated with a cluster of other substantiating symptomatology. Some patients with obsessive-compulsive disorder may exhibit what appears to be bizarre behavior around food, eating, or meal preparation, but, on further exploration, their behavior is in response to an obsession unrelated to body image disturbance (e.g., fear of contamination). Such patients, in contrast to those with AN, generally admit their discomfort with the need to engage in these behaviors. Although comorbid psychopathology may be encountered in patients with AN, including symptoms of depression, anxiety, or OCD, the hallmark of AN (the fear of becoming fat and the relentless pursuit of thinness) is absent in other psychiatric syndromes. The term *anorexia*, which itself refers to absence of appetite, is a misnomer in the case of the syndrome of AN. True anorexia, such as that encountered in many medical conditions or diseases, would be accompanied by other signs or symptoms of those illnesses (as in gastrointestinal disease or many cancers).

Avoidant/Restrictive Food Intake Disorder

ARFID is the newest eating disorder described in the DSM-5, and not unlike AN, is associated with restrictive eating patterns. The absence of body image concerns is the core feature that differentiates ARFID from AN. Individuals with ARFID avoid food for reasons unrelated to body image disturbance. There are three types of ARFID specified in the DSM-5, including individuals with an aversion to the sensory characteristics of food (e.g., textures, smells, and visual appearance), those with a lack of interest in food or with limited appetite, and those who may fear negative consequences of eating, (e.g., vomiting, choking, gastrointestinal pain, or fullness), often related to a specific traumatic incident around eating. The degree of dietary restriction must be severe enough to lead to at least one of the following consequences: failure to attain growth milestones in height or weight, or weight loss; nutritional deficiencies associated with exclusion of entire food groups; dependence on enteral feeding or nutritional supplementation, or marked interference in psychosocial functioning (e.g., inability to eat outside of the home).

Distinguishing between ARFID and other eating disorders is not always straightforward. Other eating disorders such as AN, BN, and BED most typically occur in early-late adolescence after a period of normative eating, whereas individuals with ARFID may have long-standing difficulties with eating, with the exception of those who fear negative consequences of eating. As noted, individuals with ARFID do not demonstrate body image disturbance or fear of weight gain as seen in other eating disorders. However, this core feature is not consistently expressed in other eating disorders. For this reason, DSM-5 allows the diagnosis of AN to be made in the context of persistent behavior that interferes with weight gain in the context of low weight (e.g., avoidance of high-density foods or engaging in excessive exercise). While less common, it is possible for AN to emerge out of restrictive eating and malnourishment associated with an earlier ARFID presentation (around 12% in one sample transitioned from an ARFID to AN diagnosis during treatment). Therefore, gathering a detailed history of eating and feeding behaviors, including longstanding food preferences, and other behaviors that may indicate concern about weight/shape (e.g., checking weight and/or shape, tracking intake, function of physical activity) is critical.

Bulimia Nervosa

BN is characterized by recurrent episodes of binge eating (i.e., eating objectively large quantities of food in a discrete period of time, accompanied by a feeling of losing control over eating). Binge episodes are followed by recurrent inappropriate compensatory behaviors to prevent weight gain; both occur a minimum of once a week for 3 months. Compensatory behaviors include self-induced vomiting, misuse of laxatives, diuretics, or other medications, fasting, and/or excessive exercise. Similar to AN and atypical AN, a key feature of BN is the centrality of body image in self-evaluation and extreme dissatisfaction with body weight/shape. Dietary restraint is common; however, the level of dietary restriction in combination with binge eating does not result in significant weight loss. BN of low frequency and/or limited duration can be specified under other specified feeding or eating disorders if all of the criteria for BN are met, with a frequency of less than once per week or a duration less than 3 months. Among those with BN, weight is within or above a normal weight range, unlike those with AN who may engage in bingeing and purging. Individuals with BN often experience their symptoms as distressing and ego-dystonic, however shame and stigma often contribute to a prolonged course prior to presentation for treatment. Primary care providers may be the first to identify bulimia, noting signs and symptoms associated with gastritis, esophagitis, dehydration, or electrolyte disturbances. Physical exam may uncover enamel decay and parotid gland enlargement due to recurrent vomiting. Discussing findings from physical exam and laboratory values with individuals may prompt exploration of self-induced vomiting, use of diuretics or laxatives, and disordered eating patterns even when an individual does not initially bring forward these concerns. These symptoms should be further assessed in a psychiatric evaluation. Co-occurring psychiatric diagnoses include mood and anxiety disorders, substance use disorders, and personality disorders (specifically borderline personality disorder).

Binge Eating Disorder

Binge eating disorder is characterized by recurrent episodes of binge eating that occur on average at least once a week for 3 months and are associated with significant distress. Binge episodes are characterized by eating much more rapidly than normal, eating until feeling uncomfortably full, eating large amounts of food when not feeling physically hungry, eating alone because of feeling embarrassed by how much one is eating, and/or feeling disgusted with oneself, depressed or guilty afterward. Unlike BN, binge eating is not followed by recurrent compensatory behaviors. Binge eating is distinguished from overeating in that it is associated with a sense of loss of control over eating, which is highly distressing and associated with other co-occurring psychological problems. The prevalence of BED increases as BMI increases, so BED frequently occurs in the context of obesity. Although not part of the diagnostic criteria, individuals with BED typically have weight loss as their primary goal, often associated with high weight/shape dissatisfaction. Among those seeking bariatric surgery, approximately one-third have BED, with prevalence rates near 10% in community samples of individuals with obesity. Similar to BN, BED of low frequency and/or limited duration can be specified if the symptoms are less frequent or have a shorter duration but cause clinically significant distress and impairment. BED can emerge in adolescence but typically onsets in early adulthood.

Purging Disorder

Purging disorder is characterized by recurrent purging behavior intended to influence weight or shape in the absence of binge eating. Should significant weight loss occur, these symptoms would more likely be indicative of AN or atypical AN. However, this disorder appropriately captures individuals with recurrent purging (i.e., self-induced vomiting, misuse of laxatives, diuretics, or other medications) in the absence of low weight, significant weight loss, or binge episodes.

MULTIDIMENSIONAL MODEL

A comprehensive multidimensional model best illustrates the role various factors play in the genesis of clinically significant eating disturbances. Referred to as a stress–diathesis model, psychological, biological, and sociocultural stressors contribute to the development of the syndrome (see Chapter 36). Much is still unknown about the causes of eating disorders, but the dynamic interplay of multiple factors is evident in the development and maintenance of these complex disorders.

Psychological factors include personality features, such as obsessive-compulsive traits, cognitive rigidity, emotion sensitivity, and impulsivity. They also include the influence of developmental stressors or trauma and interpersonal relationships. Body dissatisfaction, combined with other psychological, behavioral (in particular, dieting), or biological vulnerabilities, appears to be an important contributor and is known to increase risk.

Biological factors are highly contributory in the development and maintenance of eating disorders. Data suggest that greater than 50% of the variance in eating disorders and disordered eating behaviors can be accounted for by additive genetic effects. A preexisting biological vulnerability is supported by neurophysiologic investigations showing dysfunction of neurotransmitter systems, including serotonin, dopamine, and norepinephrine neuromodulator systems, as well as opioids and cholecystokinin (CCK). Rationale for the examination of these hormones and other substances derives from our understanding of the pathways modulating appetitive behavior, including hypothalamic regulation and the known connection between the gastrointestinal tract and the central nervous system. Individuals with AN can develop amenorrhea preceding significant weight loss suggestive of hypothalamic dysregulation. The additional contribution of components of the peripheral satiety network is being elucidated. Further, biology is influenced by the adverse effects of starvation, malnutrition, and purging behaviors, including vomiting and the misuse of laxatives and diuretics. Restrictive dieting and subsequent malnourishment may contribute to the development or exacerbation of comorbid psychiatric conditions, such as anxiety and depression.

Sociocultural factors figure prominently in the etiology of eating disorders. The idealization of thinness and subsequent body dissatisfaction contributes to dieting behavior, often beginning in early adolescence. Of note, dieting is frequently a precipitant to the development of an eating disorder. Adoption of Western ideals of beauty and accompanying dieting behavior is contributing to an increased prevalence of eating disorders in ethnically diverse populations both in the United States and globally. Other precipitants include periods of illness leading to weight loss; in fact, for those with AN, low BMI was shown to be the most potent predictor of development of the disorder and degree of risk was amplified by elevated body dissatisfaction.

TREATMENT CONSIDERATIONS

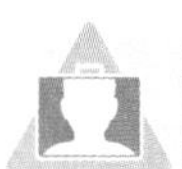

CASE ILLUSTRATION 1

Anna, a 15-year-old high school sophomore, presented to her pediatrician at her mother's insistence with vague complaints of abdominal pain and bloating, particularly after meals. Though she answered all questions posed, she was rather reserved and hesitant to embellish her responses. A review of systems revealed infrequent constipation and a history of two nonconsecutive missed periods over the last 6 months, a departure from her generally regular periods since onset of menses at the age of 13 years. Vital signs were notable for a pulse of 54 and a sitting BP of 85/60 mm Hg. She was 5 ft. 4 in. tall and weighed 102 lb, 9 lb less than what was recorded at the time of her annual examination, approximately 8 months ago. Physical examination was without significant findings. In particular, there were no findings suggesting focal abdominal pathology.

In private, Anna's mother told the pediatrician that she was less socially engaged over the last several months, preferring solitary activities such as studying to going out with friends. She also noted that Anna appeared to be using a treadmill in the basement for extended periods of time, and was concerned that she may have lost "a few pounds" recently. This would not ordinarily concern her, but Anna was also skipping meals with the family and had become "so picky" with regards to food choices. She was concerned that Anna was establishing unhealthy eating and exercise habits.

When presented with her mother's concerns and the clinical information by her pediatrician, Anna insisted that there was nothing to worry about, and denied voluntary attempts to lose weight. She did admit, though, that she was concerned about the amount of food her mother was serving at dinner, and that she had begun to avoid "fattening" foods and desserts, insisting that it was for health reasons. She reluctantly added that she was concerned that her hips were "too large" for her frame, and was hoping that continued exercise might minimize this perceived defect. She was unconcerned about her irregular periods, even though the pediatrician explained that it was unhealthy and likely due to her recent changes in weight, exercise, and eating habits. Following discussion with Anna and her mother, the pediatrician referred her for an evaluation by a psychologist with expertise in diagnosing and treating eating disorders, given his concern that she had likely developed anorexia nervosa.

ANOREXIA NERVOSA & ATYPICAL ANOREXIA NERVOSA

Treatment

ADOLESCENTS

Outpatient management that includes family members is considered best practice provided the adolescent is medically stable. Family-based treatment (FBT) has the strongest evidence for the treatment of adolescents with AN, and preliminary data suggest that this approach can be extended successfully to treat adolescents with atypical AN. FBT posits that AN is not under the control of the adolescent, and therefore it empowers parents to directly manage eating disorder behaviors (e.g., dietary restriction, excessive exercise, binge eating, and purging). Caregivers are placed in charge of providing their child "medicine" in the form of food. FBT first prioritizes renourishment and weight restoration in order to restore healthy organ functioning and cognition, or at least to minimize medical consequences (e.g., growth stunting and osteopenia). Because of severe cognitive disturbances secondary to self-starvation, individuals with AN are generally unable to engage in meaningful therapeutic work, and therefore individual therapy is not indicated. An important component of family therapy is psychoeducation about eating disorders. First and foremost, families are taught that eating disorder behaviors reflect emotional and social consequences of the disorder, rather than manifestations of other problems or their child's personality. This stance is very helpful in reducing any guilt or blame related to the development of the eating disorder in the family, as well as reducing criticism, which is not uncommon in the context of caregivers making extraordinary efforts to help their child recover in the face of the adolescent demonstrating great resistance or behavioral challenges in this process. As health is restored, greater adolescent autonomy is negotiated so that the adolescent is able to manage food/eating in a developmentally appropriate way and return to their normal activities, including physical activity, in a healthy manner. FBT leads to higher remission rates, fewer hospitalizations, and lower rates of relapse than individual therapy.

ADULTS

Therapy is generally more effective when the patient has begun to gain weight and is beyond acute medical risk. Cognitive behavior therapy (CBT) focuses on erroneous and rigid beliefs (i.e., cognitive distortions) that prompt and maintain maladaptive behaviors that arise out of negative experiences associated with eating, food, or body image. CBT helps the patient to establish more effective behavioral alternatives and may also be effective in dealing with the central psychological features of AN, such as disturbance in body image. For young adults who are willing to allow their caregivers and/or a significant other to support them in treatment, an adapted version of FBT for young adults (FBT-TAY) is also a promising approach. Following stabilization and resolution of the acute crisis, including achievement of weight restoration, patients often require longer-term psychotherapeutic interventions.

Unfortunately, approximately 20–25% of patients with AN do not recover over the long term, and outcomes are poor for those with severe and enduring AN. Treatments for severe and enduring AN generally use a harm reduction perspective, minimizing the importance of weight gain, and instead focusing on improving quality of life. A multidisciplinary team is fundamental for providing support and stability in the treatment of severe and enduring AN, including a mental health professional, a physician to monitor medical stability, and a psychiatrist and/or dietician as needed. This work requires a strong therapeutic alliance between the therapist and patient, which is achieved by establishing a therapeutic environment of patience, respect, and autonomy, validation and empathy, and acceptance. Finally, therapeutic goals should be collaboratively determined based on achievable, realistic changes, rather than "ideal" outcomes that may not be attainable and could increase likelihood of treatment dropout. Nevertheless, setting clear limits from the outset of treatment is critical, particularly requirements for medical safety monitoring and the establishment of clear criteria for medical stabilization.

ATYPICAL AN

The treatment of atypical AN is complicated by the fact that significant weight loss in the absence of underweight status is not alarming to patients, their families, and often their medical providers. This raises controversial questions in the field about healthy weight in the context of premorbid overweight or obesity after the onset of an eating disorder. Given the metabolic reduction from dieting, individuals with atypical AN would need to continue to engage in restrictive eating patterns and/or excessive exercise in order to maintain their weight. This arguably would keep them trapped in disordered eating behaviors and prevent full recovery and/or increase risk of relapse.

PHARMACOTHERAPY

Pharmacological therapy can play an adjunctive role in the management of both primary eating symptoms and their co-occurring psychiatric features, including anxiety and depression. Such treatments should focus on particular target symptoms or behaviors. No single medication is consistently effective in managing the primary psychiatric disturbances of AN. Psychotherapy and nutritional rehabilitation often resolve mild to moderate co-occurring depressive or anxiety symptoms. Antidepressants are generally ineffective in the context of AN, particularly while individuals remain underweight. There is some research to suggest that low doses of atypical antipsychotics (e.g., olanzapine) may possibly enhance weight gain, with particular benefit for patients who are severely obsessional or agitated. Anxiolytics, especially benzodiazepines, should generally not be given due to lack of evidence to support their efficacy and risk of addiction.

Medical Complications

The mortality rate of individuals with AN is 5–10 times higher than that in the general population, and more than half of the deaths in AN are attributable to medical complications. All major organ systems can be affected by the progressive malnutrition that characterizes AN, often accompanied by physiologic disturbances, such as bradycardia, hypotension, orthostasis, and hypothermia. Medical hospitalization for these problems is indicated and must ensure prevention of purging behaviors. An electrocardiogram should also be obtained, since emaciation and associated electrolyte disturbances can contribute to significant cardiac abnormalities, particularly for those who purge. Laboratory screening should include tests for electrolytes, liver function, amylase (elevated in patients who purge), thyroid function, a complete blood count with differential, and a urinalysis. Common laboratory findings include leukopenia with a relative lymphocytosis, metabolic alkalosis with associated hypokalemia, hypochloremia, elevated serum bicarbonate levels, and occasionally, metabolic acidosis in patients who abuse large amounts of stimulant-type laxatives. Purging can also be associated with esophageal tears, intractable vomiting, and hematemesis. Although most medical complications resolve with weight restoration, cessation of purging behaviors, and nutritional rehabilitation, some can have permanent adverse effects, including persistent osteopenic changes in those who have experienced extended periods of malnourishment and suppression of growth in adolescence. In most cases, initiating oral intake of fluids and food reverses minor disturbances in electrolytes and establishes adequate hydration. More severe cases may require intravenous hydration and parenteral replacement of depleted electrolytes. Care should be taken to avoid overhydration and the consequences of excess fluid retention in vulnerable individuals. In the case of food refusal, nasogastric tubes are also sometimes needed. However, the goal is for all intake to be in the form of solid food for normalization of eating behavior.

AVOIDANT-RESTRICTIVE FOOD INTAKE DISORDER

Treatment

Current treatment protocols for ARFID are mostly informed by historical practices described in the pediatric feeding literature, and case series describing adaptation of evidence-based models like CBT and FBT for adolescent eating disorders. Exposures in CBT are critical to encourage corrective experiences that inhibit previously held beliefs about food (e.g., "If I eat that oatmeal, I will vomit"). Exposures may be graded using an individual's rating of associated anxiety and willingness to confront the challenge and are often conducted both in and out of the therapy session. For individuals with sensory sensitivities, exposures may involve engaging with food (touching, smelling, licking, examining visually), before one is encouraged to even taste a small quantity of the food. Both FBT and CBT are well-positioned to treat the maintaining features of food avoidance through use of exposure-based practices with prioritization of renourishment to reverse potential health consequences as needed. For the pediatric population, involvement of caregivers is indicated to interrupt familial patterns of accommodation (e.g., only buying preferred foods) in an effort to help their child eat a broader range of foods and support weight restoration.

For individuals who are experiencing significant physiological consequences of restrictive eating, treatment should prioritize their reversal. Medical hospitalization or specialized feeding within an eating disorder program may be required, with availability of nasogastric feeding, nutritional supplementation, and individualized nutritional plans that are closely monitored to reverse the physical consequences of ARFID. It appears that individuals with ARFID requiring medical hospitalization were twice as likely to require NGT feeding than those with other eating disorders. Providers caring for these patients highlight the importance of expeditious tube weaning to avoid potential longer-term reliance on NGT and reinforcement of ongoing avoidance of eating. There are no evidence-based medication treatments for ARFID. Mirtazapine may be indicated due to its known positive impact on appetite and weight gain. In a small clinical case series of young patients treated in an eating disorder specialty program, the medication was well-tolerated and was associated with a faster rate of weight gain.

Medical Complications

The medical complications seen in ARFID are associated with malnutrition and its physiologic disturbances as described above. Vitamin and mineral deficiencies may be seen in those with an extremely limited variety of nutrition (i.e., vitamins A, E, B12, D, K, and folate), and can occur independent of weight status. Individuals with picky eating across the lifespan may exhibit growth stunting or extremely low BMI percentiles (<1%ile). Those avoiding eating due to fear of pain or other aversive consequences may limit intake to the point that gastric motility is impacted, thus resulting in increased discomfort and pain, further reinforcing avoidance behaviors. The cycle of avoidance may be effectively addressed in tertiary care settings where nutritional supplementation, customized meal-plans, and nasogastric feeding are utilized while the individual is relearning to eat without fear.

CASE ILLUSTRATION 2

Evan, a 28-year-old biracial single attorney with no significant medical history, presented to his primary care physician with complaints consistent with gastroesophageal reflux. Symptoms included substernal burning sensations and regurgitation occurring several times a week, particularly following a large meal. He also reported occasional sharp chest pains lasting only a few seconds, not associated with shortness of breath or other signs or symptoms suggestive of cardiac origin. Other complaints noted on review of symptoms were general myalgia and fatigue, both experienced "a few days a week." He stated that he took the suggested dose of an over-the-counter (OTC) laxative for constipation one or two times a week. Vital signs were normal, and he was afebrile. The only positive finding on physical examination was bilateral, nonpainful enlargement of the parotid glands. An electrocardiogram showed normal rate and rhythm, with nonspecific T-wave changes. Routine blood work was drawn, and a prescription for a proton pump inhibitor was given for symptoms of gastroesophageal reflux. His habitus was muscular with a BMI in the "normal" range. He reported running approximately 50 miles per week, and weight training 3 days per week.

A review of Evan's laboratory values the next day revealed an elevated amylase and a serum potassium of 2.7. The laboratory abnormalities, together with the enlarged parotids and his presenting complaints, suggested self-induced vomiting. During a telephone call to Evan that day, his physician expressed concern and asked directly about engagement in purging and other eating disorder behaviors. Evan hesitantly admitted to having a 5-year history of bingeing and purging by self-induced vomiting that followed graduation from college, when he stopped running competitively. He agreed to return to the office for repeat electrolytes, given his concern about his physical health. Reviewing the labs during the follow-up visit allowed his primary care physician to objectively discuss the medical risks associated with bulimia nervosa and provide psychoeducation about evidence-based psychological treatment. Although Evan was uncertain about whether he wanted to engage in therapy, he agreed to schedule an assessment at nearby eating disorders clinic. At the conclusion of the initial assessment with the psychologist, and with the help of motivational interviewing techniques, he decided to engage in treatment.

BULIMIA NERVOSA

Treatment

Early interventions such as increasing awareness of the negative consequences of binge/purge behaviors and dispelling myths about the inefficacy and risks of laxatives, diuretics, and self-induced vomiting, may be enough to motivate a decrease in their frequency. Education coupled with minimizing shame can encourage individuals to seek specialty care that often includes psychotherapy, nutrition counseling and medical management.

ADOLESCENTS

Compared to the adult literature, there are only four randomized treatment trials for adolescent BN suggesting that both FBT and CBT are viable treatment options, although FBT appears to bring about more rapid reduction in bingeing and purging behaviors, with higher rates of abstinence at the end of treatment. FBT for BN is very similar to FBT for AN and Atypical AN in that parents are charged with normalizing their child's eating behavior and preventing inappropriate compensatory behavior, including incorporating avoided foods in appropriate quantities. Unique features of BN inform modifications to the model as initially developed for adolescent AN. Individuals with BN experience bingeing and purging behaviors as ego-dystonic, and thus highly distressing. Therefore, in FBT, the adolescent with BN is engaged more collaboratively with their parents to disrupt disordered eating patterns, and where there is lack of motivation to change problematic behaviors, increased parental intervention is encouraged.

In contrast, CBT for BN is an individual therapy, although caregivers are still engaged in treatment, including being updated about progress and supporting their child outside of therapy (e.g., temporarily locking up food prior to bedtime if the adolescent has identified that restricted access to these foods at night would help to curb late night binge eating). CBT may include challenging individuals to modify unhelpful and distorted thinking patterns through cognitive restructuring techniques. For example, a common cue that frequently leads to eating disorder behavior is the normal sensation of fullness. Rather than recognizing satiety as a normal physiologic response, an individual with BN commonly misinterprets this cue to mean, "I am fat." This cognitive distortion, unchallenged, is associated with emotional distress, leading to attempts to "fix" perceived reality by ridding themselves of the meal through purging or compensatory exercise. This cycle would be interrupted in part through use of education about physiology, monitoring weight fluctuations over time, exploration of alternative means of describing the experience, and teaching skills to encourage tolerating distress associated with fullness.

ADULTS

CBT is much more established as a treatment for adults with BN, having demonstrated greater effectiveness than nondirective supportive counseling, nutritional counseling, stress management, and antidepressant medication. The primary target is interruption of illness-maintaining behaviors. An enhanced version of CBT for eating disorders (CBT-E) is designed to address other maintaining features of BN, including interpersonal difficulties, perfectionism, and low self-worth. The establishment of a regular pattern of eating and use of self-monitoring to identify vulnerabilities or cues to eating disorder behaviors is a goal of early phases of treatment. The aim here is to increase one's awareness of cues so that they may respond to them deliberately rather than automatically. Cues are both internal and external. Internal cues can be physiologic (hunger or fullness), as well as cognitive and emotional. External cues encompass a broad array of experiences from sensual, such as sight or smell, to situational (certain environments or interpersonal situations). The relationship between cues and one's response (automatic interpretations, emotions, and urges or behaviors) are explored with the aim of developing alternative more adaptive responses. Patients are taught to recognize that behaviors follow cues and that responses to cues can be broken down into thoughts, emotions, and behaviors.

PHARMACOTHERAPY

Pharmacological management may play a significant role in treatment and, unlike in AN, can more predictably affect outcome. Antidepressants (SSRIs) have the most evidence of efficacy in treating BN and can reduce symptoms of depression and anxiety as well as the frequency of bingeing and purging. For adults, fluoxetine (60 mg) is indicated for the treatment of binge eating, purging and related cognitions, and a small pilot study found it to be acceptable among adolescents. Bupropion is the only antidepressant that is contraindicated, as the metabolic imbalances precipitated by purging can make the patient more prone to seizures. Antidepressants are not as effective as CBT and are more effective when combined with therapy.

Medical Complications

All-cause mortality is two to five times higher in individuals with BN than the general population. The majority of medical complications due to BN are consequences of purging behaviors (See "Medical Complications" of Anorexia Nervosa & Atypical Anorexia Nervosa section). In addition, long-term use of the emetic ipecac can lead to myopathies, including cardiomyopathy, the latter a rare cause of death in patients with bulimia. Individuals with an acute medical condition, such as dehydration or symptomatic hypokalemia accompanied by electrocardiographic changes, require hospitalization for medical stabilization. Similarly, inpatient treatment may be required for those with significant depression and acute suicidal ideation, but otherwise outpatient treatment as described above is indicated.

BINGE EATING DISORDER

Treatment

Binge eating is the initial target of CBT for BED, which focuses on modifying unrealistic weight loss expectations and promoting acceptance of a larger than average body size. The cognitive work primarily involves identifying and challenging maladaptive cognitions regarding eating, weight, and shape, as well as other thoughts that serve as triggers for binge eating. This treatment approach conveys a firm stance toward first eliminating binge eating and establishing healthier eating patterns before engaging in weight loss attempts. While CBT does provide psychoeducation about nutrition and incorporates regular exercise, the target of the treatment is to improve control over binge eating rather than to reduce weight. It would seem critical to address binge eating prior to weight loss, given that restrictive eating patterns (sometimes associated with weight loss) are tied to increased binge eating in the CBT conceptual framework. However, research has found that behavioral weight loss (BWL) treatment is also a viable treatment and requires less specialist training than CBT. BWL specifically targets eating behavior to establish regular eating habits, thereby reducing disorganized eating and binge eating. It incorporates various behavioral strategies to promote weight loss, such as restricting caloric intake and increasing physical activity. Outcomes are comparable with respect to reductions in binge eating between CBT and BWL (although some studies favor CBT with respect to binge abstinence).

PHARMACOTHERAPY

Although some have endorsed medication monotherapy as sufficient for certain individuals with BED, medication is most often considered as an adjunctive therapy. The various medications examined in the treatment of BED include anticonvulsants (topiramate and lamotrigine), antiobesity agents (orlistat), central nervous system stimulants (lisdexamfetamine), several second-generation antidepressants (e.g., citalopram, fluoxetine, and sertraline), and other medications (including acamprosate and armodafinil). In 2015, lisdexamfetamine (originally marketed for attention deficit hyperactivity disorder) became the first medication that the U.S. Food and Drug Administration approved for BED. Lisdexamfetamine, topiramate, and antidepressants are all associated with reductions in binge eating and eating disorder psychopathology, with lisdexamfetamine being superior to antidepressants with respect to achieving abstinence from binge eating. Whereas lisdexamfetamine and topiramate result in greater weight loss (compared to placebo), antidepressants do not. Further, the effects of lisdexamfetamine on those with a history of substance use disorder, suicide attempt, mania, or cardiac abnormality are unknown given that these individuals are excluded from trials given it is classified as a Schedule II drug.

Medical Complications

Overweight and obesity is prevalent among individuals with BED. While individuals with BED often endorse somatic symptoms and general dissatisfaction with health, research does not support the idea that medical complications can be directly attributed to binge eating but rather that obesity-associated comorbidity accounts for medical complications including metabolic syndrome and type 2 diabetes mellitus. Certainly, bariatric surgery is contraindicated when binge eating is present, as binge episodes would interfere with adherence to postsurgical nutritional recommendations and diminish the efficacy of the surgical intervention for weight loss. Indeed, the evidence suggests that individuals with obesity and BED have more postoperative complications, less weight loss, and more weight regain than those with obesity alone.

SUMMARY

Eating disorders represent a broad spectrum of psychopathologic features, and their development is influenced by an interplay of multiple etiologic factors. Specialized psychological treatment is indicated across diagnoses, with the initial focus of treatment to normalize eating behavior and minimize medical consequences. One potential exception is severe and enduring anorexia nervosa, which initially focuses on engaging patients through a collaborative therapeutic relationship. Medical management is also essential given serious medical risks that may require inpatient medical stabilization. Disruption of eating disorder behaviors may also be augmented through pharmacological management that may improve co-occurring symptomatology. Caregiver involvement is critical in the treatment of children and adolescents and often leveraged in the treatment of young adults as well. Across disciplines, most practitioners do not receive sufficient training to be competent in specialized psychological treatments or medical management for eating disorders. Given the high risks of elevated suicidality, life-threatening medical consequences, and potential chronicity, treatment for these complex psychiatric disorders is best delivered in specialty settings.

SUGGESTED READINGS

Brownell KD, Walsh BT. *Eating Disorders and Obesity: A Comprehensive Handbook*, 3rd ed. New York, NY: Guilford Press; 2017.

Grilo CM, Mitchell JE, eds. *The Treatment of Eating Disorders: A Clinical Handbook*. New York, NY: Guilford Press; 2010.

Kaye W, Strober M, Jimmerson D. The neurobiology of eating disorders. In: Charney DF, Nestler EJ, eds. *The Neurobiology of Mental Illness*. New York, NY: Oxford University Press; 2004, pp. 1112–1128.

Le Grange D, Lock J, eds. *Eating Disorders in Children and Adolescents: A Clinical Handbook*. New York, NY: Guilford Press; 2011.

Thomas JJ, Lawson EA, Micali N, et al. Avoidant/ Restrictive Food Intake Disorder: a three-dimensional model of neurobiology with implications for etiology and treatment. *Curr Psychiatry Rep* 19:54, 2017.

WEBSITE

Academy for Eating Disorders. http://www.aedweb.org Reston, VA, 2018.

Unhealthy Alcohol & Other Substance Use

24

Derek D. Satre, PhD; J. Carlo Hojilla, RN, PhD; Kelly C. Young-Wolff, PhD, MPH; & E. Jennifer Edelman, MD, MHS

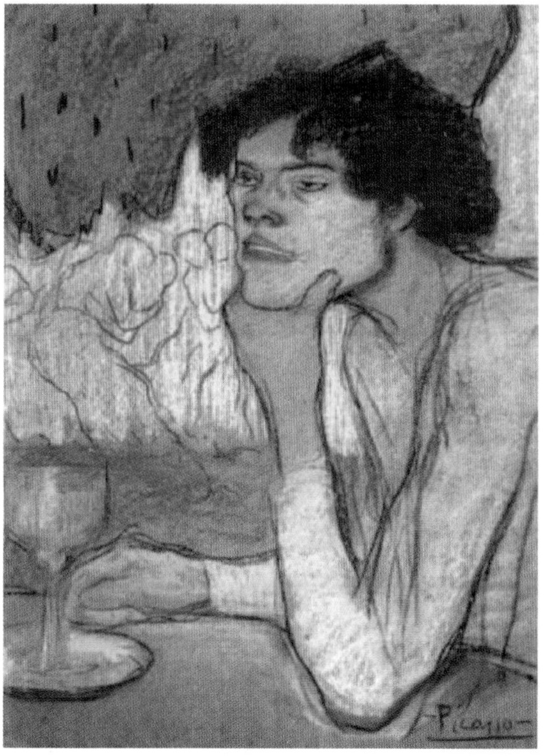

Picasso's "Absinthe drinker." Pablo Picasso: "L'Absinthe," 1901.

INTRODUCTION

Unhealthy alcohol and other substance use, defined as the spectrum of use that includes "at-risk" levels of use and substance use disorders, is common among patients presenting to primary care settings. The prevalence of substance use disorders exceeds 20% in ambulatory practices and is even higher in hospitalized patients. Those affected include everyone from adolescents to older adults, including clinicians themselves. Even though alcohol and other substance use have a major impact on health and function, they often go unaddressed in routine health care settings, as clinicians often lack the language, knowledge, and skills to identify unhealthy substance use and treat it.

Evidence from many sources provides reason for optimism, however, and shows that clinicians who take a few moments to thoughtfully structure their interventions with patients and offer indicated treatments can reduce harm, lower medical care costs, lessen morbidity and mortality, strengthen patients' family and social relationships, and enhance patient self-esteem and emotional stability. Indeed, the rate of successful treatment (i.e., achievement of abstinence) is about 30–40% of treated patients, which exceeds that for most other chronic illnesses. These relationships can be very satisfying for patients and providers alike, akin to the treatment of other life-threatening medical conditions such as cancer.

Primary care medicine is increasing its role in addressing alcohol and other substance-related problems, since the majority of individuals with such problems may be reluctant to seek care from specialized addiction treatment programs. Several important developments are significant in this regard. One is a push for early identification and treatment of alcohol and other substance use before those problems become severe. The Screening, Brief Intervention and Referral to Treatment (SBIRT) model is a public health approach promoted by the National Institutes of Health (NIH) and the Substance Abuse and Mental Health Services Administration (SAMHSA) to encourage universal primary care screening and intervention when needed. This screening qualifies for Medicare reimbursement and has been further encouraged by changes in reimbursement structure associated with the Affordable Care Act. In addition, primary care is a natural place to address substance use because patients frequently present with medical and psychiatric conditions that are related to their use. Primary care providers are already trained in providing care for chronic conditions such as diabetes mellitus that involve referral to specialty care as needed. Specialty care capacity is also limited, and it is important both to build workforce skill in primary care and to de-stigmatize substance use interventions by integrating them into routine health services.

Physicians and other primary care clinicians, including nurse practitioners and physician assistants, have a key role to play in this process. In this chapter, we discuss identification and management of substance use problems, and how clinician interactions with patients can enhance patients' coping with these problems. We note that this chapter will focus on strategies for addressing unhealthy alcohol and other commonly used substances, including cannabis and stimulants. Problems related to opioid use are addressed separately in Chapter 25, and tobacco use is addressed in Chapter 21.

Substance use disorders (alcohol and drug) are chronic, progressive illnesses affecting 25–29% of Americans at some time in their lives (lifetime prevalence) and approximately 8% of Americans at any given point in time. Unhealthy alcohol or drug use has the potential to precipitate a vicious cycle of increased use associated with medical, behavioral, and social problems. Unhealthy alcohol use is associated with elevated risk for a range of medical problems, including hypertension, gastrointestinal bleeding, sleep disorders, major depression, hemorrhagic stroke, cirrhosis of the liver, HIV acquisition, and several cancers. Similarly, numerous health problems are associated with use of other substances. For example, regular cannabis use, especially among adolescents, impairs short-term memory and performance in school, has the potential to impact psychiatric symptoms and cognitive development, and increases risk of psychosis and psychotic disorders. Stimulants, such as methamphetamine and cocaine, are associated with cardiovascular complications, mental health problems, sexual risk taking, and poor health care engagement. The insidious development of tolerance to intoxication, cognitive deficits from high doses, and dysphoria leads to social impairment. Relationship problems are exacerbated when friends and family experience the consequences of substance use. Further, emotional isolation may develop when those suffering from addiction make excuses for their behavior, direct blame onto others, and show hostility when lower limits of substance use are discussed. Clinicians have an important role to play in preventing and mitigating these adverse consequences.

CASE ILLUSTRATION

Jim is a 50-year-old factory worker with high blood pressure. He has a follow-up visit with the doctor who has been his primary care physician for the past decade. He mentions that he recently received his second "driving under the influence" (DUI) citation and considers it unfair. His probation officer ordered Jim to undergo alcohol counseling at the local alcohol treatment center. Jim has no interest in counseling but he thinks he must attend to keep his driver's license, which he needs to get to his job.

Jim cannot remember his father, but knows he had serious drinking problems and left the family when Jim was 4 years old.

Jim began drinking as a teenager, up to a 12-pack of beer per day. He cut back once he got out of his twenties, since "that was going nowhere" but he still drinks four to six beers daily—at his club or playing pool or cards with his buddies, and up to two six-packs per day on the weekend. (Based on his self-report and national survey data, only 3% of American men drink more than Jim.)

You have asked Jim the Alcohol Use Disorder Identification Test—Consumption (AUDIT-C) questions (Table 24-1) in the past, and at that time he said that when he was a lot younger he needed to cut down. He reports drinking four or more times a week, with a usual quantity of three or four drinks, and having six or more drinks in a day about once per month. Now, as you ask questions, he seems irritated.

You decide to begin your assessment of Jim's current situation by asking him the AUDIT-C questions again. You ask about cutting down:

***Jim:** Look, doc, my father may have had problems with alcohol, and many of my buddies drink a lot more than me, but I don't—I can take it or leave it.*

Rather than confronting him with the considerable evidence already available that indicates he likely has an alcohol use disorder, you decide to use an empathic style and reflect his apparent feeling state as well as the content of his declaration.

***Doctor:** Jim, I see this is a sensitive topic, as it is for most people, and I get it that you are convinced that drinking is not a problem for you.*

***Jim:** I quit several times when my wife complained, no problem. But 2 years ago, she took the kids and left, saying that they couldn't live with me unless I quit drinking. I don't understand women!*

You have important new data about drinking and about Jim's life, and Jim feels understood rather than interrogated.

On repeated checks over the past couple of years, Jim has had an elevated mean corpuscular volume

Table 24-1. Alcohol Use Disorder Identification Test—Consumption (AUDIT-C) screening test for unhealthy alcohol use.

Questions	0	1	2	3	4
How often do you have a drink containing alcohol?	Never	Monthly or less	2–4 times a month	2–3 times a week	4 or more times a week
How many standard drinks containing alcohol do you have on a typical day?	1–2	3–4	5–6	7–9	10 or more
How often do you have six or more drinks on one occasion?	Never	Less than monthly	Monthly	Weekly	Daily or almost daily

Each response choice has a point allotted. Scores ≥ 4 in men and ≥ 3 in women are considered positive and warrant further investigation to identify hazardous drinking or an alcohol use disorder.

(MCV), but the rest of his complete blood count, metabolic panel, and liver function panel are repeatedly normal. He tells you his blood alcohol concentration was 0.22% (220 mg/dL, 0.08%, is now the "legal limit" in all U.S. states) when he was cited.

Your physical examination shows Jim's blood pressure is controlled, and you find no evidence for new medical problems or active withdrawal from alcohol.

Doctor: *We have talked about alcohol quite a bit today, Jim. On a scale of 0–10, how interested are you in making a change in your drinking at this time, where 0 means not at all and 10 means quitting is a top priority?*

Jim: *I'm quitting until I get my license back, no problem.*

Doctor: *You feel you are in full control of your alcohol intake.*

Jim: *I'm fine, doc, and thanks for checking.*

Doctor: *I am pleased that you are ready to quit now, and I know you have been successful in the past. Also, I'm concerned, because I think you may have an alcohol use disorder that will require your attention even after you get the license back . . . What are your thoughts about that?*

SUBSTANCE USE TERMINOLOGY & DIAGNOSTIC CATEGORIES

Alcohol and drug problems exist on a continuum (Figure 24-1). At times, diagnosis may require multiple visits with an individual patient and/or additional information from family members, friends, or other clinicians. Nevertheless, experts agree on an evidence-based classification system that is useful in guiding clinician actions. Substance use disorders in the Diagnostic and Statistical Manual of Mental Disorders, Fifth Edition (DSM-5) are categorized as Mild: meeting 2–3 criteria; Moderate: 4–5 criteria; or Severe: 6–11 criteria. **Physical dependence** and **withdrawal syndromes** are key hallmarks of substance use disorders, along with manifestations of **loss of control** over substance use and **adverse consequences**. These conditions are sometimes referred to as *alcoholism* or *drug addiction,* but the terms can often be stigmatizing for patients. Using appropriate patient-centered terminology can help facilitate frank discussions but still ensure that patients feel respected.

The extreme end of the continuum is diagnostically classified as *severe alcohol or drug use disorder*, which is the level of substance use associated with the most severe medical, behavioral, and social consequences. People toward the center of the continuum, with problems of modest severity, have mild–moderate drug or alcohol use disorder, a maladaptive pattern that leads to impairment or distress. Note that what distinguishes the patient with a mild–moderate substance use disorder from the patient with severe drug use disorder is not the **nature** of the problems, but the **frequency, persistence, and pervasiveness** of the problems. Thus, both severe and mild–moderate drug use disorders may be associated with health problems (e.g., stroke from cocaine use, hypertension from alcohol use, and oversedation from benzodiazepines), family dysfunction, and performance problems at school or work.

At the milder end of the continuum, conceptualization of alcohol and drug use problems has been broadened to include patterns of substance use that do not meet strict diagnostic criteria, but which put patients at risk for adverse health consequences. These patients have been described as "at-risk," or "hazardous" users. These people use above recommended limits but may not have developed significant negative consequences. Clinicians should tailor their treatment response based on the patient's level of use, their underlying health status, and the associated potential and experienced consequences. For instance, while a college student who reports binge drinking should reduce their alcohol consumption due to risk for accidental injury, an older adult who reports falling and/or takes multiple medications likely should avoid alcohol completely.

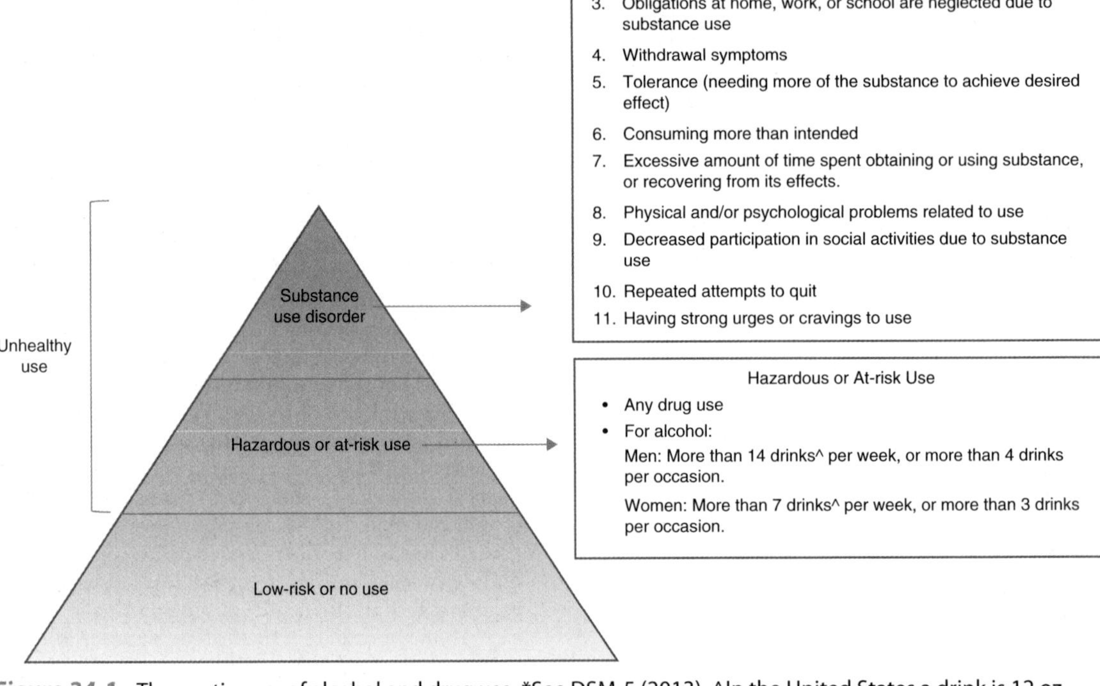

Figure 24-1. The continuum of alcohol and drug use. *See DSM-5 (2013). ^In the United States a drink is 12 oz beer, 5 oz wine, or 1.5 oz (bar shot) of hard liquor. Figure adapted from Pace & Samet. Substance use disorders. *Ann Intern Med. 2016;164(7):ITC49-ITC64.*

Regarding alcohol, expert consensus is that *lower risk* or *moderate drinking* is defined by quantity of intake (not more than 14 drinks per week for men and 7 for women), and amount consumed at one time (not more than four drinks per occasion for men and three for women). Drinking above these limits, when criteria for a substance use disorder is not met, is called *at-risk* or *hazardous*, and is likely to cause harm, according to long-term studies. *At-risk* drinking is very common. According to the National Institute on Alcohol Abuse and Alcoholism (NIAAA), approximately 3 out of 10 adults in the United States drink at levels that put them at risk for physical and mental health problems.

At-risk drug use includes any use of mood-altering illicit drugs (e.g., heroin and cocaine) or medications in a manner other than as prescribed (e.g., prescription opioids, benzodiazepines, stimulants, anxiolytics, sedatives, and even antivirals). This may occur in the context of being prescribed such medications (e.g., *nonmedical use:* taking more than prescribed or for a different purpose than prescribed) or outside the context of a prescribed medication (i.e., obtaining medications from a friend or family member or from the street). Although a full discussion of psychotropic medication misuse is beyond the scope of this chapter, clinicians should carefully follow published guidelines for safe prescribing. For additional information regarding risky use of opioids, see Chapter 25.

While cannabis use disorder and cannabis withdrawal may be less widely recognized by clinicians, cannabis use disorders are prevalent, with recent data from a national survey indicating that nearly 20% of people with lifetime cannabis use met criteria for a cannabis use disorder. Clinicians are likely to see an increase in the number of patients with a cannabis use disorder, as the potency of cannabis, the number of routes of administration (e.g., vaping and edibles), and the perception that cannabis is harmless increase over time. At-risk use of cannabis may include using before the age of 16 years, using high potency products, using synthetic cannabinoids, driving while under the influence of cannabis, and near-daily or daily use. Patients who endorse any such behavior warrant further assessment. Synthetic cannabinoids (e.g., K2 and Spice) are particularly dangerous given the great variability of the ingredients and potential for contamination, and have been associated with a number of severe medical and psychiatric problems as well as death.

WORKING EFFECTIVELY WITH PATIENTS

Discussing alcohol and drug use with patients is an important, and often sensitive, topic largely because of the stigma around substance use. The language we use, whether intentional or not, can perpetuate that stigma, further marginalize individuals, and discourage persons from seeking medical care. Terms like "addict," "alcoholic," "drug abuser," and "dirty urine" are common in the medical literature and lay press but promote the perception that the individual is flawed and that they deserve punishment instead of treatment. We encourage clinicians to avoid stigmatizing language and instead use person-first terminology, such as a "person who uses substances," "urine with evidence of cocaine use," that more accurately captures the medical nature of substance use disorders and acknowledges the dignity of individuals. Utilizing appropriate patient-centered terminology can help facilitate frank discussions and encourage patients to seek care.

Although the brain effects of addictive drugs vary in neurochemical mechanisms, timing, intensity, and potential toxicity, severe substance use disorders are similar across the various drug classes and specific drugs. For example, dopamine is the final pathway involved with substance use, and as a result, patients with addiction may feel that they need a specific substance in order to feel normal. However, different treatment strategies have been found to be effective depending on levels of use and substance. Regardless of the specific substance used, engaging in a patient-centered approach and developing a trusting relationship and using destigmatizing language is an important first step.

Promoting Behavior Change

Several methods for promoting behavior change in patients with substance use problems have emerged from research. A key first step is screening all patients for unhealthy substance use. For those with indications of unhealthy substance use, several approaches may be utilized depending on the severity of the problem. These include *brief intervention, motivational interviewing, shared decision making, relationship-centered care,* and *autonomy support* (see Chapter 19 for a full discussion on behavior change). The fundamental **principles** derived from this research are as follows:

- Generally speaking, the clinician takes responsibility for calibrating and adjusting interventions so that patients can hear information and feedback that create or amplify differences between the way life is now and the goals and values patients espouse. Using an empathic and caring style, the clinician shows that discrepancies between actual behavior and patients' values might be minimized if patients change their alcohol and drug use patterns.
- Patients will not change until they are ready, and ambivalence about change and/or resistance to change is normal.
- Clinicians can best promote change by maintaining an empathic and relationship-centered style. Taking a strongly persuasive stand usually fails to promote change.
- Only the patient can take responsibility for change and effect change. Clinicians can promote change by providing information (both feedback about the patient's health and information about resources), by showing attentiveness and listening carefully to the patient's ideas about both the pros and the cons of possible changes, and by helping boost the patient's self-confidence about change.

The fundamental **content messages** clinicians should include in interviews are as follows:

- I am concerned that your substance use may be hurting you and others you care about.
- Most people use a lot less than you do or abstain completely.
- For better health, you should curb (or cease) your substance use.
- The key choices are up to you.
- I will give you my best advice, which is based on expert consensus and my experience with other patients with similar problems.
- I want to collaborate with you, even if progress is slow or intermittent.

The fundamental **process strategies** clinicians should follow are as follows:

- Maintain dialogue when giving information and recommendations; use a *tell, ask, tell* strategy.
- Make clear recommendations, but do not try to persuade patients.
- State explicitly that you will advise, but that the patient decides.
- Establish the patient's commitment to any plans on which you agree.

- Never argue with patients and do not try to overcome resistance, reluctance, rebellion, or rationalization. Use reflection to respond to these manifestations of ambivalence.
- Support the patient's self-confidence.

Two key steps can assist clinicians in doing a better job with patients who have substance use disorders. The first is to intervene as soon as any clue suggests that an alcohol or drug use problem might be present; do not wait until the evidence is glaring or a patient's health has begun to suffer. Clinicians can better limit serious consequences of substance use by broadening their focus from the detection of substance use disorders to include the detection of at-risk patterns of use.

The second key step is to conduct those interventions using techniques specifically structured to promote behavior change, as described below. We will discuss first the process of deciding which patients require interventions, and then discuss principles, content, and strategies of effective clinician–patient interactions.

IDENTIFYING SUBSTANCE USE PROBLEMS

"Brief interventions" can be structured for "at-risk" users as well as those who have developed mild, moderate, or severe substance use disorders. However, studies suggest that brief interventions are most effective when targeted toward at-risk drinkers and when reinforced over multiple visits. Evidence has been less consistent on the effectiveness of brief interventions in addressing alcohol and drug use disorders.

Adjusting interventions to problem severity is necessary, and consequently we suggest simple strategies that separate healthy users from potentially problematic ones and help clinicians assess severity. Subsequent sections advise clinicians what to do in each case. In the steps below, we incorporate the NIAAA *Clinician's Guide: Helping Patients Who Drink Too Much,* which is a very useful reference and includes procedures also relevant to screening and treatment of drug use. These steps can be recalled using the "**4 A's**"—**A**sk, **A**ssess, **A**dvise, and **A**ssist.

Step One: Ask About Alcohol and Drug Use

Step one is to ask **about alcohol and drug use**. Prescreen every new patient with two questions: "Do you sometimes drink beer, wine, or other alcoholic beverages?" and "How many times in the past year have you used a prescription medication for nonmedical reasons or illegal drugs?" If the answer is "No," "Never," or "Years ago," leave this topic after reinforcing that this is important for patients' health. If patients belong to an abstinent subgroup with past problems, they often disclose this spontaneously.

Table 24-2. Single item screening questions for unhealthy substance use⁺.

How many times in the past year have you had five or more drinks in 1 day (men); four or more drinks in 1 day (women)?
How many times in the past year have you used illicit drugs or prescription drugs for nonmedical reasons?

⁺Patients who screen positive (i.e., one or more drinking days or report of any drug use) should receive brief intervention.
(Data from National Institute on Alcohol Abuse and Alcoholism. *Helping patients who drink too much: A clinician's guide.* Available at: https://www.niaaa.nih.gov/sites/default/files/publications/guide.pdf; National Institute on Drug Use. *Screening for drug use in general medical settings.* Available at: https://www.drugabuse.gov/sites/default/files/resource_guide.pdf; Smith PC, et al. A Single-Question Screening Test for Drug Use in Primary Care. *Arch Intern Med* 2010; 170(3):1155–1160).

For patients who report any alcohol use, ask the NIAAA recommended **single question about hazardous drinking** (Table 24-2). If positive (five or more drinks in a day for men; four or more in a day for women), quantify the drinking behavior. Determine a weekly average by asking: "On average, how many days a week do you have a drink?" and "On a typical day, how many drinks do you have?" Drinking above "safe limits" (Figure 24-1) means the person is at least an at-risk user.

The National Institute on Drug Abuse (NIDA) has developed a similar stepped screening approach (see Table 24-2). The first step is to ask patients which drugs they have used in the past year (including major categories of illicit drugs as well as prescription psychotropics used other than as prescribed); and of these, which if any have been used in the past 3 months.

Step Two: Assess for Substance Use Disorders & Substance-Related Problems

For patients who drink alcohol over recommended limits or who report drug use in the past 3 months, the next step is to determine if patients meet criteria for a substance use disorder. See Figure 24-1 for a summary of diagnostic criteria.

If there is any evidence of physiologic substance dependence, or if intake exceeds safe limits, or if another clue from examination or the family suggests a drinking or drug problem, the clinician needs more detail to clarify the extent of the problems. A search for characteristic negative consequences is warranted and can be effectively completed within the context of a routine medical visit. The provider decides when to conduct this inquiry based on priorities for the present encounter; however, because alcohol and drug use produces many symptoms and affects many other illness conditions, at least a brief

Table 24-3. Examples of possible alcohol- and drug-related problems.

- Medical conditions: Gastritis, hypertension, viral infections (HIV, Hepatitis C), cirrhosis, new-onset seizure, respiratory depression and overdose, trauma, falls.
- Psychosocial: Symptoms of anxiety, depression, insomnia, sexual risk behaviors, unemployment.
- Legal: motor vehicle accidents, arrests for driving while intoxicated or under the influence.
- Alcohol-specific: Any spontaneous mention of drinking behavior, such as "partying" or hangover, withdrawal symptoms, tolerance, blackouts.

Table 24-4. Potential menu of treatment options for patients with unhealthy alcohol or drug use.

Cut down on amount and/or frequency of drinking or substance use
Quit completely
Use online and mobile application-based resources (e.g., Addiction-Comprehensive Health Enhancement Support System; A-CHESS)
Attend mutual help meetings (e.g., Alcoholics Anonymous, Narcotics Anonymous)
Addiction counseling
Seek clinical treatment (e.g., behavioral or medical interventions)
Enroll in short-term residential program
Enroll in an addiction treatment program

inventory when the issue initially surfaces is imperative. Asking patients about the symptoms in Table 24-3 as they relate to alcohol use provides ample data for the primary assessment, and the NIAAA Clinician's Guide organizes this inquiry very well. Protocols for drug use assessment are less well developed than those for alcohol, but the NIDA *Screening for Drug Use in General Medical Settings Resource Guide* provides helpful information. Patients can be assessed further by inquiring how much money they spend per week on drugs, the frequency of use, consequences of use, and how many days or weeks they have abstained in the past 12 months.

Interviews with others, including family, close friends, or social workers, enlarge the inquiry if the patient furnishes insufficient data. Such interviews require consent as well as buy-in from the patient, in order to maintain rapport. Records from other clinicians or hospitals may contain unanticipated information that helps determine a diagnosis. Obtaining a thorough evaluation allows the clinician to discuss impressions in a compassionate manner. In fact, experimental data show that thoughtful diagnostic conversation itself produces beneficial therapeutic effects. Additional assessment approaches, including laboratory testing, are described below.

A helpful tool that can be used to gather greater information about alcohol use patterns is the Alcohol Use Disorders Identification Test (AUDIT) (Appendix 24-A). The AUDIT is a 10-item instrument developed by the World Health Organization to screen for alcohol-related problems and to quantify severity. The NIAAA Clinician's Guide also includes the AUDIT Questionnaire, with suggestions for its use and scoring in clinical practice. An abbreviated version of the scale, the AUDIT-C, which includes only the first three questions of the AUDIT, has comparable psychometric properties, and may be more suitable in the primary care setting because it can be more easily administered (see Table 24-1). To screen for hazardous drug use, the NIDA resource guide includes a modified version of the alcohol, smoking and substance involvement screening test (ASSIST). The scale is an eight-item questionnaire tailored for clinical use that can help identify appropriate interventions based on a patient's level of risk.

Step Three: Advise & Assist

For patients whose pattern of use indicates that they are either at risk of alcohol or drug problems or who already meet criteria for a substance use disorder, the next steps include strategies to help them reduce or eliminate drug use. In delivering brief interventions, the components we describe in this chapter can be remembered using the acronym FRAMES:

Feedback is given to the individual about personal risk or impairment, including sources for normative data such as national surveys.

Responsibility for change is placed on the patient.

Advice to change is given by the provider.

Menu of alternative self-help or treatment options is offered to the patient (Table 24-4)

Empathic style is used in counseling.

Self-efficacy or optimistic empowerment is engendered in the patient.

Responding Effectively to Challenge, Resistance, & Ambivalence

We introduce the skill of "reflection"—paraphrasing the patient's message or meaning—(Table 24-5) at this moment because as clinicians ask screening and clarifying questions, patients sometimes show resistance. Clinicians can improve the quality of the data as well as minimize tension by responding to irritation or resistance with reflections. This approach has been described extensively as "reflective listening," a key component of motivational interviewing.

Table 24-5. Reflection.

Description: Tell the patient the message you heard (or perceived nonverbally). Always statements, not questions, agreement or disagreement, judgment, and so on. Always brief: Reflector may have to choose among several messages to be brief.
Examples: "I see, you think that none of your problems is related to drug use." "Alcohol really helps you to sleep." "That I think these abnormal liver tests stem from alcohol is confusing to you, because you drink so little." "You seem irritated with my continuing to discuss drug use."

Clinicians who can gently reflect back the resistance, ambivalence, or challenge they receive from patients generate an atmosphere of alliance and partnership. Reflection shows a desire to fully understand the patient, demonstrating acceptance of the person and a willingness to listen. Reflection is neither aggressive nor defensive, and helps to minimize arguing, hostility, and negativity. Simple reflection gives the patient full choice over what to say next (whereas questions seek answers, and giving advice stakes out a position, as does agreement or disagreement, and statements of values). In fact, studies demonstrate that reflecting negative, resistant, or reluctant statements helps engage patients in dialogue (see Chapters 1–4 for additional information on reflections and other key motivational interviewing skills).

Especially when the patient seems negative or hostile, reflection is not an intuitive response. Studies show that doctors usually respond by asking questions, giving advice, persuading or arguing the point, or shifting the interview focus. With practice and attentiveness, clinicians can reflect back patients' expressions of ambivalence, resistance, or challenge.

Jim: *I drink a lot because of the neuropathy and pain in my feet, so that I can sleep.*

Doctor: *So, alcohol helps you a lot.*

Jim: *Well, it's probably not so good for my liver.*

Doctor: *You feel some conflict about getting sleep at the expense of hurting your liver.*

Jim: *The drink seems to produce nothing but problems.*

As this example illustrates, an empathic reflection that recognizes patients' reasons for using substances can allow them to move forward and admit potential downsides to their pattern of use. Clinicians can equally reflect patients' statements about feeling, thinking, attribution, choice, action, or behavior. Reflection helps the physician by encouraging patients to share more of their perspectives, feelings, and thoughts; it thus engenders more trust and a feeling of safety in both persons. As patients who initially show disinterest, hostility, a sullen demeanor, or confusion reveal more of themselves, clinicians become less judgmental and critical, more inclined to join patients and to support them. Patients who feel joined are more likely to listen to their doctors and have more strength to take responsibility for attempting change that might at first seem unimaginable. Reflection is useful in all interview stages, whether the physician seeks more information about drug use and its consequences, additional psychosocial information, or wishes to develop sensible management strategies for a patient.

PHYSICAL EXAMINATION & LABORATORY STUDIES

Physical and laboratory examinations are useful adjuncts to structured interviewing. *Odor of alcohol* is alarming, and distinctly abnormal in medical encounters. If alcohol is easily smelled in the room, the blood alcohol level (BAL) is likely greater than 0.125 mg/dL, and a less dramatic odor indicates a BAL between 0.075 and 0.125 mg/dL. The nose is a good breath analyzer. Alcohol on the breath is a convincing sign, and likely signals a serious alcohol disorder.

Intoxication (slurred speech, incoordination, and/or emotional lability) in any encounter is worrisome, and means a high likelihood of drug or alcohol disorder, even in the emergency department. To underscore this important point, assume that the 10% of the population who have an alcohol or drug use disorder are intoxicated once a week. Assume also that the 60% who do not have an alcohol or drug use disorder are intoxicated once yearly. Thus, in a year, from a population of 100, 30 abstainers yield no episodes of intoxication, 60 users (not in trouble) yield 60, and 10 people with an alcohol or drug use disorder yield 520 episodes of intoxication. Further, moderate users seldom become as intoxicated and are more likely to use in controlled environments (e.g., where someone else can drive). Intoxicated people in the emergency department are not typically healthy users or drinkers who "have had one too many."

Further, with respect to alcohol, if the odor of alcohol is apparent, and if the patient manifests no evidence of intoxication, *tolerance* to alcohol effect is likely present. Tolerance indicates brain adaptation to intoxicating alcohol levels, which is caused by heavy drinking, is inevitably toxic, and usually means that the patient is physically dependent on alcohol. Withdrawal symptoms (see Management of Withdrawal) indicate additional brain dysfunction, and are easier to discern than tolerance. The same reasoning holds for drugs other than alcohol, but our ability to quantify their use or blood levels, as well as our ability to detect intoxication (except for sedatives or opiates), is limited, so tolerance must be inferred less directly from the patient's history.

Other physical and laboratory findings (see general medicine textbooks for the multitudinous possibilities) are poor screening tests, as they have either low sensitivity or specificity, or both. Once again, more data are available about alcohol than for other drugs. Alcohol has a broad range of toxic effects and an abnormality may prove useful in context. First, an unexplained finding may begin a fruitful investigative process. For example, despite a negative response to the alcohol screening question, the concerned clinician of a young woman with palmar erythema continued the assessment, allowing the patient to reveal her alcohol problem. Second, in the presence of a clue, physical or laboratory findings substantially raise the posttest probability, and clinicians should order appropriate tests, such as MCV and liver enzymes (include alanine aminotransferase [ALT], aspartate aminotransferase [AST], and γ-glutamyl transpeptidase [GGT], the most sensitive to alcohol intake). For example, a 55-year-old man with chronic pulmonary disease was admitted for atrial fibrillation. His wife complained about his drinking, and an elevated MCV, AST, and ECG confirmed not only significant alcohol use but also "holiday heart" (alcohol-induced arrhythmia after binge drinking). Carbohydrate-deficient transferrin (CDT) is a more specific marker of heavy alcohol use and can be used to monitor abstinence for the patient needing ongoing treatment for a severe alcohol use disorder. Phosphatidylethanol (PEth), an alcohol metabolite expressed on the surface of red blood cells after alcohol use, is an alcohol biomarker that reflects that past 21 days of alcohol use. Currently, its use has generally been restricted to the research setting, though it may become more widely used in clinical practice as it is a highly specific marker of alcohol use with higher levels reflecting higher levels of use. Illicit drugs are readily detectable in urine; however, the ability to identify them varies with the technique used. Drugs that may not be included in routine panels include hydrocodone, oxycodone, methadone, fentanyl, buprenorphine, anabolic steroids, and short-acting designer drugs. Cannabis can be detected for 30 days or longer in the urine of daily smokers (for approximately 7 days in intermittent smokers) depending on factors such as the potency of the cannabis and mode of administration, but all other illicit drugs are cleared within 72 hours; for example, a positive test for cocaine indicates use within the past 2–3 days. Simply being near a cannabis smoker never produces a positive urine test (it can be detected by mass spectroscopy, but levels are well below the cutoff levels of routine urine testing). Urine drug screening for recent alcohol use (last 48–72 hours) can be determined using the ethyl glucuronide/ethyl sulfate test. This test must be specifically ordered as it is not part of a routine panel of drugs tested. Further, ethyl glucuronide and ethyl sulfate are metabolites of alcohol that result from hepatic metabolism. This test will not be positive in urine that has been contaminated by ethanol-producing bacteria and so is considered to be specific for alcohol use.

Biomarkers of alcohol and drug use can be useful tools for clinicians by providing objective measures to screen for unhealthy use and for monitoring abstinence among those in treatment. However, biomarkers should never substitute for a comprehensive assessment. Misinterpretation of false-positive results can have serious consequences for patients so the decision to use biomarkers should be made with an understanding of each test's strengths and weaknesses. All positive toxicology tests should be followed up with a confirmatory test using highly specific and sensitive methodology. For example, ethyl glucuronide/ethyl sulfate has a high sensitivity to recent alcohol use but false-positive responses from exposure to alcohol-containing products like hand sanitizers and mouthwash have been documented. Similarly, urine drug tests using immunoassays have resulted in false-positive responses for amphetamine use in patients taking antidepressants and other psychiatric medications.

MANAGEMENT OF WITHDRAWAL

Treatment of alcohol or drug withdrawal is of special concern to the medical practitioner. Other urgent complications associated with substance use, such as arrhythmia, alcohol or viral hepatitis, bleeding, gastritis, pancreatitis, skin abscess, sepsis, and overdose are covered in appropriate medical textbooks. Typical withdrawal symptoms observed in commonly used substances are summarized in Table 24-6. Alcohol and opioid withdrawal are the most common withdrawal disorders, and clinicians can manage many patients in outpatient settings if the withdrawal syndrome is mild in severity (see Chapter 25 regarding opioid withdrawal). A common misperception among clinicians and the general population is that heavy cannabis use does not lead to withdrawal. However, we now know that cannabis withdrawal exists and is relatively common. Important parameters that patients should meet for adequate treatment in the outpatient setting include a commitment to abstaining from all mood-altering drugs during withdrawal (except as prescribed for withdrawal) and an expressed willingness to engage in continuing treatment. Persons who are homeless or others not living with someone who can help monitor medication and symptoms in case of adverse events, those with significant polysubstance use, and those with important or unstable medical or psychiatric illness should not be treated as outpatients.

With regard to alcohol, when physical dependence develops, initial withdrawal symptoms of anxiety, sleep disorder, and tremor are mild, sometimes not attributed to alcohol, and easily relieved by drinking. As time passes, alcohol less reliably controls symptoms, and intoxication is fleeting, occurring only at a high blood alcohol level (BAL) (>250 mg/dL). Withdrawal is not an all-or-nothing state, and physiologically dependent

Table 24-6. Withdrawal symptoms of commonly used substances.

Drug	Action	Withdrawal Onset	Duration	Characteristics
Cocaine	Stimulant	Varies but can begin within hours of last use	3–4 days	- Insomnia or hypersomnia - Increased appetite - Depression - Paranoia - Decreased energy
Alcohol	Sedative	24–48 hours	5–7 days	- Increased blood pressure - Increased heart rate - Elevated temperature - Nausea, vomiting, diarrhea - Seizures - Delirium - Death
Opioids	Sedative, euphoriant	Within 24 hours of last use	4–7 days	- Nausea, vomiting, diarrhea - Restlessness - Muscle and bone pain - Leg movements
Cannabis	Euphoriant, hallucinogenic at high doses	Ongoing debate about cannabis withdrawal, but onset may be within the first 10 days of last use	May last up to several weeks	- Irritability - Difficulty sleeping - Decreased appetite - Anxiety

Data from Center for Substance Abuse Treatment. *Treatment Improvement Protocol (TIP): Detoxification and substance abuse treatment.* 2006. Available at: https://www.ncbi.nlm.nih.gov/books/NBK64115/. Accessed August 2018; National Institute on Drug Abuse. *Commonly abused drugs and withdrawal symptoms.* Available at: https://www.drugabuse.gov/drugs-abuse/commonly-abused-drugs-charts. Accessed August 2018.

patients experience symptoms whenever their BAL falls. The altered neurophysiology in the brain "perceives" a drop in BAL as disruptive to the new steady-state condition of addiction and expresses the disruption through withdrawal symptoms. Soon, the person drinks steadily to alleviate withdrawal, but relief is brief. The range of BAL at which the individual feels "not sick" diminishes, and severe withdrawal, even delirium tremens, may develop despite a BAL of 300 mg/dL or more.

Outpatient treatment can be attempted in mild withdrawal. Clinicians should hospitalize patients with clouded sensorium, fever, hyperventilation, a concomitant medical problem (e.g., hepatic failure and pancreatitis), or a history of alcohol withdrawal-related seizures, or if the patient has three risk factors for severe withdrawal (Table 24-7). Degree of tremor, anxiety, tachycardia, and stomach symptoms are poor predictors of need for inpatient care. When outpatient management is feasible, pharmacological support helps with symptom relief (Table 24-8) and must be integrated with patient education and referral options designed to help patients change entrenched behaviors. Medical withdrawal from alcohol should not be attempted on outpatients unless a responsible significant other has been identified who will stay with the patient and ensure that the medications for the patient are administered according to the clinician's instructions. If there is not such a support system, a patient should be admitted to the hospital or residential substance use treatment facility where 24-hour skilled staff are available.

Patients should check with their clinician face to face every 2–3 days until symptoms are minimal, and during the withdrawal process make initial contact with a professional treatment program. The patient will relapse unless support in coping with psychosocial aspects of dependence is available. We underscore this crucial point: treatment of withdrawal is not treatment of an alcohol use disorder.

Patients with an alcohol use disorder and concurrent benzodiazepine use (either nonmedically or prescribed)

Table 24-7. Risk factors for severe alcohol withdrawal.

- Daily drinking for extended period of time.
- Sedative, cocaine, or opiate opioid use.
- History of severe withdrawal.
- High alanine aminotransferase.
- High serum γ-glutamyl transpeptidase.
- Low platelet count.
- Low potassium level.

Data from Goodson CM, et al. *Alcohol Clin Exp Res* 2014;38(10): 2664–2677. Maldonado JR, et al. *Alcohol* 2014;48(4):375–390.

Table 24-8. Medication for outpatient alcohol withdrawal.

Day 1: Give 25–50 mg chlordiazepoxide initially, then 25–50 mg every 4–6 hours, if needed. Alternatively, in those with hepatic impairment, give lorazepam 1–2 mg initially; then 1 mg every 4–6 hours as needed.
Day 2: Give 25 mg chlordiazepoxide every 4–6 hours. Alternatively, give lorazepam 1 mg every 4–6 hours.
Day 3 Give 25 mg chlordiazepoxide every 6–8 hours. Alternatively, give lorazepam 1 mg every 6–8 hours.
Day 4: Give 25 mg chlordiazepoxide or lorazepam 1 mg every 12 hours.
Day 5: Give 25 mg chlordiazepoxide or lorazepam 1 mg; then discontinue.
Patients should be evaluated daily when undergoing outpatient alcohol medical withdrawal as severe withdrawal not controlled by the recommended doses can be associated with complications including seizures or the development of delirium tremens. Those with ongoing withdrawal symptoms despite medication should be admitted to the hospital to safely complete withdrawal.
Admit for inpatient withdrawal treatment if the patient drinks or uses other drugs during taper.
All patients should be prescribed a multivitamin containing thiamine and folate to reduce risk of anemia and worsening encephalopathy.

are not candidates for outpatient medical withdrawal. Their medication needs are likely to be significantly higher than for a patient physiologically dependent on alcohol alone. The use of high doses of benzodiazepines during medical withdrawal procedures can be medically dangerous and such patients should be referred for inpatient treatment.

INTERVENTION STRATEGIES

Early intervention is more important than certainty about diagnosis. Clinicians should always share their concern when they perceive a potential problem with drugs or alcohol. Effectiveness is more dependent on intervening early with the style and skills we discuss, rather than waiting to get the diagnosis exactly correct. Habits and addictive cycles are complex and entrenched, so starting earlier with effective brief interventions is better than waiting. The strategies described below are drawn from the NIDA and NIAAA Clinician's Guides for brief interventions for alcohol drug problems in primary care settings as well as the motivational interviewing treatment model of Miller and Rollnick.

Assess Patients' Current Readiness to Reduce Substance Use

As we move from data gathering to sharing information and planning, we like to begin with an assessment of interest in changing alcohol or drug use. An inquiry regarding current readiness level can also open a useful dialogue that can serve to increase motivation. For example:

> ***Doctor:*** *How interested are you in making a change in your cannabis use at this time, on a scale of 0–10?*
>
> ***Jim:*** *Well, I would say about a 2.*
>
> ***Doctor:*** *Why would you say a 2 and not 0?*
>
> ***Jim:*** *I am a little concerned about how much money I have been spending on it every week.*
>
> ***Doctor:*** *Tell me a little more about how cannabis may be impacting your finances and what your concerns are.*

As this example illustrates, it is helpful to listen carefully for what patients report as their specific reasons for change. Miller and Rollnick refer to this as "change talk." Whereas a clinician is typically most concerned about the impact of alcohol or drug use on health, often patients are more concerned about other issues that nevertheless are important sources of motivation to reduce use, as in the example here in which the patient is more concerned about the financial cost of drug use. Listening for change talk is an important strategy for clinicians to use, allowing patients to make the case for change in their own words. As shown above, the physician responds with reflection or a request for elaboration.

Support Autonomy

Patients must make commitments and decisions in an atmosphere that genuinely tolerates and respects the full expression of ambivalence, resistance, and uncertainty, with respect to both facts and feelings. Clinicians create such an atmosphere when they show they are listening to patients' perspectives without judgment by simply reflecting what they hear, and by reminding patients that they are in charge of all the important decisions, and free to take whatever action (or inaction) they choose. That is, clinicians recognize patients' autonomy, while simultaneously offering their own expertise, clear recommendations, and support. A more explicit autonomy supportive statement (to Jim, above) could have been:

> ***Jim:*** *I'm quitting until I get my license back, no problem.*
>
> ***Doctor:*** *It is your choice whether you wish to make any change in your drinking. I will always give you my best advice, and you make the final decisions.*

CREATE DIALOGUE

True dialogue is difficult in conversations that involve substantial differentials in perspectives, expertise, and/or power. Patients tend either to defend a point of view or to be passive and silent. Clinicians can encourage dialogue by consciously employing a format of "inform, ask, inform, ask," which supports taking turns and results in a dialogue. Briefly provide advice or information (i.e., "inform"), and then "ask" patients what they think about it, or how it feels to hear it, or what they intend to do about it. Keeping the "informing" brief helps clarity, and "asking" allows the patient to choose a "change-enhancing" or "change-obstructing" response. The manner in which patients respond to the "ask" also suggests which next steps will likely be helpful. Generally, "change-enhancing" responses include statements of agreement, commitment, or optimism, and these suggest that exploring the facts might be helpful. Generally, "change-obstructing" responses, such as statements of disagreement, reservation, pessimism, defensiveness, noncommittal statements, and all questions that do not ask for clarification of meaning, suggest that the clinician should reflect back the response as the next step in the conversation. Reflection invites patients to look inside themselves and encourages motivation and attention to discrepancy between patients' current situation and stated goals. Both "asking" and making reflections foster exploration and choice.

Dialogue About Information

Provide information about what is known about drug problems in an impersonal "objective" or "scientific" way. Here are some examples:

- "Research shows that treatment helps," or
- "Steady drug use changes brain function," or
- "Having a high tolerance for alcohol means that a person is deprived of the early warning system that tells him to stop drinking before the alcohol level gets so high as to be dangerous," or
- "95% of men drink less than 35 drinks per week," or
- "Many people are terrified to imagine stopping drug use," or
- "Being sick in the morning until after a drink means a person's brain has become hooked on alcohol," or
- "Men with any close relative with drinking problems have an almost 50% chance of developing serious problems themselves," or
- "Guidelines from extensive research show that drinking more than 14 drinks a week is risky."

Next, *ask* what patients think of this information, and how it might apply to their situation.

Provide information about the patient's situation as a fact, a number, or score, rather than a conclusion:

- "Three of your liver tests are abnormal," rather than "alcohol has damaged your liver," or
- "Your alcohol level when you arrived in the emergency room was 0.160," rather than "You were drinking heavily before you came into the emergency room," or
- "You have a serious infection in your arm," rather than "You got this infection because you were injecting," or
- "You mentioned three important things—that your relationship with your wife is going poorly, that you are having a lot of stomach trouble, and that you lost your license to drive," rather than "Alcohol is wrecking your marriage, your career, and your body," or
- "You are very shaky and sick to your stomach until you can get another pill," rather than "You are addicted to tranquilizers," or
- "You have quit drinking several times," rather than "Your relapses show you are addicted."

Next, *ask* what the patient thinks of this information. Think about whether the patient's response to the "*ask*" is "change-obstructing" or "change-enhancing."

Dialogue About Recommendations; *Provide* Advice Clearly, but Not Harshly

Then, after discussing relevant information, *provide* advice tentatively, as part of a search for a suitable and attainable action option before the next visit. "Wagging one's finger," actually or figuratively, tends to push patients into a corner, it highlights any feelings of shame or stigma, and it inhibits discussion. Clinicians who display a posture of "I know what is right for you," without regard to cautions that apply to science (today's truth is tomorrow's fiction, and every case is unique), make patients defensive, and encourage arguments.

Useful advice has two other characteristics. First, give an objective rationale derived from a broader database than this case; and second, make your advice consistent with your assessment of your patient's willingness to consider it. The following specific examples illustrate these ideas.

- "The option that I recommend, based on data in the medical literature, and my experience with experts who have advised me about similar patients, is that you stop drinking all alcohol. Of course, no one can be certain that this is the right thing for you to do, or that it will work for you," or
- "Most people find that talking with people in Alcoholics Anonymous (AA) is helpful. AA might or might not be right for you. I recommend you go there."

Ask what the patient thinks of the advice. Commanding or ordering instead of checking the result of giving advice ensures poor adherence, as patients will not do things that they do not choose to do. If clinicians push ahead and try persuading patients in spite of reluctance, they foster continued ambivalence, raise resistance to change, and begin an enervating downward spiral in which both participants become further demoralized and discouraged.

> **Doctor:** *Jim, one option that I recommend, based on my experience with experts who have advised me about similar patients, is that you take this opportunity to stop drinking all alcohol, and actively*

participate in the counseling. Of course, no one can be certain that this is the right thing for you to do, or that it will work for you.

Jim: *Thanks for your concern, Doc, but I know I'm OK; I'll quit for now, zoom through the stupid counseling thing, and get my license right back.*

Doctor: *We have different perspectives, Jim. Your focus is on the license, while mine is on the big picture of alcohol effects over the years.*

Jim: *Doc, you know me pretty well, so maybe there is some truth in what you say.*

Doctor: *Since alcohol can have important effects on blood pressure, let's check your pressure while you are off alcohol and then continue our conversation about your license and drinking as well.*

Here is another example of how this discussion might proceed.

Jim: *Thanks for your concern, Doc, but I know I'm OK; I'll quit for now, zoom through the stupid counseling thing, and get my license right back.*

Doctor: *Jim, I appreciate that you are thinking about this matter, but are not interested in making a longer commitment right now. Before your next appointment with me, which I will schedule for about 6 weeks, I wonder if you would be willing to take careful note of both the good things about drinking and the not-so-good things about drinking? Think a bit about the good things and the not-so-good things about NOT drinking, too. Then, I'd value the chance to seek a deeper understanding of the total picture, and help you make the best decision you can for yourself, as time goes by.*

(Jim's response might surprise you)

Jim: *You know, a fellow at work has been pushing me to go to AA, and I almost went with him after I got my DUI* (driving under the influence; suggesting that Jim is or was more worried than he declares now).

(You might act on this hypothesis)

Doctor: *It seems that we agree that it might be good to do something differently right now. Many people learn a lot about themselves when they go to a few AA meetings with an open mind. Would you be willing to go to one meeting a week until I see you again in a month or so?*

Confirm Results of Dialogue

Finally, clinicians need to be explicit that agreement has been reached on a specific plan. Check with patients that they are indeed committed to the plan and confident that they can carry it out. Set a specific timetable to follow up.

Doctor: *"So, you are going to abstain until you get your license, and we'll meet to check your pressure and talk in about a month, right?"*

Doctor: *"You plan to go to six Alcoholics Anonymous meetings in the coming month, and we will talk about what you learn at your next appointment."*

Doctor: *"You decided to seek naltrexone to help with your alcohol cravings from the city clinic. I'll send them a note about your diabetes and anemia, and I look forward to seeing you again after you get started there."*

Helping to Maintain Change Over Time

At the follow-up visit, it is important to ask about any behavior change that the patient may have agreed to in the interim, even if the patient indicates that they are not yet ready to cut back on alcohol or drug use. For example, if the patient agreed to track how much they are drinking or to consider pros and cons of cutting back (as in the example above), continue the dialogue to help continue building patient motivation for change.

Many patients come to primary health care clinicians having already made changes in drinking and drug use. These patients will benefit from thoughtful follow-up regarding those changes. Begin by acknowledging that change is difficult, and support any positive change, or efforts to change. Listen to patients' perspectives on their situation and encourage reflection about both goals and strategies. Reaffirm your willingness to assist and talk, address any co-occurring psychiatric problems such as anxiety or depression, and renegotiate the goals and plans when appropriate.

PHARMACOLOGICAL CONSIDERATIONS

Medications for Alcohol Use Disorders

Currently there are three medications approved by the U.S. Food and Drug Administration (FDA) for the treatment of alcohol dependence (moderate to severe alcohol use disorder). These include disulfiram, naltrexone (both oral and injectable formulations), and acamprosate. All can be useful treatments in selected patients in the context of an office-based practice. Medication options are summarized in Table 24-9.

Disulfiram is an aldehyde dehydrogenase inhibitor that inhibits the metabolism of acetaldehyde, a metabolite of alcohol, leading to a noxious reaction that includes flushing, palpitations, and headaches when alcohol is ingested following disulfiram administration. Disulfiram may be best reserved for those who have either failed other alcohol medications or for highly motivated individuals for whom complete abstinence is a goal. For some individuals, it can be helpful to have a family member administer the disulfiram to optimize medication adherence. Disulfiram is contraindicated in pregnancy, in those with significant liver disease, esophageal varices, a history of gastrointestinal bleeding, or in those

Table 24-9. Medication options for the management of alcohol use disorder.

	Usual Dose	Common Adverse Effects	Special Considerations
FDA approved for alcohol use disorder			
Oral naltrexone	50 mg daily	Nausea Headache Dizziness	Should not be given to patients prescribed long-term opioids for pain. Patients should be counseled that their opioid tolerance may be lowered with naltrexone; careful titration of opioids upon stopping naltrexone is necessary to avoid potentially life-threatening opioid-related harms (i.e., respiratory depression, overdose). Contraindicated in acute hepatitis or liver failure
Depot naltrexone	380 mg intramuscularly every four weeks	Nausea Fatigue Decreased appetite	Should not be given to patients prescribed long-term opioids for pain management; may be used after 7–10 days of opioid abstinence for treatment of comorbid opioid use disorder. Patients should be counseled that opioid tolerance may be lowered with naltrexone; careful titration of opioids upon stopping naltrexone is necessary to avoid potentially life-threatening opioid-related harms (i.e., respiratory depression and overdose). Contraindicated in acute hepatitis or liver failure
Acamprosate	666 mg orally three times daily	Diarrhea Nervousness Fatigue	Lower doses may be needed for patients with renal impairment or body weight < 60 kg Contraindicated in patients with renal failure
Disulfiram	250–500 mg orally daily	Fatigue Drowsiness Headache	Reserved for highly motivated patients with goal of complete abstinence; may be helpful to have family member administer the medication Monitor for hepatotoxicity
Medications not FDA approved for alcohol use disorder			
Gabapentin	300–600 mg orally three times daily	Sedation Dizziness	Can be prone to misuse by some patients with substance use disorder
Topiramate	Start at 50 mg daily and increase to maximum dose of 150 mg twice daily	Cognitive impairment Paresthesia Weight loss Headache Fatigue Dizziness Depression	Titrate dose gradually over several weeks to minimize side effects
Baclofen	30–60 mg daily	Nausea Vertigo Sleepiness	Clinical trials have found mixed results and further investigation on efficacy of drug is warranted

Data from Substance Abuse and Mental Health Services Administration. *Medication for the Treatment of Alcohol Use Disorder: A Brief Guide*. Available at: https://store.samhsa.gov/product/Medication-for-the-Treatment-of-Alcohol-Use-Disorder-A-Brief-Guide/SMA15-4907. Accessed September 2018.

with psychosis, impulse control problems, or suicidality, as well as hypersensitivity to disulfiram or to other thiuram derivatives used in pesticides and rubber vulcanization. Patients who are taking or have recently taken metronidazole, paraldehyde, alcohol, or alcohol-containing preparations (e.g., cough syrups and tonics) should not be given disulfiram. Disulfiram labeling also includes several important precautions regarding drug–drug interactions. See the package insert for specific contraindications and warnings. A once-daily dose of disulfiram 250 mg will inhibit aldehyde dehydrogenases within 12 hours to a degree at which a disulfiram/alcohol reaction will be observed should alcohol be ingested. The aldehyde dehydrogenase enzymes are fully inhibited in 3 days. Further, patients must generate new enzymes that metabolize alcohol before they can drink again without experiencing the disulfiram/alcohol reaction, and this will require at least 6 days following the last dose of disulfiram.

Naltrexone is a mu-opioid antagonist medication that, in addition to being FDA approved for the treatment of opioid use disorder, is also approved for the treatment of alcohol dependence. Notably, compared to other medications for alcohol use disorder, naltrexone has the strongest data to support its use for this indication. Naltrexone is thought to decrease craving for alcohol because it blocks some of the pleasant and reinforcing effects of alcohol by preventing the stimulation of opioid receptors and the reduction of dopamine release in the ventral tegmental area (VTA). Naltrexone is given at a dose of 50 mg orally daily, and there is also an injectable form of the medication given once monthly in the buttock at a dose of 380 mg. Naltrexone is generally well tolerated; the most common side effects with naltrexone treatment are stomach upset and headache. The medication can be started at a lower dose (12.5–25 mg/d) if this is a concern. Naltrexone has been associated with hepatotoxicity in some, usually at doses much higher than those approved by the FDA, but this has led to recommendations of baseline liver function tests and follow-up tests approximately every 3 months. Because naltrexone is an opioid antagonist, it is contraindicated in those who will need opioid medications for pain relief or who are already receiving treatment with opioid pain relievers as this may lead to precipitated opioid withdrawal. It is important, therefore, that patients are opioid free at the time of initiation of naltrexone with up to 7–10 days of abstinence recommended when injectable naltrexone is prescribed for alcohol use disorder with comorbid opioid use disorder.

Acamprosate is an anticraving medication that stabilizes excitatory glutamatergic neurotransmission that is altered during withdrawal from alcohol and is also FDA approved for the treatment of alcohol dependence. Like disulfiram and naltrexone, it does not have mood-altering effects and no sedative/hypnotic or muscle relaxant properties. One difficulty for some patients is the need to take this medication three times daily. Acamprosate is renally cleared and can be an option for patients with an alcohol use disorder complicated by serious liver disease or for patients who need ongoing opioid pain medications. Because disulfiram, naltrexone, and acamprosate are not controlled substances and have no mood-altering effects, these medications are easily prescribed by primary care clinicians who can provide medical care for alcohol use disorders in addition to other medical illnesses.

Efforts to identify additional treatment options to address alcohol use disorder are ongoing. While studies to date support a potential role for gabapentin and topiramate, the data are less consistent for baclofen.

As detailed in the SAMHSA *Medication for the Treatment of Alcohol Use Disorder: A Brief Guide,* these medications are easy to prescribe, do not require specific training, and are safe and effective for decreasing alcohol use and its consequences among patients with alcohol use disorder. Consistent with the model of care for other chronic health conditions, such as diabetes mellitus and hypertension, patients should be offered these medications when presenting for treatment across medical settings. This includes primary care-based settings (e.g. primary care and HIV treatment settings), inpatient settings, and specialty care (i.e., addiction treatment programs). Ongoing training and support for prescribing these medications is available through the Provider Clinical Support System (www.pcssnow.org).

Medications to Address Drug Use

In contrast to alcohol use disorder, there are few pharmacological options available for managing stimulant and cannabis use disorder, although a number of compounds are being explored. Early trials evaluating the efficacy of dopamine agonists, disulfiram, and doxazosin have shown some indication that these medications may help reduce cocaine use. There is also tentative evidence to support further evaluation of bupropion, modafinil, naltrexone, and mirtazapine as adjuvant pharmacotherapy for persons with problematic methamphetamine use. Gabapentin, *N*-acetylcysteine, the sleep aid zolpidem, and an antianxiety/antistress medication called buspirone have shown the most promise in reducing cannabis use, but available data are inconclusive and further studies are warranted. The FDA has not approved any medication for the treatment of either stimulant or cannabis use disorder as no medication has consistently demonstrated efficacy in randomized trials. Psychosocial interventions using modalities like cognitive behavioral therapy, motivational interviewing, and contingency management have the most robust evidence supporting efficacy and are the primary approach to managing these disorders.

Preventive Health Measures Among Patients With Alcohol & Drug Use

Primary care clinicians are well-suited to provide preventive health and harm reduction measures that can help reduce morbidity associated with alcohol and drug use. For example, current guidelines recommend pneumonia vaccination in persons with an alcohol use disorder as these individuals are at increased risk for invasive pneumococcal disease. For persons who inject drugs, the Centers of Disease Control and Prevention recommends routine screening for HIV and other sexually transmitted infections, tuberculosis, and hepatitis C. Standing orders can be used to administer hepatitis A and B vaccines for persons who have not completed the series. Patients who inject drugs may also benefit from referrals to needle exchange programs, which can help reduce HIV and hepatitis C transmission.

Persons with unhealthy alcohol or drug use may also benefit from HIV pre-exposure prophylaxis (PrEP). PrEP is a biomedical strategy proven to reduce the risk of HIV acquisition in various populations, including men who have sex with men (MSM), transgender women, and persons who inject drugs. Clinicians should discuss sexual health with all of their patients, but particularly among those with signs or symptoms indicative of unhealthy substance use. "Chemsex," or the use of drugs such as methamphetamine and poppers during sex to enhance sexual pleasure, is a growing trend among MSM. These behaviors are well-established correlates of sexual risk taking and place individuals at increased risk for HIV and other sexually transmitted infections. Currently, the only medication approved for PrEP is daily oral emtricitabine–tenofovir disoproxil fumarate (FTC–TDF). The effectiveness of PrEP is contingent on optimal adherence, and when taken daily it can reduce the risk of HIV by over 90%. The need for daily adherence may be challenging for some patients as unhealthy alcohol and substance use have been associated with poor medication adherence and care engagement in other contexts. Available data evaluating how these behaviors affect PrEP adherence are limited and findings have been mixed. Most studies have found no association between unhealthy alcohol use and poor PrEP adherence, but there is some indication that persons who use stimulant drugs experience greater difficulty adhering to PrEP and remaining engaged in care. However, substance use should not preclude the provision of PrEP in individuals with known risk factors. Studies evaluating other medications and delivery methods that have a lower patient burden (e.g., injectable long-acting formulations, implants, or nondaily dosing) are underway. Clinical practice guidelines from the U.S. Public Health Service are routinely updated with recommendations for the management and monitoring of patients on PrEP.

Referral to Specialized Treatment

Addiction treatment programs provide patients with specialized care, and clinicians should refer any patient who does not make progress on changing substance use patterns in the primary care setting. Whether patients are making progress is more important to the need for referral than the apparent level of problem. Patients with substance use disorders may benefit from access to medical withdrawal services and multidisciplinary counseling opportunities. Treatment approaches included in specialty addiction treatment often include the pharmacological approaches described above, as well as behavioral interventions such as cognitive behavioral therapy and contingency management. Treatment programs can also help patients initiate contact with community-based self-help organizations, halfway houses, and intensive counseling, sometimes in an inpatient setting. Programs with co-occurring disorders treatment capabilities (i.e., the ability to provide treatment for both substance use disorders and other mental disorders) are able to serve patients with additional psychiatric problems known to occur frequently in those with substance use problems. Clinicians in these specialized treatment programs will be more familiar with, and so better prepared to treat, patients with substance use disorders complicated by mental illness. Findings from the 2016 National Survey on Drug Use and Health underscore the need for such programs as referral centers for the primary care provider who has identified a patient with multiple disorders. This survey reported rates of mental illness in those with substance use disorders to be 43% (versus a rate of mental illness in those without substance use disorders of 16%), and the rate of substance use disorders in those with mental illness was 10–27.8% depending on the severity of the mental illness (those without mental illness have an overall rate of substance use disorders of 5.4%).

Patients may resist following through on a referral for specialized treatment. A helpful strategy is to confirm the patient's intention and commitment to follow through, as discussed in the sections above on making choices, supporting autonomy, and giving advice. An additional strategy is to emphasize your need for a second opinion from a specialist, just as might be the case with referral to a cardiologist. Set up the appointment before the patient leaves the office. Tell the patient you will send a referral letter summarizing your views and asking for advice from the specialist. Let the patient know that you will speak with the specialist after the assessment, and that you would like to participate in the treatment plan. It may also be helpful to indicate that outpatient treatment programs often have flexible options in the services they offer—for example, intensive or less intensive services, day or evening programs—and to encourage patients to get an appointment with a program even if they are not sure that they are ready for abstinence.

Many communities have programs for patients with special needs, such as adolescents, women, those who use particular drugs (methadone treatment for opioid use disorder with evidence of physical dependence on opioids is the best-known example), and patients with severe psychiatric problems. Self-help alternatives to AA and other mutual help groups exist in many communities; Rational Recovery is one example, and Women for Sobriety is another. These resources are available to help primary care clinicians provide patients a range of available interventions. The primary care clinician can play a key role in screening patients for substance use problems, raising their motivation to reduce their substance use, providing brief interventions, and connecting them with other available resources, thus serving as a critical touchpoint on patients' road to recovery.

SUGGESTED READINGS

Center for Behavioral Health Statistics and Quality. *2016 National Survey on Drug Use and Health: Detailed Tables.* 2017. https://www.samhsa.gov/data/sites/default/files/NSDUH-DetTabs-2016/NSDUH-DetTabs-2016.pdf. Accessed August 2018.

Centers for Disease Control and Prevention (2018). Pre-exposure prophylaxis for the prevention of HIV infection in the United States—2017 update: A clinical practice guideline. https://www.cdc.gov/hiv/pdf/guidelines/cdc-hiv-prep-guidelines-2017.pdf. Accessed August 2018.

Chan KK, Neighbors C, Gilson M, Larimer ME, Marlatt GA. Epidemiological trends in drinking by age and gender: providing normative feedback to adults. *Addic Behav* 2007;32(5):967–976.

Fischer B, Russell C, Sabioni P, et al. Lower-risk cannabis use guidelines: a comprehensive update of evidence and recommendations. *Am J Public Health* 2017;107(8):e1–e12.

Haile CN, Kosten, TR. Pharmacotherapy for stimulant-related disorders. *Curr Psychiatry Rep* 2013;15(11).

Han B, Gfroerer JC, Colliver JD. Associations between duration of illicit drug use and health conditions: results from the 2005–2007 national surveys on drug use and health. *Ann Epidemiol* 2010;20(4):289–297.

Jonas DE, Garbutt JC, Amrick HR, et al. Behavioral counseling after screening for alcohol misuse in primary care: a systematic review and meta-analysis for the US Preventive Services Task Force. *Ann Intern Med* 2012;157(9):645–654.

National Institute on Drug Use (NIDA). *Screening for drug use in general medical settings.* https://www.drugabuse.gov/sites/default/files/resource_guide.pdf. Accessed August 2018.

NIAAA. *Helping patients who drink too much: a clinician's guide.* 2005. https://pubs.niaaa.nih.gov/publications/practitioner/cliniciansguide2005/guide.pdf. Accessed August 2018.

Pace CA, Samet JH. Substance use disorders. *Ann Intern Med* 2016;164(7):ITC49–ITC64.

Rollnick S, Miller WR, Butler CC. *Motivational Interviewing in Health Care.* New York, NY: Guilford; 2008.

Substance Abuse and Mental Health Services Administration and National Institute on Alcohol Abuse and Alcoholism. *Medication for the Treatment of Alcohol Use Disorder: A Brief Guide.* HHS Publication No. (SMA) 15-4907. Rockville, MD: Substance Abuse and Mental Health Services Administration; 2015.

Wamsley M, Satterfield J, Curtis A, Levy E, Lundgren L, Satre DD. Alcohol and drug use screening, brief intervention and referral to treatment (SBIRT) training and implementation: perspectives from four health professions. *J AddictMed* 2018;12(4):262–272.

Willenbring ML, Massey SH, Gardner MB. Helping patients who drink too much: an evidence-based guide for primary care physicians. *Am Fam Physician* 2009;80(1):44–50.

WEBSITES

Clark WC, Parish S. *Alcohol: Interviewing and Advising. Module in Doc.com: An Interactive Learning Resource for Healthcare Communication.* American Academy on Communication in Healthcare. http://doccom.aachonline.org/dnn/Home.aspx. Accessed August 2018.

National Institute on Alcohol Abuse and Alcoholism (NIAAA). www.niaaa.nih.gov. Accessed August 2018.

Providers' Clinical Support System for Medication Assisted Treatment. www.pcssnow.org. Accessed August 2018.

Substance Abuse and Mental Health Services Administration. http://www.samhsa.gov/. Accessed August 2018.

SCORING THE AUDIT (Appendix 24-A)

Record the score for each response in the blank box at the end of each line, then total these numbers. The maximum possible total is 40. Total scores of 8 or more for men up to the age of 60 years or 4 or more for women, adolescents, and men over the age of 60 years are considered positive screens. For patients with totals near the cut-points, clinicians may wish to examine individual responses to questions and clarify them during the clinical examination.

Note: The AUDIT's sensitivity and specificity for detecting heavy drinking and alcohol use disorders varies across different populations. Lowering the cut-points increases sensitivity (the proportion of "true positive" cases), whereas increasing the number of false positives. Thus, it may be easier to use a cut-point of 4 for all patients, recognizing that more false positives may be identified among men.

Appendix 24-A. The Alcohol Use Disorders Identification Test (AUDIT).

AUDIT

PATIENT: Because alcohol use can affect your health and can interfere with certain medications and treatments, it is important that we ask some questions about your use of alcohol. Your answers will remain confidential, so please be honest.

For each question in the chart below, place an X in one box that best describes your answer.

NOTE: In the United States, a single drink serving contains about 14 g of ethanol or "pure" alcohol. Although the drinks below are different sizes, each one contains the same amount of pure alcohol and counts as a single drink:

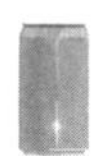

12 oz. of beer (about 5% alcohol) =

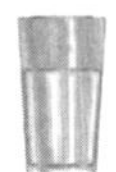

8-9 oz. of malt liquor (about 7% alcohol) =

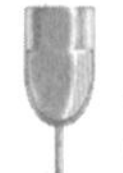

5 oz. of wine (about 12% alcohol) =

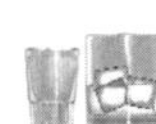

1.5 oz. of hard liquor (about 40% alcohol)

Questions	0	1	2	3	4	
1. How often do you have a drink containing alcohol?	Never	Monthly or less	2 to 4 times a month	2 to 3 times a week	4 or more times a week	
2. How many drinks containing alcohol do you have on a typical day when you are drinking?	1 or 2	3 or 4	5 or 6	7 to 9	10 or more	
3. How often do you have 5 or more drinks on one occasion?	Never	Less than monthly	Monthly	Weekly	Daily or almost daily	
4. How often during the last year have you found that you were not able to stop drinking once you had started?	Never	Less than monthly	Monthly	Weekly	Daily or almost daily	
5. How often during the last year have you failed to do what was normally expected of you because of drinking?	Never	Less than monthly	Monthly	Weekly	Daily or almost daily	
6. How often during the last year have you needed a first drink in the morning to get yourself going after a heavy drinking session?	Never	Less than monthly	Monthly	Weekly	Daily or almost daily	
7. How often during the last year have you had a feeling of guilt or remorse after drinking?	Never	Less than monthly	Monthly	Weekly	Daily or almost daily	
8. How often during the last year have you been unable to remember what happened the night before because of your drinking?	Never	Less than monthly	Monthly	Weekly	Daily or almost daily	
9. Have you or someone else been injured because of your drinking?	No		Yes, but not in the last year		Yes, during the last year	
10. Has a relative, friend, doctor, or other health care worker been concerned about your drinking or suggested you cut down?	No		Yes, but not in the last year		Yes, during the last year	
					Total	

Note: This questionnaire (the AUDIT) is reprinted with permission from the World Health Organization. To reflect drink serving sizes in the United States (14 g of pure alcohol), the number of drinks in question 3 was changed from 6 to 5. A free AUDIT manual with guidelines for use in primary care settings is available online at www.who.org.

Excerpted from NIH Publication No. 07-3769 National Institute on Alcohol and Alcoholism www.niaaa.nih.gov/guide

Opioids

25

Stephen G. Henry, MD, MSc

INTRODUCTION

Opioid analgesics play a central role in pain management; hydrocodone-acetaminophen is the most commonly prescribed medication the United States. At the same time, widespread use of opioid analgesics to treat chronic pain in the 1990s and 2000s contributed to a rapid rise in opioid-related deaths and patients diagnosed with opioid use disorder. In 2016 more than 42,000 deaths in the United States were associated with prescription opioids, including 1 in 5 deaths among adults between 25 and 34 years old. Encouraging behavioral change related to pain and opioids can be especially challenging; both clinicians and patients report that conversations about opioids, especially opioids prescribed for chronic pain, are frequently frustrating and unproductive.

Because of the rise in opioid-related deaths, opioid analgesics are currently the focus of intense clinical and health services research. Laws, policies, and regulations related to opioid prescribing are also rapidly changing. In most cases these changes involve increasing regulations and restrictions around opioid prescribing.

This chapter provides practical strategies clinicians can use to encourage behavior change related to managing opioids, with a focus on opioid prescribing for chronic pain. Two overarching principles should be kept in mind when managing prescription opioids:

1. Decisions to prescribe opioids should be based on the overall balance of opioid-related risks and benefits for individual patients. Assessing risks and benefits requires attention to both patients' perspectives and objective evaluation of patients' functional status and opioid-related risks, particularly overdose and substance use disorder.
2. Effective communication is critical for managing prescription opioids. Effective communication requires taking the patient's pain seriously, managing the unpleasant emotions that often arise (for both patients and clinicians) during discussions about opioids, and navigating disagreements, all while maintaining a therapeutic relationship.

Skillful opioid prescribing and effective communication require clinical knowledge of both pain management and management of substance use disorders. These important topics are discussed in more detail in Chapters 38 and 24, respectively. This chapter focuses on challenges that are relatively unique to prescription opioids.

HISTORICAL PERSPECTIVE ON OPIOIDS

The attitude of organized medicine and society towards opioid analgesics has shifted over time, sometimes emphasizing opioids' ability to reduce pain and relieve suffering, and other times emphasizing opioids' addictive, destructive potential (Table 25-1). Opioids are chemical derivatives of opium, which is harvested from the seed pods of the opium poppy, *Papaver somniferum.* Opium has been cultivated and used for thousands of years for both therapeutic and recreational purposes. Processed opium is either smoked or swallowed, usually in the form of a liquid solution. Laudanum, a tincture of opium mixed with alcohol, was popularized by Thomas Sydenham in the 1660s. Morphine is a naturally-occurring component of opium that was isolated in the early nineteenth century and was commercially available in Europe and the United States by the 1820s. Morphine became extremely popular in large part due to the invention of the hypodermic needle, which made it possible to administer morphine subcutaneously and intravenously. Both the analgesic benefits and addictive potential of morphine were readily appreciated by the late nineteenth century. Diacetylmorphine, or heroin, was first synthesized in 1874 as part of a search (still ongoing today) for nonaddictive alternatives to morphine.

In 1914 the United States passed the Harrison Narcotics Tax Act, the first major federal law to regulate and tax the manufacture and sale of opioids. This law was prompted by concerns about widespread morphine addiction; its subsequent interpretation by the federal courts effectively outlawed prescribing morphine to

Table 25-1. Partial timeline of events related to opioid use in the United States.

Year	Event
1914	Harrison Narcotics Tax Act establishes federal regulation of opioids
1970	Comprehensive Drug Abuse Prevention and Control Act creates the modern regulatory framework for controlled substances
1990	California and Texas pass the first "Intractable Pain Laws" legalizing use of prescription opioids to treat chronic pain
1996	American Pain Society launches the "Fifth Vital Sign" public health campaign
2000	Drug Addiction Treatment Act allows qualified physicians to prescribe Schedule III-IV opioids (i.e., buprenorphine) to treat opioid use disorder in the office setting
2007	Perdue Pharmaceuticals executives convicted of criminally misbranding OxyContin© (long-acting oxycodone)
2010	First large study published showing an association between higher opioid doses and increased overdose risk
2016	CDC publishes opioid prescribing guidelines that discourage use of opioids as first line treatment for chronic pain
2017	President Trump declares the "opioid crisis" to be a national public health emergency

patients with active opioid use disorder. These changes led to prosecution of thousands of clinicians and forced many patients with opioid use disorder to consume illicit opioids, including heroin, instead. During the mid-twentieth century, clinical use of opioids was largely confined to treating acute or postsurgical pain.

In the late 1970s, clinicians began to advocate for the use of opioids as a part of palliative care for patients with terminal cancer pain. Opioids appeared to successfully relieve pain and suffering for these patients, and so in the mid-1980s, clinicians began to advocate for the use of opioids to treat chronic, noncancer pain. During the 1990s, many states passed laws explicitly legalizing the prescription of opioids to treat "intractable pain"; these laws typically excluded patients with active substance use disorders. The passage of these laws indicates the degree to which prescribing opioids for chronic pain was a departure from the clinical standards of care that developed after the Harrison Act. In 1996 the American Pain Society launched a successful public health campaign to treat pain as the "Fifth Vital Sign" in order to highlight patients' ethical right to pain treatment and to encourage the use of opioids to treat chronic pain. Both the Joint Commission and the Veterans Health Administration adopted the "Fifth Vital Sign" policy, effectively mandating regular pain assessment in both the inpatient and outpatient settings.

As a result of these changes, opioid prescribing nearly quadrupled between 1999 and 2010, largely because of increased use for chronic pain. Most clinicians and patients who advocated for increased use of opioids were motivated by a sincere desire to provide patient-centered, compassionate care to patients suffering from chronic pain. In hindsight, it is clear that many pharmaceutical companies intentionally minimized or hid the addictive potential of long-term opioid use. In 2007, executives from Perdue Pharmaceuticals pled guilty to criminally misbranding OxyContin© (long-acting oxycodone).

In the 2010s, evidence of increases in opioid-related overdoses began to emerge, and cohort studies established a dose-response relationship between prescribed opioid dose and overdose risk. The continual rise in opioid-related overdose deaths eventually prompted the Centers for Disease Control and Prevention (CDC) to issue clinical guidelines for opioid prescribing (Table 25-2) that emphasized opioid-related risks and discouraged the use of opioids as a first-line treatment for chronic pain. Nationwide, opioid prescribing peaked between 2010 and 2012 and began to decline thereafter. The CDC guidelines accelerated this decline; however, there is substantial geographic variation in opioid prescribing across the United States.

A small proportion (5–10%) of high-risk patients account for most prescription opioid-related overdoses. The rate of heroin-related overdose deaths, which had been stable for many years, began to rise in 2010, likely due to high-risk patients starting to use heroin when they could no longer obtain prescription opioids. In 2018, most heroin users reported using prescription opioids before transitioning to heroin; however, the vast majority of patients prescribed opioids do not become heroin users. In 2014, deaths related to use of illicit fentanyl began to increase dramatically, and by 2017 overdose deaths associated with illicit opioids outnumbered deaths associated with prescription opioids. Illicit fentanyl is extremely potent and much cheaper to manufacture than heroin. It is typically packaged and sold mixed with or disguised as heroin or prescription opioids, and can be fatal to first-time users.

PHYSIOLOGIC EFFECTS OF OPIOIDS

The term *opiate* refers to compounds structurally related to opium; *opioid* refers to any substance that acts on an opioid receptor, including endogenous opioids present in the central nervous system. Both terms are used interchangeably in clinical contexts. The physiologic effects of opioids are mediated primarily through activation of the mu opioid receptor, which is associated with the brain's pain and reward pathways. Thus, opioid use

Table 25-2. CDC recommendations for prescribing opioids for chronic pain.

1. Nonpharmacologic therapy and nonopioid pharmacologic therapy are preferred for chronic pain. Clinicians should consider opioid therapy only if expected benefits for both pain and function are anticipated to outweigh risks to the patient. If opioids are used, they should be combined with nonpharmacologic therapy and nonopioid pharmacologic therapy, as appropriate.
2. Before starting opioid therapy for chronic pain, clinicians should establish treatment goals with all patients, including realistic goals for pain and function, and should consider how therapy will be discontinued if benefits do not outweigh risks. Clinicians should continue opioid therapy only if there is clinically meaningful improvement in pain and function that outweighs risks to patient safety.
3. Before starting and periodically during opioid therapy, clinicians should discuss with patients known risks and realistic benefits of opioid therapy and patient and clinician responsibilities for managing therapy.
4. When starting opioid therapy for chronic pain, clinicians should prescribe immediate-release opioids instead of extended-release/long-acting (ER/LA) opioids.
5. When opioids are started, clinicians should prescribe the lowest effective dosage. Clinicians should use caution when prescribing opioids at any dosage, should carefully reassess evidence of individual benefits and risks when increasing dosage to 50 morphine milligram equivalents (MME) or more per day, and should avoid increasing dosage to 90 MME or more per day or carefully justify a decision to titrate dosage to 90 MME or more per day.
6. Long-term opioid use often begins with treatment of acute pain. When opioids are used for acute pain, clinicians should prescribe the lowest effective dose of immediate-release opioids and should prescribe no greater quantity than needed for the expected duration of pain severe enough to require opioids. Three days or less will often be sufficient; >7 days will rarely be needed.
7. Clinicians should evaluate benefits and harms with patients within 1–4 weeks of starting opioid therapy for chronic pain or of dose escalation. Clinicians should evaluate benefits and harms of continued therapy with patients every 3 months or more frequently. If benefits do not outweigh harms of continued opioid therapy, clinicians should optimize therapies and work with patients to taper opioids to lower dosages or to taper and discontinue opioids.
8. Before starting and periodically during continuation of opioid therapy, clinicians should evaluate risk factors for opioid-related harms. Clinicians should incorporate into the management plan strategies to mitigate risk, including considering offering naloxone when factors that increase risk for opioid overdose, such as history of overdose, history of substance use disorder, higher opioid dosages (≥50 MME/d), or concurrent benzodiazepine use are present.
9. Clinicians should review the patient's history of controlled substance prescriptions using state prescription drug monitoring program (PDMP) data to determine whether the patient is receiving opioid dosages or dangerous combinations that put him or her at high risk for overdose. Clinicians should review PDMP data when starting opioid therapy for chronic pain and periodically during opioid therapy for chronic pain, ranging from every prescription to every 3 months.
10. When prescribing opioids for chronic pain, clinicians should use urine drug testing before starting opioid therapy and consider urine drug testing at least annually to assess for prescribed medications as well as other controlled prescription drugs and illicit drugs.
11. Clinicians should avoid prescribing opioid pain medication and benzodiazepines concurrently whenever possible.
12. Clinicians should offer or arrange evidence-based treatment (usually medication-assisted treatment with buprenorphine or methadone in combination with behavioral therapies) for patients with opioid use disorder.

Adapted from Dowell D, Haegerich TM, Chou R. CDC Guideline for Prescribing Opioids for Chronic Pain—United States, 2016. *JAMA.* 2016;315(15):1624–1645.

reliably leads to pain relief as well as euphoria, which can range from decreased anxiety to a physiologic "high." Regular use of opioid analgesics results in tolerance (i.e., higher doses are required to achieve the same analgesic or euphoric effects) and physiologic dependence (i.e., stopping or decreasing opioids causes withdrawal symptoms). Acute opioid withdrawal is often very uncomfortable but, unlike alcohol or benzodiazepine withdrawal, is not physiologically dangerous.

Table 25-3 lists commonly used opioid analgesics. Opioids' potency is measured relative to morphine, and is expressed in morphine milligram equivalents (MME). The conversion factors listed in Table 25-3 are widely accepted approximations based on clinical consensus. The relative potency of methadone is variable, and increases with both higher doses and prolonged use. Cross-tolerance between different opioids is incomplete, so replacing one opioid with another, or "opioid rotation," is a common clinical strategy for avoiding dose escalation among patients who have developed opioid tolerance after long-term use. When rotating opioids, start with a dose of the new medication that decreases the patient's overall daily MME to avoid inadvertent oversedation.

OPIOID EFFICACY

The analgesia, euphoria, and side effects caused by particular opioids vary substantially from patient to patient, so the risks and benefits of each medication should be assessed for each patient individually. For example, a

Table 25-3. Relative potency of commonly used opioid analgesics.

	Oral Morphine Equivalents
Natural opiates	
morphine	1.0
codeine	0.15
Semisynthetic opiates	
hydrocodone	1.0
oxycodone	1.5
oxymorphone	3.0
hydromorphone	4.0
Synthetic opioids	
fentanyl (transdermal), mcg/h	2.4
methadone	4–12
tramadol	0.1–0.2
tapentadol	0.4
Partial opioid agonists	
buprenorphine	10–13

patient who gets excellent pain relief from hydrocodone may experience minimal pain relief and intolerable sedation from oxycodone.

Acute Pain

Opioids play a central role in acute pain treatment in the hospital and emergency department settings; 80% of patients undergoing common ambulatory surgical procedures are prescribed opioids at discharge. However, 3–6% of patients prescribed opioids after major surgery, and 10% of patients prescribed opioids after cancer surgery become long-term opioid users who are still taking opioids a year after surgery. Similarly, a small proportion of patients prescribed opioids for acute pain in the emergency department or primary care setting become long-term opioid users. Long-term opioid use is defined as using opioids for more than 90 days, because most patients prescribed opioids for more than 90 days tend to stay on opioids for years. The CDC recommendation to limit opioid prescribing for acute and postoperative pain to 7 days' supply or less (see Table 25-2) is an effort to prevent patients prescribed opioids for acute pain from becoming long-term opioid users due to automatic refills or clinical inertia.

Many emergency departments have developed pain management protocols to minimize opioid use and, by extension, the number of patients discharged from the emergency department with short-term opioid prescriptions. There is increasing evidence that suggests nonsteroidal anti-inflammatory drugs (NSAIDs) are reasonable alternatives to opioids for acute pain relief. A recent clinical trial found that ibuprofen, oxycodone, hydrocodone, and codeine all provided similar short-term pain relief for patients presenting to an emergency department with extremity pain. However, a substantial minority of study patients treated with ibuprofen required opioids to achieve sufficient pain control, and the study excluded patients with prior analgesic use or contraindications to non-opioid medications. Nevertheless, nonopioid analgesics should be used as first-line treatments for acute pain when feasible.

Chronic Pain

The widespread adoption of opioids to treat chronic pain in the 1990s and 2000s was not supported by robust empirical evidence. Few studies of long-term opioid use have followed patients for more than 12 weeks, many studies were sponsored by pharmaceutical companies, and a large proportion of study patients dropped out due to intolerable opioid side effects or lack of efficacy. The SPACE trial, the first randomized study of opioid use for chronic pain that followed patients for at least 1 year, was published in 2018. This study compared an opioid-intensive versus an opioid-sparing analgesic treatment protocol among veterans with back, neck, or hip pain who had not previously tried opioids. It found that opioid-intensive and opioid-sparing analgesic protocols were associated with clinically similar levels of pain relief for hip, knee, or back pain after 1 year, though patients in the opioid-intensive regimen reported more side effects. Additional clinical trials evaluating opioid use for chronic pain are ongoing and will eventually expand the evidence available for clinical decision making. In the meantime, the SPACE study is consistent with the CDC recommendations that opioids should not be considered first-line treatments for chronic pain.

For all patients, opioids should be considered as one component of a comprehensive pain treatment plan; opioids alone are not sufficient to treat chronic pain. Clinicians should avoid a one-size-fits-all approach to prescribing opioids for chronic pain. Some patients with chronic opioids do benefit from long-term opioid use; other patients have contraindications to NSAIDs and other nonopioid analgesics. Patients who benefit from long-term opioid use typically experience these benefits at low or moderate opioid doses. Most patients with chronic pain who do not experience clinical benefit from taking 60 to 90 daily MME will not obtain benefit with further dose escalation. *Evaluation of clinical benefits of long-term opioid use should be based on patients' functional improvement with opioids, and not on changes in numeric pain rating scores.* Numeric pain rating scales have limited value for evaluating chronic pain; high scores often indicated psychosocial distress or other factors that are correlated with but distinct from pain intensity.

Cancer Pain

Opioids are the mainstay of pain treatment for patients in active cancer treatment. However, there is minimal evidence about the safety or efficacy of long-term opioid use among cancer patients or cancer survivors, and the CDC guidelines exclude patients being treated for cancer. Patients taking opioids for cancer pain are much less stigmatized than patients taking opioids for chronic noncancer pain, because cancer can be objectively diagnosed and so is considered a more "legitimate" reason to have pain in Western culture.

Neuropathic Pain

Opioids are not recommended to treat pain due to nerve damage or dysfunction, including pain from diabetic neuropathy, fibromyalgia, or sciatica.

OPIOID SIDE EFFECTS

In addition to analgesia and euphoria, opioid analgesics produce many clinically important side effects. Opioid-naïve patients often describe their first experience with opioids as unpleasant, and bothersome side effects are a major reason that patients elect to discontinue opioids. Knowledge of clinically important opioid side effects is necessary in order to ask, and when necessary, educate patients about them. Patients may not connect less obvious side effects, such as hypogonadism or hyperalgesia, with their opioid use. Explaining the link between opioid use and bothersome symptoms is often an effective way to encourage patients to reduce their opioid dose.

Developing an "Opioid Review of Systems," such as the one shown in Table 25-4, is a useful way to remember and ask about the full range of opioid-related side effects. Patients are more likely to notice side effects when they first start taking opioids and when they increase their opioid dose. Patients develop tolerance to different effects of opioids at different rates. Tolerance to opioids' analgesic and euphoric effects develops faster than does tolerance to opioid-related respiratory depression; patients taking higher opioid doses to maintain pain relief or euphoria are thus at heightened risk for inadvertent overdose. Clinicians should counsel patients about these risks before increasing their opioid dose.

The physiologic basis for opioid-induced hyperalgesia is poorly understood, but it is common with long-term use of opioids at doses more than 90 MME. Hyperalgesia manifests as diffuse, generalized pain and an abnormally low pain threshold; patients with hyperalgesia report severe pain with minor trauma or with normal movements during daily activities. Hyperalgesia can be reversed by reducing patients' opioid dose and is one reason that most patients report their pain intensity decreases or does not change after they taper down from high opioid doses.

Table 25-4. "Opioid Review of Systems" for clinically important side effects associated with oral opioid consumption or opioid withdrawal.

General	Fatigue, sedation, euphoria, inability to drive, falls, opioid-induced hyperalgesia
HEENT	Miosis, dry mouth, watery eyes,* allergy symptoms,* rhinorrhea*
Cardiac	Increased blood pressure,* tachycardia*
Pulmonary	Decreased respiratory drive, central sleep apnea
Gastrointestinal	Nausea, vomiting, constipation, diarrhea*
Skin	Pruritus, flushing
Genitourinary	Urinary retention
Endocrine	Hypogonadism, decreased libido, menstrual irregularities, osteoporosis
Rheumatologic	Muscle or joint aches,* inability to get out of bed in the morning without opioids*
Psychiatric	Social isolation, anhedonia, increased time and energy spent thinking about opioids, anxiety,* restlessness,* insomnia*

*Symptoms associated with opioid withdrawal.

Decreased respiratory drive due to opioid use is the major cause of opioid overdose. Patients do not perceive the effects of opioids on their breathing. Patients taking opioids for chronic pain should be screened for obstructive sleep apnea and should undergo a sleep study when there is clinical suspicion for obstructive or central sleep apnea. Elderly patients on long-term opioids should be evaluated for fall risk. Opioid-related endocrine dysfunction is most common among patients taking long-acting or extended-release opioids, such as methadone or transdermal fentanyl. When patients endorse decreased libido or menstrual irregularities, laboratory testing for the relevant sex hormones should be performed. Dual-energy x-ray absorptiometry (DEXA) scans can be obtained to evaluate patients on long-acting opioids for osteoporosis, especially for patients with additional osteoporosis risk factors.

Some unpleasant symptoms associated with long-term opioid use indicate mild or moderate opioid withdrawal. Most patients can easily identify severe withdrawal, which is marked by diarrhea, arthralgia, and flu-like symptoms. However, they may not recognize mild withdrawal symptoms, such as rhinorrhea, insomnia, and anxiety. For patients who have been on opioids for months or years, it is important to distinguish uncontrolled pain from opioid withdrawal. These two categories are not always mutually exclusive.

Table 25-5. Distinguishing uncontrolled pain from opioid withdrawal.

Useful questions
- What happens when you miss or are late for a dose of your pain medicine?
- Walk me through a typical day, including how and when you take your pain medication.

Patterns that suggest uncontrolled pain
- Increased pain is reliably associated with increased physical activities.
- Patient increases opioid use prior to planned activities.
- Patient decreases opioid use when not working or not physically active.
- Stable monthly opioid dose over time.

Patterns that suggest withdrawal
- Rhinorrhea, restlessness, or other nonpain symptoms just before the next opioid dose.
- Patient needs opioids to get out of bed in the morning.
- Patient takes opioids to avoid getting sick or to "stay normal."
- Patient takes opioids to help with sleep or anxiety.
- Pain when missing opioids is different than pain for which opioids are prescribed.

For example, patients may take short-acting opioids primarily to relieve pain but take long-acting opioids primarily to avoid withdrawal symptoms. Table 25-5 describes questions and activity patterns that are useful for making this distinction.

In addition to the side effects listed in Table 25-4, clinicians should be mindful of drug-drug interactions that increase patients' risk for opioid-related overdose. Sedating medication—especially benzodiazepines—increase overdose risk and should be used with caution in patients on long-term opioids. Methadone has fallen out of favor for treating chronic pain because it interacts with more drugs than prototypical opioids, is associated with prolonged QT intervals on electrocardiograms, and has metabolites that build up with prolonged use. Meperidine and tramadol are both contraindicated in patients taking monoamine oxidase inhibitors (MAOIs) inhibitors and increase the risk of serotonin syndrome in patients taking selective serotonin reuptake inhibitors (SSRIs) such as paroxetine.

OVERDOSE RISK

Opioid-related overdose is the most serious and publicly visible complication of opioid use, but it is also very rare relative to the number of patients prescribed opioids. The vast majority of patients prescribed opioids have a very low absolute risk for overdose; 5–10% of high-risk patients account for most fatal and nonfatal overdoses. *Decisions about prescribing and tapering opioids should be based on patients' absolute overdose risk, rather than their relative overdose risk.* Table 25-6 lists major clinical risk factors for opioid overdose.

Table 25-6. Major risk factors for opioid-related overdose.

History of opioid-related overdose
Current or prior substance use disorder, especially opioid use disorder
Higher prescribed opioid dose
Concurrent use of benzodiazepines or other sedatives
Obtaining opioids from multiple prescribers and/or pharmacies
Posttraumatic stress disorder
Clinical evidence of loss of control over opioid use
Conditions impairing lung function or respiratory drive

Substance Use Disorder

Past or current substance use disorder is the most important single risk factors for overdose (other than prior opioid overdose), so a careful substance use history (see Chapter 24) is essential when considering opioid prescribing. *Opioids should not be prescribed to patients actively misusing alcohol or using illicit drugs.* Patients should be asked specifically about use of opioids obtained from nonmedical sources.

Opioid Dose

Multiple large cohort studies have demonstrated that overdose risk increases with higher prescribed opioid doses. However, there is no single threshold that delineates safe from unsafe opioid doses. Table 25-7 shows the sensitivity, specificity, and positive likelihood ratio for unintentional fatal opioid dose associated with different dosage thresholds. These estimates are based on analysis of nationwide data from the Veterans Health Administration, controlling for all available comorbid diagnoses and clinical characteristics. At best, opioid dose is a moderate predictor of overdose risk; the CDC-recommended threshold of 50 MME (see Table 25-2) has a sensitivity of only 59%. *Patients prescribed high opioid doses may have a high relative risk of overdose, but high-dose opioid use in the absence of other risk factors does not convey high absolute overdose risk because the baseline risk of overdose is very low.* In the data used to create Table 25-7, fewer than 1 in 1000 patients prescribed opioids experienced a fatal overdose over multiple years of follow up. Nationwide, the top 10% of patients taking opioids account for more than 50% of all the MMEs prescribed. In most large studies, the mean dose for patients on long-term opioids is less than 30 MME, and the median dose, about 20 MME. Thus, clinicians should not focus on prescribed opioid dose to the exclusion of other risks factors when evaluating patients' overdose risk.

Table 25-7. Sensitivity, specificity, and positive likelihood ratio associated with prescribed opioid dose thresholds for predicting fatal opioid overdose.

Daily Dose (MME)	Sensitivity (%)	Specificity (%)	Likelihood Ratio (+)
10	97	14	1.12
20	87	41	1.47
30	71	63	1.94
40	66	71	2.27
50	59	76	2.50
60	48	81	2.50
70	45	82	2.50
80	41	84	2.60
90	33	88	2.67
100	31	89	2.83
110	28	90	2.82
120	21	93	3.06
130	20	95	3.67
140	17	95	3.70
150	15	96	3.67
160	15	96	3.67
170	14	96	3.45
180	12	97	3.71
190	11	97	3.43
200	10	97	3.28

MME = morphine milligram equivalents.
Adapted from Bohnert AS et al. A Detailed Exploration Into the Association of Prescribed Opioid Dosage and Overdose Deaths Among Patients With Chronic Pain. *Medical Care*. 2016;54:435–441.

Benzodiazepine Use

Concurrent use of benzodiazepines and opioids substantially increases patients' risk of opioid overdose and should be avoided whenever possible. Patients are at greatest risk during the first 3–6 months of concurrent use and after a benzodiazepine or opioid dose escalation. Patients with clinical indications for both long-term opioids and benzodiazepines should be monitored closely and undergo evaluation by pain specialists and other relevant specialty clinicians. Concurrent use of opioids and non-benzodiazepine sedatives should also be avoided.

Medical Comorbidities

Patients with chronic hypoxemia or impaired lung function due to conditions such as chronic obstructive pulmonary disease (COPD), muscular dystrophy, and pulmonary hypertension are at increased overdose risk due to respiratory depression. Opioid use among patients with pulmonary comorbidities should be minimized. When opioids are prescribed to these patients, they should be closely monitored for respiratory compromise and screened for sleep apnea before long-term opioid use is initiated.

Other Risk Factors

Patients getting opioid prescriptions from multiple prescribers or filling prescriptions for multiple pharmacies have increased risk of overdose. Posttraumatic stress disorder (PTSD) is also an independent risk factor for overdose, though data on other mental health diagnoses are inconclusive. Patients with severe mental health disorders, such as schizophrenia, bipolar disorder, or severe depression, should be considered at higher risk of overdose. Nationally, overdoses are more common among men than women, among non-Hispanic white patients than minority patients, and among patients age 20–40. However, most overdoses among young adults are due to nonmedical opioid use rather than prescribed opioids.

Clinical History

Patients' clinical history of opioid use should also be considered when evaluating overdose risk. Patients who routinely request early refills, have multiple unexpected findings on urine drug screens, or refuse to consider nonopioid or nonpharmacologic pain management strategies are at higher overdose risk. Rapid dose escalation is also a risk factor for overdose. A patient who has been taking 180 mg of extended-release morphine for 2 years is at lower overdose risk than a similar patient who escalated to that same dose within 1 year of starting opioids.

OPIOID MISUSE & OPIOID USE DISORDER

Risk factors for opioid use disorder are less well defined than those for overdose, largely because the Diagnostic and Statistical Manual of Mental Disorders, Fifth Edition (DSM-5) criteria for diagnosing substance use disorder are often unhelpful for assessing disorders involving iatrogenic physical dependence. Many risk factors for opioid overdose are also risk factors for opioid use disorder. The most important risk factor for developing opioid use disorder is prior history of opioid use disorder or some other substance use disorder.

Approximately 25% of patients on long-term opioids will sometimes take opioids other than how they are prescribed, and 1 in 10 will develop addiction (i.e., continued use of prescription opioids despite adverse consequences). Clinicians should assess patients' risk for misuse and opioid use disorder before starting opioids for chronic pain, because it is much easier to avoid starting opioids than it is to discontinue opioids after patients have been taking opioids for months or years. Several risk assessment tools have been developed to help clinicians evaluate patients' risk of opioid misuse or abuse. The Opioid Risk Tool and the short form of the Screener and Opioid Assessment for Patients with Pain (SOAPP-SF) are two brief screening tools that may help identify high-risk patients before opioids are started. These tools were developed for use in pain clinics but are also useful in primary care settings. The Current Opioid Misuse Measure (COMM) is a screening tool for patients already taking opioids that has been validated in primary care populations but is too long for routine clinical use.

A careful history and clinical assessment are essential for evaluating patients' overall risk for opioid use disorder. Hallmarks of opioid use disorder include repeated consumption of more opioids than prescribed, substantial time and effort spent worrying about and obtaining opioids, and inability to curtail opioid use despite adverse consequences (e.g., inability to work or fulfill family roles, adverse health consequences). Evaluating patients for opioid use disorder requires asking not just about their pain but about their everyday life, including their work, social relationships, daily activities, and patterns of opioid use. *Tolerance and physical dependence are predictable consequences of long-term prescription opioid use and do not by themselves constitute opioid use disorder.* Chapter 24 provides more detail on assessing patients for substance use disorder.

MONITORING PATIENTS ON LONG-TERM OPIOIDS

Prescription drug monitoring programs, urine toxicology screens, and patient–clinician agreements are three tools that should be used to monitor patients taking opioids. Each of these tools has important limitations and must be accompanied by a careful patient history and clinical assessment. An unexpected test result or "violation" of a patient–clinician agreement should prompt additional discussion and closer monitoring rather than automatic cessation of opioid prescribing.

Prescription drug monitoring programs are electronic statewide databases that record all controlled substances (in most cases, Schedules II, III, and IV) dispensed by outpatient pharmacies in a given state. Physicians, pharmacists, and other clinicians can use web-based interfaces to look up patients' prescription histories at the point of care when deciding whether to prescribe an opioid. Clinicians should check a patient's prescription history using their state's prescription drug monitoring program before starting a new opioid prescription and should check patients taking long-term opioids every 3–6 months. Patients receiving controlled substances from multiple prescribers or multiple pharmacies are at increased risk for opioid overdose. Since the mid-2010s, many states have passed laws requiring clinicians to register with their state's prescription drug monitoring program or to check patients' prescription history before prescribing opioids. Legal requirements related to prescription drug monitoring programs vary from state to state; clinicians should know the requirements for the state in which they are practicing. Currently, there is insufficient evidence to determine whether implementing prescription drug monitoring programs reduce prescription-opioid related overdose rates.

Urine toxicology screens are helpful tools for monitoring patients on long-term opioids. These tests can be used to identify whether patients have recently used illicit drugs (e.g., methamphetamine, cocaine) or prescription opioids other than those they are prescribed. Clinicians should communicate with their local laboratory to understand the types of toxicology screens available and their limitations. For example, urine toxicology assays designed to detect illegal drugs often do not reliably detect hydrocodone or oxycodone. More sophisticated assays that use mass spectroscopy can detect a wider array of opioids but are more expensive. Determining the appropriate urine toxicology screen depends on what tests are available, what the patient is being prescribed, and the clinicians' suspicion for use of illicit substances. A negative test result for a prescribed opioid may indicate diversion (i.e., selling rather than consuming prescription opioids). Urine toxicology screens should be checked at least annually for patients on opioids for chronic pain and, more frequently, if there is concern for opioid misuse or use of illicit substances. No high-quality studies or clinical trials have shown that routine use of urine toxicology screens reduces overdose rates.

Patient–clinician agreements are written documents signed by both the patient and clinician that detail the risks, benefits, and expectations for patients on long-term opioid therapy. These documents typically outline patients' treatment goals and the expectations that patients will only get opioids from one clinician and pharmacy at a time. These agreements are essentially written documentation of informed consent to take prescription opioids; they are not legal contracts. Deviations from agreements should not be used as a pretext for stopping opioids but should instead prompt further discussion and reevaluation of the risks and benefits of continued opioid use.

A PRACTICAL APPROACH FOR ASSESSING OVERDOSE & ABUSE RISK

Scholarship on risks for opioid overdose and opioid use disorder is expanding, but validated risk scores or algorithms for assessing risk do not yet exist. Table 25-8 summarizes a straightforward, practical approach for evaluating patients' overdose risk that categorizes patients taking long-term opioids as low, intermediate, or high risk.

Low-risk patients are those taking 50 MME or less who have no other overdose or substance use risk factors.

Table 25-8. Practical approach for classifying patients by overdose risk.

Low-risk patients
Must meet all the following criteria:
- Taking ≤50 MME
- No history of substance use disorder or PTSD
- Not taking benzodiazepines or other sedatives
- No impaired lung function
- No behaviors concerning for opioid misuse or abuse

Intermediate-risk patients
- Patients who are not high or low risk

High-risk patients
Taking >50 MME and one or more of the following:
- Active substance use disorder
- Persistent evidence of impaired opioid control despite remedial discussions
- Severely impaired lung function or comorbidity associated with high absolute overdose risk

These patients should be carefully monitored for signs of opioid misuse, but they have negligible risk of overdose, so overdose risk should not factor into opioid prescribing decisions.

High-risk patients are those taking greater than 50 MME who have at least one additional major overdose risk factor. The most common major risk factors are repeated red flags indicating misuse or diversion and active substance use disorder. A few patients with severely impaired lung function (marked by hypoxemia and or severe restrictive lung disease) are also high risk. High-risk patients typically comprise 5–10% of primary care patients on opioids and should be easy to identify clinically if the CDC's recommendations for routine monitoring and evaluation are followed. By definition, high-risk patients should not be on long-term opioids. For high-risk patients with active substance use disorders, clinicians should prioritize getting patients to initiate appropriate treatment (see Chapter 24). Concerns about overdose and reasons for tapering should be explained to high-risk patients using objective, nonjudgmental language. Even with high-risk patients, clinicians should work to obtain some degree of patient buy-in prior to tapering and should continue to pursue nonopioid pain treatment strategies.

Intermediate-risk patients are those that do not fall into either the high- or low-risk categories; they make up the majority of primary care patients taking opioids for chronic pain. For intermediate-risk patients, careful assessment and discussion about the risks and benefits of opioid use are required to determine whether opioid treatment should be continued.

The remainder of this chapter covers strategies for communicating effectively with patients about opioids and chronic pain; these strategies are primarily designed for intermediate risk patients, but are applicable to all patients taking opioids. Specific communication techniques for handling angry and demanding patients are reviewed in Chapter 4.

STIGMA

Patients taking opioids for chronic pain may face stigma from clinicians, clinic staff, and family members. First, patients with chronic pain, especially those without an obvious source of pain visible on imaging studies, must often work to convince skeptical clinicians that their pain is "real" and worthy of treatment. Effective, patient-centered discussions about chronic pain require clinicians to take patients' pain (and patients' pain-related concerns) seriously. Taking a patient's pain seriously requires exploring and taking an active interest in their experience of pain and suffering. It does not preclude challenging a patient who is fixated on numeric pain rating scales or denying a patient's request.

Second, many clinicians suspect (either consciously or unconsciously) that patients taking opioids for chronic pain are misusing opioids or are focused on obtaining opioids rather than treating pain. These clinicians often interpret slight deviations from patient–clinician agreements and seemingly common-sense behaviors (e.g., switching pharmacies for convenience, taking a few extra opioid pills due to a newly twisted ankle) as evidence of "aberrancy" and use these deviations to justify stopping opioids. Careful monitoring is always appropriate when prescribing opioids; however, only about 1 in 10 patients taking long-term opioids develops opioid use disorder. Most patients genuinely want better pain control and many are willing to consider nonopioid treatments. Clinicians should always obtain additional information from patients who demonstrate "aberrant" behaviors before deciding about further opioid prescribing.

A third source of stigma is the common presumption that chronic pain, especially comorbid pain and substance use disorder, is evidence of "weak character" or moral failure rather than a chronic medical problem with biologic origins that requires long-term management. Clinicians should approach chronic pain and substance use disorder in the same way that they approach hypertension, diabetes, and other chronic medical problems.

The stigma associated with chronic pain and opioid use is especially harmful for minority patients, particularly black patients, due to racial stereotypes and biases common in American culture that serve to reinforce stereotypes about pain among minority patients. For example, while clinicians tend to underestimate pain relative to their patients, they underestimate pain for black patients to a greater degree than for white patients.

Communicating effectively with patients taking opioids for chronic pain requires attention to and awareness of one's assumptions and biases about chronic pain and opioids. Clinicians who tend to emphasize compassion and ensuring adequate pain relief must remember to monitor patients for evidence of opioid dependence and misuse. Clinicians who find patients with chronic pain tiresome and frustrating should remind themselves that they have an obligation to comprehensively evaluate and treat pain, and that most patients taking opioids are taking low doses and do not develop opioid use disorder.

CASE ILLUSTRATION 1

Mrs. Park is a 58–year-old woman coming to clinic for a routine refill on her pain medications. She takes 60 mg morphine extended-release every 8 hours along with hydrocodone-acetaminophen 10 mg/325 mg for "breakthrough pain." She is frustrated that her pain is not getting any better. She has been coming to this clinic for 2 years, since her previous primary care clinician retired, and has been on the same opioid dose for 3 years.

Her pain is primarily in her lower back. She describes it as constant, aching, and 8 out of 10 in severity. Her pain gets worse with activity and improves with lying down. She occasionally has pain that radiates down her right leg and gets 3-4 unpredictable "pain attacks" during the day for which she takes hydrocodone.

She does some cleaning around the house but is often unable to cook and rarely leaves the house due to her pain. Her husband does the shopping and most of the cooking.

TALKING ABOUT PAIN & OPIOIDS

Table 25-9 summarizes a practical, step-by-step approach for effectively communicating with patients taking opioids. Communicating with patients who have been taking opioids for months and years is often more challenging than communicating with patients who are taking opioids for acute pain; however, the approach in Table 25-9 is applicable to all patients.

Step 1: Mentally Prepare for the Visit

Difficult conversations and challenging visits are unavoidable in clinical medicine. Primary care clinicians rate approximately 40% of visits involving patients taking opioids for chronic pain as "difficult," (i.e., challenging or engendering negative clinician emotions) compared to 15–18% of all primary care visits. So, it is normal to feel apprehensive or nervous when seeing patients with chronic pain. Unfortunately, approaching a visit feeling defensive or nervous can hinder open, effective communication. Thus, when preparing to discuss opioids and chronic pain, clinicians should be *mindful* of their own emotions—both before and during the visit—to ensure that these emotions do not adversely affect their behavior or decision making.

Mindfulness refers to clinicians' capacity for self-awareness and reflection during patient–clinician interactions (see Chapter 7). Many clinicians report that they are fearful or apprehensive about seeing patients with chronic pain, so one effective approach for cultivating mindfulness is to bring to mind one's biggest fear about a visit, and then to state this fear in a complete sentence (either to oneself or to a colleague). For example:

- I'm afraid this patient is going to ask for more hydromorphone, then I'll refuse and he'll start yelling at me.
- I'm afraid this patient will resist when I tell her she needs to take less oxycodone, and she'll make me feel like I'm a terrible person and a bad doctor.

Explicitly identifying fears in this way helps to reduce their effect on one's own emotions and actions. Overt conflict about pain and opioids is actually uncommon; analysis of audio-recorded visits indicates that overt conflict occurs in fewer than 10% of visits. The majority of discussions about chronic pain and opioids are marked by relative agreement and civil discussion between patients and clinicians.

Table 25-9. Steps for communicating effectively about opioids and chronic pain.

1. **Mentally prepare for the visit.**
   Be mindful—monitor your emotions
   Be curious—approach the visit with an open mind
2. **Show patients that you take their pain seriously**
   Ask open-ended questions about the patient's pain, medication use, and functional status
   Elicit the patient's perspective on pain and opioids
   Use empathetic statements to build rapport and convey commitment
3. **Establish shared pain treatment goals**
   Identify realistic treatment goals based on patient function
   When patients resist functional goals, emphasize effectiveness and life goals
4. **Develop a goal-directed treatment plan**
   Offer multiple treatment options
   Commit to listening, being flexible, and working with the patient long-term
   When discussing opioid tapering, focus on better pain management, not counting pills
   When patients insist on opioid-focused treatment, emphasize observable treatment goals

When negative emotions surface *during* a visit, clinicians should develop strategies for recognizing and partially detaching from these emotions. Strategies that many clinicians find effective include taking slow, deep breaths, tightening or relaxing leg or arm muscles, and, in extreme cases, leaving the room briefly in order to calm down.

Clinicians may assume the worst about patients with chronic pain, especially patients on long-term opioids. It can be easy to take a patient's response for granted (e.g., "I know this patient will resist if I suggest taking less hydrocodone.") without checking whether these assumptions are correct. Similarly, entering a visit with predetermined goals or treatment plans, such as decreasing a patient's hydromorphone dose, can make clinicians defensive and engender unnecessary conflict. *Actively listening for the patient's perspective on pain and opioids is an important tool for avoiding these common pitfalls when discussing chronic pain.* Listening is important even when you disagree with the patient's perspective or desired treatment. By actively trying to understand why a patient is requesting a specific treatment, it is often possible to discern the goals, concerns, and beliefs underlying the request, and so identify an opening to engage the patient in a dialog about treatment alternatives.

A useful strategy for keeping an open mind about opioids and chronic pain is to identify something unknown about the patient's beliefs about pain and opioids and then ask about this during the visit. This exercise helps to remind clinicians to consider the patient's perspective about pain and helps to avoid mistaken assumptions. The following previsit questions might be helpful when preparing to see Mrs. Park, the patient in the case illustration:

- Does she think she will be on opioids forever?
- How much time during the day does she spend thinking about opioids?
- What does she think is the cause of her pain?
- Are there stresses or problems in her life that are making her pain worse?

Step 2: Show Patients That You Take Their Pain Seriously

The most important way to show patients that you take their pain seriously is to ask open-ended questions about their pain, medication use, and functional status. In interviews about patient–clinician communication, patients with chronic pain reported that clinicians often do not seem to take their pain seriously and identified asking detailed questions as an important way that clinicians can demonstrate that they take patients' pain seriously and care about treating it. Table 25-10 lists useful questions for patients with chronic pain. Asking open-ended questions may seem too time consuming, especially during a busy visit with patients who have multiple problems. However, when done skillfully, asking questions and actively listening to the answers is efficient over the long run because it simultaneously furthers all the following communication goals:

- Elicits information needed to set treatment goals and to tailor pain treatment plans to the patient's individual needs
- Shows the patient the clinician takes their pain seriously and is treating them as an individual rather than a generic "back pain" patient
- Produces opportunities to build rapport by demonstrating empathy
- Elicits information about opioid effectiveness (or lack thereof) that can often provide openings for discussing opioid tapering

Table 25-10. Useful questions for eliciting patients' perspective on pain.

Tell me about your pain.
How does the pain affect you/your life?
Walk me through a typical day for you, starting with when you get up in the morning. Include details about when and how you take your pain medications.
Thinking about your pain, what are you most worried about?
How are your pain medications working for you?
What problems are you having with your pain medications?
What happens when you miss or are late for a dose of pain medication?
How much time do you spend thinking about opioid medications during the day?
What activities, if any, can you do after you take your pain medication that you couldn't do without your medications?
When do you delay or avoid taking your pain medication?

In addition to the questions in Table 25-10, it is often useful to clarify the extent to which patients on long-term opioids are taking opioids to maintain functionality versus to cope with pain-related distress and prevent withdrawal. Making this distinction requires careful questioning and listening, sometimes over several visits, and these two categories are not mutually exclusive. Table 25-11 shows patterns of opioid use that can help make this distinction. It is often reasonable to continue prescribing opioids when taking opioids helps patients keep their jobs or perform daily activities. On the other hand, patients who are taking opioids primarily to relieve distress or cope with stressful life circumstances tend to be less functional when taking opioids. These patients should be encouraged to use nonopioid strategies, such as SSRIs, cognitive behavioral therapy, and mindfulness exercises instead of opioids.

Table 25-11. Distinguishing opioid use to maintain function from opioid use to cope with pain-related distress.

Patterns that suggest patients are taking opioids to maintain function
Patient takes opioids prior to planned activities, such as gardening or shopping
Patient takes opioids to stay functional at work
Patient takes fewer opioids during nights, weekends, or other times associated with fewer required activities
Patterns that suggest patients are taking opioids to cope with pain-related distress
Patient takes opioids to recover or relax after planned activities
Patient does not take opioids when working or cannot work when taking opioids
Patient takes more opioids during nights, weekends, or other times associated with fewer required activities
Patient avoids using opioids when driving
Patient uses opioids to help with sleep or anxiety

Eliciting patients' perspective also shows patients that the clinician takes their pain seriously. As mentioned above, one benefit of the questions listed in Table 25-10 is that they prompt patients to volunteer their perspective on these topics. In many cases, skillful use of open-ended questions will be sufficient to elicit the patient's perspective on pain, including their understanding about what is causing their pain, their attitudes about opioids, and the activities and social roles that are important to them. Preparing a question to ask before the visit (see Step 1) also helps to ensure that clinicians elicit the patient's perspective.

Another way to determine the patient's perspective is to ask the patient directly. The "ask-tell-ask" approach is one simple, effective strategy for eliciting patients' perspective while also suggesting a potential treatment approach. In this approach, the clinician elicits the patient's perspective and/or willingness to engage (ASK) before providing information (TELL) and then follows up with a question to assess the patients' understanding or reaction (ASK).

ASK	**Clinician**: Sounds as if you're worried about your pain. What do you think might be going on? **Patient**: I'm not sure, but the pain is really making it hard to work because I can't sit at my desk. And then my back is so sore that I'm not sleeping very well either.
TELL	**Clinician**: In your situation, I think your trouble sleeping is making your pain worse. So if we can find a way to help you sleep better, your pain should improve as well.
ASK	**Clinician**: What do you think about that plan?

ASK	**Clinician**: It doesn't seem like your pain is under good control right now. What do you think? **Patient**: My pain is terrible! I've tried taking the extra Percocets that you gave me last time, but it hasn't made much difference.
TELL	**Clinician**: Relying just on opioids doesn't seem to be working for you. We need to try something else. I think we should start by giving physical therapy and daily stretching another try.
ASK	**Clinician**: What do you think about that idea?

Conveying empathy is another important tool that, when used properly, shows the patient that the clinician takes their pain seriously and cares about relieving their suffering. Many different strategies and frameworks for conveying empathy have been developed, such as the reflective listening technique of motivational interviewing (see Chapter 19). Chapter 2 summarizes the importance of empathy as a clinical tool and discusses specific strategies for conveying empathy in more detail. All of these techniques include some or all of the following components:

- Actively listening to recognize a patient's underlying emotion
- Acknowledging or referencing that emotion explicitly
- Normalizing the patient's experience
- Providing support or encouragement
- Committing to working together with the patient to address the problem

Table 25-12 provides example questions and statements for conveying empathy around chronic pain.

Tone and nonverbal behavior are critically important for effectively conveying empathy. Facing and focusing on the patient (instead of talking while typing on the computer) can effectively convey empathy and support without any words. On the other hand, when clinicians feel frustrated or exasperated, these feelings often manifest through nonverbal communication and can cause the patient to interpret potentially empathetic statements as condescending. Thus, monitoring one's own emotions (see Step 1) is an important prerequisite for effectively conveying empathy.

Step 3: Establish Shared Pain Treatment Goals

Pain treatment goals should be observable, realistic, meaningful to the patient, and specific. As much as possible, use insights gained from the patient's history and perspective on opioids to identify target goals. *Avoid goals focused on pain rating scales or opioid dosage targets.* Pain scores are entirely subjective, mean different things to different patients, and, in the case of chronic pain,

Table 25-12. Useful questions for conveying empathy about chronic pain.

Acknowledging emotions
It sounds like you've been having a really hard time.
It sounds as if you feel trapped by the pain and don't know what to do about it.
You've really been suffering over the past 2 weeks.
Well, you're worried that the back pain is a signal of nerve damage.
You might be worried that you'll have to quit your job because of these headaches.

Normalizing the patient's experience
It's understandable that you've had so much trouble with your pain.
It's normal to worry that you might not be able to drive because of this pain.
Anybody who had to go through as much as you have would be frustrated.

Supportive statements
Most people in your situation wouldn't be holding up as well as you are.
You've really worked hard to take care of your children despite your pain.
You've been suffering from this pain for a long time.
It sounds like you're really uncomfortable; I'm sorry you've been hurting so much.
I want to treat your pain well; I take it seriously.

Committing to work with the patient
It's scary to make these changes, but I will be with you every step of the way.
I know you're in pain. Let's see what we can do to help you.
I know you're suffering from real physical pain, and I am committed to working with you to help you manage your pain so you can get your life back.
We're going to work on relieving your pain together, as long as it takes.
Treating your pain well and safely is a priority for me.
I will keep working with you to treat your pain; I will not abandon you.

often reflect emotional distress or frustration rather than pain intensity. Specific opioid dosage targets may be reasonable for reducing patients' risk of opioid overdose but do not relate directly to the patient's pain. It is important not to conflate opioid management and pain management; effective chronic pain management requires a multipronged approach of which opioids are only one component. Chapter 38 provides more details about pain management. Table 25-13 lists common domains for setting pain treatment goals with patients.

Patients who have been taking opioids for years often have difficulty articulating functional pain treatment goals. After all, until the early 2010s, patients on opioids were instructed and trained by clinicians to focus

Table 25-13. Common domains for functional pain treatment goals.

Domain	Examples
Ability to perform daily activities	Walking around the house, getting the mail, going to the store, playing with grandchildren, doing yardwork
Ability to work or perform social roles	Avoiding pain-related work absences, preparing meals, caring for family members, taking children to school
Better management of medical comorbidities	Reaching hemoglobin A_{1C} goals, losing weight, controlling blood pressure, exercising regularly
Better management of mental health comorbidities	Improved control of depression or anxiety, engaging with counselors, better medication adherence
Improved sleep	Decreased daytime sleepiness, improved sleep hygiene

on reducing their numerical pain score as the primary goal of pain treatment. Characterizing the association between opioid use and function (see Table 25-11) is particularly important for patients who resist functional treatment goals. In rare cases, patients do get functional benefit from high-dose opioids; however, for most patients the benefits of high-dose opioids diminish over time. Patients such as Mrs. Park from the case illustration who are taking very high opioid doses (>180 MME) often lead very sedentary lives due to a combination of opioid-induced hyperalgesia and sedation. Tolerance to opioids' analgesic effects develops faster than tolerance to their sedating effects, so patients taking high opioid doses often experience both uncontrolled pain and substantial sedation. Patients do not always recognize their degree of sedation, so it is important to obtain collateral information from friends or family members. Collateral information about daily activities is also helpful when treating patients with impaired mobility for whom standard assessments of functional status are less useful.

Table 25-14 lists some questions that can help broach the subject of functional treatment goals with patients who are resistant or unable to articulate them. These questions can be used to steer the conversation away from pain ratings scales and engage patients in a discussion about their day-to-day lives.

Step 4: Develop a Goal-Directed Treatment Plan

Unfortunately, simple, highly effective treatments for chronic pain do not exist for the most common chronic pain syndromes. Patients with chronic pain typically need to use multiple treatments simultaneously (each of which has small to moderate effects by itself) to achieve optimal pain control. The dearth of simple, highly

Table 25-14. Useful questions for discussing pain treatment goals.

What would successful pain management look like to you?

Can you state your goal for pain management without using the word *pain*?

I know your pain is terrible, but how are *you* doing? How is your life?

What do your "good" days look like? What are some things you'd like to do if we could increase the number of "good" days you have?

It sounds like you're frustrated because you're not getting out of the house much due to pain. How would you feel if you could get to the point where you could walk your dog around the block once a day?

You said that your diabetes control is not where you want it to be. How much is your pain interfering with your ability to manage your diabetes?

effective treatments is a major source of frustration for clinicians and patients. Clinicians' desire for a "silver bullet" to treat chronic pain was one reason they embraced opioids during the 1990s and 2000s. Table 25-15 lists common treatment categories for chronic pain; Chapter 38 provides more detail about pain management.

When formulating treatment plans, clinicians should propose multiple different options and give patients a choice about which ones to pursue. When possible, clinicians should tell patients that many different options are available for treating pain and that the clinician will keep trying different options until treatments that work for the patient are identified. Giving patients treatments options promotes buy-in to the treatment plan. Telling patients that multiple options are available and conveying confidence about the prospects for eventual success conveys hope and optimism to the patient.

Table 25-15. Nonopioid treatment categories for chronic pain.

Category	Examples
Nonopioid oral analgesics	NSAIDs, gabapentin, acetaminophen
Topical analgesics	Lidocaine, capsaicin
Antidepressants	SSRIs, SNRIs, tricyclic antidepressants
Exercise-based treatments	Physical therapy, stretching
Manipulation therapies	Osteopathic manipulation, massage
Procedures	Trigger point injections, surgery
Integrative treatments	Biofeedback, meditation, acupuncture

Communicating nonabandonment to patients on long-term opioids is critical for building patient rapport. Managing long-term opioid therapy requires a therapeutic patient–clinician relationship; patients are more likely to agree with treatment recommendations, including opioid tapering, when they believe clinicians have their best interest at heart. Thus, clinicians should explicitly tell patients that they are committed to working with them over time and are willing to listen and adjust treatment plans based on their response. Clinicians should make plans to check in regularly with patients. Scheduling follow-up communication shows patients that clinicians are treating patients as individuals rather than generic "pain patients." The following phrases provide examples for conveying commitment and flexibility when discussing treatment plans:

> **Clinician**: For most patients, we need to combine multiple different treatments to achieve the best possible pain control. There are a lot of different treatments out there, and every patient's situation is different. I know this pain is frustrating, but I will keep working with you until we find the right combination of treatments for your situation.
>
> **Clinician**: Okay, I think we have a good plan set for today. I want you to contact me in 2 weeks and let me know how things are going. When we're making changes, it's important that I know how you're doing so that we can make changes to the plan if needed.
>
> **Clinician**: Tapering down on opioids is scary. We're only going down by one pill per day, so I don't think that withdrawal is going to be a problem. But if you *are* having problems, let the clinic know right away. There is no reason for you to suffer through withdrawal. We'll talk through the problems and find a way to get things under better control.
>
> **Clinician**: You've been living with your pain for a long time; we are not going to fix this overnight or even in 1 or 2 months, but I want you to know that as long as you are willing to work with me, I want us to be a team working together to figure out everything we can possibly do to better understand your pain and to help you live the life you want to be able to live despite your pain.

OPIOID TAPERING

Clinicians often approach communicating about opioid tapering defensively; however, using the communication approach outlined in this chapter will help to build a patient–clinician relationship within which productive discussions about tapering can take place. Monitoring one's own emotions, understanding patients' perspectives and how pain affects their day-to-day life, and establishing common pain treatment goals are all important prerequisites for discussing tapering.

When discussing opioid tapering, focus on better pain management, not counting pills. Insisting on prescribing fewer pills to an unwilling patient creates a battle with no possible winner. Most patients who have been taking opioids for years perceive some benefit from them and have learned to tolerate opioid-related side effects. Thus, patients are likely to resist discussions framed around decreasing their opioid dose, especially if they think the clinician is trying to take away their pain medication without offering anything else in return. Instead, frame discussions around improving patients' functional status and quality of life. Clinicians should start by recommending additional pain treatments or strategies and giving the patient choices whenever possible. Clinicians can then advise the patient that they will likely need fewer opioids in the future, once these new strategies take effect.

It is usually unhelpful to cite risk of overdose and death as the justification for opioid tapering unless the patient has a high absolute overdose risk or has previously expressed concerns about opioid safety. Patients who have been taking opioids for years are appropriately skeptical of claims that they need to taper urgently in order to avoid death. Patients on long-term opioids are also typically aware of opioids' addictive potential and consider themselves at low risk for becoming "drug addicts." Some patients do consider themselves "addicted" to opioids but consider addiction a worthwhile price to pay for pain relief.

Clinicians should use information gleaned from the patient's history to make the case for tapering. Ongoing severe pain or poor functional status despite high-dose opioid use is *de facto* evidence that opioids are not working. When patients endorse side effects or problems with opioid dependence, this gives clinicians an opening to highlight these factors to remind patients about the downsides of long-term opioid use. Patients at intermediate or low risk of overdose (see Table 25-8) should not be tapered without their consent; doing so can seriously damage patient–clinician relationships. Patients do not need to be excited about tapering, just willing to try a lower dose.

When discussing tapering with patients who have been taking opioids for years, clinicians should acknowledge that medical practice has changed in response to new evidence. Taking some responsibility (on behalf of the medical establishment) for starting paticnts on opioids in the first place can help build trust with patients. Remind patients that research indicates that most patients who taper to lower opioid doses experience no change or even slight improvements in pain severity and that most also report better functional status and quality of life after tapering. Some examples of how to broach the topic of tapering are provided below:

> **Clinician**: You've been on high doses of fentanyl for 3 years, and your pain is still not well controlled most days. These medications aren't working. Let's work together to find other ways to get your pain under better control.

> **Clinician**: You're taking a lot of oxycodone, but you're still stuck in the house all day. You talked last time about wanting to spend more time with your grandkids, but that isn't happening. You're not making progress on these medications. Let's try some changes to see what we can do to get you more active. I know we can do better a better job of treating your pain.

Clinicians can also use the ask-tell-ask approach to broach the subject of tapering:

ASK	**Clinician**: It sounds like worrying about opioids has taken over your life. **Patient**: Sometimes it feels that way, but I've got to have something for the pain! **Clinician**: I know it's frustrating. There is new research about opioids that is relevant to your situation. Would it be okay for me to review it with you? **Patient:** Sure.
TELL	**Clinician**: Doctors used to start patients on opioids all the time for chronic pain; we thought we were helping them. Newer studies show that patients typically get less pain relief and more side effects from opioid over time. A lot of people end up feeling like their lives revolve around taking opioids. I'm really sorry that you've been taking these medications for so long. The good news is that when patients gradually take lower doses, their pain stays the same or even gets a little better, and they have a lot fewer side effects. So, I think we should try adding new treatments for your pain, and then gradually decrease your opioid dose over time.
ASK	**Clinician**: What do you think about that idea?

When patients resist tapering, keep the discussion focused on the patient's goals rather than pain intensity; do not get drawn into a fight about opioid dosages. When patients insist that they derive functional benefit from opioids, take time to clarify the relationship between their opioid use and functional status (see Table 25-11). If the patient does seem to derive functional benefit from opioids, work with the patient to establish mutually acceptable functional pain treatment goals that can be followed objectively over time. Then, advise the patient that continued opioid prescribing will be contingent on satisfactory progress towards the patient's treatment goal. Patients who insist on taking opioids while also refusing to try nonopioid treatments should be reevaluated for evidence of opioid misuse or opioid use disorder. Table 25-16 summarizes communication strategies to use and to avoid when discussing tapering.

Table 25-16. Do's and Don'ts for discussing opioid tapering with patients.

Don't	Do
Focus on reducing or taking away opioids	Focus on adding new treatments for pain
Emphasize overdose as a reason for tapering (unless patients are truly high risk)	Emphasize improving pain and quality of life
Discount patients' perception that opioids relieve pain	Highlight severe pain or poor function as evidence that opioids are not working
Ignore patients' fears and worries	Tell patients that tapering is not associated with worse pain
Force patients to taper without some level of agreement	Take responsibility (on behalf of the medical establishment) for starting patients on opioids in the past
Adopt a rigid tapering schedule	Slow or pause tapering to mitigate withdrawal symptoms
Insist on tapering off opioids completely	Reevaluate tapering goals once patient has tapered to <90 MME

TAPERING PROTOCOLS

There are scant empirical data to support specific tapering protocols, largely because patients' psychological and physiologic responses to tapering vary tremendously. Thus, tapering plans should be flexible and tailored to patients' individual needs. Some patients can taper off relatively rapidly without noticeable withdrawal symptoms. Patients with substantial physiologic dependence will experience both withdrawal symptoms and opioid cravings when tapering; these patients must be tapered off very gradually over months or even years. In general, patients who have been taking opioids for longer periods of time require more gradual tapering schedules. Clinicians and patients should agree ahead of time on procedures for regular clinic visits and for obtaining refills. Clinicians have a responsibility to arrange coverage during usual business hours when they are on vacation or not available to communicate with the patient for some other reason.

When starting a taper, a good rule of thumb is to decrease the patient's opioid dose by about 10% during the first month and then adjust further tapering based on the patient's clinical response. An initial decrease of 15–20% during the first month is reasonable for patients taking greater than 200 MME. If a patient experiences withdrawal symptoms, there is little clinical downside to pausing the taper for a few months or slowing the rate of subsequent dose reductions. Continuing to taper patients who are suffering from withdrawal is dangerous and may prompt patients to seek opioids from nonmedical sources. Whenever feasible, give patients options and control over how they taper. For example, clinicians can allow patients taking both long-acting and immediate-release opioid formulations to decide which formulation to taper first. Tapering protocols are affected by the opioid formulations and tablet strengths available for the opioids that patients are taking; converting patients to a single immediate-release opioid formulation without acetaminophen (to avoid potential acetaminophen toxicity) often simplifies tapering for both patients and clinicians. Morphine, oxycodone, and hydromorphone are all available in a wide range of tablet strengths that facilitate gradual reductions in patients' overall opioid dose. Advise patients about what to expect when tapering, including potential withdrawal symptoms. Most patients on high-dose opioids are aware of common withdrawal symptoms. Advise patients to call if they experience withdrawal, so that adjustments to the treatment plan can be considered.

Patients on high-dose opioids can almost always taper down to lower doses. However, some patients reach a point at which they cannot reduce their opioid dose further without intolerable withdrawal symptoms. Patients who cannot tolerate further reduction in their opioid consumption despite coordination with their clinician are at high risk for developing opioid use disorder. Thus, these patients should be formally evaluated for possible opioid use disorder, including assessment of opioid cravings, adverse social consequences related to opioid use, and use of opioids from non-medical sources. The most common treatment for opioid use disorder is buprenorphine. Chapter 24 provides more details about treatment options for substance use disorder. Prescribing buprenorphine to treat substance use disorder requires special training and a Drug Addiction Treatment Act 2000 (DATA) waiver (also known as an "x-waiver") from the federal government. *Primary care clinicians without a DATA waiver should not prescribe buprenorphine to facilitate tapering for patients who are unable to further taper using typical opioids*; doing so could be construed as unlicensed treatment of opioid use disorder. Instead, clinicians should refer such patients to pain and/or addiction specialists for further evaluation and management.

CONCLUSION

Opioid analgesics are among the most controversial medications in the United States today. Primary care clinicians are at the center of the "opioid crisis" and prescribe the majority of opioids for patients suffering from chronic pain. They face the challenge of working to prevent opioid-related deaths and facilitating treatment for opioid use disorder, while at the same time effectively and compassionately treating patients suffering from pain. With a mindful, evidence-based approach, clinicians can successfully treat patient's suffering from pain while maintaining a trusting, therapeutic relationship.

SUGGESTED READINGS

Dowell D, Haegerich TM, Chou R. CDC guideline for prescribing opioids for chronic pain—United States. *JAMA* 2016;315:1624–1645.

Krebs EE, Gravely A, Nugent S, et al. Effect of opioid vs nonopioid medications on pain-related function in patients with chronic back pain or hip or knee osteoarthritis pain: the SPACE randomized clinical trial. *JAMA* 2018;319:872–882.

Providers Clinical Support System (PCSS). Substance Abuse and Mental Health Services Administration (SAMHSA). https://pcssnow.org/. Accessed August 2018.

SECTION V
Mental & Behavioral Disorders

Depression

26

Y. Pritham Raj, MD; John F. Christensen, PhD; & Mitchell D. Feldman, MD, MPhil, FACP

INTRODUCTION

Depression is common, disabling, and often underrecognized in general medical practice. More than 300 million people are affected by depression worldwide. Stigma of mental illness and other psychosocial barriers such as negative expectations often diminish the motivation of individuals with depression to seek care. Even when recognized, depression is often inadequately addressed by practitioners who lack either the time or training to provide timely, effective, evidence-based treatment. Despite evidence that depression is quite treatable, and the widespread availability of evidence-based assessment and treatment guidelines, overall outcomes remain poor.

About 3/4 of patients seeking care for depression are treated in primary care rather than by mental health professionals. This chapter focuses on the core knowledge and skills needed by general medical practitioners to effectively assess and manage major depressive disorder (MDD). We also review other related depressive disorders as updated in the DSM-5 including: disruptive mood dysregulation disorder, persistent depressive disorder (dysthymia), premenstrual dysphoric disorder (PMDD), adjustment disorder with depressed mood, substance/medication-induced depressive disorder, depressive disorder due to another medical condition, bipolar disorder/bipolar depression, and other specified and unspecified depressive disorders.

In diagnosing depression, we emphasize the routine use of brief patient self-assessment tools such as the nine-item Patient Health Questionnaire (PHQ-9). The U.S. Preventive Services Task Force (USPSTF) guidelines recommend screening the general adult population "when adequate systems are in place to ensure accurate diagnosis, effective treatment, and appropriate follow-up." Unfortunately, despite the publication of such screening recommendations, adoption of the use of rating scales by providers has been poor. The national depression screening rate was less than 5% of all adult ambulatory care visits according to the National Ambulatory Medical Care Survey (2005–2015). Increased use of screening and rating instruments in depression should provide pivotal leverage needed to improve outcomes for depression, especially since measurement-based care (MBC) is the new standard in the management of MDD and has been shown to improve clinical outcomes.

DEPRESSIVE DISORDERS: MAJOR DEPRESSION & RELATED CONDITIONS

Major depressive disorder (MDD) is associated with considerable disability, morbidity, and mortality. Epidemiologic studies demonstrate that MDD causes as much or more disability and social and role impairment than other chronic illnesses such as diabetes, arthritis, hypertension, and coronary artery disease. The hallmark of MDD is when five or more of nine cardinal symptoms of depression are present during the same 2-week period with at least one of the symptoms being either depressed mood or loss of interest or pleasure (anhedonia). The symptoms must cause clinically significant distress and not be attributable to the effects of a substance or another medical condition (see Table 26-1).

MDD is a well-documented and common comorbidity in many medical conditions, especially severe physical disorders such as cancer, stroke, and acute coronary syndrome. A large 1-year U.S. prevalence study

Table 26-1. Diagnosis of major depression.

1. Depressed mood
2. Anhedonia (lack of interest or pleasure in almost all activities)
3. Sleep disorder (insomnia or hypersomnia)
4. Appetite loss, weight loss; appetite gain, weight gain
5. Fatigue or loss of energy
6. Psychomotor retardation or agitation
7. Trouble concentrating or trouble making decisions
8. Low self-esteem or guilt
9. Recurrent thoughts of death or suicidal ideation

Five symptoms from the above are required to make the diagnosis of depression and must include depressed mood and/or anhedonia. The symptoms must have been present most of the day, nearly every day, for 2 weeks.

found that patients with chronic medical diseases were nearly three times as likely to get depressed compared to healthy controls. When present as a comorbidity, depression accounts for significant increases in disability, morbidity, and mortality.

The etiologic and sustaining relationships between depression and many other medical conditions appear to be bidirectional. For example, preexisting depression is a predictor of future atherosclerotic coronary artery disease (CAD), and CAD is associated with MDD. In several studies, 17–44% of patients with CAD have a comorbid diagnosis of major depression which in turn puts them at greater risk for sudden cardiac death. Depressed patients with heart disease (coronary artery disease and congestive heart failure) have increased risk of reinfarction after myocardial infarction (MI) and up to a threefold increase in all-cause mortality, even after controlling for all other identifiable and measurable cardiac risk factors. Diabetes mellitus (DM) and depression also have a bidirectional relationship. The relative risk for developing type 2 diabetes mellitus in depressed patients is reported as high as 1.6, while the relative risk for developing depression in a patient with DM is around 1.2. Patients with comorbid diabetes and depression have worse glycemic control, more microvascular and macrovascular complications and greater all-cause mortality. High inflammatory states (e.g., high plasma c-reactive protein levels) in patients with depression are associated with metabolic alterations that predict responses to both traditional antidepressants as well as some experimental anti-inflammatory therapies such as infliximab that will be briefly discussed later in this chapter.

Major depression is associated with adverse health habits, such as addictions (tobacco and alcohol use disorders in particular), poor diet, overeating, and sedentary lifestyle, which in turn can contribute to the development of metabolic syndrome and other general medical illnesses. Conversely, functional impairment stemming from these chronic illnesses predispose to development of new depression. From an etiologic perspective, variables such as genetic vulnerability, childhood adversity (neglect and abuse), and stressful life events all contribute to the development of depression itself as well as to lifestyle risks such as obesity, sedentary behavior, and smoking that themselves predispose to chronic general medical illnesses.

Chronic care of general medical illness requires self-management behaviors to optimize treatment. In fact, much of primary care medicine involves lifestyle modification counseling, including diet modification, promotion of physical activity, regulation of substances (especially alcohol and caffeine), tobacco cessation, and medication adherence for maintenance of health. Studies show that depression adversely impacts self-management, at least partly due to the fact that depressed patients are less likely to be adherent with lifestyle modification plans than nondepressed patients. Depressed diabetic patients have decreased adherence to diet and suffer more lapses in refills of oral hypoglycemic medications. Depressed patients with heart disease or stroke show decreased adherence to treatment recommendations such as taking daily aspirin and participating in exercise rehabilitation programs. This nonadherence in post-MI patients predicts increased rehospitalization rates and overall mortality. Major depressive disorder, with or without general medical comorbidity generally is a chronic, recurring illness, with varying cycles of exacerbation and remission. Furthermore, these exacerbations or new episodes of depression tend to occur more frequently and with greater severity as the patient ages.

Disruptive mood dysregulation disorder is a depressive disorder highlighted by severe recurrent temper outbursts manifested verbally and/or behaviorally that are out of proportion to a situation or provocation. The outbursts, such as verbal rages or physical aggression, occur on average, three or more times per week and are often accompanied by persistently irritable mood most of the day, nearly every day—a feature that makes it challenging to differentiate from the episodic irritability often seen in bipolar disorder as a manic-equivalent feature. The diagnosis should not be made for the first time before age 6 years or after age 18, which also presents a challenge when teasing out this disorder from bipolar disorder, where symptoms typically emerge earlier than age 25.

Persistent depressive disorder (dysthymia) represents a consolidation of DSM-IV defined chronic MDD and dysthymic disorder—a less severe but more chronic form of depressive illness that is also associated with significant disability. This disorder is diagnosed when depressed mood and at least two other symptoms of depression have been present "more than half the days" during the previous 2 years (or 1 year for children or adolescents). Persistent depressive disorder has been shown to respond to treatment with antidepressant medication. If full criteria for a major depressive episode are ever met (five of nine criteria) during the course of illness, the patient should be given a diagnosis of major depressive disorder.

Premenstrual dysphoric disorder (PMDD) is a condition affecting 3–8% of menstruating women. It is diagnosed when in the majority of menstrual cycles at least five symptoms of affective, behavioral and/or somatic dysregulation are present in the week antecedent to the onset of menses (luteal phase), start to improve within a few days after the onset of menses, and attenuate or resolve in the week post-menses. One or more of the following symptoms must be present: mood swings (affective lability), irritability/anger, depressed mood, or marked anxiety. As with other mood disorders, the symptoms must cause significant distress or interference with usual activities. It may be considered a severe form of premenstrual syndrome (PMS) and is treated best by serotonin reuptake inhibitors or ovulation suppression via contraception.

Substance/medication-induced depressive disorder is a disturbance in mood characterized by depression (not delirium) that develops during or soon after substance intoxication or withdrawal (e.g., amphetamine) or after exposure to a medication (e.g., interferon). It is well known that illicit substances can lead to depression. Alcohol is a prototypical substance that acts as a depressant. In fact, nearly one-third of people with major depression also have a pattern of problem drinking, making substance-induced depressive disorder difficult to separate from MDD. Many providers overlook substances as an etiology of depression either because of lack of screening or underreporting of use by the patient. We recommend evidence-based screening programs such as the Screening, Brief Intervention, and Referral to Treatment (SBIRT) practice to aid in the assessment of the severity of substance use (screening forms available at: http://www.sbirtoregon.org/screening-forms/). Specifically, the Alcohol Use Disorders Identification Test (AUDIT) and the Drug Abuse Screening Test (DAST-10) should be administered to adult patients who screen positive for substance abuse to identify, reduce, and prevent problematic use of substances that contribute to myriad disorders including depression.

Several medications have been implicated in the development of depression or suicidal ideation. According to one study, more than a third of all Americans were prescribed one or more drugs that have been tied to depression or suicidal ideation. In general, high-quality studies in this area are lacking, often making it difficult to ascertain causal relationships between medications and medication-induced depression. Some experts suggest that isotretinoin and alpha-interferons pose the highest risk of medication-induced depressive disorder, while corticosteroids, varenicline, progesterone inserts, and finasteride pose a moderately high risk.

Depressive disorders due to another medical condition refers to psychiatric syndromes thought to result from the direct physiological consequence of a general medical condition (e.g., hypothyroidism). Treatment focuses on resolution of the underlying general medical problem or withdrawal of the offending medication, although specific psychiatric treatment may also be useful. For example, in the case of hypothyroidism, it is paramount to treat with levothyroxine to a TSH around 1.5 mU/L (perhaps slightly higher in elderly adults) to target both the medical and depressive symptoms. The use of antidepressants alone would be inappropriate.

Other specified and unspecified depressive disorders are categories for presentations in which symptoms of depression are either not of adequate duration or symptom severity to meet diagnostic criteria of other depressive disorders but yet cause clinically significant distress.

Adjustment disorder with depressed mood is now listed under the trauma- and stressor-related disorders such as posttraumatic stress disorder (PTSD). It is a commonly occurring disorder following an identifiable stressor, such as divorce or job loss, when marked distress and emotional or behavioral symptoms occur within 3 months of the onset of the stressor. It may occur with mixed anxiety symptoms. The symptoms must not represent normal bereavement, and thus a "normal" reaction to a distressing life event should not be diagnosed as an adjustment disorder. Once the stressor or its consequences have terminated, the symptoms do not persist for more than an additional 6 months. When a stressor precipitates a depressive condition that meets the severity and symptom criteria for major depression, the diagnosis of major depression is made, regardless of the condition's etiologic relationship to an identifiable stressor.

One of the controversies with the DSM-5 definition of MDD surrounded the elimination of the bereavement exclusion criterion, suggesting that grief might not be considered a normal process. The revision makes it easier to diagnose MDD in patients who would have previously been considered to be grieving a loss. Ultimately, careful clinical judgment is required to separate MDD from bereavement based on the patient's history and cultural norms of expressing grief, much of which may still fall well within the normal range for the grieving patient.

Bipolar disorder is a common and severe mental illness, occurring in about 3–4% of the general population, causing significant disability, and carrying 80–85% genetic heritability. Up to 30% of primary care patients treated for depression actually have bipolar disorder. Bipolar I disorder refers to patients with a history of at least one episode meeting full criteria for major depression and at least one other distinct episode meeting criteria for mania. Other bipolar spectrum disorders such as bipolar II disorder (a condition marked by episodes of major depression and at least one documented episode of hypomania, not mania) and cyclothymic disorder (no episodes meeting full criteria for either major depression or mania/hypomania) are probably much more common, thought to occur in approximately 4–6% of the population.

Bipolar depression refers to an episode of illness meeting criteria for major depression/major depressive episode (MDE) in a patient with a history of either mania or hypomania. Studies in general medicine indicate that 60% of people with bipolar disorder are in the depressed phase when they go to their primary care provider for help. In bipolar II disorder, symptomatic patients are almost always in the depressed phase rather than the hypomanic phase. Few patients actually seek care during periods of hypomania since these are often pleasant periods of respite from the more prominent, frequent depressive episodes.

It can be very difficult for providers to differentiate an episode of major depression from an episode of bipolar depression because the two conditions are phenotypically identical. Thus, bipolar II disorder is arguably one of the most challenging disorders to diagnose in all of psychiatry. It is extremely important, however, to distinguish between major depression and bipolar depression, because although the two conditions present with similar, mostly overlapping symptoms, they are treated very differently.

Evidence for the best treatment of bipolar depression, however, is still somewhat limited and controversial. Only three medications, quetiapine, lurasidone, and a combination product (olanzapine and fluoxetine) have received Food and Drug Administration (FDA) approval for the treatment of acute bipolar depression. Lamotrigine has FDA approval for maintenance treatment of bipolar depression, but it is not yet approved for acute bipolar depression. Many experts recommend adding an antidepressant for bipolar depression only when combined with two mood stabilizers (e.g., lithium, valproate, carbamazepine, or atypical antipsychotic) at maximum dose as augmentation for residual symptoms of depression. Bipolar depression should *not* be treated with an antidepressant alone. Such "unopposed" treatment (i.e., antidepressant without mood stabilizer) increases the likelihood of precipitating an affective "switch" from depression to mania. Failure to elicit a history of mania or hypomania by the medical practitioner can lead, therefore, to such a switch occurring after treatment with an antidepressant, with attendant risks of erratic or irrational behavior; poor judgment in social, occupational, economic, or interpersonal situations; psychosis; and even suicide. The section on differential diagnosis offers guidelines to help providers make the diagnosis of bipolar depression in patients presenting with the symptom profile of major depression.

Peripartum depression encompasses the period during pregnancy or in the 4 weeks following delivery, a period fraught with hormonal and psychological variability. The USPSTF recommends screening all pregnant and postpartum women for perinatal depression, but still it is frequently overlooked in the postpartum period as "baby blues" can also be seen during the adjustment period. Between 3% and 6% of women will experience the onset of a major depressive episode in the peripartum period with 50% of "postpartum" major depressive episodes beginning prior to delivery. Postpartum depression occurs in about 10–20% of childbearing women. A major debate in psychiatry involves whether antidepressants should be used in pregnant or postpartum women who may be breastfeeding. Most experts suggest that SSRI and SNRI antidepressants (other than paroxetine in the first trimester due to congenital heart defect risk), if used during pregnancy, should be continued if the benefits outweigh the risks, since birth defects and other risks such as persistent pulmonary hypertension of the newborn (PPHN) or discontinuation syndrome are thought to be small. Thus far there are no FDA-approved medications for peripartum depression, although the new intravenous medication option, brexanolone (a neuroactive steroid and positive allosteric modulator of GABA-A receptors), has pending approval for moderate-to-severe postpartum depression after successful phase 3 trials. Sertraline and paroxetine have the lowest expression in breast milk among the SSRI medications.

In addition to the premenstrual and peripartum stages previously mentioned, the perimenopausal (menopause transition and early postmenopausal) reproductive stage is also associated with increased risk for MDE and subthreshold depressive symptoms. Evidence generally suggests that most midlife women who experience a major depressive episode during perimenopause have experienced a prior episode of depression. Midlife depression presents with classic depressive symptoms commonly in combination with menopause symptoms (i.e., vasomotor symptoms and sleep disturbance), and psychosocial challenges. Diagnosis involves identification of menopausal stage, assessment of co-occurring psychiatric and menopause symptoms, appreciation of the psychosocial factors common in midlife, differential diagnoses, and the use of validated screening instruments. Proven therapeutic options for depression (i.e., antidepressants and psychotherapy) are the frontline treatments for perimenopausal depression. Although estrogen therapy is not approved to treat perimenopausal depression, there is evidence that it has antidepressant effects in perimenopausal women, particularly those with concomitant vasomotor symptoms.

Seasonal pattern depression occurs when onset and remission of episodes of depression are temporally related to a particular time of the year, occurring at least over a 2-year cycle without any nonseasonal depressive episodes during that time. One of the main reasons for the change in nomenclature from seasonal affective disorder (SAD) to depression with seasonal pattern is the misconception that SAD was a disorder unto itself. It is simply a specifier for the underlying mood disorder (depression or bipolar disorder) as one cannot have SAD in isolation.

The prevalence of depression with seasonal pattern is 4–6% in the United States with most experiencing their symptoms in the fall-winter months, although this can vary with latitude, age, and sex. Latitudes far north or south of the equator are more at risk. For example, 1% of Florida residents and 9% of those who live in New England or Alaska suffer from seasonal depression. About 10% of patients with seasonal pattern depression experience symptoms during spring–summer months, although this too can vary. Younger persons and women tend to have a higher burden of winter depressive episodes (4:1 ratio of women to men). The treatment of this condition can involve light therapy (see "Light Therapy" section) especially in winter months when the days are shorter. In summer months, the focus is often on preserving proper sleep–wake schedules and avoiding disruptions that longer days and perhaps summer vacations can pose.

Burnout, while not a DSM disorder, is an important issue when discussing depression (see Chapters 6, 36, & 49). Burnout rates among medical professionals are increasing with rates now twice as high as in other professions even after adjusting for factors such as age, sex, level of education, and hours worked in the past week. A good working definition for burnout is a long-term stress reaction characterized by depersonalization, including cynical or negative attitudes toward patients; emotional exhaustion; a feeling of decreased personal achievement; and a lack of empathy for patients. Burnout is thought to have at least a 15% overlap with symptoms of depression. Many experts suggest that burnout is basically a depressive syndrome caused by chronic stressors found in the workplace.

EPIDEMIOLOGY

The prevalence of major depression is 6.7% of all U.S. adults and the estimated lifetime risk of a major depressive episode is around 30%. The prevalence of major depressive episode (MDE) among adult females is almost two times that seen in males. Reasons for gender differences in the prevalence of depression have not been fully elucidated, but both biological and sociocultural factors are thought to contribute. The prevalence rates of depression (and suicide) are far higher in transgender individuals with rates hovering around 50%. Key factors implicated in these markedly elevated rates for transgender individuals include discrimination, stigma, lack of acceptance, and abuse compared to gender binary individuals. In addition, MDD rates are highest among adults reporting two or more races. Among the protective factors in the prevention of depression are high education and socioeconomic advantage.

In ambulatory medical settings, numerous studies report a 10–15% prevalence of major depression, with a substantially higher rate (20–40%) in patients with coexisting medical problems, particularly in those with diseases associated with strong biological or psychological predispositions to depression (e.g., stroke, Parkinson disease, traumatic brain injury, diabetes, coronary atherosclerotic disease, pancreatic cancer, and other terminal illnesses). Individuals aged 18–25 (10.9%) have the highest prevalence, and depression-related suicide is the second leading cause of death for this group. Because the mean age at onset of MDD is 32.5 years old, an apparent first episode of depression in an older patient should prompt a thorough evaluation to exclude underlying disease and/or medication effects.

While MDD occurs in no more than about 5% of community dwelling older adults, rates of up to 10% are found in primary care settings and are much higher in nursing homes and after an acute hospitalization. In addition to genetic vulnerabilities, cognitive diathesis, and stress, a common pathway to depression in older adults is thought to be curtailment of daily activities. Major depression is often misdiagnosed in elderly primary care patients as a sign of aging, and cognitive impairment may also complicate accurate diagnosis. Some medications commonly prescribed in the elderly population may actually precipitate the onset of depression or cause symptoms like fatigue and poor concentration, which may mimic depressive symptoms.

ETIOLOGY

MDD represents a heterogeneous group of disorders. It is likely that future research will eventually provide diagnostic specificity to these disorders, leading to more targeted and effective treatments. For present purposes, however, the clinical manifestation of a major depressive episode should be considered a final common psychobiological pathway among multiple candidate etiologic determinants. Advances in genetic, anatomic, physiologic, and immunologic studies already point the way toward a more precise biological understanding of this common and disabling condition.

THE EMERGING BIOLOGY OF DEPRESSION: ADVANCES IN GENETICS, ANATOMY, PHYSIOLOGY, & IMMUNOLOGY

Recurrent major depression has been shown to have a heritability of 35–40%, and genetic linkage and twin studies have begun to identify specific regions of the genome thought to be candidates for carrying depression susceptibility. One interesting candidate gene is the serotonin transporter gene (*5-HTT*), which makes functional sense since many antidepressants seem to work through binding to the *5-HTT* protein. Case-control association studies of the serotonin receptor gene *HTR2A* and major depression have yielded similar mixed results as for the *5HTT* gene. More recently, researchers at the University of Maryland School of Medicine identified another gene of interest, the *Slc6a15* gene in the D2 neurons of the nucleus accumbens (the "reward center" of the brain).

Postmortem pathologic studies, along with functional and structural imaging studies, have converged to help identify key anatomic loci of depressive illness, including the hippocampus, the dorsolateral prefrontal cortex, the anterior cingulate cortex, and the amygdala. Animal and human studies confirm volumetric decreases in the hippocampus in depressive illness in individuals with a history of adverse childhood events. Antidepressant medications appear to induce neurogenesis (increases in volume) in the hippocampus, possibly through increases in brain-derived neurotrophic factor (BDNF).

From the physiologic point of view, a considerable body of emerging evidence conceptually and experimentally points to dysregulation of distributed brain networks and second messenger abnormalities as the underlying neurobiological abnormalities in recurrent mood disorders. This contrasts with earlier theories postulating that neurotransmitter deficiencies (e.g., decreases in norepinephrine, serotonin, and/or dopamine) serve as the biological substrate of depression. Clinically, it is important that patients with depression not have an impression that they somehow have a brain "deficiency." It is more appropriate to discuss the physiology of depression as a state where the brain may be using the neurotransmitters it produces in an inefficient manner, which is what pharmacotherapy and even psychotherapy targets.

Lastly, immunologic studies have consistently found abnormalities of cytokines associated with depressive illness. High levels of several proinflammatory components of the immune system, such as interleukin-6, C-reactive protein, tumor necrosis factor (TNF)-α, or neopterin, in patients suffering from depression point to the involvement of an inflammatory process in the pathophysiology of MDD (see Chapter 36). A large-scale epidemiological study in MDD clearly demonstrated that severe infections and autoimmune disorders are lifetime risk factors for development of MDD. Advances in all these biological correlates of depression hold great promise for the development of more specific and more effective treatments of depressive disorders in the not too distant future.

SOCIAL & PSYCHOLOGICAL FACTORS

High Stress & Low Support

From a societal perspective, significant life stress and/or lack of social support predisposes to development of MDD. Life stress that involves loss, for example, death of a parent or spouse, the end of a relationship, and events involving loss of self-esteem, such as termination from a job, create particular vulnerability for depression. Low social support, both independently and in the face of significant stress also predisposes to depressive disorder. Low *perceived* social support, that is, the extent to which an individual *believes* himself or herself to lack a supportive social network, creates a higher risk than any absolute or objective measure. (It is worth noting that these same risk factors of high stress and low support tend to increase risk for all illnesses, whether psychiatric or general medical illnesses.)

The stress caused by natural disasters also increases the vulnerability of survivors to depression. While the psychiatric impact of such disasters includes increased prevalence rates of PTSD, substance abuse, and other conditions, the increased rate of depression itself is significant and measurable. For example, children and adults in the tsunami-affected areas of southwestern Thailand showed significantly increased and persistent rates of depression—ranging from 6% to 30% depending upon level of exposure and level of life disruption. Similarly, war has always been a stressor with major mental health consequences. Key drivers of vulnerability to stress include: any personal or family psychiatric history, history of previous trauma (including childhood sexual abuse), low intelligence, limited social supports, and childhood separation from parents or divorce of parents in early childhood.

With increased life expectancy and the aging of the population in the United States, spousal caregiving of persons with disability, including dementia, is increasing. Caregivers (most often the female partner) of spouses with major neurocognitive disorder (e.g., Alzheimer disease) experience extreme physical and emotional burden. The role of caregiver presents a situation of both high stress and increasingly low support (as the caregiver progressively loses any emotionally meaningful relationship with the patient). Up to 40% of caregivers of patients with progressive dementia suffer from significant depressive symptoms or major depression.

Postpartum "baby blues" typically occurs in 50–80% of women within 1–5 days of childbirth and lasts up to 1 week. As discussed earlier, this "normal" reaction should be distinguished from depression with peripartum onset (previously postpartum depression), which occurs in 10–15% of women in the first 3–6 months after childbirth. Postpartum psychosis, which occurs in 0.5–2.0/1000 deliveries and typically begins 2–3 days after delivery, is most common in individuals with a personal or family history of bipolar disorder. The tragic case of Andrea Yates, who drowned her five young children in Houston, Texas in 2001 during a period of postpartum depression and psychosis, highlights the depth of psychosis that can accompany underlying bipolar disorder. Postpartum psychosis is a highly acute psychiatric illness that usually requires mood stabilizers such as neuroleptic medications or lithium, and psychiatric referral (see Chapter 16).

DIAGNOSIS

The criteria for major depression require that five of nine symptoms be present for a 2-week period (see Table 26-1). One of these nine symptoms must be either a persistent depressed mood (present most of the day, nearly every day) **or** pervasive anhedonia (from the Greek meaning "without pleasure").

Clinicians should realize that a depressed mood is not synonymous with major depression and is neither necessary nor sufficient for a diagnosis of major depression. Sadness (or tearfulness) does not constitute major depression and, conversely, major depression can be diagnosed without the presence of depressed mood (if pervasive anhedonia is present), a presentation that is more common in the elderly.

Organizing these nine symptoms into clusters of four hallmarks can facilitate clinical evaluation: (1) depressed mood; (2) anhedonia; (3) physical symptoms (sleep disorder, appetite problem, fatigue, and psychomotor changes); and (4) psychological symptoms (difficulty concentrating or indecisiveness, guilt or low self-esteem, and thoughts of death). Physical symptoms predict a favorable response to biological intervention. For example, when middle insomnia is present (awaking at 3 or 4 A.M. with an inability to return to sleep) and when a diurnal variation in mood is present (feeling more depressed in the morning), patients are more likely to respond to biological interventions.

The Fallacy of "Good Reasons"

Depression is often mistakenly believed to be an "expected" result of stressful life events. Studies of individuals under stress (e.g., terminal cancer or natural disaster) show rates of major depression above the general population rate, but these rates do not typically exceed 50%. Although sad or depressed affect is an expected accompaniment of a stressful event, the full syndrome of major depression does not appear in everyone. Thus, life stressors including bereavement may seem to provide "good reasons" for sadness, but a stressful event, in itself, should not be considered a rationale to withhold depression treatment. If a major depressive syndrome emerges following a stressful life situation, the medical provider should treat it appropriately.

The Confound of Overlapping Etiology

A comorbid general medical condition (such as cancer or Parkinson disease) may seemingly "cause" many of the physical symptoms of major depression, such as fatigue, anorexia, or psychomotor retardation. These symptoms may lead clinicians to discount their relevance and thus disregard the possibility of a treatable depression. However, it is important to ***include*** these symptoms in the initial diagnostic approach to depression in the medically ill and to exclude them *only if they are clearly and fully accounted for by the physical illness.* Although this "inclusive" approach might seem to result in the overdiagnosis of MDD or depressive disorder due to a medical disorder; studies in stroke, Parkinson disease, hospitalized elderly, and traumatic brain injury indicate that the problem of overdiagnosis is quite low when compared with the underdiagnosis of depression.

THE MEDICAL INTERVIEW

Build Trust by Responding to Distress

The medical interview holds the key to the assessment of major depression. Efficient assessment involves attention to data-gathering as well as rapport-building with the patient. Physicians should be alert for nonverbal cues of depression: for example, a sad mood may be communicated by downcast eyes, slow speech, wrinkled brow, or a tearful affect. When a depressed mood is detected or emotional distress is suspected, clinicians should first respond empathically to this distress, by demonstrating a caring attitude, and using attentive silence or direct reflective and empathic statements, such as "I can see you're having some trouble," or "It sounds like you've been under a lot of stress lately," or "You seem down right now." Responding directly to the patient's distress builds trust and encourages the patient to share the feelings that may underlie a depressive illness.

Use Direct, Open-Ended Questioning

Use open-ended questions and facilitation techniques to provide patients with the opportunity to discuss the issues that may be troubling (see Chapter 1). In gathering data for assessment, clinicians should focus on *anhedonia* (e.g., "What do you enjoy doing these days?") and *depressed mood* (e.g., "How has your mood been the last few weeks?" or "Have you been feeling sad, blue, or down in the dumps?"). These simple questions can effectively uncover an underlying depression in most patients, despite the fact that many depressed patients in the general medical setting initially present with physical and bodily symptoms (e.g., headache, fatigue, and insomnia).

Involve the Family

Optimal assessment and management of the depressed patient is enhanced by involvement of one or more significant other(s). A spouse, partner, parent, or others can help the physician gather useful information regarding the patient's mood, activities, behaviors, and history.

In fact, because of stigma, denial, and other psychosocial barriers, other persons often provide much more accurate information regarding depressive illness than the self-report of the patient. Additionally, clinical changes (improvement or worsening) are often more quickly recognized by loved ones than the patient herself due in large part to habituation to the symptoms of depression.

The Patient Health Questionnaire: Screening, Assessment, Engagement, & Monitoring

The PHQ-2 consists of the first two items of the PHQ-9 and is a convenient and evidence-based approach to depression screening in primary care. PHQ-2 scores can range from 0 to 6; a cut-point of ≥3 is considered positive and should prompt administration of the full PHQ-9. Some experts advocate use of the full PHQ-9 (Appendix 26-A) to screen "red flag" patients, that is, those likely to be at high risk of major depression. "Red flag" patients generally include those with chronic medical illness (e.g., diabetes), and patients with persistent unexplained medical complaints. This one-step approach, combining screening and assessment, can simplify operational strategies.

The PHQ-9 is an assessment and severity tool that has been validated for use in general medical as well as specialty psychiatric settings. A score of 10 or more has an 88% sensitivity and specificity for the diagnosis of major depression. Furthermore, the tool also can be used effectively to track patients' symptom severity and improvement over time. The instrument and scoring key are in Appendices 26-A and 26-B.

BARRIERS TO DIAGNOSIS

Patient Barriers: Somatic Presentations & Stigma

Primary care patients with major depression often present with physical complaints, such as pain (headache, backache), fatigue, insomnia, dizziness, or gastrointestinal (GI) problems rather than mood complaints. Many of these patients are willing to acknowledge feelings of depressed mood and to consider the possibility that biologically mediated depression may also cause or exacerbate their physical problems. Some somatically preoccupied patients, however, are reluctant to consider that depression may contribute to their physical symptoms. In these patients, evaluating both general medical and psychiatric problems simultaneously saves time, expense, and frustration for both clinician and patient.

Many patients and families (particularly in some cultures) are reluctant to accept the diagnosis of depression because of associated social stigma. Providers can help overcome this barrier by explaining to patients and families that depression is a common and treatable illness, like other medical illnesses. The hope is that with more awareness and destigmatization of depression, the societal burden of the disorder may diminish.

Clinician Barriers

Depression is often undetected or is not adequately treated in the medical setting. Some providers avoid depression diagnoses because they harbor the same stigmatizing attitudes toward depression that many of their patients feel. In addition, inadequate knowledge and skill, lack of time, reluctance to "open up" new domains of emotional distress, habits leading to low value care (e.g., failing to titrate antidepressant medications in a timely fashion), and misaligned financial incentives all operate as barriers to physician recognition and treatment. However, early recognition of behavioral and psychiatric disorders is ultimately time efficient, while minimizing the cost and risk of extended, unnecessary workups for nonspecific physical complaints.

SUICIDE

There is one death by suicide every 12 minutes in the United States, making suicide one of the top 10 causes of death in all age groups. Roughly 90% of suicide deaths can be traced back to mental illness, most often depression. Suicide risk must be evaluated in all patients with symptoms of depression. Risk factors for completed suicide include gender (elderly white males are at highest risk), alcoholism, psychosis, chronic physical illness, lack of social support, recent humiliation, descent from mania, and use of lethal methods (e.g., gun rather than overdose of pills). Increased risk of suicide has also been noted among depressed adolescents and among LGBTQ (lesbian, gay, bisexual, transgender, and questioning) patients. Explicit suicidal intent, hopelessness, and a well-formulated plan indicate relatively higher risk. Many patients who eventually commit suicide visit a primary care provider in the weeks or months before they take their lives. PCPs are sometimes reluctant to explore suicidal ideation in the mistaken belief that asking about suicide may actually increase a patient's risk. However, assessment of suicidal tendencies usually reassures patients, reduces anxiety for both patient and provider, and facilitates partnership in suicide prevention.

The assessment of suicidal ideation is best approached gradually albeit *systematically* after an examination of Question 9 of the PHQ-9 (or other pertinent suicide questions from alternative depression screening tools), with general questions like, "I notice you marked positive the question about having thoughts about death or hurting yourself in some way on the depression screening tool. When did you last have such thoughts or feel that life is not worth living?" These questions should be followed by asking more specifically about a history of suicide attempts, any specific current plans, hopelessness, impulsivity, and any specific current intentions. Once a patient reveals suicidal ideation, the medical provider should always consider psychiatric consultation and/or hospitalization if the suicidal thoughts are active. However, if there is no intent to act on these thoughts and outpatient management is being considered as a next step, the clinician should assess the following: delirium (using a cognitive screening test), psychosis (screening for auditory and visual hallucinations are considered the standard of care for the nonpsychiatrist), and of course, depression. To complete the assessment, it is often helpful to restate what the patient plans to do next (and perhaps offer a suggestion if needed) after the evaluation. It is also important to gather collateral information on the safety of the patient from a third party either in person or by phone.

A time-honored summary statement that would appropriately capture the key elements of a systematic inpatient safety evaluation that can also be adapted for the outpatient setting is: "Patient says that she is no longer feeling suicidal. There is no evidence of delirium or psychotic features. She acknowledges her family problems and says that counseling makes sense. She has agreed to a follow-up appointment at the mental health center tomorrow and plans to call her employer today to say she will be back at work next week. She has discussed these plans with her husband who agrees to be seen with her at the initial psychiatric assessment following discharge. Patient no longer needs constant observation."

The use of a "no suicide contract" is controversial. The contract was formally recommended in 1973 and involves asking the patient to promise that he or she will contact the physician (or other appropriate caregiver) if there is a danger of losing control of a suicidal impulse. In using such a "contract" however, providers need to realize that there is no convincing empirical evidence to support its validity. In fact, most experts specifically advise against its use, arguing that a mechanistic pursuit of obtaining a "contract" can functionally undermine an open relationship and lead providers into a false sense of security. The main utility of the "contract" may be as a tool to discuss the strength of the individual's suicidal ideas.

In all cases when treating depression, providers must evaluate suicidality at the initiation of treatment and throughout the treatment program. Routine use of the PHQ-9 can aid in assessing suicide risk at the initiation of treatment and, of equal importance, can also aid in the recognition of any subsequent or treatment-emergent suicide risk. Because the risk of suicide sometimes increases within the first few weeks of treatment and can emerge at any point in the subsequent treatment, regular and routine use of the PHQ-9 can function as an efficient and effective suicide reassessment tool. The Columbia-Suicide Severity Rating Scale is also a useful clinician-administered instrument (http://www.cssrs.columbia.edu/about_cssrs.html).

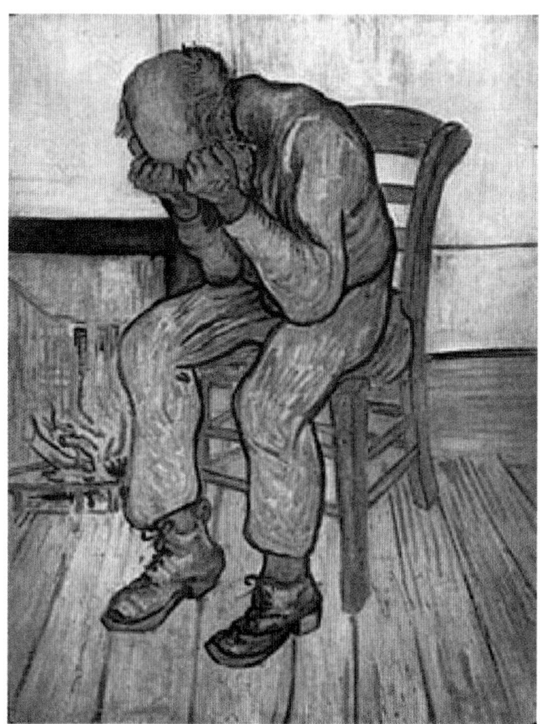

Vincent Van Gogh—At Eternity's Gate

PHYSICAL EXAMINATION

There are no specific diagnostic signs of depression in the physical exam. A careful medical history and physical examination are required for the evaluation of depression at all ages, but especially in the elderly. Some medical "mimics" of depression (e.g., hypothyroidism and Cushing syndrome) present with classic physical signs.

LABORATORY STUDIES

No laboratory studies can be used to diagnose major depression reliably or specifically. A general but targeted laboratory screen may be useful in selected patients to rule out other conditions that may mimic or exacerbate depression: chemistry profile (the highest value test), TSH, urine drug screen, and perhaps a complete blood count in patients reporting bleeding (such as menstruating women) or when treating with medication that can affect hematological lines. In treatment-resistant cases, or when indicated, vitamin levels, urinalysis, brain imaging, or even electroencephalogram (EEG) or lumbar puncture (LP) can be considered, particularly if there are fluctuations in mental status, but these studies are not part of the standard workup. Patients over age 40 usually require an electrocardiogram (ECG) to rule out conduction disturbances or bradycardia when considering treatment with a tricyclic antidepressant (TCA), certain antipsychotics, or citalopram at doses greater than 40 mg/d, since those doses may be associated with prolonged QT intervals and arrhythmias.

DIFFERENTIAL DIAGNOSIS

Mental Disorders

Other mental disorders often present with symptoms similar to depression; in addition, depression often presents in combination with other mental disorders. In the presence of psychiatric comorbidity, effective treatment of depression may lead to improvement in the other condition as well. Modifications of treatment, however, may be necessary depending on the particular comorbidity present.

Major Depressive Disorder Versus Bipolar Depression

It is critically important to distinguish MDD from bipolar depression. The signs and symptoms of the two disorders are identical. One key historical question helps to differentiate the two conditions: *Did the patient ever experience clinical mania or hypomania?* The symptoms of a manic episode are listed in Table 26-2, the most common of which include an elated or irritable mood, racing thoughts, poor judgment in interpersonal, sexual, or financial situations, and excess energy for 1 week (or less if hospitalization is required). Criteria for hypomania are the same but are less intense and not disruptive of normal functioning but last at least 4 days. To uncover a possible history of mania/hypomania, the provider should ask about any personal or family history of treatment of mania/hypomania/bipolar disorder and consider asking a 2-question screen for mood lability that may help distinguish patients with bipolar II disorder from patients with unipolar major depression. The 2 questions are: "Are you a person who frequently experiences ups and downs in mood over life?" and "Do these mood swings occur without cause?" A positive response to at least 1 question indicates mood lability and an increased likelihood of bipolar disorder.

The Mood Disorders Questionnaire (MDQ) may be helpful in making a diagnosis of bipolar disorder (Table 26-3), though its sensitivity and specificity are not high enough to be used as a stand-alone tool. Even if there is no history of mania/hypomania, if the individual has a strong family history of bipolar disorder, the clinician must consider that at least one-third of bipolar patients have depression as their index mood episode. Such a history should help make the clinician alert to potential mood switches with antidepressant treatment.

Table 26-2. Criteria for manic episode.

A. A distinct period of abnormally and persistently elevated, expansive, or irritable mood, lasting at least 1 week (or any duration if hospitalization is necessary).
B. During the period of mood disturbance, three (or more) of the following symptoms have persisted (four if the mood is only irritable) and have been present to a significant degree:
   1. Inflated self-esteem or grandiosity
   2. Decreased need for sleep (e.g., feels rested after only 3 hours of sleep)
   3. More talkative than usual or pressure to keep talking
   4. Flight of ideas or subjective experience that thoughts are racing
   5. Distractibility (i.e., attention too easily drawn to unimportant or irrelevant external stimuli)
   6. Increase in goal-directed activity (either socially, at work or school, or sexually) or psychomotor agitation
   7. Excessive involvement in pleasurable activities that have a high potential for painful consequences (e.g., engaging in unrestrained buying sprees, sexual indiscretions, or foolish business investments)

The mood disturbance is sufficiently severe to cause marked impairment in occupational functioning or in usual social activities or relationships with others, or to necessitate hospitalization to prevent harm to self or others, or there are psychotic features.

Anxiety Disorders

Anxiety and depression commonly co-occur in medical patients. Most patients with depression suffer from anxiety symptoms or an anxiety disorder, and most patients with an anxiety disorder have depressive symptoms or meet criteria for major depression. The most common anxiety disorders in medical outpatients are generalized anxiety disorder (GAD), panic disorder (PD), and social anxiety disorder (social phobia). Treatment of the major depression by itself, however, often helps to resolve or improve these other coexisting conditions (see Chapter 27), especially since many antidepressant medications have proven safe and effective for treating many of the anxiety disorders, PTSD, and OCD.

Somatic Symptom & Related Disorders

Depression often presents with unexplained bodily complaints. It can therefore be challenging to differentiate between a depressive illness and somatic symptom disorder, which includes previously used terms such as medically unexplained symptoms (see Chapter 29). Depressive

Table 26-3. The MDQ and scoring guide.

THE MOOD DISORDER QUESTIONNAIRE		
Instructions: Please answer each question as best you can.		
1 Has there ever been a period of time when you were not your usual self and ...	YES	NO
... you felt so good or so hyper that other people thought you were not your normal self or you were so hyper that you got into trouble?	❍	❍
... you were so irritable that you shouted at people or started fights or arguments?	❍	❍
... you felt much more self-confident than usual?	❍	❍
... you got much less sleep than usual and found you didn't really miss it?	❍	❍
... you were much more talkative or spoke much faster than usual?	❍	❍
... thoughts raced through your head or you couldn't slow your mind down?	❍	❍
... you were so easily distracted by things around you that you had trouble concentrating or staying on track?	❍	❍
... you had much more energy than usual?	❍	❍
... you were much more active or did many more things than usual?	❍	❍
... you were much more social or outgoing than usual, for example, you telephoned friends in the middle of the night?	❍	❍
... you were much more interested in sex than usual?	❍	❍
... you did things that were unusual for you or that other people might have thought were excessive, foolish or risky?	❍	❍
... spending money got you or your family into trouble?	❍	❍
2 If you checked YES to more than one of the above, have several of these ever happened during the same period of time?	❍	❍
3 How much of a problem did any of these cause you—like being unable to work; having family, money or legal troubles; getting into arguments or fights? Please circle one response only. No problem Minor problem Moderate problem Serious problem	❍	❍
4 Have any of your blood relatives (i.e., children, siblings, parents, grandparents, aunts, uncles) had manic-depressive illness or bipolar disorder?	❍	❍
5 Has a health professional ever told you that you have manic-depressive illness or bipolar disorder?	❍	❍
Positive Screen (all three of the following criteria must be met) Question 1: 7 of 13 positive (yes) responses + Question 2: positive (yes) response + Question 3: "moderate" or "serious" response		

Adapted from Hirschfeld RM, Williams JB, Spitzer RL, et al. Development and validation of a screening instrument for bipolar spectrum disorder: The Mood Disorder Questionnaire. *Am J Psychiatry* 2000;157(11):1873-1875. This instrument is designed for screening purposes only and is not to be used as a diagnostic tool.

disorders are highly treatable, but somatic symptom disorders can be more chronic and refractory to treatment. Somatic symptom disorders are usually best managed conservatively with a focus on improved functioning, whereas depression should be treated aggressively with the goal of complete recovery/remission. Any of the somatic symptom disorders (illness anxiety disorder, conversion disorder, factitious disorder, etc.) can present comorbidly with major depression. Approximately 50% of patients with persistent unexplained physical complaints suffer from depression. Effective treatment of major depression as well as short, focused, regular visits to talk about the somatic complaints usually improves the severity, intensity, and functional impairment of a comorbid somatic symptom disorder.

Substance-Related & Addictive Disorders

The substance-related disorders encompass 10 separate classes of drugs that are not fully distinct. Patients with alcohol use disorder or other substance use disorders commonly have comorbid major depression. Unfortunately, a recent study found that only a small fraction (2.4%) of primary care adult patients with depression and severe alcohol use were screened for depression (given a PHQ-9 within 30 days of alcohol screening). Conversely, all patients diagnosed with depression should be screened for comorbid substance use disorders.

Major depression, even in the context of substance dependence, deserves treatment in its own right, as long as the treatment plan attends to potential complications from continuing substance abuse. Furthermore, effective treatment of depression (especially nonpharmacological therapies such as cognitive behavioral therapy) may help ameliorate the alcohol and/or other substance use problems and does not generally lead to increased complications. However, in most cases, treating the substance use disorder first is a key to addressing the depressive symptoms. Some patients will benefit from referral to specialty mental health or substance abuse treatment facilities for their addiction issues, and some severely ill patients will need treatment in settings with the capacity to treat "dual diagnosis" patients (those with both a substance use disorder and a primary mood or thought disorder).

Personality Disorders

Personality disorders represent enduring character patterns that are deeply ingrained and are not generally amenable to alteration (see Chapter 30). They often complicate the diagnosis and management of mood disorders. Because patients with certain personality disorders can be difficult and demanding, providers often try to minimize contact and, in some cases, lose empathy with such individuals. Unfortunately, this may lead to failure to diagnose depression. What often helps the most when interacting with a personality-disordered patient is acknowledging any countertransference issues that may be present by pausing to imagine what the patient's life is like and to then listen empathically without judgement. In the words of Dr. Morton Swartz from Massachusetts General Hospital, "the patient wants to know the doctor cares before he cares what the doctor knows." Beyond these techniques, effective treatment of major depression often improves functioning when the depression coexists with a personality disorder, even if the underlying personality disorder is itself not fundamentally changed.

Neurocognitive Disorders (Formerly Dementia)

In its early stages, mild neurocognitive disorder can be often difficult to distinguish from depression. Depression often leads to reversible cognitive impairment in the form of decreased concentration, memory difficulties, impaired decision-making ability, difficulty planning and organizing, and difficulty getting started on tasks. These are also impairments that can result from an insidious and irreversible neurodegenerative process. Likewise, the effect of neurocognitive disorder on a person's functioning can lead to depressed mood. When diagnostic uncertainty exists, the Cornell Scale for Depression in Dementia (CSDD) is considered the gold standard in the assessment. Because the cognitive impairments of MDD are reversible, clinicians should treat the depressive component (with both medication and counseling) and observe for changes in the patient's cognitive symptom cluster.

The term "pseudodementia" is used to describe treatable depression presenting with features of cognitive impairment. While it is useful for clinicians to understand that depression may be associated with cognitive impairment, clinicians should avoid use of this terminology. In actual practice, some patients for whom the concept of "pseudodementia" is considered may actually suffer from both conditions. Furthermore, late-onset depression (even reversible late-onset depression) is itself predictive of future dementia.

Table 26-4. General medical conditions with high prevalence of depression.

Disease/Condition
Lewy body disease
End-stage renal failure
Parkinson disease
Stroke
Cancer or AIDS
Chronic fatigue
Diabetes mellitus
Chronic pain
Heart disease
Chronic lung disease
Following CABG surgery

Depression due to General Medical Conditions or Medications

Approximately 10–15% of all depression is considered to be the direct physiologic result of a medical illness, such as hypothyroidism, pancreatic cancer, Parkinson disease, or stroke (Table 26-4). Because there are no clear criteria to help guide clinicians in their evaluation, this diagnosis is ultimately made by clinical inference, considering the timing of the depression in relation to the physical illness. Limited data seem to indicate that standard treatments for major depression are effective in these cases.

Similarly, depression can be caused by exogenous medications (Table 26-5). Approximately 50% of

Table 26-5. Medications that can cause depression.

- Interferon
- Antihypertensives
- Hormones
- Anticonvulsants
- Steroids
- Digitalis
- Antiparkinsonian agents
- Antineoplastic agents

patients treated with interferon develop a full major depressive episode, and a history of previous depression or the presence of even mild current depressive symptoms can reliably predict the development of subsequent depression during treatment with interferon. Evidence now supports the prophylactic use of antidepressants before initiating interferon treatment, especially in patients with histories of depression. No medication has been noted to "cause" depression in all patients, so it is therefore crucial to carefully evaluate the patient's clinical history and link the onset of depressive symptoms to the initiation of new medications or changes in the current regimen as well as considering psychosocial stressors to obtain the clearest picture of depression causation.

TREATMENT

Use Communication Skills, PHQ-9 Scores, & the Family for Engagement

Building on the patient's trust, the working alliance, and the doctor–patient relationship, the clinician should integrate his or her understanding of the patient's symptoms and life situation into a clear presentation of the diagnosis to engage the patient for collaborative management.

In addition, the process of the clinician's communication with a depressed patient should be informed by an appreciation of the patient's slower rate of cognitive processing. Information should be given in small chunks, allowing adequate attentive silence for the patient to assimilate and respond. In addition, the clinician should verify adequate assimilation of information by asking the patient to summarize what has just been communicated. The following statement would be appropriate:

"Doctors sometimes have a hard time communicating clearly with their patients. Just to be sure I have been able to make my thoughts clear to you; would you mind summarizing what we just went over?"

By using the PHQ-9, practitioners can integrate these results into the engagement process. The first step is to check some of the symptoms with the patient to verify the validity of specific responses. Then discuss the diagnosis and engage the patient for collaborative treatment planning. Because some patients may feel shame or embarrassment with a diagnosis of depression, it may be helpful to explain that major depression is a common *biological* disorder. Drawing a picture of a synapse and neurotransmitters also may be helpful for some in terms of illustrating how serotonin and norepinephrine are passed most efficiently in the brain (one construct in treating depression).

A crucial part of the engagement process involves instilling hope that this painful illness is treatable. The treatment involves mobilizing patient resources and/or external resources such as medication and social support. Indicate that depressive symptoms can be relieved and note that "others may notice improvements in you before you notice the change yourself." When adverse life circumstances contribute to the depression, the clinician can acknowledge the role played by the stressors but must also help the patient understand that treatment of the depression can help in coping better with life's adversities.

The clinician should attempt to involve the family or other support systems in treatment planning to help ensure adherence to the collaborative plans. Keep in mind, however, that family and/or friends may at times undermine treatment and impede recovery. Approximately 40% of depressed patients suffer from some degree of discord in their relationships that contributes to illness onset and/or becomes a barrier to recovery. When discord is detected, it should be acknowledged and included in the overall treatment.

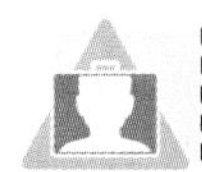

CASE ILLUSTRATION

The following case illustrates many of the principles discussed earlier.

Mrs. Gladstone, a 45-year-old single woman, presents complaining of abdominal pain and fatigue. The abdominal pain is similar to episodes in the past of irritable bowel syndrome, and after a very brief history the primary care provider is convinced that conservative management with added fiber in the diet and antispasmodic medication is appropriate.

Within the first 5 minutes of the interview, however, her PCP also notes that her affect is flat and that she speaks with long latencies. She also complains of having trouble sleeping, frequently awakening after 4 hours with inability to get back to sleep because of worries that she is not qualified for her new managerial position. Things are not going well at home either. Her husband complains that her work keeps her from her responsibilities to her adolescent children, to the household, and to him.

The PCP then asks her to fill out the PHQ-9 and notes that the patient scores 16 on the PHQ-9, with significant symptoms including sleep problems, energy problems, low self-esteem, anhedonia, and sad mood. She does not endorse suicidal ideation. Knowing that this score is associated with a high probability of moderate-to-severe major depression, the following dialogue represents one possible method for presenting the diagnosis and engaging the patient in treatment planning.

Provider: I see you answered affirmatively to several questions on this form. I wonder what you think about the questions.

Mrs. Gladstone: I kind of surprised myself. I'm having trouble with almost everything on that form.

Provider: It seems like you're under some stress.

Mrs. Gladstone: (Tearful) I am. When I go to bed, I dread the next day . . . I know I won't get enough rest and I get this sinking feeling I just can't do it—I'm not good at anything anymore—my work, my home, my marriage. And the stomach pain isn't going away.

Provider: I have some ideas for the stomach pain, but I wanted to check a few of your answers on this form before we come up with a plan for your stomach. It seems like you are feeling very sad almost all the time and there's not much fun in your life.

Mrs. Gladstone: (nods positively—with tears again). And I'm crying by myself a lot. I don't want the kids or my husband to see me.

Provider: It sounds like you're really struggling. The good news is that I think I know what is going on and I think I can help. Your score on this questionnaire is 16—which tells me you're probably suffering from depression—on top of everything else.

Mrs. Gladstone: Well, with the stress of the job, no sleep, the kids' constant whining, and my husband's criticism, who wouldn't be depressed?

Provider: You're right. A lot of people would get depressed with this kind of stress. But now you've got a depression that reflects a chemical imbalance in your brain. And the good news is that there's a lot we can do to help you feel better. If that makes sense to you, we can start talking about different ways we might begin to treat this problem and help you feel a lot better.

Treatment Goals: Defining Clinically Significant Improvement, Response, & Remission

A wide variety of biological and psychological therapies have been shown in randomized clinical trials to be effective for treatment of depression. The concept of "effectiveness," however, hinges on the demonstration of a "response" to treatment defined as "50% improvement in symptoms." A 50% improvement is important clinically, but this criterion is broad enough to leave significant residual symptoms unresolved. The concept of "remission," therefore, has been introduced to underscore the importance of helping the depressed patient reach full return of function and achieve relative absence of all depressive symptoms (in research terms also defined as "70% improvement in symptoms").

The following sections review broad treatment guidelines, psychotherapies, biological treatments, self-management support (SMS), and the need for objective monitoring of symptoms to help the patient attain full remission. Using the Case Illustration of Mrs. Gladstone, a 5-point decrease in her PHQ score from 16 to 11 would be considered a *clinically significant improvement* (the "minimally important clinical difference"). A decrease of 50%, from 16 to 8, would be considered a treatment "*response*," but the score of 8 reflects the persistence of residual symptoms of depression. Not until her PHQ score goes below 5, can Mrs. Gladstone be considered to be in *remission*.

General Treatment Guidelines: Close Monitoring, Persistence in Treatment Trials, & Chronic Reassessment

Research indicates a 50% response rate and a 33% remission rate for the first antidepressant a physician selects for the treatment of depression. Using logical strategies to switch or combine antidepressants after the first failure, about 70% of all patients will eventually respond to treatment. At least 50% of patients with a major depressive episode will have a second episode, and patients who have had two or more episodes of major depression have a 75–90% likelihood of recurrence.

These results suggest the following 7-point treatment program to encourage close monitoring, persistence of treatment trials, and chronic care for patients suffering from major depression. These points are all aligned with current evidence-based guidelines.

1. Use the PHQ-9 to help confirm the diagnosis and establish baseline severity.
2. For those treated with medication, patients should have an "early follow-up" contact, visit or phone call (within 1–3 weeks) to check on adherence to treatment, side effects, or potential change in symptoms for better or worse (e.g., emergent suicidality).
3. The first goal of treatment should be a 5-point decrease in PHQ-9, which is considered a clinically significant improvement. A general target goal (which is difficult to attain) should be a 5-point decrease in PHQ-9 score every month until a score below 5 is attained.
4. Patients should be evaluated with a repeat PHQ-9 once per month until remission is achieved (PHQ-9 <5). In general, the treatment approach should be modified if the patient does not show continuing improvement in PHQ-9 scores. (Modifications could include, e.g., adding medication to psychotherapy or the converse, increasing the dose of a medication, switching medication, augmenting medication, and reevaluating the diagnosis.)
5. Once patients reach remission, treatment should be continued (at the current dose of medication(s), or decreased frequency of psychotherapy) for at least 6–12 months.

6. For patients achieving remission with medications, evidence is clear that maintenance therapy requires the same dose of medication used for recovery. For patients achieving remission with psychotherapy, evidence is less clear, but there is some indication that intermittent "refresher" maintenance psychotherapy sessions can help prevent recurrences.
7. Patients with a history of depression should receive PHQ-9 "check-ups" every 6–12 months for the rest of their lives.

Choosing Initial Treatments: Respect Patient Preferences

Evidence-based treatment for depression includes antidepressant medication, several forms of psychotherapy, a combination of medication and psychotherapy, and, in refractory cases, procedure-based treatments such as electroconvulsive therapy (ECT) or transcranial magnetic stimulation (TMS), or ketamine. ECT remains the gold standard for severe depression, and it can be lifesaving.

Management of depressive illness, like any other chronic illness, should be collaborative. After providing basic education, providers should offer patients realistic treatment options and respect patient preferences. Patients tend to be more adherent to a treatment if they have selected it. Patients may need to be reminded that, if they can stick with the treatment, they have an excellent chance of responding to it. They should also be told that without treatment, they are likely to continue to suffer from depressive symptoms with potential premature brain atrophy.

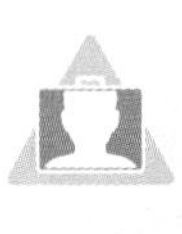

CASE ILLUSTRATION: MRS. GLADSTONE CONTINUED

Let's consider the way the physician and Mrs. Gladstone might collaboratively agree on a management strategy and self-management plan.

Provider: *OK, let's review the treatment options. The kind of depression you're struggling with responds well to antidepressant medication, counseling, or a combination of both medication and counseling. Often the combination works best, but if you are interested in either medication or counseling alone, that should work fine. Do you have any preferences?*

Mrs. Gladstone: *Well, I don't really like the idea of taking medication, but I have no time and no interest in psychobabble stuff. I'm OK with giving the medication a try, if you think it will help.*

Provider: *OK. That's fine. I'll get to the medication recommendation in another moment, but first I wonder if we could talk about some things you might want to do for yourself, to help manage your own illness.*

Mrs. Gladstone: *Sure, but I'm not sure what you mean.*

Provider: *Ok, let me explain. We have found that there are lots of things depressed patients can actually do themselves that can help them feel better . . . and I wonder if you would be interested in doing something specifically that might help your depression.*

Mrs. Gladstone: *Sure, why not. I don't have anything to lose—but I don't have any time for anything anymore.*

Provider: *Ok, let me tell you a little about some things that have worked for other people with depression and then you can let me know if any one of them sounds like something you might want to do.*

Mrs. Gladstone: *OK.*

Provider: *Well, taking your medication regularly helps, of course. Getting some physical activity helps. Planning a schedule and including things you enjoy are helpful. Getting together with friends and family helps. These are some of the things that have worked for others. Would you like to make a plan to do one of these, or perhaps something else you think might help?*

Mrs. Gladstone: *Well, I already said I'm going to take the medication. The other things sound great, but I don't think I'm ready to do anything like that—I just don't have the time or energy for any of them. Can we start with the medication first—maybe later I'll think of something else I can do.*

Provider: *Sure, that's fine. Let's see how the medication works for you. You will need to take it every day, once a day. Lots of people find it difficult to take their medication every day as prescribed. On a scale of 1 to 10, where 10 means you're sure you will take it every day, and 1 means you're not at all sure, how confident do you feel that you will actually take your medication every day.*

Mrs. Gladstone: *I want to get better. I am sure I'll take it—at least an 8 or 9.*

Individual Office Counseling by the Medical Provider

Counseling by the medical provider anchors all treatment modalities (pharmacotherapy, care management, psychotherapy) and provides the relational framework for continuity with the patient's other health care needs. PCP counseling provides the context for discussing the diagnosis, instilling hope for change, mobilizing the patient's self-management, and planning treatment. The time frame for such counseling can be a few minutes to an extended 30-minute visit.

Some providers may want to engage in more specific counseling. The patient, however, should be notified that this interaction should not be considered formal psychotherapy, unless the provider has been adequately trained. Psychotherapeutic situations invariably arouse strong emotions in both patients and providers. When complex interpersonal issues or strong feelings emerge during office counseling, the medical provider should seek supervision from a trained therapist or consultation from a colleague.

The acronym SPEAK was developed by one of the authors (JFC) to help providers in counseling depressed patients (Table 26-6). The five components of **SPEAK** (**S**chedule, **P**leasurable activities, **E**xercise, **A**ssertiveness, and **K**ind thoughts about oneself) are grounded in core elements of evidence-based psychotherapies of depression, including behavioral, interpersonal, and cognitive approaches. They provide a framework both for patient education and for ongoing supportive counseling by the clinician. The SPEAK summary in Table 26-6 can be given to the patient as a handout to use as a component of *guided self-help* (see below).

Table 26-6. SPEAK approach to clinician counseling for depression.

S Schedule **P** Pleasurable activities **E** Exercise **A** Assertiveness **K** Kind thoughts about oneself
S Schedule:
Make a weekly schedule for yourself, with columns for each day of the week and rows for the hours of the day. Using a pencil (so you can make changes) make a plan for activities you will do each hour. Some of the times will already be structured for you, e.g., at work. Focus especially on the times that are currently unstructured. Start with things you know you usually do, e.g., eating meals, preparing meals. Include on the schedule time to do household chores and errands, but also include times for fun activities and exercise. Because temporarily you may not feel the motivation or desire to do any of these things, follow what the schedule says **whether or not you feel like doing it**. Sometimes you might feel like you are just going through the motions. When the time comes to switch to another activity, do so **whether or not you have completed the previous task**. You are making progress by putting in time on all these activities, not by getting through your "to do" list. Proceeding in this way will help you move out of depression by getting yourself moving through the day.
P Pleasurable activities:
Some of the items on your schedule should be activities that previously were fun for you before you became depressed. For the time being, you may feel you are just going through the motions in these activities. When we are depressed the part of the brain that allows us to feel pleasure is not functioning smoothly, so it is important to have a "jump start." You should plan something each day that would normally be fun and make yourself do it.
E Exercise:
Aerobic exercise increases oxygen and circulation to the brain and counteracts the hormonal changes caused by depression. It helps activate the natural pharmacy in your brain that will work with other parts of your treatment to help you come out of depression. Times for daily exercise should be included on your schedule. Running, swimming, bicycling, aerobic dancing, and walking are all forms of exercise that will help.
A Assertiveness:
This involves being **direct** with other people in your communication. Practice letting others know your feelings, needs, wants, opinions, and choices. This is more difficult when we are depressed, because we tend to doubt our own judgment. Or we might hold back because we are afraid others will think poorly of us. These thoughts are a product of depression, so it is necessary to act as if you were confident, even though inside you don't feel it. It takes more energy to hold in feelings than to express them. You might find that by stating clearly what you need or by saying "No" to what you don't want will help increase your energy and confidence. Read *Your Perfect Right* by Alberti and Emmons.
K Kind thoughts about yourself:
Since depression leads us to think self-punishing thoughts, it is very important to increase your awareness of when this is happening and to replace the negative thoughts with positive ones. Most of the time these negative thoughts are strongly held opinions that are not based on evidence. It is like carrying a negative, opinionated relative with you wherever you go. Once you become aware of this pattern of thoughts, begin to analyze them. You might write the most persistent negative thought on a 3 × 5 card. Then turn the card over and write three positive thoughts with which you could replace it. Carry this card with you and refer to it frequently. It takes about three positive statements to counteract the effect of one negative statement.

Source: Courtesy of John F. Christensen, PhD.

Including the Patient's Partner

For patients in a significant relationship, including the partner in conjoint counseling can place the patient's symptoms and recovery within a relational context. Engaging the partner as an ally in the patient's self-management activities can increase adherence as well as external motivation in the context of a caring relationship. It can also help the partner understand the patient's symptoms as part of the illness being treated. In working with couples, practitioners can utilize some of the following interventions, all of which now have an emerging evidence base. Again, make it clear to patient and partner that these interventions are not a substitute for therapy by a mental health specialist. When involving the partner in assessment or management of depression, it is essential to obtain informed consent from the patient first.

1. *Listen attentively* to the patient and their partner; discuss their current life stresses and emotional difficulties. Allowing straightforward "ventilation" can be therapeutic in itself, and you will learn the extent to which discord in the relationship may be a factor in the depression. In addition, by expressing empathy to each partner, the clinician can model appropriate interpersonal behavior for the discordant couple and build mutual support and trust.
2. *Straightforward education about the biological nature of depression* is a necessary component of all treatment, but in the context of discord in a couple it can help both partners view the depression in a more "forgiving" manner. In a common, but painful and maladaptive "dance," the discordant partner typically expresses a blaming attitude toward the depressed partner, which the patient accepts wholeheartedly because it resonates with his or her own highly negative cognitive self-appraisal. Similarly, an educated spouse is more likely to be able to view the depressed individual's depressive irritability as a symptom needing to be addressed, rather than a personal attack. By reframing the illness as a biological condition, the practitioner helps build the relationship and aids medication adherence (if antidepressants are part of the treatment plan).
3. *Encourage or facilitate joint problem solving.* Helping the depressed patient and their partner identify two or three troubling life problems they face and helping them develop a shared, concrete behavioral solution can help build their alliance and contribute to recovery. However, continuing or persistent discord may undermine treatment or recovery and should be referred for formal couple counseling.

Psychotherapy

The psychotherapy strategies commonly used in treating depression include cognitive behavioral therapy (CBT), interpersonal therapy (IPT), psychodynamic therapy (PDT), problem-solving therapy (PST), and family therapy (including couple therapy). Some of these therapies can be administered in individual or group sessions (CBT, IPT, and PST). In addition, some therapies can be offered via the Internet (real-time text messaging, email, or video conference) or by telephone. Psychotherapy is typically provided by a licensed mental health therapist (psychiatrist, clinical psychologist, clinical social worker, psychiatric nurse practitioner).

Cognitive behavioral therapy attempts to identify and challenge cognitive distortions (e.g., "I fail at everything") that are pessimistic or self-critical thoughts which contribute to and maintain the depressed mood. Once these negative cognitive patterns are identified, the patient learns to challenge them and to develop countermessages that are more evidence based and positive. In addition, CBT teaches "behavioral activation" to counter the inertia of depression (e.g., engaging in pleasurable activities in the presence of anhedonia, or engaging in physical exercise in the absence of motivation). Evidence supports the effectiveness of CBT in treating depression, both as a single problem and as a comorbidity with somatic illnesses. Cognitive behavioral therapy combined with pharmacotherapy has higher effectiveness than CBT alone in treating older adults, particularly in patients with chronic, treatment-resistant depression.

There is also evidence that several variants of CBT, such as mindfulness-based cognitive therapy (MBCT) and cognitive behavioral analysis system of psychotherapy (CBASP) may be effective in the treatment of depression. Mindfulness-based cognitive therapy utilizes mindfulness meditation to teach patients to recognize and let go of ruminative thinking by enhancing "metacognitive awareness," which is a nonjudgmental observation of the passage of thoughts and feelings and how they are constructed. Patients undergoing this approach learn to experience negative thoughts and feelings as mental events, rather than as the self (see Chapter 7).

Within the domain of CBT, two methods of therapy have emerged in recent decades with a good evidence base for treatment of depression: dialectical behavior therapy (DBT) and acceptance and commitment therapy (ACT). Dialectical behavior therapy was originally developed to treat the parasuicidal behavior of patients suffering from borderline personality disorder. The treatment is dialectical in that its goal is to synthesize the alternative principles of acceptance and change. Acceptance strategies are similar to the notion of unconditional positive regard in client-centered therapy. Change strategies have the objective of changing thoughts and overt behavior. Dialectical behavior therapy addresses four skill sets: mindfulness, interpersonal effectiveness, emotion regulation, and distress tolerance. Group DBT treatment has shown positive effects in reducing symptoms in patients with treatment-resistant depression.

Acceptance and commitment therapy conceptualizes psychopathology as stemming from unhealthy efforts to control emotions, thoughts, memories, and other private experiences and a lack of clarity about one's core values and the ability to act in accordance with them. The goal of ACT is to diminish the role of thought while encouraging the patient to embrace experience directly without suppression. At the same time, it encourages behavior consistent with one's chosen values. Compared to traditional cognitive therapy, ACT has shown equal effectiveness in reducing symptoms of depression.

Interpersonal therapy focuses on one or more of several interpersonal situations that may relate to initiating or sustaining depression: interpersonal conflict, role transition, grief, or social skills deficits. Assertiveness training is one component of IPT that develops patients' capacity to be direct in communicating feelings, thoughts, and preferences in their current relationships. In the treatment of depression, IPT has been shown to be more effective than placebo and equivalent to medication in adults. In late life depression, medication was more effective. Overall, CBT and IPT have the broadest evidence base for effectiveness in treatment of depression.

Psychodynamic therapy focuses on interpersonal relationships and unconscious feelings, desires, strivings, and thoughts to treat symptom disorders. It involves using the therapeutic alliance to gain an understanding of the ways maladaptive defense mechanisms have developed and contribute to depression and then working through these mechanisms in an effort to build more adaptive and less punishing defense mechanisms. A meta-analysis of short-term dynamic psychotherapy (STDP) found that it had significant effects for depressive symptoms and that these changes endured at 1-year follow-up. Although other forms of psychotherapy showed a greater effect immediately posttreatment, there were no differences at 1-year follow-up.

Problem-solving therapy teaches patients to break down larger life problems into smaller elements and to identify specific steps to address these elements. It has been shown to be as effective as antidepressant medication in the treatment of depressed primary care patients. Meta-analysis has shown a modest effect of PST on depression, with greater effects noted in group treatment with PST.

The evidence from many randomized clinical trials is that these psychotherapies are as effective as antidepressant medication (in mild-to-moderate MDD) in achieving a significant reduction of symptoms (over 50% response rate) after 10–16 weeks of treatment. Although the response to antidepressants is generally evident in the first 4 weeks, response to psychotherapy catches up and by 12 weeks the efficacy of medication and psychotherapy are comparable. There is some reason to believe that antidepressant medication and psychotherapy of depression achieve their benefits through different neurobiological mechanisms, so it is not surprising that combination treatments (medication and psychotherapy) have generally been found to be more effective than either one alone. For individuals with severe depression, antidepressants are the mainstays of treatment and are more effective than psychotherapy alone.

Cognitive behavioral therapy is generally considered the treatment of choice for depression in children and adolescents, though one medication (fluoxetine) is FDA approved for this age group. The clinical benefits of psychotherapy are usually seen in 8–12 weeks, and the duration of treatment is typically 6–16 sessions. Meta-analysis has shown that psychotherapy is moderately effective in the short run, especially for adolescents aged 12–18 years, but that after 6 months psychotherapy does not show enduring effects.

Guided self-help involves the patient working at home with a standardized psychological treatment, such as CBT, with guidance from a physician or mental health therapist, who provides initial support and occasional coaching. Therapist support can be face-to-face or via telephone or email. The standardized treatment can be in various formats—book, audio CD, video, or Internet. Remote psychotherapy via phone or Internet also has shown promise for the treatment of depression.

Considerations for choosing psychotherapy in the acute phase of treatment are shown in Table 26-7. Besides being an adjunct to medication for the treatment of depression, psychotherapy may also have a role in prophylactic maintenance therapy for the prevention or delay of future depressive episodes in patients susceptible to recurrences. For example, MBCT has been shown to reduce depressive relapse rates at levels similar to maintenance antidepressants in several randomized controlled trials. Psychotherapy can also be useful for women with major depression who want to become pregnant and bear a child in a medication-free condition or for other patients with major depression who must be medication free for limited periods. In mild-to-moderate depressions, psychotherapy alone may be as effective as psychotherapy combined with antidepressants.

Marital & Couple Therapy

Couple therapy may be an appropriate choice of psychotherapy, especially when relationship problems are

Table 26-7. Considerations for acute-phase treatment with psychotherapy.

- Less severe depression
- Prior response to psychotherapy
- Incomplete response to treatment with medication alone
- Chronic psychosocial problems
- Availability of trained, competent therapist
- Patient preference

entwined with depression. Although individual therapy for depression can be effective in decreasing depressive symptoms even in the presence of marital discord, if the discord in the relationship is not addressed, relapse into depression is more likely.

Exercise & Physical Activity

Although previous evidence from randomized clinical trials has been inconclusive on the benefits of moderate exercise in the treatment of depression, recent meta-analyses with more rigorous selection methodologies suggest a positive effect of exercise on depression. One meta-analysis found that compared with nonactive controls, moderate to vigorous aerobic exercise, especially when supervised by exercise professionals, had a large and significant antidepressant effect in MDD. Another meta-analysis concluded that exercise has a moderate antidepressant effect compared with no treatment and placebo, and that it may be recommended for people with mild and moderate depression. These findings are consistent with a large cross-sectional study of 1.2 million adults in the United States, which found that physical exercise was significantly and meaningfully associated with a reduced self-reported mental health burden.

Self-Help Books

For motivated patients, self-help books that increase understanding of depression and provide guidance on self-management strategies can be an effective adjunct to treatment. For patients without access to psychotherapy, the use of self-help materials can be a beneficial substitute. A meta-analysis of studies examining the use of self-help books in the United Kingdom found that one book, *Feeling Good*, had a large treatment effect compared to delayed treatment.

ANTIDEPRESSANT PHARMACOTHERAPY

Evidence from large trials, especially "real world" studies such as the Sequenced Treatment Alternatives to Relieve Depression (STAR*D) trial, demonstrates that antidepressant medications are effective for the treatment of major depression and persistent depressive disorder (dysthymia). There are no compelling data, however, to support the use of antidepressant medication for patients with adjustment disorders or other minor depressive disorders. The initial treatment of choice for most patients with an adjustment disorder or other minor depressive episode is "watchful waiting," which consists of provider support, office counseling, and close observation, with repeat assessment to document improvement, remission, lack of improvement, or possible transformation into major depression. Patients with sub-syndromal depression who do not improve after 3–6 months of watchful waiting can be treated empirically with a trial of antidepressant medication or referred for psychotherapy.

Communicating With Patients About Medication

Patients initiating antidepressant medication for the first time sometimes are concerned about the stigma associated with their use or potential adverse effects. Some fear becoming dependent on the medicine or that it will change their personality in some way. It is important to explain that antidepressants are generally nonaddictive medicines that can make the brain more efficient in how it uses the neurotransmitters that it produces to combat depression and actually work to restore neural pathways and connections. It can be helpful to inform the patient about the possibility of experiencing some of the known side effects of the particular antidepressant—most commonly headache and upset stomach with serotonergic medication during the first 7–10 days. It can allay fears to refer to those potential adverse effects as an indicator of the drug's potency to achieve the desired results, especially since serotonin is found most abundantly in the brain and gut.

Despite the STAR*D data showing that antidepressants work (66% aggregate remission rate), 2/3s of patients *stopped* prescribed meds within the first 3 months. Thus, it is important to build a realistic expectation about the tempo of therapeutic effectiveness by letting the patient know that even though the symptoms of depression may persist for several weeks after starting the antidepressant, the healing process has already begun. Adherence to treatment has been shown to be enhanced when the physician–patient alliance is optimized, when the patient's attitudes toward and experience with treatment are thoroughly explored, and when the patient's opinion in treatment decisions is explicitly valued through a spirit of shared decision making.

Pharmacotherapy Options

According to many practice guidelines, selective serotonin reuptake inhibitors (SSRIs), serotonin norepinephrine reuptake inhibitors (SNRIs), and several antidepressants classified separately (such as bupropion, mirtazapine, and vortioxetine) are considered appropriate initial treatment options for MDD. Many factors must be considered when individualizing a pharmacotherapy plan. Two important studies by Cipriani and colleagues (see "Suggested Readings") highlight the value of assessing not just efficacy but also tolerability (or acceptability) of a drug. Figure 26-1 shows a ranking of the most commonly prescribed antidepressants according to their efficacy and acceptability.

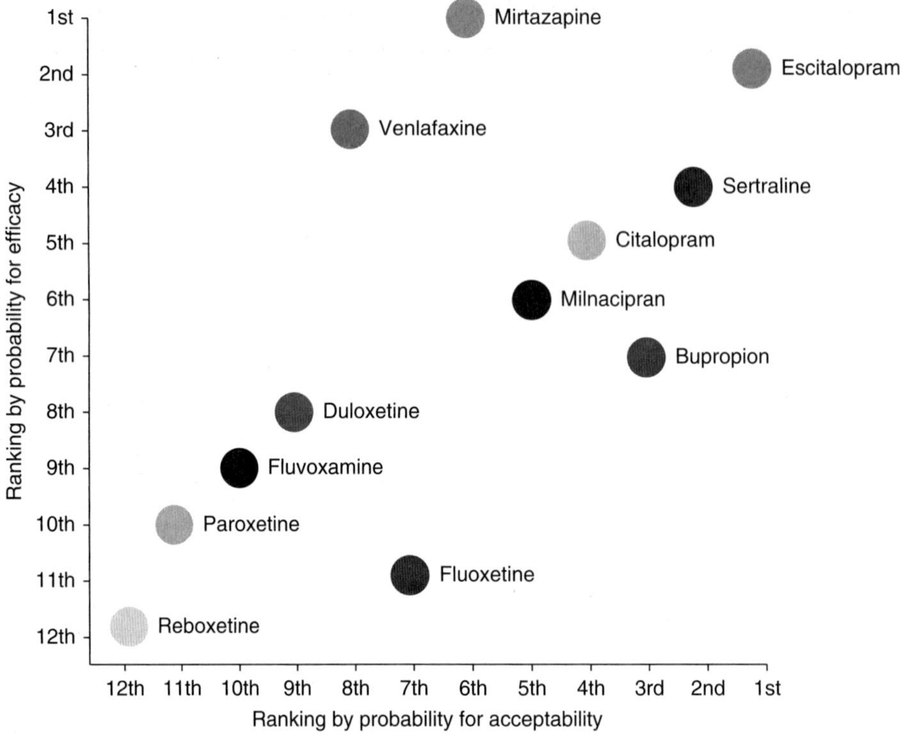

Figure 26-1. Ranking of commonly used antidepressants by efficacy and acceptability. Reprinted from Cipriani A, Furukawa TA, Salanti G, et al (2009). Comparative efficacy and acceptability of 12 new-generation antidepressants: a multiple-treatments meta-analysis. *The Lancet* 373:746-758.

Antidepressants elicit immediate first-dose pharmacological effects on the catecholamine reuptake system; however, these agents only begin to provide some symptom improvement after 1–2 weeks of treatment. An adequate trial of an antidepressant requires a minimum of 4–6 weeks at appropriate doses. Cyclic antidepressant response rates approximate 50–70%; hence, physicians should expect that up to half of the patients they treat with the first antidepressant may not respond. Patients with no response or minimal response should be switched to another agent. Patients with partial response can be managed with augmenting agents. If the first SSRI trial fails, patients may be switched to another SSRI or a drug of another class (e.g., bupropion, venlafaxine, mirtazapine, or a TCA). Of note, 25–50% of patients who fail to respond to the first trial of an SSRI will respond to a different SSRI on a second trial. A list of current antidepressants, adverse effects, mechanisms of action, and dosages is listed in Table 26-8.

Selective Serotonin Reuptake Inhibitors

There are five SSRIs approved for major depression in the United States—fluoxetine, paroxetine, sertraline, citalopram, and escitalopram. The SSRIs are first-line agents for major depression because they are generally better tolerated and are not life-threatening in overdose. Selective serotonin reuptake inhibitors are virtually free of antimuscarinic, antihistaminic, and antiadrenergic side effects. As previously noted, all SSRIs were thought to be equally effective per the STAR*D trial; therefore, choice of any particular SSRI is generally based on side effect profiles, pharmacokinetics, drug interactions, dosage forms, cost, formulary availability, and so on. Table 26-9 demonstrates comparative SSRI adverse effects.

As a class, many SSRIs have also been shown to be effective for PD, GAD, OCD, social anxiety disorder, PTSD, premenstrual dysphoric disorder, and bulimia nervosa. Fluoxetine is the only SSRI with an FDA indication for the treatment of childhood or adolescent depression, and fluoxetine, paroxetine, and sertraline have FDA indications for the treatment of childhood and adolescent OCD. Vilazodone is also a partial agonist at the 5-HT1A receptors and appears to have less sexual dysfunction and potential for weight gain. Vortioxetine is an SSRI that also has serotonin receptor modulator activity. In addition to its antidepressant effect, vortioxetine has been shown to have positive effects on cognitive function in adults with recurrent MDD.

Table 26-8. Commonly used antidepressants (listed in alphabetical order within classes).

Medication	Usual Daily Oral Dose (mg)	Usual Daily Maximum Dose (mg)	Sedative Effects[1]	Anticholinergic Effects[1]	Cost per Unit	Cost for 30 Days Treatment Based on Maximum Dosage[2]
SSRIs						
Citalopram (Celexa)	20	40	< 1	1	$2.53/40 mg	$75.90
Escitalopram (Lexapro)	10	20	< 1	1	$4.51/20 mg	$135.30
Fluoxetine (Prozac, Sarafem)	5–40	80	< 1	< 1	$2.48/20 mg	$297.60
Fluvoxamine (Luvox)	100–300	300	1	< 1	$2.64/100 mg	$237.60
Paroxetine (Paxil)	20–30	50	1	1	$2.64/20 mg	$161.10
Sertraline (Zoloft)	50–150	200	< 1	< 1	$2.85/100 mg	$171.00
SNRIs						
Desvenlafaxine (Pristiq)	50	100	1	< 1	$11.47/100 mg	$344.10
Duloxetine (Cymbalta)	40	60	2	3	$5.93/60 mg	$177.90
Levomilnacipran (Fetzima)	40	120	1	1	$14.35/80 mg	$430.50
Milnacipran (Savella)	100	200	1	1	$6.98/100 mg	$418.80
Venlafaxine XR (Effexor)	150–225	225	1	< 1	$4.67/75 mg	$420.30
Tricyclic and Clinically Similar Compounds						
Amitriptyline (Elavil)	150–250	300	4	4	$2.14/150 mg	$128.40
Amoxapine (Asendin)	150–200	400	2	2	$1.98/100 mg	$237.60
Clomipramine (Anafranil)	100	250	3	3	$11.24/75 mg	$1348.80
Desipramine (Norpramin)	100–250	300	1	1	$5.74/100 mg	$498.60
Doxepin (Sinequan)	150–200	300	4	3	$1.97/100 mg	$177.30
Imipramine (Tofranil)	150–200	300	3	3	$1.22/50 mg	$219.60
Maprotiline (Ludiomil)	100–200	300	4	2	$2.34/75 mg	$280.80
Nortriptyline (Aventyl, Pamelor)	100–150	150	2	2	$0.29/75 mg	$17.40
Protriptyline (Vivactil)	15–40	60	1	3	$3.30/10 mg	$594.00
Trimipramine (Surmontil)	75–200	200	4	4	$9.44/100 mg	$566.40
Monoamine Oxidase Inhibitors						
Phenelzine (Nardil)	45–60	90	…	…	$0.84/15 mg	$151.20
Selegiline transdermal (Emsam)	6 (skin patch)	12	…	…	$65.98/6 mg patch	$1979.50
Tranylcypromine (Parnate)	20–30	50	…	…	$8.41/10 mg	$1261.50

(Continued)

Table 26-8. Commonly used antidepressants (listed in alphabetical order within classes). (*Continued*)

Medication	Usual Daily Oral Dose (mg)	Usual Daily Maximum Dose (mg)	Sedative Effects[1]	Anticholinergic Effects[1]	Cost per Unit	Cost for 30 Days Treatment Based on Maximum Dosage[2]
			Other Compounds			
Bupropion SR (Wellbutrin SR)	300	400[3]	< 1	< 1	$3.38/200 mg	$202.80
Bupropion XL (Wellbutrin XL)	300[4]	450[4]	< 1	< 1	$0.55/300 mg	$32.10
Mirtazapine (Remeron)	15–45	45	4	2	$2.80/30 mg	$84.90
Nefazodone (Serzone)	150–600	600	3	1	$4.98/200 mg	$448.20
Trazodone (Desyrel)	100–300	400	4	< 1	$0.50/100 mg	$60.00
Vilazodone (Viibryd)	10–40	40	1	1	$9.94/40 mg	$298.20
Vortioxetine (Brintellix)	10	20	<1	< 1	$15.12/20 mg	$453.60

[1]1, weak effect; 4, strong effect.
[2]Average wholesale price (AWP, for AB-rated generic when available) for quantity listed. *Source: Red Book* (electronic version), Truven Health Analytics, Information, http://www.micormedexsolutions.com, accessed April 10, 2018. AWP may not accurately represent the actual pharmacy cost because wide contractual variations exist among institutions.
[3]200 mg twice daily.
[4]Wellbutrin XL is a once-daily form of bupropion. Bupropion is still available as immediate release, and, if used, no single dose should exceed 150 mg.
SSRIs, selective serotonin reuptake inhibitors; SNRIs, serotonin norepinephrin reuptake inhibitors.
Reproduced with permission from Raj KS, Williams N, DeBattista C. *Psychiatric Disorders.* In: Papadakis MA, McPhee SJ, Rabow MW, eds. *Current Medical Diagnosis and Treatment 2019*, 58th ed. New York: McGraw-Hill; 2019.

With the exception of fluoxetine and paroxetine, SSRIs show very little inhibition of liver isoenzyme systems. Because of a common SSRI discontinuation syndrome, marked by GI and autonomic signs and symptoms, providers taking patients off these medications should taper them slowly. Withdrawal from paroxetine seems to be more problematic than other SSRIs due to its short half-life. Although without strong evidence, brief use of the long-acting SSRI fluoxetine has been proposed for use to help mitigate SSRI withdrawal effects when discontinuing other SSRIs. In the overdose setting, SSRIs can cause dose-related toxicity, manifesting with nausea and vomiting, tremor, myoclonus, dysrhythmias, and seizures—plausibly all manifestations of the serotonin syndrome.

Gastrointestinal Adverse Effects

The SSRIs inhibit serotonin reuptake, thereby activating 5-HT$_3$ receptors, which can cause nausea and vomiting in 10–15% of patients. Due to desensitization of the 5-HT$_3$ receptors, tolerance to nausea and vomiting usually occurs within 1–2 weeks. Short-term use of cyproheptadine (5-HT$_3$ receptor antagonist) may decrease

Table 26-9. Comparative adverse effects of SSRIs.*

Drug	Nausea/GI Upset	Insomnia	Somnolence	Weight Gain	Sexual Dysfunction	Anticholinergic Effects
Fluoxetine	+++	++++	+	+	+++	0
Sertraline	+++	++	+	+	+++	0
Paroxetine	+++	++	++	+++	++++	+
Citalopram	+++	++	+	Unknown	+++	0
Escitalopram	+++	++	+	Unknown	+++	0

*0, none; +, minimal; ++, mild; +++, moderate; ++++, severe.

uncomfortable nausea and vomiting, although any number of anti-emetics can be employed to mitigate symptoms. To minimize GI irritation, nausea, and vomiting, it is useful to administer the SSRIs with food. Dose-related diarrhea is also a common adverse effect of the SSRIs.

Weight Gain & Weight Loss

Both weight gain and weight loss have been reported with the SSRIs, often corresponding to the type of depression. In classic MDD where weight loss is common, antidepressant-associated weight gain can occur sometimes as a natural result of eating more normally again. In contrast, depression with atypical features is typically associated with significant weight gain or increase in appetite that may reduce as the patient improves on antidepressant therapy. Addition of bupropion may decrease SSRI-induced weight gain. Anorexia and weight loss have also been reported during early treatment, especially in overweight individuals with carbohydrate cravings, underweight depressed patients, bulimics, or patients using fluoxetine.

Syndrome of Inappropriate Antidiuretic Hormone Secretion

A clinically relevant and underappreciated adverse effect of the cyclic antidepressants is the syndrome of inappropriate antidiuretic hormone secretion (SIADH). Syndrome of inappropriate antidiuretic hormone secretion presents with serum hyponatremia (<135 mmol/L) and hypoosmolality (<275 mOsm/Kg), and urinary hypernatremia (usually >20 mmol/L) and hyperosmolality (>100 and usually >280 mOsm/kg). This syndrome is caused by an excessive release of antidiuretic hormone, presenting with signs and symptoms such as nausea, vomiting, weakness, fatigue, confusion, and seizures. SIADH has been reported with most antidepressants and is reversible upon dose reduction or discontinuation. Management also includes fluid restriction and sometimes the combination of saline with loop diuretics. SIADH is more common in the context of tobacco use.

Bleeding Diatheses

Studies have shown an association between serotonergic antidepressants and both upper GI and dysfunctional uterine bleeding in particular. Epistaxis, petechiae, purpura, and ecchymosis can also be seen, because approximately 95% of serotonin is stored in platelets, and serotonin is one of many chemotactic factors responsible for platelet aggregation. SSRIs possess an aspirin-like effect and inhibit platelet aggregation, but the potency and duration of this effect is not yet well elucidated. When SSRIs are coadministered with nonsteroidal anti-inflammatory drugs (NSAIDs), the risk of NSAID-induced gastropathy/erosions increases significantly. Physicians should be cautious when prescribing an SSRI in patients with a history of GI bleeding and in patients who are already taking other antiplatelet medications. In the context of concurrent NSAIDs, aspirin, or other antiplatelet therapy, physicians should consider adding a gastroprotective medication (e.g., proton pump inhibitor) for prophylaxis to prevent GI bleeding.

Sexual Dysfunction

Decreased libido, orgasmic difficulties or anorgasmia, penile anesthesia, and erectile dysfunction (impotence) are common adverse effects associated with the SSRIs in men and women. Sexual side effects occur in 25–75% of all patients, a higher prevalence than reported in package inserts because of underreporting and the short duration of clinical trials. The true incidence of SRI antidepressant-associated sexual dysfunction (SRI-AASD) itself has been difficult to pin down, but it is usually dose-related, occurs early in treatment, and rarely remits spontaneously.

Bupropion and mirtazapine are less likely to cause sexual dysfunction. The prevailing thought regarding the physiological cause of SRI-AASD is the stimulation of 5-HT_{2A} receptors. Mirtazapine actually does the opposite through antagonism at the 5-HT_{2A} and 5-HT_{2C} receptors, both of which are thought to protect sexual functioning.

Sexual dysfunction in males, especially erectile dysfunction, has been successfully managed with phosphodiesterase type-5 antagonists, such as sildenafil, tadalafil, and vardenafil. Other medications such as yohimbine, amantadine, buspirone, bethanechol, neostigmine, cyproheptadine, and *Ginkgo biloba* do not have clear evidence of efficacy from randomized controlled clinical trials. Some clinicians will suggest a *drug holiday*, recommending skipping the dose of the SSRI 24 hours prior to sexual activity (not effective with fluoxetine because of its long half-life). Because sexual dysfunction has such a significant impact on quality of life, this problem may be the most common limiting factor in the use of SSRIs.

Serotonin Syndrome

Poison control centers report over 27,000 toxic exposures to SSRIs annually, with 15% of these reporting a serotonin syndrome. The serotonin syndrome can occur in overdose or when two or more serotonergic agents are combined. Table 26-9 lists common serotonergic agents and their adverse effects. The serotonin syndrome presents as a clinical triad of autonomic dysfunction (e.g., hyperthermia and labile blood pressure), neuromuscular dysfunction (e.g., clonus and hyperreflexia), and mental status changes (e.g., agitation and delirium). This spectrum of clinical findings can be mild and transient and include akathisia, tremor, and altered mental status; however, it can progress to life-threatening symptoms, such as sustained clonus, muscular hypertonicity, and hyperthermia approaching 40°C. Severe serotonin syndrome is a medical emergency with a mortality rate ranging from 2% to 12%. Bupropion does not have serotonin effects, which makes it a safer and effective augmentation strategy in combination with serotonergic medications.

Serotonin Norepinephrine Reuptake Inhibitors

Venlafaxine is a bicyclic antidepressant, approved in 1994 as the first *dual-acting* antidepressant agent to inhibit the reuptake of both norepinephrine and serotonin. These agents are often referred to as SNRIs. At lower doses, venlafaxine exhibits relatively more serotoninergic activity; however, at doses above 150 mg daily the adrenergic and serotonergic effects become more balanced. Venlafaxine is also FDA approved for the management of generalized and social anxiety disorder and PD. The extended release form of the product (XR) has become preferred because it can be used once daily and has much lower propensity to cause nausea, vomiting, and increases in blood pressure (3% of patients on doses of 375 mg experience sustained elevation in blood pressure). Venlafaxine shows very low inhibition of liver isoenzyme systems and has much lower protein binding (about 30%) than most other antidepressants that are very highly protein bound. Discontinuation of venlafaxine is associated with an SSRI-like discontinuation syndrome, requiring gradual taper (or "covering" for withdrawal effects with fluoxetine). Desvenlafaxine is a newer preparation consisting of a metabolite of the desmethyl metabolite of venlafaxine. It offers simpler dosing starting at 50 mg, which is the same as the full continuation dose. This is a modest advantage in that venlafaxine typically requires gradual increases in dosing to avoid GI side effects.

Duloxetine is a bicyclic SNRI antidepressant indicated for MDD, GAD, diabetic peripheral neuropathic pain, fibromyalgia, and chronic musculoskeletal pain. Duloxetine, like venlafaxine, can produce modest increases in blood pressure, nausea, sweating, insomnia, dizziness, and sexual dysfunction. Duloxetine is metabolized by CYP-1A2 and 2D6, and is a 2D6 inhibitor. Of clinical importance, physicians should be aware that when duloxetine is administered with 1A2 inhibitors, such as fluvoxamine or ciprofloxacin, or 2D6 inhibitors, such as paroxetine, duloxetine serum concentrations can increase considerably. Duloxetine should not be used in patients with a creatinine clearance less than 30 mL/min due to significant accumulation of the parent (twofold) and numerous metabolites (ninefold). Duloxetine has been associated with hepatotoxicity; in controlled trials 1% of the patients experienced elevations in liver enzyme tests three times the upper limit of normal. Duloxetine is best avoided in patients with a history of alcohol abuse or hepatic disease, and in patients receiving concomitant hepatotoxic agents.

Levomilnacipran was FDA approved in 2013 for MDD. Levomilnacipran is unique among the SNRI medications because its serotonin:norepinephrine ratio is 1:2; none of the other SNRIs on the market have a ratio favoring norepinephrine.

Other First-Line Antidepressants

Mirtazapine, a tetracyclic noradrenaline and specific serotonin antidepressant (an NaSSa agent), is a potent serotonin-2 (5-HT_2), serotonin-3 (5-HT_3), and central alpha-2-adrenergic receptor antagonist. Advantages of mirtazapine include the following: it is less likely to cause sexual dysfunction, may reduce sleep latency and prolong sleep duration, may have anxiolytic effects, is relatively devoid of alpha-1 blocking effects such as orthostatic hypotension, and may cause less GI adverse effects than the SSRIs. Mirtazapine is a potent appetite stimulant, causing substantial weight gain in many patients. This can be advantageous in patients who are cachectic and nutritionally deficient, such as debilitated elderly and patients with cancer and HIV/AIDS. However, in obese, diabetic, and patients with cardiovascular diseases, mirtazapine-induced weight gain is undesirable and has been associated with deleterious effects on the lipoprotein profile (increased cholesterol and triglycerides). Mirtazapine possesses significant antihistaminergic and minimal antimuscarinic effects, with the potential for considerable drowsiness, dry mouth, and constipation. Mirtazapine has a very low incidence of transient rise in liver enzymes (2%) and severe neutropenia or reversible agranulocytosis (0.1% incidence). It may be prudent for physicians to check white counts at initiation of the medication, semiannually, and with occurrence of infectious illnesses. Mirtazapine is unlikely to have clinically significant effects on the metabolism of other medications through liver enzyme systems.

Bupropion is a monocyclic antidepressant that inhibits the reuptake of norepinephrine and dopamine into presynaptic neurons and is referred to as a norepinephrine dopamine reuptake inhibitor (NDRI). Bupropion does not inhibit serotonin reuptake and does not cause the serotonin syndrome, which is why it is the most frequently used augmentation strategy in combination with SSRI medications. Bupropion is also indicated for smoking cessation under the trade name Zyban. Bupropion may enhance energy and motivation due to norepinephrine- and dopamine-induced activating effects. However, bupropion's activating effect can also cause agitation, irritability, aggression, vivid dreams, nightmares, and insomnia. Despite this pro-norepinephrine and pro-dopamine effect, only 2% of patients on this medication demonstrate elevations in blood pressure. Bupropion may be used for sexual dysfunction. Bupropion is contraindicated in patients with seizure disorders, bulimia, anorexia, and alcohol withdrawal. Bupropion-induced seizure disorders are dose related, and total daily doses above 450 mg, single doses above 150 mg of immediate-release dosage, or 200 mg of the sustained-release dosage forms increase the risk of seizures and should be avoided. Up to 450 mg of the XL form of the medication can be prescribed once a day, which is a major advantage for improving adherence.

Tricyclic Antidepressants

The TCAs have fallen out of favor predominantly because of their adverse effects and toxicity profile in the overdose setting. Common antimuscarinic effects include dry mouth, blurred vision, constipation, urinary retention, and sinus tachycardia; histamine receptor blockade effects include sedation, drowsiness, and weight gain; and alpha-1 receptor blockade effects include orthostatic hypotension and sedation. The TCAs also possess quinidine-like effects, such as QRS and QTc prolongation, which can predispose to ventricular dysrhythmias and torsades de pointes—especially in overdoses or in patients with preexisting cardiac disease. A TCA overdose is a medical emergency, with significant risk of lethality. Tricyclic antidepressants lower the seizure threshold, with the potential for refractory seizures in overdose. To minimize the risk of lethal overdose in patients with suicidal ideation, principles of prudent care suggest that only limited amounts of TCAs should be prescribed at any one time (e.g., 7–10 days' supply, especially in higher doses). Secondary amines, such as desipramine and nortriptyline, are favored over tertiary amines, such as amitriptyline and imipramine, because of a lower propensity to induce antimuscarinic adverse effects, less orthostatic hypotension, and less sedation. The adverse effects of the TCAs are dose related and can be minimized by starting patients on low doses, then titrating upward slowly. Though the newer antidepressants seem to be generally as effective as the TCAs for the broad category of major depression, these older agents may be more effective for the more severe depressive disorders, especially depression with melancholic features.

Second-Generation (Atypical) Antipsychotics

Four second-generation antipsychotics (SGAs) have been approved by the United States Food and Drug Administration (USFDA) as augmentation therapy to antidepressants for treating MDD. These include aripiprazole, quetiapine extended release, olanzapine, and most recently brexpiprazole. Olanzapine specifically was approved as a combined agent with fluoxetine for treatment-resistant depression (TRD), defined as MDD patients who do not respond to two separate trials of two or more antidepressants after an appropriate duration and dose. The antidepressant effects of SGAs are thought to be related to several possible pathways that vary depending on the drug and include (among others): rapid disengagement and/or reduced activation of dopamine (DA) receptors, reduced activation of 5-HT$_{1A}$ receptors, a decrease in cortisol levels, and an increase in Brain-derived neurotrophic factor (BDNF) levels. Clinicians should monitor patients for the emergence of adverse effects, including extrapyramidal symptoms (EPS), weight gain, hyperglycemia, akathisia, and somnolence.

Ketamine

Ketamine has received interest as an antidepressant option for treatment-resistant depression (TRD). Ketamine is an anesthetic developed in the 1960s that works by increasing the activity of the neurotransmitter glutamate in the frontal cortex of the brain, allowing new synapses to form in the same area. It works quickly in terms of antidepressant effect because it bypasses serotonin and instead acts as a noncompetitive *N*-methyl-D-aspartate (NMDA) receptor antagonist to activate the glutamate system in the brain. In addition to the NMDA antagonism, ketamine is thought to act on several other brain receptors including opioid system activation. The FDA has approved esketamine (the *S*-enantiomer of ketamine) as an intranasal spray, to be used with an oral antidepressant for patients with treatment resistant depression. Because of its abuse potential and other side-affects, esketamine must be administered in a health care facility under the supervision of a physician. Side effects may include dissociation, dizziness, vertigo, nausea, sedation, anxiety, lethargy, and increased blood pressure.

Black Box Warning on Antidepressant-Induced Suicide Ideation in Children & Adolescents

The FDA has issued a "black box" warning that the use of antidepressant medication in children, adolescents and young adults up to age 24 may be associated with an increase in suicide ideation and suicide attempts. The black box recommends that when prescribing antidepressant medication in children, adolescents, and young adults, physicians should warn patients and families to report immediately any increase in agitation or thoughts of suicide, and physicians should monitor patients through regular and frequent follow-up visits. The warning results from a pooled analysis of 4400 subjects in 24 placebo-controlled drug trials that found prevalence rates of treatment-emergent suicidal thoughts or suicide attempts in 4% of all patients in the active medication group, compared to 2% of patients taking placebo (a statistically significant difference). *There were no completed suicides in any of the studies.* Similar pooled analyses in adults found no difference between active drug and placebo in studies totaling more than 50,000 patients.

In the decade before this warning was issued, suicide attempts and completed suicides decreased significantly in children and adolescents, somewhat paralleling the increased use of antidepressant medications in the population. Since 2004, however, use of these medications in children and adolescents has decreased by 25%, and of interest and concern, rates of suicide attempts and completions in children and adolescents have increased for the first time in over a decade. Furthermore, large observational studies have documented that the risk of a suicide attempt actually decreases after patients begin taking medication and that communities with higher rates of antidepressant use have, on average, lower rates of suicide.

Drug Interactions

Clinicians should routinely use an electronic database such as Micromedex to check potential drug interactions whenever they prescribe a new medication for depression. They should understand the basic principles of enzyme substrates and enzyme inhibitors to be able to better interpret the results they receive from such an electronic database.

All antidepressant medications are metabolized by cytochrome P450 liver enzyme subsystems. That is, they are *substrates* for one or more major P450 isoenzyme systems 1A2, 2C9, 2C19, 2D6, and 3A4. While all antidepressants are metabolized in the liver, only some of the SSRIs are moderate inhibitors of either 2C19 (fluoxetine and sertraline) or 2D6 (fluoxetine and paroxetine). Fluoxetine and paroxetine, for example, are moderate 2D6 inhibitors. As such, these drugs inhibit the metabolism of drugs metabolized by the 2D6 subsystem, for example, several beta-blockers, some antipsychotic medications, most TCAs, some benzodiazepines, and the over-the-counter cough suppressant dextromethorphan. When dextromethorphan is combined with fluoxetine or paroxetine, its plasma levels can increase significantly, which could theoretically increase the likelihood of a serotonin syndrome. Also, some SSRIs may inhibit the hepatic 2D6-mediated conversion of several prodrug-like opioids into their active analgesic metabolites, such as codeine to morphine, oxycodone to oxymorphone, and hydrocodone to hydromorphone. Clinically, this inhibition could theoretically decrease the analgesic effect of the opiates listed above. Among the SSRIs, sertraline, citalopram, and escitalopram present the least inhibition of 2D6, while mirtazapine and venlafaxine also have little effect on 2D6.

Pharmacogenomics

Pharmacogenomics refers to the interaction of multiple genes in determining drug response. For example, genetic polymorphisms in the serotonin transporter gene have been associated with differential SSRI response rates. Some individuals have been shown to have differential activity levels of 2C19 and 2D6 isoenzymes—some patients are "extensive" metabolizers (high activity) and some are "poor" metabolizers (low enzyme activity). Of interest to researchers is that the prevalence rates of "poor metabolizers" vary by ethnicity: 30% of Asians, 10% of African Americans, and 5% of whites are poor metabolizers. From a clinical perspective, given the same dose of drug, poor metabolizers are likely to have much higher blood levels of the medication than extensive metabolizers. Why some individuals are more sensitive to lower doses of medication and/or respond better to lower doses, may be secondary to this genetically determined rate of metabolism, though how to apply this information clinically has not been clearly established.

The FDA has licensed and accredited several laboratories to provide DNA testing as well as blood tests for determination of CYP-2C9, -2C19, -2D6, and -1A2 genotypes. Although these tests are currently available, they have not yet gained widespread acceptance due to questions about cost-effectiveness and overall utility. The next decade will probably witness great progress in pharmacogenomics, such that testing and genomic-based medication algorithms will become part of the routine practice of medicine.

Antidepressant Withdrawal

Abrupt withdrawal of SSRIs may cause a *discontinuation syndrome* consisting of a constellation of somatic, neurologic, and psychological symptoms—usually within 24–48 hours of discontinuation. These symptoms include GI complaints, headache, fever, malaise, vivid dreams, myalgias, paresthesias, "electric shock-like" sensations, worsened mood, irritability, anxiety, confusion, and forgetfulness. These symptoms can be extremely uncomfortable, even leading to emergency room visits, but they are not life threatening. The incidence of the SSRI *discontinuation syndrome* may be as high as 40%, but the most common and most severe withdrawal syndrome is associated with paroxetine, probably due to its short half-life (21 hours) and the absence of any active metabolites. Fluoxetine is unlikely to cause the discontinuation syndrome because of its long half-life (4–14 days, plus its active metabolite norfluoxetine), and hence has a self-tapering discontinuation mechanism. Venlafaxine, duloxetine, trazodone, and mirtazapine have also been associated with the discontinuation syndrome. Treatment of the discontinuation syndrome consists of reinstituting the SSRI and tapering more slowly or substituting the SSRI with one or two doses of fluoxetine (10–20 mg). In summary, all known antidepressants, with the possible exception of fluoxetine and bupropion should be withdrawn gradually to avoid the discontinuation syndrome.

Antidepressant "Tolerance"

Despite the absence of clear evidence, clinicians commonly observe a tolerance phenomenon or *poop-out syndrome* that may occur in 10–20% of patients who have successfully responded to antidepressant therapy and remain compliant. Possible mechanisms for this observed tachyphylaxis include adaptation of central nervous system receptors via upregulation and decreased receptor density, disease severity or exacerbation, loss of a placebo effect, unrecognized rapid cycling, accumulation of a less potent or competitively antagonistic metabolite, or drug interactions. Enzyme-inducing medications, such as St. John's wort, phenytoin, barbiturates, carbamazepine, oxcarbazepine, rifampin, and rifabutin, may increase the hepatic metabolism of non-CYP-2D6 substrate antidepressants, thus decreasing plasma levels. For example, phenobarbital has been associated with a 25% decrease in the area under the paroxetine serum concentration–time curve; St. John's wort has been associated with a 22% decrease in the area under the serum concentration–time curve of amitriptyline and a 41% decrease in its metabolite nortriptyline; and phenobarbital can decrease the plasma levels of mirtazapine by 60%. Additionally, clinicians should be suspicious of a lack of compliance in all patients with the poop-out syndrome. Management of the poop-out syndrome includes increasing antidepressant doses, switching to an alternative agent, or adding augmentation therapy.

Augmentation Therapy

After an antidepressant at maximal doses has produced only a partial response, with persistent residual symptoms, experts usually recommend consideration of augmentation therapy, which consists of adding another agent to the antidepressant currently in use. Quantitative assessment with the PHQ-9 can help clinicians make decisions about when to initiate augmentation therapy.

Clinicians can use the following guideline.

When a depressed patient experiences a significant clinical improvement (as manifested by a drop in PHQ-9 score by 5 points or more), but *fails* to reach remission (PHQ <5) within a minimum of 1 month after the dose of the initial antidepressant is raised to its maximum, then consider augmentation therapy.

The most commonly used augmentation agents include use of a second antidepressant from a different class (e.g., bupropion, venlafaxine, mirtazapine, or buspirone [approved for GAD]), lithium carbonate, an atypical antipsychotic (see SGA section), lamotrigine, and triiodothyronine (T3). In rarer circumstances, psychostimulants (e.g., methylphenidate, dextroamphetamine, and modafinil) can be considered.

Deprescribing

The rate of long-term antidepressant use has more than tripled in the United States since 2000 such that nearly 7% of American adults have taken prescription antidepressants for at least 5 years (see Figure 26-2). Older white women account for 58% of those on antidepressants long term. Similar statistics are seen in other parts of the world. Depression is a relapsing-remitting illness that makes it challenging to know how long to treat with antidepressants. Often in primary care there is reluctance on the part of both the patient and the prescriber to stop treatment when things appear "stable." However, there are few research studies that guide decisions on long-term treatment (beyond 2 years).

The idea of deprescribing, or "the planned and supervised process of dose reduction or stopping of medications that may be causing harm or no longer providing benefit" is one that has become especially important with older patients. One of the founding fathers of modern psychiatry, Philippe Pinel, wrote in 1809, "It is an art of no little importance to administer medicines properly; but it is an art of much greater and more difficult acquisition to know when to suspend or altogether omit them."

Evidence-based guidelines for deprescribing are being developed and are most robustly published in psychiatry when it comes to benzodiazepine receptor agonists (BZRA). However, when it comes to antidepressant therapy, it is still very much an "art" that involves shared decision making. Most experts agree that there is a subset of patients who benefit from lifelong prescriptions, especially those that have had two or more episodes of MDD within a few years or three or more episodes in their lifetime. Careful prescribing and deprescribing practices are the mandate of all prescribers—especially with antidepressant drugs such as venlafaxine and sertraline, which are known to be more challenging for patients when coming off of them as discussed earlier.

ANTIDEPRESSANTS IN THE ELDERLY & MEDICALLY ILL

There have been surprisingly few randomized-controlled trials supporting the safety and efficacy of antidepressant medication in the medically ill and elderly. However, a systematic review of studies in specific medical populations, such as post-MI, poststroke, cancer, diabetes, cancer, Alzheimer disease, as well as other recent studies in general medical populations and elderly medical populations, suggest that the use of antidepressant medications in these populations is safe and efficacious. Physicians should be aware, however, that most studies

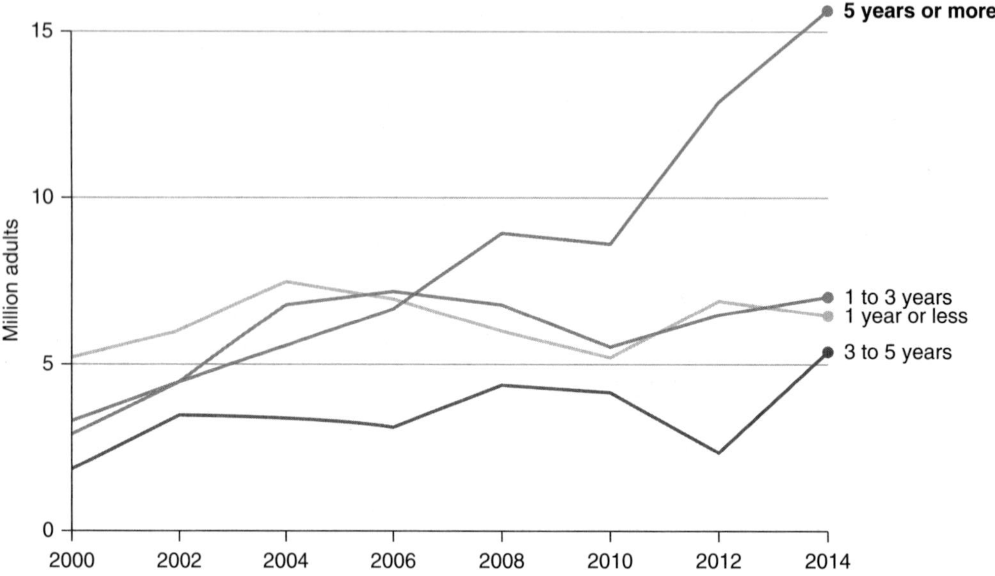

Figure 26-2. Long-term Antidepressant Use among American Adults.

indicate that a concurrent general medical illness is associated with somewhat lower overall depression response and remission rates compared to patients without concurrent medical illness. Of particular importance, the SADHART study (Sertraline Antidepressant Heart Attack Trial) documented the safety of SSRI use (sertraline) immediately after a heart attack, even in patients with severe cardiac disease and in patients using multiple other medications. Other recent studies now also document the safety and effectiveness of citalopram, escitalopram and mirtazapine for depression after acute coronary syndrome. For many of the reasons enumerated earlier, the SSRIs and other new agents have become the agents of choice in the elderly and in the medically ill.

Dosing strategies in the elderly and medically ill should adhere to the general guideline "start low and go slow." Pharmacokinetically, antidepressant agents are metabolized more slowly, resulting in accumulation and toxicity. Increased pharmacodynamic effects in the elderly may result from lower albumin levels, leading to higher levels of unbound drug.

Because depression is associated with increased morbidity, mortality, and cost in patients with concurrent general medical illness, it is reasonable to ask whether improvement in depression in medical patients leads to improvements in these other domains. There are limited and somewhat conflicting data on these questions, but some recent and notable studies point to potential decreases in morbidity, mortality, and overall health care costs with adequate treatment of depression. The SADHART study showed a trend (but not statistically significant) toward decreased rate of incident severe cardiac events and death in the sertraline group compared to placebo. A naturalistic outcome report of patients in the Enhancing Recovery in Coronary Heart Disease (ENRICHD) psychotherapy study noted that depressed patients treated with SSRIs (at physician/patient discretion, outside of protocol) had a statistically significant decrease in cardiac morbidity and mortality compared with the depressed patients who did not receive this treatment. A 2-year study of the collaborative care of patients with both depression and diabetes has shown an overall decrease in total health costs (general medical and psychiatric) in patients successfully treated for depression.

Electroconvulsive Therapy

Electroconvulsive therapy (ECT) is still the most effective means available for the treatment of refractory depression with classic data suggesting that the percentage of total improvement with ECT reaches 90%. ECT uses an electric current passed through the brain to induce a brief, controlled seizure while the patient is sedated with general anesthesia and given a muscle relaxant to prevent movement during the procedure. It remains the treatment of choice for patients with depression (with or without psychotic features) refractory to pharmacotherapy, and for some patients who are acutely suicidal. It can also be used in other conditions such as bipolar disorder and psychotic disorders (especially with catatonia).

Despite the negative cinematic portrayal of ECT (especially older versions of convulsive therapy), social prejudices, and general fear about ECT, new methods of administration such as unilateral placement of the electrodes on the scalp have proven it to be a safe and effective treatment. Two major advantages of ECT over medication are that ECT begins to work quicker, and older individuals respond especially quickly. In fact, ECT can be safer than antidepressant medication in the elderly despite the anesthesia-related mortality risk which previously stood at 1/1000 and has now fallen to 0.4/100,000. Some short-term memory loss is common, but research indicates that this reverts to normal in most patients. In some cases, ECT can be lifesaving and should not be denied to patients because of poor understanding or unrealistic fear. A full "index" course of ECT is usually delivered 3 days a week over a period of about 4 weeks. If this does not lead to remission, patients with recurrent depression should receive either maintenance ECT ranging from one session per week to one session every few months, often in addition to antidepressant medication.

Light Therapy

Light therapy of at least 10,000 lux, where the light box is kept at a distance of about 16–24 inches from the face typically in daily sessions of about 20–30 minutes, has been used successfully in the treatment of depression with winter-type seasonal pattern (previously seasonal affective disorder or SAD). For most people, light therapy is most effective when done early in the morning after waking and when it is used consistently. Phototherapy is based on the principle that the presentation of artificial light at a similar strength to natural sunlight will prevent the biological changes that mediate seasonal depression during the winter. The light must enter the eyes to be effective (not the skin) but must be indirect so as not to cause damage to the eyes. Light therapy may trigger mania in patients with bipolar disorder, so screening remains an important part of this treatment as well.

Repetitive Transcranial Magnetic Stimulation

Repetitive transcranial magnetic stimulation (rTMS) is approved for use in individuals with treatment resistant depression without psychotic features. Although its mechanism is unclear, an electromagnetic pulse is introduced into the left dorsolateral prefrontal cortex of the brain which has shown to improve depressive symptoms. About one-third of patients achieve remission and two-thirds respond to treatment. The only real adverse effect (AE) is scalp pain or sensitivity during the procedure that abates quickly once the treatment concludes—an attractive AE profile compared to pharmacotherapy. The typical course of treatment is 6 weeks, during which patients undergo five sessions per week of less than half an hour in duration, depending on the protocol.

Vagus Nerve Stimulation

Originally developed as a treatment for epilepsy, with the first human implant in 1989, Vagus Nerve Stimulation (VNS) was approved by the FDA for treatment-resistant depression in 2005. It works through a device implanted under the skin that sends electrical pulses through the left vagus nerve, which carries signals from systemic organs to the cortical-limbic-thalamic-striatal neural circuit thought to be pertinent to emotional and cognitive functions relevant in depression. Despite FDA approval, VNS is infrequently used compared to the other brain stimulation therapies, largely based on mixed data regarding the efficacy.

Other Brain Stimulation Interventions

With increasing awareness of alterations in brain networks, a number of other direct brain stimulation interventions have been explored recently. These include approaches such as deep brain stimulation (DBS) and magnetic seizure therapy (MST). Deep brain stimulation, first developed as a treatment for Parkinson's disease, is available on an experimental basis for refractory depression (there is a Humanitarian Device Exemption for the use of DBS to treat obsessive compulsive disorder). It focuses on decreasing activation of Brodmann Area 25 in the subgenual cingulate gyrus using a pair of electrodes implanted in the brain and controlled by a generator in the chest. This intervention can have immediate effects, but it is a neurosurgical procedure with attendant risks, so that its application appears limited. Magnetic seizure therapy is being researched as an alternative to ECT and shows preliminary promise carrying fewer memory side effects, shorter seizures, and shorter recovery time compared to ECT.

COLLABORATIVE CARE MODELS OF DEPRESSION

A generation of randomized, controlled health services trials indicates that systematic implementation of a "collaborative care model," or "chronic illness care" (or "chronic disease management") model of health care for depressed medical outpatients improves key processes and outcomes of care such as detection of depression; adequacy of depression treatment; patient adherence with treatment; improved clinical outcomes as assessed by measures such as PHQ-9 scores; and improved patient satisfaction. Key components of most of these new models generally include use of structured tools for assessment and management; utilization of care managers to help educate patients, support self-management, coordinate care and ensure follow-up; use of formal evidence-based guidelines and decision support tools; and finally, integration of behavioral health specialists into the medical team for consultation and ongoing support.

WHEN TO REFER

The criteria for referral to a mental health specialist depend a great deal on the experience and expertise of the primary treating physician and the availability of expert mental health consultants. The key is not to wait too long to refer to specialty care, because the chance of remission declines rapidly the more failed treatment trials the patient receives. Patients should be informed that consultation with a mental health specialist may be necessary if the depression does not fully remit. This advanced warning can make referral at a later stage much easier and better received.

Because partial remission is a common occurrence, medical providers should make every effort to establish clear indications of predepression functioning, and if full return to baseline functioning does not occur, referral to a specialist should be made. A baseline pretreatment PHQ-9 should be obtained and repeated at regular intervals to ensure that the patient is responding appropriately to treatment. Patients with persistently elevated PHQ-9 scores (20 or above), or whose scores are not reduced to at least 50% of pretreatment levels, should be evaluated by a mental health specialist. Other indications for referral include active suicidality, most bipolar disorder and psychosis, diagnostic uncertainty, and for advice about pharmacological management of treatment-resistant depression. The medical provider should communicate with the mental health specialist and provide the following information: the nature of the depressive symptoms, baseline premorbid functioning, baseline and follow-up PHQ-9 scores, other treatments (including medications) that have been tried previously or are concurrent, and patient understanding and expectations about the pending referral. Communication with the specialist should always be bidirectional, which is why care models (e.g., the primary care medical home) that involve integrated care for both mental and physical needs, often have the best results. Unfortunately, failure to follow through on a referral and/or premature discontinuation of psychotherapy is even more common than failure to adhere to a pharmacotherapy treatment plan.

CONCLUSION

Of all the psychiatric conditions relevant to the general medical practitioner, major depression is arguably the most common and most important. Major depression is a serious, often disabling condition associated with increased morbidity and mortality especially when co-occurring with general medical conditions. Teasing unipolar depression from bipolar depression is one of the most challenging diagnostic dilemmas even for the most seasoned practitioner. Despite suboptimal rates of recognition and treatment of depression, especially in general medical settings, newer standards such as measurement-based care will hopefully usher in a new era in the recognition and effective management of depression. Newer psychiatric care models, such as partial hospitalization or intensive outpatient programs, and newer technologies, such as repetitive transcranial magnetic stimulation, are also poised to add to the historical gains of psychotherapy, pharmacotherapy, and even traditional inpatient care in the treatment of depression. Ultimately, close collaboration between medical and mental health care delivery systems is key to improving outcomes in this debilitating condition.

SUGGESTED READINGS

Benazzi F, Akiskal HS. A downscaled practical measure of mood lability as a screening tool for bipolar II. *J Affect Disord* 2005;84:225–232.

Cheng-Ta L, et al. Association between antidepressant resistance in unipolar depression and subsequent bipolar disorder: cohort study. *Brit J Psychiatr* 2012;200:45–51.

Chekroud SR, Gueorguieva R, Zheutlin AB, et al. Association between physical exercise and mental health in 1.2 million individuals in the USA between 2011 and 2015: a cross-sectional study. *Lancet Psychiatry* 2018;5:739–746.

Cipriani A, Furukawa TA, Salanti G, et al. Comparative efficacy and acceptability of 21 antidepressant drugs for the acute treatment of adults with major depressive disorder: a systematic review and network meta-analysis. *Lancet* 2018;391:1357–1366.

Hollon SD, Javrett RB, Nierenberg AA, Thase ME, Trivedi M, Rush AJ. Psychotherapy and medication in the treatment of adult and geriatric depression: which monotherapy or combined treatment? *J Clin Psychiatry* 2005;66:455–468.

Josefsson T, Lindwall M, Archer T. Physical exercise intervention in depressive disorders: meta-analysis and systematic review. *Scand J Med Sci Sports* 2014;24:259–272.

Kim JM, Stewart R, Lee YS, et al. Effect of escitalopram vs placebo treatment for depression on long-term cardiac outcomes in patients with acute coronary syndrome: a randomized clinical trial. *JAMA* 2018;320:350–358.

Maki PM, Kornstein SG, Joffe H, et al. Guidelines for the evaluation and treatment of perimenopausal depression: summary and recommendations. *Menopause* 2018;25:1069–1085.

Park LT, Zarate CA. Depression in the primary care setting. *N Engl J Med* 2019;380;6:559–568.

Qato DM, Ozenberger K, Olfson M. Prevalence of prescription medications with depression as a potential adverse effect among adults in the United States. *JAMA* 2018;319:2289–2298.

Raj YP, Parker J, Safani D, Nam K. Psychiatric disorders: bipolar and related disorders in *Primary Care Psychiatry*, 2nd ed. Wolters Kluwer: Philadelphia, PA; 2018.

Rush AJ. STAR*D: what have we learned? *Am J Psychiatry* 2007;164:201–204.

Schuch FB, Vancampfort D, Richards J, et al. Exercise as a treatment for depression: a meta-analysis adjusting for publication bias. *J Psychiatr Res* 2016;77:42–51.

Taylor WD. Depression in the elderly. *N Engl J Med* 2014;37:1228–1236.

Van der Velden AM, Kuyken W, Wattar U, et al. A systematic review of mechanisms of change in mindfulness-based cognitive therapy in the treatment of recurrent major depressive disorder. *Clin Psychol Rev* 2015;37:26–39.

PATIENT BIBLIOGRAPHY

Alberti RE, Emmons ML. *Your Perfect Right: Assertiveness and Equality in Your Life and Relationships,* 9th ed. Atascadero, CA: Impact Publishers; 2008.

Burns DD. *Feeling Good—The New Mood Therapy.* New York, NY: Avon Books; 1999.

Greenberger D, Padesky C. *Mind over Mood: Change How You Feel by Changing the Way You Think.* New York, NY: The Guilford Press; 1995.

Hayes SC, Smith S. *Get Out of Your Mind and into Your Life.* Oakland, CA: New Harbinger Press; 2005.

Solomon A. *The Noonday Demon: An Atlas of Depression.* New York, NY: Scribner; 2011.

Williams M, Teasdale J, Segal Z, Kabat-Zinn J. *The Mindful Way through Depression: Freeing Yourself from Chronic Unhappiness.* New York, NY: Guilford Press; 2007.

WEBSITES

Columbia Lighthouse Project (website provides the Columbia Suicide Severity Rating Scale, which can be downloaded, along with supportive research.) http://cssrs.columbia.edu/the-columbia-scale-c-ssrs/evidence/. Accessed May 2019.

National Institute of Mental Health Depression Information Website. http://www.nimh.nih.gov/health/topics/depression/index.shtml. Accessed August 2019.

National Alliance on Mental Illness Website. https://www.nami.org/Learn-More/Mental-Health-Conditions/Depression. Accessed August 2019.

NIH statistics on major depression. https://www.nimh.nih.gov/health/statistics/major-depression.shtml. Accessed May 2019.

NIMH website on brain stimulation therapies: https://www.nimh.nih.gov/health/topics/brain-stimulation-therapies/brain-stimulation-therapies.shtml. Accessed May 2019.

Screening, Brief Intervention, and Referral to Treatment (SBIRT) (assessment instruments for substance use). http://www.sbirtoregon.org/screening-forms/. Accessed May 2019.

US Preventive Services Task Force recommendation for depression screening in adults. https://www.uspreventiveservicestaskforce.org/Page/Document/RecommendationStatementFinal/depression-in-adults-screening1. Accessed August 2019.

Appendix 26-A. Patient Health Questionnaire—PHQ-9.

Name ____________ Physician ____________ Date ____________

Over the last 2 *weeks*, how often have you been bothered by any of the following problems?

	Not At All (0)	Several Days (1)	More Than Half the Days (2)	Nearly Every Day (3)
1. Feeling down, depressed, or hopeless?	☐	☐	☐	☐
2. Little interest or pleasure in doing things?	☐	☐	☐	☐
3. Trouble falling or staying asleep, or sleeping too much?	☐	☐	☐	☐
4. Feeling tired or having little energy?	☐	☐	☐	☐
5. Poor appetite or overeating?	☐	☐	☐	☐
6. Feeling bad about yourself—or that you are a failure or have let yourself or your family down?	☐	☐	☐	☐
7. Trouble concentrating on things, such as reading the newspaper or watching television?	☐	☐	☐	☐
8. Moving or speaking so slowly that other people could have noticed? Or the opposite—being so fidgety or restless that you have been moving around a lot more than usual?	☐	☐	☐	☐
9. Thoughts that you would be better off dead or of hurting yourself in some way?*	☐	☐	☐	☐

10. If you are experiencing any of the problems on this form, how ***difficult*** have these problems made it for you to do your work, take care of things at home, or get along with other people?
☐ Not difficult at all ☐ Somewhat difficult ☐ Very difficult ☐ Extremely difficult

Office Use Only

Number of Symptoms: ____________ **Severity Score:** ____________

**If you have had thoughts that you would be better off dead or of hurting yourself in some way, please discuss this with your doctor, go to a hospital emergency room, or call 911.*

Appendix 26-B. Scoring the PHQ-9.

How to Score the Patient Health Questionnaire (PHQ-9)

The PHQ-9 can assist in diagnosing depression, as well as planning and monitoring depression treatment. There are three steps to scoring the PHQ-9: Number of Depressive Symptoms, Severity Score, and Functional Assessment. The Number of Depressive Symptoms is used to aid in making the diagnosis of Depression. The PHQ-9 Severity Score and Functional Assessment are measured at initial assessment and regularly after treatment begins to determine the severity of depression and to evaluate patient progress.

Number of Depressive Symptoms (Diagnosis)

1. For questions 1–8, count the number of symptoms the patient checked as "More than half the days" or "Nearly every day." For question 9, count the question positive if the patient checks "Several days," "More than half the days," or "Nearly every day."
2. Use the following interpretation grid to diagnose depression subtypes:

0–2 PHQ symptoms	Not clinically depressed
3–4 PHQ symptoms*	Other depressive syndrome
5 or more PHQ symptoms*	Major depression

Severity Score

1. Assign a score to each response by the number value under the answer headings (Not at all = 0; Several days = 1; More than half the days = 2; and Nearly every day = 3).
2. Total the values for each response to obtain the severity score.
3. Use the following interpretation grid:

0–4	Not clinically depressed
5–9	Mild depression
10–14	Moderate depression
≥15	Severe depression

Functional Assessment

The final question on the PHQ-9 asks the patient how emotional difficulties or problems impact work, things at home, or relationships with other people and if this has caused difficulty for 2 years or more. Patient responses can be one of four: "Not difficult at all"; "Somewhat difficult"; "Very difficult"; or "Extremely difficult."

- If the patient selects one of the last two responses, "Very difficult" or "Extremely difficult," his or her functionality at work, at home, or in relationships with other people is significantly impaired.
- If the patient has had difficulty with these problems for 2 years or more, consider the diagnosis of dysthymia (chronic depression).

**PHQ-9 items #1 or #2 must be one of the symptoms checked.*

PHQ-9 is adapted from PRIME-MD Today. Developed by Drs. Robert L. Spitzer, Janet B.W. Williams, Kurt Kroenke and colleagues, with an educational grant from Pfizer Inc. No permission required to reproduce, translate, display or distribute.

Anxiety

27

Jason M. Satterfield, PhD & Mitchell D. Feldman, MD, MPhil, FACP

INTRODUCTION

Anxiety disorders are common and disabling conditions and as a group are the most common disorders seen in the general medical setting. Anxiety is a common, normal emotion; most people experience occasional trepidation, fear, nervousness, "jitters," or at times, even panic. Mild anxiety may aid mental sharpness as uncertainty or pressure mounts. For some individuals, however, anxiety occurs as part of an anxiety disorder that is a prominent, persistent, and disruptive aspect of their daily lives. Among the general population in the United States, lifetime prevalence of an anxiety disorder is up to 29%, making anxiety more common than depressive disorders. Because these disorders often present first during childhood or adolescence, early identification and treatment is important to prevent unnecessary morbidity and decreased quality of life. In addition, the direct and indirect annual costs associated with anxiety disorders in the United States are similar to, and may even surpass, the economic burdens attributed to mood disorders.

Anxiety disorders are often comorbid with depression and with one another (e.g., panic disorder [PD] and agoraphobia). Similar to depression, patients with an unrecognized anxiety disorder often present to general medical or specialist settings rather than to specialty mental health. As up to half of patients present with somatic complaints associated with the anxiety disorder rather than its emotional symptoms, many patients are undiagnosed and untreated.

It is important to distinguish among the various anxiety disorders and identify possible comorbidities because of differences in treatment, complications, and prognoses. Although cross-cultural epidemiologic research has shown that anxiety disorders are present in all cultures, ethnicities, and age groups, providers also must be alert to a variety of common medical conditions and medication side effects that can have symptoms resembling an anxiety disorder (Table 27-1).

SCREENING & DIAGNOSIS

Office-based screening instruments can improve the detection of anxiety disorders and can be used to evaluate treatment response. The Generalized Anxiety Disorder-7 (GAD-7) is the most common screener used in primary care and has been validated for generalized anxiety disorder (GAD) as well as for panic disorder (Figure 27-1). A two-question screener, the GAD-2 subscale of the GAD-7, performs well as a rapid screening tool for GAD. The GAD-2 questions consist of the first two questions of the GAD-7: *Over the last 2 weeks how often have you been bothered by the following problems: (1) Feeling nervous, anxious, or on edge; and (2) Not being able to stop or control worrying.* This is calculated by assigning scores of 0, 1, 2, and 3, to the response categories of *not at all (0), several days (1), more than half the days (2), and nearly every day (3)*, respectively. GAD-2 scores can range from 0 to 6. A score of 3 or greater is considered positive and should prompt administration of the full GAD-7 and other diagnostic evaluations as indicated. The GAD-7 total score for the seven items ranges from 0 to 21. Scores of 5, 10, and 15 represent cut-points for mild, moderate, and severe anxiety, respectively. Though designed primarily as a screening and severity measure for generalized anxiety disorder, the GAD-7 also has moderately good operating characteristics for three other common disorders: panic disorder, social anxiety disorder, and posttraumatic stress disorder. When screening for anxiety disorders, a recommended cut-point for further evaluation is a score of 10 or greater.

Other clinically useful screening questions are listed in Table 27-2.

Table 27-1. Selected medical conditions that can simulate an anxiety disorder.

- Cardiac
  Ischemic heart disease, mitral valve prolapse, arrhythmias
- Endocrine/metabolic
  Hyperthyroidism, hypoglycemia, pheochromocytoma, carcinoid
- Gynecologic
  Menopause, premenstrual syndrome
- Neurologic
  Transient ischemic attacks, seizure disorders
- Pharmacologic
  Caffeine, alcohol, sympathomimetic agents, amphetamines, corticosteroids, theophylline, illicit drugs
- Respiratory
  Asthma, chronic obstructive pulmonary disease

Early recognition of anxiety disorders can help identify patients suffering from treatable problems and provide the patient and the clinician with a formal diagnosis to better explain the patient's symptoms. It may also reduce the risk of iatrogenic complications by decreasing or eliminating unnecessary medical testing, "treatment" trials of pharmacological agents, and referrals to specialists to evaluate unexplained physical and somatic symptoms.

Symptoms & Signs

Understanding the signs, symptoms, and epidemiologic features of the various anxiety disorders can help the clinician make an accurate diagnosis and initiate timely, appropriate treatment while avoiding invasive or unnecessary testing.

Anxiety disorders typically manifest with *emotional symptoms* (e.g., fear and nervousness), *cognitive symptoms* (e.g., worry, a sense of doom, or derealization), and *physical symptoms* (e.g., muscular tension, tachycardia, dizziness, and insomnia). Up to half of patients with medically unexplained symptoms are suffering from an underlying anxiety disorder. As the number of symptoms increases, the likelihood that there is a comorbid anxiety disorder also increases. Clinicians must decide how much diagnostic investigation is both feasible and necessary to rule out other important nonpsychiatric diseases. For example, when should a patient with palpitations undergo cardiac monitoring, thyroid function studies, evaluation for pheochromocytoma, or referral for cardiac catheterization? When does a patient with episodic nausea and abdominal pain require upper and lower endoscopy?

GAD-7

Over the last 2 weeks, how often have you been bothered by the following problems? *(Use "√" to indicate your answer)*	**Not at all**	**Several days**	**More than half the days**	**Nearly every day**
1. Feeling nervous, anxious, or on edge	0	1	2	3
2. Not being able to stop or control worrying	0	1	2	3
3. Worrying too much about different things	0	1	2	3
4. Trouble relaxing	0	1	2	3
5. Being so restless that it is hard to sit still	0	1	2	3
6. Becoming easily annoyed or irritable	0	1	2	3
7. Feeling afraid as if something awful might happen	0	1	2	3
	(For office coding: Total Score T____ = ____ + ____ + ____)			

Figure 27-1. Generalized Anxiety Disorder-7 Screener (GAD-7). (Developed by Drs. Robert L. Spitzer, Janet B.W. Williams, Kurt Kroenke, and colleagues, with an educational grant from Pfizer Inc. No permission required to reproduce, translate, display, or distribute.)

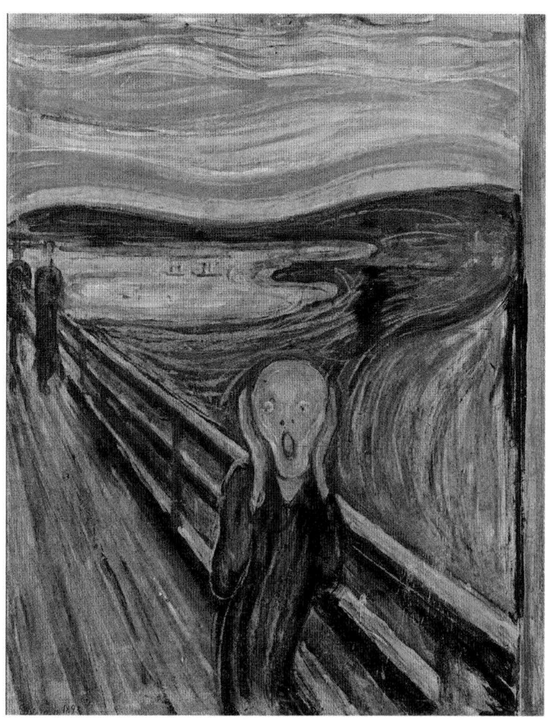

Edvard Munch (The Scream)

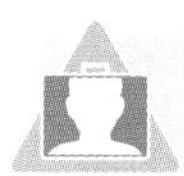

CASE ILLUSTRATION 1

Gwen is a 28-year-old woman who was admitted for a "rule out" and evaluation of syncope after presenting to the emergency department (ED) with shortness of breath, tachycardia, and a sensation that she is going to faint. The episodes are not associated with activity and started approximately 4 months ago, shortly after her husband was temporarily laid off from his job. She is now experiencing as many as four episodes per week lasting approximately 5–10 minutes each. Gwen is fearful that she may faint while driving or when out with her child. She is also worried about her heart, as her mother had heart disease in her early fifties.

Gwen was monitored overnight and had several tests, including thyroid function studies and a Holter monitor. She was told those test results were all "normal" and to follow-up with her primary care provider who after reviewing the history and test results recognizes that the symptoms are consistent with panic disorder. Further historical details eliminate other medical or substance-related illness, comorbid depression, or new use of caffeine or over-the-counter herbal or other remedies. The physician then reassures Gwen that her symptoms are common and that 2–4% of all people suffer from PD. Sensing Gwen might be embarrassed by a psychological diagnosis, the doctor

Table 27-2. Suggested screening questions for anxiety.

Disorder	Question
GAD	Would you describe yourself generally as a nervous person? Are you a worrier? Do you feel nervous or tense?
PD	Have you ever had a sudden attack of rapid heartbeat or rush of intense fear, anxiety, or nervousness? Did anything seem to trigger it?
Agoraphobia	Have you ever avoided important activities because you were afraid you would have a sudden attack like the one I just asked you about?
Social anxiety disorder	Some people have strong fears of being watched or evaluated by others. For example, some people don't want to eat, speak, or write in front of people for fear of embarrassing themselves. Is anything like this a problem for you?
Specific phobia	Some people have strong fears or phobias about things like heights, flying, bugs, or snakes? Do you have any strong fears or phobias?
Obsession	Some people are bothered by intrusive, silly, unpleasant, or horrible thoughts that keep repeating over and over. For example, some people have repeated thoughts of hurting someone they love even though they don't want to; that a loved one has been seriously hurt; that they will yell obscenities in public; or that they are contaminated by germs. Has anything like this troubled you?
Compulsion	Some people are bothered by doing something over and over that they can't resist, even when they try. They might wash their hands every few minutes, or repeatedly check to see that the stove is off or the door is locked, or count things excessively. Has anything like this been a problem for you?

explains the nature of PD, emphasizing its biological basis, and asks her if she thinks the new onset of her symptoms are possibly related to her concerns regarding her family's financial security. To help Gwen learn more about PD, the doctor gives her a booklet and a website address to read about self managing her anxiety symptoms and schedules a follow-up visit in 2 weeks to review this information and see how she is doing.

At their follow-up encounter, Gwen asks about medication for her panic symptoms as she has become worried about experiencing new attacks. Her physician recommends a selective serotonin reuptake inhibitor (SSRI) and advises that she use one-half of a tablet for the first week and then increase to a full tablet in 7–10 days. The doctor also advises Gwen that it may take 4–6 weeks before she notices any improvement from the medication, and recommends another follow-up visit in 2 weeks to see how she is feeling, review the self-help recommendations, and answer any new questions she may have. After a month on the medication Gwen's symptoms are much improved.

Differential Diagnosis

Symptoms resembling an anxiety disorder can be triggered by use of or intoxication from over-the-counter cold medications, caffeine, cocaine, theophylline preparations, amphetamines, and marijuana or withdrawal from alcohol, benzodiazepines, barbiturates, sedative–hypnotic agents, and other central nervous system (CNS) depressants. These conditions are commonly referred to as "substance-induced anxiety disorder" (see Table 27-1). Therefore, the astute clinician must review the patient's list of medications and inquire about the use of over-the-counter medications, including "herbal supplements" and performance-enhancing preparations (anabolic steroids), legal (alcohol, tobacco, and caffeine) and illegal substances (cocaine).

Many medical conditions also have symptoms resembling those of anxiety (see Table 27-1). Some are relatively common and obvious to practitioners (arrhythmias and asthma) and others are less so (insulinoma, pheochromocytoma, and carcinoid). Anxiety symptoms may also develop as a consequence of a medical condition. Examples include patients who experience anxiety symptoms following a myocardial infarction or following a pulmonary embolism. Clues to help guide diagnostic testing when sorting medical from psychiatric presentations include patient age and gender, past medical and psychiatric history, family history, and social history. Indeed, people who have been in excellent physical health and develop new-onset anxiety symptoms after the age of 50 years are more likely to have medical etiologies explaining their anxiety symptoms than those under the age of 25 years who have presented previously to several physicians and undergone extensive medical testing for evaluation of multiple unexplained somatic symptoms.

Etiology

The development of anxiety disorders involves multiple factors, including biological abnormalities, past and present psychological stressors, maladaptive cognitions, and environmentally conditioned behaviors. Abnormalities in the CNS associated with anxiety disorders relate to the gamma-aminobutyric acid (GABA) receptor as well as to the locus ceruleus. Animal studies have shown that stimulation of the locus ceruleus produces hyperarousal states similar to those seen in anxious humans. GABA is an inhibitory neurotransmitter found throughout most of the CNS. It may decrease anxiety by inhibiting locus ceruleus activity and modulating the reticular activating system, another area of the brainstem thought to affect alertness and fear. Benzodiazepines, a class of medications commonly used to treat anxiety, bind to specific sites on the GABA receptor. When the benzodiazepine molecule binds the GABA receptor, the effect of GABA on the GABA receptor is enhanced, reducing anxiety. Two other neurotransmitters, serotonin and norepinephrine, are also under investigation based on therapeutic responses to medications that affect these systems (e.g., SSRIs and serotonin–norepinephrine reuptake inhibitors [SNRIs]). Poor regulation of the adrenergic system is also suspected, as beta-adrenergic agonists induce symptoms of panic and alpha-adrenergic agonists decrease symptoms of anxiety.

Genetic factors also likely play a role in anxiety disorders, as evidenced by twin studies showing a higher concordance for PD and obsessive–compulsive disorder (OCD) among monozygotic twins than among dizygotic twins. In addition, for unclear reasons, women are at increased risk of suffering from an anxiety disorder.

Cognitive behavioral therapy (CBT) holds that emotions and behavior are driven by underlying beliefs or *cognitions.* Patients with anxiety typically overestimate danger or threats and underestimate their ability to effectively cope. These patients subsequently feel "stressed" or anxious and select avoidant or other maladaptive coping strategies.

Conditioned learning may also play a pivotal role in the development of anxiety disorders, and the resulting avoidance often seriously compounds patients' anxiety-related functional impairment. For example, patients may notice some unusual autonomic arousal or physical sensation while driving a car. They may misinterpret this initially random and benign sensation as a life-threatening event (e.g., "I'm having a heart attack!"), which further intensifies the autonomic response, fuels the misinterpretation, and snowballs into a full-blown panic attack. They may learn to associate the physical sensation and the subsequent attack with the act of driving and feel heightened anxiety—fueled by catastrophic thinking—when they drive or anticipate driving. Initially, the association between driving and panic is coincidental (driving is not the event provoking the initial sensation or the panic attack). Eventually, however, a patient may completely stop driving for fear that another panic attack will occur. This conditioned learning between driving and panic may gradually become so strong that driving becomes a precipitant of panic attacks. Thus, the driver mistakenly becomes conditioned to fear driving.

Traumatic, highly stressful, and catastrophic life events are also key factors leading to anxiety disorders. Childhood maltreatment and trauma, sexual assault, or exposure to overly protective or overly harsh parenting styles can predispose individuals to develop hyperactive physiologic responses to everyday stressors, placing them at greater risk for developing anxiety and mood disorders.

SPECIFIC DISORDERS

Panic Attacks

A panic attack is characterized by a discrete period of intense fear accompanied by the abrupt onset of several cognitive and somatic symptoms. Cognitive symptoms may include but are not limited to racing thoughts, preoccupation with health concerns, catastrophic misinterpretation of somatic symptoms, or believing one is going insane. Somatic symptoms may include a choking sensation, racing heartbeat, sweating, "jelly" legs, nausea, shaking, chest pain, numbness, or feeling detached or unreal. Frightening physical symptoms are commonly prominent and scare many patients into seeking urgent medical care. Primary care providers can usually be reassuring, as panic attacks are often infrequent, self-limited, and not related to any serious mental or physical disorder. Panic attacks are categorized as follows:

- Unexpected (untriggered or uncued);
- Situationally bound (always environmentally or psychologically cued); or
- Situationally predisposed (sometimes, but not invariably, cued).

Panic attacks can be comorbid with a number of other anxiety disorders including social and specific phobias, OCD, and PTSD. The presence and type of a panic trigger help clinicians make a correct diagnosis. Uncued panic attacks are characteristic of PD, whereas cued attacks suggest other psychiatric conditions such as the following:

- Social phobia (attack triggered by fear of embarrassment in social situations);
- Specific phobia (fear of places or things);
- OCD (triggered by exposure to the object of an obsession, such as contamination); or
- PTSD (triggered by an event resembling the original trauma).

Panic attacks are quite common; most people experience a subclinical or limited-symptom attack at some time. Only about 9% of the general population ever experiences a full-blown panic attack.

Panic Disorder

Diagnosis

Panic disorder is diagnosed when a person experiences *panic attacks* that are uncued and recurrent and are followed by a month or more of persistent fear of another attack or avoidance of situations because of fear of having another attack. Lifetime prevalence in the community is 2–4%, and about 3–8% of patients who present to primary care physicians meet current criteria. Panic disorder is approximately twice as common in women as among men. Community-based studies also reveal that suicide attempts are more common among patients with PD than among patients with major depression.

Panic disorder (PD) is a potentially debilitating disease with major complications. PD sometimes leads to agoraphobia, a fear of being in a place or a situation where escape or rescue might be difficult if another attack occurs, most often within 6 months of the first panic attack. This fear may cause many patients to avoid important activities of daily living, such as shopping or using public transportation. Patients who develop PD as adolescents often develop depressive disorders in early adulthood.

Management

Effective treatment exists for PD and for many of the other anxiety disorders and has been shown to be effective in clinical trials at reducing anxiety symptoms and in improving health-related quality of life and employment patterns. Appropriate treatment may also reduce substance use among patients who self-medicate with alcohol, benzodiazepines, or other substances in an effort to ameliorate their symptoms.

Initial management of PD and other anxiety disorders begins with providing the patient with a clear understanding of the problem. This tends to ease anxiety, increase the strength of the therapeutic alliance, and the subsequent likelihood that the patient will adhere with the treatment plan. It may be helpful to emphasize the biological nature of PD, as most patients find it reassuring and destigmatizing to know that they have a recognized, treatable biological syndrome that typically has a good prognosis. Patients should also be referred to self-help books, support groups, and cognitive behavioral resources, which are widely available (see "Suggested Readings").

In tailoring the treatment of PD to the patient, several factors should be weighed, including the degree of avoidance, the severity of physical manifestations, and the comorbidity of other psychiatric disorders. The clinician must balance patient education and supportive counseling with patients' beliefs about the cause of their symptoms. For example, if the physical symptoms are attributed to a cardiac problem, correcting this misinterpretation and emphasizing the biological basis of PD may help the patient accept the diagnosis and thus improve adherence to treatment. The provider has a vital role to play in many of the treatments, such as patient education, advice to avoid possible triggering substances (such as caffeine and cold medicines), supportive counseling, and initial pharmacotherapy, which can appropriately be incorporated into routine office visits.

Patients with PD often focus on the somatic symptoms of the disorder, thus presenting to medical settings with chest pain, dizziness, abdominal concerns, and other unexplained complaints. Iatrogenesis and avoidable medical costs can and often do result from unnecessary procedures and treatments. The dilemma for clinicians, therefore, is to decide whether and how extensively to evaluate the patient's specific symptoms.

One clinical strategy is to evaluate conservatively those symptoms that are potentially catastrophic, involve objective findings, or present as a classic constellation of symptoms. While the investigation is proceeding, the patient can be treated for PD and the symptoms periodically reassessed. Effective pharmacological treatment can reduce the cognitive and physical symptoms of panic and lessen the patient's belief that the problem is caused by an undiscovered medical condition.

Medications used to treat PD include antidepressants, most commonly SSRIs and SNRIs, but tricyclic antidepressants (TCAs) and monoamine oxidase inhibitors (MAOIs) can also be used. Benzodiazepines (alprazolam, clonazepam) relieve symptoms rapidly, usually within the first week of treatment, and they have a relatively wide therapeutic index. Their main disadvantages are their potential for misuse and dependence, a high incidence of rebound panic attacks when the medication is discontinued, and interference with exposure-based CBT. In contrast, SSRIs and SNRIs are not associated with dependence and may have a synergistic effect with CBT, but generally take 3–4 weeks or longer before reaching maximum effectiveness. In addition, some antidepressants may exacerbate symptoms of anxiety during the first 1–2 weeks of administration.

A benzodiazepine can also be used in combination with either an SSRI or an SNRI (to avoid a "serotonin syndrome," SSRIs and SNRIs should not be used in combination). Given the availability of several potential first-line agents believed to be of similar efficacy (Table 27-3), the clinician is advised to first inquire about past personal and family experience with pharmacotherapy, side effects, brand preference, and insurance formulary restrictions before suggesting a particular medication.

A common practice is to initiate treatment with a low daily dose of a generically available SSRI (e.g., escitalopram, 5 mg orally each day), titrating the dose slowly upward to 20 mg daily over several weeks as tolerated until symptom relief or the maximum dosage is attained, whichever arrives first. If the panic symptoms are particularly troublesome or if they worsen in the initial week of therapy, a benzodiazepine such as alprazolam or clonazepam can be added for more rapid control of symptoms and then tapered off and discontinued when the SSRI or SNRI commences effect. As with treatment of major depression, to avoid symptom relapse, experts recommend that anxiolytic pharmacotherapy be continued for a minimum of 9–12 months, and longer if the symptoms are particularly disabling or recurrent.

Adjunctive cognitive behavioral interventions (e.g., relaxation training, challenging catastrophic thinking, and gradual exposures) can treat both the physical manifestations and avoidance behaviors and substantially decrease the likelihood of symptom relapse following discontinuation of pharmacotherapy. Patients should be helped to gradually face the situations and activities they feared and fully experience the physical sensations they once believed indicated a serious medical problem. For example, the patient in Case Illustration 1 would be encouraged to drive, shop, and manage other tasks outside her home while experiencing and eventually managing her shortness of breath, racing heartbeat, and sensation of fainting. If patients are at first overwhelmed by the prospect of doing this, they can first initiate exposure mentally, using relaxation techniques and guided imagery. The patient should be instructed to imagine a frightening but tolerable aspect of the activity (in this case, driving) while doing a relaxation exercise and to repeatedly visualize successfully coping with the activity. In some cases, it may be necessary to enlist the assistance of a cognitive behavioral therapist who can design and manage successive "exposure" exercises for overly frightened patients. Cognitive behavioral therapy and antidepressant medications have been found equally efficacious, with combined CBT and antidepressants showing a modest advantage.

Phobias

Diagnosis

Specific phobias and social anxiety disorder are characterized by episodic anxiety in response to specific precipitants. Stimuli for specific phobias include places, things, or events, such as airplane flights, heights, insects, snakes, or rodents. Affected individuals are aware that their fears are exaggerated or unreasonable; nonetheless, when exposed to the precipitant, patients experience intense, excessive fear leading to avoidance behaviors. Specific phobias are perhaps the most common but least disabling of the various anxiety disorders. Although many individuals have at least one, most experience

Table 27-3. Preferred anxiolytic medications for use in medical outpatients.

Generic Name	Class	Starting Dosage	Step-Up Dose	Target Dose	Top Dose/Day	Comment
First-Line Agent						
Citalopram	SSRI	10 mg qd	10–20 mg/qd	20–40 mg/d	40 mg	Possibly fewer cytochrome P450 drug interactions
Duloxetine	SNRI	20 mg qd	20 mg/d	30 mg bid or 60 mg qd	60 mg bid	FDA-approved for depression
Escitalopram	SSRI	5 mg qd	5–10 mg qd	10–20 mg/d	20 mg	Enantiomer of citalopram; possibly fewer cytochrome P450 drug interactions; FDA-approved for GAD
Fluoxetine	SSRI	10 mg qd	10 mg/d	20–40 mg/d	80 mg	Most activating of SSRI class; slower onset of action; FDA-approved for depression, PD, OCD, and bulimia
Paroxetine	SSRI	10 mg qd	10–20 mg/d	40 mg/d	40 mg	FDA-approved for depression, PD, GAD, PTSD, OCD, social anxiety; slightly sedating
Sertraline	SSRI	25 mg qd	25 mg/d	100 mg/d	200 mg	FDA-approved for depression, PD, OCD, PTSD, social anxiety
Venlafaxine XR	SNRI	37.5 mg qd	37.5 mg qd	75–150 mg qd	225 mg	FDA-approved for depression, PD, GAD. Social anxiety; may increase blood pressure at higher doses
Second-Line Agent						
Fluvoxamine	SSRI	50 mg qd	50 mg bid	50 mg bid	300 mg	FDA-approved for OCD, social anxiety (extended release)
Bupropion SR	NDRI	100 mg/d	50 mg bid	150 mg bid	450 mg	FDA-approved for depression; favored if comorbid depression; may induce seizures at higher doses in seizure-prone individuals
Nefazodone	SARI	100 mg bid	50 mg bid	150 mg bid	600 mg	Sedation prominent at start; FDA-approved for depression; possible hepatotoxicity
Alprazolam	BZD	0.25 mg bid-tid	0.25 mg bid	0.25 mg prn	4 mg	Short onset and duration of action; FDA-approved for anxiety and PD
Lorazepam	BZD	0.5 mg tid-qid	0.5 mg qd	1.0 mg tid	10 mg	Short onset and duration of action; FDA-approved for anxiety
Clonazapine	BZD	0.5 mg bid	0.5 mg qd	1.0 mg bid	4 mg	Longer onset and duration of action; FDA-approved for PD and anxiety
Third-Line Agent						
Buspirone	Other	5 mg tid	5 mg qd	20–30 mg bid	60 mg	Moderate efficacy compared to SSRIs; no antidepressant effect; FDA-approved for GAD only
Mirtazapine	NaSSA	15 mg qHS	7.5-15 mg qd	45-60 mg qd	60 mg	Approved for treatment of depression. Commonly used for comorbid depression and anxiety; common adjunct with other antidepressants; inverse relationship between dose and sedation

Abreviations: BZD, benzodiazepine; NDRI, norepinephrine and dopamine reuptake inhibitor; NaSSA, noradrenergic and specific serotonergic antidepressants; SARI, serotonin agonist and reuptake inhibitor.

only minor related dysfunction, and therefore seldom seek medical care. Indeed, when care is sought, the diagnosis is usually evident from the history and requires no further testing.

Social anxiety disorder involves excessive fear of embarrassment, failure, or humiliation before others. Social anxiety disorder is classified into one of the two subtypes—nongeneralized and generalized. The more common nongeneralized subtype may be manifested as a fear of speaking, performing, eating, or writing in public. Less often, it presents as a generalized type of anxiety that disables the patient in a wide range of social situations. Its physical symptoms include blushing, profuse sweating, trembling, nausea, and difficulty talking. Marked anticipatory anxiety can also cause avoidance behaviors that significantly disrupt patients' functioning.

CASE ILLUSTRATION 2

Charlie, a man in his mid-thirties, presents to his primary care provider complaining of palpitations, sweating, and tremulousness. The symptoms occur when he is waiting in the customs line. As he approaches the front of the line, fear of evaluation and fear of talking with the customs official intensifies until the symptoms occur. Sometimes he flees to the end of the long line before he feels ready to face the customs official. Charlie realizes this cycle is silly and laughs anxiously as he describes it. This symptom is a major problem for him because his occupation is writing travel books. He has begun avoiding travel and is increasingly worried about his ability to meet writing deadlines and to continue working. A medical workup is unrevealing, and the primary care provider makes the diagnosis of specific social anxiety disorder, prescribing a trial of alprazolam to be used a short time before standing in the customs line. Charlie is also given a self-help book and a recording on relaxation techniques and the use of guided imagery as a way of visualizing success in the customs line. Charlie uses these treatment approaches successfully on his next trip and realizes that the problem is controllable. He incorporates them into his routine work schedule, and within 2 months has returned to full occupational functioning.

MANAGEMENT

Treatment of specific phobias and social anxiety disorder almost always involves some form of CBT, such as systematic desensitization, in which the patient is gradually exposed to the feared object or situation. Generally accepted pharmacotherapy guidelines have not been established for specific phobias. As noted in Case Illustration 2, patients with phobia and specific social anxiety disorder are often prescribed short-acting benzodiazepines (or beta-blockers in the case of performance anxiety) to be taken prior to an anticipated exposure to the phobic stimulus. Benzodiazepines are often given for exposures to infrequent events that have no complex performance requirements (e.g., traveling by commercial airplane). Patients should be informed of the risk of anterograde amnesia, or blackouts, associated with some of these drugs. Sertraline, paroxetine, fluvoxamine (extended release), and venlafaxine have all been Food and Drug Administration (FDA)-approved for the treatment of social anxiety disorder. Therapeutic effects typically occur within 2–6 weeks but may take up to 12 weeks. Although less data are presently available, the other SSRI and SNRI medications may be similarly effective at treating this disorder.

Obsessive–Compulsive Disorder

DIAGNOSIS

OCD is no longer categorized as an anxiety disorder in the Diagnostic and Statistical Manual of Mental Disorders, Fifth Edition (DSM-5); it is listed under the heading of "Obsessive–Compulsive and Related Disorder." However, as OCD is commonly seen in general medical settings, we will review the diagnosis and treatment here.

Patients with OCD experience regular, intrusive, thoughts—called obsessions—or are driven to repeatedly perform seemingly unnecessary and at times odd or unusual rituals—called compulsions. Aggression, sex, and religion are common obsessional themes. Compulsions may involve mental tasks, such as counting or praying, or they may involve physical rituals, such as repeated hand-washing or checking the state of an object. In patients with both obsessions and compulsions, the ritualized compulsions are usually performed to control the anxiety generated by the obsessive thoughts (e.g., obsessive fear about germs is eased by compulsive hand-washing). Although patients' level of insight is typically high—they generally experience obsessions and compulsions as intrusive, upsetting, and silly—such insight may diminish acutely when they are faced with the focus of an obsession. They may also become so preoccupied with their obsessions and compulsions that they become extremely anxious, slow, and disabled. In one instance, a patient wrung her hands so constantly she could not cook, work, or sleep. Another washed his hands every 10–15 minutes, which interfered significantly with his normal business and social activities.

Until the introduction of effective pharmacotherapies for OCD, the disorder was markedly underrecognized in both primary care and psychiatric practice. About 1–3% of the general population develops OCD during their lives. The disorder has been found to have a distinct biological component, a finding supported by the efficacy of biological therapies that selectively inhibit the reuptake of serotonin at CNS neurosynapses, and twin studies that show a significantly higher percentage of monozygotic twins with diagnostic concordance than dizygotic twins. Additionally, there is a distinct and reciprocal association between OCD and Tourette syndrome, a neurologic disorder involving persistent motor and verbal tics.

MANAGEMENT

Psychotherapy for OCD often involves a form of CBT called "exposure with response prevention" in which the patient is exposed to the anxiety-provoking obsessions or situation but does not engage in the subsequent compulsions or other maladaptive strategies to manage the anxiety. Patients are taught alternate ways of coping with the anxiety, including diaphragmatic breathing and progressive muscle relaxation. The cognitive behavioral therapist may also guide the patient in identifying faulty beliefs and assist the patient in testing those beliefs. The belief, "something terrible will happen if I don't check my lock a hundred times a day," is first rationally examined, then a behavioral test of that belief is collaboratively designed and executed—much as a scientist would design and run a test for any hypothesis.

SSRIs inhibit presynaptic reuptake of serotonin and are effective in treating OCD. In addition, clomipramine, the only TCA with this quality, is also effective. SSRIs have the advantages of ease of dosing and low toxicity in overdose. FDA-approved SSRIs for treatment of OCD include fluoxetine (Prozac), fluvoxamine (Luvox), paroxetine (Paxil), citalopram (Celexa), escitalopram (Lexapro), and sertraline (Zoloft). The dual SNRIs (venlafaxine and duloxetine) may also have efficacy in OCD. However, neither has yet been FDA-approved specifically for treatment of OCD. A recent meta-analysis recommends antipsychotic (haloperidol and risperidone) augmentation of SSRIs for treatment-refractory OCD.

Generalized Anxiety Disorder

DIAGNOSIS

GAD consists of chronic, persistent worry that affects patients for more days than not for at least 6 months and interferes with normal functioning. The worry and anxiety are difficult for the patient to control and are associated with edginess or restlessness, easy fatigability, difficulty concentrating, irritability, muscle tension, or sleep disturbance. Worries typically involve multiple domains and may include concern about routine life circumstances, with the magnitude of worry being out of proportion to the severity of the situation. Symptoms must not be due to the physiologic effects of a medical problem, such as hyperthyroidism or abuse of a medication or drug. Patients with GAD usually complain of feeling "up-tight" or constantly nervous. Physical symptoms, such as muscle aches, twitching, trembling, sweating, dry mouth, headaches, gastrointestinal symptoms, urinary frequency, and exaggerated startle, often accompany the disorder and are often the patient's presenting complaint.

GAD has a lifetime prevalence of 4–6%, and two-thirds of those affected are women. It is commonly associated with depression, alcohol and substance use. In fact, approximately half of all cases of GAD are comorbid with depression. The disorder tends to have a chronic, fluctuating course that worsens under stress. Patients with GAD will often respond affirmatively to the question: "Do you worry excessively about minor matters?" Patients can be further assessed with the GAD-2 and GAD-7 (see Figure 27-1).

MANAGEMENT

Results from randomized trials suggest that a stepped care approach to treatment of GAD is recommended. First, the patient can be educated about GAD and lifestyle changes, such as adequate sleep, aerobic exercise, and cutting back on caffeine and alcohol. Basic primary care strategies include empathic listening; encouragement; and assisting patients to identify problems, discuss possible solutions, and solve the problem. Second, depending on patient preference, pharmacotherapy, psychotherapy, or both can then be initiated for more severe and/or persistent symptoms. Many patients with GAD have focal life conflicts or stressors for which short-term psychotherapy may be helpful. Cognitive behavioral techniques can be used to help patients examine the catastrophic beliefs that underlie their unrealistic worries. Biofeedback and relaxation techniques are useful for improving patient control over muscle tension and other physiologic signs of anxiety.

Several SSRIs, SNRIs, benzodiazepines, and the non-benzodiazepine anxiolytic buspirone are approved for treatment of GAD. SSRIs are given at the same dose as is used for depression and generally take 4–6 weeks before a response is seen. Benzodiazepine therapy at doses lower than those required for PD is usually rapidly effective with few adverse effects. Sedation is the most common side effect but diminishes over time. Tolerance to therapeutic effects is minimal. Minimum effective doses should be used, but only for 3–6 months before tapering them off. As with benzodiazepine treatment for other anxiety disorders, rebound symptoms of anxiety are the rule as medication is discontinued. Often a lengthy (a month or more) taper is required. SSRIs are preferred as first-line agents over benzodiazepines because of concerns about misuse and dependence.

Buspirone is a nonsedating medication specifically indicated for patients with GAD. It alleviates the symptoms of this anxiety disorder but like the SSRIs and venlafaxine has a slow onset of action to reach efficacy.

Unlike these other medications, buspirone also requires twice daily dosing, which may adversely affect patient adherence. Importantly, it only has moderate efficacy compared with the SSRIs, and it lacks an antidepressant effect, placing it at a disadvantage for patients with comorbid depression.

Adjustment Disorder With Anxiety

DIAGNOSIS

Adjustment disorder with anxiety should be considered in patients who are responding with maladaptive anxiety to a recent situational stressor but who do not meet the criteria for another mental disorder. The stressor may be a medical event (e.g., surgery, hospitalization, or onset of an illness), but most often is a personal crisis such as a divorce, financial problems, or a job change. Symptoms usually begin within 2 months of the onset of the stressor and significantly impair social or occupational functioning. If symptoms persist for more than 6 months, then another diagnosis, such as GAD, is usually more appropriate. Sleeplessness and the physiologic aspects of anxiety predominate, and the patient may seek care for somatic complaints. Eliciting the history of the stressful life event and ascertaining the relationship of symptoms to that event help to establish this diagnosis.

MANAGEMENT

The fundamental management of adjustment disorder with anxious mood is supportive counseling, in which the patient discusses the stressful event and the provider helps the patient actively identify and solve problems and/or find ways to more effectively manage the stress (e.g., more effectively access social supports or engage in pleasant activities). Patients with adjustment disorder are generally well cared for by a primary care physician who has learned the details of the precipitating event and can incorporate brief supportive strategies into the office visit. Structured relaxation exercises and stress management or other support groups may also be helpful. Sometimes a brief trial of benzodiazepine (less than 3 weeks) can help improve patient coping by reducing the debilitating stress-related symptoms (e.g., insomnia or overwhelming fear). Referral to mental health professionals may help if patients do not respond quickly, are severely incapacitated, show a repetitive pattern of maladaptive coping, or specifically request a therapist.

Many studies suggest that there is a substantial group of primary care patients who present with relatively minor complaints of anxiety and depression. Although they do not satisfy criteria for a mental disorder, they do experience associated poor functioning. Often psychosocial stressors or chronic medical problems exacerbate the emotional symptoms. Generally speaking, effective management should emphasize supportive psychosocial rather than pharmacological interventions.

MANAGEMENT OF ANXIETY: GENERAL PRINCIPLES

Several general principles pertaining to the primary care treatment of anxiety disorders are worthy of note.

Psychosocial Therapies

Primary care providers should not underestimate the importance of basic supportive measures that can easily be performed in the general medical setting. The relationship between the clinician and patient usually plays a pivotal role for anxious patients in need of reassurance. Patient–provider trust is especially important for anxious patients, enhancing timely and accurate history taking, physical examination, diagnosis, and treatment adherence.

Symptoms of anxiety are extremely distressing to patients, who often fear that occult disease is causing their symptoms. Clinicians must try to view the symptoms through the eyes and perceptions of the affected patient—what seems trivial to a provider may be overwhelming for the patient. Listening to patients, expressing empathy for their feelings and concerns, and providing information about anxiety disorders are crucial ways to improve patient rapport (see Chapters 1 and 2) and should be routine in the course of care.

Equipping patients with basic information about anxiety disorders is essential ("bibliotherapy"). Patients with anxiety are common in medical settings, so hospitals and clinics should be prepared and knowledgeable with patient education resources such as brochures and relevant websites to enable patients to find high-quality information. Most patients find such explanations and self-management strategies from appropriate lay publications reassuring. A number of well-validated and available psychosocial treatments can be recommended (Table 27-4).

Pharmacotherapy

Pharmacological treatment (see Table 27-3) is appropriate when the patient's symptoms are severe enough to significantly interfere with functioning, and the benefits of medication outweigh the risks for a given patient. The treatment must be carefully individualized, based on the patient's prior experiences with pharmacotherapy—such as family experiences, brand name preference, insurance formulary restrictions, symptom severity, complicating medical or substance-abuse problems, vulnerability to various side effects, and willingness to collaborate in a psychopharmacological approach to treatment.

When medications are prescribed, it is important to recognize, track, and document specific target symptoms. We generally recommend treatment with a generically available SSRI or SNRI for treatment-naïve patients unless there is a compelling reason to

Table 27-4. Nonpharmacologic management of anxiety disorders.

Type of Treatment	Description	Indication
Education	Provides basic information and reassurance	Appropriate in all disorders Lay publications useful
Cognitive-behavioral therapy (e.g., systematic desensitization)	Gradually increases exposure to feared stimulus using relaxation techniques Helps patient reorganize way of thinking about symptoms	Useful in all disorders Particularly effective for PD and OCD
Relaxation techniques	Uses muscle-relaxation therapy, including hypnosis, biofeedback, meditation	Particularly useful in PD, GAD, adjustment disorder with anxious mood

use a branded medication, as no medication within these classes has been proved to be more effective than another. The medication should be initiated at half the typical starting dosage for unipolar major depression, and then titrated upward at 1- to 3-week intervals so as to minimize both the target symptoms and bothersome side effects. Lower starting dosages are recommended for those aged 60 years and older, because these drugs have longer half-lives in this age group, accumulation can easily occur, and sensitivity to unwanted cognitive and other toxic effects is greater. In addition, for this age group we recommend against use of TCAs to avoid the potential for cardiac side effects, and against use of benzodiazepines to avert cognitive and physical impairment (e.g., falls).

It is critically important to speak to the patient by telephone or in the office within 1–2 weeks and then again approximately every 2–4 weeks after the start of pharmacotherapy until symptoms remit. The purpose of these follow-up contacts is to: (1) promote medication adherence, (2) monitor for potential side effects, (3) assess for emerging suicidality, (4) monitor treatment response, and (5) answer any new questions or concerns the patient may have. Following complete symptom remission, patients should be seen or contacted every few months over the first year of treatment.

Although monotherapy is almost always preferable to medication combinations, a common exception is prescribing both ongoing antidepressants and 2–4 weeks of minor tranquilizers for patients with PD. This strategy achieves rapid reduction of symptoms, avoids the intensification of anxiety sometimes seen in early antidepressant treatment of anxiety disorders, and allows discontinuation of benzodiazepines before dependence occurs. If patients are being referred to CBT, a benzodiazepine taper, typically a reduction by 25% of the daily dose every week, and discontinuation are recommended. Benzodiazepines should seldom be used in patients with a history of substance abuse.

INDICATIONS FOR REFERRAL

Multiple randomized, controlled trials have shown that pharmacotherapy and/or CBT are effective treatments for most anxiety disorders. Patients should be considered for referral to a mental health professional under the following circumstances:

1. The patient has suicidal or homicidal thoughts or exhibits intended suicidal or homicidal behavior.
2. The treatment does not lead to improvement in the patient's symptoms within the expected time frame.
3. Diagnostic uncertainty. It is particularly important to differentiate patients who have bipolar disorder, alcohol abuse/dependence, or personality disorders from those with an anxiety disorder. Mental health consultation is appropriate if the primary care clinician is uncertain and the distinction has therapeutic implications.
4. Comorbid substance abuse is suspected.
5. The provider has questions about appropriate administration or tapering of benzodiazepines and questions regarding possible dependence.
6. The patient has an especially complicated set of ongoing psychosocial stressors, whose resolution requires greater time and expertise than can be provided in primary care.
7. When a multidisciplinary or more specialized treatment approach is indicated. Such conditions include, but are not limited to acute stress disorder (ASD), PTSD, and desensitization therapy for specific or social phobia.

In some circumstances, the primary care physician may be uncertain about whether a patient has another medical illness and believes a specialist is necessary to consider that possibility. It is helpful to select a specialist who understands anxiety disorders and will work with the referring physician to explain the nature of the specific anxiety disorder to the patient. It is imperative that the specialist bring a conservative approach to diagnostic studies, an understanding of the many physical manifestations of anxiety, and a respectful approach to treatment of the anxiety-disordered patient.

The accurate and prompt diagnosis of anxiety disorders can prevent unnecessary diagnostic testing, specialty referral, and iatrogenic harm. The primary care physician who is knowledgeable and skilled in the diagnosis and management of anxiety disorders can make an important contribution to the quality of patient care and to the appropriate use of health resources, particularly in the managed care environment. Nevertheless, providing appropriate care can be difficult in typical practice settings. To overcome patient, physician, and system barriers to provision of guideline-based treatment and provide sustained patient follow-up, "collaborative care" models have been developed and subsequently proved to be effective at improving clinical outcomes for panic and GAD. They typically involve a nurse or other allied health professional who follows an evidence-based protocol under the direction of a primary care physician with specialty back-up when necessary, who has the time to educate the patient about his or her disorder, monitor use of pharmacotherapy, and impart self-management skills either in person or via telephone.

SUGGESTED READINGS

Craske MG, Stein MB. Anxiety. *Lancet* 2016;388:3048–3059.

Metzler DH, Mahoney D, Freedy JR. Anxiety disorders in primary care. *Prim Care Clin Office Pract* 2016;43:245–261.

Slee A, Nazareth I, Bondaroneck P, et al. Pharmacological treatments for generalized anxiety disorder: a systematic review and network meta-analysis. *Lancet* 2019;393:768–777.

Stein MB, Sareen J. Generalized anxiety disorder. *N Engl J Med* 2015;373:2059–2068.

PATIENT BIBLIOGRAPHY (REFERENCE BOOKS FOR PATIENTS)

Bourne EJ. *The Anxiety and Phobia Workbook,* 4th ed. Oakland, CA: New Harbinger Press; 2005.

Craske MG, Barlow DH. *Mastery of Your Anxiety and Worry,* 2nd ed. New York, NY: Oxford University Press; 2006.

Davis M, McKay M, Eshelman ER. *The Relaxation and Stress Reduction Workbook,* 5th ed. Oakland, CA: New Harbinger Press; 2000.

Foa E, Wilson R. *Stop Obsessing! How to Overcome Your Obsessions and Compulsions.* New York, NY: Bantam; 2001.

Zuercher-White E. *An End to Panic: Breakthrough Techniques for Overcoming Panic Disorder,* 2nd ed. Oakland, CA: New Harbinger Press; 1998.

WEBSITES

Anxiety Disorders Association of America Website. http://www.adaa.org. Accessed May 2019.

Cognitive Behavioral Therapy Website. http://www.abct.org/Home/. Accessed May 2019.

Attention Deficit Hyperactivity Disorder

28

H. Russell Searight, PhD, MPH & Taylor Severance, BS

INTRODUCTION

Attention deficit hyperactivity disorder (ADHD) is a condition typically first evident in early childhood. Symptoms include difficulties with attention, concentration, and short-term memory as well as impulsivity. Children with ADHD are overly active (as if "driven by a motor") and cannot control ongoing activity ranging from fidgeting to difficulty remaining seated for 5 minutes to inappropriately running, jumping, and yelling in public places. Since these deficits significantly impair academic performance and are disruptive in a typical classroom, concerns about ADHD usually arise during kindergarten or first grade. However, ADHD is a lifelong condition with functional impairment extending throughout adulthood.

Recent data from the Centers for Disease Control (CDC) suggest a prevalence of ADHD between 9% and 10% of children. There is debate about whether ADHD's incidence is increasing historically. To date, the majority of epidemiologic studies have been conducted in North America and Europe. However, available data suggest that the condition has similar prevalence rates internationally. Even within the United States, there is also considerable variability in prevalence rates that may reflect differing diagnostic practices, differing definitions of the condition, or both. A recent U.S. study by the CDC reported state-based prevalence rates ranging from 5.6% (Nevada) to 15.6% (North Carolina). ADHD disproportionately affects males with a sex ratio between 3:1 and 9:1, with more conservative figures in clinical rather than community samples. Lower socioeconomic status (SES) has been associated with increased ADHD rates.

Diagnostic criteria for ADHD include two symptom clusters: **inattention** (failing to give attention to detail, problems maintaining attention, not appearing to listen when spoken to directly, failure to follow through on instructions for completion of schoolwork or other tasks, problems with organization, avoiding activities requiring sustained concentration, losing important items, being easily distracted, and forgetfulness), or **hyperactivity/impulsivity** (fidgeting, inability to remain seated, inappropriate running and climbing, difficulty playing quietly, acting as if "driven by a motor," excessive talking, blurting out answers before questions are finished, difficulty taking turns, and intruding upon others' activities and/or conversations). Children must have at least six symptoms from either (or both) the inattention group of criteria and the hyperactivity/impulsivity criteria, whereas older adolescents and adults (over the age of 17 years) must present with five criteria with some symptoms present before age 12.

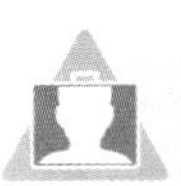

CASE ILLUSTRATION 1: EARLY CHILDHOOD

Five-and-a-half-year-old Joey has been repeatedly sent home early during the first month of his all-day kindergarten because of disruptive behavior. Joey's mother brings a teacher's note chronicling his recent behavior:

- *9/25 = "Ran out of classroom and was on his way out of the building before I stopped him."*
- *9/28 = "Became frustrated with an assignment and dumped a whole box of crayons on the floor. When asked to pick them up, he refused."*
- *10/02 = "Joey would not stay seated during story hour. Threw milk cartons during lunch time."*

In your examination room, Joey is lying across your stool face down yelling, "I'm flying," while pushing off from the walls with his feet. His mother, appearing exhausted, makes a few half-hearted attempts to get Joey to settle down but quickly gives up saying, "You see, doctor, this is what it's like."

Although there are no precise figures, ADHD is increasingly accepted as a lifelong condition for many, if not most, patients. Development, however, does affect the symptom picture. Research indicates that at around the age of 9 years, hyperactivity and impulsivity begin to become less pronounced, whereas inattention and other cognitive deficits persist, with hyperactivity being replaced by restlessness and fidgeting.

With children referred in preschool or the early grades, there is typically a high level of parental distress and urgency. Hyperactivity may take the form of an inability to remain seated for more than 5 minutes at school or during family meals. Even when seated, the child may be swinging their legs, rocking, or picking up nearby objects. By the time they reach first grade, children may also have a number of scars on their legs, arms, and head, and can provide a number of stories about jumping off the garage roof, rear-ending a car with their bicycle, and running into countless pieces of furniture. Among older adolescents and adults, household chores may be initiated but not completed, bills are forgotten, sitting through a movie or presentation is extremely difficult, and others complain about the patient's frequent conversational interruptions. The phrase "as if driven by a motor" captures the quality of the child's activity level. Although the child, with adult urging, may sit relatively still for 2–3 minutes, they will soon begin moving again as if they cannot stop themselves. The hyperactive/impulsive behavior is not experienced as under the patient's control. In many instances, when older children with ADHD are reminded of a recent reminder to stay seated, they will be apologetic.

CASE ILLUSTRATION 2: EARLY ELEMENTARY SCHOOL CHILD

Christopher is an 8-year-old boy in the second grade, who is accompanied to your office by both parents. They bring several notes that the teacher has sent home since school began several months ago. The parents also bring samples of Christopher's schoolwork. The teacher's notes describe situations in which Chris got up from his seat to sharpen his pencil 20 times in the course of a day, he was repeatedly told to stop playing with the hair of the girl who sits in front of him, and he continued to yell out answers to the teacher's questions before she finished speaking. Christopher's parents say that his reading and spelling skills are below grade level because he is easily distracted and cannot follow the lessons. At home, they describe mealtime as a "hit and run" experience where Chris eats while alternately sitting and standing at the table for no more than 10 minutes, during which he frequently knocks over his milk. Christopher's mother says she no longer takes him shopping because he runs off from her in the store and she is afraid he will get lost or unintentionally break items.

Among both children and adults, impaired attention and concentration, distractibility, and short-term memory deficits are often misattributed to "laziness," poor motivation, or "not caring" rather than a central nervous system disorder. Parents frequently complain about having to tell their child "a hundred times" to do something before the request "seems to register." Multistep directions are particularly challenging for those of all ages with ADHD. A mother tells her teenaged son to go upstairs and get his new pants to be hemmed, the sewing kit, and a piece of chalk. Fifteen minutes later, when he has not appeared, his mother goes upstairs to find him. He is in his room, trying on a shirt with his new pants in his hand, having forgotten what he was asked to do.

CASE ILLUSTRATION 3: MIDDLE ELEMENTARY SCHOOL CHILD

Miranda, an 11-year-old fourth grader, is seen because of poor grades. Her teacher describes Miranda as "spacey" with difficulty concentrating, paying attention, and remembering. However, she and Miranda's mother both describe Miranda as a "sweet, sensitive, and helpful girl" without any disruptive behavior. A Vanderbilt Scale confirms this picture. The teacher's version includes a comment that Miranda may have to repeat the grade unless her academic performance improves.

At school, inattention and poor concentration impair academic performance. Much of school success is still based on memorization. To encode material into longer-term memory for a test, it is necessary to pay attention to relevant information, relate it to existing knowledge, and rehearse it in short-term memory. When this process is disrupted, retaining information from textbooks and classroom presentations is extremely challenging. In elementary school, a typical didactic process is that the teacher will present a lesson (e.g., steps involved in long division and identifying adverbs) with several examples of the concept and then students will individually work on exercises applying that particular concept. In the later elementary years through college, there is much greater emphasis on independent reading and retaining what is read. College students with untreated ADHD often report that despite rereading material multiple times, they cannot remember it.

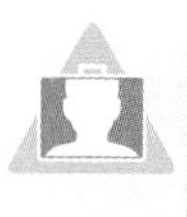

CASE ILLUSTRATION 4: ADOLESCENT

Josh, a 16-year-old, is brought in by his father for a drug test. Yesterday, Josh was suspended from school after a baggie of marijuana was found in his locker. He readily admitted smoking it several times a week for the past 6 months to "help calm me down." Josh has also been smoking cigarettes regularly for the past year. Josh was diagnosed with ADHD-combined type at the age of 7 years and responded well to stimulant pharmacotherapy until about a year ago. At that time, Josh's grades declined—largely because of missing assignments—and he has had several school detentions because of being late to class. His father describes his son as fidgety, disorganized, and forgetful. During the seventh grade, Josh said he felt embarrassed about going to the school nurse's office for his second methylphenidate dose. Josh was then switched from short-acting methylphenidate to an extended-release formulation that he only took once, in the morning, before school. When asked about how he was tolerating the current medication, Josh responded: "I don't like taking that stuff; it doesn't do anything for me. My friends don't have to take it." Josh's father adds, "Now that I think about it, we have at least two extra bottles full of pills at home. I don't think Josh is taking it every day."

Up to 80% of adolescents initially diagnosed with ADHD in childhood continue to exhibit symptoms with a comparable adult prevalence of 60–70%. In addition to elevated rates of psychiatric disorders, use of cigarettes at an earlier age and the rapid development of nicotine dependency are also more common among youth with ADHD. Noncompletion of high school, auto accidents, and both nonviolent and violent legal offenses are also higher among teenagers with childhood ADHD histories.

Among adults with ADHD, work and family are affected by inattention and poor short-term memory. Birthdays and anniversaries are forgotten, as are commitments to attend children's school activities. Multiple auto accidents are also common. At work, projects may be initiated but remain uncompleted. Phone calls, coworkers, and email all pose distractions that make it particularly difficult to get back "on track." Task switching has been found to lead to poorer performance among all adults but is particularly challenging for those with ADHD.

Even when adolescents no longer meet formal DSM-5 diagnostic criteria, deficits are often present along with comorbid conditions, such as oppositional defiant disorder (ODD) or conduct disorder (CD) as well as substance abuse in adolescents. Among adults with ADHD, mood and anxiety disorders and substance abuse are common. Among those adults with childhood ADHD symptoms that appear to remit, other psychiatric conditions are likely to emerge. Although findings have been mixed, there are indications that stimulant treatment during childhood reduces the likelihood of grade retention in school as well as cigarette and marijuana use in adolescence and early adulthood.

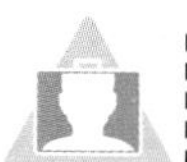

CASE ILLUSTRATION 5: ADULT

Jim, a 35-year-old man, comes to see you after a particularly poor performance evaluation at work. Jim is an auto salesman who was recently promoted to manager of a small group of junior sales people. On his evaluation, Jim's supervisor describes Jim as ". . . scattered, unable to set priorities; starts projects but doesn't finish them; paperwork late or lost." His supervisors describe him as a "nice guy" but "it's hard to know what he wants; he contradicts himself a lot."

At home, Jim's wife took over the family's schedule after Jim forgot several important dates, including her birthday. Many mornings, he dashes around the house looking for misplaced car keys. Jim's wife has also become the primary disciplinarian of their two children because Jim had difficulty being consistent and following through with consequences.

Jim describes having had a hard time getting through high school: "I did really badly on tests; I just couldn't memorize." Even in elementary school, "I was sent to the principal's office for being the class clown." College was a greater challenge. Jim had to repeat several classes and required an extra three semesters to graduate.

ETIOLOGY

Studies of monozygotic twins suggest that ADHD's heritability is between 0.70 and 0.80. Adoption studies further support the strong role of genetics in the condition. Seven candidate genes for ADHD have been implicated. Of these, the largest number of genes are involved in dopamine transport. Specifically, genes coding for dopaminergic (*DAT1*, *DRD4*, and *DRD5*), serotonergic (*5HTT*), and axonal growth and synaptic activity (*SNAP-25*) have been implicated. Recent studies have linked some of these genetic variations to specific ADHD symptoms. For example, 5HTT variations have been linked to impulsivity. These neurogenetic patterns are consistent with the action of stimulant drugs that block dopamine transport. Altered dopaminergic genetic activity is also likely to be a factor in the predisposition to cigarette smoking among youth with ADHD. Finally, new investigations suggest that, in some cases, emergence of the ADHD phenotype may result from the interaction between environmental factors such as parental inconsistency and specific dopaminergic genes. Reduced dopaminergic activity in the frontal brain region has been conceptually linked to core deficits of disinhibition and poor self-monitoring.

Certain environmental exposures, although not specific to ADHD, have been associated with increased prevalence. Lead exposure appears to be associated with hyperactivity and cognitive difficulties; however, most ADHD children do not have elevated lead and, conversely, most children with elevated lead do not develop ADHD. Pregnancy and delivery complications, including toxemia, maternal age, fetal post maturity, low birth weight, long duration of labor, fetal distress, hemorrhage, and prematurity are all ADHD risk factors. Alcohol use and maternal smoking during pregnancy also elevate ADHD risk. Recent research has been examining environmental chemical exposures during pregnancy with some evidence of a modest association between mercury and fluoride and the development of ADHD symptoms. It is likely that these factors, both directly and indirectly, are associated with subtle central nervous system abnormalities in regions associated with the condition.

Among structural brain anomalies that have been associated with ADHD, the thalamus as well as circuits involving the frontal lobe, basal ganglia, and central cerebellum have been implicated. Structurally, reduced cerebral and cerebellar volumes have been noted. There are suggestions that stimulant treatment is associated with fewer structural central nervous system abnormalities and greater total white matter and brain volume as compared with that of untreated children and adolescents.

THE CLINICAL HISTORY

In obtaining a clinical history, there are several essential features regardless of the patient's age. First, the symptoms must be persistent and evident in at least two settings. Typically, parents report that hyperactivity was first evident at the age of 3–4 years. Inattention may not be apparent until a child is in elementary school. In many instances, when evaluating ADHD-inattentive type, the child's difficulties may not be apparent in school for several years—until the child is 9 or 10 years old. A recent onset of hyperactivity and inattention in an older child, adolescent, or adult is usually inconsistent with ADHD, and other diagnostic possibilities should be considered.

In the past, critics argued that strict adherence to the DSM IV-TR ADHD symptoms as well as the wording of the criteria did not capture adults with the condition. These issues were addressed in the DSM-5 through changes in the number of symptoms required (5 rather than 6 for those ages 18 and above) and evidence of some symptoms before the age of 12 (rather than a cutoff of age 7) with symptom descriptions more appropriate for adults (e.g., for "easily distracted by extraneous stimuli"; this phrase was added "... for older adolescents and adults, may include unrelated thoughts.")

Recently, there has been debate about the existence of adult-onset ADHD. Several studies involving large longitudinal data sets have reported subsets of patients who, despite repeated assessments beginning in early childhood, did not meet diagnostic criteria until late adolescence or adulthood. While there are multiple explanations that can account for this symptom history without creating a new diagnostic category, this phenomenon highlights a pattern among adults consulting a physician for the first time for ADHD symptoms. Adults with predominant inattention, who are intellectually gifted, and who had previously been in structured educational and work settings, may not manifest symptoms until having to perform with less external structure. There do not appear to be differences in treatment response or prognosis among patients with later versus earlier age of onset.

Among children, ADHD symptoms are almost always evident in school. If a parent reports that inattention and/or hyperactivity are only demonstrated at home, an ADHD diagnosis is unlikely. The physician's office cannot be used as one of the two environmental settings required to meet diagnostic criteria. Moreover, the diagnosis cannot be ruled out from a parental report that the child can focus on video games for hours at a time. The constantly changing visual and auditory feedback unique to video games often engages the child with ADHD.

Eliciting specific behavioral examples is important—particularly in evaluating hyperactivity/impulsivity. Parents and, at times, teachers, often conceptually group all externalizing behavior under ADHD. Significant, repeated aggression and/or property destruction, talking back, theft, lying, or refusal to do schoolwork are not core ADHD symptoms. These behaviors suggest other diagnoses (CD or ODD) instead of, or possibly comorbid with, ADHD. For example, in the first vignette, it would be important to determine if Joey's episodes of throwing objects were reactions to task-related frustration versus intentional aggressive acts toward others. Developmentally, aggressive behavior should be declining at age four; when it persists beyond this age, aggression predicts later conduct disorder. Additionally, during the preschool years, 30% of children with ADHD have comorbid ODD.

Children with poor academic performance may be seen because school personnel and/or parents attribute a child's poor grades to ADHD. Because of budgetary issues and the large number of children with learning and/or behavioral problems, adequate special education services are often not readily available. School personnel,

Table 28-1. Process of ADHD evaluation.

1. What are the symptoms?
   - Are they core ADHD symptoms?
   - In self-diagnosed patients, are there other clinical conditions that could be contributing to the symptoms?
2. How long have symptoms been present?
   - Some symptoms must be consistently present prior to age 12
3. Do the symptoms impair daily functioning?
4. Use rating scales (e.g. Connors, Vanderbilt, and Child Behavior Checklist)
5. Screen mental status in office with particular attention to attention (digits forward), concentration (digits backwards or serial "7"s), and short-term recall (recall of four words or a brief story at 5–10 minute delay)
6. Do symptoms seem to be better explained by another condition (e.g., sleep apnea and elevated lead level)? If yes, treat that condition and reassess at later date.
7. If information is generally consistent with ADHD diagnosis, initiate treatment.
8. If information is ambiguous, there is a complicated differential diagnosis, or significant comorbidities, refer to psychologist or psychiatrist for further assessment.

hoping that if there is a problem it can be managed without additional educational resources, may encourage parents to seek an ADHD evaluation (Table 28-1). Reviewing academic testing, report cards, schoolwork samples, as well as the developmental history may suggest a learning disability. Again, learning disabilities are frequently comorbid with reading impairment, the most common specific learning disability accompanying ADHD.

MENTAL STATUS TESTING

Although detailed neuropsychological assessments are beyond the scope of the typical primary care setting, there are several cognitive tasks that, when used along with other information, may be helpful. Attention and immediate memory may be assessed by saying a sentence (in the case of preschool children) or string of random numbers and asking the patient to repeat them. A task assessing concentration requires the patient to say the numbers immediately afterward but in reverse order. Words can also be used as the auditory stimulus with the request to spell them forward and backward. Vigilance may be evaluated by asking the patient to tap their finger every time they hear the letter "A." The examiner then says a string of random letters and frequently, yet at unexpected intervals, says "A." The ability to recall four words after a 5- to 10-minute delay tests short-term memory. While not commonly used in the primary care setting, computerized continuous performance tasks may be useful in assessing response to stimulant pharmacotherapy.

MEDICAL TESTING

There is no agreed upon set of laboratory tests to aid in diagnosing ADHD. In geographic regions with high levels of lead exposure, lead levels should be obtained, since elevations have been associated with hyperactivity. Since hyperthyroidism may present with inattention, decreased recent memory, and increased motor activity, thyroid function tests are occasionally obtained—particularly with adults.

Obstructive sleep apnea is associated with impaired attention and concentration. A sleep study should be considered when other indications are present (loud snoring, brief breathing cessation, etc.).

RATING SCALES & CHECKLISTS

Children and adolescents with ADHD do not reliably report their own symptoms and typically do not recognize their hyperactivity, impulsivity, inattention, or distractibility. Because parents, teachers, and spouses, rather than patients, often notice symptoms, standardized behavioral ratings should be obtained. Although these scales vary somewhat according to the instrument's developer and, more importantly, the age group to which they are applied, most instruments share basic properties. All require the respondent's judgment about symptom frequency. The cognitive or behavioral symptoms must be nearly always present (observable everyday) to be considered positive. Scales may simply list the DSM-5 symptoms, or ADHD criteria may be intermingled with symptoms of other disorders including oppositional defiant, conduct, major depressive, or substance use disorders.

The Conners Rating Scales-Revised (CRS-R) and the Conners-3 includes forms for parents, teachers, and a self-report version for older children and adolescents. The Conners-3 assesses oppositional and conduct disordered behavior, cognitive difficulties, and hyperactivity; it also includes a Global ADHD Index. The long versions of these scales require approximately 20 minutes for completion while the brief versions require approximately 10 minutes. The Conners Scales have a large reference population for interpreting scores. The Vanderbilt Scale, while including all DSM ADHD criteria, also includes pediatric mood and anxiety disorder symptoms, as well as a section for teachers and parents to rate the level of impairment created by the symptoms. The teachers' Vanderbilt has been used successfully to monitor response to treatment.

The Child Behavior Checklist (CBCL) is a broadband rating scale that may be particularly useful in differential diagnosis and detecting comorbid conditions. Several of the CBCL's subscales form the basis of a "Dysregulation Profile" assessing self-regulation which, when deficient, is associated with greater ADHD symptom severity.

Since the classroom places demands on attention, concentration, organizational skills, and impulse inhibition, teacher ratings should always be obtained, if possible. Maternal child behavior ratings have been found to be strongly influenced by the mother's level of emotional distress. Depressed mothers rate their children as having more behavioral problems.

Adult rating scales demonstrate more heterogeneity, reflecting the greater emphasis placed on cognitive DSM-5 symptoms and more subtle forms of hyperactivity among older ADHD patients. The Conners Adult ADHD Rating Scale (CAARS) assesses current symptoms. The CAARS is a self-report measure but can be completed by a collateral informant such as a spouse or parent. The Adult Self-Report Scale-V1.1 is a brief screening tool that can help primary care providers identify adult patients at risk for having ADHD. Finally, the Adult ADHD Investigator Symptom Rating Scale (AISRS) is a clinician-administered instrument covering the diagnostic criteria for ADHD but with adult versions of symptoms.

Rating scales, while providing important information about core ADHD symptoms and the possible presence of comorbid conditions, should not be used in isolation or weighed too heavily in making an ADHD diagnosis. An issue that arises with childrens' ratings, which is more pronounced with adults, is the high number of false positives. These scales are generally sensitive but diagnostic specificity is less consistent. Among adults, ADHD's cognitive symptoms also characterize mood and anxiety disorders.

TREATMENT

Pharmacotherapy

STIMULANTS

Stimulant medications, specifically methylphenidate and amphetamine-based formulations, are the mainstays of ADHD therapy. Their mode of action appears to be blocking of dopamine transporters. Historically, the most commonly prescribed treatment has been immediate-release methylphenidate given two to three times per day in doses of 5–20 mg. Methylphenidate typically begins working in 30–60 minutes, with effects peaking at 1–2 hours and an overall duration of 2–5 hours. The somewhat longer-acting *d*- or *l*-amphetamine salts (Adderall) are equally effective in treating core ADHD symptoms and are an alternative for patients who do not respond to methylphenidate.

In the past decade, the major pharmacotherapeutic innovation has been in the delivery systems for these two stimulants. Whereas the initial mode of release was immediate, more recent long-acting stimulants in a continuous-release (CR) form, permit once-a-day dosing. Medications such as lisdexamfetamine dimesylate (Vyvanse) as well as methylphenidate (Concerta), dexmethylphenidate (Focalin-XR), and amphetamine preparations (Adderall XR) are examples of "second-generation" CR delivery systems. Delivery systems also include a transdermal patch (Daytrana) and more recently, extended release oral suspensions such as amphetamine in liquid form (Dyanavel) and methylphenidate extended-release oral suspensions (Quillivant-XR) as well as chewing gum (QuilliChew-ER). These medications are typically taken once, and on occasion twice, per day. Stimulants appear to have their most pronounced benefits for symptoms of hyperactivity/impulsivity and are less effective in addressing cognitive symptoms, including attention, concentration, and short-term recall.

Stimulants' adverse effects include appetite suppression, insomnia, and weight loss. Reduced appetite may occur in up to 50% of children and is considered a significant side effect for about 10% of treated patients. Less common side effects include headaches and nervousness. Ritalin "rebound" is frequently experienced when the stimulant wears off and is characterized by fatigue and irritability. In some patients, irritability is less pronounced with longer-acting stimulants. Side effects occurring within 2 hours of ingestion are probably best addressed by reducing the dose. The stimulants, particularly amphetamine and methylphenidate, may have some cardiovascular risk, prompting the Drug, Safety and Risk Management Advisory Committee of the Food and Drug Administration (FDA) to issue a black box warning for these medications. Subsequent research with adults has found stimulants to be associated with increased heart rate and systolic blood pressure and longer post-exercise recovery time for these cardiovascular indices. However, recent reviews have suggested that despite these effects, appropriately prescribed stimulants are not associated with increased rates of cardiovascular disease among adults. In pediatric populations, while rare, stimulant medications do appear to be associated with increased risk of cardiovascular events.

Stimulant therapies appear to be less effective with preschool children with ADHD. Up to a third of these younger patients demonstrate pronounced side effects with methylphenidate, leading to a higher discontinuation rate compared with school-aged children. Evidence-based guidelines for treating ADHD in children ages 6 and under indicate behavior therapy as first-line treatment with stimulant medication reserved for nonresponders.

NONSTIMULANT MEDICATIONS

Nonstimulants are second-line therapies to be considered under certain circumstances such as: difficulty with stimulant side effects; comorbid conditions such as anxiety disorders, Tourette syndrome, or seizure disorders; concerns about stimulant abuse; or parents philosophically opposed to stimulant use.

Atomoxetine (Strattera), a norepinephrine reuptake inhibitor, has demonstrated efficacy relative to a placebo in reducing ADHD symptoms. As a nonstimulant, atomoxetine is not associated with growth suppression, tics, or insomnia. Adverse effects may include nausea, vomiting, weight loss, and sleep problems. After reports of serious liver damage, the FDA required a written warning that it should be discontinued when jaundice is present or there is laboratory evidence of liver disease. Atomoxetine does not appear to demonstrate any abuse potential and is unscheduled. Because atomoxetine is an antidepressant, it has the standard black box warning about risk of suicide accompanying antidepressant medication, including the possibility of increased suicidal ideation. To date, suicide risk has not been a significant clinical concern with atomoxetine.

Extended-release guanfacine in 1-, 2-, 3-, and 4-mg doses (INTUNIV) is marketed both as monotherapy as well as adjunctive treatment with a stimulant. A timed-release clonidine preparation (KAPVAY) is another non-stimulant for ADHD. The alpha-2 agonists have been helpful with comorbid conduct disturbance, particularly when angry outbursts and aggression are present. In addition, they may reduce motor tics that may accompany stimulant treatment and also may reduce headaches and "jitteriness" that are common stimulant side effects. Patients should be closely monitored for hypotension and sedation.

Atomoxetine, clonidine, and guanfacine all appear to be less effective in reducing ADHD symptoms than stimulants.

Other antidepressants, such as bupropion and tricyclic agents, have demonstrated some efficacy with ADHD in open-label studies. Presently, these agents are more commonly used with adult rather than childhood ADHD. The TCAs have associated cardiovascular risk, and adult patients with preexisting cardiac disease should generally avoid these medications. Bupropion should be avoided in patients with seizure histories as well as in patients with eating disorders.

Once pharmacotherapy has been titrated to optimal effectiveness, patients' comorbid conditions and residual difficulties are often more apparent. Learning disabilities, social skills deficits, and in adult patients, communication and organizational skills may become a treatment focus.

Nonpharmacological Treatment

Recently, the FDA approved the first medical device for treating ADHD. The external Trigeminal Nerve Stimulation system (eTNS), in a four week blinded sham placebo trial, with children ages 8-12 years old, was associated with a statistically significant reduction in ADHD symptom ratings. The investigators indicated that the magnitude of the symptom reduction was comparable to that of "non stimulant" ADHD medication. The treatment is reportedly well tolerated with side effects including increased appetite, teeth clenching, and drowsiness.

Psychoeducational approaches for parents of ADHD children may be beneficial for increased medication adherence, as well as decreasing school and family stress. Key components include: (1) an explanation of ADHD's etiology as a biologically based condition; (2) reassurance to parents that they are not at fault or responsible for ADHD; (3) distinguishing between impulsive, uncontrollable behavior and volitional acts; (4) explaining the role of pharmacotherapy—specifically, the type of symptoms addressed and not treated by medication; (5) description of common medication side effects; and (6) discussing the likelihood that medication doses may be changed and that trying different agents and doses may be necessary before achieving optimal symptom control.

Encouraging parents to communicate frequently with their child's teacher helps identify problems early, before they have significant academic consequences. If possible, a daily note-to-home system should be established between the school and parents.

At home, high levels of structure and predictability will make ADHD more manageable. Bedtimes, meals, and homework should ideally occur at preplanned times that rarely vary from day to day. Encouraging children to lay out all material needed for the next day, including wardrobe, will make mornings run more smoothly. Older children should keep their desk or homework completion area free of distracting clutter, whereas younger children should pick up all of their play items before moving to another activity.

For children with ADHD alone, the addition of behavior therapy to stimulant medication may not appear to add further benefit. However, for the high proportion of ADHD children with comorbid CD or ODD, behavioral intervention is strongly indicated. Key elements of parent training include: (1) specifying no more than two to three target behaviors to address at one time; (2) establishing positive reinforcement for appropriately prosocial behavior; (3) developing a reasonable time frame and frequency of target behavior so that the child will realistically receive early positive reinforcement; (4) responding to inappropriate behavior through ignoring or time out; and (5) clear communication of requests and expectations.

Several recent studies have shown that among adolescents and adults, cognitive behavioral therapy (CBT) as an adjunct to pharmacotherapy augments outcomes. Self-esteem and organization skills, in particular, improved with the addition of CBT. An educational approach with demonstrated efficacy for adult ADHD is meta-cognitive therapy emphasizing effective self-management, including time awareness, breaking down larger tasks into manageable parts, self-reward, and disputing depressionogenic thoughts.

At a practical level, adults with ADHD benefit from making frequent lists, using planners and calendars, as well as smartphones, to help organize activities and remember important events and deadlines. For those employed in office settings, going into work early before most coworkers arrive will allow task completion without interruption.

Adult ADHD can wreak havoc on intimate relationships. In many instances, marriage counseling may be valuable for addressing effects of long-standing forgetfulness and the inability to actively listen and be psychologically present to one's spouse or partner. For the spouse without ADHD, it is important to recognize that this pattern of neglect does not indicate a lack of loving concern but is a by-product of the condition that can be improved.

A number of complementary and alternative therapies have been promoted for both childhood and adult ADHD. EEG neurofeedback involves learning to regulate a signal derived from neural electrical activity. While demonstrating some effectiveness, sham feedback is equally efficacious as actual EEG neurofeedback. Benefits appear to derive from attending 30–40 weekly visits with a clinician in which patients practice sitting attentively. Omega-3 oils' impact on core ADHD symptoms appears, at best, equivocal. However, the addition of Omega 3 to standard ADHD pharmacotherapy may reduce associated mood instability and angry outbursts.

CONCLUSIONS: THE COST OF ADHD

In addition to health care expenditures, ADHD has economic, legal, and social costs. Youth with ADHD have more outpatient physician office visits—even exceeding those for children and adolescents with asthma. Adults with ADHD as well as parents of children with the condition have greater health care costs, more lost workdays, and greater job turnover. Rates of accidental poisoning, as well as injuries, are also higher among children with ADHD. In addition to greater health care utilization, the high comorbidity of ADHD with learning disabilities leads to more costly special education services.

By adolescence, there is also a marked rise in comorbidity. Conduct Disorder, when together with ADHD, is particularly pronounced and contributes to property damage, theft, and harm to others. High school is particularly challenging for youth with ADHD. Approximately one-third of adolescents with ADHD do not complete high school; a disproportionate number are expelled compared with teens without ADHD. The high drop-out rate may, in part, reflect the fact that by high school nearly half of adolescents with ADHD have repeated at least one grade. A significant percentage of teens with ADHD are having sexual intercourse by the age of 15 years and with multiple partners, reflecting the brevity of their relationships. In examining this association in more detail, risky sexual behavior characterizes a subgroup of ADHD adolescents with comorbid conduct disorder and significant cannabis use.

By the time adulthood is reached, ADHD has adversely impacted most significant life arenas. In the workplace, adults with ADHD change jobs and are fired at a rate two to three times greater than those without the condition. These outcomes likely stem from reduced productivity, interpersonal issues, and increased work-related accidental injuries and illness-related absences. Annual medical costs are two to three times higher than for those without ADHD. A 30-year longitudinal study found elevated mortality associated with ADHD.

Adults with ADHD have three times as many sexual partners and are significantly more likely to have unplanned pregnancies, as well as to contract a sexually transmitted disease. A disproportionate number of parents with ADHD no longer have custody of their children. Rates of vehicular accidents are greater among persons with ADHD; pharmacotherapy reduced the risk by 50%. While there is often concern among parents about whether treatment with a stimulant medication will increase the risk of later psychiatric and behavioral problems, the opposite appears to be the case. Several longitudinal studies have found that when compared with those not treated with stimulant medication, adolescents and young adults with ADHD who had stimulant treatment as children were less likely to develop mood and anxiety disorders and more likely to perform better academically.

SUGGESTED READINGS

Barkley R. *Attention Deficit Hyperactivity Disorder: A Handbook for Diagnosis and Treatment.* 4th ed. New York: Guilford Press; 2018.

Chorozoglou M, Smith E, Koerting J, et al. Preschool hyperactivity is associated with long-term economic burden: evidence from a longitudinal health economic analysis of costs incurred across childhood, adolescence and young adulthood. *J Child Psychol Psychiatry* 2015;56(9):966–975.

Conners CK. *Conners 3rd Edition Multi-Health Systems.* Toronto, Ontario, Canada: 2008.

Cortese S, D'Acunto G, Konofal E, et al. New formulations of methylphenidate for the treatment of attention-deficit/hyperactivity disorder: pharmacokinetics, efficacy, and tolerability. *CNS Drugs* 2017;31(2):149–160.

Faraone SV, Larsson H. Genetics of attention deficit hyperactivity disorder. *Mol Psychiatry* 2018;11:1.

Hinshaw SP. Attention deficit hyperactivity disorder (ADHD): controversy, developmental mechanisms, and multiple levels of analysis. *Annu Rev Clin Psychol* 2018;14:291–316.

McGough JJ, Sturm A, Cowen J, et al. Double-blind, sham-controlled, pilot study of trigeminal nerve stimulation for attention-deficit/hyperactivity disorder. *Journal of the American Academy of Child & Adolescent Psychiatry* 2019;58:403–411.

Sarver DE, McCart MR, Sheidow AJ, Letourneau EJ. ADHD and risky sexual behavior in adolescents: conduct problems and substance use as mediators of risk. *J Child Psychol Psychiatry* 2014;55(12):1345–1353.

Searight HR, Evans SL, Gafford J. Attention deficit hyperactivity disorder. In: Smith A, Shimp L, Schrager S, eds. *Family Medicine: Ambulatory Care and Prevention*. 5th ed. New York, NY: Appleton and Lange; 2014.

Sibley MH, Rohde LA, Swanson JM, et al. Late-onset ADHD reconsidered with comprehensive repeated assessments between ages 10 and 25. *Am J Psychiatry* 2017;175(2):140–149.

Solanto MV, Marks DJ, Wasserstein J, et al. Efficacy of meta-cognitive therapy for adult ADHD. *Am J Psychiatry* 2010;167:958–968.

Spencer TJ, Adler LA, Qiao M, et al. Validation of the adult ADHD investigator symptom rating scale (AISRS). *J Atten Disord* 2010;14:57–68.

Sprich SE, Safren SA, Finkelstein D, Remmert JE, Hammerness P. A randomized controlled trial of cognitive behavioral therapy for ADHD in medication-treated adolescents. *J Child Psychol Psychiatry* 2016;57(11):1218–1226.

Tervo T, Michelsson K, Launes J, Hokkanen L. A prospective 30-year follow-up of ADHD associated with perinatal risks. *J Atten Disord* 2017;21(10):799–810.

Thibault RT, Raz A. The psychology of neurofeedback: clinical intervention even if applied placebo. *Am Psychol* 2017;72(7):679.

Somatic Symptom & Related Disorders

29

Y. Pritham Raj, MD

INTRODUCTION

CASE ILLUSTRATION 1

Ms. A, a 57-year-old woman, makes an appointment with a new clinician. She presents with a 10-year history of multiple, unexplained symptoms. She has seen many physicians over the past decade, including several primary care physicians and numerous subspecialists. Her principal complaints today include abdominal pain, chest pain, headache, palpitations, fatigue, and intermittent dizziness. She brings a thick stack of records from some of her prior physicians. These records include multiple laboratory tests and diagnostic procedures, none of which has identified any cause for her symptoms.

Clinician: How can I help you today, Ms. A?

Patient (sighing): I don't know. A friend of mine saw you a few months ago and said you were very good. I hope you can help me. I've had these problems for years now, and no one seems to be able to figure them out. Maybe you can. I know there's something wrong. I've been so sick.

Clinician: Why don't you tell me about your symptoms?

Patient: Well, it all began about 10 years ago. . . .

Clinicians are taught that patients will present with symptoms (subjective complaints) and signs (objective findings) that suggest the presence of a pathophysiological process. They are trained to recognize these presentations and to diagnose the underlying disease so that they may institute the appropriate treatment. Satisfaction for the care provider arises from the ability to perform these tasks proficiently and ameliorate suffering. Patients typically come to the clinician's office seeking an explanation for and relief from their symptoms. Difficulties arise in the relationship when the patient presents with symptoms and the clinician can find no disease to explain them. Complications can also arise when clinicians focus too much on somatic symptoms and not the underlying etiology of the symptoms, which in many cases can be psychological rather than physical. Symptoms that lack discernible physical pathology, which can be seen in up to 40% of primary care patients, have been referred to variously as medically unexplained, functional, or related to "somatization." The term somatization has had changing definitions over the years, and is now best defined under the umbrella of the somatic symptom and related disorders.

The term *somatic symptom disorder* (SSD) as defined in the Diagnostic and Statistical Manual of Mental Disorders, Fifth Edition (DSM-5), is broadly characterized by somatic (physical) symptoms that are either very distressing or result in significant disruption of functioning, as well as excessive and disproportionate thoughts, feelings, and behaviors regarding those symptoms. Many patients who experience and report physical symptoms that cause distress but lack a corresponding level of tissue damage or pathology meet criteria for SSD. The previous *DSM-IV* diagnostic labels including somatization disorder, hypochondriasis, pain disorder and undifferentiated somatoform disorder have been removed, partly due to their pejorative connotations. Collectively, the somatic symptom and related disorders have replaced the somatoform disorders of the *DSM-IV.* Regardless of the terminology, it is much more common, especially in primary care, to encounter patients who have somatic symptoms but do not meet the full criteria for a psychiatric diagnosis.

In many individuals, prominent somatic symptoms might be a transient phenomenon during a particularly stressful period such as divorce proceedings, consisting of an exaggeration of common physical symptoms such as headache. In other patients, the process may be more persistent, and the symptoms may be disabling. In yet others, somatic symptoms may be a more culturally appropriate expression of other psychiatric disorders like depression or generalized anxiety. For example, in many Asian countries it is rare for patients with depressive disorders to directly report symptoms of low or depressed mood. However, subjective symptoms of vague abdominal pain or headache may much more commonly suggest underlying depression and must be approached with a broad differential diagnosis (see Chapter 26).

Patients with chronic somatic symptoms can be particularly difficult for clinicians. Although their symptoms may suggest an underlying medical or neurologic condition, no such etiology is discovered upon appropriate diagnostic evaluation. Some patients do find reassurance in the provider's statements that no medical cause for their symptoms has been found. Other patients may become upset and accuse the clinician of not believing them or of being incompetent. Some patients, especially those concerned that their symptoms are not being taken seriously, will even invent symptoms or exaggerate the severity of those already present. In a 2018 survey of patients, 47% admitted that they often or sometimes lie to their doctors, and another 30% said they also lied, but only rarely. When patients lie about their symptoms for no apparent benefit, this is most consistent with factitious disorder (Table 29-1). But if they lie for some form of financial or material gain, this is considered "malingering" (now a V code rather than a formal diagnosis in the DSM-5). Some patients insist on continued diagnostic testing or referral to specialists. The symptoms often fail to respond to standard medical treatments; this therapeutic failure can lead to requests for more testing, referrals, or different treatment regimens. The combination of increasing demands made by patients and their lack of response to treatment can be very frustrating for clinicians and patients alike.

HISTORICAL CONCEPTS

The existence of medically unexplained symptoms has been recognized throughout the history of medicine. Before the Renaissance, medical theories were based on limited understanding of anatomy or physiology and, as a result, seem quite primitive to modern practitioners. Diseases lacking an apparent cause were believed to result from gross disturbances in the function and behavior of bodily organs. For example, hysteria, an earlier conceptualization of somatization and somatic symptom disorder, was attributed to a "wandering uterus" as early as 1900 BCE. The treatments for hysteria flowed from

Table 29-1. Somatic symptom and related disorders.

Disorder	Definition
Somatic symptom disorder	• Distressing somatic symptoms that result in significant disruption of daily life • Abnormal thoughts, feelings, or behaviors related to the somatic symptoms
Illness anxiety disorder (formerly hypochondriasis)	• Preoccupation with having or acquiring a serious illness • High level of anxiety about health disproportional to the real threat to health • Excessive health-related behaviors or maladaptive avoidance
Conversion disorder (also known as functional neurologic symptom disorder)	• Altered voluntary motor or sensory function • Symptoms are not due to a recognized neurologic or medical condition
Psychological factors affecting other medical conditions	• Psychological or behavioral factors adversely influence the course, treatment, or underlying pathophysiology of an existing medical condition
Factitious disorder	• Falsification of physical or physiological signs or symptoms (or induction of injury or disease) • There is no obvious external reward for the deception
Other specified somatic symptom and related disorder	• Diagnosis is used when full criteria for one of the abovementioned disorders is not met • Reason for not meeting full criteria is added as a specifier • Pseudocyesis (false in belief in being pregnant with signs/symptoms of pregnancy) is one specifier for this diagnosis
Unspecified somatic symptom and related disorder	• Diagnosis is used when full criteria for one of the abovementioned disorders is not met *and* the reason for not meeting the diagnosis is not specified

The abovementioned disorders (1) cause clinically significant distress or impairment in social or occupational functioning and (2) are not due to other general medical or psychiatric conditions.
Reprinted with permission from Reed M, et al. Somatic Symptom and Related Disorders. In: McCarron, RM, eds. *Primary Care Psychiatry*, 2nd ed. Philadelphia, PA: Wolters Kluwer; 2018.

this conceptual model and included the application of ointments to the labia or manipulation of the uterus to return it to its "natural" position. It was not until after the Renaissance that medical practitioners began to implicate disturbances of the nervous system in the genesis of medically unexplained symptoms.

By the end of the seventeenth century, and continuing into the eighteenth century, clinicians increasingly recognized the role psychological factors played in the origin and maintenance of somatic symptoms. Medical authorities no longer focused exclusively on somatic therapies in the care of afflicted individuals. Instead, practitioners were encouraged to inquire about and demonstrate an active interest in their patients' mental state and welfare. Further, clinicians recognized the need to attempt to promote optimism about recovery in their patients.

In the nineteenth century, there was awareness that despite many advances in the understanding of pathology, patients suffering from somatization syndromes lacked discernible anatomic abnormalities. As a result, the medically unexplained disorders were attributed to a subtle or "functional" pathological disturbance. This explanatory model of illness was associated with a return to predominantly somatic interventions for treating the symptoms. However, some practitioners maintained that psychological treatments were important for managing these patients. These clinicians also recognized that unless the therapy was delivered in a way that was consistent with the patients' belief that their illness had a physical etiology, the intervention would be rejected. Paul Briquet, in his seminal *Treatise on Hysteria* (1859) described the in-depth study of over 400 patients with "hysteria" during a 10-year period and emphasized that the treatment of such patients should address social and environmental problems.

At the turn of the twentieth century, an exclusively psychological model for these disorders was developed. The idea of a functional pathological lesion of the nervous system was replaced with the concept of psychogenesis (i.e., the somatization symptoms arose from the mind). Somatization was viewed as the means by which unconscious mental conflicts could be manifested in the form of physical symptoms. As a result, mental health practitioners became responsible for the diagnosis and treatment of these disorders. However, the idea of physical complaints originating from the mind was also associated with implications that the symptoms were not "real." Further, many patients were not convinced of the value of this interpretation of illness.

Medically unexplained syndromes have persisted as clinical problems for practitioners. Patients often present with many symptoms that are not associated with abnormalities demonstrable by physical examination or laboratory or radiological studies. The symptoms are often clustered together as syndromes with a variety of proposed etiologies, including environmental exposures, infections (e.g., chronic Lyme (*Borrelia burgdorferi*) disease, *Candida*, Epstein–Barr virus), or multiple chemical sensitivity. In addition, the broad range of advocacy and educational groups that try to promote various agendas with regard to the disorders can make the evaluation of these syndromes difficult.

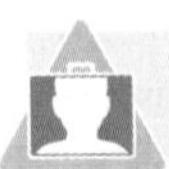

CASE ILLUSTRATION 2

Mr. B is a 32-year-old man presented to his primary care physician with complaints about being tired, weak, and nauseated. He also complained about intermittent abdominal and chest pain as well as a feeling of "dizziness." He noted that he lived in an old building and was worried he had been exposed to lead or some other toxin. His physical examination and laboratory values were all normal. However, he was not relieved by these results and his complaints persisted. He began to phone frequently with questions about chronic Candida infections, postviral syndromes, and multiple chemical sensitivity syndromes. His physician would discuss each process with him and continued to perform appropriate medical evaluations of Mr. B's symptoms. The patient began to research his symptoms on the Internet. He was convinced that he suffered from sensitivity to multiple compounds in his home and became involved in a number of online support groups. He resisted other explanations for his symptoms and gradually became dissatisfied with his primary care physician and chose to seek care from "experts" on his disorder.

ETIOLOGY

Somatic symptom and related disorders can be understood from a number of different perspectives, each of which proposes a cause for the symptoms. However, because the precise cause of these symptoms is not known, none of the following theories are fully explanatory. Rather, each view provides practitioners with insight into the genesis of somatic symptoms and suggests possible treatments as well. Unfortunately, each model is able to explain the symptoms of only a select group of patients. A more comprehensive understanding of patients comes from incorporating more than one perspective.

Neurobiological

According to the neurobiological perspective, SSD (previously somatization disorder) is the result of dysfunction in the neuroendocrine systems responsible for processing peripheral sensory and central emotional information. As a result, the affected individual misinterprets normal bodily sensations or emotional signals as indicating a dangerous somatic process. For example, researchers have suggested that hypocortisolism plays a role in posttraumatic stress disorder, fibromyalgia, chronic fatigue syndrome, and some chronic pain disorders. Although hypocortisolism has been found in groups of individuals with the above diagnoses, the relationship between a deficiency of cortisol and the production of these symptoms is not well understood. Additional research has examined the inability of individuals with somatic symptoms to habituate to novel stimuli. Individuals with somatic symptom and related disorders reported higher levels of tension in novel situations and were less likely to habituate to the situation over time. In addition, the affected individuals had a slower return to baseline heart rate upon leaving stressful situations. These studies suggest a relationship between physiologic mechanisms involved in adapting to novel or stressful stimuli and the apparently psychological symptoms of individuals with somatic symptom disorders.

Psychodynamic

According to psychodynamic theory, somatic symptoms arise solely from the mind. They are believed to represent the outward expression of underlying, internal psychological conflicts. Studies have demonstrated that individuals with somatic symptom and related disorders have higher rates of prior emotional and physical abuse, depression, and anxiety than nonaffected populations. It is hypothesized that abuse places individuals at risk for the types of internal conflicts that result in somatic symptom disorders. For example, women who have suffered sexual abuse in childhood have increased rates of chronic pelvic pain when compared with those without a history of abuse. Depression and anxiety may be both a product and cause of these internal conflicts. Patients with somatic symptom disorders may be less able to correctly interpret emotional arousal and instead identify these signals as physical symptoms. This is further supported by studies that demonstrate a link between alexithymia, or the inability to identify and verbally describe emotions and feelings in oneself or others, and somatic symptom disorders. Other findings suggest that childhood trauma in women is associated with higher levels of somatic symptom disorders, mediated by the development of insecure attachment. Attachment theory predicts how individuals' interactions in interpersonal relationships are influenced by early experiences with caregivers. A four-category model has been proposed, which describes four different types of attachment: *secure*, *preoccupied*, *dismissive*, and *fearful*. In particular, research examining the role of attachment style and its link to somatic symptom disorder and subsequent health care utilization has found that patients with *preoccupied* attachment (where the individual tends to idealize others, is less self-reliant and needs more reassurance) and *fearful* attachment (where the individual may be less trusting of others as well as less self-reliant) are more likely to be high in somatic symptom reporting and are higher users of medical resources.

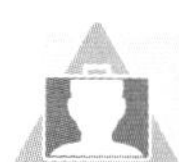

CASE ILLUSTRATION 3

Mrs. G is a 51-year-old woman who had suffered from abdominal pain and progressive loss of function over the last 1 ½ years. She had failed conservative management and was admitted to the hospital for an exploratory laparotomy. However, there were no organic findings to explain her symptoms. Psychiatric consultation was requested to evaluate for a psychological component to her pain. At evaluation, Mrs. G denied any psychological stressors, but her husband shared that around the time of the onset of her symptoms, Mrs. G's mother, with whom she is very close, had moved out of state to care for another daughter who had become ill. Mrs. G was referred for psychotherapy to explore this perceived loss and to explore alternatives for support. Over the course of this treatment, Mrs. G's abdominal pain resolved.

Cognitive Behavioral

According to cognitive behavioral theorists, symptoms of somatic symptom disorders arise from incorrect beliefs about bodily sensations, for example, the belief that mild gastroesophageal reflux (or panic symptoms) represents myocardial ischemia. These misinterpretations, in turn, result in certain maladaptive behaviors, such as going from one emergency room to another seeking evaluation of the symptom and reassurance that the heart is functioning normally. These symptoms are reinforced by factors in the individual's environment such as the responses of other people to the perceived illness. For instance, the affected individual may be excused from work or social obligations. As an example of this process, some researchers proposed that learning about a disease may lead certain individuals to attribute previously overlooked symptoms to the illness. The affected person seeks out confirmatory evidence of additional symptoms that both reinforce the belief in the illness and amplify the somatic symptoms. The person's self-validating review of symptoms may be augmented by contact with advocacy or educational groups that promote awareness of the disease. The processing of bodily information gradually becomes colored by the belief that the person has a disease, and this can result in the affected individual embracing the sick role.

CASE ILLUSTRATION 4

Mr. C is a 53-year-old man who worked as a manual laborer. He had always been in good health. One day, while lifting a particularly heavy item, he experienced pain on the right side of his chest. A colleague said that his father had a similar experience and died of a heart attack shortly thereafter. Mr. C became focused on the idea that he has heart disease, and began visiting a number of emergency rooms, primary care physicians, and cardiologists. His evaluations were always completely negative. However, his concern has persisted and he now presents to a new clinician.

Clinician: How are you doing today Mr. C?

Patient: Doc, I know that I have a problem with my heart.

Clinician: What makes you think it is a problem with your heart?

Patient: Well, I sometimes feel like I am more out of breath, and if I lift heavy things I can feel some pain in the muscle over my chest. Other times, I start to breathe fast and my fingers get tingly. I've watched programs on TV, and they say those are the things that can mean I have angina. I've stopped working because I don't want to stress myself out and have a heart attack.

Sociocultural

According to the sociocultural perspective, individuals learn to express disease and distress in culturally sanctioned ways. In any culture, the expression of certain bodily symptoms and illness behaviors are encouraged whereas others are discouraged. Although somatic complaints are a universal process, an individual's culture can affect the manner in which somatic representations of emotional distress are utilized. Further, this theory maintains that because the patient and the clinician are often from different backgrounds, the cultural interaction between clinician and patient is important. This interaction often determines how the patient's symptoms are experienced, interpreted, and reported. The clinician's task in these meetings is to correctly recognize which of the patient's somatic complaints represent cultural idioms of emotional distress. Failure to correctly assess somatic symptoms can lead to misdiagnosis, unnecessary medical treatment, frustration on the part of the provider when the patient does not respond as expected, and patient dissatisfaction.

A DIFFERENT PARADIGM

Although the theoretical models discussed above have evidence to support them and have been used as the basis for treatment in cases of somatic symptom disorders, there is another way to conceptualize the somatic symptom and related disorders. This view begins with the clinician abandoning the either–or categories of "physical" and "psychological." This dichotomous framework leads to interactions in which patients feel that they and their symptoms are being discounted by the clinician and conclude, "The doctor's saying it's all in my head." Instead, the new paradigm adopts a more comprehensive view of disease based on the *biopsychosocial* model of illness that includes key elements from other explanatory models. In this paradigm, all illnesses are understood to have biological, psychological, and sociocultural dimensions.

Although the western medical model focuses on the biological aspects of disease, it often ignores the psychological and sociocultural facets of the patient's experience. In addition, this model, often very effective for understanding and treating acute disease processes, may fail to explain much of the complexity of chronic illness. For example, pain researchers have found that psychological factors are more important than physical factors in predicting future disability. Such research has led to the development of new treatment paradigms that recognize the interplay between the biological disease process and the psychosocial impact of symptoms. Treatment is focused on both relieving the biomedical symptoms and modifying the thoughts, feelings, and behaviors associated with the pain and disability.

Using the biopsychosocial model, illness can be understood as occurring along a spectrum with disorders characterized by predominantly somatic problems at one end and disorders with predominantly psychological or social manifestations at the other (see Chapter 36). Therefore, evaluation of patients should routinely include inquiries into both the physical and psychosocial dimensions of their illness. With this biopsychosocial framework, the somatic symptom disorders stem from patients' neglect of the psychosocial components of their illness in favor of a somatic perspective. For example, an individual with a history of chronic pelvic pain who has undergone multiple thorough evaluations with no identified anatomic etiology but who insists on repeating the workup rather than discussing psychosocial facets of the symptoms may be experiencing somatic symptom disorder or illness anxiety disorder. According to this model, symptom amplification, a phenomenon seen commonly in somatic symptom and related disorders, may arise when the experience of these symptoms is modified by psychosocial factors. This is illustrated in Figure 29-1, where these factors are represented by a psychosocial lens, which alters the "image" of the stimulus (somatic symptoms), resulting in a magnified image (effect), or

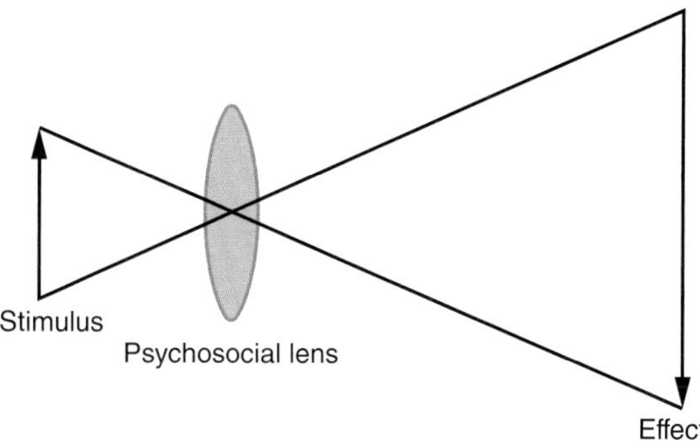

Figure 29-1. Symptom amplification.

increased experience of these symptoms. The spectrum of the somatic symptom and related disorders are not a single entity. Like most illnesses they can be understood to have a continuum of expression. At one end is the transient, stress-related exaggeration of common physical symptoms and at the other are the serious, persistent complaints that leave the patient disabled.

> **Patient:** I don't know. Maybe I am crazy . . . that's what everyone else seems to think.
>
> **Clinician:** Let me assure you that you're not crazy. I hear your concern. Why don't we talk about this a little bit?
>
> **Patient:** Well, a friend of mine had a disease called Cushing's. Do you think I might have that?
>
> **Clinician:** That's a good question. There are a great many diseases that can present with symptoms like yours. I want you to know that as I've listened to you and examined you, I've tried to think of rare diseases, not just the more common. I don't believe any of them are very likely, especially since you've had your symptoms for so long. I do want to be honest with you, though. There's no way to be absolutely certain. There are so many different diseases that it would be impossible to get tested for all of them. Let's get a few higher-yield laboratory tests done, though. If they're normal, let's not do any more tests, but I'll keep an open mind regarding all possibilities as we get to know each other during the course of the next few months. If you develop symptoms later that suggest one of these rare diseases to me, I'll certainly order more tests. How does that sound to you?
>
> **Patient:** Okay, that sounds like it could work.
>
> **Clinician:** Are there other things going on that add stress to your life?
>
> **Patient:** Now that you mention it, there are some stressful things going on...

In this brief dialogue, the practitioner acknowledges uncertainty while communicating a sense of honesty and trustworthiness. By reinforcing the continuity of the relationship and the willingness to entertain different possibilities in the future, the provider helps the patient feel cared for without the need for multiple, and most likely unnecessary, diagnostic tests. Moreover, the clinician has helped the patient to entertain the idea of a connection between psychosocial and somatic factors in illness.

PREVALENCE

The somatic symptom disorder spectrum is frequently encountered in primary care clinics with estimates of prevalence between 25% and 75%. Other studies have found that somatic symptom disorders can be diagnosed in up to 22% of patients in primary care outpatient clinics. One study found an absence of organic cause in 80% of primary care visits scheduled for the evaluation of common symptoms such as dizziness, chest pain, and fatigue. Research has also shown that 50–80% of patients who have an anxiety or depressive disorder initially present to health care providers with physical symptoms. Another study found that somatic symptom disorders were the most common psychiatric diagnoses in a population of medical inpatients.

Worldwide, medically unexplained symptoms are more common in females and individuals of lower socioeconomic status. In the United States, there is higher prevalence among Latinos. While rates of somatic symptom disorder are relatively low (0.1% in the United States, 0.8% in Germany), these numbers increase as the inclusion criteria for somatic symptom disorders are broadened, ranging from 22% to 80% in some European countries. Although studies have demonstrated there is no systematic pattern of cultures which are more or less likely to have somatic symptom disorders, it appears that patients who lack an ongoing relationship with a stable provider are more likely to have a greater number of somatic symptoms. In other words, the "culture" of the clinician–patient encounter also has significant impact on the presence of somatic symptom disorder. Overall these results indicate that the phenomenon of somatization, as well as more rigorously defined somatic symptom and related disorders, is very common among patients presenting for medical services.

IMPACT & OUTCOMES

Somatic symptom disorders are not only common, but also expensive. One study estimated that patients with somatic symptom disorders generate medical costs nine times those of the average medical patient. Other work has calculated total annual health care costs attributable to somatic symptom and related disorders in the United States to be over $250 billion, even after adjusting for comorbid psychiatric disorders. In addition, these patients often require a great deal of time and attention but frequently do not respond to the prescribed treatment. This can eventually lead to frustration for the practitioner and even feelings of incompetence or inadequacy. A patient's seemingly unending complaints can lead to feelings of anger at the individual or dread when the patient's name appears on the appointment list. Thus, patients with somatic symptom disorders not only tax the health care system by disproportionately utilizing limited resources, but also burden health care providers who can feel overwhelmed by the needs of these individuals.

Research has consistently demonstrated that individuals with somatic symptom disorders have worse health outcomes, physical functioning, and psychological well-being than those patients who do not manifest these symptoms. Patients with somatic symptom disorders have ongoing difficulties not only with their somatic complaints and concerns about physical illness, but also with emotional and social impairment and reduced quality of life. It is important to accurately diagnose these individuals so that appropriate management can be instituted.

DIFFERENTIAL DIAGNOSIS

Patients with somatic symptoms should be evaluated for a biomedical etiology that could explain the presenting complaints. The nature of the evaluation will depend on the patient's medical history, presenting symptoms, and age. In evaluating patients, it is important to remember that the onset of multiple physical symptoms late in life is almost always due to a general medical condition; somatic symptom disorders generally start decades earlier.

The somatic symptom and related disorders classification is based on the common feature of prominent somatic symptoms and related significant distress and functional impairment. In addition, the somatic complaints in these disorders are produced unconsciously and are not under the voluntary control of the patient (see Table 29-1). A number of functional syndromes have also been identified, such as irritable bowel syndrome, fibromyalgia, chronic fatigue syndrome, and noncardiac chest pain. These disorders may fall under the "other specified somatic symptom and related disorder" diagnosis.

Criticism of the taxonomy and nomenclature of what were previously called the somatoform disorders suggested that the various disorders in this category were quite disparate, had limited validity, and the diagnoses did little to inform an effective treatment approach. As noted earlier, the term "somatoform" was felt to be pejorative; the absence of a clear medical etiology did not rightly categorize the cause as psychological. This "either/or" approach also set up an unintended mind–body dualism. Ultimately patients were made to feel their symptoms were not "real" and overlooked their very real experience of physical symptoms. For this reason, attempts were made to revise the criteria for these disorders in the *DSM*-5. A further problem was that a considerable number of patients who presented for care with medically unexplained symptoms did not meet criteria for the somatoform disorders (10–15% prevalence in primary care).

Several psychiatric disorders have been associated with somatic symptoms and should be considered when evaluating a patient who has physical complaints. For example, anxiety in the form of panic attacks often involves symptoms in multiple organ systems, such as palpitations, nausea, shortness of breath, and tingling in the extremities. Unlike symptoms of somatic symptom disorders, however, the symptoms of a panic attack have an abrupt onset and are limited to the episode. A careful history can often elicit this time course and prove to be helpful in making the diagnosis. Patients with generalized anxiety disorder may also present with multiple somatic complaints, such as fatigue and muscle tension. Excessive worrying about multiple domains in life is the key feature of this disorder and helps to separate it from the somatic symptom disorders. Depressed patients often present to medical practitioners with unexplained physical symptoms, especially headache, pain, and gastrointestinal problems. Whereas the somatic symptoms of the somatic symptom and related disorders tend to be chronic, the physical complaints in depression exist only in the presence of the mood symptoms. In such cases, the depression and the somatic complaints resolve contemporaneously. Studies have demonstrated a high level of comorbidity between depression and somatic symptom disorders, so clinically both disorders may be present (see Chapter 26). Patients with obsessive–compulsive disorder whose beliefs focus on bodily functions or organs can appear to be suffering from a somatic symptom disorder. The key to diagnosis is a careful history about the presence of the obsessions and compulsions. Patients with psychotic disorders, such as schizophrenia, may also present with multiple somatic complaints. In contrast to the concerns in the somatic symptom disorders, psychotic symptoms tend to be bizarre or completely irrational (e.g., "My insides are rotting" or "I have pain from the dinosaur eggs in my stomach"). It is important to remember, however, that the patients may have both a diagnosable mental disorder as well as a somatic symptom disorder. Conversely, patients with clear medical conditions may simultaneously qualify for a diagnosis of a somatic symptom and related disorder.

In contrast to the psychiatric disorders described above, there are conditions in which the individual's symptoms are consciously produced. Factitious disorder is included in the category of somatic symptom and related disorders. It is diagnosed when the clinician

Table 29-2. Abnormal illness-affirming states.

	Symptom Production	Motivation
Malingering	conscious	conscious
Factitious disorder	conscious	unconscious
Somatic symptom disorder	unconscious	unconscious
Illness anxiety disorder	unconscious	unconscious
Conversion disorder (functional neurological symptom disorder)	unconscious	unconscious
Other specified somatic symptom and related disorder	unconscious	unconscious
Unspecified somatic symptom and related disorder	unconscious	unconscious

Adapted from Eisendrath SJ, Lichtmacher J. Psychiatric disorders. In: *Current Medical Diagnosis and Treatment* 2007, S. McPhee et al (ed); Appleton and Lange; 2006.

determines that the symptoms are consciously or voluntarily induced or exaggerated. However, in these individuals there is no discernible external incentive, such as financial compensation, to produce the symptoms. The patient's primary goal is to assume the sick role. Malingering, on the other hand, is diagnosed when the clinician determines that the individual has consciously produced the symptoms for clear external gain, such as obtaining a monetary award, acquiring drugs, or avoiding a noxious situation such as military duty or incarceration. Malingering is not considered a mental disorder (Table 29-2).

EVALUATION

Most patients do not meet criteria for a formal diagnosis of a somatic symptom disorder, yet somatic symptoms are quite frequent. As these patients present overwhelmingly to primary care settings (not mental health providers), it is useful for medical clinicians to have a systematic method of elucidating the presence of somatic symptoms without a clear medical basis by first trying to get to the heart of the symptoms while also excluding the presence of organic disease. Providers have a tendency to focus too much on symptom inquiry during diagnostic evaluations with a typical provider-centered line of questioning going as follows:

Clinician: What brought you to the clinic (or hospital) today?

Patient: I have headaches.

Clinician: Where are the headaches? How long do they last? What do you do to relieve them?

The questions posed in this scenario are all reasonable but tend to focus too much on symptomatology. Contrast this with a more patient-centered line of questioning that can allow a provider to more efficiently and accurately get to the heart of a clinical situation.

Clinician: What brought you here today?

Patient: I have headaches.

Clinician: What else?

Patient: Well, I have problems sleeping.

Clinician: Is there something else?*

Patient: I am very worried about my son. He is using drugs.

Ultimately, a stepwise, evidence-based approach is invaluable to the evaluation of patients with suspected somatic symptom disorder spectrum. This framework can help the clinician avoid unnecessary and costly diagnostic procedures or referrals to specialists. In addition, it can spare the patient potential iatrogenic complications from any of the evaluation procedures. As with all of medicine, the first step in evaluating the patient with multiple somatic complaints is a detailed and thorough history of the presenting problem. The clinician should, of course, include review of pertinent medical records in the history-gathering phase of the evaluation. The practitioner should then perform appropriate physical and neurologic examinations. The provider may then consider what tests are indicated to confirm the diagnosis or rule out a predominantly biomedical disease based on the information obtained. The urge to order a wide variety of tests should be resisted. Instead, a rational determination of the patient's needs is more helpful in clarifying the treatment plan. Obtaining an informal consultation from a colleague can be useful in appropriately evaluating these individuals.

Once the provider determines that the patient's physical symptoms are not explained by any underlying pathological abnormalities, the focus can turn to more predominantly psychological disorders. The assessment of psychiatric disorders can be accomplished through the use of a careful clinical interview, a semi-structured interview tool, or by referral to a mental health clinician. The clinical interview can be helpful in establishing the presence of psychiatric illness as well as in communicating to the patient that the clinician is taking an active interest in the individual's life. Instruments such as the self-administered Patient Health Questionnaire (PHQ), which are designed for use in primary care settings, can help the provider diagnose somatic symptom disorders as well as depression, anxiety, eating disorders, and substance use disorder. Such instruments have the advantages of rapid administration and established validity.

*Experts suggest that the phrase "Is there something else?" is preferred over "Is there anything else?"

The PHQ-15 is a subscale of the PHQ that assesses somatic symptoms, and it can be used to monitor symptom severity as well as symptom improvement. Such instruments are useful as many patients decline referral to a mental health specialist as an option, because they fear that their complaints are being dismissed. Above all, when evaluating a patient the clinician should recognize and articulate the interplay between the physical and psychosocial realms.

Clinician: Today I would like to talk about how you are doing.

Patient: Well, my chest has been hurting again and I have been really worn down.

Clinician: (after several pertinent questions about the symptoms) It sounds like this is the same pain you've had before, although I do understand that it's a little worse. I wonder if there is anything else that has changed in your life recently besides the intensity of the pain?

Patient: Nothing . . . really. Well my wife and I are arguing about the mortgage again.

Clinician: Oh, I remember that's been a problem before when you've been having pain.

Patient: Yeah. I just get tired of her nagging and the stress of barely making ends meet.

Clinician: I think it's possible that the stress you've been under may be taking its toll on your body and your sense of well-being.

TREATMENT

The following treatment strategies are not specific to a certain somatic symptom disorder diagnosis. In most cases, it is less important to make a specific psychiatric diagnosis of a somatic symptom disorder than it is to recognize that the patient's symptoms represent the spectrum in general. However, if a psychiatric disorder such as anxiety, depression, or psychosis is present, specific treatments for the identified disorder should be utilized.

Treatments Designed for Primary Care Providers

A management plan with an emphasis on nonsomatic interventions is useful for treating somatic symptom disorders. Patients with somatic symptoms most often present to the primary care setting and are resistant to psychiatric referrals. Techniques are required that are effective, acceptable to primary care clinicians, and useful in busy primary care settings. Finally, the intervention must be congruent with patients' beliefs about the nature of their illness so that they are willing to engage in the treatment.

The most important aspect of managing patients with somatic symptom disorders is the development of a stable, empathic, trusting relationship. Although it is not easy to form such a relationship with these individuals, establishing a therapeutic alliance is critical to both diagnosis and treatment. It can be helpful to remember that patients with somatic symptom disorders are reacting in the best and, without treatment, only way available to them. Before considering specific therapies for these individuals, it is useful to consider basic techniques for interacting with them.

The practitioner should never challenge the reality of the patient's physical symptoms. Somatic symptom disorder is an unconscious process, and therefore the somatic complaints are very real to the patient. Further, because most of the symptoms are subjective in nature, there is no means to verify or dispute them. It can be helpful to explicitly acknowledge and validate the patient's suffering to bolster the therapeutic relationship.

Clinician: I can see how much you've suffered with all of these symptoms.

Patient: You're the only one who seems to understand that.

Medical providers should avoid trying to convince the patient that the symptoms are psychological in origin. They should also avoid the use of psychological labels (e.g., depression, anxiety). Instead, they should try to use easily understandable and mutually acceptable language to discuss symptoms without focusing too much on them. Each appointment should begin with a discussion of the somatic complaint. The provider can then use descriptive physiologic explanations, which are more acceptable to these individuals, to describe the symptoms (e.g., "abnormally tense muscles in your neck go into painful spasm"). It is important to note that although such descriptors imply a physiologic component to the symptoms, they do not provide an etiology. Over time (often months or years), the patient and clinician may begin to explore possible explanations for the symptoms that integrate somatic and psychosocial aspects of the problem.

Patient: I just don't get why my neck keeps getting spasms.

Clinician: I have noticed that sometimes you mention this happening after your supervisor criticizes you. Sometimes our muscles react to emotions like anger or stress by tightening up. When this becomes extreme, they can spasm.

Patient: You know that makes some sense. When he comes around, I can feel myself grit my teeth and begin to feel stiff.

Another management suggestion is to have the provider evaluate the patient in an appropriate manner to rule out somatic causes of their symptoms. Once a somatic symptom disorder is identified, the clinician continues to schedule the individual for brief appointments at regularly spaced intervals. These visits are time contingent; patients need not have new symptoms to be able to meet regularly with their medical practitioner. These visits allow for an initial brief check-in regarding the somatic symptoms followed by discussions of events in the patient's life and the patient's emotional well-being and relationships. The clinician can adopt a conservative approach toward new treatments or diagnostic workups when the patient presents with new or worsening symptoms. The goal is to focus patients on behaviors that promote well-being and help them discuss the psychosocial aspects of their life and illness. Patients are redirected from pursuing new therapies or evaluations for their symptoms. At the same time, they are shown that the provider is taking an active interest in their problems. Moreover, patients learn that they will receive this care and attention even without new symptoms or exacerbations of existing symptoms. The clinician may also ask patients when they want to return for the next visit. This provides them with a sense of control, and over time many patients will suggest lengthening the interval between appointments.

Establishing appropriate goals is also important when working with patients with somatic symptom disorders. These disorders, like any chronic disease, are often not curable. However, clinicians often hope that another medication will relieve the symptoms or that one more diagnostic procedure will elucidate the cause of the patient's problem. However, these beliefs can lead to disappointment for both patient and clinician. Rather than aiming for complete resolution of the symptoms, it is better to set more realistic goals. For the primary care practitioner, these might include reducing the number of phone calls and visits with new symptoms, the number of requests for medications or referrals to specialists, and the number of emergency room visits. For patients, these goals might include an increased sense of control in their lives, improved social functioning, better coping with day-to-day symptoms, and overall enhanced functioning.

Clinician: Today I would like to talk about what we should expect from each other in this relationship. From your perspective, I suspect that the best thing I could do would be to figure out what's causing these symptoms and make them go away completely. Given all of your years of suffering and the many doctors you've seen and the limited success of treatments so far, it might be more realistic for us not to focus so much on pursuing a cure but to look at how to improve how you feel and maximize your functioning. What do you think?

Patient: Well, of course I was hoping that you could find a cure. So—does this mean that you can't help me?

Clinician: No, I didn't mean to imply that. I do think I can help. First, I'd like to work on helping you learn to cope more effectively with your symptoms. We could also work to improve how you function from day to day. Whether or not we are immediately successful, I'm committed to helping you in the best way I can.

A novel treatment for somatic symptom disorders involves the use of a "written self-disclosure protocol." This therapy involves having the patient periodically write in a journal format. The clinician invites the patient to spend 20 minutes one time per week at home writing about distressing experiences in his/her life. The patients do the writing outside of the office visit. They are specifically encouraged to think about experiences involving relationships with others. The patients are also instructed to write about how these experiences have affected them in the past and how they may continue to affect them in the future. The journal may be shared with others if the patient wishes, but it does not have to be shared to have a benefit. This technique has been found to be acceptable by both patients and providers. It has also been found to be helpful, as well as time- and cost-effective. Studies of this management strategy have demonstrated decreases in health care utilization.

Another method for treating patients with somatic symptom disorders in the primary care setting is for practitioners to teach patients to reattribute and relate physical symptoms to psychosocial problems. The clinician is encouraged to take a history of the patient's illness, including related physical, mood, and social factors. The clinician then broadens the view of the problem and the necessary treatment by reframing the complaint using the biopsychosocial information provided by the patient (see Chapter 36). The practitioner then links the patient's distress and the physical complaint using a coherent explanation of how psychosocial factors can give rise to and contribute to physical symptoms. This intervention model has been found to be both clinically and cost-effective.

Despite all of these interventions, it may be necessary to refer the patient to a mental health specialist. Many individuals with somatic symptom disorders will resist such a referral. Although this reluctance on the patient's part can be frustrating, the primary care provider should remember that many of these patients have experienced such a referral as the first step in the termination of the relationship with a health care provider. The primary care provider can address this concern by making a follow-up appointment with the patient prior to the referral. Once the continuity of the relationship is ensured, the referral can be discussed. Further, a consultation model in which the patient is asked to see the mental health provider for one or a few visits to "advise and help the primary care provider do a better job" is often more acceptable to patients than a referral for ongoing treatment. The consultation can be useful in confirming a diagnosis or in providing advice on the use of psychotropic medications.

Clinician: I'd like to see you in a month. In the meantime, I'd like you to consider seeing Dr. R, the psychiatrist we've talked about. I know that you don't think that your chest pain is caused by your depression. But we've both agreed to try to treat the depression. I still don't know if we've found the right antidepressant, and I'd really value Dr. R's opinion. What do you think?

Psychotherapy

Cognitive behavioral therapy (CBT) has been studied as a means of addressing medically unexplained somatic symptoms. This treatment is based on the theory that incorrect beliefs about bodily functioning underlie these symptoms or produce much of the dysfunction. The first task in therapy is to identify these beliefs and behaviors. Next, the patient is encouraged to challenge the beliefs and is taught to formulate more accurate ideas about bodily functioning. This change is paired with adoption of more appropriate behaviors. An analysis of randomized trials of specific treatments for patients with somatic symptom disorders indicated that CBT had the strongest and most consistent evidence of effectiveness. A subsequent review of intervention studies in patients with somatic symptom disorders, functional somatic symptoms, somatization, or medically unexplained symptoms corroborated this finding. Furthermore, a growing body of evidence supports the benefit of mindfulness-based cognitive therapy in treating associated stress, depression, and anxiety in patients with multiple somatic complaints, as well as in patients with medically unexplained symptoms. Although early results of these studies are promising, there is a need for larger, controlled trials. Overall, this research suggests that CBT approaches are effective in patients with somatic symptom and other related disorders.

Psychodynamic psychotherapy is based on the assumption that the individual is experiencing internal emotional conflicts and that the associated emotions cannot be identified or expressed. As a result, the conflict is manifested through somatic symptoms. The therapy focuses on attempting to uncover and resolve these conflicts by having the patient identify associated emotions and express them openly in the therapy sessions. As the patient does this work, the somatic symptoms become unnecessary and remit. A meta-analysis of short-term therapy for somatic symptom disorders found benefits for subjects in multiple areas, including physical symptom reduction, improvement in social and occupational functioning and psychological symptoms, and decrease in health care utilization. Unfortunately, many patients with somatic symptom disorders may not be enthusiastic about exploring unconscious conflicts. In general, psychodynamic psychotherapy is a longer-term, time-intensive approach that requires a referral to a specialist and a significant commitment from the patient.

In *family-oriented approaches to therapy*, therapists must integrate the biological and psychosocial aspects of the patient's illness. The care provider must collaborate with the patient and the patient's family in treating the illness. Further, the clinician must demonstrate true interest in and curiosity about the patient's symptoms, family, relationships, and life. These therapies attempt to help patients and their families break down the distinction between physical and psychological and move their thinking from "either–or" (e.g., it is either a physical problem or a mental problem) to "both–and" (e.g., the problem has both physical and mental facets). Relational therapists argue that effective therapy involves validating the illness, involving the family, working closely with the health care team, and enhancing the patient's curiosity about symptoms. They also emphasize demonstrating interest in the patient's somatic symptoms, helping the patient to see the relationship between the somatic symptoms and psychosocial stressors, and using physical interventions (e.g., biofeedback and relaxation techniques) to form an alliance with the patient to deal with the illness.

Medication

Data on the efficacy of using medications to treat somatic symptom disorders is limited; to date there are few randomized, controlled studies. However, there have been several small, open studies demonstrating the effectiveness of selective serotonin reuptake inhibitors (SSRIs) such as fluoxetine, sertraline, and escitalopram; serotonin norepinephrine reuptake inhibitors (SNRIs) such as venlafaxine; and other antidepressants classified separately (mirtazapine) in reducing somatic complaints, depressive symptoms, and improving overall assessment of health. There is also evidence that St. John's wort is effective in treating somatic symptom disorders, with reduction in somatic symptoms and improvement in patients' self-assessments of health. However, information on the long-term effectiveness of such treatments is yet to be elucidated. Moreover, investigations into the benefits of treatment of comorbid anxiety and depression have yielded mixed results depending on the specific somatic condition, with less success in patients with chronic pain and fibromyalgia.

A summary of recommendations for managing patients with somatic symptoms is found in Table 29-3.

CLINICIAN–PATIENT RELATIONSHIP

Caring for individuals with somatic symptom disorders is difficult. Patients present with symptoms suggestive of a medical or neurologic illness and require an appropriate evaluation. However, at the completion of the evaluation the clinician is faced with an individual who, by definition, does not have a physical condition

Table 29-3. Management of somatic symptom disorder.

Interventions
1. Take a detailed history, perform a physical examination, and order appropriate diagnostic studies.
2. Screen individuals with multiple somatic complaints for psychiatric disorders.
3. Integrate the patient's physical and psychosocial concerns by inquiring not only about somatic symptoms but also about other events in the person's life.
4. Develop an empathic relationship.
5. Never challenge the validity of the patient's somatic symptoms.
6. Do not utilize psychological labels for the patient's symptoms.
7. Schedule the patient for appointments at regular intervals.
8. Establish realistic expectations.
9. Care for yourself.

Adapted from Eisendrath SJ, Lichtmacher J. Psychiatric disorders. In *Current Medical Diagnosis and Treatment* 2007, S. McPhee et al (ed); Appleton and Lange, 2006.

or who has a condition that cannot account for the level of symptoms or disability experienced. In contrast, the patient views the symptoms as somatic and strenuously resists the idea that the symptoms have a psychological component. As a result, neither party is satisfied with the interaction.

Why is dealing with patients who experience somatic symptom disorders so difficult? One theory is that clinicians use terminology that was developed to promote communication with other health care providers or used for billing purposes. It is not meant to provide patients with an explanation of or validation of their illness experience. Health providers focus on understanding the pathophysiology of disease in a scientific manner. Laypersons have different explanatory models of disease, and therefore when they present to the clinician's office they may already have a theory about the origin of their symptoms. In the case of patients with somatic symptom and related disorders, this theory involves a physical cause. In contrast, the practitioner may feel that a physical cause for the symptoms is less likely than a psychological etiology. As a result, the patient and clinician possess models of illness that are not only competing but also conflicting. To work effectively with the patient, the provider must reconcile these theories.

Patient: So you think I have "depression"? How is that causing me to be tired all the time? I don't understand how you can say that. I don't cry and I don't feel sad.

Clinician: Depression is not just feeling sad. It is a medical illness, just like diabetes or heart disease. It is caused by inefficiencies in how the brain uses chemicals called neurotransmitters that help brain cells communicate with each other. When those neurotransmitters, such as serotonin, norepinephrine, and dopamine, are used inefficiently the brain does not function optimally, and people develop symptoms such as fatigue, sadness, changes in sleep and appetite, and changes in their ability to concentrate.

Patient: Well what can be done?

Clinician: The good news is there are a number of treatments. Medications can be very helpful by directly affecting how efficiently the brain uses the transmitters it produces. Other treatments involve working with someone to help you train your brain to function better without medications.

Working with these patients is difficult because they do not share the clinician's explanatory models and may resist giving up their own ideas about their illness. When providers are able to explain the patient's symptoms in a way that provides a holistic and empowering perspective, they are viewed as a positive and helpful influence. As a result, the patient is satisfied, an alliance is formed to address the symptoms in a collaborative manner, and the practitioner may feel more positive about the patient.

Research has also focused on the reasons clinicians experience certain patients as difficult. Patients who are rated as difficult by health providers have twice the prevalence of psychiatric disorders (see Chapter 4). Further, the presence of more physical symptoms, both those judged to result from medical causes and those judged to be related to a somatic symptom disorder, contributes to the sense that the patient is difficult. In addition, clinicians expect physical symptoms to be associated with medical diagnoses, and the lack of such an association leads to frustration over the "vagueness" of the symptoms and their own inability to make a diagnosis. The practitioner may feel that the patient is consciously faking symptoms. However, patients may have reasons, conscious or unconscious, for holding onto the symptoms. The assumption of the sick role may confer some benefits, through changes in social and family systems that are difficult for the provider to discern or understand. Clinicians should attempt to understand the role that the symptoms play in the patient's family and social systems to gain insight into why the symptoms persist despite the lack of a somatic etiology.

CARING FOR THE CLINICIAN

The care of patients with somatic symptom disorders can be a draining experience, and the clinician must take care to avoid burnout (see Chapters 6, 26, 36, & 49). The patient's seemingly unending physical concerns, resistance to recommended treatments, and complaints that the clinician is not doing enough can easily overwhelm the provider. The practitioner needs to remember that these are chronic disorders. As a consequence, it is most helpful to set collaborative, realistic goals for treatment using a "care and not cure" approach. Clinicians must understand that they can provide support and effective treatment but that the patient will likely have some residual symptoms. The practitioner should feel comfortable setting limits with their patients with somatic symptom and related disorders. Once the clinician and patient have committed to short, regular follow-up appointments, it is appropriate to set limits on telephone calls and drop-in visits. For example, the patient can be asked to reserve all but emergency complaints for the regular visits. If the patient calls between scheduled sessions, the discussion should be limited to ascertaining if there is an emergency. If there is none, then the patient can be gently urged to defer further discussion until the next visit. This strategy works best if all practice partners (especially those who take call for the primary provider) maintain a similar stance and avoid attempts to "rescue" the patient by way of lengthy phone conversations, etc.

Outside of work, practitioners should take time for physical activity, family, friends, and other interests to avoid the trappings of a negative physical and psychological "energy account." Practitioners may also wish to discuss difficult cases with colleagues to manage the powerful feelings these patients can elicit. In this way, they can maintain a healthy work–life balance. Clinicians must keep in mind that the illness belongs to the patient and not to them. They must not allow the patient's frustration or demands make them forget this key fact. The combination of empathic listening, conservative (but appropriate) evaluation, and gentle limit setting can not only benefit these patients, but also improve the provider's satisfaction with these relationships.

ACKNOWLEDGMENTS

J. Jewel Shim, MD and Stuart J. Eisendrath, MD contributed to this chapter in the fourth edition and some material from that chapter has been retained here.

SUGGESTED READINGS

Abbas A, Kisely S, Kroenke K. Short-term psychodynamic psychotherapy for somatic disorders. *Psychother Psychosom* 2009; 78:265–274.

Allen LA, Woolfolk RL, Escobar JI, et al. Cognitive-behavioral therapy for somatization disorder: a randomized controlled trial. *Arch Intern Med* 2006;166:512.

Cosci F, Fava GA, Sonino N. Mood and anxiety disorders as early manifestations of medical illness: a systematic review. *Psychother Psychosom* 2015;84(1):22–29.

Creed FH, Davies I, Jackson J. The epidemiology of multiple somatic symptoms. *J Psychosom Res* 2012:72;311–317.

Heritage J, Robinson JD, Elliott MN, et al. Reducing patients' unmet concerns in primary care: the difference one word can make. *J Gen Intern Med* 2007;22:1429–1433.

Kirmayer LJ, Sartorius, NS. Cultural models and somatic syndromes. *Psychosom Med* 2007;69:832–840.

Kroenke K. Efficacy of treatment for somatoform disorders: a review of randomized controlled trials. *Psychosom Med* 2007;69:881–888.

Kroenke K, Spitzer RL, Williams JB. The PHQ-15: validity of a new measure for evaluating the severity of somatic symptoms. *Psychosom Med* 2002;64:258.

Reed M, Sampathi BR, McCarron RM, Xiong GL. Somatic symptom and related disorders. In: *Primary Care Psychiatry*, 2nd ed. Philadelphia, PA: Wolters Kluwer; 2018.

Rizzo M, Creed F, Goldberg D, Meader N, Pilling S. A systematic review of non-pharmacological treatments for depression in people with chronic physical health problems. *J Psychsom Res* 2011:71;18–27.

Sadock BJ, Sadock VA. *Synopsis of Psychiatry.* Philadelphia: Lippincott Williams & Wilkins; 2015.

Sirri, L, Fava, GA. Diagnostic criteria for psychosomatic research and somatic symptom disorders. *Int Rev Psychiatry* 2013;25(1):19–30.

Sumithipala A. What is the evidence for the efficacy of treatments for somatoform disorders? A critical review of previous intervention studies. *Psychosom Med* 2007;69:889–900.

Somatic Symptom and Related Disorders. *Diagnostic and Statistical Manual of Mental Disorders,* 5th ed. Arlington, VA: American Psychiatric Association; 2013.

Someshekar B, Jainer A, Wuntakal B. Psychopharmacotherapy of somatic symptoms disorders. *Int Rev Psychiatry* 2013;25:107–115.

WEBSITES

Medicare Advantage. The lies patients and doctors tell. TZ Insurance Solutions. https://www.medicareadvantage.com/patient-doctor-lies-survey. Accessed June 2019.

Medscape. Somatic Symptom and Related Disorders. https://emedicine.medscape.com/article/294908-overview. Accessed June 2019.

Merck Manual Online. Somatic Symptom and Related Disorders. https://www.merckmanuals.com/professional/psychiatric-disorders/somatic-symptom-and-related-disorders/overview-of-somatization. Accessed June 2019.

Patient Health Questionnaire Physical Symptoms (PHQ-15). Screening instrument and scoring. file:///C:/Users/nagar/Downloads/APA_DSM5_Level-2-Somatic-Symptom-Adult%20(1).pdf. Accessed June 2019.

Personality Disorders

30

John Q. Young, MD, MPP, PhD & Timothy R. Kreider, MD, PhD

INTRODUCTION

Patients with personality disorders are common in medical practice and have worse medical outcomes than patients without personality disorders. A personality disorder interferes with the therapeutic alliance between patient and clinician and as a result, clinicians face challenges in multiple critical dimensions of patient care: eliciting an accurate symptom history, explaining the assessment, reaching agreement over a treatment plan, and motivating behavior change. As a consequence of this impairment in the patient–clinician relationship, patients with personality disorders often experience suboptimal utilization of medical care (both over- and under-use) leading to worse medical outcomes and higher hospitalization rates. Furthermore, such patients are often experienced as "difficult" by clinicians, who in turn, may feel increasingly unsatisfied and frustrated themselves, leading to risk of burnout (see Chapter 4).

This chapter provides a framework to help recognize, understand, and manage the common personality disorders and styles encountered in medical practice. Applying this framework can help clinicians anticipate the challenging interpersonal, behavioral, and medical problems that may arise in working with these patients and enable clinicians to work through their own negative emotions that these patients may engender. These skills will lead to more appropriate treatment plans, improved alliance between patient and clinician, and better outcomes.

The Diagnostic and Statistical Manual of Mental Disorders (DSM-5) defines a personality disorder as: *an enduring pattern of inner experience and behavior that deviates markedly from the expectations of the individual's culture, is pervasive and inflexible, has an onset in adolescence or early adulthood, is stable over time, and leads to distress or impairment.* People suffering from personality disorders have dysfunctional beliefs about self and others. These dysfunctional beliefs and the resulting maladaptive interpersonal behaviors impair their capacity to establish and maintain intimate relationships, function at work, and experience pleasure in life. These patients have difficulty negotiating complex situations and coping with stress and anxiety. The sick role and the demands of medical care can be particularly problematic for them. The stress of illness is often extreme and sets into motion defensive and inflexible emotions, cognitions, and behaviors—with negative consequences for their medical treatment. In addition, these patients' difficulties in relating to others typically manifest in the clinician–patient relationship. They may be quite demanding or disrespectful of the needs of others, or the need to trust or confide in others may trigger so much anxiety that they avoid building relationships.

DIAGNOSTIC CLASSIFICATION OF PERSONALITY DISORDERS

Personality theorists have long debated how best to understand and classify personality disorders, with debate centering on two models. The categorical model, used in the DSM-5, views personality disorders as entities that are distinct from one another—that is, classified in separate categories—and also distinct from normalcy. This model is contrasted with the dimensional model, which views personality disorders as entities that overlap each other and that are on a spectrum with normalcy so that the maladaptive traits of patients with personality disorders represent normal traits that are exaggerated. The DSM-5 describes personality disorders according to a categorical model, and indeed this approach blends more easily with traditional medical diagnosis. Nevertheless, the dimensional model is alternately presented in a DSM-5 provisional section, meant to encourage continued study on the strengths of this alternate approach. Regardless of the diagnostic system used, clinicians can usefully understand and recognize that a patient may have specific personality "traits" even if the symptoms and impairment do not rise to the diagnostic threshold for the full syndrome.

DSM-5 lists 10 personality disorder diagnoses and groups them into three clusters based on descriptive

Table 30-1. DSM-5 personality disorders and their prevalence.

Cluster	Personality Disorder	Discriminating Feature	Prevalence in General Population (%)[1]
A: Odd or eccentric	Paranoid	Suspicious	4.4
	Schizoid	Socially indifferent	3.1
	Schizotypal	Eccentric	3.9
B: Dramatic, emotional, or erratic	Antisocial	Disagreeable	3.6
	Borderline	Unstable	5.9
	Histrionic	Attention-seeking	1.8
	Narcissistic	Self-centered	6.2
C: Anxious or fearful	Avoidant	Inhibited	2.4
	Dependent	Submissive	0.5
	Obsessive–compulsive	Perfectionistic	7.9

[1]Prevalence data from National Epidemiologic Survey of Alcohol and Related Conditions (NESARC).

similarities (Table 30-1). Given the unique nature of any individual personality, a patient can exhibit traits of two or more personality disorders, or meet the full diagnostic criteria for more than one disorder. Co-occurrence is very common. National survey data suggest that approximately 15% of the general population have at least one personality disorder. Table 30-1 indicates the prevalence of each personality disorder within the general U.S. population; the prevalence in medical patients is likely higher.

Diagnosing a personality disorder can be difficult. To make an accurate diagnosis, it is usually necessary for the clinician to get to know the patient over time, to learn how the patient reacts and relates to people in a variety of contexts, and to obtain collateral information from family and friends. Clinicians should attend to four key issues.

First, *it is important to differentiate a true personality disorder from personality traits* that become exaggerated under stress, such as during acute medical illness. The stress of illness often causes a patient to behave in maladaptive ways; many patients, at one time or another, may appear to have a personality disorder. Patients who do not suffer from a true personality disorder, however, are usually capable of more adaptive functioning. The maladaptive behavior itself is less "enduring" and "engrained" and more situational and modifiable. In these cases, the clinician can successfully intervene by supporting and strengthening these patients' own natural coping skills, resulting in much more rapid improvement than will be observed for a patient with a personality disorder.

Second, it is *important to differentiate personality disorders from psychiatric disorders* such as major depression or generalized anxiety disorder. For example, patients with panic disorder may—out of sheer terror—become extremely dependent on their clinician. If their panic disorder is diagnosed and treated, they may reveal an underlying independent and self-sufficient personality. Similarly, a patient's grandiosity and arrogance may stem largely from a manic episode of bipolar disorder rather than from a narcissistic personality disorder. In addition, patients who do have a personality disorder may also have comorbid other psychiatric disorders, such as major depressive disorder, and recognizing such comorbidity is crucial for management. Treating an episode of major depression in a patient with borderline personality disorder, for example, can alleviate suffering and lead to much better coping with their other illnesses and broader life.

Third, personality disorders *should be distinguished from personality changes* caused by general medical conditions, such as traumatic brain injury, stroke, epilepsy, or endocrine disorders. Patients with one of these problems may exhibit many of the characteristics of a personality disorder, such as suspiciousness, impulsivity, or obsessiveness. These behaviors can be distinguished from a true personality disorder in that they typically represent a relatively acute or subacute change from baseline personality characteristics. Medical conditions may also exacerbate preexisting personality traits (e.g., obsessive mannerisms). Treatment of the underlying medical problem may bring about reversal of the personality changes.

Finally, personality disorder diagnoses, like other mental disorder diagnoses, are often misunderstood and *may serve to stigmatize the patient*, even among clinicians. These diagnoses should therefore be made carefully, deferred in cases of uncertainty, and noted in medical records and correspondence in respectful terms and only so as to be helpful in enhancing patient care.

Clinician–Patient Relationship Issues

The primary care provider may find many challenges in working with patients with personality disorders.

Personality disorders often significantly impair the quality of interpersonal relationships. Because the clinician–patient relationship requires effective communication about important health issues of a personal nature, tensions and at times overt conflict may develop between patients with personality disorders and their providers. These tensions may also affect other members of the health care team and may be especially pronounced in the context of acute illness or crisis situations. In fact, the first diagnostic clues suggesting personality dysfunction or disorder may appear as difficulties in the clinician–patient relationship.

For patients with personality disorders, physical illness can cause exaggerated degrees of emotional distress, not always expressed to the provider. Although some patients tell their providers about their emotional distress, others may instead manifest distress as nonadherence with the agreed-upon plan of evaluation or treatment or as changed, unexpected, or undesirable behavior (as judged by the clinician) toward the clinician.

In response to these patient's actions or statements, clinicians may have strong emotional reactions that change their behavior toward the patient. Even when experiencing no subjective distress from a medical condition or the clinician–patient relationship, patients with personality dysfunction may have such aberrant expectations of others that their statements or behaviors are troubling or burdensome to the clinician. Clinicians must be aware of their own emotional responses to such patients or they may fail to recognize a personality disorder or other psychiatric diagnosis or fail to address the diagnostic and treatment needs of the patient with compassion and thoroughness. When clinicians recognize and deal with their negative feelings, they will minimize the emotional strain for both patient and clinician and optimize the quality of the medical outcome.

Appreciating the unique vulnerabilities associated with each personality disorder can aid in identifying problematic behaviors and can help to maintain the necessary degree of cooperation and collaboration, even when the patient has significant personality dysfunction. Table 30-2 outlines typical responses to illness by patients with each of the most common personality disorders, details troublesome reactions by clinicians, and suggests strategies to avoid further problems with these challenging patients.

Management of Patients With Personality Disorders

In most cases, a stable therapeutic alliance with patients who have personality disorders can be maintained by implementing the behavioral strategies suggested in the following sections. Sometimes other factors must also be addressed. Pharmacotherapy and psychotherapy are often more complex for patients with comorbid disorders. This is particularly evident when patients with personality disorders have concurrent substance-abuse problems or psychotic symptoms (e.g., hallucinations, delusions, and paranoid ideation). In such cases, mental health consultation can be particularly helpful.

When a primary care clinician feels unable to continue productive work with a patient with a personality disorder, it may be appropriate to transfer the patient to another clinician. Although such transfers of care may be both necessary and helpful, they require consideration of the impact of the transfer on the well-being of the patient. Patients with certain personality disorders may experience such transfers as rejection or abandonment, perceptions that may exacerbate their emotional distress and potentially disrupt their medical treatment. Prior consultation with a mental health clinician can be useful in determining whether such a transfer might be helpful and can aid in carrying it out smoothly.

The remainder of this chapter discusses the 10 personality disorders as they manifest in the medical setting, and, for each, presents management recommendations.

PARANOID PERSONALITY DISORDER

Symptoms & Signs

Patients with paranoid personality disorder have a long-standing pattern of distrust and suspiciousness. They perceive the behavior and motives of others as malevolent in nature and expect others, in many situations, to disappoint or take advantage of them. They are reluctant to confide in others and can be preoccupied with unwarranted doubts about the loyalty or trustworthiness of friends and associates. They may perceive seemingly benign or innocuous statements or behavior by others as threatening, insulting, or hurtful. To defend against their perceived vulnerability, they usually adopt a rigid, distanced, or guarded position. In general, persons with this personality structure find intimate relationships undesirable and difficult, which often leave them without any significant social supports.

Differential Diagnosis

Long-standing psychotic symptoms, such as delusions and hallucinations, suggest a diagnosis of paranoid delusional disorder or paranoid schizophrenia. Although persons with paranoid personality disorder usually do not have frank paranoid delusions, at times of extreme stress they may develop such symptoms for brief periods. Paranoid ideation may also be associated with medical causes or with alcohol or substance abuse or withdrawal.

Illness Experience & Illness Behavior

Illness is difficult for individuals with paranoid personality disorder because illness makes them more dependent,

Table 30-2. Common manifestations of the DSM-5 personality disorders and management strategies.

Personality Disorder	Paranoid	Schizoid	Schizotypal	Antisocial	Borderline
Prominent features of disorder	Distrust and suspiciousness of others, such that their motives are interpreted as malevolent	Pattern of detachment from social relationships and a restricted range of emotional expression	Odd beliefs, inappropriate affect, perceptual distortions, and desire for social isolation	Disregard for and violation of the rights of others, beginning in adolescence	Pattern of instability in interpersonal relationships, self-image, and affect, with marked impulsivity
Patient's experience of medical illness	Heightened sense of fear and vulnerability	Threat to personal integrity; increased anxiety because illness forces interaction with others	May have odd interpretations of illness, increased anxiety because of interactions with others, may become overtly psychotic	Sense of fear may be masked by increased hostility or entitled stance	Terrifying fantasies about illness; feels either completely well or deathly ill
Problematic behavior in the medical care setting	Fear that clinician or others may harm them Misinterpretation of innocuous or even helpful behaviors Increased likelihood of argument or conflict with staff	May delay seeking care until symptoms become severe, out of fear of interacting with others May appear detached and unappreciative of help	May delay care because of odd and magical beliefs about symptoms, may not recognize symptoms as a sign of illness May appear odd and eccentric and paranoid toward others	Irresponsible, impulsive, or dangerous health behavior, without regard for consequences to self or others Angry, deceitful, or manipulative behavior	Mistrust of clinicians and delay in seeking treatment Intense fear of rejection and abandonment Abrupt shifts from idealizing to devaluing clinician; splitting Self-destructive threats and acts
Problematic reactions to patient by clinician	Defensive, argumentative, or angry response that "confirms" patient's suspicions Ignoring the patient's suspicious or angry stance	Overzealous attempts to connect with patient Frustration at feeling unappreciated	Frustration about patient's misinterpretation of illness Not wanting to connect with an odd and eccentric patient	Succumbing to patient's manipulation Angry, punitive reaction when manipulation is discovered	Succumbing to patient's idealization and splitting Getting too close to patient, causing overstimulation for patient Despair at patient's self-destructive behaviors Temptation to punish patient angrily

Management strategies	Attend to and be empathic toward patient fears, even when irrational in appearance Carefully detail care plan for patient with advance information about risks of procedures/treatments Maintain patient's independence when possible and optimize the patient's control Not overly friendly, but with a professional, objective stance	Appreciate need for privacy and maintain a low-key approach Focus on technical elements of treatment; these are better tolerated Encourage patient to maintain daily routines Do not become overly personally involved or too zealous in trying to provide social supports	Try not to be turned off by patient's odd appearance Try to educate patient about the illness and its treatment Do not become overly involved in trying to provide social support	Carefully, respectfully investigate patient's concerns and motives Communicate directly; avoid punitive reactions to patient Set clear limits in context of medically indicated interventions	Don't get too close to patient Schedule frequent periodic check-ups even if patient is doing well Provide clear, nontechnical answers to questions to counter scary fantasies Tolerate periodic angry outbursts, but set limits Be aware of patient's potential for self-destructive behavior Discuss feelings with coworkers and multidisciplinary team

Personality Disorder	Histrionic	Narcissistic	Avoidant	Dependent	Obsessive–Compulsive
Prominent features of disorder	Pattern of excessive attention seeking and emotionality	Pervasive pattern of grandiosity, need for admiration, and lack of empathy for others	Pattern of social inhibition because of fears of being rejected or humiliated by others	Pervasive and excessive need to be taken care of that leads to submissive and clinging behavior, and fears of separation	Pattern of preoccupation with orderliness, perfectionism, control
Patient's experience of medical illness	Threatened sense of attractiveness and self-esteem	Illness may increase anxiety related to doubts about personal adequacy and disrupts image of self as resilient and superior	Illness may heighten sense of inadequacy and worsen low self-esteem	Fear that illness will lead to abandonment and helplessness	Fear of losing control over bodily functions and over emotions generated by illness; feelings of shame and vulnerability
Problematic behavior in the medical care setting	Overly dramatic, attention-seeking behavior, with tendency to draw clinician into excessively familiar relationship Inadequate focus on symptoms and their management, with overemphasis on feeling states May provide answers they believe clinician wants to hear Tendency for somatization	Demanding, entitled attitude Excessive praise toward clinician may turn to devaluation, in effort to maintain sense of superiority Denial of illness or minimization of symptoms	May not be forthcoming about symptom severity, may easily agree with clinician out of fear of not being liked	Dramatic and urgent demands for medical attention Angry outbursts at clinician if not responded to Patient may act to prolong illness or encourage medical procedures in order to get attention May abuse substances and medications	Anger about disruption of routines Repetitive questions and excessive attention to detail Fear of relinquishing control to health care team

(*Continued*)

Table 30-2. Common manifestations of the DSM-5 personality disorders and management strategies. (*Continued*)

Personality Disorder	Histrionic	Narcissistic	Avoidant	Dependent	Obsessive–Compulsive
Problematic reactions to patient by clinician	Performing excessive workup (when patient is dramatic) or inadequate workup (when patient is vague) Allowing too much emotional closeness, thereby losing objectivity Frustration with patient's dramatic or vague presentation	Outright rejection of patient's demands, resulting in patient distancing self from clinician Excessive submission to patient's grandiose stance	Feeling overly concerned for the patient, taking on a paternalistic role that may increase patient's sense of inadequacy Anger if the patient's symptoms turn out to be more extensive than initially reported	Inability to set limits to availability, thus leading to burnout Hostile rejection of patient	Impatience and cutting answers short Attempts to control treatment planning
Management strategies	Show respectful and professional concern for feelings, with emphasis on objective issues Avoid excessive familiarity	Generous validation of patient's concerns, with attentive but factual response to questions Allow patients to maintain sense of competence by rechanneling their "skills" to deal with illness, obviating need for devaluation of clinician Present treatment recommendations in the context of their right to the best care	Provide reassurance, validate patient's concerns Encourage reporting of symptoms and concerns	Provide reassurance and schedule frequent periodic check-ups Be consistently available but provide firm realistic limits to availability Enlist other members of the health care team in providing support for patient Help patient obtain outside support Avoid hostile rejection of patient	Thorough history taking and careful diagnostic workups are reassuring Give clear and thorough explanation of diagnosis and treatment options Do not overemphasize uncertainties about treatments Avoid vague and impressionistic explanations Treat patient as an equal partner; encourage self-monitoring and allow patient participation in treatment

and, hence, more vulnerable. Communicating personal information to the clinician may challenge the self-protective, rigid way they approach social interactions. Patients may experience a heightened sense of vulnerability and fear of harm by the clinician. In their fearful state, they may perceive innocuous or even overtly helpful behavior as threatening. They may then question or challenge the clinician about the content of an intervention or the motives behind it. This can lead to conflict and argument between patient and clinician or to the patient disengaging from care.

The Clinician–Patient Relationship

Clinicians confronted with such a paranoid stance may react in ways that exacerbate the situation. If they feel that their intentions are inappropriately suspect they might argue with the patient or become defensive, perhaps using an angry tone. This kind of reaction may frighten the patient and may be perceived as confirmation of the patient's suspicion. Although such a response should be avoided, ignoring the patient's distrustful or angry behavior can also be problematic; the patient's concerns, however irrational, may increase if not addressed.

Specific Management Strategies

It is essential to address the patient's concerns and fears empathically, however irrational they seem. Although the clinician may see the patient's concern as unrealistic, for the patient the fear is real. Dismissing these patients' concerns or calling them paranoid will not address their emotional needs and may instead create distance in the clinician–patient relationship. A professional, "matter-of-fact" or objective stance is most reassuring to these patients. Excessive friendliness or reassurance may be misinterpreted and may intensify their paranoia. It is important to give these patients detailed information about their proposed treatment plan, allowing them to feel they are in control of the treatment and can make independent decisions. Provide factual information about risks associated with the treatment, whenever possible, before any major procedures or changes in treatment.

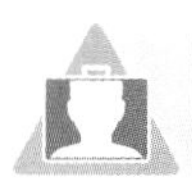

CASE ILLUSTRATION 1

Simon, a 42-year-old, single, male parking lot attendant, presents to the urgent care clinic complaining of 3 months of tension headaches and fatigue in the context of what he calls "job stress." The only notable finding on physical examination is a mild elevation of blood pressure. The clinician also observes that Simon seems angry and anxious. When asked about his job stress, Simon reveals anxieties about not being able to trust two new coworkers, along with fears that his supervisors are conspiring to dismiss him from his job. He also mentions, hesitantly, that he had not sought evaluation of his headaches sooner because he worried that the clinician would dismiss his fears as unfounded or "crazy." Additional social history reveals difficulty with close relationships and recurrent problems adjusting to changes in the workplace.

The clinician listens in a nonjudgmental and empathic manner. She responds with scientific curiosity asking specific and thorough questions in order to define the nature of the complaint. An over-the-counter analgesic for the headaches and a selective serotonin reuptake inhibitor for anxiety are prescribed after a discussion of the likely diagnosis and the pros and cons of each treatment option, including the option of cognitive behavior therapy to help him cope with anxiety and anger at work. The clinician plans follow-up measurements of the blood pressure and suggests that Simon see a psychiatrist for further evaluation of his very stressful job situation.

Simon feels that his concerns have been taken seriously. He finds the referral to a psychiatrist acceptable because it has been proposed in a way that offers support and does not dismiss his fears as pathological. The clinician's matter-of-fact responses to Simon's somatic complaints help increase the patient's trust in the clinician.

SCHIZOID PERSONALITY DISORDER

Symptoms & Signs

Individuals with schizoid personality disorder remain detached from social relationships and exhibit a restricted range of emotional expression in their interactions with others, often appearing cold or indifferent. Patients with this disorder experience intense emotions, intimacy, and interpersonal conflict as highly threatening, and as a result they tend to isolate themselves and avoid close relationships. They prefer dealing with technical or abstract concepts rather than people, and so they may devote their time to pursuits such as mathematical games. Work can be problematic if it involves interactions with others, but many individuals can perform quite well if they work with some degree of independence.

Differential Diagnosis

Patients with schizoid personality disorder do not exhibit prolonged psychotic symptoms. They may, however, suffer a brief psychotic decompensation during times of extreme stress. In addition, schizoid personality disorder may in some cases precede the development of psychotic conditions, such as schizophrenia or delusional disorder. It can also coexist with schizotypal, paranoid, or avoidant personality disorders.

Illness Experience & Illness Behavior

Illness can be especially stressful for these patients because it gives rise to strong emotions with which they are not prepared to cope. The necessity of interacting with caregivers when ill, often around quite intimate issues, forces them to do the very thing they systematically avoid. They may therefore delay seeking care until their symptoms become more serious. When they finally present for medical attention, they may appear indifferent or detached as a way of protecting themselves from overwhelming emotion. They may show little facial expression and may not respond in kind to caregivers' empathic nods or comments—which may make establishing a therapeutic relationship difficult.

THE CLINICIAN–PATIENT RELATIONSHIP

Because these patients often appear cold or indifferent, clinicians may consider them as unappreciative of help. They may also be puzzled or frustrated by their patients' delay in seeking medical care and their apparent passivity in the face of illness. As a result, caregivers may make overzealous attempts to connect with patients by trying to be especially empathic, a tactic that may instead frighten them away. On the other hand, providers may themselves draw back and lose their enthusiasm for helping patients who seem so unappreciative or uninvolved in their own treatment.

Specific Management Strategies

Understanding that individuals with schizoid personality disorder have difficulty tolerating emotions and intimate interactions is important. Clinicians should appreciate their patients' need for privacy and should maintain a low-key approach, avoiding attempts to reach out by becoming too close or by insisting on providing social support. It is helpful to focus on the more technical aspects of treatment, as these are better tolerated, and encourage patients to maintain daily routines. Caregivers should remain available and provide steady but unobtrusive help.

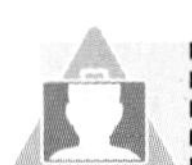

CASE ILLUSTRATION 2

Ben, a 44-year-old computer programmer, is admitted to the university hospital for evaluation of nausea, anorexia, and a 30-lb weight loss occurring over the previous several months. When asked by the admitting resident why he had not sought treatment before, Ben states that he has always been healthy and thought he would probably regain the lost weight.

Throughout the interview, Ben makes poor eye contact and gives brief answers to questions. He appears to dislike being interviewed by both a medical student and a resident. He becomes more distant when asked questions about his personal life and how he likes spending his time. Ben states that he usually keeps to himself, with the exception of visiting his sister about once a month. He spends much of his time programming and playing games on his computer.

Ben appears visibly anxious when the resident recommends a consultation by the gastroenterology service. He asks whether this is truly necessary. The resident emphasizes the importance of this consultation, and Ben seems to calm down a bit when the conversation focuses more on the possible tests that might be done to evaluate his symptoms, thereby distracting his attention from his concerns about having to see yet another clinician. The resident later explains to the medical student that it is important to minimize the number of clinicians Ben sees over time and to avoid an overfriendly style, which might frighten him.

SCHIZOTYPAL PERSONALITY DISORDER

Symptoms & Signs

Patients with schizotypal personality disorder behave in an odd and eccentric manner, are socially inept and isolated, and experience cognitive or perceptual distortions. Their cognitive distortions include magical thinking, odd beliefs, ideas of reference, bodily illusions, or telepathic and clairvoyant experiences. These beliefs and distortions are inconsistent with subcultural norms, occur frequently, and are an important and pervasive core component of the patient's experience. The patient's enduring psychotic-like symptoms may worsen under stress. Patients often dress in an odd and peculiar fashion and their affect is often inappropriate; for example, they may laugh inappropriately during the visit while talking about their problems.

These patients are socially isolated and usually have few or no close friends. Their social isolation stems from their odd behavior as well as from their persistent social anxiety due to suspiciousness or paranoia toward others.

Differential Diagnosis

Schizotypal personality disorder shares the symptom of suspiciousness and paranoia with paranoid personality disorder and that of social isolation with schizoid personality disorder. However, the latter two disorders do not present with odd and peculiar mannerisms and behaviors and also lack cognitive or perceptual distortions.

The differential diagnosis includes schizophrenia. Although patients with schizotypal personality disorder lack signs and symptoms of overt psychosis, the disorder is considered a schizophrenia spectrum disorder. This means that it may be related to schizophrenia. Family studies show an increased risk of schizophrenia in relatives of patients with schizotypal personality disorder and an increased risk of schizotypal personality disorder in families of patients with schizophrenia.

Illness Experience & Illness Behavior

Patients with schizotypal personality disorder may present late in the course of their illness because they may have odd interpretations of their illness and may, therefore, not recognize the serious nature of their symptoms. Also, like patients with schizoid personality disorder, they do not like to interact with and seek the company of others. Illness forces them to interact with health care providers and their support staff, something they may not be prepared to do. This may lead to increased paranoid ideation or overt psychotic symptoms.

The Clinician–Patient Relationship

These patients' eccentric appearance may cause the clinician to be hesitant in approaching them. Odd interpretations of illness may lead to misunderstandings between patient and clinician. It may be challenging for the clinician to improve these patients' understanding of their problems.

Specific Management Strategies

Clinicians should try to overcome their apprehension about treating these patients, often caused by their eccentric appearance. It is helpful to find out what these patients think about their symptoms and to help them obtain a better understanding of their illness. At the same time, the clinician should not get overly involved in trying to increase their patients' social support or exposure to others. Knowing that patients with schizotypal personality disorder desire social isolation is important. Occasionally, assessing decision-making capacity can be complicated by odd or magical beliefs associated with the illness. Consultation can be helpful.

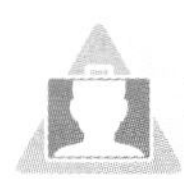

CASE ILLUSTRATION 3

Donna, a 35-year-old single female, has developed a cough, high fever, and chills and her family noticed that she started to look ill. She was brought to the emergency room by her mother. She is oddly dressed in a long and colorful country-style wraparound shirt with military-type boots. Her hair is unkempt and pinned up with a number of different hairpins. During the interview, Donna laughs in a silly manner while discussing her problem with the clinician and the nurse. She says that she does not like to see a clinician because she prefers to walk in the woods by herself and communicate with the birds and insects.

The clinician focuses on the patient's presenting symptoms and explains to her that she may suffer from pneumonia. She explains to her in simple terms what pneumonia is and that she needs sputum cultures and a chest X-ray to confirm the diagnosis.

While Donna has her chest X-ray taken, the clinician and the nurse discuss how the health care team should help the patient understand her symptoms as well as the rationale for her medical workup and treatment. The clinician also recommends focusing on the patient's problems and respecting her need for distance from others.

ANTISOCIAL PERSONALITY DISORDER

Symptoms & Signs

Persons with antisocial personality disorder demonstrate a disregard for others and behavior that violates others' rights. The diagnosis can be made only in persons over the age of 18 years, and it requires a history of conduct disorder prior to that age. Characteristics include lack of conformity to social norms and laws, using lies or other deceitfulness for personal gain, and impulsiveness and irresponsibility in many settings. These individuals may be threatening, manipulative, or harmful to others, and they are generally not remorseful. Their tendencies toward aggressive behavior may not be immediately evident, but contact with collateral sources frequently reveals a criminal record. These character traits affect relations with both strangers and family alike, as persons with antisocial personality disorder may engage in inconsiderate, angry, or harmful behaviors. These individuals may present themselves in a superficially grandiose manner, and they can also initially appear charismatic, until others recognize their charm as manipulative.

Differential Diagnosis

Antisocial personality disorder can overlap significantly with other personality disorder traits, most commonly narcissistic, histrionic, or borderline personality disorder. Because substance abuse is a frequent comorbid diagnosis, it is important to distinguish between the problems; when making the diagnosis of antisocial personality disorder, the antisocial behavior should be observed in multiple contexts, not solely in relation to substance addiction.

Illness Experience & Illness Behavior

To mask the fear that illness may cause, patients with antisocial personality disorder may unconsciously adopt an excessively self-assured, entitled, or hostile stance. Irresponsible, impulsive, or dangerous health behavior may help these patients deny their vulnerability to illness. This behavior can occur without regard for medical consequences, and many patients show blatant disregard for the health care personnel and resources from which they have benefited. Patients may assume a privileged, self-deserving stance and can become antagonistic if they fail to obtain the desired response. They may attempt to manipulate their clinician, malingering to obtain things such as drugs or inappropriate disability benefits. This behavior can be an embellishment of a real illness, or it can occur when they are not ill.

THE CLINICIAN–PATIENT RELATIONSHIP

Because these patients often behave in ways that are noncompliant, ungracious, or dishonest, they are frequently irritating to health care providers. Clinicians may become angry with these individuals or reject them if they see that the treatments in which they have invested their knowledge and time have not been followed, or if they discover these patients have manipulated them.

Specific Management Strategies

Managing manipulative patients can be particularly challenging. If the patient successfully manipulates the clinician, the outcome is usually detrimental to the patient's overall health (broadly defined). On the other hand, although recognizing the manipulative behavior may avert a detrimental health outcome, the clinician's confrontation can alienate the patient. The more authoritarian the clinician's stance, the more likely it is that the patient will become oppositional, reducing the possibility for development of an effective therapeutic alliance.

The key here is to maintain an objective, thorough, nonauthoritarian, and respectful approach to investigating the patient's presenting complaints. If the patient's presentation or motives are suspicious, the provider should gather corroborating data from collateral sources (other providers or family members) when needed. Such behavior by the provider can cause the patient to become hostile, with additional deterioration in the clinician–patient relationship. If confrontation or disagreement is necessary, it is essential to avoid humiliating the patient while identifying the attempted manipulation. Communication should be direct and factual with these patients, based on what is medically indicated, and clear limits should be set on the diagnostic or treatment plan.

CASE ILLUSTRATION 4

On returning from vacation, the nurse practitioner's (NP) first patient is Randy, an angry 42-year-old man, well known to her for his problems with longstanding recurrent low back pain. Although his back pain is generally well controlled with back exercises and as needed nonsteroidal analgesics, Randy frequently takes long motorcycle trips with friends, during which he does not exercise or take his analgesics. While the NP was away, Randy went on a motorcycle tour and had a recurrence of acute back pain. He then telephoned the clinic and became angry and abusive toward the on-call clinician, who would not submit to his demands for narcotics.

The NP, who has seen similar behavior from Randy in the past, listens carefully to his story, acknowledges his anger, and reflects empathically on how painful his back must be. She inquires, nonjudgmentally, about the reasons for his failure to exercise. She then explains the benefits of a more preventive approach–using exercise and avoiding pain-inducing behaviors–compared with the long-term risks of relying on narcotics and failing to exercise. Finally, she offers him referral to a physical therapist for a review of the exercise plan, along with a refill of his nonsteroidal analgesic, emphasizing her view that this would offer the best long-term outcome. With some bitterness, Randy acknowledges the benefits of these recommendations and agrees to try to follow through with them.

In dealing with Randy, the primary care clinician uses her past experience with him as a guide. Randy's self-destructive behavior, hostility, and disregard for others are met with clear limit setting by the NP, who responds in a calm and nonpunitive manner, emphasizing her concern for the patient's long-term well-being.

BORDERLINE PERSONALITY DISORDER

Symptoms & Signs

Patients with borderline personality disorder exhibit instability in their self-image, affect, and relationships with others. They can be quite impulsive and may engage in self-destructive behaviors, such as substance abuse, self-mutilation, and suicide attempts. These behaviors reflect a deep sense of emptiness and an intense fear of abandonment by others. On the other hand, patients with borderline personality disorder are also often fearful of closeness. They experience many contradictory emotions and feelings that are not integrated into a stable sense of who they are and that may be associated with rapid shifts in mood. This instability can cause frequent changes in goals and values. These patients usually have difficulty differentiating reality from fantasy and tend toward all-or-nothing thinking in their view of themselves and others, alternating between idealization and devaluation.

Differential Diagnosis

Some patients with borderline personality disorder may suffer brief psychotic episodes when under stress. They may, for example, become very anxious in a way that mimics paranoia, or they may experience brief dissociative episodes or auditory hallucinations. The brief duration and specific association with stressors distinguish these episodes from psychotic disorders. The affective lability of patients with borderline personality disorder may be distinguished from mood episodes of a depressive or bipolar disorder by time course: patients with borderline personality disorder often endorse multiple mood swings per day, as opposed to the days- to weeks-long episodes of mood change in depressive and bipolar disorders. Complicating the differential further, patients with borderline personality disorder often suffer from a concurrent depressive or bipolar disorder, which should, of course, be treated. Other personality disorders (e.g., histrionic or narcissistic) may co-occur or be confused with borderline personality disorder.

Illness Experience & Illness Behavior

Patients with borderline personality disorder have difficulty distinguishing reality from fantasy, and they may have terrifying fantasies about illness, such as that illness symptoms will drive away all their loved ones or that the illness is confirmation that they are "bad" or "unlovable." The complex and contradictory feelings engendered in response to illness can feel intolerable to these patients, so they may try to cope by pretending that they are completely well and denying the presence of illness. Alternatively, they may become convinced that they are deathly ill, even when suffering from a mild illness. Having felt wounded in earlier relationships, individuals with borderline personality disorder mistrust and fear caregivers. In an attempt to cope with their simultaneous intense wish for, and fear of, closeness, they tend to conceptualize caregivers as all good or all bad—a mechanism called "splitting." To complicate things further, these conceptualizations are not stable. Even an idealized caregiver can abruptly become the "bad clinician" when the patient with borderline personality disorder is disappointed by the clinician. In addition, patients with borderline personality disorder may respond to feeling overwhelmed by engaging in impulsive and self-destructive acts, such as self-mutilation, substance abuse, and suicide attempts. They may also be nonadherent with treatment in order to test the limits of the clinician's availability, devalue the clinician, or even to remain ill and thus maintain an ongoing relationship with the caregiver.

The Clinician–Patient Relationship

A common mistake clinicians make in treating patients with borderline personality disorder is getting too emotionally close or over-involved in meeting their needs. This occurs when clinicians feel intensely drawn to help patients through their suffering and spend a great deal of time with them. This usually causes overstimulation of the patient's emotions, leading to initial idealization of the clinician as "perfect" or the "friend/clinician/support they never had" followed by the inevitable devaluation. It should be noted that the patient's emotional behavior can cloud the clinician's judgment, causing the clinician to succumb to the patient's idealization and splitting and seek to stay on the 'patient's good side' even when it means becoming overly involved. It is important to remember that the idealization lasts only so long; the clinician will inevitably disappoint the patient. The borderline patient's self-destructive or often provocative behaviors can then cause despair and helplessness in caregivers. Caregivers may also feel tempted to punish the patient, for example, by becoming uncharacteristically inflexible or withholding needed (e.g., pain) medication or care (e.g., more frequent visits), or, in extreme situations, even verbally abusive.

Specific Management Strategies

While providing basic support and reassurance, clinicians should be careful not to become emotionally over-involved with the borderline personality disorder patient. It is appropriate to counter the patient's frightening fantasies about illness and "overwhelming neediness" by scheduling regular (even if brief) periodic check-ups and providing clear, nontechnical answers to questions. Clinicians may have to tolerate periodic angry outbursts, but it is appropriate to set firm limits on the patient's disruptive behavior. For example, the clinician might say that "when you raise your voice, I cannot concentrate and provide the care you need. If you cannot communicate without yelling right now, then we will have to reschedule for a time when you are able to be calmer." When a multidisciplinary team of clinicians is involved, meetings of all providers should be arranged, to allow them to vent their feelings about the patient and to reach consensus on a treatment plan. It is helpful to select a small number of caregivers to interact with the patient directly and to present the same clear and consistent plan. This approach often prevents splitting. Finally, it is essential to remain aware of these patients' potential for self-destructive or overly demanding behavior and not to retaliate by displaying anger at them when setting limits or even punishing them (e.g., not responding to valid requests for care).

CASE ILLUSTRATION 5

A primary care resident expresses concern about her patient Amanda to her clinic's attending clinician. She is scheduled to leave the clinic in 3 months and believes that Amanda will find transferring to a new clinician difficult.

Amanda is a 35-year-old temporary clerical worker with a long-standing history of migraine headaches. She often delays taking medication until her migraine headaches become severe, and then calls the resident, complaining of unbearable pain, sometimes stating that the pain is so intolerable that she wishes to die. She sometimes comes to the clinic without a scheduled appointment, demanding to be seen right away. On the other hand, she often misses regularly scheduled appointments. During her visits, she expresses a fear of becoming homeless; she house-sits at other people's homes but does not have a stable place of her own.

The resident asks for a psychiatric consultation to help her work with Amanda. She is particularly concerned about Amanda's periodic statements that she wishes to die.

Following the psychiatrist's recommendations, the resident continues to schedule regular, brief follow-up appointments, and encourages Amanda to keep these appointments. She explains that this is not a walk-in clinic, and that Amanda will have to seek treatment for acute pain at the urgent care center. She also reminds Amanda that taking medication early will likely keep the headache from becoming very intense.

Other helpful interventions include providing increased support to Amanda by referring her to a psychotherapist and asking the team social worker to assist her in finding a stable residence. It is also important to monitor Amanda for suicidal ideation. If she expresses a wish to die, the resident assesses her suicidal ideation and intent. One afternoon, Amanda presents at the clinic expressing suicidal ideation, and a nurse practitioner calls for an urgent psychiatric consultation. After talking to the psychiatrist, Amanda gradually calms down and denies any suicidal intent; however, she refuses a referral for ongoing psychiatric treatment.

Over time, Amanda continues to miss some appointments, and occasionally becomes demanding or complains bitterly about the resident to the nurse practitioner. When both the resident and the nurse practitioner, however, firmly and supportively continue to reiterate their support for the same treatment plan—to meet with the clinician for regular appointments, to treat migraines early, and to go to urgent care for acute pain—Amanda's unpredictable visits and noncompliance diminish. Periodic meetings between the resident and the nurse practitioner help them both present the same coherent plan to Amanda, thus minimizing splitting.

In planning ahead for her departure from the clinic, the resident and the attending clinician discuss some helpful strategies to facilitate this transition, such as introducing the new resident to Amanda ahead of time and involving the nurse practitioner—who is staying at the clinic—in the process.

In this case, regular meetings of all the involved clinicians and staff (e.g., trainees, the attending clinician, consultants, receptionist, and the nurse practitioner) allow them to present the same coherent plan to the patient, minimize the splitting, and reduce the patient's anxiety and unpredictable behavior. This approach successfully combines increased support and limit setting.

HISTRIONIC PERSONALITY DISORDER

Symptoms & Signs

Histrionic personality disorder is marked by excessive attention seeking and emotionalism. These patients may present with dramatic, theatrical shows of feeling, or they may dress or behave in a sexually provocative fashion in an unconscious effort to engage others and draw attention to themselves. The emotions they express may be shallow and inconsistent, but the patients may still believe that the sharing of those feelings creates a special closeness (which they often exaggerate) with the clinician. These patients tend to prefer subjective and intuitive impressions to objective, fact-driven reasoning. They often have somatic complaints, with impressive—but inconsistent—presentations.

Differential Diagnosis

Histrionic personality disorder may be difficult to distinguish from narcissistic or borderline personality disorder, and patients in each of these categories may exhibit traits common to patients in the others. Patients with histrionic personality disorder are deeply affected by perceived frailties in relationship bonds, as are patients with borderline personality disorder. The latter, however, display less emotional stability and are more impulsive and self-destructive. Patients with histrionic personality disorder may crave attention—as patients with narcissistic personality disorder crave admiration—but the former tend to be less grandiose, arrogant, and self-absorbed.

Illness Experience & Illness Behavior

Medical illness represents a particular threat to the emotional well-being of patients with histrionic personality disorder, who derive much of their sense of self-worth and personal desirability from their sense of physical attractiveness. To reduce the fear of being deemed less desirable by others, these patients may attempt to bolster and show off their physical appearance or abilities. For example, they may engage in flirtatious or seductive behavior with clinicians.

When these patients feel weak and vulnerable, they may express their emotions with more intensity, in an attempt to strengthen their bond with the clinician. In addition, because these patients focus on feelings, rather than on carefully observed physical symptoms, they may present with a collection of loosely connected somatic complaints. Their descriptions of the symptoms may reflect their desire to capture the clinician's interest.

THE CLINICIAN–PATIENT RELATIONSHIP

In working with the histrionic patient, the clinician may be drawn in by the patient's dramatic and somewhat dependent style, become overly involved, and perhaps embark on an excessive workup. As the clinician becomes increasingly engaged by the patient's style, the patient may then become anxious, distant, or noncompliant, puzzling and frustrating the clinician. Alternatively, the clinician may instead pursue too cursory an evaluation, because of a lack of objective information, or out of frustration with the patient's emotional and vague style.

Specific Management Strategies

Because the patient with histrionic personality disorder has a vague and global emotional (rather than a precise, logical) style and may display contrasting behaviors—that range from excessive anxiety about potentially minor symptoms to inappropriate indifference about significant medical problems—it is essential that the clinician maintain an objective stance. The clinician must offer a supportive and logical approach to the patient's problems. This requires being both sensitive to the patient's emotional concerns and sufficiently distanced to avoid any degree of closeness that the patient might misperceive as intimate or sexual.

CASE ILLUSTRATION 6

Rita is 38-year-old, single, unemployed actress with lupus. She is excessively friendly and flirtatious with her 45-year-old male clinician, calling him frequently with questions about her medical problems and dressing somewhat seductively for office visits. During these visits she asks for examinations of a variety of somatic complaints. Over time, the clinician becomes increasingly uncomfortable. One day, Rita complains that she would like more time to discuss her problems at each office visit, and she asks the clinician if he thinks her problems "deserve more time."

After reflecting on the chronicity of this pattern of behavior, the clinician responds that Rita's medical problems are significant and deserving of attention. He states that he intends to evaluate each of them carefully, allocating time on the basis of his impression of their medical necessity. He also says that he understands that she would like more time to discuss her concerns, but that as a primary care clinician he cannot make additional time available to her. He suggests, gently, that if he cannot provide adequate emotional support to her within the time constraints of a follow up visit, he could refer her to a local clinic's health psychologist. Although she is rather disappointed, Rita is able to accept this limit setting and continues to work with this clinician.

This approach is successful because the clinician shows positive regard for the patient and her problems—while clearly setting the limits of the clinician–patient relationship.

NARCISSISTIC PERSONALITY DISORDER

Symptoms & Signs

Narcissistic personality disorder is characterized by a long-standing pattern of grandiosity, with a need for praise and admiration that stands out in contrast to a lack of sensitivity to the feelings of others. These persons may display an exaggerated sense of self-importance and social status and require excessive admiration. They may be driven toward attaining an idealized position in terms of social, personal, romantic, or career accomplishment. In this regard, they may be envious and potentially devaluing of others whose accomplishments they perceive as exceeding their own. Beneath the grandiosity and devaluation exists an underlying view of self as inferior or inadequate. To avoid these beliefs and their associated painful affects, patients seek to convince self and others of their "specialness" or "unusual talent."

Differential Diagnosis

Narcissistic personality disorder may be difficult to distinguish from borderline, antisocial, histrionic, or obsessive–compulsive personality disorders, and in many cases it may overlap with these disorders. When the differentiation is unclear, identifying a high degree of grandiosity and a need for admiration can help clarify the diagnosis. In contrast to persons with borderline personality disorder, persons with narcissistic personality disorder have a more stable self-image and display less impulsiveness and sensitivity to relationship losses. In addition, persons with narcissistic personality disorder are generally less aggressive and deceitful than are persons with antisocial personality disorder, who also display evidence of childhood conduct disorder. Persons with histrionic personality disorder, in contrast, may be relatively more dramatic and emotional than those with narcissistic personality disorder. Although persons with narcissistic personality disorder, like those with obsessive–compulsive personality disorder, may be perfectionists, the former often have a higher self-assessment of their accomplishments.

Clinicians must be careful not to misdiagnose a person with hypomanic or manic grandiosity as having narcissistic personality disorder. Similarly, it is important to distinguish between narcissistic personality disorder and transient substance-related personality changes (e.g., from central nervous system stimulants) or personality changes caused by a general medical condition.

Illness Experience & Illness Behavior

Health problems are a particular blow to patients with narcissistic personality disorder. Illness threatens these patients' unconscious attempts to maintain an intrapsychic and external image of untarnished well-being, resiliency, and superiority. Medical problems and physical limitations may disrupt this image, threaten their public personas, and leave them fearing disruption of their (unrealistically unchallengeable) sense of self. In an attempt to defend against this threat, patients may minimize the significance of symptoms or deny the presence of the illness. More commonly, as patients try to recapture their admired, idealized status, they may demand special treatment, second opinions, or transfer of care to more "senior" or "well-known" clinicians. These patients may devalue, criticize, or question the behavior or credentials of the treating clinician, or they may fail to comply with treatment recommendations.

The Clinician–Patient Relationship

Narcissistic patients' arrogant and grandiose behavior, combined with demands for special treatment, can be extremely irritating to clinicians. Reactions to these patients can take many forms. Sometimes, in an attempt to avoid conflict, clinicians submit to the demands. With particularly critical patients, providers may feel frustration, resentment, and even anger. Alternatively, they may feel devalued and question their own competence. Frustration may be especially great if the provider expends special energy on behalf of a charismatic or demanding patient, only to later become the butt of unfair criticism. Clinicians may reject or avoid the patient, withhold treatment, or respond in an angry manner—responses that can harm both the patient and the clinician–patient relationship.

Specific Management Strategies

The most effective strategy for dealing with narcissistic patients is to be respectful and nonconfrontational about their sense of specialness and entitlement and to help them use their self-perceived talents in the service of their treatment. If narcissistic patients feel vulnerable and threatened by the illness, they are more likely to criticize and devalue the clinician. Thus, clinicians should not take this devaluation personally, and instead understand it as the patients' attempt to cope with their own intense insecurity. Providers can appeal to the patients' narcissism by explaining that they chose a particular course of action because they believe it represents the best possible care—a course of action they feel the patients deserve. Clinicians can further support the patients by validating their concerns about the illness and pointing to their patients' ability to respond competently to its challenges. This approach helps the patients feel more secure and able, allowing them to ally confidently with—rather than defensively attack—their providers.

CASE ILLUSTRATION 7

James, a 44-year-old married lawyer who is quite prominent in the community, is an unusually demanding patient. He becomes very angry with his clinician, whom he accuses of not responding adequately to his complaints. In fact, the clinician has done all the necessary laboratory tests and has answered numerous phone calls by the patient over a period of several months.

The clinician, aware of James' long-standing sense of entitlement and extreme sensitivity to slights, responds by reviewing his concerns, discussing the treatment plan and rationale, and encouraging him to discuss some of his emotional reactions to his symptoms. He then emphasizes the special consideration he has put into the evaluation and treatment plan. He arranges more frequent office visits during the next year and tells James that he predicts a relatively good response to treatment, given his active involvement in his care.

This response is reassuring to the patient, because it validates his concerns and satisfies his narcissistic feelings of entitlement.

AVOIDANT PERSONALITY DISORDER

Symptoms & Signs

Patients with avoidant personality disorder have a longstanding pattern of excessive anxiety in social situations and in intimate relationships, and extreme hypersensitivity to what other people think about them. These patients desire relationships but avoid them because of fears of being rejected, humiliated, or embarrassed. If they do engage in social situations or relationships, they are constantly preoccupied with being rejected, criticized, and not being liked by others. As a result, these patients have low self-esteem, feel socially inept, have feelings of inferiority, and are shy and inhibited.

Differential Diagnosis

Patients with schizoid personality disorder also avoid social situations and relationships but they do desire social isolation. In contrast, patients with avoidant personality disorder strongly desire relationships but avoid them because of anxiety and fears of rejection and humiliation. Patients with dependent and borderline personality disorders also strongly fear interpersonal rejection, but they do not avoid relationships but rather actively seek them.

Avoidant personality disorder should be distinguished from social phobia by how pervasive and consistent the symptoms are across time and settings. Whereas patients with avoidant personality disorder try to avoid social interactions in all situations, patients with social phobia usually have more specific concerns related to social performance in particular contexts, such as saying something inappropriate to unfamiliar people at a social gathering or during small, interactive, seminar style courses.

Illness Experience & Illness Behavior

Illness provokes anxiety and increases feelings of ineptness in patients with avoidant personality disorder. Patients may delay care or not be forthcoming about their problems out of fear of not being liked or being rejected by the caregiver. They may blame their physical discomfort on themselves and may actually not ask for appropriate pain relief. Because these patients feel that they may not deserve attention by their clinician, they may be reluctant to undergo necessary medical procedures.

THE CLINICIAN–PATIENT RELATIONSHIP

Clinicians treating patients with avoidant personality disorder may initially not realize the full extent of their patients' symptoms. Because these patients are shy and easily agreeable to what their clinicians propose, clinicians may be prone to take a more paternalistic stance with them. If they discover later that the patient's symptoms are more severe than initially reported, clinicians may react with concern or feel betrayed by the patient for withholding information and for their passive attitude.

Specific Management Strategies

Patients with avoidant personality disorder need reassurance and permission to express their distress and concerns in a nonjudgmental environment. It is helpful for health care providers to explain that they are interested in knowing about the patient's problems.

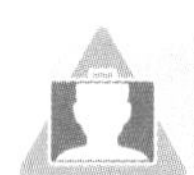

CASE ILLUSTRATION 8

Michael, a 45-year-old single office clerk, presents 45 minutes early for his annual check-up with his primary care clinician. While signing in at the reception desk, he asks whether he has arrived on time for his appointment.

The clinician finds a marked rash over the patient's elbows upon physical examination. The patient has a known history of psoriasis. Michael's face turns red out of embarrassment. He starts to explain that he applied the cream that his clinician prescribed for him last year but that he ran out of the prescription some time ago. When asked why he did not call the clinician's office for a refill, Michael states that he felt that he should not bother his clinician for just a rash.

The clinician expresses concern about the patient's rash, while trying to avoid a tone that could be interpreted as scolding. He writes a new prescription and asks Michael to call his office for a refill once he finishes the prescription. The clinician explains to the patient that he does not feel bothered by the patient's phone calls and that communication between patient and clinician is necessary to ensure appropriate medical care. He again requests that Michael call him for any refills or problems in the future.

This reassuring and supportive approach encourages the patient to communicate with his clinician and not hold back out of fear of being rejected.

DEPENDENT PERSONALITY DISORDER

Symptoms & Signs

Patients with dependent personality disorder have a pervasive and excessive need to be taken care of. They experience intense fear of separation and abandonment and feel great discomfort when they are alone. This leads to submissive and clinging behavior in their interpersonal relationships. These patients have difficulty making independent decisions without a great deal of advice and reassurance, and they are afraid of disagreeing with others.

Differential Diagnosis

It is important to distinguish dependent personality disorder from the dependency that arises from panic disorder, mood disorders, or agoraphobia. Patients suffering from medical illnesses may also become very dependent on others, without having this disorder. Dependent personality disorder can sometimes be confused with other personality disorders that involve fear of abandonment, and it can be distinguished by submissive behaviors. Dependent personality traits may be the result of chronic substance abuse; conversely, self-medication of intolerable affects may explain the high comorbidity of dependent personality disorder and substance use disorders.

Illness Experience & Illness Behavior

Patients with dependent personality disorder fear that illness will lead to both helplessness and abandonment by others. In their interactions with caregivers, they may become very needy and make dramatic demands for urgent medical attention. If the response is not what they wish, they may display angry outbursts at the clinician. They may also blame their physical discomfort on others, including their clinician. In addition, they may use addictive substances or overuse medications in a desperate attempt to obtain immediate relief from their suffering. Because receiving medical care may fulfill their wishes for attention from others, some dependent patients may unconsciously contribute to prolonging their illness, or—in some extreme cases—they may encourage unnecessary medical procedures.

The Clinician–Patient Relationship

Clinicians treating patients with dependent personality disorder may initially react with aversion to their patients' clingy and demanding behavior. Alternatively, clinicians may find it difficult to set limits on their availability and may try to provide reassurance by attempting to meet every demand, which ultimately leads to burnout or feelings of inadequacy. Eventually, caregivers may react in a hostile fashion and openly reject these patients.

Specific Management Strategies

Effective ways to provide reassurance to dependent patients and allay their fear of being abandoned include scheduling frequent periodic check-ups and being consistently available. It is nonetheless important to provide firm, realistic limits to this availability early in treatment or as soon as the patient's dependent traits become apparent. To prevent burnout, enlist other members of the health care team in providing support for the patient. In addition, clinicians should help these patients find outside support systems to lessen fears of abandonment. They must also be alert to the patients' potential contribution to prolonging their illness or to their possible abuse of substances or medications.

CASE ILLUSTRATION 9

Terry, a 50-year-old divorced secretary, repeatedly presents to her primary care clinician complaining of various somatic symptoms, including dizziness, headaches, blurred vision, and leg pains. Repeated workups of her symptoms are negative, and her evaluation for major depression is negative. Further inquiry into Terry's life reveals that after her divorce 6 years ago, her daughter became the focus of her life. Even though her history of occasional somatic symptoms goes back to her teenage years, there had been no appreciable change until 2 years ago, when her daughter got married and left her home.

Terry makes frequent phone calls to her clinician. She usually sounds nervous, expresses concern about some new symptom, and asks for medication. The clinician decides to schedule regular follow-up appointments to address Terry's concerns. Terry often complains during office visits that there is not enough time to evaluate all her symptoms and laments that her daughter no longer has much time for her. Her clinician listens in a supportive manner and acknowledges that the available appointment time is limited, explaining how he will ultimately address all the complaints. He also emphasizes the importance of continuing to meet for regular appointments. In addition, the clinician acknowledges Terry's increased sense of isolation after her daughter's marriage and evaluates her for possible major depression. He further suggests a referral to the clinic's social worker as a means of helping her pursue a volunteer activity and increase her social interactions.

This approach usually helps diminish the patient's anxiety and decreases the frequency of phone calls. If the patient's distress does not improve with such interventions, a referral for psychotherapy and evaluation for a possible comorbid anxiety disorder is indicated.

OBSESSIVE–COMPULSIVE PERSONALITY DISORDER

Symptoms & Signs

Individuals with obsessive–compulsive personality disorder are preoccupied with orderliness, perfectionism, and control. They are excessively concerned with details and rules, tend to be overly moralistic, and are usually focused on work to the exclusion of leisure. They find it difficult to adapt themselves to others and instead insist that others follow their plans. Their general inflexibility and restricted emotional expression betray an underlying fear of losing control. Because they can be indecisive, they feel distressed when faced with the need to make decisions.

Differential Diagnosis

Obsessive–compulsive disorder (see Chapter 26) is distinguished from obsessive–compulsive personality disorder by the presence of actual obsessions (repetitive intrusive thoughts) and compulsions. Sometimes, however, both disorders coexist in one patient, and obsessive–compulsive personality disorder can also be confused with other personality disorders.

Illness Experience & Illness Behavior

Illness is threatening to persons with obsessive–compulsive personality disorder because it generates an intense fear of losing control over bodily functions and emotions. Patients may experience extremely unsettling feelings of shame and vulnerability. They may also feel anger at the disruption of their usual daily routines by medical appointments and treatments. They may fear having to relinquish control to health care providers. In the clinician's office, their intense anxiety tends to drive them to ask repetitive questions and to pay excessive attention to detail.

The Clinician–Patient Relationship

Caregivers may react to patients with obsessive–compulsive personality disorder by becoming impatient at their repetitive questions, cutting their answers short. They may feel their competence challenged by their patients' insistence on knowing every single detail and reason for choosing a particular treatment. Clinicians may also inadvertently attempt to control treatment planning rather than making it a joint effort, without realizing how important it is for these patients to remain in control.

Specific Management Strategies

Helpful strategies in working with patients with obsessive–compulsive personality disorder include taking a comprehensive history, performing a careful diagnostic workup, giving patients a clear and thorough explanation of their diagnosis and treatment options, and providing and explaining laboratory test results. It is important not to overemphasize uncertainties about treatments or the patient's possible response to treatment. Patients find it reassuring when clinicians cite literature reports and avoid vague and inexact impressionistic explanations. It is helpful to treat these patients as equal partners, encourage self-monitoring, allow their participation in treatment, and give them recognition for their clear reasoning and high standards.

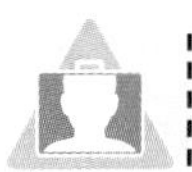

CASE ILLUSTRATION 10

Sam, a 42-year-old biochemist, requests an appointment with his primary care clinician for evaluation of an uncomfortable lump in his left groin. The clinician is familiar with Sam's mild nervousness during routine medical check-ups and his tendency to ask detailed questions about his health. After a physical examination, the clinician diagnoses an inguinal hernia and recommends a surgical consultation for further evaluation and possible surgery. Sam, in his usual formal and somewhat restricted manner—but this time appearing visibly more anxious—repeatedly asks several questions about surgical repair, whether the literature discusses any alternative treatments, and what guidelines clinicians follow to recommend one treatment over another. He then asks questions about the risks of general anesthesia and whether this procedure can be performed under local anesthesia.

When the clinician tries to reassure him that this is a routine procedure, Sam asks him whether he is sure of his diagnosis; he also asks him to list the criteria he used in diagnosing the inguinal hernia. Sam also talks at length about his responsibilities at work and expresses concern that surgery might disrupt ongoing projects at his laboratory, as several people depend on him for regular supervision. He also wants to know how long his clinician has known the recommended surgeon, and whether they have worked together in the past.

The clinician explains that the surgeon is both trustworthy and well known to him. He praises Sam for his thoroughness and initiative in finding out about treatment alternatives before making a decision. He answers basic questions in a precise manner and defers some questions to the surgeon, explaining that these will be better answered by a specialist. He reassures Sam that he will not wait for a written report but will personally contact the surgeon after the consultation to discuss treatment options. The clinician also suggests a follow-up appointment to help Sam with his decision.

Although Sam continues to express concern that the surgery will disrupt his work, his anxiety decreases somewhat after the clinician takes his concerns seriously. His questions are answered precisely, and the clinician further suggests an article in the literature that he can read to learn more about the treatment of inguinal hernias.

Reassurance is essential here. Redirection of many questions should be gentle but firm. Citing evidence-based guidelines is helpful, as it appeals to the patient's strength of using rules and structure.

TREATMENT OF PERSONALITY DISORDERS

For the primary care clinician or medical specialist, the preceding sections describe the first-line approach for managing the medical patient with a comorbid personality disorder. In addition, it is important to identify and address other comorbid behavioral health disorders. Patients with personality disorders have high rates of psychiatric comorbidity, particularly with major depressive, bipolar, substance use, posttraumatic stress, panic, social anxiety, and obsessive–compulsive disorders. The symptoms of the personality disorders will often improve, sometimes markedly, when co-morbid behavioral health disorders are adequately treated.

Regarding treatment specific for personality disorders, the treatments with the strongest evidence for efficacy are typically psychosocial in nature, rather than pharmacologic. These treatments include multiple evidence-based psychotherapies, including cognitive behavioral therapy, mentalization-based therapy, dialectal behavioral therapy, psychodynamic therapy, and acceptance and commitment therapy. Each of these treatments addresses in some way the distorted thought patterns, dysregulated emotions, maladaptive behaviors, and impaired interpersonal functioning that cause distress for these patients. The choice of which specific therapy will depend on local resources, patient preference, and the recommendation of a behavioral health clinician.

Psychopharmacological treatments are used when psychosocial treatments are not sufficient. Definitive psychopharmacological treatment does not exist for a given personality disorder and, in general, there are limited efficacy data. Nevertheless, pharmacotherapy may be initiated by the primary care clinician, ideally with support from a psychiatrist. Medications are at times helpful in targeting symptoms associated with a personality disorder cluster. For example, anxiety and fear are the most dominant symptoms for patients with cluster C disorders (avoidant, dependent, and obsessive–compulsive personality disorder), anxiety and fear are the most dominant symptoms. Symptoms in these patients may improve by treatment with selective serotonin reuptake inhibitors (e.g., escitalopram or fluoxetine). Time-limited symptomatic treatment with a benzodiazepine might be considered. For patients with cluster A disorders (paranoid, schizoid, and schizotypal personality disorder), symptoms such as paranoid ideation and suspiciousness may improve with low-dose antipsychotic treatment (e.g., risperidone or aripiprazole). Consultation with a psychiatrist is especially advised before initiating antipsychotic medication, given the high side effect burden of these medications.

Patients with cluster B disorders (antisocial, borderline, histrionic, and narcissistic personality disorder) often appear dramatic and emotional and have impulsive behaviors; these symptoms may benefit from pharmacologic treatment. Borderline personality disorder in particular has the largest evidence base supporting psychopharmacology. A reasonable first step for the patient with prominent anxiety, anger, or depression is an antidepressant medication, such as a selective serotonin reuptake inhibitor, provided that a comorbid bipolar disorder is not present. A next step is a "mood stabilizer" medication, starting with more tolerable agents (such as lamotrigine or topiramate) and subsequently if needed medicines like valproate or lithium. If symptoms of dissociation, paranoia, or transient psychosis are prominent, then low-dose second-generation antipsychotic medication may be helpful, such as quetiapine or aripiprazole. The value of psychiatric consultation for cases requiring antipsychotic or multiple medications cannot be overstressed.

When contemplating pharmacotherapy for any personality disorder, psychiatric consultation should always be considered. If a medication is initiated, repeated assessment should be used to confirm that symptom improvement has occurred to justify the cost and side effects of medication. Rating scales for target symptoms should be used whenever possible to minimize variability in reporting and recall. Careful use of mediations for off-label indications is warranted, so long as inappropriate polypharmacy is avoided by discontinuing any medication demonstrated to be ineffective. The principles of "start low, go slow" and "make one change at a time" are prudent in these cases, even though patients may advocate for a more aggressive approach.

SUMMARY

Common themes emerge from the study of specific personality disorders regarding how clinicians can manage the therapeutic alliance and treatment plan for patients with any personality disorder, or indeed for patients who have "personality traits" suggestive of a disorder but are not diagnosed with the full syndrome.

Crucially, clinicians must be mindful of their own emotions and automatic thoughts that arise in the presence of such patients. If emotions are ignored or judgmental thoughts go unchallenged, then the clinician will not be able to provide the best care possible. It is crucial that clinicians remind themselves to "not take it personally" with respect to challenging patient behaviors, whether those behaviors be avoidant, aggressive, or flattering.

Additionally, clinicians should stay grounded in objective data and standards when managing treatment.

Patients with personality disorders may explicitly or implicitly push clinicians to "bend the rules," and doing so is rarely in their best interests. Clinicians should strive to be calmly supportive and remain within professional boundaries. Consulting colleagues or specialists about patient's challenging behavior can be helpful in maintaining the right therapeutic stance.

The presence of a personality disorder (or traits of a personality disorder) has significant implications for a variety of health outcomes. Whether or not a patient accepts specialist referral to manage psychiatric symptoms—and many will not, particularly if insight is low—the value of a thoughtful primary care provider cannot be overstated. A steady, empathic authority figure who maintains firm, fair boundaries can be therapeutic above and beyond any specific medical care provided. The skillful primary care clinician may even learn to enjoy caring for such patients, who despite their challenging presentations can, with time and support, get better.

SUGGESTED READINGS

Gabbard GO. Psychotherapy of personality disorders. *J Psychother Pract Res* 2000;9:1–6.

Geringer ES, Stern TA. Coping with medical illness: the impact of personality types. *Psychosomatics* 1986;27:251–261.

Giesen-Bloo J, van Dyck R, Spinhoven P, et al. Outpatient psychotherapy for borderline personality disorder: randomized trial of schema-focused therapy vs transference-focused psychotherapy. *Arch Gen Psychiatry* 2006;63:649–658. [Erratum in: *Arch Gen Psychiatry* 2006;63:1008.]

Gross R, Olfson M, Gameroff M, et al. Borderline personality disorder in primary care. *Arch Intern Med* 2002;162:53–60.

Linehan MM, Comtois KA, Murray AM, et al. Two-year randomized controlled trial and follow-up of dialectical behavior therapy vs therapy by experts for suicidal behaviors and borderline personality disorder. *Arch Gen Psychiatry* 2006;63:757–766.

Markovitz PJ. Related articles, links: recent trends in the pharmacotherapy of personality disorders. *J Personal Disord* 2004;18: 90–101.

Psychosis

31

Olesya Pokorna, MD & Emma Samelson-Jones, MD

INTRODUCTION

Psychotic symptoms include hallucinations, delusions (fixed false beliefs, such as the belief that aliens have taken over one's body and are controlling one's thoughts and actions), and disorganized thinking (as demonstrated by illogical or incoherent speech) or behavior. In chronic form, these symptoms are most commonly associated with schizophrenia spectrum disorders, but they can occur in the context of many other illnesses, including major depression or bipolar disorder, substance intoxication or withdrawal, borderline personality disorder, and a wide range of other medical conditions, including neurodegenerative, infectious, inflammatory, and autoimmune diseases (Table 31-1).

SCHIZOPHRENIA SPECTRUM DISORDERS

The schizophrenia spectrum disorders include brief psychotic disorder, schizophreniform disorder, schizophrenia, schizoaffective disorder, and delusional disorder. They are distinguished from each other by the duration and types of psychotic symptoms, and the presence or absence of concurrent mood symptoms.

The onset of multiple types of psychotic symptoms (delusions, hallucinations, disorganized speech or behavior) in the absence of affective symptoms, a toxic exposure, or an associated medical condition defines **brief psychotic disorder** if it lasts less than a month, **schizophreniform** disorder if it lasts 1–6 months, and **schizophrenia** if it lasts at least 6 months. Schizophrenia tends to begin in late adolescence or early adulthood and affects between 0.3% and 0.9% of the population worldwide. **Schizoaffective** disorder requires the presence of multiple psychotic symptoms in addition to recurrent episodes of major depression or mania. It also commonly starts in adolescence or young adulthood, and affects an additional 0.3% of the population. **Delusional disorder** is characterized by the presence of isolated delusions (such as the belief that a neighbor has placed cameras all over one's apartment and is constantly monitoring one's conversations), without functional impairment outside of the impact of the delusion. In contrast to schizophrenia, it most commonly begins in middle age and has a lifetime prevalence of 0.2%.

Schizophrenia

The diagnosis of schizophrenia requires the presence of two of five of the following symptoms lasting at least 1 month: hallucinations, delusions, disorganized thinking, disorganized behavior, or negative symptoms. Negative symptoms are deficits of normal emotional responses or thought processes, such as reduced emotional expression, poverty of speech, anhedonia, lack of motivation, or lack of desire to form social relationships. These symptoms exist within a 6-month period of functional decline. Although not required for the diagnosis, this decline usually involves some degree of cognitive impairment, most commonly deficits in processing speed, working memory, social cognition, and executive functioning. The severity of negative and cognitive symptoms correlates more closely with reduced overall level of functioning than does the severity of the positive symptoms of hallucinations, delusions, or disorganization.

There are both genetic and environmental risk factors in the development of schizophrenia. There is a 50% concordance of schizophrenia between identical twins, and among siblings and parents of people with schizophrenia, there is a 10–15 times increased risk of the illness, compared with the general population. Schizotypal personality disorder, which is characterized by a pervasive pattern of social and interpersonal deficits as well as cognitive or perceptual distortions or eccentricities of behavior, is more prevalent among first-degree biological relatives of people with schizophrenia than among the general population. Environmental exposures, including prenatal environmental insults such as maternal infections or nutritional deficiencies, complications at the time of birth, and other types of trauma increase the risk of developing subsequent psychotic disorders.

Table 31-1. Differential diagnosis of new onset psychosis.

Schizophrenia spectrum disorders, including brief psychotic disorder, schizophreniform disorder, schizophrenia, schizoaffective disorder, and delusional disorder
Affective psychoses, including major depression with psychotic features or bipolar disorder (bipolar depression or mania) with psychotic features
Other psychiatric disorders, including PTSD, borderline personality disorder
Substance intoxication with amphetamines, cocaine, PCP, cannabis, and synthetic cannabinoids such as spice, psychedelic drugs such as LSD, psilocybin, or ayahuasca
Substance withdrawal from alcohol, benzodiazepines, barbiturates
Medication-induced psychosis from steroids, dopamine agonists, and others
Delirium, characterized by fluctuating levels of attention and confusion that often presents rapidly. Broad differential diagnosis, including electrolyte abnormalities, hypoxia or hypercapnia, infections, hepatic or uremic encephalopathy, and others
Endocrine disorders, including hypothyroidism (myxedema madness), hyperthyroidism, adrenal insufficiency, hypo- or hyperparathyroidism, Cushing's disease, or Cushing's syndrome
Inflammatory disorders, including anti-NMDA receptor encephalitis, systemic lupus erythematosus (lupus psychosis usually occurs early in the illness in context of florid clinical and serological activity), multiple sclerosis, leukodystrophies
Infectious diseases involving the brain, including HIV, neurosyphilis, herpes simplex encephalitis, prion disorders
Neurodegenerative disorders, including Alzheimer's disease, dementia with Lewy Bodies, Parkinson's disease, Huntington's disease
Neurological disorders, including traumatic brain injury (TBI), brain tumors, or other space occupying lesions in the head, stroke, seizures
Vitamin deficiency with vitamin B12
Metabolic disorders, including Wilson's disease and acute intermittent porphyria

Usually, before the onset of the psychotic symptoms of schizophrenia, there is a prodromal period of subclinical signs and symptoms that can last from weeks to years. Prodromal symptoms commonly include an increase in social isolation, decreased emotional expressivity, and a decline in performance in school or work settings. Symptoms of depression and anxiety are also common. There can also be attenuated psychotic symptoms, including illusions or other perceptual abnormalities, or odd beliefs with preserved skepticism as to the reality of these experiences. The onset of psychotic symptoms marks the beginning of the schizophrenia syndrome. Prompt treatment of the first episode of psychosis shortens the duration of psychotic episodes, reduces the risk of recurrent episodes, and reduces the degree of functional deterioration. Early intervention efforts to minimize the duration of untreated psychosis may therefore reduce the lifetime morbidity associated with schizophrenia.

Clinical Approach to Psychosis

People who suffer with psychotic symptoms have experiences or beliefs that are not part of a shared reality with others. They may be hearing the voice of God telling them what the future will bring or believe that the FBI is tracking them and that they are in physical danger. As a clinician trying to help a family, it is important to understand both the individual's perceptual experience of reality and the reality of their situation. Just as an appropriate evaluation of people with memory problems requires more information than their own account of their history, an appropriate evaluation of someone with psychosis requires both the individual's account and a parallel history from someone whose reality testing is not impaired.

The primary goal of a first visit with a person with psychosis is to develop enough of a therapeutic relationship that the person is willing to return for a second visit. If a person is distrustful or frankly paranoid, this can be challenging, so keeping problem lists short and consensual (e.g., "to help you feel less anxious") is advisable. It may be helpful to keep the interview short and to provide plenty of physical space and emotional distance, for example by using less eye contact than typical, or by seeing the patient in a larger room. Neutral, calm body language and straightforward verbal communication can go a long way toward putting a fearful patient at ease. Be mindful of signs of physical agitation, including hand wringing, fist clenching, or pacing, and stop the interview early if the level of agitation is rising.

HISTORY

A reasonable screen for psychosis in someone with depression or mania, for whom your suspicion for psychosis is low, could include the questions: "Do you ever hear voices that other people do not hear?" and, "Do you ever feel like your mind is playing tricks on you?" If your suspicion for psychosis is higher, based on prior

Table 31-2. Asking about psychotic symptoms.

Screening Questions:
Do you ever hear voices that other people do not hear?
Do you ever see things that other people do not see?
Do your thoughts ever feel strange to you in some way?
Do you ever feel like your mind is playing tricks on you?
Do you ever feel as if someone were out to get you or trying to harm you? (paranoid ideation)
Do you ever feel as if things online or on TV were written especially for you? (ideas of reference)
Do you ever feel as if you have special abilities or powers? (grandiosity)
Do you ever feel that someone is putting thoughts or feelings into your mind? (thought insertion)
Do you ever have thoughts that are so vivid that you worry that someone else could hear them? (thought broadcasting)

Further evaluation of voices:
Can you tell me more about your experience of hearing voices?
How many voices do you hear? Can you tell if the voice is a man or a woman? Many people I've spoken with have thought that their voice might be a person they know, or some kind of God or devil. Have you ever thought something similar? What makes you think the voice is (specific name)?
Can you tell me what kinds of things the voice says? Does it ever talk to you or about you? Does the voice ever tell you to do anything? Give you advice or suggestions? Comment on what you are doing or thinking? Threaten to harm you or someone else?
Are there certain times or occasions when your voices are more active? (time of day, when doing certain activities, or feeling a certain way). Are there times when you don't hear voices? Is there anything you have found that makes the voices go away or seem less intense (talking with someone, talking with the voice, watching TV, drugs, or medications)
How do you feel when the voice speaks?
When the voice talks, what do you usually do?
(If the voice tells you to do something)—Do you do what the voice commands? Do you ever resist the voice's commands?

Further evaluation of delusional experiences:
Tell me more about this experience.
Do you remember the first time that you had this experience? What triggered it?
How does this experience make you feel?
What do you do when you have this experience?
How much time did you spend thinking about this experience in the past month?
What do you make of this experience (i.e., how do you explain your experience)? What do other people make of this experience?
How sure are you about your explanation of this experience?

history or a positive screen in the first two questions, it may be useful to expand screening questions to include all those listed in Table 31-2.

The goal of further history gathering is to understand patients' psychotic experiences, reducing their sense of isolation by helping them talk about them within a safe space. Because talking about psychotic experiences requires a high degree of vulnerability on the part of the patient, it is important to use a gentle approach, bring an attitude of genuine curiosity, and start with open-ended questions. The evaluation of hearing voices involves learning what the experience is, what exacerbates or alleviates it, and how the experience of hearing voices affects the patient's feelings and behavior. The evaluation of delusional experiences involves understanding how the belief developed, how preoccupying the belief is, how it affects the patient's feelings and behaviors, and how the person makes sense of the belief. Specific questions for further exploring auditory hallucinations and delusional beliefs are listed in Table 31-2.

PHYSICAL EXAMINATION & LABORATORY STUDIES

In the case of new onset psychosis, the differential diagnosis is broad (see Table 31-1). It is therefore important to complete a full medical history and exam, with particular emphasis on the endocrine, rheumatologic, and neurologic review of systems and exam. Any change in level of consciousness, new onset seizures, focal neurologic signs, rapid decline in cognitive status, or a history or exam suggestive of systemic autoimmune or neurological illness should prompt further medical workup, including relevant labs and head imaging. Additionally, if the onset of psychosis is rapid and without a prodromal period, or otherwise atypical for a schizophrenia spectrum disorder (e.g., the presence of visual hallucinations without auditory hallucinations), further medical workup would also be indicated. Table 31-3 describes the risk factors that increase the probability of a medical or neurological cause of new onset psychosis.

Table 31-3. Risk factors for medical or neurologic cause of psychosis.

- Onset of psychosis > age 50
- Acute onset of symptoms (over days to weeks)
- Visual or tactile hallucinations without co-occurring auditory hallucinations
- Any olfactory or gustatory hallucinations
- Intellectual disability or developmental disability
- History of head trauma, loss of consciousness or fluctuating levels of consciousness, or seizures
- History of cancer or cancer risk factors (smoking, genetic predisposition)
- Personal or family history of autoimmune, neurologic, endocrine, metabolic, or genetic disorders

Toxicology screening and a few basic labs should be routinely ordered in the setting of otherwise unexplained new psychotic symptoms (Table 31-4). Head imaging is not recommended in the workup of new onset psychosis in people under the age of 50 with no significant findings on history or exam.

MANAGEMENT OF PSYCHOSIS

If psychotic symptoms are secondary to a medical or neurologic etiology, treatment is directed toward the underlying disorder, with antipsychotic medications used as adjunctive treatments only. For example, treatment of lupus psychosis would center on appropriate immunosuppression. The pharmacologic management of the affective psychoses (depression, mania, or a mixed episode with psychotic features) involves the addition of an antipsychotic medication to either an antidepressant (in the case of unipolar depression), or a mood stabilizer such as lithium or valproate (in the case of bipolar disorder). In people with schizophrenia spectrum disorders, antipsychotic medications may reduce the symptoms of hallucinations, delusions, and disorganized thinking or behaviors. These medications unfortunately do not improve negative symptoms or cognitive deficits associated with psychotic disorders.

Table 31-4. First-line medical assessment of new onset psychosis.

- Detailed medical and neurologic history and exam, with special attention to endocrine, rheumatologic, and neurologic systems.
- Routine labs should include a complete blood count with differential to evaluate for evidence of infection, electrolytes with calcium, liver function tests, urine drug screen, thyroid stimulating hormone, treponemal screen for syphilis (fluorescent treponemal absorption test or other), HIV, and vitamin B12.
- Consider head imaging in someone with new onset psychosis over the age of 50 or with risk factors for medical or neurologic causes of psychosis.
- If the patient is not currently taking an antipsychotic medication but planning to start, obtain baseline cholesterol panel, HgA1c or fasting glucose, and consider baseline prolactin if starting a medication associated with a high risk of hyperprolactinemia (risperidone, haloperidol).

Several converging lines of scientific evidence have shown that heavy marijuana use during early adolescence increases later risk of schizophrenia. A dose–response relationship also exists, in that the use of more potent strains of marijuana, that is those with higher THC content, confers a higher risk of developing schizophrenia than use of less potent strains. After the age of 21, susceptible individuals may still develop psychotic symptoms in response to marijuana, but the strength of the causal association between marijuana and schizophrenia diminishes. Individuals who present with psychosis and who are also using cannabis or other pro-psychotic drugs, including stimulants, PCP, and hallucinogens, should be educated about the association between the use of certain drugs and psychosis, and a trial of abstinence should be recommended.

Comprehensive care for psychotic disorders aims to both reduce psychotic symptoms, and, more importantly, to help a patient recover. Treatments focused on psychosocial recovery aim to help an individual maintain or regain the ability to form and maintain social relationships, and to participate in work or school. Early intervention programs that offer individual psychotherapy, family psychoeducation, supported employment or education, and medication management within a multidisciplinary team of providers reduce the morbidity and disability associated with psychotic disorders. Additional treatments that can support recovery include social skills training, multiple family groups, membership in social organizations for people with mental illness (sometimes referred to as clubhouses), and appropriate treatment for co-morbid addiction, mood, or anxiety disorders.

ANTIPSYCHOTIC MEDICATIONS

Among people with schizophrenia, 30–40% have a good response to antipsychotic medications, 40% have a partial response, and 20–30% have no significant response. If an individual is going to respond to a medication, typically the initial response will be within 1–2 weeks, a significant response within 2–4 weeks, and most of the expected response by 10 weeks. Clozapine is a notable exception to this expected response time course among antipsychotics. It can take up to 6 months to achieve a full therapeutic response from a given dose of clozapine.

The choice of which antipsychotic medications to use involves balancing the risks, benefits, and costs of the available medications. On the whole, first-generation antipsychotic medications (FGAs) and second-generation antipsychotic medications (SGAs) have similar efficacy and dropout rates, but different side effect profiles. The FGAs are associated with a higher rate of extrapyramidal side effects, including dystonia, akathisia, parkinsonism, and tardive dyskinesia. The SGAs are more commonly associated with weight gain, dyslipidemia, and an increased risk for diabetes. For people who are "treatment resistant," meaning that they fail to respond to adequate trials of two antipsychotic medications, clozapine has superior efficacy, as compared with other antipsychotic medications. Clozapine also reduces suicidal behaviors in patients with schizophrenia and schizoaffective disorder.

Because all antipsychotic medications carry significant risks with long-term exposure, clinicians should always aim for minimal effective dosing. Table 31-5 provides details about dosing and side effect considerations for many of the commonly used antipsychotic medications.

Long-acting injectable (LAIs) formulations of several antipsychotic medications are available and are administered intramuscularly every 2–12 weeks depending on the medication. They are an effective alternative to oral medications for patients who have responded well to antipsychotic medications, but are at high risk for relapse due to medication nonadherence. Tolerance to an oral formulation of a medication is necessary prior to administering a LAI to avoid ongoing adverse responses. Haloperidol, paliperidone, risperidone, and aripiprazole all have long-acting injectable formulation and should be considered for patients with a history of treatment nonadherence. As compared to the corresponding oral medication, LAIs have similar side effect profiles and do not appear to confer additional risks of adverse outcomes.

There are also short-acting injectable forms of several antipsychotic medications that are used in emergency situations to treat acutely agitated psychotic patients. When verbal de-escalation fails, oral medication should be offered first to give a patient a sense of agency and control over the situation. To ensure drug ingestion, liquid or disintegrating tablet formulations are often preferred. If the patient is unwilling or unable to take oral medications, clinicians may administer medications intramuscularly. Parenteral haloperidol, olanzapine, aripiprazole, and ziprasidone are frequently used for managing acute psychosis emergently. One common combination treatment for agitation includes haloperidol (PO/IM) 0.5–5mg, lorazepam (PO/IM/IV) 0.5–2 mg, along with either diphenhydramine 25–50 mg or benztropine 0.5–2 mg to prevent dystonic reactions or other extrapyramidal side effects.

Antipsychotic medications are also used in several nonpsychotic conditions, including bipolar disorder, refractory anxiety disorders, obsessive compulsive disorder, unipolar depression, tics and Tourette's disorder, autism-related irritability, and agitated delirium. Lower doses of antipsychotic medications are usually sufficient to treat these conditions as compared to doses required to treat schizophrenia spectrum disorders.

It can seem complicated to talk with patients about antipsychotic medications when they have impaired reality testing, or trouble with attention and cognition. Tailor the information about the potential risks and benefits to the patient's ability to comprehend the information. For someone who is suffering with auditory hallucinations without any insight into the nonreality of the situation, telling the patient "It sounds like the voices are interfering with your sleep. This medication should help with your sleep," may be sufficient informed consent at the beginning of treatment. As the patient's condition improves with treatment, more nuanced conversations become possible, and the discussion about risks and benefits can continue in more depth. Informed consent for antipsychotic medications should be understood as an ongoing process, rather than a one-time conversation.

PSYCHOSOCIAL INTERVENTIONS

A combination of appropriate antipsychotic medications and psychosocial interventions can significantly improve clinical outcomes and make a positive impact on the patient's overall functioning, social integration, quality of life, and treatment compliance. The following psychosocial interventions have been shown to be effective in multiple research studies.

Therapy

CBT adapted for psychosis (CBTp) focuses on optimizing functioning, understanding psychotic experiences, and reducing distress associated with delusions or hallucinations. It is most commonly provided on an individual basis, but can also be delivered in a group setting. Therapeutic work starts with identifying the most troubling symptoms and setting achievable goals to motivate treatment. A therapist then gently leads that patient to develop alternative explanations, test the evidence for and against maladaptive beliefs, and identify effective coping strategies.

Family Interventions

Due to the chronic and disabling nature of psychotic illnesses, family members often carry a significant burden of care. There is evidence to suggest that people living in family environments that include a high level of hostility, criticism, and emotional over-involvement are at higher risk for a psychotic relapse. The main goals of family interventions for psychotic illness is to prevent relapse, promote medication compliance, reduce caretaker stress, and help patients function more independently. Table 31-6 details initial psychoeducation interventions

Table 31-5. Antipsychotic medications.

Name	Formulations	Starting Dose	Step-up Dose	Target Daily Dose	Maximum Daily dose	Unique Side Effects	Comments
First-generation Antipsychotics							
Haloperidol	tabs, oral concentrate, IM, LAI (every 4 weeks), IV	0.5–5 mg BID	5 mg	5–20 mg/d	30 mg/d	High risk of EPS	High potency IV formulation carries highest risk of QTc prolongation, consider continuous EKG
Trifluoperazine	tabs	5 mg daily	5 mg	10–20 mg/d	40 mg	High risk of EPS	High potency
Perphenazine	tabs	4–8 mg PO TID	4–8 mg	24–48 mg in divided doses	64 mg/d		Mid potency Once a target dose is reached, can be given BID or at bedtime
Second-generation Antipsychotics							
Clozapine	PO, ODT	12.5 mg at bedtime	See below*	200–400 mg/d	900 mg/d	High risk for: sedation, weight gain, metabolic syndrome, orthostasis, anticholinergic SEs *Risk for*: agranulocytosis, seizures, myocarditis	-Indicated for treatment resistant schizophrenia (failed 2 prior antipsychotic trials) -Reduces risk of suicide -Requires weekly lab monitoring** and careful dose titration when starting
Olanzapine	tabs, ODT, IM	2.5–5 mg at bedtime	5 mg	10–20 mg	30 mg/d	High risk for: weight gain, metabolic syndrome, sedation, anticholinergic SEs	-Most efficacious antipsychotic other than clozapine (CATIE study***) -Not recommended as first-line treatment in young people due to significant metabolic side effects
Risperidone	tab, solution, ODT (M-Tab), LAI (every 2 weeks)	0.5–1 mg BID	1–2 mg	4–6 mg/d	16 mg/d	High risk for: Hyperprolactinemia orthostasis EPS	-Can be dosed once daily when at target dose -Paliperidone, the active metabolite of risperidone, is available in a LAI given every 4–12 weeks. Oral tolerance can be established with risperidone prior to use of paliperidone LAI.
Quetiapine	Tabs: IR, XR	25 mg daily or BID	25–50 mg	300–600 mg	800 mg	High risk for: orthostasis, weight gain, metabolic syndrome. Associated with cataracts. Low risk of EPS	-Initial slower dose titration is required to avoid significant orthostasis -XR formulation can be started at 200mg bedtime

(*Continued*)

Table 31-5. Antipsychotic medications. (*Continued*)

Name	Formulations	Starting Dose	Step-up Dose	Target Daily Dose	Maximum Daily dose	Unique Side Effects	Comments
Aripiprazole	PO tabs, PO solution, IM, LAI every 4–10 weeks	5 mg daily	5–10 mg	10–20 mg/d	30 mg/d	Moderate risk of akathisia or insomnia early in treatment. Lower risk of metabolic syndrome, QTc prolongation	Can be used to treat hyperprolactinemia
Ziprasidone	PO, IM	20 mg daily or BID with food	20–40 mg	40 mg BID	80 mg BID	High risk for QTc prolongation. Moderate risk of sedation. Low risk of weight gain and metabolic syndrome	Bioavailability is increased when taken with food
Lurasidone	PO	20–40 mg daily with food	20–40 mg/d	60–120 mg/d	160 mg/d	Favorable metabolic profile Moderate risk of EPS, in particular akathisia	Bioavailability is increased when taken with at least 350 cal of food

Clozapine titration*: Start at 12.5–25 mg at bedtime. Increase by 25–50 mg every few days, either at bedtime or in twice daily dosing, up to a target dose of 300 mg a day. Slow titration minimizes risk of orthostasis, seizures, and oversedation.
Clozapine lab monitoring**: Baseline EKG, ANC (absolute neutrophil count) every week for 6 months, then every other week for 6 months, then monthly. Consider troponin/CRP for first 4–8 weeks. HgA1c or fasting glucose and lipids, at baseline, 3 months, then yearly.
CATIE study***: Clinical Antipsychotic Trials of Intervention Effectiveness.
Abbreviations: BID = twice daily; IM = intramuscular; IR = immediate release; LAI = long acting injectable; ODT = oral disintegrating tablet; PO = oral; QID = four times a day; tab = tablet; TID = three times a day; XR = extended release.

Table 31-6. Psychoeducation for families struggling with new onset psychosis.

- Psychosis refers to changes in the brain that interfere with a person's experience of the world. Symptoms may include hearing voices or seeing visions (hallucinations), false beliefs or marked suspicions of others (delusions), jumbled thoughts or speech (disorganized thinking), and difficulty concentrating or making sense of social situations (cognitive symptoms). People who experience psychosis have a heightened sensitivity to incoming sensory information (sights, sounds, smells, touch, movement); stress; rapid changes in expectations, events, or routines; illicit drugs; and criticism or lack of warmth.
- The symptoms of psychosis are treatable.
- Psychosis is no one's fault—neither the symptomatic person nor the family is to blame for this sensitivity.
- Symptoms of psychosis should not be ignored. The longer that they exist, the less chance there is for treatment effectiveness and complete recovery. If you look up psychosis, you will find all sorts of things, much of which will not be useful as you navigate this illness. A certain number of people recover completely. A certain number of people have serious trouble for a long time. Most people end up in between these two options. We know that the sooner that we intervene, the better people do.
- The early experience of psychosis is extremely confusing and traumatic for both the person and her family. In addition to the use of medications to reduce the vulnerability to psychotic symptoms (i.e., hallucinations, delusions, or disorganized thinking), comprehensive care for psychotic disorders involves support, counseling, and education that aims to reduce stress and teach effective coping strategies for both the individual and family.
- The aim of treatment is psychosocial recovery, meaning a return to premorbid abilities to form and maintain social relationships, and to participate in work or school. Early intervention programs that offer individual psychotherapy, family psychoeducation, supported employment or education, and medication management within a multidisciplinary team of providers help reduce the disability associated with psychotic disorders.

for families. Family interventions provide psychoeducation about the nature and the course of the psychotic illness, help reduce stigma, emphasize the role of medication adherence, help family members recognize signs of psychotic relapse, and teach effective communication skills and problem solving. These interventions usually last 6–9 months and take place in a group setting.

Social Skills Training

Most patients with psychotic disorders experience some degree of social impairment, which further limits their social and occupational functioning, contributes to overall distress, and leads to psychosocial isolation. Social skills training aims at remediating deficits in areas of social communication.

Supported Employment

The goal of supported employment is to optimize vocational functioning in people with serious mental illnesses. One model, Individual Placement and Support (IPS), integrates employment support with mental health services. Supported employment interventions start with identifying a patient's strengths, professional experiences, and personal preferences, and assists with a job search in the community. Once a participant finds a suitable position, IPS provides open-ended individual support to ensure job retention.

Clubhouses

The clubhouse model of psychosocial rehabilitation helps people whose lives have been interrupted by serious mental illness rejoin the worlds of friendships, family, employment and education, and gain access to the services and support that they may individually need to continue their recovery. Unlike mental health clinics, clubhouses are open in the evenings and on holidays. Members are closely involved with all the tasks of running a clubhouse.

Assertive Community Treatment

Assertive community treatment (ACT) teams provide intensive case-management and mental health treatment in the community. The interdisciplinary teams include a psychiatrist, nurse, case managers, and employment specialists; and they provide services in a community, including home visits, medication delivery, therapy, and supported employment.

CASE ILLUSTRATION 1: NEW ONSET PSYCHOSIS

A 19-year-old man, Jim, is brought to his primary care provider's office by his parents for the new onset of "hearing voices." Jim is sitting slumped in the waiting room chair, wearing sunglasses and headphones. Both his parents are with him and they look very anxious.

You speak with Jim alone first. He tells you that he is frequently distracted by two voices. For the past 3 months, he has been hearing a man's voice, who narrates what he is doing in the third person (e.g.,

"He's walking through the door. He's getting into the car.") He finds this annoying and distracting but is not emotionally upset by it. For the past month, however, he has also been hearing a woman's voice that calls to him directly and tells him that she is in trouble and that only he can save her. Sometimes he hears her scream, "as though she is being tortured." Sometimes she yells at him that he is taking too long to help her. He is highly distressed when he hears her talking to him. He thinks the woman is real, although he hasn't seen her. Maybe he is "connected to the woman through a spiritual connection." He's not sure. He tends to hear her voice more often at night, when he is alone in bed, and it keeps him from falling asleep. He thinks that whoever is torturing her is also monitoring him, maybe through the control of cameras on electronic devices. He has taped over the cameras on his phone and laptop and has been keeping the shades in his bedroom drawn at all times. He is confused about what is happening to him, and highly distressed. He denies any medical history, drug use, or other symptoms. There is no history of loss of consciousness, seizures, changes in vision, or weakness. He has not been sick recently, has no new sexual contacts, and has not had any rashes or pain. His last HIV test was a year ago. He denies hot or cold intolerance, changes in hair or nails, fatigue, or changes in his vision. A complete physical exam is normal.

You ask if you can talk with his parents, and he says ok. You ask him to wait in the waiting room, so that you can talk with his parents alone. His parents say that Jim met all of his developmental milestones as a child. He was mildly anxious in middle school but more social and outgoing in high school, and he graduated from high school with honors. He went to college last year. His first semester went well—he made friends, received As & Bs in his classes, and participated in several clubs. Starting about 6 months ago, he withdrew from the clubs and seemed to spend more time alone on his computer, but he continued to go to class. His parents worried that he might be depressed. He finished the last semester with a C average and then came home for the summer. He has been home for about a month and spends most of his time in his room over the past several weeks. He has been yelling in his room on occasion, telling someone to leave him alone, that he can't help them. He eats dinner with the family but doesn't talk much and seems distracted much of the time. Two weeks ago, he started putting duct tape on various electronics in the house, and he lowers all of the shades in the house if he is left home alone. His maternal aunt was diagnosed with schizophrenia when she was 23; there is no family history of depression, anxiety, bipolar disorder, or suicide. His maternal grandmother has diabetes, but there is no history of autoimmune, rheumatologic, sudden death, or cancer in the family. He has not threatened anyone or talked about hurting himself or not wanting to be alive anymore. His parents are not concerned about his safety or the safety of anyone else.

You bring the whole family together to discuss a plan. You highlight that Jim has shared some distressing experiences with you, including hearing voices and thinking that people are monitoring him. You are glad that they came to talk with you, and you think that you can likely be helpful. You recommend that Jim start taking a medication that may quiet the voices and help him sleep better at night. You would also like to refer him to a clinic that specializes in working with people who have similar experiences, if he is up for it. With Jim's assent, you prescribe aripiprazole 5mg daily, and tell him to break the pill in half for the first 6 days. You let him know to call if he becomes restless or has any side effects from the medication. You ask him to get baseline labs drawn, including lipids, HgA1c, and the routine labs listed in Table 31-4. You refer him to an early psychosis program at the local university for multidisciplinary care and arrange a follow-up appointment with you in 2 weeks.

CASE ILLUSTRATION 2: CHRONIC SCHIZOPHRENIA

Mr. R. is a 54-year-old man with a long history of schizophrenia, recently well controlled with olanzapine 15 mg daily. He has multiple medical comorbidities, including hypertension, dyslipidemia, and obesity. He has a history of drug and alcohol use, but he has been sober for several years now. He is single, lives by himself in a supported housing facility, and works as a part time landscaping assistant. He was psychiatrically hospitalized many times in the past and was trialed on multiple first- and second-generation antipsychotics, but he could not tolerate most of them due to side effects. When he was started on olanzapine during his last inpatient psychiatric admission 2 years ago, his symptoms improved significantly, and he has tolerated the medication well, albeit with significant weight gain. Mr. R. has a significant distrust of all psychiatrists and refuses to go to a mental health clinic, despite frequent encouragement. He has been getting his psychiatric medications prescribed by a primary care provider. In general, he presents as mildly anxious, with intermittent eye contact and fair grooming.

Today he comes in for his regular medical check-up. He is unshaven, mildly malodorous, smelling strongly of cigarette smoke, wearing dirty clothing, and appears tired and very anxious. During the appointment, he looks suspiciously around the exam room, and avoids eye contact with the physician. When asked about how he was doing, he responds that he is "fine," but has been having difficulty sleeping; he asks for a sleeping medication.

His PCP suspects that this patient's psychotic symptoms are worsening. He seems to be responding to internal stimuli, and the PCP suspects that the voices are becoming more persistent. His thought process is also moderately more disorganized, although it is possible to follow the train of thought most of the time. The patient reports full adherence with olanzapine. He does not have any suicidal or homicidal thoughts, but on further questioning he discloses that the CIA has been following him everywhere and has installed cameras in his bedroom to monitor him in his sleep. He has no insight into the delusional nature of these beliefs. Mr. R has been eating and drinking normally, and his PCP concludes that he is still able to take care of himself at home. The clinician determines Mr. R. can be treated in an outpatient setting with close follow up, but he will need a higher dose of his antipsychotic medication.

***Clinician:** Sounds like you are going through a very rough time and are under a lot of stress now. It must be very tiring to be on your guard all the time.*

Directly challenging a delusion is counterproductive and will only alienate the patient, making him feel lonely and misunderstood. One approach is to empathize with the feeling without attempting to either agree with or disprove a delusional belief.

***Clinician:** What makes you think they are spying on you? Did you see cameras installed in your room?*

By asking simple, factual questions in a neutral, nonaccusatory manner, a clinician can establish how fixed the delusions are and whether the patient is able to logically examine evidence for his beliefs. Mr. R. says that he never saw anyone enter his room and did not notice any cameras but was nevertheless certain they were there. The clinician realizes that further discussion around the delusions will not be productive at this time and chooses to focus on addressing the symptoms that are troubling the patient.

***Clinician:** I wonder if these fears make it difficult for you to fall asleep?*

***Mr. R:** Absolutely. Could you sleep if someone were watching you all the time?*

***Clinician:** I can understand why it's a struggle. I worry about you. You are not getting enough sleep, and feel constantly stressed, overwhelmed, and fatigued during the day. I agree with you that improving your sleep is important. I suggest that instead of adding a new sleeping medication, we increase the dose of your olanzapine at bedtime. I think it will help with anxiety and let you sleep better. I will see you in 2 weeks, and at that point we can decide if there is something else we need to do to make you feel better. What do you think about this plan?*

Mr. R. admits that it would be nice to get rest and feel less anxious, and he agrees to the change in medication and the plan for follow-up.

MONITORING AND MANAGING SIDE EFFECTS OF ANTIPSYCHOTIC MEDICATIONS

Extrapyramidal Side Effects

Extrapyramidal side effects (EPS), including dystonia, akathisia, parkinsonism, and tardive dyskinesia (TD), can occur with any dopamine-blocking drug, including antipsychotic medications. Table 31-7 defines these side effects and summarizes treatment options for each. Acute extrapyramidal side effects, including dystonic reactions, akathisia, and parkinsonian symptoms, usually occur in the first days or weeks of antipsychotic treatment. These can be ameliorated with dose reduction or discontinuation, switching to another agent with lower propensity to cause EPS, or adding a medication to treat the symptoms. In contrast, chronic extrapyramidal side effects, such as tardive dyskinesia, occur after months or years of medication therapy and may not be reversed with dose reduction or drug discontinuation.

Although EPS can occur with any antipsychotic medications, the FGAs and the SGA risperidone confer the highest risk. Aripiprazole and lurasidone confer a moderate risk of EPS, particularly akathisia. The SGAs quetiapine, olanzapine, and clozapine confer the lowest risk. Risk factors for developing EPS include being over age 65, having a prior history of EPS or another movement disorder, and having a history of TBI or other neurologic injury, as well as using high dose medications, parenteral administration, and rapid dose titration schedules. Minimizing cumulative exposure to antipsychotic medications and careful monitoring for early signs of TD are strongly recommended.

To monitor for acute EPS symptoms, the guidelines of the American Psychiatric Association recommend screening for restlessness, slowed movements, muscle stiffness, or tremor at baseline, then weekly during dose titration, and at each visit thereafter. For TD symptoms, the current recommendation is to screen at baseline, then every 6 months for patients taking first-generation antipsychotics and every 12 months for patients taking second-generation antipsychotics. For patients deemed to be at high risk for developing EPS, screening should be performed every 3 and 6 months for first- and second-generation antipsychotics, respectively. The Abnormal Involuntary Movement Scale (AIMS) can be used for screening and monitoring (see suggested websites for link).

Cardiovascular effects—QTc prolongation is a common side effect of antipsychotic medications and is

Table 31-7. Pharmacologic management of acute and tardive extrapyramidal side effects.

EPS	Symptoms	Treatment
	Acute	
Akathisia	Restlessness, strong urge to move, pacing, inability to remain still	**First line:** **Beta blockers** • Propranolol: 10mg BID, can increase incrementally to 40mg BID, max 90 mg/d **Second line:** **Benzodiazepines** • Lorazepam: 0.5–2 mg BID
Parkinsonism	Mask-like facies, resting tremor, cogwheel rigidity, shuffling gait, psychomotor retardation	**First line:** Benztropine: 1 mg BID, increase to 2 mg BID, max 6 mg/daily **Second line** (if taking anticholinergic, antipsychotic, or cannot tolerate first line) Amantadine: 100 mg BID/TID
Dystonia	Acute muscle spasm: torticollis, oculogyric crisis, laryngospasms	**Acute treatment:** Benztropine: 1–2 mg IM/IV/PO, q10 min Diphenhydramine: 25–50 mg IM/IV, q10 min **Prophylactic treatment:** Benztropine: 1–2 mg BID
	Chronic	
Tardive dyskinesia	Mostly orofacial muscles: sucking, lip smacking, tongue movements, grimacing, lateral jaw movement. Other body parts can also be involved.	Discontinue the drug, switch to another agent. Valbenazine 40mg daily, increase to 80 mg in 1 week.

dose dependent. Ziprasidone, thioridazine, and pimozide carry the highest risk of QTc prolongation, while lurasidone and aripiprazole are the least likely to cause QTc prolongation. Preexisting prolonged QT syndrome (QTc interval >500 ms), history of arrhythmia, recent acute myocardial infarction, or uncompensated heart failure are contraindications to the use of high risk agents. Current guidelines recommend obtaining a baseline EKG and serum potassium prior to treatment with high-risk agents and a repeat EKG when the drug is at a therapeutic level. Routine EKGs are not recommended as a screening tool for patients who do not carry cardiac risk factors and are taking lower risk medications.

Sedation

All antipsychotic medications can cause sedation, particularly at higher doses and during the first several weeks of treatment. Many but not all patients become tolerant to this side effect with continued treatment. Low potency medications, including chlorpromazine, clozapine, olanzapine, and quetiapine, tend to be the most sedating. Many people with psychotic disorders struggle with low energy, cognitive blunting, and amotivation, which can be further compounded by the sedating properties of medications. Sedation can be mitigated by starting at a low dose, titrating the medication slowly, using the minimum effective dose, dosing the medication once daily at bedtime, and choosing an antipsychotic medication that is less likely to be sedating.

Orthostasis

Orthostatic hypotension is a common side effect of antipsychotic medications and is caused by alpha-1 adrenoreceptor antagonism. It is sometimes accompanied by reflex tachycardia and is most commonly seen at the beginning of the treatment or during rapid dose titration. Chlorpromazine, clozapine, and quetiapine are most likely to cause orthostasis; olanzapine and risperidone carry an intermediate risk; aripiprazole and lurasidone are rarely implicated in producing orthostasis. No specific monitoring is recommended, but low initial doses, slow titration, and divided dosing, particularly during titration, can minimize orthostasis. For symptomatic cases, supportive management can include counseling to sit up and stand up slowly, increase dietary salt and fluid intake, and wear support stockings; or treatment with fludrocortisone.

Anticholinergic Side Effects

Anticholinergic side effects, including constipation, urinary retention, dry mouth, blurred vision due to inhibition of accommodation, and cognitive impairment, are due to the blockade of muscarinic receptors by antipsychotic medications. Clozapine and olanzapine are the most anticholinergic among the antipsychotic medications, followed closely by quetiapine. Careful monitoring, dose reduction, switching agents to a lower risk drug, eliminating other anticholinergic medications, and symptomatic treatment (for example of constipation) are all strategies for managing anticholinergic side effects. Uncontrolled narrow-angle glaucoma and prostatic hypertrophy are contraindications to antipsychotic treatment with a medication that is strongly anticholinergic.

Metabolic Syndrome

Weight gain from antipsychotic medications is common, occurring in up to 85% of patients. While the exact mechanism is unclear, significant weight gain has been associated with both increased appetite and with changes in metabolic pathways. Most of the weight gain appears to occur in the first 6 months, is not dose dependent, and plateaus at about 2–3 years of treatment.

The SGAs clozapine and olanzapine confer the highest risk of weight gain. Ziprasidone, lurasidone, and high potency FGAs are the least likely to cause weight gain. In addition to adverse medical outcomes, antipsychotic induced weight gain negatively affects quality of life and self-esteem, leading to poor adherence. Evidence-based interventions aimed at weight loss and weight gain prevention may include cognitive and behavioral strategies, such as understanding eating behaviors; training in problem solving, goal setting, and monitoring eating habits; nutritional counseling; and exercise programs. Among pharmacological interventions, dose minimization and switching to a more weight-neutral agent is the first step in management. If the risk of relapse or clinical deterioration makes switching medications impractical, adjuvant agents can be tried. Treatment with **metformin**, at doses of 1500–2000 mg daily in divided doses, has been shown to help prevent antipsychotic induced weight gain, even in people without glucose abnormalities.

Although patients with schizophrenia are at increased independent risk for developing **diabetes**, treatment with SGAs further compounds this risk. Weight gain can contribute to insulin resistance and indirectly lead to diabetes mellitus (DM). SGAs are also linked to glucose metabolism abnormalities and new onset of type 2 diabetes in individuals with a normal body mass index (BMI). Clozapine and olanzapine carry the highest risk for causing hyperglycemia and DM, both of which usually occur during the first year of treatment. Quetiapine and risperidone also carry a moderate risk for the development of glucose abnormalities.

Dyslipidemia, in particular hypertriglyceridemia, is another common side effect of SGAs. Here again, the highest risk medications are clozapine and olanzapine, with quetiapine and low-potency FGAs conferring an intermediate risk. Aripiprazole and high-potency FGAs are the least likely to cause dyslipidemias.

Patients receiving treatment with all antipsychotics should be screened for metabolic abnormalities (lipid panel, fasting glucose of HgA1c) at baseline, 3 months, 6 months, 1 year, and annually thereafter.

Prolactin Elevation

Antipsychotic-induced prolactin elevation is common in treatment with antipsychotic drugs that are strongly dopamine-blocking, in particular the FGAs and risperidone. Common manifestations of hyperprolactinemia include menstrual abnormalities in women and sexual dysfunction, fertility problems, breast engorgement, and galactorrhea in both genders. Women of reproductive age are more susceptible to the adverse effects of elevated prolactin. Women with breast cancer should not be prescribed high potency FGAs or risperidone.

Hyperprolactinemia can be managed by lowering the medication dose or by switching to an agent with a lower incidence of prolactin elevation, such as aripiprazole or quetiapine. There is also evidence for using adjuvant aripiprazole, if switching antipsychotics is not appropriate. Routine measurement of prolactin is not recommended in asymptomatic patients, but patients on high risk medications should be regularly asked about the symptoms of hyperprolactinemia. In symptomatic patients, prolactin levels should be obtained. Due to concern about decreased bone mineralization and osteoporosis associated with low levels of gonadal hormones, women of reproductive age may be prescribed a combined oral contraceptive to counteract the effects of estrogen deficiency if the medication cannot be changed.

Cataracts

First-generation antipsychotics, particularly chlorpromazine, are associated with increased incidence of cataract formation. Among the SGAs, quetiapine carries a manufacturer recommendation for a slit-lamp examination at baseline and every 6 months for the duration of treatment.

Seizures

All antipsychotics lower the seizure threshold in a dose-dependent manner. First-generation antipsychotics and clozapine confer the highest risk of seizures.

Neuroleptic Malignant Syndrome

Neuroleptic malignant syndrome (NMS) is a life-threatening idiosyncratic reaction to medications that block dopamine receptors. It is characterized by a tetrad of fever, altered mental status, muscle rigidity, and autonomic dysfunction. All antipsychotic medications can cause NMS, but the risk is highest with high-potency FGAs, such as haloperidol. The symptoms can occur at any time during treatment, although higher doses of antipsychotics and polypharmacy are associated with an increased risk of developing NMS. Treatment is supportive and usually requires ICU admission.

SIDE EFFECTS OF CLOZAPINE

Shared Side Effects

Clozapine carries a low incidence of acute and chronic extrapyramidal side effects, prolactin elevation, or QTc prolongation. It is associated with a high risk of **sedation**, **anticholinergic effects**, **orthostatic hypotension**, and **metabolic syndrome,** as are olanzapine and several other antipsychotic medications. It also confers unique side effects, as described below.

Common Side Effects

Constipation occurs in up to 60% of treated patients. Constipation can be severe and can progress to paralytic ileus and intestinal obstruction. Risk factors include concurrent treatment with other anticholinergic medications, recent initiation of clozapine, and higher medication doses. Constipation should be carefully monitored and promptly treated in all patients.

Hypersalivation, particularly when sleeping, is a common side effect of clozapine. Patients may be advised to place a towel over the pillow at night and to mitigate symptoms during the day by using sugar-free gum or lozenges to stimulate swallowing. Pharmacological interventions include sublingual application of atropine eye drops or ipratropium spray up to three times daily.

Sinus tachycardia is a common side effect of clozapine, occurring in up to 25% of all treated patients. If clinically significant, it can be treated with a beta-blocker, such as metoprolol.

Serious Side Effects

Clozapine is also associated with several potentially lethal side effects, including severe neutropenia and agranulocytosis, seizures, myocarditis, and cardiomyopathy. The FDA mandates that all prescribers in the United States, dispensing pharmacies, and patients register with the Clozapine Risk Evaluation and Mitigation Strategy (REMS) to ensure appropriate prescription practices and monitoring. Before prescribing clozapine, providers must complete an enrollment form, course, and quiz online, all of which can be found at www.clozapinerems.com. The entire process usually takes less than an hour.

A transient neutropenia [absolute neutrophil count (ANC)<1500] develops in some clozapine-treated patients, which can progress to **agranulocytosis**, defined as an ANC<500, which occurs in 1–2% of treated patients. Due to this risk, close hematologic monitoring of ANC is required weekly for the first 6 months of treatment, then every 2 weeks between 6 and 12 months, and monthly afterward. In cases of mild neutropenia, with an ANC>1000, treatment can be continued with ANC monitoring 3 times weekly until neutropenia resolves. If ANC drops below 1000, treatment should be discontinued, and providers are encouraged to seek hematology consultation.

In general, clozapine should not be initiated for patients with ANC<1500. However, certain ethnic groups, such as people of African and Jewish descent, have chronically lower neutrophil counts (ANC ranging between 1000 and 1500) without any clinically significant effects. Patients with benign ethnic neutropenia are not at higher risk for developing blood dyscrasias and can be safely treated with clozapine at ANC>1000, with the same monitoring as people with a baseline ANC>1500.

Clozapine is associated with several adverse cardiovascular outcomes, including **dilated cardiomyopathy, myocarditis, and pericarditis**. Myocarditis occurs in about 3% of treated patients in a dose-independent manner, most commonly within 4–8 weeks of the treatment initiation. If myocarditis is diagnosed, clozapine should be promptly discontinued. Symptoms of myocarditis include unexplained fever, chest pain, palpitations, and shortness of breath; and they require weekly monitoring. Baseline EKG and weekly vital signs are also recommended to monitor for early signs of myocarditis. Some providers will check weekly c-reactive protein (CRP) and troponin levels for the first 4–8 weeks of treatment for additional monitoring.

Clozapine treatment increases the risk for generalized tonic-clonic **seizures** in a dose-dependent way. Myoclonic jerks may be an early warning sign preceding eventual seizure. Lower total doses and slow rates of titration can reduce the risk of seizures. Patients who develop seizures, or who require high doses of clozapine (above 600 mg) should be treated with valproate or another antiseizure medication.

MEDICAL COMORBIDITIES

Medical comorbidities are highly prevalent in patients with psychotic illnesses. Schizophrenia is "a life-shortening disease," with an expected life-span reduction of 12 and 15 years for women and men, respectively. Cardiovascular disease is the major contributing factor to increased mortality.

People with schizophrenia have a higher prevalence of cardiovascular and pulmonary disease; thromboembolic events; reproductive disorders; inflammatory, autoimmune and infectious diseases; metabolic abnormalities, including diabetes mellitus and hypercholesterolemia; and dental disease. Sedentary lifestyle; poverty; poor diet; higher incidence of alcohol, tobacco, and substance use; as well as iatrogenic factors, mostly related to the chronic use of antipsychotic medication, further compound poor health outcomes in this population.

Despite the high prevalence of medical comorbidities, patients with psychotic conditions have overall poorer access to medical care, higher rates of preventable hospitalizations, and more often go underdiagnosed and undertreated for their medical conditions. On the one hand, disorganized thought processes, paranoia, cognitive impairment, and amotivation may make it particularly difficult for these patients to recognize and describe their physical symptoms, take medications as prescribed, keep appointments, or seek medical care in the first place. On the other hand, "therapeutic nihilism" among providers may result in lower rates of specialist referrals, fewer prescriptions, and less frequent appointments.

ACKNOWLEDGMENT

The authors wish to thank Dr. Demian Rose for his editorial assistance.

SUGGESTED READINGS

Lehman AF, Lieberman JA, Dixon LB, et al. Practice guideline for the treatment of patients with schizophrenia. *Am J Psychiatry* 2004;161: SUPPL.

Lieberman JA, First MB. Psychotic disorders. *N Engl J Med* 2018;379:270–280.

Lieberman JA, Stroup TS, McEvoy JP, et al. Effectiveness of antipsychotic drugs in patients with chronic schizophrenia. *N Engl J Med* 2005;353:1209–1223.

Saks E. *The Center Cannot Hold: My Journey Through Madness*. NY: Hyperion; 2007.

Torrey EF. *Surviving Schizophrenia: A Family Manual*, 6th ed. NY: Harper Perennial; 2013.

WEBSITES

Abnormal Involuntary Movement Scale, AIMS (Word document can be downloaded from first link at this website). https://searchapp.mo.gov/search-missouri/dmh?q=AIMS. Accessed August 2019.

Australian mental health information and resource center for 12–25-year-olds. Headspace.org.au. Accessed August 2019.

Center for Practice Innovations, Columbia Psychiatry. http://practiceinnovations.org/CPI-Resources/First-Episode-Psychosis-Recovery-Stories. Accessed August 2019.

Center for Practice Innovations, Columbia Psychiatry. http://practiceinnovations.org/CPI-Resources/Medication-and-Medication-Side-Effects. Accessed August 2019.

Clozapine Risk Evaluation and Mitigation. https://www.clozapinerems.com. Accessed August 2019.

Clubhouse International. http://clubhouse-intl.org/. Accessed August 2019.

National Alliance on Mental Illness; runs family-to-family groups. www.nami.org. Accessed August 2019.

PEPPNET, Stanford Medicine; includes directory of early psychosis programs in the United States. http://med.stanford.edu/peppnet.html. Accessed August 2019.

Schizophrenia and Related Disorders Alliance of America. www.sardaa.org. Accessed August 2019.

Sleep Disorders

32

David Claman, MD; Karli Okeson, DO; & Clifford Singer, MD

INTRODUCTION

Thirty-five percent of adults experience sleep-related symptoms over the course of a year, making them among the most common complaints in clinical practice. Ten to fifteen percent of adults suffer chronic insomnia and they account for the largest proportion of sleep-related problems. Insomnia increases risk for other chronic diseases, including hypertension, diabetes, depression, and dementia. Daytime sleepiness impairs work performance and increases the risk of industrial and motor vehicle accidents. Sleep loss due to sleep-related breathing problems leads to profound fatigue and life-threatening cardiovascular and pulmonary diseases. Sleep medications themselves carry morbidity such as falls, daytime anxiety, and worsened sleep apnea. In this chapter, we review normal sleep, disorders of both sleep and wakefulness, and a logical clinical approach to these disorders.

SLEEP THROUGH THE LIFE CYCLE

Sleep has a structure, or architecture, that consists of non-rapid eye movement (non-REM) and rapid eye movement (REM) sleep cycles. The wake electroencephalogram (EEG) contains low-voltage, high-frequency waveforms that become dominated by alpha waveforms (8–12 cps) as a person becomes drowsy. There are four stages of non-REM sleep. Stage 1 is defined by the disappearance of the alpha pattern, the appearance of slower theta waveforms (2–7 cps) along with slow, rolling eye movements. Stage 2 is defined by the appearance of low-frequency, high-amplitude discharges (K complexes) and brief high frequency (12–14 cps), variable-amplitude discharges (sleep spindles) on a background of theta waveforms similar to stage 1. The majority of sleep time is spent in stage 2 non-REM. The emergence of slow waves (high-amplitude, low-frequency [0.5–2 cps] delta waveforms) heralds stage 3 sleep, when they make up at least 20% of sleep time, and stage 4 sleep when they comprise more than 50% of sleep time. These two stages of "slow wave sleep" are also known as the "deep" sleep, because they are associated with high-arousal thresholds and persistent grogginess ("sleep inertia") on awakening. The percentage of deep sleep can increase with sleep following sleep deprivation. Deep sleep has been shown to be important for growth, tissue repair, immune function, and daytime alertness. REM sleep is a distinct state of sleep characterized by wake-pattern EEG, skeletal muscle paralysis, and rapid, conjugate eye movements. The central nervous system (CNS) is predominantly active during REM sleep, and this is when a majority of dreams occur.

With the initiation of sleep, the healthy adult will descend through the non-REM stages within 45–60 minutes before beginning the first REM cycle, which tends to be brief. As the night progresses, less time is spent in slow-wave sleep, and REM cycle duration increases, eventually comprising 20–25% of total sleep time. The non-REM/REM cycle typically lasts 90–110 minutes, with about four complete cycles per night.

The timing and duration of sleep are controlled by many factors, including genetics. Many people are genetically determined "chronotypes" with strong tendencies to be either early risers ("larks") or late sleepers ("owls"). Although most adults are flexible in their sleep times and have some control over when they go to bed and when they get up, they have less control over how much sleep they need and the quality of the sleep they get. Although stimulants such as caffeine and habituation to a state of chronic fatigue can help people cope with inadequate sleep, they must ultimately pay the price of diminished energy and mental efficiency. Individual sleep requirements vary; although most people need 6–9 hours of sleep per night, the human range is greater than that. Children generally need more sleep than adults, but after adolescence, daily sleep requirement remains fairly stable until late life. In old age, sleep need may increase or decrease, but the most dramatic changes are in sleep quality and duration. There is a gradual reduction in the amount of time spent in deep sleep as we age, which is associated with reduced growth hormone secretion and changes in memory consolidation during sleep. The age-related reduction in slow wave sleep begins early in middle-age and is much more pronounced in men than women, although women have higher rates of insomnia. As we age, both men and women show a tendency to have more awakenings at night and more naps during the day. Most sleep experts agree that people of all ages tend to be sleep deprived. A recent poll by the National Sleep Foundation (NSF) found that only 10% of Americans rank sleep among their top five priorities even though most acknowledge that adequate sleep makes them more effective in work and in life. The NSF offers useful information with recommended sleep duration through the lifespan: (https://www.sleepfoundation.org/excessive-sleepiness/support/how-much-sleep-do-we-really-need). The timing of sleep is strongly influenced by the body clock (hypothalamic suprachiasmatic nucleus or SCN), which functions as the circadian pacemaker. It superimposes a rhythm of sleepiness and alertness to days and nights and determines whether a person is a night owl, morning lark, or somewhere in between. The light–dark cycle and nightly rhythm of melatonin secretion by the pineal gland act synergistically to keep the body clock synchronized with the day–night cycle, allowing alertness during the day and sleepiness at night for people who are entrained to a conventional diurnal schedule. The interaction of the SCN, melatonin cycle, and exposure to dawn and dusk time cues determines how well a person adapts to changes in sleep schedule in order to accommodate travel across time zones, seasonal changes in photoperiod, or work and social schedules that keep people active during the night. Blindness imposes special challenges in adaptation of sleep to the light–dark cycle. The majority of patients with complete blindness have circadian rhythm effects, specifically non-24-hour sleep disorder. Patients with partial visual impairment may also be affected.

Yawning is a phenomenon that has intrigued humans for decades. Yawning is thought to be an arousal mechanism that provides signals to the diencephalon to remain awake. It may also serve a social function. "Contagious" yawning is seen in most mammalian species and most commonly occurs between individuals that are closely related to each other or engaged in collaborative activity.

Newborns

Newborns have a distinct sleep pattern and architecture for the first few months of life. They typically will sleep for 2–3 hour stretches and awake to feed. Sixteen to eighteen hours a day are spent sleeping and this comprises day and nighttime hours. Interestingly, they have an equal amount of REM and non-REM sleep, with REM sleep initiating their cycle. It is thought that newborns need more REM sleep to aid with neurologic development.

At about 2 months of age, infants begin to develop a circadian rhythm with release of melatonin and growth hormone regulation. This causes them to sleep for longer stretches at night and take shorter naps during the day, a phenomenon called sleep consolidation and regulation. Sleeping through the night is one of the first maturational milestones, and this development is of great interest to fatigued parents. When infants are about 2 months old, most experts advise parents to let their baby "cry it out" during awakenings, allowing the child to learn to self-soothe and return back to sleep on their own. They have the ability to sleep for 5–6 hours at this stage, so sleep training should be fostered as long as the baby is not in distress.

There is ongoing debate over household arrangements for children's sleep. Some anthropologists point out that isolating a newborn in a separate bedroom is unique to western cultures and that co-sleeping with infants is more natural and may be beneficial. Recent studies have linked bed sharing with sudden infant death syndrome (SIDS), however, and the current recommendation of the American Academy of Pediatrics is to place infants in a separate sleeping area in the same room with the parent.

The American Academy of Pediatrics also recommends that all infants be placed on their back on a firm surface while sleeping. Their bassinet or crib should be in the parents' room without bed-sharing or co-sleeping. Families should avoid soft bedding and overheating. A proper safe sleep environment is crucial to reduce the risk of sleep-related infant deaths (SIDS, ill-defined deaths, and accidental suffocation and strangulation in bed) that cause 3500 deaths in the United States annually.

Childhood

As children become older, their sleep patterns become more comparable to adults. Daytime napping becomes less frequent as the child turns 4 or 5 years old. From the age of 5–10 years, children are usually consummate nocturnal sleepers with few arousals. Total sleep time gradually decreases throughout childhood, but for hormonal and psychosocial reasons, the amount and quality of sleep drops sharply with puberty. It is important to implement proper sleep hygiene at this age with routine bedtimes and awakenings. The recommended sleep duration for children ages 3–6 years old is 10–13 hours and for ages 6–12 years old is 9–12 hours.

Children who do not get adequate sleep are more fatigued and have a harder time learning than well-rested kids. Sleep deprivation affects brain function in many ways, and daytime restlessness, impulsive behaviors, and the full spectrum of attention deficit hyperactivity disorder (ADHD) should prompt consideration of poor sleep hygiene or other medical issues such as obstructive sleep apnea (OSA) syndrome, often due to enlarged tonsils and adenoids in children (see Chapter 28).

Adolescence & Young Adulthood

Adolescents are generally able to maintain the high sleep efficiency of childhood, with few nighttime arousals and little daytime sleepiness, although they do have a decrease in slow-wave sleep. In practice, adolescents frequently become more night-oriented, staying up late to do homework, work part-time jobs, chat with friends via text or phone, using Internet social media sites, or socializing away from home. Many adolescents and young adults develop strong tendencies to being "night owls" (see delayed sleep phase disorder in the "Chronobiological" section). Getting up for school may become an extreme challenge for some, and overall sleep deprivation with daytime sleepiness (especially in the morning) is endemic in high schools. Not only is a psychosocial change occurring in this age group, but adolescents also have an altered release of melatonin that perpetuates these tendencies to delay sleep. Also, high prevalence rates of mood and anxiety disorders with the normal emotional highs and lows of this period of life make transient insomnia more common, with difficulty falling asleep, staying asleep, or both. Early experiences with various substances affecting sleep, such as caffeine, nicotine, alcohol, marijuana, hallucinogens, and stimulants, can also be strong factors. Serious mental illnesses such as schizophrenia and bipolar spectrum mood disorders, start to express themselves with significant prevalence in adolescence and young adulthood, sometimes manifesting initially as sleep disorders. Physical illnesses producing inflammation, pain, endocrine, and metabolic imbalances can all impact sleep and need to be ruled out by clinical assessment.

Excessive daytime sleepiness at this age is usually due to sleep deprivation, but substance abuse, infection, and narcolepsy need to be considered. Infectious mononucleosis from Epstein–Barr Virus (EBV) is prevalent in adolescents. This leads to fever, pharyngitis, adenopathy, atypical lymphocytosis, and fatigue. Most of these symptoms improve within a month, but the fatigue can be severe and persistent. A prospective study of 150 EBV patients showed that 13% had persistent fatigue at 6 months after initial presentation of illness. Narcolepsy should be considered in anyone with spells of sleepiness off and on during the day, especially if a very brief nap is very helpful for an hour or two. People may suffer for many years with narcolepsy before the diagnosis is made.

Middle Adulthood & Old Age

Sleep tends to be lighter as people age, with more frequent awakenings. Healthy elderly women maintain slow-wave sleep, but elderly men show reduced slow-wave sleep. Sleep timing may "phase advance" with earlier bedtimes and early morning awakenings as people age. Whereas younger insomniacs typically struggle with sleep onset, older people with insomnia may just as likely complain of sleep maintenance problems due to this tendency toward phase-advanced sleep–wake cycle. More frequent daytime napping, either through boredom or need, is very common in older adults. This, along with decreased daytime physical activity, further erodes nighttime sleep efficiency. Frequent nocturia and esophageal reflux can make a bad situation worse with regard to sleep. Clinical sleep disorders also increase with age. Obstructive sleep apnea, periodic leg movements, restless legs syndrome (RLS), depression, anxiety, alcohol, and pain all affect the restorative qualities of sleep. Little wonder, then, that insomnia becomes more prevalent in midlife, especially in women and people with multiple chronic diseases.

CLINICAL ASSESSMENT

Clinical Assessment in the Office Setting

Every review of systems should include screening for daytime sleepiness and nighttime sleep symptoms. Four basic questions give clinicians a head start in diagnosing sleep disorders and determining whether they warrant treatment:

- *How are you sleeping?*
- *How much sleep do you get in a typical night?*
- *How much sleep do you typically need to feel your best?*
- *Do you feel alert during the day?*

Follow-up questions should sharpen the differential diagnosis of specific disorders of either sleep or wakefulness. In both pediatrics and geriatrics, it is often the parent, spouse, or caregiver who notices a problem. With children, ascertain whether the parent or caregiver is knowledgeable about normal sleep patterns for children. If the behavior is outside of the norm, then further questioning is necessary for diagnosis.

Although most clinicians, especially in primary care practice, rely on a few questions to the patient and possibly caregiver, use of more objective measures can improve diagnosis and assess treatment response. People's memory for sleep quality is short-lived and their subjective report of sleep symptoms may not be accurate. Sleep diaries maintained over days or weeks can improve clinical assessment. The National Sleep Foundation has one available for downloading (https://sleepfoundation.org/sites/default/files/SleepDiaryv6.pdf) but one can easily make one up to record the basic data of time in bed, "lights out," estimated sleep duration and sleep quality. Sleep quality rating scales, such as the Pittsburgh Sleep Quality Index or Insomnia Severity Index, are in the public domain and add accuracy to diagnosis. Wearable technology, such as fitness watches that have sleep tracking software, provide reasonable accuracy when compared to standard clinical assessment with wrist actigraphs or sleep EEG. Thin electronic pads containing pressure sensors placed under the bedsheet have been shown to document sleep time and breathing rhythms and will soon be on the market, offering clinicians another way to get accurate, longitudinal data on sleep for both diagnosis and assessment of treatment response. These methodologies are focused on insomnia. Clinical assessment of other disorders will be addressed in subsequent sections.

Clinical Assessment by Polysomnography

The sleep–wake cycle is a complex electrophysiologic process consisting of alternating periods of wakefulness, REM sleep, and non-REM sleep. Each of these periods has a characteristic EEG, peripheral muscle, and autonomic nervous system pattern that can be documented by polysomnographic (PSG) recording in hospital and clinic-based sleep laboratories or in the home, using technologies that allow for unattended in-home recordings. PSG allows clinicians to make specific diagnoses based on electrophysiologic monitoring of EEG, electrooculogram, electromyogram, nasal airflow, ear oximetry, and electrocardiogram. Most patients with insomnia can be assessed without PSG, but people with suspected disorders other than insomnia will likely need referral and comprehensive assessment with PSG.

CLINICAL SLEEP DISORDERS

Sleep disorders are generally grouped into three categories: disorders of initiating and maintaining sleep (insomnia), disorders of excessive daytime sleepiness (hypersomnia), and abnormal sleep behaviors (parasomnia) (Table 32-1).

Table 32-1. Common clinical sleep disorders.

Category	Clinical Diagnoses
Insomnia	Transient and chronic insomnia, chronobiologic insomnia, comorbid insomnia secondary to other conditions (RLS, periodic leg movements, mood and anxiety disorders, alcohol and drugs, medications, caffeine and stimulants, pain, and medical disorders affecting sleep)
Hypersomnia or excessive daytime sleepiness	Sleep apnea syndrome, narcolepsy, idiopathic CNS hypersomnolence, delirium, advanced dementia, and traumatic brain injury
Parasomnia	Pavor nocturnus (sleep terrors), nightmares, somnambulism (sleep walking), and REM behavior disorder

Insomnia: Insufficient & Nonrestorative Sleep

Insomnia is one of the most common complaints in primary care practice. It is diagnosed when there is either insufficient or nonrestorative sleep. It is essentially a subjective diagnosis, although more objective means of assessment will be discussed later in the chapter. One of the first diagnostic tasks is to confirm deficient sleep quantity or quality relative to normal sleep requirement for that person. Sleep requirement is best defined by how much sleep a person needs to be alert through the day, with perhaps a brief dip in alertness at midday. Sleep requirement is genetically determined and also influenced by age, activity, and health. Eight hours is the adult mean sleep requirement with a range of 6–9 hours for most people. There can also be seasonal variation at high latitudes. Nonrestorative sleep diagnoses (e.g., sleep apnea, periodic leg movements, pain, depression, and nightmares) should be pursued when there is adequate sleep time but poor daytime function.

It is best to think of insomnia as a symptom rather than a diagnosis. Many factors combine to produce insomnia, which often occurs when a delicate balance is tipped; for example, a constitutionally light sleeper may be fine until he or she enters a period of stress or uses a medication that has alerting effects. It may be necessary to deal with several causative factors concurrently to restore a natural sleep cycle.

Insomnia is often described as initial insomnia (trouble falling asleep), and middle or terminal insomnia (trouble staying asleep or early awakening). Insomnia may be transient (self-limited) or chronic (persistent or relapsing). Transient insomnia caused by stress, environment (cold, noise, new baby), acute illness, or pain is easy to identify and usually needs no special intervention other than addressing the underlying problem. A brief course of sedative–hypnotic medication is occasionally warranted and may reduce the risk of developing long-term insomnia. Travel across time zones can cause a mismatch between the body clock and the day–night cycle, resulting in transient insomnia known as "jet lag." Combined with fatigue from travel, jet lag can ruin the first few days of a trip. Shift workers may experience the same phenomenon and can suffer severe health and social consequences because of it.

Transient insomnia can evolve into chronic insomnia by perpetuating factors. Persistent or chronic insomnia accounts for 40–88% of patients who present with a primary complaint of insomnia. Chronic insomnia is a diagnosis of exclusion and must be differentiated from the many other causes of long-term sleep disruption. Chronic insomnia may be due to persistence of the stress that initially caused transient insomnia. Occasionally, the insomnia continues even when the precipitating factors have resolved, presumably through a process of operant conditioning to an arousal state incompatible with sustained, restful sleep. "Conditioned" or learned insomnia may persist secondary to poor sleep hygiene, such as erratic sleep schedules, alcohol, caffeine, nicotine, work on finances, nighttime television or Internet, and other habits that can prevent achieving the peaceful state of mind that is important to overcome sleep resistance. Apart from the online content on electronic devices that might unsettle one's mind before bedtime, recent research tells us that the light spectrum of cell phone and tablet screens is chronobiologically active, capable of suppressing melatonin production, phase delaying sleep propensity rhythm, and contributing to delayed sleep onset. Growing frustration with failed attempts to sleep increases the psychophysiologic arousal that is the underlying cause of sleeplessness. In fact, this type of insomnia, developing over time in association with stress, worry, and frustration over sleep, is often called "psychophysiologic" insomnia. People with this type of insomnia show high levels of physiologic stress markers (hormonal, autonomic, and cognitive). Despite severe sleep deprivation and pent up sleep drive, the arousal mechanisms of the stress response create too much sleep resistance to be overcome. Occasionally, this psychophysiologic arousal may be seen early in life in a form of "primary insomnia" due to intrinsic biological variation in either sleep drive (reduced) or stress response (increased). In contrast to people with transient insomnia and sleep deprivation, patients with the psychophysiologic and primary forms of chronic insomnia report inability to nap. The DSM-5 criteria for insomnia diagnosis are shown in Table 32-2.

As a model psychosomatic illness, chronic insomnia requires a holistic approach that can include use of medication as well as cognitive and behavioral strategies to reduce anxiety and changes to improve sleep hygiene (Table 32-3). Short-term use of sedative–hypnotic medications is appropriate to break the cycle of anxiety, arousal, and insomnia (see "Medical Treatment"). In some patients, the symptoms suggest another disorder that can be targeted separately (depression, RLS, pain, etc.).

Table 32-2. DSM-5 diagnostic criteria for insomnia.

A. A predominant complaint of dissatisfaction with sleep quality, associated with one (or more) of the following symptoms:
   1. Difficulty initiating sleep. (In children, this may manifest as difficulty initiating sleep without caregiver intervention.)
   2. Difficulty maintaining sleep, characterized by frequent awakenings or problems returning to sleep after awakenings. (In children, this may manifest as difficulty returning to sleep without caregiver intervention.)
   3. Early-morning awakening with inability to return to sleep.

B. The sleep disturbance causes clinically significant distress or impairment in social, occupational, education, academic, behavioral, or other important areas of functioning.

C. The sleep difficulty occurs at least three nights per week.

D. The sleep difficulty is present for at least 3 months.

E. The sleep difficulty occurs despite adequate opportunity for sleep.

F. The insomnia is not better explained by and does not occur exclusively during the course of another sleep-wake disorder (e.g., narcolepsy, a breathing-related sleep disorder, a circadian rhythm sleep-wake disorder, and a parasomnia).

G. The insomnia is not attributable to the physiological effects of a substance (e.g., a drug of abuse or a medication).

H. Coexisting mental disorders and medical conditions do not adequately explain the predominant complaint of insomnia.

Reprinted with permission from Insomnia Disorder. In: The *Diagnostic and Statistical Manual of Mental Disorders*, Fifth Edition, (Copyright ©2013). American Psychiatric Association.

CHRONOBIOLOGICAL DISORDERS

CASE ILLUSTRATION 1

Greg is a 27-year-old man who presents with a complaint of insomnia. He describes having trouble getting up in the morning. He is chronically late for work and his job is in jeopardy. No matter what time he goes to bed, Greg cannot fall asleep until about 2:00 A.M. and then sleeps through the alarm set for 7:00 A.M. His wife has given up trying to wake him, and although he has arranged for an answering service to call him, the ringing telephone does not awaken him either. He is often tired and sleepy during the day, but in the evening gets his "second wind" just as his wife goes to bed. He craves weekends and vacations when he sleeps until noon and feels alert the rest of the day.

The keys to Greg's diagnosis of ***delayed sleep phase syndrome*** *are his very strong drive to stay up late and sleep late, a relative inability to adjust to a conventional sleep schedule, and normal sleep when able to sleep on his internal biological schedule. Adjusting his sleep–wake schedule will take discipline but can improve his health, marriage, and career. The strategic use of low-dose melatonin in the early evening, bright light exposure in the early morning, and resisting the temptations of late night activities will be necessary.*

Table 32-3. Basic cognitive behavioral treatment (CBT) for insomnia.

Essential Cognitive Technique	Essential Behavioral Change
Discuss the frustration of not falling asleep and practice reaching a perspective of calm acceptance.	*Bed or sleep restriction:* time in bed limited to period of time the person can sleep; gradually increasing as sleep duration increases.
Provide education about insomnia as a potential chronic or recurrent condition that may require behavioral adaptations.	*Stimulus control:* go to bed only when sleepy, use bedroom only for sleep and sex, out of bed if awake more than 30 minutes, remove items of stress and clutter from bedroom, limit TV and screen time in bed.
Teach technique of suppressing thoughts: mindful practice or putting disturbing thoughts aside while trying to rest.	*Improve sleep hygiene:* no caffeine within 6–8 hours of bed; no meals, alcohol or nicotine before bedtime; physical activity/exercise in afternoon not at night; naps OK if short (<1 hr) and not in late afternoon.

Many cases of both transient and chronic insomnia are due to underlying chronobiological or circadian rhythm disturbances. If there is a mismatch between a person's attempts to sleep and their endogenous circadian rhythm for sleep, insomnia may result. The circadian rhythm of the sleep–wake cycle is driven by the hypothalamic circadian pacemaker or "body clock." Disturbances in the circadian timing of sleep may be transient, as in jet lag and shift work syndromes, or chronic, as in delayed sleep phase syndrome (DSPS), advanced sleep phase syndrome, irregular sleep wake cycle, and free-running sleep syndrome. The last is most common in blind persons, who lack the critical input of the light–dark cycle in regulating circadian rhythms. Diagnosis of chronobiological disorders is based on the understanding that except for its timing, sleep is normal in these conditions.

In DSPS, patients are "obligate" night owls, staying up late into the night through varying proportions of choice and biological drive. Patients with this condition struggle to awaken in the morning for school or work. They tend to have more energy as the day progresses and may "come alive" in the evening. Attempts to fall asleep before midnight can result in hours of tossing and turning. Sleep efficiency is usually normal when they are free to choose their own bedtimes. The condition is common in young people but can persist into middle adulthood and even old age, although it does tend to moderate with time. Adults with DSPS typically migrate to jobs in which they can work swing or night shifts, or keep totally flexible hours. They may have particular difficulty flying east across time zones, as they are relatively resistant to circadian "phase advance." Most "night owls" have flexibility in their circadian pacemaker and can adapt to earlier sleep hours with effort. Those with true DSPS cannot adjust to conventional hours at all, or only with great effort and treatment.

Children and adolescents with DSPS may be thought of as "lazy" because of how difficult it is for them to get out of bed in the morning and their tendency to "sleep in" on weekends. When school is in session, Sunday night bedtime and Monday morning awakenings are particularly challenging. With a late sleep-onset, the child has trouble waking up Monday mornings, and this starts the week off "on the wrong side of the bed." This may lead to disruptive behavior, hyperactivity, distractibility, failure to attend, and learning problems in school. Parents and teachers must recognize that DSPS is not a behavioral problem but a circadian rhythm disorder that can improve with proper treatment. A phase-shift approach by the whole family of consistent bed times 7 days a week is very helpful. Practicing good sleep hygiene, bright light therapy, and melatonin have been shown to be effective (see "Treatment of Insomnia").

Other forms of chronobiological sleep disorders are seen in practice. Shift workers often try to live on a conventional schedule to spend days off with friends or family. This can result in failure to adapt to either day or night and leads to poor sleep, poor energy, and chronically elevated risk for chronic illness and premature death. Scheduled exposure to bright light and melatonin can accelerate adaptation to shift work schedules.

Many completely blind individuals also have problems maintaining synchronicity between sleep and the day–night cycle. Lacking photic input to the circadian pacemaker via the retinohypothalamic tract, blind individuals can have an internal sleep propensity rhythm that is chronically out of phase with the day–night cycle, leading to frequent bouts of insomnia. Chronobiological insomnia from "free-running" circadian rhythms in blind patients is treatable with properly timed melatonin administration, but this and other chronobiological disorders should be treated in consultation with a sleep disorder specialist.

NEUROPSYCHIATRIC DISORDERS

CASE ILLUSTRATION 2

Francine is a 47-year-old woman complaining of anxiety. She feels restless and fidgety during the day, but she is also tired. She cries easily and has trouble concentrating, making decisions, and getting things done. Although quite fatigued, it can take her an hour to fall asleep. When sleep finally comes, it is restless and interrupted by many awakenings, filled with worried thoughts. She has experienced similar symptoms before, but this time they are more persistent, having lasted more than 2 months.

Francine's diagnosis is likely to be major depression, presenting with prominent symptoms of anxiety and insomnia. Medical or neurologic disease presenting with comorbid depression also needs to be considered, but Francine is at an age of higher risk for depression in women. If depression is the primary disorder, disease education, emotional support, and antidepressant medication are indicated. Short-term CBT can be very helpful both for the depression as well as the insomnia. Short-term use (several days to weeks) of a sedative–hypnotic can be offered if a less-sedating antidepressant is chosen as the primary agent.

Sleep disturbances are among the most common symptoms of mental illnesses, particularly mood and anxiety disorders. Depression should always be considered in patients complaining of frequent nighttime awakenings and early morning arousal, particularly when those arousals are accompanied by anxiety and worry. On the other hand, many depressed patients complain of hypersomnia with fatigue and difficulty getting going in the morning. This symptom is especially characteristic of seasonal affective disorder (SAD) and so-called "atypical depression." Both are common in young and middle-aged adults. Depressed patients find the sleep changes of their mood disorder very distressing, in contrast to manic patients. Bipolar patients in manic or less severe hypomanic states, typically experience less sleep drive and will enjoy their round-the-clock energy even as it impairs their judgment and physical health (see Chapter 26).

Sedating antidepressant medications (e.g., mirtazapine) may help with the insomnia secondary to depression, but can also lead to daytime sedation. Trazodone and the more sedating tricyclic antidepressants (TCAs)—for example, doxepin, amitriptyline, and nortriptyline—may be considered. The TCAs combine moderate-to-severe sedation with effective antidepressant activity but must be used with caution due to overdose toxicity and anticholinergic effects. Selective serotonin reuptake inhibitors (either SSRIs or SNRIs) generally will not improve sleep immediately, and can even increase leg movements and arousals. A brief course of a sedative–hypnotic agent for help with sleep is a comforting strategy for some patients. The sleep medication can be tapered and discontinued as the depression and secondary insomnia improve.

Anxiety disorders can also present with initial and middle insomnia (see Chapter 27). Nightmares, particularly in posttraumatic stress disorder (PTSD), frequently complicate the picture. Antidepressant medications, prazosin, and clonidine have been reported to be helpful with the sleep-related symptoms. Bereavement is usually accompanied by anxiety and insomnia. Short-term use of sedative–hypnotic medications may help patients who struggle to get through long nights.

Attention deficit disorder (ADD) and ADHD may be associated with disturbances in REM sleep as well as frequent myoclonic or periodic movements throughout the night. Insomnia is common; many patients with the condition report difficulty controlling racing thoughts and restlessness day or night. Snoring and obstructive apneas are frequently present in children who have mild symptoms of ADD–ADHD. In these cases, the cognitive and behavioral syndrome of ADD–ADHD can improve with treatment of the sleep-related breathing disorder by tonsillectomy or dental appliances.

Traumatic brain injuries and stroke impair alertness more often than sleep, but disruption of circadian rhythms with daytime sleep and nighttime awakenings are common. Neurodegenerative diseases such as Alzheimer disease (AD) and Parkinson disease (PD) disrupt sleep. Alzheimer disease can erode normal diurnal sleep–wake patterns, resulting in long nighttime awakenings and increased daytime sleep. This can be stressful for caregivers, who must be vigilant during these nocturnal wanderings. Sleep disruption is among the most stressful aspects of caring for a person with dementia at home. Severe insomnia can develop in some patients with AD, with little sleep day or night. Others may sleep off and on day and night with persistently impaired arousal as the disease progresses into late stages. Structured daytime activity can help reduce daytime sleepiness, especially if boredom appears to be one of the contributing factors. Antihistamines and benzodiazepines should be avoided given the risk for confusion and paradoxical excitement. Cautious use of melatonin, trazodone, or quetiapine may be helpful, although the data are limited. However, given how stressful sleep disruption is for families and patients, trials of sleep-promoting medications at low doses can be justified.

Parkinson disease patients can also have severe sleep problems. Akinesia causes physical discomfort over pressure points that normally would be relieved by tossing and turning in sleep. Medications used to treat PD can also impair sleep. Furthermore, the neurodegenerative and neurotransmitter changes caused by the disease adversely affect sleep quality. Dementia from PD and Lewy Body disease are associated both with impaired nighttime sleep, poor daytime alertness, and increased motor activity during REM sleep (see "REM Behavior Disorder" section).

ALCOHOL AND DRUGS

Alcohol has variable influence on sleep patterns, but it generally impairs both alertness and sleep. Like other sedatives, alcohol suppresses slow-wave sleep, making sleep lighter. With its short half-life, alcohol also tends to produce a rebound arousal in the second half of the night and can reduce total sleep time.

Other drugs can affect sleep. Amphetamines and cocaine cause marked reduction in sleep during acute intoxication and profound hypersomnia during the withdrawal phase. Opioids have acute tranquilizing effects and improve sleep when nighttime pain contributes to insomnia. Caffeine causes longer sleep latency (time needed to fall asleep) and increased wakefulness during the night. Some people do not perceive the effects of caffeine on sleep even when they are documented on sleep EEG; others are very aware of these effects. Caffeine has a half-life of 4–6 hours, so it can clearly affect sleep unless ingested many hours before bedtime.

Both prescription and over-the-counter (OTC) sedative–hypnotic medications can contribute to rebound insomnia when doses are missed. Medication with short half-lives can lead to rebound insomnia in the second half of the night, whereas drugs with long half-lives can cause daytime sedation. Although they are common geriatric problems, memory impairment and unexplained falls should cue the physician to consider alcohol or sedative–hypnotic abuse in elderly patients. For example, the antihistamine diphenhydramine, a component of many OTC sleep-promoting products, has potent anticholinergic effects and can cause mild cognitive impairment and, rarely, frank delirium in older people.

Education about the effects of these substances on sleep may motivate patients to reduce their intake. Patients with more severe dependency and abuse problems need referral to specific treatment programs for chemical dependency (see Chapters 24 & 25).

Medical Disorders

Cardiac and pulmonary diseases, dyspepsia, inflammatory bowel diseases, and nocturia may all contribute to insomnia. Gastroesophageal reflux disease (GERD) is an extremely common cause of nighttime awakening. Limiting nighttime meals and eating no later than 2 hours before bedtime can be helpful. Acquired immunodeficiency syndrome (AIDS) has been associated with daytime sleepiness, decreased total slow-wave sleep with alpha wave intrusions, increasing arousals, and frequent nightmares. The high comorbidity of major depression in patients with many chronic diseases should lead the clinician to consider using sedating antidepressants to improve sleep in this population.

Sleep disturbances are common in persons with diabetes, possibly due to the disease itself or from secondary problems of depression, sleep apnea, peripheral neuropathy, or polyuria. In a classic vicious cycle, insomnia worsens insulin sensitivity and glucose regulation.

Acute illness may cause diffuse cerebral dysfunction in the frail elderly. The resulting delirium is almost always accompanied by disruption of sleep and alertness. Medications can also cause insomnia and daytime drowsiness. Bronchodilators, activating antidepressants, and steroids, for example, often interfere with sleep, whereas many psychotropic medications, opioid analgesics, and clonidine can cause daytime drowsiness.

Pain and rheumatological disorders deserve special mention (see Chapter 38). Pain perception tends to be greater at night, and more time in bed may increase certain types of musculoskeletal pain. One of the classic medical syndromes affecting sleep is fibromyalgia syndrome (FMS), a condition characterized by nonrestorative sleep; patients complain of feeling tired despite sleep duration in the normal range. In overnight PSG recordings, the EEG of fibromyalgia patients reveals alpha wave intrusions into stages 2, 3, and 4 of non-REM sleep. This alpha–delta sleep may signify cortical arousals that impair sleep continuity. Sleep may be additionally fragmented in FMS patients by RLS (20% of patients) and OSA (5% of patients). Fibromyalgia syndrome patients have decreased slow wave and REM sleep duration. In addition to nonrestorative sleep, FMS is characterized by widespread muscle pain, focal tender points, and chronic fatigue. The common complaint of patients with fibromyalgia is the restless sleep pattern that blunts their daytime energy and vigor. In studies with normal human adult subjects, it has been shown that sleep deprivation lowers the pain threshold. Investigators have documented increases in generalized body pain, back pain, abdominal pain, and a heightened hyperalgesic state the following day after a night of disrupted sleep. Improved sleep can produce significant remission in pain.

Restless Legs Syndrome

RLS comes on with rest and produces an irresistible need to move, stretch, or rub the lower extremities. Severe dysesthesia may occur, which can variably be described as "creepy-crawling sensations," aching, tension, tingling, or prickling. The restless need to move makes it difficult to fall asleep, so the most common symptom of RLS is insomnia, particularly at sleep onset. The vast majority (80–90%) of people with RLS also have periodic limb movements during sleep, potentially causing further sleep disruption. Beyond sleep initiation, RLS can also interfere with any sedentary activity, such as plane travel, driving, theaters and concerts, deskwork, video media, and reading.

RLS is common, affecting 3–10% of the population (prevalence varies with ethnicity), and may be even more common as an intermittent cause of symptoms. In women it sometimes first appears during pregnancy, but in both genders it can run in families and worsen with age. It is especially common in patients with renal failure and PD. Many physicians do not think to ask about this symptom and hence fail to recognize it as a cause of discomfort and insomnia.

Diagnosis of RLS is based on four essential clinical criteria: (1) an urge to move; (2) onset or exacerbation with rest; (3) relief with movement; and (4) nighttime onset or worsening of symptoms. The differential diagnosis includes neuropathy, nocturnal leg cramps, and akathisia induced by dopamine antagonists. RLS can be exacerbated by drugs and medications, especially caffeine, alcohol, and antidepressants. Iron appears to play an important role in RLS. Reduced iron levels, particularly in the substantia nigra, can contribute to worsening symptoms. This mechanism may contribute to the higher prevalence of RLS in women, since menstrual blood loss and pregnancy can worsen iron deficiency. It is recommended that ferritin and transferrin saturation be measured in all RLS patients. If the ferritin is less than 75 mcg/L, iron supplementation for 3 months is recommended with a goal of raising ferritin above 100 mcg/L.

The first-line treatment of RLS involves the use of the newer nonergotamine dopamine agonists (e.g., pramipexole and ropinirole). Dopamine precursor treatment levadopa/carbidopa is effective as well, but more frequently causes "rebound" or "augmentation" effects, with a tendency for the symptoms to develop earlier in the day. Benzodiazepines (clonazepam) and anticonvulsants (gabapentin) are second-line agents. Combination therapy can be effective for more severe symptoms, and opiates can also be considered in refractory cases. The syndrome is so distressful for some of its sufferers that there is a national support group and newsletter (see website www.rls.org).

PERIODIC LIMB MOVEMENTS OF SLEEP

Periodic limb movements of sleep (PLMS) are repetitive myoclonic movements of the extremities, most commonly in the legs, that occur every 5–90 seconds over many hours; they are more common in, but not limited to, the first half of the night. The movements can be associated with brief EEG arousals and potentially cause nonrestorative sleep and daytime somnolence (although larger studies have failed to show a consistent association with excessive daytime sleepiness). Prevalence estimates range from 5% in people aged 30–50 years, to 29% in those aged 50–65 years, and 44% in those over the age of 65 years. PLMS are often seen in metabolic and neurodegenerative diseases. PLMS should be distinguished from nocturnal leg cramps, which are painful, prolonged involuntary contractions of the muscles of the lower legs. Antidepressants, lithium carbonate, and withdrawal from benzodiazepines and alcohol can induce or worsen PLMS. It is often asymptomatic, but in severe cases patients may have sleep-onset insomnia, nonrestorative sleep, or frequent arousals during the night from more robust myoclonic movements. Not infrequently, the bed partner is the one complaining about the jerking leg movements at night.

Whereas RLS is primarily a clinical diagnosis based on patient-reported symptoms, PLMS are best documented by PSG in the home or sleep laboratory. PLMS are treated similarly to RLS. Dopaminergic agents are the treatment of choice, since they reduce the frequency of leg kicking, but rebound of symptoms in the second half of the night or during the following day can complicate treatment. Sedative–hypnotics can improve sleep continuity in PLMS patients, but do not reduce the number of leg movements. Opiates, such as a bedtime dose of codeine, work well in PLMS (as in RLS), but should be reserved for patients with severe symptoms.

TREATMENT OF INSOMNIA

Reframing the Psychosocial Context of Sleep Disturbance

Sleep problems in children and adolescents usually affect the rest of the family, causing sleep loss in parents and siblings who may in some respects suffer as much as the patient. Because misinformation and inappropriate blaming may confound the problem, the disturbed sleep of such patients needs to be addressed as a problem for the whole family.

Modifying family routines may be helpful. Good sleep hygiene, including well-maintained bedtime rituals such as bathing, storytelling, and rocking a small child can facilitate the winding-down process that is an important prelude to sleep. Occasionally, a child becomes overly dependent on a particular routine (e.g., repeated drinks of water every time he or she wakes up) and the parents must set limits. After an expected period of protest, most children relinquish the need for unnecessary attention. These benign disruptions must be differentiated from the more serious panic that some children experience with separation. For this latter kind of anxiety, parental access through the night may be necessary, at least for some time.

In adolescence, sleep is often shortened at both ends by social demands. In the evening, there is homework, socializing, school athletic events, and family life. In the morning, high school schedules often begin quite early, sometimes preceded by an even earlier bus ride. For many teenagers, the morning includes a formidable grooming ritual. Add to this the increasing tendency for teenagers to take part-time jobs after school, and the result is an epidemic of chronic sleep deprivation that is of increasing societal concern. Weekend sleeping-in may recover some of the lost sleep, but it tends to produce a phase delay that reinforces the tendency to stay up late during the week. In one experiment, high school students increased their IQ scores by 20 points after a week in which they systematically extended their sleep time.

In counseling teenagers, some flexibility and compromise are usually most effective. Adding naps during the day may improve alertness. A warning about the dangers of driving while sleepy, intoxicated, or both is important. Chronobiological interventions, such as light therapy, may be needed to counteract extremely delayed sleep. Outside the office, informed physicians may be able to influence public policy to help alleviate the problem, such as adopting sensible work rules for teens and scheduling school activities at reasonable hours.

Adults are not immune to the effects of social and occupational demands on sleep. Many working adults become progressively more sleep deprived as the workweek progresses. Educating patients about appropriate sleep hygiene and cognitive measures helps them regain some sense of control over their symptoms of fatigue (see Table 32-3). New knowledge of the health consequences of sleep deprivation can help motivate people to prioritize sleep as an important health behavior.

Persons with more persistent insomnia or those who appear to have severe emotional distress (as a result or cause of the sleep disturbance) may warrant evaluation by a mental health specialist. As in children, sleep disorders in adults can affect family members. Partners and caregivers of patients with severe sleep disorders may need both emotional support and education about the nature of the sleep disturbance. Understanding the problem can help them to support the patient in following treatment recommendations.

Cognitive Behavioral Therapy

There is now ample evidence that cognitive behavioral therapy (CBT) for primary insomnia, especially over the long term, is at least as effective as sleep medication. The basic approach is to counsel patients to change critical beliefs that induce anxiety around falling asleep and to motivate them to change bedtime behaviors that may be perpetuating insomnia. The basic approach is to motivate patients to practice cognitive skills that will help minimize the worry and frustration that induces the physiologic stress response and impedes sleep. With time, patients can learn to suppress intrusive, unwanted thoughts and activate calming ones. Certain audio books or meditation CDs can help this practice. The "behavioral" component of CBT is the application of sleep hygiene measures. The National Sleep Foundation website (www.sleepfoundation.org) has many helpful suggestions for people interested in improving sleep hygiene.

Medical Treatment

Insomnia has a good prognosis acutely, but can become chronic and recurrent. Acute insomnia can be treated with sedative–hypnotic drugs (Table 32-4) in conjunction with a sleep-hygiene program to maximize efficacy and reduce the dosage and duration of treatment. These medications should not be used in pregnancy. People with secondary insomnia from depression, pain, substance abuse, medications, or circadian rhythm disorders are at risk for chronic insomnia if the acute symptoms do not resolve, and they may need specific sleep therapies in addition to treating the underlying cause of sleeplessness.

Benzodiazepines

All benzodiazepines have sleep-promoting effects, although only five are currently marketed as sedative–hypnotics. These drugs work well for short-term treatment of insomnia; tolerance and dependence can develop quickly in some patients. However, some patients, especially those with an anxiety component to their insomnia, may benefit from long-term use. Benzodiazepines alter sleep structure, reducing both REM and slow-wave sleep, but the clinical significance of this is unknown. They are generally safe for younger adults, even in overdose, although combining them with alcohol and other depressants can produce potentially catastrophic synergistic effects. In older individuals, the safety profile is less benign; amnesia, ataxia, falls, confusion, and worsening sleep apnea may develop.

Table 32-4. Sedative hypnotic medications.

	Trade Name	Type	Half-Life (hours)	Dosing Range (mg)
Temazepam	Restoril	Benzodiazepine	8–15	7.5–30
Triazolam	Halcion	Benzodiazepine	2–5	2–5
Zolpidem	Ambien	Benzodiazepine agonist	3	5–10
Zolpidem CR	Ambien CR	Benzodiazepine agonist	3	6.25–12.5
Zaleplon	Sonata	Benzodiazepine agonist	1	5–10
Eszopiclone	Lunesta	Benzodiazepine agonist	5–7	1–3
Ramelteon	Rozerem	Melatonin agonist	2–5	8
Suvorexant	Belsomra	Hypocretin (orexin) antagonist	12–15	5–20

Choosing one benzodiazepine over another for a specific patient is partly based on drug half-life, and this will require prioritizing goals. Short-acting drugs such as triazolam are useful for the treatment of sleep-onset insomnia, but many individuals will have rebound insomnia in the second half of the night or anxiety the following day. Longer-acting drugs may work better for middle-of-the-night insomnia, but some persons will have morning "hangover" effects. Longer-acting drugs can be particularly troublesome in older adults, as drug accumulation will lead to ataxia, confusion, and daytime sedation. Temazepam and estazolam are intermediate in half-life and represent reasonable compromises for patients with sleep maintenance insomnia who get hangover effects from the longer-acting drugs.

These drugs should not be prescribed for patients with sleep apnea, severe respiratory disease, gait and balance problems, or alcohol abuse. Doses should be kept low in elderly patients and those with hepatic insufficiency. Rebound insomnia can complicate withdrawal from these drugs, causing patients to return to their use.

Benzodiazepine Receptor Agonists

These drugs are structurally unrelated to benzodiazepines but share some characteristics with them due to the fact that they have agonist activity at more sleep-specific benzodiazepine receptors (GABAα). They have varying half-lives (eszopiclone and zolpidem, 1.4–3.8 hours; zaleplon, 1.0 hours), so they are most suitable for patients with sleep-onset or initial sleep maintenance problems. These medications preserve natural sleep architecture, which provides at least a theoretical advantage over benzodiazepines. Precautions similar to benzodiazepines apply to these medications in terms of dependency, abuse, and adverse effects. Eszopiclone (Lunesta) and zolpidem in continuous-release formulation (Ambien CR) have been shown to retain efficacy over 6 months, and they are the only benzodiazepine or benzodiazepine receptor agonists (BZRA) that are FDA-approved for chronic insomnia (see Table 32-4). Even so, in clinical practice, tolerance develops and limits efficacy over time.

Orexin/Hypocretin Inhibitors

Belsomra (suvorexant) is the first in this class of insomnia medications to the U.S. market. Suvorexant inhibits the action of the neuropeptide orexin (aka hypocretin), which promotes wakefulness. There are two orexin receptors (OX1R and OX2R) and since suvorexant blocks both, it is considered a dual-orexin receptor antagonist (DORA). Orexin inhibitors such as suvorexant promote sleep not through direct sedation but by inhibiting wakefulness or the processes that increase arousal in patients with chronic insomnia. It is considered a schedule IV controlled substance by the U.S. Drug Enforement Administration. Suvorexant should be taken 30 minutes before bedtime at doses ranging from 5 to 20 mg. Half-life is 12–15 hours and is slowed in obese individuals, but dose reductions are not necessary with mild to moderate hepatic or renal insufficiency. Narcolepsy is a contraindication but old age is not. Safety with pregnancy or lactation is unknown. Suvorexant shows modest benefits versus placebo (about the same as other sleep medications) in shortening sleep onset latency and improving sleep maintenance. It has not been tested against active controls such as BZRA. It is generally well tolerated at recommended doses with daytime somnolence being the most common side effect. High doses of suvorexant can induce narcolepsy-like symptoms, including cataplexy. Suvorexant has minimal effect on memory or balance at lower doses and is probably a safer alternative to benzodiazepines and BZRAs for people with sleep apnea.

Melatonin Agonist

Ramelteon (rozerem) is a potent melatonin agonist that is the first nonscheduled, prescription sedative–hypnotic. It has the capacity to shorten sleep latency in people with sleep-onset insomnia, but it does not help people stay asleep. It has no potential for abuse, tolerance, or physical dependency, and does not cause ataxia, confusion, or worsen sleep-related breathing disorders. In the clinical trials, the drug was associated with an increase in prolactin in a few subjects. Ramelteon is prescribed at 8 mg before bedtime. Higher doses have not been shown to improve response, but there is some evidence that the response improves over several weeks. Combining ramelteon with CBT or sleep hygiene measures seems a benign and potentially effective long-term strategy for many insomnia patients.

Sedating Antidepressants

Many clinicians use sedating antidepressants such as trazodone, mirtazapine, doxepin, and amitriptyline for long-term treatment of insomnia, especially when chronic pain, depression, or anxiety are comorbid conditions. Theoretical advantages over benzodiazepines include less slow-wave sleep alteration and treatment of underlying depression if present. Tolerance to the sedating effects of antidepressants develops in some patients. Side effects are numerous, and special care must be taken in elderly patients, especially with amitriptyline, because of its potent anticholinergic effects that can impair cognition (especially memory and concentration) as well as bowel and bladder function. There are data indicating efficacy of doxepin and mirtazapine at very low doses (under 10 mg) that may enhance sleep while minimizing side effects.

Antihistamines

Diphenhydramine is sedating and is found in many OTC preparations. It is generally safe and effective for short-term use, although tolerance develops very quickly after nightly ingestion. Diphenhydramine has some anticholinergic properties and can cause confusion and urinary retention in elderly persons.

COMPLEMENTARY AND ALTERNATIVE MEDICINES

The pineal hormone melatonin, sold in this country as a food supplement, has sleep-promoting effects in some people. Melatonin is the best studied of the food supplements and OTC remedies for insomnia and is commonly available at health food stores and pharmacies. Patients should be cautioned that melatonin is a naturally occurring hormone with potential neuroendocrine, immunologic, and reproductive effects, although it appears to be quite safe with short-term administration. Results from placebo-controlled trials of melatonin for insomnia in various populations suggest it has only modest efficacy, though some individuals respond quite well. Moreover, when taken at the correct point in the circadian cycle, melatonin can be an effective remedy for jet lag and can help people adapt to shift work. Commercial preparations may contain 0.5–5 mg of melatonin per capsule (sometimes in combination with vitamins). The most effective dose is unknown, and it may vary from person to person. It is in widespread use, especially for children, sometimes at high doses (6–12 mg), with great popular belief in efficacy despite the challenges at proving robust effects beyond placebo in controlled trials.

CHRONOBIOLOGICAL THERAPIES

Sleep–wake cycle disorders can be treated with scheduled exposure to bright natural or artificial light. Patients with advanced sleep-phase syndrome need to have a corrective phase delay with exposure to bright light in the evening. Bright light exposure must be carefully timed so that the circadian pacemaker is phase shifted to move sleep propensity to later hours, allowing these patients to be more alert in the evening. For the more common delayed sleep-phase syndrome (DSPS), patients need to force themselves awake by receiving appropriately timed light exposure, which should begin around the time they want to wake up. The first few days are very difficult, but after several mornings of 30-minute light exposure, patients can begin falling asleep before midnight and wake up for morning classes or work. For safety and efficacy, patients should use special fixtures marketed to treat SAD ("SAD lights"). Light fixtures are available from numerous commercial vendors.

Melatonin may achieve this same goal with greater convenience, although probably with less robustness and with opposite timing. For example, people with DSPS who want to advance the timing of their sleep might take synthetic melatonin (0.5–1 mg) in the evening at 9:00 or 10:00 P.M.—hours before their own phase-delayed melatonin secretion begins and more synchronous with the timing of melatonin onset in people with earlier sleep—to reset their body clock to the desired phase position. Ramelteon can be effective when used in this same way. These treatments may also be of value in helping shift workers, time zone travelers and persons with visual impairments adapt to a new sleep–wake schedule. Shift workers should be counseled to try to maintain their workweek sleep schedule on their days off work, although this can be difficult because of family and social demands. Some cases may require referral to a sleep specialist.

The Sleepy Patient: Disorders of Excessive Somnolence

Patients are more likely to complain about insomnia than about excessive daytime sleepiness. They may complain of fatigue or feeling tired, but sleepiness per se may not be acknowledged without specific inquiry by the clinician. Two questions that should be included in every sleep-related "review of systems" are:

- *Do you struggle to stay awake while driving, reading, watching television and movies, or listening to lectures during daytime hours?*
- *Do you feel tired, fatigued, and lacking in energy during the day, especially in the morning?*

If the answer is "yes" to either question, follow-up questions should determine if the problem is inadequate nighttime sleep, drowsiness from medications, narcolepsy, or sleep-related breathing problems. The Epworth Sleepiness Scale (Table 32-5) is a validated instrument used to assess pathological sleepiness in patients. It is

Table 32-5. Epworth Sleepiness Scale.

How often are you likely to doze off or fall asleep in the following situations, in contrast to feeling just tired? This refers to your usual way of life in recent times. Even if you have not done some of these things recently, try to work out how they would have affected you. Use the following scale to choose the *most appropriate number* for each situation: **0** = would *never* doze **1** = *slight* chance of dozing **2** = *moderate* chance of dozing **3** = *high* chance of dozing
Sitting and reading
Watching TV
Sitting inactive in a public place (e.g., a theater or meeting)
As a passenger in a car for an hour without a break
Lying down to rest in the afternoon when circumstances permit
Sitting and talking to someone
Sitting quietly after lunch without alcohol
In a car, while stopped for a few minutes in traffic
TOTAL

Reprinted with permission from Johns MW. A New Method for Measuring Daytime Sleepiness: The Epworth Sleepiness Scale. *Sleep* 1991: 14:540.

a questionnaire that scores a patient's tendency to fall asleep in eight hypothetical situations on a 0–3 scale, with zero scored for "not at all likely to doze" and three for "extremely likely to doze" in each situation. A cumulative score above 10 suggests the need for referral to a sleep disorders specialist. A discussion of driving or operating machinery while sleepy should also be initiated. Excessive daytime sleepiness requires a thoughtful diagnostic approach.

Sleep-Related Breathing Problems

OBSTRUCTIVE SLEEP APNEA SYNDROME AND SNORING

CASE ILLUSTRATION 3

Jim is 64 years old and visits his primary care physician for a follow-up of his hypertension treatment. His wife has accompanied him to the office to ask whether there is any medical explanation for her husband's fatigue. Close questioning reveals that the fatigue predates the antihypertensive medication and is not clearly attributable to the drug. The tiredness is accompanied by true sleepiness; Jim can fall asleep anytime during the day while reading or driving. He scores 12 on the Epworth Sleepiness Scale, indicating significant daytime sleepiness. He minimizes the problem, yet he acknowledges having trouble with memory and concentration. He falls asleep easily after getting into bed at night, but his wife describes him as a restless sleeper who snores loudly.

As a late middle-aged man with hypertension and daytime sleepiness, Jim needs to be referred to a sleep laboratory to rule out obstructive sleep apnea (OSA), which would be the most likely diagnosis in a sleepy middle-aged man.

Obstructive sleep apnea is increasingly recognized as a common, important, and treatable disease (see Concise Review http://annals.org/aim/fullarticle/1742606/management-obstructive-sleep-apnea-adults-clinical-practice-guideline-from-american). Originally thought of as a relatively rare disturbance in severely obese patients with the classic "Pickwickian Syndrome" of somnolence, hypoventilation, and polycythemia, OSA is now known to represent a range of upper airway narrowing in sleep. Epidemiologic studies in middle-aged adults show a prevalence of 2% of women and 4% of men, but these are likely underestimates given recent trends in increased body weight. Increasing BMI into the range of morbid obesity (BMI ≥ 40) also increases risk of obesity hypoventilation syndrome as a complication of OSA. Although more common in men, the incidence of OSA increases in middle-aged women, especially with higher body mass indices. Fatigue, rather than sleepiness, is more likely to be the chief complaint in women with OSA.

Obstructive sleep apnea is a significant cause of fatigue, daytime somnolence, and cardiovascular morbidity in adults. Nighttime symptoms of OSA include loud snoring (often beginning early in adulthood and worsening with age and increased weight), apnea witnessed by the sleeping partner, snorting or gagging sounds, restlessness, night sweats, and abrupt awakenings with a feeling of choking. Arousals triggered by the apneic episodes cause interrupted sleep quality, excessive daytime sleepiness, and subjective fatigue. There is also mounting evidence of objective deficits in cognitive processing, attention, and executive functions. Although less common, insomnia may be the presenting complaint. Validated screening instruments include the Berlin and STOPBANG questionnaires, developed for primary care and anesthesia respectively.

Patients are often unaware of the severity of the sleep disruption and may attribute their sleepiness to some other cause, such as working too hard. Although the degree of sleepiness is variable, it is a key symptom of OSA. Questions about dozing while reading or watching television, nodding off at the wheel, or poor concentration need to be posed directly to patients. Assessment with a standardized scale measuring daytime sleepiness, such as the Epworth Sleepiness Scale, may be helpful (see Table 32-5).

One way of rating the severity of OSA is with the Apnea-Hypopnea Index (AHI), which represents the number of apnea and hypopnea events per hour of sleep. Severe OSA (AHI > 30) is associated with cardiovascular morbidity and mortality, which may manifest as hypertension, heart failure, stroke, and possibly myocardial infarction.

Diagnosis of OSA begins with a clinical assessment, but a sleep study is necessary to confirm the diagnosis and severity of OSA. A formal PSG in a sleep laboratory remains the gold standard for diagnosis, but less-detailed home testing using portable technology that does not require a sleep technician to be in attendance is becoming more common. When PSG in the sleep laboratory confirms the diagnosis of OSA, there is an opportunity for a good first impression since the patient can try CPAP treatment with a supervised mask fitting by an experienced sleep technologist. If the diagnosis is made with a home-based study, Auto CPAP has been effective in short-term trials of obese patients with mostly severe OSA and no comorbidities, but CPAP is still optimally titrated during follow-up PSG. Treatment options should be individualized depending on the severity of OSA, as well as patient symptoms and comorbidities. Initial treatments to reduce OSA include weight loss, avoidance of sedating medications or alcohol for at least 3 hours before bed, and appliances to prevent back sleeping (tennis balls sewn in the back of nightshirt are an inexpensive option). Continuous positive airway pressure (with either mask or nasal pillow) remains the most common and effective treatment for improving sleep quality, reducing daytime symptoms, and reducing cardiovascular risk. In patients who cannot tolerate CPAP, other treatment options are typically ENT surgery or oral (dental) devices. A variety of surgical techniques are available, but the low success rates make surgery a less appealing initial treatment in most cases. Some adults will have significant tonsillar hypertrophy and be better surgical candidates. A new FDA-approved hypoglossal nerve stimulator is available for highly selected patients who fail CPAP but require detailed ENT evaluation. Tracheotomy has a very high success rate, but it is a morbid procedure that has been less frequently performed since CPAP has a high success rate. Oral appliances fitted and adjusted by an experienced dentist can maintain the tongue in a more forward position to improve airway patency in mild-to-moderate cases of OSA or for those who cannot tolerate CPAP (Figure 32-1). Patients who have surgical or dental treatments should have a follow-up sleep study to document the efficacy of those treatments. The correct diagnosis and effective treatment of OSA can help improve quality of life, prevent serious accidents, and reduce cardiovascular risk.

Snoring is a common sleep symptom. Apart from being a nuisance to bed partners, snoring may herald the development of serious respiratory obstruction during sleep along a continuum of partial to complete airway closure. Men snore more than women, but the prevalence increases in women after menopause. Aside from male gender, other factors associated with snoring include anatomic narrowing of the airway, body habitus (obesity), supine sleep position, use of alcohol and sedative–hypnotics near bedtime, endocrinopathy (hypothyroidism, acromegaly), and possibly, genetic factors. Since snoring is a common presenting symptom of OSA, it is important to ask questions regarding apnea and OSA symptoms in any patient who complains of snoring. Similar to OSA, initial treatments to reduce snoring include weight loss, the avoidance of sedating medications and alcohol, and appliances to prevent back sleeping. If a sleep study confirms the absence of apnea, but snoring remains disruptive, then potential interventions include oral (dental) appliances, surgery, and nasal valve resistors. Oral appliances thrust the tongue or mandible forward during sleep and are best fitted by an experienced dental provider. ENT surgical techniques to reduce the uvula and soft palate are available, but the long-term effects are unknown. Because surgery can eliminate the noise of snoring without relieving

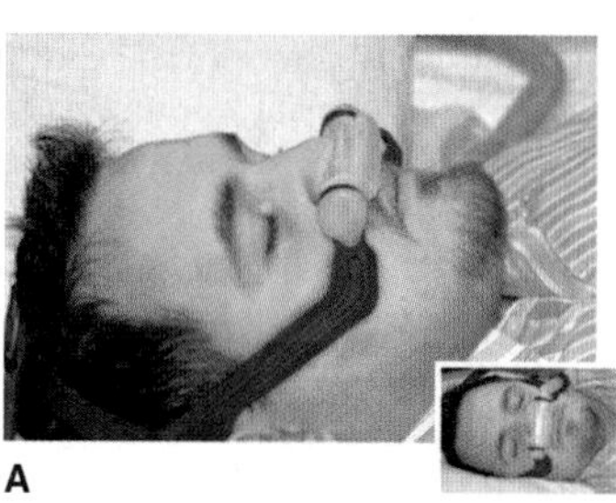

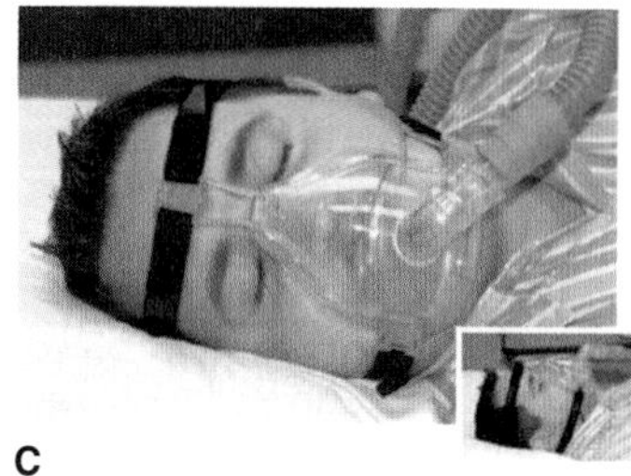

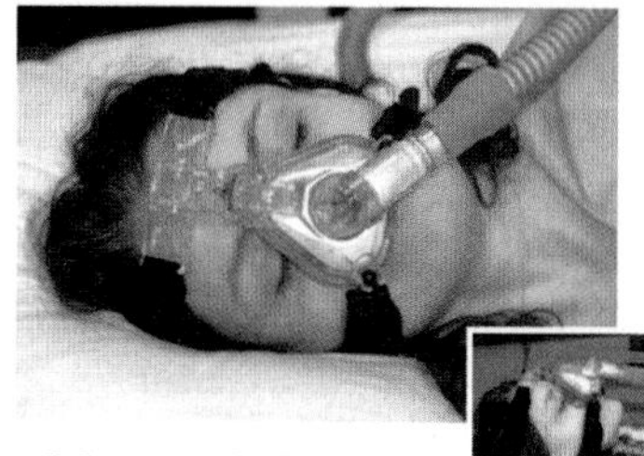

Figure 32-1. Various positive airway pressure interfaces for patients who are CPAP-intolerant. (Reproduced with permission from Lee J, Schulman DA. Sleep Apnea and Obesity Hypoventilation Syndrome. In: McKean SC, et al., eds. *Principles and Practice of Hospital Medicine,* 2e New York, NY: McGraw-Hill; 2017.)

airway obstruction, a diagnostic sleep study should be performed to rule out OSA prior to surgery.

Obstructive sleep apnea also occurs in 1–3% of younger children. Tonsil and adenoid hypertrophy are thought to contribute, since resection of these results in relief from OSA for most patients. Obstructive sleep apnea should also be considered in children with craniofacial abnormalities, macroglossia, neuromuscular disease, and obesity. As in adults, loud snoring, restless sleep, and witnessed pauses in breathing are symptomatic. Children with OSA may not complain of sleepiness; instead they may manifest daytime irritability, hyperactivity, decreased attention, or declining school performance. Secondary nocturnal enuresis is another important symptom of OSA. Parents should be asked about snoring and breath-holding during sleep. Consultation with an ENT specialist is advised whenever OSA is suspected. Tonsillectomy is curative in up to 90% of cases and should be the first step in treatment. Other causes of OSA can be treated with CPAP, though careful monitoring for midface hypoplasia should be undertaken in children aged less than 12 years. Surgical approaches such as tracheostomy or craniofacial reconstruction may be necessary in rare cases.

CENTRAL SLEEP APNEA

Central sleep apnea (CSA) is defined as the cessation of airflow for at least 10 seconds with no ventilatory effort. In adults, central apnea accounts for approximately 5% of apnea cases, so CSA is much less common than OSA. Patients with predominantly central apnea tend to complain more of insomnia than of hypersomnolence, which may be a helpful distinguishing feature from OSA. The differential diagnosis of CSA includes high altitude, congestive heart failure (CHF), hypoventilation (from chest wall, neuromuscular, or CNS disease), stroke, nasal obstruction, GERD, postnasal drip, and opiates.

In patients with hypoventilation due to neuromuscular disease, chest wall disease or neurodegenerative diseases that affect the CNS respiratory control, bilevel treatment can address both the central apnea and hypoventilation. Gastroesophageal reflux disease and postnasal drip are infrequent causes of CSA, but they should be addressed if no other causes are present. Opiates can cause CSA in a minority of patients, and the risk appears to be dose related; these cases may be more frequently seen because more patients are being treated for chronic pain issues. Lastly, the term "complex" sleep apnea has been used to describe OSA patients who develop central apnea when they are treated with CPAP. Complex sleep apnea has been estimated to occur in 6–15% of OSA patients treated with CPAP, but it usually resolves over time with continued CPAP treatment. If necessary, both opiate-induced CSA and complex apnea can be treated with a bilevel device that delivers a back-up rate. Although much less common than OSA, complex sleep apnea remains difficult and challenging.

Central sleep apnea can also be seen in prematurity, neonates, and children, but the differential diagnosis is broad and complex. A detailed discussion is beyond the scope of this chapter. The differential diagnosis includes apnea of premature infants, GERD, neurologic syndromes, and hypoventilation syndromes such as congenital central hypoventilation syndrome. Pediatric CSA may contribute to sudden infant death syndrome (SIDS). The cause of SIDS remains a mystery, but a wide variety of intrinsic and extrinsic factors are thought to play a role. A public information campaign to encourage mothers to avoid placing infants prone face down ("Back to Sleep") has been ongoing since 1995, and subsequent epidemiologic assessments have shown a dramatic decrease in the number of SIDS cases.

NARCOLEPSY

Narcolepsy is a disorder in which elements of sleep intrude into wakefulness, and wakefulness intrudes into sleep. It consists of four primary symptoms: excessive daytime sleepiness, cataplexy, and less frequently, sleep paralysis and hypnagogic hallucinations. Many narcoleptic patients also report sleep disruption. Estimated prevalence is approximately 1 in 2000 people. Narcolepsy usually begins in the teens or early twenties, but onset as old as the eighth decade has been reported. Prevalence is roughly equal in men and women, and a formal diagnosis is frequently not made until 5 or 10 years after the onset of symptoms.

The cardinal symptom is sleepiness that comes on suddenly and irresistibly in what are called "sleep attacks." Low-grade, persistent sleepiness affecting concentration, thinking, and memory may also occur. Sleep episodes may be brief (several minutes to an hour), but the person usually awakens feeling more alert, and the next sleep episode usually does not come on for at least an hour. Cataplexy, the brief, sudden loss of muscle tone leading to neck muscle weakness, buckling of the knees, or rarely, complete collapse, occurs in 60–70% of patients, and is triggered by strong emotional reactions such as laughter or anger. Narcolepsy with cataplexy (type 1) is almost always associated with reduced CSF hypocretin, in contrast to narcolepsy without cataplexy (type 2). Narcolepsy can impair nighttime sleep with frequent awakenings, vivid nightmares, and intense, realistic hallucinations prior to sleep onset (hypnagogic images). The hallucinations are usually visual, but they may involve any sensory modality. Sleep paralysis is transient immobility on awakening, often accompanied by the vivid hallucinations of REM dreaming, all while the patient is lying in bed perfectly alert. The spells are brief, lasting several minutes at most. If the syndrome is not diagnosed and treated, people with the disorder may be perceived as lazy and unmotivated due to persistence of significant symptoms. Additional sequelae of a missed diagnosis include poor school and work performance, social stigma, and accidents.

Hypocretin-1 (orexin), an alerting neuropeptide secreted by the hypothalamus, has been shown to play an important role in narcolepsy with cataplexy (type 1); a low CSF hypocretin-1 concentration below 110 pg/mL can be used as a diagnostic criterion. A combination of infectious, immune, and genetic factors appears to play a role in narcolepsy. Confirmation of the diagnosis should be undertaken with overnight PSG followed by a multiple sleep latency test (MSLT). The finding of mean sleep latency less than 8 minutes and REM periods during at least two naps confirms the diagnosis. Since diagnosis can be challenging in atypical cases, the testing should be supervised by a sleep disorders specialist who can integrate both clinical history and sleep testing data. Without the symptoms of cataplexy, the diagnosis is more difficult. An accurate diagnosis is advisable, since narcolepsy is a life-long condition that often requires a commitment to long-term treatment.

Excessive daytime somnolence (EDS) of narcolepsy may be treated with modafinil (200–400 mg) or armodafinil (150–250 mg) each morning, which can significantly improve daytime function. Sodium oxybate (Xyrem), the sodium salt of gamma-hydroxybutyrate (GHB), is FDA-approved to treat cataplexy and is used by some clinicians to treat EDS. The older CNS stimulants, dextroamphetamine (5–60 mg/d), methamphetamine (20–25 mg/d), and methylphenidate (10–60 mg/d), can also be used. Scheduling brief naps into one's daily routine is important and can be very helpful in improving function and reducing sleep attacks. Cataplexy and sleep paralysis can also be treated with REM-suppressant drugs such as TCAs and SSRIs. Joining a narcolepsy support group can help patients cope with the psychological sequelae, which result from the social and occupational stigma of having little control over sleep onset.

Kleine–Levin Syndrome

Kleine–Levin Syndrome is a condition characterized by periods of excessive hypersomnia and increased sleep time with frequent recurrences of the symptoms. The peculiar disorder is usually seen in people in their late adolescent years. These episodes can last from less than a week to 30 days. While the disease is active, some people experience other symptoms of excessive eating and hypersexuality. Social aspects of the patient's life will suffer during the active periods, such as not attending school or work. In between the flare-ups, the patient functions normally in all respects, but recurring symptomatic periods will begin to show sporadically. In most cases, the frequency and intensity of the spells decreases as the adolescent matures and eventually will resolve. It is thought to be caused by a virus or local encephalitis in the diencephalon region. Amphetamines, methylphenidates, and modafinil have been used as treatment, but usually they are only effective for a few hours.

Patients With Abnormal Nighttime Behavior: The Parasomnias

An accurate diagnosis of the underlying cause of bizarre nighttime behavior can be challenging. Diagnostic considerations include seizure disorders, psychosis, delirium, and intoxication. Parasomnias, the least common class of sleep disorders, but perhaps the most dramatic in their presentation, need to be included in the differential.

Pavor Nocturnus

Sleep terrors (pavor nocturnus) are very disconcerting to parents but are usually quite benign. The child (usually aged 3–6 years) awakens with a scream and appears terrified, with signs of autonomic arousal: eyes bulging, heart racing, and sweating. Most episodes last only a few minutes. Attempts at comfort are to no avail and may exacerbate or prolong the episode. In the morning, the child is amnestic for the episode or may have a fragmentary memory of a bad dream. Sleep terrors involve partial arousals from stage 4 (deep) sleep. Reassurance of the parents is the usual treatment; in persistent night terrors, however, benzodiazepines may be justified.

Nightmares

True nightmares typically occur in REM sleep but occasionally occur in stage 1 or 2 sleep. The nightmares involve a narrative story people can often relate once awake. This story is not necessarily a recall of actual events but a stressful episodic account that can be linked to recent or remote events. Nightmares are usually a transient problem, presumably triggered by a stressful personal incident. Persistent nightmares are a serious concern, however, and may require referral to a mental health specialist.

Posttraumatic stress disorder has many accompanying symptoms, and one indication the patient is suffering from the disorder is persistent recurring nightmares (see Chapter 27). The nightmares of PTSD patients are distinguished from other nightmares because they are narratives of the actual traumatic event, usually set in a previous time, and mimic the memory of the experience. For example, many wartime veterans have persistent nightmares that they are on the battlefield, and they feel all the fear and terror they felt when they were actually taking part in the war. When a person is stressed from normal life expectancies, dreaming can be cathartic and help to sort out feelings. For people with PTSD, dreaming about what had caused them so much stress is detrimental and just reinforces the traumatic events they experienced. The other dreams they have that do not relate directly to the trauma also have negative emotional contents of threat and aggression, and they are extremely vivid compared with control populations. There is no specific treatment for the nightmares that patients with PTSD experience, but by treating the disorder with medications and cognitive behavior therapy, the nightmare frequency will reduce. Controlled trial data and clinical experience supports the use of alpha-1 adrenergic receptor antagonists (e.g., prazosin) in reducing the intensity and frequency of nightmares in PTSD. Alpha-2 receptor agonists (e.g., clonidine and guanfacine) may help sleep and other autonomic arousal symptoms in PTSD. Antidepressant and mood-stabilizing atypical antipsychotic medications are generally used to help with daytime symptoms but can sometimes help sleep as well.

Somnambulism

Like sleep terrors, sleepwalking is a partial arousal from stage 4 sleep. Occasional sleepwalking is very common in childhood and may follow a period of stress or sleep deprivation. The main concern is accidental injury, and protective measures, such as placing gates in front of a stairwell, may be needed.

REM Behavior Disorder

In this syndrome, loss of normal REM sleep muscle atonia leads to dream-enactment behavior. The diagnosis is made in patients with sudden bursts of excited, intense, sometimes violent activity during sleep. The syndrome may be subtle, in the form of leg movements and talking, or dramatic, with punching, kicking, grabbing, strangling, running, and moving about the bedroom. Dreams of an intense, violent nature are typical. REM behavior disorder is seen frequently in toxic or metabolic delirium, but the most persistent forms of the syndrome occur in old age, and are presumed to be idiopathic, ischemic, or neurodegenerative in etiology. Antidepressant medications can also cause episodes. The syndrome is especially common in patients with PD and dementia with Lewy Bodies and can start to develop even before other signs of the diseases. In patients who present without other causes of REM Behavior Disorder, the risk of PD is approximately 40% at 10 years. Once documented by PSG, the condition can be effectively treated with clonazepam, although there are reports of other agents, such as cholinesterase inhibitors, working as well.

Movement Disorders in Children

Other movement disorders such as rhythmic sleep disorders (head banging, body rocking, and head rolling) interestingly do not cause insomnia, but are usually brought to the examiner's attention by the caregiver for hazardous concerns. Rhythmic movements are observed in normal children at 9 months of age, and the occurrence decreases 50% by the age of 18 months. By 4 years of age, the prevalence is only 8%. These movement disorders are usually seen on PSGs just before sleep onset and can persist into stage 1 non-REM sleep or after spontaneous arousal. Because these various movements can disrupt sleep, the child experiences excessive daytime sleepiness. Fortunately, between the ages of 2 and 4 years, the intensity decreases and usually resolves spontaneously. Rarely is this disorder observed in healthy adolescents or adults.

Epilepsy

Epileptic discharges often occur during sleep and may be misinterpreted as other sleep arousal phenomena, such as somnambulism or pavor nocturnus. Onset of a seizure disorder can be at any age, but most commonly will begin in adolescence. Epileptic events generally occur in the non-REM stages of sleep and rarely in the REM stages. Nocturnal seizures may produce arousals that may or may not be remembered by the patient, and depending on the frequency and duration of arousals, they can cause daytime sleepiness. Postictal sleepiness can also persist into daytime. In fact, daytime sleepiness in patients with epilepsy is not always attributable to antiepileptic medications.

There are particular types of seizures more prone to occur during sleep. Benign childhood epilepsy with centrotemporal spikes (BECTS), or benign Rolandic epilepsy, is triggered by sleep and is recognized by unilateral facial paresthesias with tonic or tonic–clonic movement. If the pharyngeal muscles are involved, these symptoms will be coupled with drooling.

Seizures that involve the frontal lobe present themselves as peculiar behavior involving motor activity and unusual vocalizations. Autosomal dominant nocturnal frontal lobe epilepsy (ADNFLE) involves thrashing activity with spastic posture and speaking vociferously. These patients may also sleep walk and become violent. Nocturnal paroxysmal dystonia involves tonic spasms of the limbs and laughter as the vocalization. Pure tonic seizures also involve the frontal lobes and appear as insomnia or hypersomnia because of periodic arousals.

Diagnosis of seizure disorder involves routine EEGs or prolonged video EEGs combined with clinical symptoms to classify the seizure type. Anticonvulsant medications are given to prevent further electrical discharges.

DIAGNOSTIC EVALUATION & REFERRAL

Most types of insomnia are diagnosed by history, and PSG evaluation of insomnia is rarely necessary or reimbursed. Clinicians should be able to accurately diagnose and treat transient insomnia without referral or consultation. Referral to a sleep specialist should be considered for patients with persistent symptoms who do not respond to initial treatment. Patients with severe RLS and chronobiological sleep disorders should usually be referred. Sleep-related breathing problems, periodic leg movements, narcolepsy, and the adult parasomnias all require PSG validation and expert management by a sleep specialist to validate the diagnosis and initial treatment plans.

SUGGESTED READINGS

Besteiro González JL, Suárez Fernández TV, Arboleya Rodríguez L, et al. Sleep architecture in patients with fibromyalgia. *Psicothema* 2011;23:368–373.

Chung F, Abdullah HR, Liao P. Stop-bang questionnaire: a practical approach to screen for obstructive sleep apnea. *Chest* 2016;149(3):631–638.

Ip S, D'Ambrosio C, Patel K, et al. Auto-titrating versus fixed continuous positive airway pressure for the treatment of obstructive sleep apnea: a systematic review with meta-analyses. *Syst Rev* 2012;1:20.

Maness DL, Khan M. Nonpharmacologic management of chronic insomnia. *Am Fam Physician* 2015;92(12):1058–1064.

Marin JM, Carrizo SJ, Vicente E, Agusti AG. Long-term cardiovascular outcomes in men with obstructive sleep apnoea-hypopnoea with or without treatment with continuous positive airward pressure: an observational study. *Lancet* 2005;365(9464):1046–1053.

McEvoy RD, Antic NA, Heeley E, et al. CPAP for prevention of cardiovascular events in obstructive sleep apnea. *N Engl J Med* 2016;375:919–931.

Moon R. *Sleep: What Every Parent Needs to Know*. AAP EBooks, American Academy of Pediatrics, 5 July 2013, ebooks .aappublications.org/content/sleep.

Morin AK. Strategies for treating chronic insomnia. *Am J Manag Care* 2006;12:S2230–S2245.

Morin CM, Bellville G, Belanger L, Ivers H. The Insomnia Severity Index: psychometric indicators to detect insomnia cases and evaluate treatment response. *Sleep* 2011;34(5):601–608.

National Sleep Foundation Sleep in America Poll® 2018: https://www .sleepfoundation.org/press-release/national-sleep-foundations-2018-sleep-americar-poll-shows-americans-failing.

Pearson NJ, Johnson LL, Nahin RL. Insomnia, trouble sleeping, and complementary and alternative medicine. *Arch Intern Med* 2006;166:1775–1782.

Rhyne DN, Anderson SL. Suvorexant in insomnia: efficacy, safety and place in therapy. *Ther Adv Drug Safety* 2015;6(5):189–195.

Senaratna CV, Perret JL, Matheson MC, et al. Validity of the Berlin questionnaire in detecting obstructive sleep apnea: a systematic review and meta-analysis. *Sleep Med Rev* 2017;36:116–124.

Silber MH. Chronic insomnia. *N Engl J Med* 2005;353:803–810.

Task Force on Sudden Infant Death Syndrome. SIDS and Other Sleep-Related Infant Deaths: Updated 2016 Recommendations for a Safe Infant Sleeping Environment. *Pediatrics*, American Academy of Pediatrics, November 1, 2016.

Vitiello MV, Rybarczyk B, Von Korff M, Stepanski EJ. Cognitive behavioral therapy for insomnia improves sleep and decreases pain in older adults with co-morbid insomnia and osteoarthritis. *J Clin Sleep Med* 2009;5:355–362.

Wickwire EM, Collop NA. Insomnia and sleep-related breathing disorders. *Chest* 2010;137:1449–1463.

Winkelman JW. Insomnia disorder. *N Engl J Med* 2015;373:1437–1444.

WEBSITES

American Academy of Sleep Medicine. www.aasmnet.org. Accessed September 2019.

The National Sleep Foundation. www.sleepfoundation.org. Accessed September 2019.

Pittsburgh Sleep Quality Index. https://consultgeri.org/try-this/general-assessment/issue-6.1.pdf. Accessed August 2019.

Restless Legs Syndrome Foundation. www.rls.org. Accessed September 2019.

The Society of Behavioral Sleep Medicine. www.behavioralsleep.org. Accessed September 2019.

Sexual Problems

33

David G. Bullard, PhD & Christine Derzko, MD

Sex is a problem for everyone.... Indeed, for a couple of weeks or a couple of months, or maybe even for a couple of years, if we are lucky, we may feel that we have solved the problem of sex. But then, of course, we change or our partners change, or the whole ball-game changes, and once again we are left trying to scramble over that obstacle with this built-in feeling that we can get over it, when actually we never can. However, in the process of trying to get over it, we learn a great deal about vulnerability and intimacy and love.... (Peck, 1993, Further Along the Road Less Traveled)

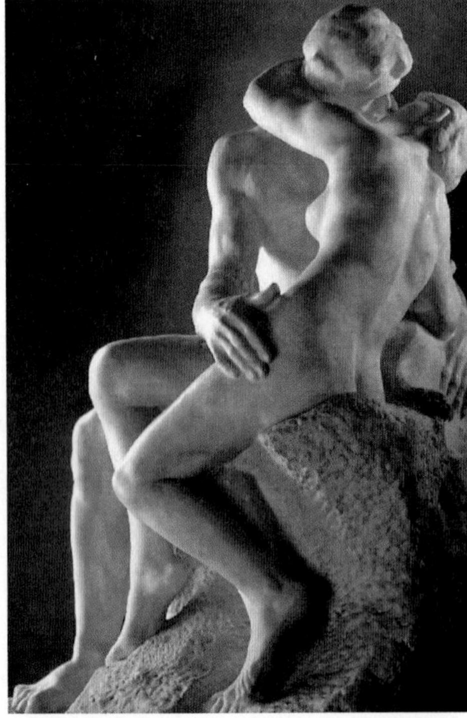

Rodin, "The Kiss". Accessed at http://theroyalist10.wordpress.com/2010/10/.

INTRODUCTION

Sexuality encompasses an enormous range of behaviors, beliefs, desires, experiences, and fantasies that patients may want to discuss with their health care providers. Sexuality also may have legal, medical, moral, political, spiritual, and religious aspects. This chapter intends to give the practicing clinician basic practical knowledge of human sexuality and useful tools for managing common problems.

Patients with sexual concerns report feeling most comfortable discussing these issues with their primary care provider and expect to receive advice and suggestions. In large studies of adult patients, more than 70% considered sexual matters to be an appropriate topic for the primary care provider to discuss. Yet, evidence of discussion about sexual problems has been found in as few as 2% of the notes of such providers. Primary care practitioners are in an optimal position to evaluate sexual problems, as they often have the most comprehensive and long-lasting relationship with the patient.

The health care provider's assessment of problems related to sexual function requires a consideration of all relevant potential etiological factors in order that any appropriate therapeutic measures may be instituted, be they psychosocial, physical, and/or pharmacological. Medical diagnoses of sexual problems are still evolving. The Consensus Statement from the 2016 Fourth International Consultation on Sexual Medicine recommended combining some DSM-5, DSM-1V-TR, and ICD-10 definitions, together with some newly developed ones.

In contrast to most other medical diagnoses, however, it is the patient who usually defines when a sexual problem exists. That is to say, a "problem" exists only if and when the patient or the partner is troubled by his or her level of sexual desire, response, or function.

Most primary care providers will find Levine's (2010) conceptualization of three broad categories useful: sexual worries, problems, and disorders. Although referral

Table 33-1. Sexual concerns of patients.

- **Common sexual worries about normalcy,** such as: Am I OK? What is a "healthy" sex life? How do I compare? Is my sex life satisfactory?
- **Sexual identity questions** relevant to lifestyle, orientation, and preference.
- **Developmental issues of sexuality** for children, adolescents, parents, and the elderly, including the development of gender identity, masturbation, genital exploration, child sex play, sexuality and the single life, marriage, divorce, and death of a partner.
- **Reproductive concerns** covering infertility, family planning, contraception, pregnancy, and abortion.
- **Sexual desire, satisfaction, and other problems,** such as a couple's differing levels of desire, and problems with vaginal lubrication, erections, orgasm, and pain.
- **Sexual changes** due to physical disability, medical illness, and treatment.
- **Sexual trauma** resulting from molestation, incest, and rape.
- **Safe sex practices:** AIDS and STDs.
- **Paraphilias and sexual compulsions.**

to medical or mental health specialists (or both) may be indicated in more severe disorders and dysfunctions, many worries and problems can be successfully addressed by the primary care practitioner. When questions about sexuality are approached in an open, matter-of-fact manner, most people are relieved and respond positively. They appreciate the affirmation that these issues are valid and important, whether or not they have current sexual concerns or are sexually active (Table 33-1).

CHALLENGE FOR CLINICIANS

To provide patients with helpful responses to their sexual health concerns, health professionals need the following:

- Willingness and ability to discuss sexual topics comfortably.
- Awareness of the range and diversity of human sexual practices and concerns across and within cultures, as well as awareness of the importance of the circumstances or conditions under which individuals function best.
- Ability to separate their own personal beliefs and values from those of patients. Unless the practitioner encounters information indicating objective harm to someone involved, it is important to maintain a nonjudgmental demeanor.
- Skill at taking a history of sex problems in appropriate detail.
- Knowledge of simple interventions such as permission-giving, transmitting accurate information, providing specific suggestions (e.g., for making sex less pressured and more pleasurable), and making referrals to other resources, when appropriate.

As health professionals, we may personally have had limited sexual experience, as well as questions and problems of our own. Consequently, we may be uncomfortable in discussing particular sexual material. Time, thought, and experience, however, can build confidence and expertise in talking about sexual problems. Health care providers can increase their comfort level by examining their own attitudes, beliefs, assumptions, and experiences; reading the literature; discussing sexual issues with friends and colleagues; and routinely incorporating sexual health questions into the general health assessment of patients.

Of course, no one—patients *or* caregivers—should be forced to talk about sexuality. It is important for everyone to recognize the limits of their own interest, comfort, and competency. However, sexual health is an integral part of health care. All who deal with patients should be alert to the possibility of sexual concerns and, at a minimum, be able to respond with nonjudgmental listening and reassurance. When in the best interest of the patient, health care providers can refer to a colleague who is comfortable and competent in discussing sexual issues.

PERSPECTIVES ON HUMAN SEXUALITY

Knowledge of human sexuality has expanded remarkably since the modern pioneering efforts of Kinsey and Masters and Johnson—who published some of the earliest evidence-based treatment of sexual problems. While initially focusing on the range of sexual behaviors and the treatment of dysfunctional mechanical problems, the field has grown to include and to better understand sexual motivations, the critical importance of sexual excitement and desire, and of the contexts required to produce sexual fulfillment.

Research in human sexuality has burgeoned, as has knowledge of the often-negative effects of long-accepted sex roles. We are also learning more about variations among individuals in terms of the role sexuality plays in life. A particular sexual problem may be perceived as central and significant to one patient, yet be seen by another to be peripheral or minor. Clinicians must be cautious not to make assumptions about the significance of various sexual problems, but rather assess and discover whatever meaning the issue has for that individual or within a particular couple.

Motivations for human sexual expression are complex and numerous. Different motivations exist throughout the life cycle, including variations in times of illness or periods of health. Motivations vary from culture to culture and from individual to individual. They may include the need to express love; the need for physical release, reproduction, or recreation; the need to increase self-esteem—or combinations of all the above. Conversely, sexuality can also be used to coerce, control, or degrade others. Sexuality may be the focus of addictive or compulsive behavior.

Sexual worries or difficulties are likely experienced by most people at some period of life and may result from developmental growth and changes in life circumstances rather than from pathology alone. Sexual problems are sometimes a blessing, such as when they compel a person to get help for symptoms that indicate underlying medical, self-esteem, or relationship problems. Surprisingly, for some people, seeking help for problems involving erection or orgasm may be more acceptable than seeking help for issues involving self-esteem.

Because the language of sex is broad and varied, primary care practitioners will find it helpful to become familiar and comfortable with the vernacular and to be able to discuss calmly and in detail matters such as masturbation, sexual positions, oral sex, anal sex, penis size, and breast size. The following section discusses a few of the areas in which misconceptions about these subjects can be resolved.

COMMON SEXUAL ISSUES

From a medical viewpoint, masturbation is "normal," universal, and physically harmless at all ages. It is highly correlated with self-acceptance and sexual adjustment, and is often suggested as "homework" in sex therapy to further sexual self-awareness. Some people freely choose not to masturbate, perhaps following personal or religious tenets. Guilt about masturbation, however, continues to affect many patients. Some may use masturbation compulsively to avoid personal or relationship issues. Sex offenders may reinforce their antisocial fantasies via masturbation. Those who are truly addicted to some sexual behaviors may suffer from a variety of life difficulties common to other addictions.

There is no standard for what constitutes acceptable sexual frequency. Individuals who are celibate may still consider themselves sexual beings, whereas others may have sex rarely but find it satisfying and enjoyable when they do. Compulsive, frequent sex can become unrewarding for some, whereas others thrive on a frequent and active sex life. What is "right" for a particular individual or couple must be determined based on the various meanings and expectations they associate with sexuality.

Sexual fantasies are limited only by human imagination and may be enjoyed for their own sake. Fantasies may be exciting to a person who would never want to experience them in real life, or they may be objects of yearning. Obsessive and intrusive images that cause discomfort may need to be addressed with psychotherapy.

The majority of women enjoy and need direct **clitoral stimulation** manually or orally to reach orgasm. Unfortunately, many men assume that their female partners are fully satisfied with only intercourse. A result of this overemphasis on intercourse is that many women and men are uncomfortable with genital caressing alone. Couples can benefit from encouragement and permission to learn about and enjoy noncoital sex.

Most gay, lesbian, bisexual, or transgender patients do not wish to have their sexual orientation or gender changed or challenged any more than do heterosexuals, and often present the same concerns as heterosexuals about normalcy, dysfunction, and intimacy.

Life Changes: Menopause, Aging, & Sexuality

Sexuality is an all-encompassing term that includes ***sexual identity, sexual function***, and ***sexual relationships***, *all of which* may be modified by a number of factors including both female ***menopause*** and ***aging***. **Gender** is a social and legal status, as well as a set of expectations from society, about behaviors, characteristics, and thoughts.

Aging brings with it a number of recognized and normal changes in sexual response. These include the following:

1. In both men and women, more direct genital stimulation and more time are needed for arousal (lubrication or erection).
2. Women may experience irritation and pain with intercourse, especially after menopause or periods of abstinence.
3. Erections may become less rigid.
4. Orgasm may not occur with each sexual encounter and the urge to ejaculate may become less intense.
5. The refractory period (the time interval between a man's ejaculation and his next erection) increases.

Many adults in their 70s, 80s, and even later years are willing to experiment in response to changes in their interest, sexual physiology, and partner status. Some older men and women become less focused on intercourse, finding increased enjoyment in petting, oral sex, and masturbation. Others may be happy to have retired from an active sexual life.

Phosphodiesterase type-5 inhibitor (PDE5) oral medications such as tadalafil (Cialis), sildenafil (Viagra), and vardenafil (Levitra) enhance erectile functioning in many men. In women, results of studies looking for positive effects of these medications on sexuality, in general, have been inconsistent, in part because different end points have been used. However, some data show benefit with PDE5 therapy in those women with previously normal sexual function who developed low libido after starting antidepressant therapy. In the future, it may be found to benefit other select groups of women as well.

Testosterone or estrogen replacement may also be beneficial to correct decreases due to aging, and they are discussed in greater detail below.

DISCUSSING SEXUALITY IN THE GENERAL MEDICAL EXAMINATION

Reasons given by health care providers who are reluctant to address sexual health issues include embarrassment, feeling ill-prepared, belief that the sexual history is not relevant to the chief complaint, and time constraints.

The prevalence of sexual concerns is consistently underestimated by physicians. Hypoactive sexual desire disorder (HSDD) is reported to be the most common sexual disorder. It affects both adult females and males, and is associated with negative emotional, psychological, and medical conditions. Lack of recognition of the widespread prevalence of sexual dysfunction in the population contributes to minimizing the importance of sexual health care.

Some patients may be more reluctant to discuss their diet or exercise patterns than the details of their sexual life, whereas others may feel they risk disapproval or judgment when talking with a medical authority about sexuality, and particularly about their sexual practices. Patients report that provider discomfort and anticipated nonempathetic responses to sexual problems are the primary barriers to discussing sexual health.

When the health care provider introduces the topic of sexuality, it is often helpful to acknowledge right away that the patient may feel some embarrassment. By routinely asking questions about sexual health in an initial history taking, a caregiver shows acceptance of sexual health as an integral part of a person's wellbeing.

Also, the provider can explain that some diseases and conditions can be major factors in the etiology of sexual dysfunction, among them diabetes mellitus, cardiovascular disease, hypertension, immunologic issues, arthritis, chronic back pain, and current and previously treated cancers.

The following is one way to initiate a discussion about sexuality:

> **Doctor**: *One area of health care that is often neglected is sexual health, yet it can be important to people. Do you have any questions about your sex life that you would like to discuss?*

A "no" response can be accepted, without ruling out possible future discussion.

> **Doctor:** *If you have any questions later on, I'd be glad to talk with you or help you find someone with whom you would be comfortable talking.*

When providers are uncomfortable about a sexual topic, they can make comments such as "I feel somewhat awkward bringing this up," or "I haven't had that experience, but let me find out," or "Can you educate me about that?" These phrases are acceptable to most patients and can extricate the clinician from some difficult situations, as well as foster patient rapport.

As part of the psychosocial component of the general medical examination, a brief sex history should cover the following:

- "How do you like to be called? By which personal pronoun?" This should be asked in the initial part of the first meeting.
- "Are you sexually active now?" "How many current partners do you have?" If none, "When was the last time you had sex?" "Is that O.K. for you at this point in your life?"
- "Are you sexually active with men, women, both, or neither?" To encourage the confidence of lesbian, gay, or bisexual patients, ask about the patient's "partner" rather than using the gender-specific terms "wife," "husband," "boyfriend," or "girlfriend." And ask about "sexual encounters" rather than "intercourse."
- "How satisfied are you with your sexual experiences and functioning?" (Frequency, variety, who initiates, etc.)
- "Do you experience any problems with lubrication, orgasm, erection, or ejaculation?"
- Rather than assuming contraception is necessary, ask, "Do you have a need for contraception?" Follow-up questions may include asking about the efficacy of or level of satisfaction with any current contraception method in use.
- "Have you ever been diagnosed and treated for sexually transmitted diseases (STDs)?" Discussion of human papillomavirus (HPV) vaccine and its relevance to cancer prevention of cervical and oral cancers can then be included.
- "Have you ever been tested for human immunodeficiency virus (HIV), and if so do you know if you are positive?" "Are you aware of safer sex precautions,

such as the use of condoms and barrier protection, even when there is no risk of pregnancy or when other contraceptives (e.g., intrauterine device [IUD] or "the pill") are used?"

- "Have you ever been/or are you currently in a relationship in which you have been/or are being abused emotionally, physically, or sexually?"

Use questions that show openness to other than the modal heterosexual preferences. Making assumptions about a person's sexuality based on age, gender, race, ethnicity, marital status, or sexual orientation may be diagnostically misleading and send damaging messages to the individual. For instance, an elderly patient assumed to be sexually inactive may in fact have multiple sexual partners, and important risk factors for STDs and acquired immunodeficiency syndrome (AIDS) may be missed; or a monogamous gay male may feel stereotyped or misunderstood if it is assumed that he has multiple partners.

Make sure that the terminology is mutually understood. Overly general or euphemistic terms such as "having sex," "getting it on," "making out," "making love," or "losing one's nature" may obscure important details. Terms that are too technical ("coitus," "copulation," and "cunnilingus") or too colloquial ("cunt," "cock," and "fucking") may be inappropriate for use in the professional relationship.

Avoid words that convey moral judgments or indicate little about what an individual is actually experiencing (e.g., "adultery," "frigid," "impotent," "nymphomaniac," and "perversion"). Clinicians can help patients discard demeaning labels by substituting behavioral descriptions such as "having sex outside of your primary relationship," "difficulty getting erections or getting aroused," or "trouble learning to have orgasms." Again, time and experience with a variety of patients provide a sense of what terms are most useful in conveying information to a given patient.

Patients may bring up vague or psychosomatic-like complaints (e.g., insomnia, fatigue, musculoskeletal aches, indigestion, headaches, or any specific symptoms of depression or anxiety) as a veiled request to talk about sexual concerns. Others mention a sexual concern at the end of a visit in an offhand manner, when there is little time for the problem to be adequately evaluated. *The provider may then choose to assess the problem briefly and validate the importance of investigating this as soon as a new appointment can be scheduled.*

Because sexual problems are often the result of a distressing gap between the patient's expectations and experiences, the effective sexual interview aims to elucidate both sides of the equation. *If expectations are unrealistic, the treatment is education; if the experience fails to meet realistic expectations, intervention or referral is indicated.* Often education and other clinical interventions are combined.

CASE ILLUSTRATION 1* VALIDATION OF EXISTING SEXUAL PRACTICES

One couple sought help from a sex therapist because, after 30 years of enjoyable and satisfying sex (involving intercourse that would last less than 5 minutes), they had read an article extolling the virtues of extended intercourse and began to feel inadequate. When encouraged to value their own unique sexual patterns, versus what might be right for someone else, they were relieved and decided they did not have a problem after all. They then felt freer to build upon what was already satisfying to them in a spirit of exploration, rather than of attempting to be more "normal."

SEX PROBLEM INTERVIEW

When getting a sex problem history and before proposing solutions, health care professionals need to ask questions about the relative importance of sex in the patient's life and their expectations for a fulfilling sex life.

The language of medicine is clinical, whereas issues of sexuality are associated with feelings and emotional vulnerabilities. Pay special attention to the case reports. They illustrate how cool clinical material can be translated to a warmer clinician–patient approach that allows for better trust and engagement with these vital human issues.

As with any other medical problem, five basic areas need to be addressed for the patient presenting with a sex problem (Table 33-2):

1. Explicit symptom or question
2. Onset and course of the symptom
3. Patient's perception of the cause and maintenance of the problem
4. Medical evaluation, including medical history, past treatment, and outcome—*(Specifically exclude such chronic health problems as diabetes mellitus, cardiovascular disease, hyperlipidemia, hypertension, the arthritides, past or current history of cancer.)*
5. Current expectations and goals for treatment

*Cases 1–10 described in this chapter were of actual patients seen in primary care settings as reported in consultation with the first author. Although some identifying characteristics of the patients have been changed to ensure confidentiality, the essential clinical issues presented are accurately portrayed. We thank all the patients and their health providers who helped us gather these examples.

Table 33-2. Sex problem interview.

Description of Current Symptom in Detail
• Signal that you are glad the patient brought up the problem (to give approval, counteract shame, and encourage the patient). • Help the patient specify exactly what the problem is, being careful to use understandable language—low desire, not getting wet or lubricating, difficulty getting or losing a "hard-on" or erection, difficulty "coming" or having orgasm, "coming too quickly" or rapid ejaculation, and so on. • *I'd like to ask a few questions to help us sort it out.* • *Tell me what happens.* • *How is that a problem for you?* • *Anything else that has changed?*
Onset and Course
• *Does it happen alone with self-pleasuring or masturbation, with a specific partner, or with any partner?* • *How does your partner respond when the problem occurs?* • *Was there a time it was more enjoyable and then changed?* • *Any situations when it's not a problem?*
Patient's Perception of Cause and Maintenance of Problem
• *Anything you think might be causing it or that you worry might be causing the problem or keeping it going?*
Medical Evaluation, Past Treatment, and Outcome
• *Do you smoke or use prescription or over-the-counter medications, drugs, or alcohol?* • *Do you have any medical illnesses or treatments, depression, anxiety, or relationship problems?* • *For women: Are your menses normal, regular? Have you had any children? Were any problems associated with pregnancy, delivery, breast-feeding?* • *For men: Do you notice morning or nocturnal erections? Are they firm enough for penetration?* • *Do you have a need for birth control? If so, what method do you (as a couple) use? Are you satisfied/happy with this choice? Are you anxious about the efficacy of this method? Are you concerned that this method could fail?* • *Are you concerned you might have gotten an STD? Has your current partner given you or do you fear that your current partner might give you an STD (e.g., he won't use a condom?)* • *Any history of physical, emotional, or sexual abuse? (In your current relationship, or in one in the past?)* • *What have you already tried to help change the problem?* • *Have you ever had psychotherapy, couple, or sex therapy? If yes, was this sexual problem addressed in the treatment?* • *Have you discussed this problem openly with your partner?*
Current Expectations and Goals for Treatment
• *How important is it to you to get help with this problem, and are you interested in trying to change it now?* • *What would be the minimum improvement you would need in order to feel it was worth your time and effort in dealing with this problem?* • *Almost everyone has sexual concerns at one time or another. Talking about them is the most important first step. I'm glad you've felt comfortable talking with me, and I suggest... (or will suggest some things after I've had a chance to review the best resources for you). Many people have been helped with these issues.*

An assessment of problems related to sexual function requires the consideration of all relevant potential etiological factors in order that any appropriate therapeutic measures may be instituted, be they psychosocial, physical, and/or pharmacological. Answers to the preceding inquiries can help guide the clinician to specific interventions.

PHYSICAL EXAMINATION

The detailed examination of the genitourinary system should include checking for signs of androgen or estrogen deficiency or excess, neurologic dysfunction, genital abnormalities, genital trauma, infections, condylomata (warts), and vascular disease.

For men, the examination should include the penis (to exclude conditions such as Peyronie's disease, penile discharge, warts, other lesions, and hypospadias); testes and scrotum (for masses, atrophy, hernia, or varicoceles); and skin, prostate, and rectum. Testing should be conducted for evidence of gynecomastia, peripheral vascular disease, and neuropathy. Testicular self-examination can also be taught and information about prostate issues provided.

For women, look for evidence of atrophic changes, skin disorders (infectious or otherwise), developmental changes, urinary tract disorders, and general evidence of genital (internal and external) physical abnormalities, pelvic floor weaknesses, and postsurgical conditions. In case of genital pain, the woman should be encouraged to point out specific sites of pain, using a mirror to localize it, if necessary.

The gynecologic examination provides an excellent opportunity for teaching patients about breast self-examination, discussing safe sex practices, importance of HPV vaccination for protection against HPV and its consequences, and, if appropriate, contraception.

Sexual symptoms are rarely as clear-cut as a factual medical approach might yield. Generally, any condition or medication that is debilitating or energy depleting can be a contributory cause of sexual problems. Debilitation and/or anxiety are most frequently the final common denominators resulting in a sex problem. When going through the steps of Annon's P-LI-SS-IT model below, look for evidence of these final common pathways as a guide to making the best use of the model.

When readily treatable conditions have been addressed and overall pathology can be excluded, patients can be reassured that their genitals look "quite healthy" and are in the normal range. This can help counter the shame that many people feel about these vulnerable areas of the body. Naming specific genital parts, such as the foreskin and glans of the penis and the clitoris and labia as you examine them, may give increased permission for the patient to ask any questions or express any concerns they may have about them. Men concerned about the size of their penis or women with worries that their genitals are somehow abnormal are more likely to voice these concerns after the clinician has comfortably used these words.

LABORATORY TESTS

In general, few laboratory tests are necessary for patients presenting with the most common sexual problems. For complaints of low sexual desire, patients should be screened for depression and fatigue; tested for anemia, abnormal thyroid hormone levels, and liver and renal disease; or any other debilitating medical problems suggested by the history and physical examinations. Negative sexual side effects may be caused by gonadotropin-releasing hormone (GnRH) agonists, and narcotics (see "Medications").

Recommended screening tests for women presenting with low libido may include TSH (thyroid stimulating hormone) and prolactin. However, it is important to recognize that there are no specific laboratory markers that "confirm or exclude" the diagnosis of low libido. In women, measurement of testosterone is not recommended, as low testosterone is neither supportive nor diagnostic of the condition.

For male patients with erectile failure or low libido, some authorities recommend evaluation of serum testosterone, TSH, and prolactin levels. Elevated prolactin levels can be the result of many medical conditions, including pituitary tumors; renal dysfunction; sarcoidosis; thyroid disease; trauma; pelvic surgery; or use of medications such as cimetidine, haloperidol, and phenothiazine. If any of these tests are abnormal or other endocrine problems are suggested by the history or physical examination, specific, relevant additional tests should be performed as indicated.

For some men with erectile concerns, testing by a urologist may be indicated. These may include monitoring of nocturnal penile tumescence (NPT) in a sleep laboratory or, more commonly and less expensively, with a home monitoring unit or simple snap gauge. Increasingly, a trial with a PDE5, such as tadalafil (Cialis), sildenafil (Viagra), or vardenafil (Levitra), is recommended for both diagnosis and treatment.

ORGANIC & PSYCHOGENIC FACTORS

Rather than describing sexual problems with a simple differential diagnosis of either organic or psychogenic etiology, it is useful to identify both categories of causal factors. These can be assessed with the psychosocial history, sex problem interview, physical examination, and laboratory testing. A symptom that is generalized (occurring in all circumstances) may indicate major organic or psychogenic involvement, whereas situational symptoms tend to be psychogenic (Table 33-3).

ORGANIC FACTORS

Organic factors may be suspected when a man reports an absence of nocturnal or morning erections or is unable to get erect with masturbation. In women who find intercourse painful, important situational variables to identify include whether she has been adequately stimulated and aroused prior to penetration, whether precoital lubricants have been used if needed, whether she feels pain with masturbation or when having sex with a partner, and whether she is able to direct the extent and timing of thrusting or is passive. Adequate vaginal estrogenization

Table 33-3. Symptom patterns and etiology.

Symptom Patterns Suggestive of Principally Organic Etiology
• Generalized (Especially for absent desire, erectile problems, rapid ejaculation, and painful intercourse. Even when generalized, however, rapid ejaculation and primary female orgasmic problems in otherwise healthy individuals are rarely organic.) • Gradual onset • Rapid onset when associated with certain medications
Symptom Patterns Suggestive of Principally Psychological Etiology
• Situational • Rapid onset (unless medications are suspected) • Sexual phobia and aversion

with local (estrogen) therapy, unless specifically contraindicated, should be ensured. Questioning should include possibilities that the problem is not physiological, but psychological, as is sometimes the case with vaginismus. Asking "under what circumstances have you felt pain?" might elicit "with one partner but not with another," "since I was raped," or "it has always been painful." Organic factors should also be considered when a patient has not responded to an adequate course of sex therapy.

MEDICAL CONDITIONS & TREATMENTS

Medical conditions and treatments affecting sexuality are listed in Table 33-4.

As we address the sexual needs of our patients, general health issues such as thyroid dysfunction, cardiovascular disease, diabetes, hypertriglyceridemia, hypertension, neurological disease, and genitourinary disease all need to be kept in mind, as do hormonal factors.

Testosterone Deficiency

Adequate testosterone is important for sexual drive and arousal in both genders. It also determines genital health and function in males. According to the traditional medical perspective, testosterone levels falling within the "normal range" are not indicative of clinically insufficient testosterone levels. However, there have been recent suggestions that men who test within the normal range may indeed benefit from testosterone supplementation.

In women, testosterone also has been shown to be important in HSDD. However, a measured "low" serum testosterone level (not total, free, or bioavailable testosterone) is neither diagnostic of nor confirmatory of the diagnosis.

Nonetheless, studies have shown that a bilateral oophorectomy, particularly premenopausally but also postmenopausally, removes the major androgen source and increases the likelihood of HSDD, as does pelvic trauma, pelvic radiation, and other surgeries that cause pelvic pain and dyspareunia. Hyperprolactinemia, hypopituitarism, hypothalamic amenorrhea, adrenal insufficiency, primary ovarian insufficiency, and ovarian suppression therapy all reduce ovarian androgen secretion as well, thus increasing the likelihood of HSDD. Also, conditions, circumstances, and disorders that increase the level of sex hormone binding globulin (SHBG) may increase the likelihood of HSDD. For example, SHBG levels may be increased by hyperthyroidism and hypothyroidism; HIV; estrogen-containing medications, such as oral contraceptives; and oral (not transdermal) menopausal hormone medications that lower free testosterone levels.

Table 33-4. Medical conditions commonly associated with sexual problems.

- Anxiety disorders
- Arthritis/joint disease
- Diabetes mellitus
- Endocrine problems
- Injury to autonomic nervous system by surgery or radiation
- Liver or renal failure
- Mood disorders, including depression
- Multiple sclerosis
- Peripheral neuropathy
- Radical pelvic surgery
- Respiratory disorders (e.g., COPD)
- Spinal cord injury
- Vascular disease

Abbreviation: COPD, chronic obstructive pulmonary disease.

TESTOSTERONE THERAPY IN WOMEN

No testosterone product specifically formulated for women is approved or available in North America, and a testosterone patch (Intrinsa) previously available in Europe now has been withdrawn from the market. A transdermal testosterone preparation approved for treatment of menopausal women with symptoms arising from testosterone deficiency currently is available only in Australia. In multiple placebo-controlled clinical trials using Intrinsa (a 300 μg transdermal testosterone patch), efficacy has been shown in the management of HSDD both in naturally and in surgically postmenopausal women. This dose, which raised serum testosterone levels only to the upper limit of normal, resulted in significantly improved libido, increased sexually satisfying experiences, and reduced sexually related distress. While no serious adverse events were reported in studies lasting up to 24 months, authorities withdrew or withheld approvals citing lack of long-term breast cancer and cardiovascular safety data.

Transdermal testosterone therapy is preferred because significant differences in absorption of oral testosterone therapy have been shown, resulting in supraphysiological levels in circulation and a resulting risk of hepatotoxicity. Concerns for cardiac and lipid effects have also been raised. Measurement of free testosterone levels is preferred.

Recommendation is that when prescribing (off-label) testosterone therapy, a transdermal route is preferred; an amount equivalent to approximately 1/10th of the male dose may be tried. Serum testosterone levels need to be monitored and dose adjusted to maintain levels within the female physiological range, to avoid virilization and toxicity effects. If a 6-month trial of testosterone therapy is not successful, therapy should be discontinued.

Estrogen Deficiency in Women

The atrophic changes in the vagina and external genital tissues caused by estrogen deficiency—genitourinary syndrome of menopause (GSM)—are reported in up to 60% of postmenopausal women and result in a multitude of problems, commonly including local dyspareunia.

ESTROGEN TREATMENT

Unless contraindicated, local vaginal estrogen preparations for estrogen therapy are recommended. They are very effective in reversing and correcting atrophic changes that occur at times of "low estrogen," such as menopause, premenopause, postpartum, during lactation/breast feeding, premature ovarian failure (early menopause), and anorexia nervosa. All local estrogen therapies are effective, such as vaginal creams, vaginal tablets, and vaginal estradiol rings.

Importantly, estrogen therapy is likely to improve libido, the sexual experience, and satisfaction by correcting atrophy and dryness, improving lubrication, and reducing dyspareunia.

ALTERNATIVES TO ESTROGEN THERAPY

Estrogen sensitive cancers (e.g., most breast cancers) are usually treated with estrogen lowering drugs ("antiestrogens" such as aromatase inhibitors). Under these circumstances estrogen therapy should not be prescribed; rather, nonestrogenic alternatives are recommended. (Note that these alternative therapies can also be combined with estrogen treatment—local or systemic.) Nonestrogenic alternatives include precoital lubricants (e.g., KY Jelly and Astroglide) and vaginal moisturizers (e.g., Replens). Particularly notable among nonestrogenic alternatives are hyaluronic acid (HA) containing products.

Hyaluronic acid is ubiquitous throughout the body, where it is responsible for maintaining tissue hydration (HA can hold >100× its weight in water). It also has been proven to be an effective vaginal moisturizer. In addition, recent studies have shown that HA has antibacterial properties and also promotes healing of mucosal lesions.

OSPEMIFENE

Ospemifene is a selective estrogen receptor modulator (SERM) that has predominantly estrogenic effects on vulvovaginal tissues and treats dyspareunia and GSM. What makes it particularly attractive for many women is that it is taken orally each day and, despite its excellent estrogenic efficacy in the vagina, it does not stimulate either the breasts or the endometrium. However, it should not be combined with other estrogens.

While the effects of estrogen deficiency have focused on vaginal genital changes, it should be noted that these changes can also lead to serious pain with oral sex and clitoral masturbation.

Centrally Acting Agents

Although the intricacy of sexual functioning in women is not yet completely understood, hormones do play an important role. Centrally, two major neurotransmitters, oxytocin and dopamine, are known to be involved in sexual desire and response in women.

Oxytocin, which rises with sexual activity, results in relaxation and bonding, increasing a woman's interest in sexual activity and reducing her anxiety, as does dopamine, which acts centrally also to reduce anxiety about sexual activity. Both are said to act like an "on/off switch."

The sexual problems of women may be complicated by the physical and emotional changes of aging and menopause, especially surgical or premature menopause. Although hormone replacement therapy may be useful, especially with surgical or premature menopause, there is serious controversy about estrogen replacement post natural menopause. In any case, it is most often necessary to address the serious emotional and life crisis issues along with the medical treatment.

Medications Associated with Sexual Dysfuntion

Medications of many kinds have been implicated in sexual dysfunction (Table 33-5). Older antidepressants such as amitriptyline (Elavil) and doxepin (Sinequan) have anticholinergic properties that undermine sexual arousal. The widely used SSRIs—antidepressants such as escitalopram (Lexapro), sertraline (Zoloft), and paroxetine (Paxil)—may inhibit orgasm for women and ejaculation and orgasm for men, while decreasing sexual desire for both. Certain cardiovascular and antihypertensive medications have been notorious for causing sexual dysfunction, as can any medication resulting in sedation or depressive effects.

Table 33-5. Medication and drug categories commonly associated with sexual problems.

- Alcohol
- Anticancer drugs and hormones
- Anticonvulsants
- Antihypertensives, including beta-blockers (at high dosage), excluding ACE inhibitors
- Carbonic anhydrase inhibitors
- Cytotoxic drugs
- Digitalis family
- Diuretics
- H_2 receptor antagonists
- Nonsteroidal anti-inflammatory agents
- Opiates
- Pain medications
- Psychedelic and hallucinogenic drugs
- Psychiatric medications (benzodiazepines, tricyclic antidepressants, monoamine oxidase inhibitors, SSRIs, antipsychotics, lithium carbonate)
- Recreational drugs (tobacco, alcohol, and opiates)
- Sleep medications
- Tranquilizers

Abbreviation: ACE, angiotensin-converting enzyme inhibitors.

MEDICATIONS TO TREAT SEXUAL DYSFUNCTION

Flibanserin (Addyi) is a nonhormonal, centrally acting daily oral multifunctional serotonin agonist and antagonist, and is the only drug currently FDA-approved for the treatment of distress-causing HSDD. It is provided as a 100 mg tablet for premenopausal women and is to be taken daily at bedtime to minimize somnolence. Concomitant alcohol use is to be avoided.

Clinical studies have shown flibanserin to be efficacious also in the treatment of postmenopausal women with HSDD, however, FDA approval for this indication has not (yet) been granted.

Other Recommendations for Patient Management

In the case of antidepressants, strategies to alleviate such dysfunction include: (1) reducing the dosage; (2) taking a weekend "holiday" in which the last dose for the week is taken on Thursday morning and the medication is resumed at noon on Sunday; (3) switching to another medication; or (4) coadministering other medications, such as bupropion-SR (Wellbutrin-SR), neostigmine (Prostigmin), cyproheptadine (Periactin), bethanechol (Duvoid), and yohimbine (Yohimex) 1–2 hours prior to sexual activity. It is hoped that antidepressants currently in development will have fewer negative sexual side effects.

PSYCHOLOGICAL FACTORS

Psychological factors often play a causal role in maintaining sexual dysfunction. This possibility should be considered even in cases when a medical condition or use of a medication that is known to cause a problem has been identified as a cause (Table 33-6). For example, a female patient experiencing difficulty reaching orgasm since being treated with an SSRI antidepressant may continue to have this problem even after discontinuing the SSRI because she is now conditioned to performance anxiety.

Following hysterectomy, some women report increased sexual enjoyment because of the relief from uncomfortable physical symptoms and bleeding, whereas others find the surgery difficult and have a psychological response to the loss of these organs and to the loss of their reproductive capacity. These women may then experience a decrease in sexual desire, arousal, or orgasmic responsiveness. This is particularly so when concomitant oophorectomy is done, notably in premenopausal women.

The research is mixed as to the effects of hysterectomy on orgasm in women. It has been proposed that women differ in the extent to which they perceive uterine and cervical contractions during orgasm, with differing sense of loss after the surgery. There is similar variability in men after prostatectomy. For many, orgasm may feel satisfactory even with a "dry" or retrograde ejaculation, with semen going into the bladder, but others may complain of a loss of orgasmic sensation.

Table 33-6. Psychological conditions commonly associated with sexual problems.

I. Immediate causes (of most concern for the general medical practitioner)
   A. Performance anxiety—fear of inadequate performance
   B. Spectatoring—critically monitoring one's own sexual performance
   C. Inadequate communication with partner regarding sex
   D. Fantasy—absence of fantasy, fantasy incompatible with sexual arousal, or distracting thoughts
II. Deeper causes (for referral)
   A. Intrapsychic issues—early conditioning, sexual trauma, depression, anxiety, guilt, fear of intimacy, or separation anxiety
   B. Relationship issues—lack of trust, power and control issues, anger at partner
   C. Sociocultural factors—attitudes and values, religious beliefs
   D. Educational and cognitive factors—sexual myths or expectations (gender roles, age and appearance, proper sexual activity, performance expectations), sexual ignorance

Adapted from Plaut SM, Lehne GK. Sexual dysfunction, gender identity disorders, and paraphilias. In: Goldman HH, ed. *Review of General Psychiatry*, 5th ed. New York, NY: McGraw-Hill; 2000.

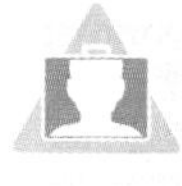

CASE ILLUSTRATION 2 ERECTILE PROBLEM

Juan, a 38-year-old male patient, believing his erection problem was caused entirely by his type II diabetes, was helped to understand that he also had performance anxiety. Declining treatment with PDE5 inhibitors such as tadalafil (Cialis), he wanted to get help without more medication. By quitting smoking cigarettes and learning to engage in noncoital caressing (sensate focusing) with his partner to decrease his pressure to perform, he was able to experience satisfying erections firm enough for intercourse. In this case, the diabetes by itself was not the determining factor in maintaining the problem.

Some medical illnesses and treatments are believed to decrease sexual desire or to cause sexual dysfunction directly. Psychosocial adaptations to virtually any medical condition, however, can indirectly affect sexual desire or functioning. For example, fears of rejection by a sexual partner because of a stoma or mastectomy or concerns about sexual functioning may lead to a suppression of sexual feelings and avoidance of sexual opportunities. Of course, many medically healthy men and women either choose to be sexually inactive or refrain out of a sense of inadequacy. The capacity to enjoy one's sexuality, therefore, cannot be predicted on the basis of medical diagnosis alone.

Psychological problems such as depression or anxiety can be either the cause or the effect of diminished sexual desire or functioning. Both may be true to some degree. In other instances, depression and sexual problems may both be the result of a third underlying factor, such as an endocrine disorder.

Sexual problems might have remote psychological causes, such as childhood trauma or prohibitions about sexual pleasure, but almost all such problems can be seen as having current maintaining variables of anxiety or depression. In general, psychological etiology is primarily suggested when the problem is situational; seems related to performance anxiety, depression, or guilt; is associated with significant relationship and communication problems; or there are indications of trauma from earlier sexual experiences.

PSYCHOLOGICAL MANAGEMENT & BRIEF SEX COUNSELING

A paradigm shift occurred in the treatment of sexual dysfunctions with the publication in 1970 of Masters and Johnson's signal work on sex therapy. The previous emphasis on the diagnosis and treatment of individual psychopathology, with somewhat poor treatment results for the sexual dysfunctions, gave way to an understanding of the importance of the conditions (internal variables such as attitudes, expectations, and lack of knowledge, as well as external factors related to the partner or the situation) under which people attempt to function sexually.

Education and suggestions for focusing on pleasure rather than on performance were found to lower anxiety and to promote improved sexual functioning and enjoyment.

Anxiety is considered one of the major psychological causes of the sexual dysfunctions, whether stemming from individual or relationship issues. Are patients comfortable, at ease, and feeling close to their partners? Or are they anxious due to lack of information, strained relationships, unrealistic attitudes about and focus on sexual performance goals, or other conditions? In these cases, modern sex therapy commonly provides anxiety-reduction interventions, many of which can be adapted for use by primary care providers. These include validating that most people at some time experience sexual problems and that such problems are often an understandable response to stress, worry, and concerns about performance; encouraging open communication between partners; dispelling maladaptive beliefs about sex; suggesting ways that patients can increase their level of comfort and safety and their ability to relax during sex; and encouraging the view that noncoital sex can be very satisfying and does not have to be considered "second best."

THE P-LI-SS-IT MODEL

Annon's P-LI-SS-IT model is a useful hierarchical guide to anxiety-reduction approaches to sexual problems and can be used by primary care practitioners. The letters in the acronym stand for different levels of intervention.

P = Permission

The fundamental intervention is to give patients permission to discuss their sexual concerns. Empathic listening, including verbal and nonverbal reassurance, helps give patients permission to talk openly about sexual issues and may encourage and enable them to discuss the problem more directly with a partner. Reassurance and permission can help validate that having a sexual problem is normal, rather than pathological. Inquire into positive exceptions: patients can describe those areas of sex about which they do feel good; for example, a woman can appreciate her ability to become aroused despite difficulty reaching orgasm, and a man can be a skillful lover despite his erectile problem. Permission to choose not to be sexually active may be very helpful for patients who feel pressured to have sex or who feel inadequate if they do not care to be sexually active.

LI = Limited Information

Facts can add to the effectiveness of reassurance and can be at the disposal of any clinician who has done basic reading about sexuality and keeps up through the literature or review courses. Keeping responses focused and limited to the expressed concern saves time and does not overwhelm the patient with extraneous information (Table 33-7). Such information gives the patient the choice of maintaining or changing sexual practices or attitudes. A simple explanation of the psychophysiology of sexual arousal and the importance of conditions for relaxation helps "normalize" the symptoms and refocuses attention on conditions that can be changed to alleviate the problem, rather than on trying to determine what is wrong with the patient. One physician conveyed this information by the following "rhinoceros" story about sexuality:

Imagine you are lying on a blanket in a secluded meadow with a loving partner after a wonderful picnic lunch on a beautiful sunny day. You start kissing and feel arousal in your genitals, when, all of a sudden, a rhinoceros charges out of the jungle straight for you. What happens to your arousal (lubrication or erection)?

Table 33-7. Limited information: maladaptive ideas and therapeutic responses to them.

Maladaptive Idea	Therapeutic Response
My sexual problems are because I'm too old.	For those who are interested and willing to be creative, sex can be an enjoyable part of life in their 70s, 80s, and beyond!
I should be interested only in survival, not sex (for someone with terminal or chronic illness).	If sex was important to you before your illness it can remain so or become so again.
I am *asexual* because I don't have an active sex life.	We are *all* sexual beings. You can be aware of and enjoy your sexual feelings without being sexually active.
Sex equals love.	Many people have very loving relationships without being sexually active, and, of course, some people have sex without having loving feelings.
Sex equals intercourse.	There is no one *right* way to be sexual, and many people enjoy touching and caressing more than intercourse.
Having sex is the same as *enjoying sex*.	Many people have to learn to enjoy their sexuality.
It is not proper to talk about sex, either with your partner or a health care provider.	It is often a great relief when people can talk confidentially about their sexual feelings and concerns.
You shouldn't talk about sex because it will destroy the mystery.	Most people find that talking about their important feelings deepens intimacy, and trust develops when you know you can be vulnerable with another. You can create more mystery from deeper sharing.
You should be interested in having sex with any willing partner.	It is most important to be able to respect yourself. Your sexuality is a gift that you share only with those you truly want to share it with.
You should be able to enjoy sex with a partner even when you are tired, angry, or feel hurt.	We all have our own conditions for what makes a sexual encounter enjoyable, and feeling close to and loved by your partner is important to most of us.
I try not to masturbate and feel guilty when I give in, because I have a partner and shouldn't need to do that.	Most married people continue to masturbate and find it does not interfere with the pleasure they have with their partner.
Sex is a performance, and it would be grim and catastrophic to "fail."	Sexual sharing can be playful, with the goals of giving and receiving feelings of pleasure and caring. If things don't go as planned, there is always next time!
A new partner will not like the size of my (breasts/penis).	Most men and women enjoy having sex with a person, not a body part. Most men compare themselves to other men when their penises are soft . . . size differences are usually not as great when erections are compared. Vaginas accommodate different penis sizes, with the outer third and the clitoris the most responsive areas for many women.
Sex should result in orgasm every time.	Does *not* having dessert ruin a fine meal? Orgasm is only one of the pleasurable aspects of a sexual encounter. Many people find it a relief to not have "shoulds" in their sex life.
Sex should never be a problem. Experiencing a problem is not normal.	Sex is perfectly natural, but not naturally perfect. Probably everyone has "problems" with sex at some time or another.

The fight-or-flight response causes a rapid redirection of blood to the brain and large-muscle groups, with a corresponding loss of erection or genital arousal. The rhinoceros represents worrisome thoughts and anxieties about having erections, arousal, or orgasm, or fears that you won't please your partner or be seen as a good lover. Some simple suggestions can help you keep the rhinoceros out of your bedroom!

SS = Specific Suggestions

Where permission and limited information do not suffice, the patient may benefit from specific suggestions to help overcome a sexual problem. Most sex counseling interventions are designed to help the patient (and partner, if available) communicate better about sex and enjoy increased sexual pleasure by reducing performance anxiety about attaining the goals of arousal, lubrication, erection, and orgasm. Helpful interventions taken from sex therapy include: (1) temporary agreement not to have intercourse; (2) suggestions for focusing on pleasurable touch, genital caressing, Kegel exercises (tensing and relaxing the pubococcygeal [PC] muscles), and progressive muscle relaxation methods; (3) correction of cognitive distortions ("self-talk"); and (4) suggestions to improve emotional and sexual communication.

Even for couples who previously enjoyed certain patterns of lovemaking, predictable repetition over time can lead to sexual boredom. Suggesting that a couple agree, for example, to temporarily forego intercourse or otherwise change their usual sexual pattern often helps them focus on moment-to-moment pleasure. Rather than making assumptions about what the other wants, the couple can communicate their likes and dislikes. Many people remember how arousing and exciting it was when they were younger and were "making out" (sexual petting) without intercourse. If agreeable to both, they can take turns exploring other ways of caressing and pleasuring each other. The sensate focus exercise, from Masters and Johnson, is done for the interest of the person doing the touching, rather than for the pleasure of the receiver. To minimize performance anxiety, each is encouraged to take turns "savoring" the experience of touching and exploring the other's body, in contrast to worrying about "turning on" or performing for the partner. For many people, permission for genital caressing in this way increases sexual pleasure and satisfaction.

Arranging for follow-up after giving specific suggestions keeps the health care provider informed as to their effectiveness, helps the patient stay focused on problem solving, and informs the clinician about the necessity for further intervention.

IT = Intensive Therapy

This is the last step in the hierarchy and involves referral to an appropriate specialist when the previous three levels of intervention have not been effective (see "Indications for Referral").

ADDITIONAL PATIENT EDUCATION

Pamphlets detailing approaches for safe sex for the prevention of AIDS can supplement discussions and should be made readily available for patients. Many good self-help books dealing with common sexual problems enable patients to move at their own pace. Often people who are reluctant to enter counseling or who are hesitant about discussing their problems in depth are willing to read about the problems in the privacy of their home where they can be relaxed and comfortable. Several books are recommended at the end of this chapter. Educational videos are also available and useful for some patients.

INDICATIONS FOR REFERRAL

Refer patients to an appropriate medical specialist if the brief treatment suggestions in this chapter fail to help or if the history and physical examination suggest primarily an organic component. Refer patients to a mental health specialist trained in sex therapy if the problem is situational, occurring only with a certain partner; if functioning is adequate under certain conditions; or if significant emotional distress is present.

Primary care clinicians can develop a resource list of providers for sex-related problems. Colleagues, teachers, friends, and clinical societies can be asked for recommendations. Identify medical and mental health specialists with expertise in treating sexual issues. Practitioners can be licensed in psychiatry, psychology, social work, psychiatric nursing, or marriage and family counseling. Most states do not license "sex therapists" or "sex counselors."

COMMON SEXUAL PROBLEMS

Low or Absent Sexual Desire & Aversion

Symptoms & Signs

The range of issues concerning sexual desire is wide (Table 33-8). As the etiology is multifactorial, the approach to treatment will also need to be broad, ranging from counseling on basic sexual and possibly lifestyle issues, to consideration of pharmacotherapies including hormones.

It must be respected that some people normally put a low priority on sex or choose to not have any active sexual life. Others may be inhibited or find sex aversive, and some are clinically phobic. These problems can be of recent origin or reflect a long-standing pattern. Lack of desire may pertain situationally only to certain sexual partners or practices (such as oral sex). Couples with different levels of desire may disagree as to which partner's level is "abnormal." In this situation, each side has valid feelings, and it is important not to stigmatize the patient with the lower level of desire. Most couples occasionally deal with periods of discrepancy in desire or mutually low desire and feel they should have sex more often than they do. Demands of family, career, and friends often take precedence over sex.

Problems with desire or sexual aversion can derive from deeper relational power struggles or reflect childhood sexual, physical, or emotional abuse that requires couple counseling or individual psychotherapy for resolution. The following case example, however, demonstrates how permission and encouragement to talk about sex directly, together with specific suggestions, can have a powerful positive influence.

CASE ILLUSTRATION 3
LOSS OF SEXUAL DESIRE

Alice, a healthy 33-year-old primary school teacher, reported having lost her desire for sex. Her sex problem history established that although she had enjoyed sexual activity with her husband for the first 2 years of their marriage, in the past year

Table 33-8. Common sexual problems and treatment approaches. (Distress levels can be more clearly delineated by a useful three-degree scale such as *no problem*—"never," *mild problem*—"hardly ever," or *significant problem*—"rather often," "often," "nearly always," and "always.")

Problem	Diagnostic Criteria	Treatment Approach
Low sexual interest/desire	Diminished or absent sexual interest or desire in thoughts or fantasies and low or absent motivation to become sexually aroused.	After organic causes ruled out or if situational: **Permission and limited information:** Restate problem in behavioral terms. Explore patient conditions for good sex (rhinoceros story), including whether patient receives adequate direct stimulation. Validate patient's right to say "no" to sex.
Sexual aversion	Extreme aversion and avoidance of genital sexual contact with a sexual partner.	May be secondary to depression, anxiety, panic, or phobic disorder (occasionally related to childhood sexual abuse), or May be symptomatic of hidden arousal or orgasmic problems (if so, treat appropriately) **Specific suggestions:** Listening exercises to *increase communication* with partner, *Suggested readings* (Barbach, 2000; Johnson, 2008, 2013; Zilbergeld, 1999). **Intensive treatment:** Refer to mental health professional trained in sexual therapy.
Sexual arousal problems	Difficulty with adequate lubrication-swelling response of sexual arousal (female) or erection (male). Three subtypes include:	**Permission and limited information:** Give brief explanation of the physiology of arousal and the need for relaxation. Is sexual desire present? (if not, treat as desire problem).
Erectile or lubrication problems	*genital sexual arousal problems* characterized by minimal genital arousal and vaginal lubrication despite subjective excitement from nongenital sexual stimulation; *subjective sexual arousal problems* with absent or diminished sexual feelings despite vaginal lubrication and other signs of physiologic response; *combined genital and subjective arousal problems* with absent or diminished feelings of sexual excitement and pleasure as well as absent or diminished vulval swelling, lubrication, or erection.	**Specific suggestions:** Is there enough and the desired kind of direct stimulation by partner? Use of lubricants (Astroglide, K-Y, and so on) or vaginal moisturizers (Replens). For males: PDE5 inhibitors tadalafil (Cialis), sildenafil (Viagra), and vardenafil (Levitra). Suggest progressive muscle relaxation and Kegel exercises, explore ways other than intercourse of pleasuring the partner, temporary intercourse ban, genital caressing/sensate focus (nondemand pleasuring), hormonal therapy, low-dose beta-blocker (10 mg Propranolol) if high-performance anxiety. **Intensive treatment:** Sexuality oriented psychotherapy, vacuum device (older male with organic etiology), intracorporeal penile injection or intraurethral application of PGE_1, penile implant.
Persistent genital arousal (female)	Spontaneous, intrusive, and unwanted genital arousal. Can be secondary to neurologic pathology, onset or discontinuation of treatment with SSRIs and other mood stabilizers, beginning menopause, severe stress, and inactivity.	**Permission and limited information:** Psychoeducation and support that this is a physiologic and psychologically distressing experience, but one many women suffer and get help with. **Specific suggestions:** Anesthetizing agents or ice, pelvic massage and stretching, SNRIs. **Intensive treatment**: Mindfulness, body awareness, and cognitive behavioral exercises.
Persistent genital arousal (male) Priapism	Full or partial erection more than 4 hours after sexual stimulation and orgasm and unrelated to sexual stimulation.	**Intensive treatment**: May need penile blood aspiration.

(*Continued*)

Table 33-8. Common sexual problems and treatment approaches. (Distress levels can be more clearly delineated by a useful three-degree scale such as *no problem*—"never," *mild problem*—"hardly ever," or *significant problem*—"rather often," "often," "nearly always," and "always.") (*Continued*)

Problem	Diagnostic Criteria	Treatment Approach
Rapid ejaculation	Lifelong rapid ejaculation occurring prior to or within about 1 minute of vaginal or anal penetration after minimal sexual stimulation, with subjective distress, bother, frustration, or avoidance of sexual situation. (Occasional or temporary rapid ejaculation is not considered problematic when age, novelty, and frequency of sexual activity increase excitement to ejaculation.)	**Permission and limited information:** As above, plus discuss masturbation patterns—he may have conditioned himself to ejaculate rapidly. Explain connection between rapid ejaculation and anxiety versus relaxation and longer-lasting erections. **Specific suggestions:** Above, plus increase frequency of ejaculation, stop–start exercises (Zilbergeld, 1999), clomipramine (Anafranil 25 mg as needed) or SSRI antidepressant medication, prilocaine–lidocaine cream with condom.
Orgasm problems	Difficulty or inability to reach orgasm, greatly diminished orgasmic sensations, or significant delay of orgasm despite significant sexual stimulation. Clinician should consider the age, sexual experience, and the adequacy of sexual stimulation received.	**Permission and limited information:** As above. **Specific suggestions:** For primary preorgasmic woman, recommend Barbach (2000); for male, Zilbergeld (1999). If orgasmic problem is secondary (at one time patient was orgasmic), then evaluate and treat for desire or arousal problem or relationship problems.
Delayed ejaculation	Unwanted delay in or difficulty reaching ejaculation (and usually orgasm) despite arousal and excitement.	**Permission and limited information:** As above, plus inquire about masturbation patterns—he may have conditioned himself to ejaculate to idiosyncratic fantasies, or with more vigorous stimulation than intercourse provides. Performance anxiety may exacerbate it. Rule out medications causing delayed ejaculation such as SSRIs. **Specific suggestions:** Encourage explicit communication with patient's partner about his need to have enough stimulation prior to ejaculation and orgasm. **Intensive treatment:** Sex therapy may be useful, focusing on sexual behaviors, fantasies, and relationship issues.
Genital pain Dyspareunia	Recurrent or persistent genital pain associated with sexual stimulation, such as intercourse, in either a man or a woman.	**Permission and limited information:** As above. **Specific suggestions:** As above, plus encourage explicit communication with patient's partner about her need to have enough stimulation prior to penetration, with the partner experiencing pain having control to choose when penetration occurs and timing of thrusting.
Vaginismus	Persistent and recurring involuntary muscle spasm of the outer third of the vagina making penetration by a penis, finger, or other object difficult.	**Intensive treatment:** Sex therapy may be useful for long-standing dyspareunia and vaginismus, due to conditioned expectation of pain.

it had become a chore that she never put on her extensive "to do" list. Because sex was seen as a bedtime activity, when she was usually tired, their sexual frequency dropped from weekly to once every several months. They did not address the problem directly, and Alice and her husband's feelings of estrangement from each other continued to grow.

When asked what steps they had taken to address these problems, Alice disclosed that she and her husband had never had an open discussion about sex. Her primary care physician validated that this was common among couples and that most people have to learn to talk more comfortably about their sexual needs (Permission and Limited Information). The physician also explained that everyone has certain conditions that need to be met to be interested in sexual activity (P and LI) and encouraged Alice to think about her conditions and then, with her husband, to "set some private time aside outside of the bedroom to let yourselves have a discussion about this, even if it is awkward" (Specific Suggestions).

Doctor: *It can be good for relationships when people risk being a little uneasy. You don't have to have the same perspective. You are each entitled to your own separate feelings about the situation, but together you can talk it out, try to understand each other, and see what other choices you have (P, LI, and SS).*

At her 1-month follow-up appointment, Alice reported significant progress. When the couple set time aside to discuss their sex life, they had a very meaningful and tender talk. The husband was relieved to learn about the major sources of Alice's lack of desire, and she acknowledged feeling resentful that he seemed unresponsive to her needs. He admitted that he had taken her lack of desire very personally, secretly, and painfully interpreting the problem as her lack of desire for him. With these hidden resentments expressed, they could set aside their power struggles and cooperate in addressing these issues. Recognizing how they had both felt lonely and uncared for allowed them to take specific actions, such as planning a regular evening each week just for the two of them to talk and nurture their intimacy.

The physician also recommended a self-help book and offered to refer the couple to a therapist who treats couples, should their attempts to communicate falter.

MANAGEMENT: PERMISSION & LIMITED INFORMATION

For many individuals and couples, not being sexually active can be a choice and, if acceptable to the people involved, should not be judged by others to be dysfunctional.

Others may learn to accept that low desire may be understandable given their immediate circumstances (e.g., the months prior to and after childbirth, recovering from illness) and that their previous levels of desire can be expected to return over time. Validate the patient's right to say "no" to sex.

When a person presents diminished or lacking sex drive as a problem, questions can explore the conditions under which the person has previously felt the desire for sexual contact and release and help her or him think about ways to reestablish some of those circumstances.

People raised within traditional sex roles can be helped to identify issues arising from sexual "suppression," wherein neither women nor men experience their sexual potentials. Questions about desire open the door to sexual fantasies and scripts, and they can form reference points for reestablishing desire where it is low or absent. For example, if a woman has experienced desire and excitement during courtship, but none after marriage, the doctor might help her understand why these changes have occurred and suggest potentially simple solutions.

SPECIFIC SUGGESTIONS

A "prescription" to go away on a weekend or to arrange a sleepover for children with relatives may help couples "break the ice" and reexperience intimacy. Suggest that patient and partner set aside time to talk about each other's feelings and discuss conditions for more enjoyable sex, with each taking an uninterrupted amount of time for self-expression. Self-help books may also be recommended.

INTENSIVE THERAPY

An assessment for couple or individual psychotherapy may be indicated when simpler discussions and behavioral changes have been unsuccessful.

OTHER MEDICAL INTERVENTIONS

Clearly, comorbid conditions should be excluded and consideration given to readjusting current medications, if appropriate. Positive results in several domains have been obtained in some studies of postmenopausal women with sexual problems, treated with transdermal testosterone, usually in addition to menopausal hormone therapy (i.e., estrogen ± progestin). (See the discussion above under "Testosterone Therapy in Women.")

Sexual Arousal Problems

SYMPTOMS & SIGNS

Problems with female arousal are primarily manifested as vaginal dryness and may be reported separately from or together with lack of desire, difficulty reaching orgasm, or pain experienced during intercourse. The most common medical cause in older women is estrogen deficiency with resulting signs of vulvar irritation and atrophic vaginitis. Arousal may be inhibited by anxiety, depression, or shame resulting from early conditioning; it may also be a side effect of antidepressant medication. These possibilities should be explored (see Tables 33-4 to 33-6).

Male arousal problems are manifested by erectile problems physically, but also include subjective inhibitions and performance anxiety as well.

CASE ILLUSTRATION 4

Betty, a 78-year-old patient, had an appointment with her female physician. She brought along her 82-year-old husband because she wanted to discuss what she called her "sexual problems." Betty said she did not care about sex, that her husband was often angry at her lack of enthusiasm, and that this pattern had existed throughout the 50 years of their marriage. She believed she was not "a sexual person" because she had never been very excited by intercourse. She did enjoy kissing and caressing and mentioned that on several occasions she had been able to have orgasm when he stroked her labia and clitoris, but that she had never had orgasm from the "real sex" (intercourse) that he preferred. The physician responded that there really is no one way to be a "sexual person," that many people cherish the sensual and emotional aspects of sex, and that Betty did not need to consider herself asexual just because she preferred different aspects of sexual intimacy than her husband (**P** and **LI**). The physician further explained that the majority of women reach orgasm more often from manual caressing than from coitus, and that many couples enjoy bringing each other to orgasm without intercourse (**P** and **LI**). The couple was relieved and admitted to having curiosity about trying this petting more. They were given brief instructions to take turns at home touching and stroking each other without the goal of orgasm (sensate focus), to get reacquainted with each other's body, and to refrain from any attempts at intercourse for 2 weeks (**SS**).

A follow-up telephone call confirmed that they were enjoying taking turns caressing each other, that orgasm often happened for each, and that they occasionally progressed to intercourse. A 1½-year follow-up was especially poignant—the husband reported that Betty had recently died from a stroke, and, although grieving her loss, he expressed profound appreciation for having gotten help for their sexual conflicts from the physician.

Husband: *Settling those old battles over sex made our last year together more loving and caring than ever before in our marriage.*

MANAGEMENT: PERMISSION & LIMITED INFORMATION

Is the patient getting stimulation in the way that works best for her? Feeling distant from or angry with a partner can inhibit sexual arousal, and such relationship concerns need to be addressed.

SPECIFIC SUGGESTIONS

Homework may be suggested for her to identify what stimulation works best. The goal is to experience the pleasure of arousal in that mode—not to reach orgasm. Inquiry should be made into the quality of the patient's relationship. Commercial lubricants (Astroglide, KY Jelly, and so on) and vaginal moisturizers (such as Replens) can be suggested and, if vaginal atrophy is present, a low-dose intravaginal estrogen preparation (cream, pill, or suppository) should be prescribed unless contraindicated.

Self-help books also can be recommended, such as ones by Barbach (2000) and Johnson (2008, 2013).

INTENSIVE THERAPY

Recommend individual or couple therapy with a clinician skilled in human sexuality issues (where appropriate).

OTHER MEDICAL INTERVENTIONS

Referral to an ob–gyn or other women's health specialist.

Erectile Problems

SYMPTOMS & SIGNS

There have been more than a dozen studies in the past 12 years or so showing a growing link between erectile problems and cardiovascular disease in men, including younger populations. If a man presents in a primary care setting with erectile complaints, the health care provider should always assess cardiovascular risk factors as potential contributing factors and recommend aggressive risk factor reduction (e.g., weight loss and exercise) if relevant.

Generally, a man with a significant psychological component is aware of nocturnal or morning erections, is able to maintain his erection for a reasonable time and then ejaculate with masturbation, or has good erections in some situations but not in others. He may be able to get a firm erection but lose it after penetration or may not get an erection with a partner at any time. The original cause of the problem is often distinct from the maintaining variable, which is generally anxiety. Consider possibilities such as performance anxiety, lack of direct physical stimulation of the penis, conscious or unconscious guilt (e.g., "widower's syndrome"), anger at his partner or other relationship issues, or childhood issues such as sexual abuse.

CASE ILLUSTRATION 5

Carl, a 58-year-old HIV-negative gay male, confided to his nurse practitioner that he had been "impotent" since the death of his partner of 17 years, with whom he had had an active and monogamous sexual life. Attributing this problem to aging and worries about HIV infection, Carl nonetheless asked for any help the practitioner could provide. A full session was scheduled for talking only. His partner had died suddenly from cardiac arrest a year before. In the past month, Carl had attempted sex on four occasions with two different men and was unable to get an erection. After a thorough sociosexual history, Carl was seen to fit the "widowers' syndrome." Clearly, he was still grieving the loss of his partner but attempted to control his tears with statements such as "I should be over this by now" and "Life has to go on; he wanted me to go on." Carl then revealed that he was very afraid of feeling such loss, fearing that he would never be able to come out of the sadness. His grieving was acknowledged and validated (**P**), and it was explained to him that temporary sexual problems were common after such loss because of a number of factors: performance pressure of being with a new partner, continuing feelings of loyalty to a deceased partner, subsequent guilt at having sex with new people, and concerns about HIV infection with a new partner (**LI**). The nurse practitioner encouraged Carl to join a grief support group or to contact a psychotherapist comfortable with gay sexuality (**SS**). In addition, she referred Carl to a book on male sexuality, with suggestions on how to talk to a potential partner about both safer sex practices and ways they could reduce the pressure to have erections (**LI** and **SS**). At a follow-up visit 4 months later, Carl reported he had been able to cry more about his loss and was enjoying sex and intimacy with a new friend who had also lost a partner.

MANAGEMENT: PERMISSION & LIMITED INFORMATION

Many patients over 40 years old report previous successful sexual encounters when they were younger, in which they became erect without direct physical stimulation of the penis. If their pattern for sexual interaction has rarely or never included direct touching by a partner, it might help them to learn that such touching becomes more necessary as men age, and that it can be an enjoyable part of sex.

SPECIFIC SUGGESTIONS

Institute a temporary ban on penetration and suggest sensate focus, progressive relaxation, and Kegel exercises. The couple should agree not to attempt penetration or intercourse even if the patient gets an improved erection.

Doctor: *For every minute you are relaxing with your partner and have an erection, your body is remembering just what it needs to do to get and maintain an erection. Your mind can be free to enjoy the pleasurable feelings and sensations of being caressed and kissing your partner. You might even allow your erection to go away. If you stay relaxed, it likely will return again with resumed stimulation.*

INTENSIVE THERAPY

Recommend individual or couple therapy with a clinician skilled in human sexuality issues (where appropriate).

OTHER MEDICAL INTERVENTIONS

Referral to a urologist interested in male sexual functioning.

PDE5 inhibitors. Tadalafil (Cialis), sildenafil (Viagra), and vardenafil (Levitra) are three oral medications popularly known to have revolutionized the medical treatment of male erectile problems. Although contraindicated in men taking organic nitrate medication for angina, these medications have been found to have broad-spectrum effectiveness across men of all ages and medical conditions, including diabetes, hypertension, neuropathy, post-prostatectomy, and depression.

An important caveat is that, in spite of the evidence of PDE5 medications' demonstrated safety and efficacy, approximately 50% of men do not refill their prescriptions. Underlying psychological and interpersonal factors may need to be explored with these patients at follow-up visits.

Testosterone replacement therapy. For men with demonstrated low levels of serum testosterone, hormone replacement therapy may be helpful. This does not seem to benefit men whose serum testosterone is within normal limits, although recent work suggests there may be more subtleties to this. Side effects can be serious, including increase of any existing prostatic cancer, enlargement of the prostate, retention of fluids, and liver damage. Careful monitoring and follow-up prostate-specific antigen (PSA) screening and prostate examinations are necessary.

Antidepressant medication. Antidepressants, especially bupropion-SR (Wellbutrin-SR), can be effective treatment for some, but other patients may find that SSRI antidepressants hinder erection and ejaculation.

External penile vacuum device. With the aid of a vacuum cylinder, a tension ring is placed around the base of the penis after it has become erect. This device may work better for men who clearly have a major organic component to their erectile problem, such as severe diabetes, multiple sclerosis, or spinal cord injury. Although this device can create erections functional for intercourse, men with a more psychogenic etiology may be disappointed when the erections are not as firm as they had been expecting. Side effects may include bruising of the penis.

Intracorporeal penile injections or intraurethral delivery of prostaglandin E1 (PGE1). These methods were originally used diagnostically by urologists. However, patients can now be taught to inject themselves prior to sexual encounters, resulting in firmer erections that often do not disappear at orgasm or ejaculation and last about an hour. Side effects are priapism in less than 3% of patients and pain. In addition, scarring may be a concern with repeated injections over time.

Penile implant surgery. Since the advent of effective oral medications, implants with semirigid silicone rods or inflatable cylinders are less commonly utilized. Total costs are high, usually over $20,000. Complications include device failure (requiring additional surgery) and infection. However, for some men, this has been an effective and helpful treatment.

Rapid Ejaculation (Premature Ejaculation)

SYMPTOMS & SIGNS

Terms such as "rapid" or "early" ejaculation are clinically preferable to the established "premature ejaculation," as they highlight the subjective nature of the problem and are less pejorative. No absolute measure—either in number of minutes or thrusts—is applicable to the diverse numbers of men presenting with this problem. Factors to be assessed include a patient's subjective evaluation, degree of sexual satisfaction, and sense of control.

CASE ILLUSTRATION 6

Donald, a 45-year-old divorced man, reported ejaculating after 1 minute or less of intercourse. This had been his pattern since becoming sexually active in his late teens. He reported proudly that he never masturbated but had a high sex drive, which led him to multiple sexual partners including prostitutes. His primary care physician gave Donald a supportive talk about how he could teach himself to last longer with certain physical exercises (**P**, **LI**, and **SS**). The patient was willing to do "self-stimulation" or "self-pleasuring" exercises for this "medical reason" and was comforted that as with the physical fitness regimen that he valued, he could tone up his PC muscles and learn to relax the pelvic muscles during sexual stimulation. Donald was advised to increase his frequency of ejaculation, was told about the importance of relaxation for maintaining an erection, and was encouraged to read Klein's (2012) self-help section on exercises for lasting longer (**P**, **LI**, and **SS**). As his confidence grew through the solo exercises, and as he increased the frequency of ejaculation, Donald was able to try the stop–start exercises with a partner with increasing success. He said that it also helped him to read about the experiences of other men (getting validation from the universality of sexual concerns) and about how many women enjoy a variety of forms of sexual stimulation in addition to intercourse.

MANAGEMENT: PERMISSION & LIMITED INFORMATION

Point out that early ejaculation is a very common problem—one study found that 35% of married males reported that they ejaculated too quickly. Tell the patient that men with this problem have a high success rate when they try one or more specific suggestions for this problem. Give a brief explanation of the psychophysiological mechanism.

Doctor: *Men aren't supposed to be able to have long-lasting erections if they are too nervous or distracted. The fight-or-flight response generally makes men more likely to ejaculate. Most men have trained themselves through rapid masturbation to get erect and ejaculate quickly; so it makes sense that they would continue to ejaculate quickly when they are with a partner.*

Assure the patient that men often report more intense orgasms after they have learned to last longer and that it is highly likely that he will gain greater ejaculatory control by following these suggestions.

SPECIFIC SUGGESTIONS

The patient may need to increase his frequency of ejaculations, alone or with a partner, perhaps masturbating to orgasm earlier on a day that a sexual encounter with a partner is anticipated. Discuss other ways he can please his partner, so he does not feel pressure to do it all with an erect penis. Discuss the importance of muscle relaxation in achieving a prolonged erection. Suggest breathing exercises and progressive muscle relaxation exercises, targeting the PC muscles or those in the buttocks.

In contrast to common attempts by men to diminish sensations in hope of lasting longer, they actually need to increase their tolerance for the good sensations and feelings and can best do this by concentrating on their feelings and getting more "turned on." Focusing on these feelings in a relaxed "practice" atmosphere can increase the threshold of enjoyment before ejaculation and orgasm.

He and his partner can read about and practice the "stop–start technique." Encourage the patient to change positions and to go from intercourse to oral or manual stimulation of his partner, and then back to intercourse (following the desires of his partner); changing positions and pleasuring a partner to orgasm without intercourse helps many men last longer.

INTENSIVE THERAPY

Recommend individual or couple therapy with a clinician skilled in human sexuality issues (where appropriate).

OTHER MEDICAL INTERVENTIONS

Clomipramine (Anafranil, 25 mg as needed) or SSRI antidepressants help men prolong their erections prior to ejaculation.

Prilocaine–lidocaine cream applied to the penis and then used with a condom has been recommended by some clinicians (although "numbing" of the genitals may detract from enjoyment for both partners).

Orgasm Problems

Symptoms & Signs

Many women do not learn to have orgasms until they are in their 20s, 30s, or even later. A primary anorgasmic or preorgasmic woman is not yet able to reach orgasm reliably either with a partner or by herself. A woman with secondary orgasmic problems was previously able to reach orgasm but is no longer able to do so. Situational orgasmic problem refers to a condition in which a woman can have orgasm with masturbation but not with a partner, or with one partner but not with another. She may reach moderate-to-high levels of arousal without experiencing the pleasure and release of climax. If no arousal or interest is present, she should be evaluated for a desire or arousal problem.

Some males might report delayed or absent ejaculation despite prolonged intercourse or other stimulation. Some report ejaculation without the sensation of orgasm.

CASE ILLUSTRATION 7

Ethyl's complaint of low sexual desire and difficulty feeling aroused led the nurse practitioner to do a brief sex problem interview. With this more open discussion, Ethyl revealed that she had never been able to climax, but had been highly aroused in the first year of her 5-year marriage. Their lovemaking style was focused on intercourse, and Ethyl's husband did not seem to understand why she did not enjoy it as much as he did. She had not faked orgasm but had never told him about her feelings of frustration about not reaching orgasm. Ethyl had never masturbated and remembered vague attitudes conveyed by her parents and her church that masturbation was not a correct thing to do. The nurse practitioner then validated that many women first learn about self-pleasuring as adults and that the information she could get about how her own body worked would then be useful in her sexual relationship with her husband. It was suggested that Ethyl read a self-help book for women who want to learn to have orgasms (**P**, **LI**, and **SS**). At a visit 3 months later, Ethyl reported that she had proudly experienced her first orgasm by herself and felt so encouraged by this that she was able to talk more openly with her husband, who then agreed to go with her to see a marital/sex therapist to discuss ways they could bring more pleasure into their own lovemaking.

CASE ILLUSTRATION 8

Frank, a 24-year-old man, confided that he had never reached orgasm with a partner. A sex problem history revealed that he had never ejaculated during intercourse and that his partners had never tried to bring him to orgasm manually or orally. Frank was able to ejaculate with masturbation, describing a vivid sexual fantasy (which he did not allow himself to have when with a partner) and a lifelong pattern of stimulation in which he rubbed his penis back and forth against a pillow without using his hands. He was congratulated for bringing this problem to his physician's attention (**P**) and was told that anxiety was often a cause of this problem, together with a masturbation pattern that did not simulate the type of sensations he would have during intercourse (**LI**). The physician encouraged Frank to take a stepwise approach to the problem by enlisting the help of a willing partner and starting with those elements that had been successful for him. He was also encouraged to expand on the kind of physical stimulation he received during masturbation by gripping his penis with his hand and stroking it. With his partner, Frank was to focus on the goal of having high arousal while his partner stimulated his penis manually and he was imagining his "tried-and-true" fantasy. The next step was to reach higher levels of arousal in this manner and to stimulate an orgasmic response (**SS**). Frank was also referred to a self-help book (**P**, **LI**, and **SS**). Follow-up indicated that Frank had successfully reached orgasm with manual stimulation with a partner in 3 weeks and was following suggestions in the book on his goal toward ejaculation during intercourse.

Management: Permission, Limited Information, & Specific Suggestions

Both men and women may present with difficulties in achieving orgasm because of a repeated pattern of masturbation that does not approximate the stimulation they receive from a partner. Although physical arousal may be apparent (erection or lubrication), these patients may not be feeling excited if they have to forego the fantasies or kinds of stimulation that had worked for them while masturbating. Encouraging them to incorporate the conditions under which they can reach orgasm when alone into their sexual play with a partner is the first step in their expanding their sexual enjoyment. In some instances, use of a vibrator may be recommended to provide the more intense stimulation needed for some people. Explicit communication with the patient's partner should be encouraged about the need to have enough stimulation prior to ejaculation and orgasm.

INTENSIVE THERAPY

Recommend individual or couple therapy with a clinician skilled in human sexuality issues (where appropriate).

OTHER MEDICAL INTERVENTIONS

The usual treatment of problems related to female orgasm is a combination of a good sex and psychosocial history, demythologizing, educating, behavioral treatments, and couples work where needed. There is no medication treatment available, since anorgasmia is rarely a physically caused problem.

Sexual Pain: Dyspareunia & Vaginismus

SYMPTOMS & SIGNS

Dyspareunia—pain for women or men associated with genital sex of all kinds may be one of the most common and perhaps most underreported of the sexual dysfunctions. Vaginismus, a specific cause of female dyspareunia, involves the involuntary spasm of muscles around the vagina. Vaginismus can usually be treated by teaching the patient exercises to establish personal vaginal control and remove sources of contributing associated anxieties, such as conditioning to previous genital trauma, fear of penetration, anatomical ignorance, and others.

A gentle, sensitive genital examination and demonstration should always be a part of the evaluation of vaginismus. The use of progressively sized vaginal dilators has been helpful in some cases, but treatment can often be successful without them.

CASE ILLUSTRATION 9

Nineteen-year-old Gina complained to her primary care provider that she had dyspareunia, was losing interest in sex, and was worried that her boyfriend was becoming impatient with her avoidance of sex. The physician then encouraged her to describe this problem behaviorally and in detail (**P**). Gina said that she had enjoyed intercourse since the age of 17 years and always used latex condoms, but on one occasion 6 months ago she suddenly felt as if her vagina "was being rubbed with sandpaper" when her partner penetrated her. Although the physical pain had not actually returned in subsequent lovemaking sessions, Gina's fear of the pain recurring diminished both her interest in and her enjoyment of sex. When asked what she would do if the pain happened again during intercourse, Gina replied that she "would have to ask him to hurry up, but sometimes he lasts longer then." The physician asked how she would feel about telling him to stop all movement immediately and to withdraw when she felt discomfort or pain. Gina expressed concern that an abrupt withdrawal from intercourse might result in her boyfriend having testicular pain. She was reassured that this would create no lasting discomfort for him, and that there were alternatives for reaching ejaculation and orgasm, either with her or alone (**P**, **LI**, and **SS**). She was also offered some suggestions for reading about how couples learn to increase their enjoyment of sex (**SS**). The physician also praised Gina for having shown the courage to discuss this personal issue and encouraged her to bring up any future concerns (**P**, **LI**).

MANAGEMENT: SPECIFIC SUGGESTIONS

These issues can be approached gradually, by encouraging the woman to speak with her partner about her needs and to be a full participant in the sexual encounter. She and her partner should be educated about the need for sufficient stimulation and arousal prior to attempted penetration, and about the importance of her being in control of the sexual movement, so that she can stop it instantly if pain is felt. Instruction in Kegel's PC muscle exercises increases the woman's awareness and control of her vaginal muscles. Vaginal self-dilatation can be accomplished with graduated cylinders or with fingers, from the little finger to multiple fingers, while practicing muscle relaxation and calming mental imagery. The patient should be encouraged to be the one in control by bearing down on the finger(s) or penis as if pushing something out of the vagina, then relaxing. It helps for some women to imagine "capturing" the penis or other object in this manner, instead of being "penetrated."

OTHER MEDICAL INTERVENTIONS

Other medical suggestions include the use of artificial lubricants, such as Astroglide, Gyne-Moistrin, or KY Jelly (not good with latex); vaginal moisturizers, such as Replens; and vaginal and vulvar application of estrogen creams. Further evaluation of vaginismus includes assessment for developmental anatomical abnormalities; if deemed appropriate, surgical revision of the vulvovaginal region and/or excision of abnormal growths in the genital area may prove helpful. Diseases thought to cause the pain, such as vaginitis, condylomata, endometriosis, pelvic inflammatory disease, and other gynecologic or pelvic diseases, may all be treated directly. When painful intercourse has been a long-standing problem, however, medical intervention alone is seldom adequate and should be followed by sex therapy directed at the probable fear and expectation of pain that have been conditioned.

SEXUAL PROBLEMS DUE TO A GENERAL MEDICAL CONDITION

Many sexual issues of those with impactful medical conditions and physical disabilities may be treated like those persons who are nondisabled and healthy. In other cases, culturally competent health practitioners knowledgeable about the social and physical issues of disability may be most effective. Some studies, such as with women following gynecologic cancer surgery, suggest that Internet support groups can be as beneficial as actual group meetings. Other online resources that are appropriately monitored and proctored by health professionals may become available in the near future.

CASE ILLUSTRATION 10

When Hannah was 22 years old, she was diagnosed with clear cell adenocarcinoma of the vagina and had surgery that removed one ovary, her uterus, tubes, the upper two-thirds of her vagina, and her bilateral pelvic lymph nodes. None of her health care team was able to comfortably discuss sexuality with her. She was completely unprepared for the first attempts at intercourse several months following the surgery and was shocked and distraught to discover how little genital sensation she had left. She sought help from a male psychiatrist who listened as she expressed her grief and fears that she would never find a man because of her sense of diminished sexual self-worth. After rapport was established, he acknowledged her fears by saying that she might never have a "clitoral" orgasm again, but that there were other routes to orgasm and sexual pleasure. He discussed with her ideas that have been helpful to others who have sustained the loss of genital sensation: that her brain knew how to feel pleasure and have orgasms, that men and women can learn to focus on sensations from other, nongenital parts of the body, such as breasts, neck, ears, and lips, and that with or without accompanying fantasy, one can thus relearn to enjoy a sense of orgasmic release and pleasure. Twelve years after her surgery, Hannah wrote, "The growth in my ideas and experiments with sexuality have increased manifold since my surgery. What was most helpful was being able to share my experiences with people who could understand and be accepting, and finding people who were trained and had accurate information on how I could help myself. Health professionals don't have to have all the answers, but they should know their own limitations and be able to refer when necessary."

For those patients who have undergone treatment for significant medical conditions such as cancer—with a potential altered body image and an understandable interruption or cessation of their sexual life—the following attitudes may be helpfully communicated to patients by their health care provider(s):

Whenever you are ready to become sexually active again, there are a few things you can keep in mind:

- ***You are loved for who you are, not just for your appearance.*** If you felt lovable or sexually desirable before you became ill, chances are that you will be afterward too.
- ***We are all sexual beings.*** Sexuality is part of who we are, whether we are sexually active or not. It is not defined just by what we do or how often we do it.
- ***Survival overshadows sexuality.*** It is normal and natural for stress, depression, worry, and fatigue to lower your interest in sex after major medical issues. Just coping with basic everyday decisions can seem like a burden. But take one day at a time and be patient. Sexual interest and feelings often come back when the immediate crisis has passed.
- ***Share your feelings.*** You may find yourself in the position of having to share your sexual feelings with someone, perhaps for the first time. This may be awkward at first, and learning how and when to talk about sexual issues may not come easily. You may feel shy or nervous about exploring new and different ways of finding sexual pleasure. You may each wait for the other to make the first move to resume sexual activities. This familiar waiting game is easily misunderstood and experienced as rejection by both people. It also may be frightening to think of breaking the silence yourself. Yet, a good move is to make the first move. Try sharing some of the myths or expectations you grew up with about sexuality. This can be humorous and may break the ice in starting a frank discussion about your sexual needs and concerns. Try not to make broad, generalized statements. Talk about what is important to you and about how you feel. The payoff is greater understanding of each other's needs and concerns, and that is worth the effort.
- ***Expect the unexpected.*** When you first have sex after a long time without it, physical limitations or fears about your performance, appearance, or rejection may keep you from focusing on the sheer pleasure of physical contact. On the other hand, you may be surprised by unfamiliar pleasurable sensations. If you expect some changes as part of the natural recovery process, they will be less likely to distract you from sexual pleasure if they do happen.
- ***Give yourself time.*** You and your partner may be frightened of, or even repulsed by, scars, unfamiliar appliances, or other physical changes. That's natural, too.

But such feelings are usually temporary. Talking about them is often the first step to mutual support and acceptance. Don't pressure yourself about having to "work on sex." A satisfactory and enjoyable sex life will happen one step at a time. You may want to spend some time by yourself exploring your body, becoming familiar with changes, and rediscovering your unique body texture and sensations. Once you feel relaxed doing this, move on to mutual body exploration with a partner.

- ***Take the pressure off intercourse.*** Almost all of us were brought up to believe that intercourse is the only real or appropriate way of expressing ourselves sexually. Yet sexual expression can encompass many forms of touching and pleasuring that are satisfying psychologically and physically.

Try spending some time in pleasurable activities—touching, fondling, kissing, and being close—without having intercourse. Reexperience the pleasure of playing, of holding and of being held without having to worry about erections and orgasms. When you feel comfortable, proceed at your own pace to other ways of being sexual, including intercourse if you like.

Experiment and explore to discover what feels best and what is acceptable. If radiation therapy, for example, has made intercourse painful, try oral or manual stimulation to orgasm, or intercourse between thighs or breasts. If you are exhausted by the disease or movement is painful, just cuddling or lying quietly next to your partner can be a wonderfully satisfying form of intimacy.

- ***Your sexuality cannot be "diagnosed."*** You will never know what pleasures you are capable of experiencing if you don't explore. Try new positions, new touches, and above all new attitudes.

OTHER SEXUAL PROBLEMS NOT OTHERWISE SPECIFIED

Serious sex-related problems may be best dealt with by a psychotherapist or health professional trained in sexual issues. A patient with compulsive sexual behavior or sexual addiction may be suffering from a form of obsessive–compulsive disorder and may require intensive psychotherapy, use of support groups, and medications such as SSRI antidepressants. Patients with gender identity disorders, patients who have experienced spousal abuse, incest, and rape, and patients troubled by paraphilias require referral for specialized treatment. Internet support groups for some people with some sexual problems can provide new possibilities for hope and validation. Infidelity can be an extremely painful issue that affects many couples, yet many of them can be helped by couple therapy to address the pain, anger, and loss of trust.

CONCLUSION

For every human being, sexuality—like health—is a challenge at some point. Feelings of personal vulnerability are inherent in sexual interactions and help to make sexuality a powerful and unique part of life. Problems of sexual desire, arousal, or functioning can lead us to confront and overcome our fears of not being lovable and to seek better communication and increased intimacy with others. The deepest expressions of love often result from just sharing our vulnerabilities or problems.

ACKNOWLEDGMENTS

The authors thank the late Linda Perlin Alperstein, LCSW; Jean M. Bullard, RN, MS; Melissa A. Bullard, PhD; Lisa Capaldini, MD; Deborah Grady, MD, MPH; Susan Knight, LCSW; Mary Rodocker, PhD, RN; & William B. Shore, MD, for reviewing earlier drafts of this chapter, and especially thank the Rev. Dr. Becca F. Barnett for her editing skill. We also benefitted from the comments on this chapter by Raymond C. Rosen, PhD and Linda J. Rosen, PhD; their career-long contributions to the study of human sexuality have been inspiring to us. Finally, we honor and remember our previous coauthor, the late Harvey Caplan, MD, for his friendship and for his pioneering and humanizing impact upon the field of sex therapy.

SUGGESTED READINGS

Readings for Patients

Barbach L. *For Yourself—Revised*. New York, NY: Signet; 2000. (A revised classic that empowers women to enjoy their own sexuality, with suggestions for women who want to learn to become orgasmic.)

Johnson S. *Hold Me Tight: Seven Conversations for a Lifetime of Love*. New York, NY: Little, Brown; 2008. (Excellent suggestions for helping couples to have deeper conversations.)

Johnson S. *Love Sense: The Revolutionary New Science of Romantic Relationships*. New York, NY: Little, Brown; 2013.

Klein M. *Sexual Intelligence: What We Really Want from Sex—and How to Get It*. New York, NY: Harper Collins; 2012.

Perel E. *Mating in Captivity: Reconciling the Erotic and the Domestic*. New York, NY: Harper Collins; 2006. (Fresh, provocative, and intelligent exploration of the erotic imagination versus the sexless marriage.)

Perel E. *The State of Affairs: Rethinking Infidelity*. New York, NY: HarperCollins; 2017.

Schover LR. *Sexuality and Fertility after Cancer*. New York, NY: Wiley & Sons; 1997. (Compassionate and hopeful resource for women and men who have had cancer.)

Spring J (with Spring M). *After the Affair: Healing the Pain and Rebuilding Trust When a Partner Has Been Unfaithful*. Updated Second Edition. New York, NY: HarperCollins; 2013. (A compassionate and hopeful resource for people grappling with the betrayal of infidelity.)

Zilbergeld B. *The New Male Sexuality—Revised.* New York, NY: Bantam; 1999. (A common sense, practical, and sane antidote to media pressures on males to be sexual superstars. Excellent discussion of the fantasy model of sex and myths of male sexuality, the importance of an individual's conditions for good sex, and specific self-help chapters dealing with common male sexual problems.)

Zilbergeld B, Zilbergeld G. *Sex and Love at Midlife.* Bethel, CT: Crown House; 2010. (Issues on aging and sexuality with a positive focus.)

Readings for Health Professionals

Al-Azzawi F, Bitzer J, Brandenburg U, et al. Therapeutic options for postmenopausal female sexual dysfunction. *Climacteric* 2010;13:103–120.

Caplan HW. An effective clinical approach to vaginismus—putting the patient in charge. *West J Med* 1988;149:769–770.

Clayton AH, Goldstein I, Kim NN, et al. The International Society for the Study of Women's Sexual Health Process of Care for Management of Hypoactive Sexual Desire Disorder in Women. *Mayo Clin Proc* 2018;93(4):467–487.

Davis SR. Editorial: understanding female sexual function. *Menopause* 2009;16:425–426.

Derzko C, Bullard D, Rosenbaum E. Changes in sexuality and sexual dysfunction. In: Rosenbaum E, Spiegel D, Fobair P, Gautier H, eds. *Cancer Survivorship.* New York, NY: Andrews McMeel; 2007.

Derzko C, Elliott S, Lam W. Management of sexual dysfunction in postmenopausal breast cancer patients taking adjuvant aromatase inhibitor therapy. *Curr Oncol* 2007;14:S20–S40.

Goldstein I, Kim NN, Clayton AH, et al. Hypoactive sexual desire disorder: International Society for the Study of Women's Sexual Health (ISSWSH), expert consensus panel review. *Mayo Clin Proc* 2017;92(1):114–128.

Levine KB, Williams RE, Hartmann KE. Vulvovaginal atrophy is strongly associated with female sexual dysfunction among sexually active postmenopausal women. *Menopause* 2008;15(4):661–666.

Levine SB. *Handbook of Clinical Sexuality for Mental Health Professionals*, 2nd ed. New York, NY: Routledge; 2010.

McCabe MP, Sharlip ID, Atalla E, et al. Definitions of Sexual Dysfunctions in Women and Men: A Consensus Sexual Statement From the Fourth International Consultation on Medicine 2015. *J Sex Med* 2016;13:135–143.

Montorsi F, Basson R, Adaikan G, et al., eds. Sexual Dysfunctions in Men and Women: 3rd International Consultation on Sexual Medicine—Paris. Health Publication Ltd; 2010: 403–495.

Mulhall JP, Incrocci L, Goldstein I, Rosen RC, eds. *Cancer and Sexual Health.* New York, NY: Humana Press; 2011.

Portman DJ, Gass ML. Genitourinary syndrome of menopause: new terminology for vulvovaginal atrophy from the International Society for the Study of Women's Sexual Health and The North American Menopause Society. *Menopause* 2014;21(10):1063–1068.

WEBSITES

American Association of Sexuality Educator Counselors and Therapists. https://www.aasect.org. Accessed January 2019.

Journal of Sexual Medicine. https://www.jsm.jsexmed.org/. Accessed September 2019.

International Society for Sexual Medicine. http://www.issm.info. Accessed January 2019.

Kinsey Institute. https://kinseyinstitute.org. Accessed January 2019.

MyPronouns.org. https://www.mypronouns.org. Accessed January 2019.

North American Menopause Society (NAMS). https://www.menopause.org/ Accessed September 2019.

Sexuality Information and Education Council of the United States. https://siecus.org. Accessed January 2019.

Society for the Scientific Study of Sexuality. http://sexscience.org. Accessed January 2019.

Dementia & Delirium

34

Leah Kalin, MD; Nicholas Kinder, MSN, APN, AGNP-C; & Elizabeth Eckstrom, MD, MPH

DEMENTIA

Dementia is an acquired, persistent, and usually progressive impairment in multiple cognitive domains, usually including memory. There must also be a significant decline in function that is severe enough to interfere with work or social life. As the disorder progresses, individuals with dementia often fail to recognize family members, are unable to express themselves clearly and meaningfully, and often undergo dramatic personality changes. In the Diagnostic and Statistical Manual of Mental Disorders, Fifth Edition (DSM-5), dementia has been relabeled Major Neurocognitive Disorder. Mild cognitive impairment has been relabeled Minor Neurocognitive Disorder. Because this newer terminology has not been widely disseminated through the clinical world, we will continue to use the names dementia and mild cognitive impairment throughout this chapter.

Dementia is a common disorder with a prevalence that doubles every 5 years after the age of 60 years, affecting up to 45% of those aged 85 years and older. Today, over 5 million Americans are living with Alzheimer disease (AD) and related dementias. By 2050, up to 16 million will have dementia. Dementia is the sixth leading cause of death in the United States. In 2014, the direct costs of caring for those with dementia totaled an estimated $214 billion, including $150 billion in costs to Medicare and Medicaid. By 2050, these costs could rise as high as $12 trillion. Nearly one in every five dollars of Medicare spending is spent on people with Alzheimer and related dementias. Two-thirds of the 5 million seniors with Alzheimer disease are women. Women in their 60s are twice as likely to develop Alzheimer disease over the rest of their lives as they are to develop breast cancer.

Despite the high prevalence of dementia, the diagnosis is often missed by clinicians, particularly in the early stages. The primary care practitioner can play an important role in diagnosing and treating dementia. An early diagnosis can offer the opportunity to involve patients in meaningful advance care planning while they are still able to express their preferences clearly. In addition, potentially treatable causes, though rare, are more likely to be partially or fully reversed if diagnosed early. Later in the disease, the practitioner can work with other team members to manage difficult behaviors, ensure that the patient is as comfortable and safe as possible, recognize when referral for specialist care is needed, educate caregivers about the condition, and support caregivers in coping with their situations to the best of their abilities.

TYPES OF DEMENTIA

Alzheimer Disease

Alzheimer disease is the most common form of dementia, accounting for about 60–70% of cases. The age of onset varies considerably, but most commonly symptoms arise after the age of 70 years. Incidence of the disease increases with age. Women may be at a slightly higher risk of developing the disorder than men. The rare patient with early onset of AD (before the age of 60 years) may have a genetic disorder with an autosomal dominant pattern of inheritance, so a thorough family history is important in these cases.

Alzheimer disease usually follows a slow but progressive course (Table 34-1). Life expectancy following the appearance of the disorder ranges from 3 to 15 years. Memory deficits are prominent in all dementias, but especially so in AD. Typically, short-term episodic memory problems are the first and most obvious manifestation of the disorder. AD affects both the encoding and retrieval of new information to a profound degree, such that these patients do not appear to benefit from cueing and prompting of memory. For example, a patient asked to remember the words "piano," "carrot," and "green" may not be helped by hints such as "musical instrument," "vegetable," or "color." Careful clinical and neuropsychological evaluation results in a reliable diagnosis of the disease in most instances. A computed tomography (CT) or magnetic resonance imaging (MRI) scan often shows

Table 34-1. Stages of Alzheimer disease.

Stage	General Change	Specific Change
Early	Patients show relatively subtle changes in memory, along with declining clarity of thought and ability to perform everyday tasks. These changes may go largely unnoticed by the patient and significant others. Patients typically retain some ability to compensate for the cognitive changes.	• Mild memory problems such as missed appointments, failure to pay bills. • Occasional mild and transitory confusion and disorientation. • A "slowed-down" quality to thinking, personality, and lifestyle. • An increase in personal rigidity and intolerance of changes. • Social isolation, loss of interest in usual activities. • Possible increase in restlessness and impulsivity.
Middle	Cognitive deficits become more prominent during this stage and the loss of functioning becomes obvious to others.	• Severe memory impairment. • Frank and persistent confusion and disorientation. • Aphasia, apraxia, and visuospatial disturbances. • Serious difficulties in the ability to manage everyday activities. • Agitation, simple paranoia, other delusions.
Late	In the third, and terminal, stage of the disorder, the patient becomes very inactive, is extremely withdrawn, and loses nearly all ability to engage in purposeful activities.	• Profound loss of short- and long-term memory. • Severe confusion and disorientation. • Bladder and bowel incontinence. • Patient eventually is bedridden and nonresponsive. • Primitive reflexes such as grasping, rooting, and sucking are present. • Seizures. • Signs of gross neurologic impairment, such as hemiplegia, tremor, pronounced rigidity. • Bodily wasting despite adequate nourishment weeks to months prior to death.

Note: The signs and symptoms of dementia include the progressive loss of cognitive abilities, especially memory, and a decline in everyday functioning. Dementia is generally a deteriorating condition, and its progression is best described in terms of several stages. The stages outlined above are based on the most common form of dementia, AD.

cerebral atrophy and hippocampal volume loss; the electroencephalogram (EEG) may show diffuse slowing.

Dementia With Lewy Bodies

Dementia with Lewy Bodies (DLB) is the second most common cause of dementia in autopsy studies, accounting for 15–30% of cases. It is defined by the presence of cognitive impairment, movement dysfunction resembling parkinsonism, prominent visual hallucinations or other psychotic symptoms, and fluctuations in alertness. Patients may not have all of these symptoms. Patients with DLB are often intolerant of traditional antipsychotic medications, and their use can induce severe parkinsonism or even death. Meta-analyses of randomized controlled trials suggest that cholinesterase inhibitors may be useful in treating the disorder.

Vascular Dementia

Vascular dementia is characterized by the development of cognitive impairment in association with single or multiple areas of infarction and/or subcortical ischemia. Not surprisingly, the risk factors for vascular dementia are identical to the risk factors for cerebrovascular disease, including smoking, hypertension, diabetes mellitus, coronary artery disease, and previous history of stroke. A patchy and inconsistent pattern of deficits may be seen initially, with relative preservation of some cognitive areas. Because vascular dementia can result from insults to a variety of cortical or subcortical areas, the neuropsychological profile of patients with vascular dementia can be quite varied.

Focal neurologic signs are more common in vascular dementia than in AD, and lateralized motor and sensory findings may be seen. CT and MRI scans frequently reveal multiple areas of infarction in the brain, often with diffuse subcortical white matter changes. Later in the course of the disorder, atrophy from loss of brain tissue may be seen.

A number of diagnostic criteria for vascular dementia have been proposed, but none are sensitive or specific enough to rule the diagnosis in or out with certainty. Many older adults show diffuse white matter changes on brain imaging, and yet are cognitively intact. Others who were thought by their clinicians to have vascular dementia because of cognitive decline following cerebral infarcts are subsequently found to have Alzheimer's pathology at autopsy in addition to the known infarcts. Such individuals, with elements of both AD and vascular dementia, are considered to have mixed dementia. In short, current diagnostic instruments and criteria are often inadequate for clinicians confidently to employ or reject the "vascular dementia" label.

Other Causes of Dementia

Frontotemporal dementias (FTDs) are a group of disorders characterized by personality change (e.g., apathy or socially inappropriate behavior), hyperorality, and cognitive decline especially involving language and executive function. Primary progressive aphasia is a variant of FTD that primarily affects language. Frontotemporal dementia tends to affect individuals at a younger age than AD, with many persons receiving the diagnosis in their 50s or 60s. Imaging studies may show marked atrophy in frontal and temporal lobes.

Advanced Parkinson disease commonly results in dementia. These patients frequently display mental sluggishness and a general lack of spontaneity. Language functions (compared with those of AD patients) are relatively preserved.

Chronic alcohol abuse can result in serious cognitive deficits if drinking is severe and prolonged, although it is not clear whether dementia occurs in the absence of coexisting thiamine deficiency.

Human immunodeficiency virus (HIV-1)-associated neurocognitive disorder (HAND) is caused by the direct infection of the brain by the HIV-1 virus. It is associated with late-stage AIDS and is generally seen in individuals whose T-cell count has fallen below 200. HIV-1-associated neurocognitive disorder is discussed further in Chapter 37.

Creutzfeldt–Jakob disease is a rare infectious cause that should be suspected when a younger person develops a rapidly dementing illness associated with other neurologic deficits such as myoclonus.

Reversible Conditions

A number of medical conditions can result in cognitive impairment including: chronic subdural hematoma; CNS infection (meningitis, encephalitis, abscess); medication side effects or toxicity; vitamin B_{12}, thiamine, or niacin deficiency; metabolic disorders such as myxedema, hepatic encephalopathy, hypercalcemia, hyper- and hypoglycemia, hyper- and hyponatremia; delirium; depression; and CNS malignancy. These may be treatable, but full or partial reversal of dementia is relatively rare, even with appropriate treatment. Assessing the patient for relevant medical conditions is an important part of the dementia workup.

Mild Cognitive Impairment

Mild cognitive impairment (MCI) is an increasingly recognized condition in which a patient complains of memory problems and demonstrates mild deficits (most commonly in short-term memory) on formal testing, but does not meet criteria for dementia as they do not display any functional loss. Dementia will develop in roughly 10% of people with MCI each year. Amnestic MCI, in which the deficit is primarily episodic memory, is more likely to progress to AD than nonamnestic MCI, which may be more pathophysiologically heterogeneous. At the time of this writing, no medication intended for the treatment of MCI has been approved by the FDA. Acetylcholinesterase inhibitors have shown mixed results in clinical trials. Any potentially reversible conditions, including depression, hearing loss, or B_{12} deficiency, should be addressed in patients with MCI. They also should be advised to complete advance care planning and followed with serial clinical evaluation at least every year.

DIAGNOSTIC WORKUP

History

A complete history should be elicited from both patients and their families. In many cases, it is helpful to ask both about the same topics. Although many individuals with dementia are unreliable historians, they may be able to provide much useful information, including symptoms of which family members are not aware.

A complete social and family history that includes native language; family history of dementia; and educational, marital, and employment background can also be useful. An educational and occupational history, for example, may provide information about a patient's previous level of functioning. Particular attention should be paid to patients' accounts of more recent events. Individuals with mild or moderate dementia often show intact recall for older, overlearned information (e.g., family, education, and work), but cannot provide accurate information about the immediate past.

Ask patients about their regular activities, appetite, and sleep habits, as well as any physical or cognitive complaints. Information about their mood can be gained not only by inquiring directly, but also by asking about things that they enjoy and look forward to, any worries or concerns they may have, and their plans for the future.

Family members may be able to supply a more complete and balanced impression of the patient's symptoms, behavioral changes, and level of functioning. Individuals with dementia often lack insight into their cognitive problems and minimize or deny any difficulties. In fact, it is the family that most frequently raises concerns about the patient. Because family members may feel more comfortable discussing their observations away from the presence of the patient, they should be interviewed separately. It is especially important to inquire about both current and potential safety issues, such as problems with ambulation and balance, dizziness, wandering, unsafe home behaviors (e.g., leaving the stove on) and instrumental activities of daily living (IADLs). Family members should be asked what level of supervision is currently available or possible.

Physical & Neurologic Examinations

In addition to a routine physical examination, a complete neurologic examination should be done. Parkinsonian signs may be apparent during the later course of many dementing illnesses such as dementia with Lewy Bodies. Individuals with a developing vascular dementia may show focal signs on the neurologic examination.

The Mental Status Examination

Because cognitive impairment is the hallmark of dementia, it is necessary to add additional screening items to the traditional mental status examination. Several brief dementia-screening instruments offer the advantages of both a structured format and a scoring system, including the Montreal Cognitive Assessment (MOCA), St. Louis University Mental Status Exam (SLUMS), and Mini-Cog (see Chapter 14 for full details).

Other Tests

The American Academy of Neurology recommends that structural neuroimaging (with noncontrast CT or MRI) be employed in the initial evaluation of most patients with dementia, as approximately 5% of such patients have been found to have important but clinically unexpected structural lesions. We believe that in cases of long-standing dementia that is consistent with AD, there may be instances when the burdens of neuroimaging outweigh the benefits, particularly in a patient who becomes agitated in unfamiliar settings. Laboratory testing should be tailored based on patient history and presentation and might include complete blood count, thyroid, liver, and renal function, electrolytes, nutrition and metabolic status markers, serologies for HIV and syphilis, toxicology, and serum medication levels. EEG, lumbar puncture, and brain biopsy are not indicated for most people presenting with cognitive impairment.

Neuropsychological Testing

Neuropsychological testing involves the use of psychometric tests designed to detect and characterize a wide variety of cognitive problems, addressing orientation, attention, executive function, verbal memory, spatial memory, language, conceptualization, calculations, and mental flexibility. The testing requires the patient to be able to attend for a minimum of 20–30 minutes, but can take 3–4 hours to complete. Consider referring a patient for neuropsychological testing in the following circumstances:

- When the reported deficits are subtle or equivocal, the impairment is mild, and the physician and/or patient want to understand the disease process better.
- When the differential diagnosis is difficult to resolve (e.g., distinguishing between dementia and depression).
- When a baseline is needed to measure the degree of cognitive deterioration over time.
- When a greater understanding of the patient's everyday level of functioning, limitations, potential safety issues, and the appropriate level of supervision is needed.
- When deficits or competency issues must be documented, such as in conservatorship proceedings.
- To monitor effects of treatment.

TREATMENT & MANAGEMENT ISSUES

Treatment of dementia consists of identifying and addressing a treatable basis for the underlying condition (if one exists), treating symptoms of the cognitive deficits, treating secondary disorders such as anxiety or depression, educating patients and their families as to the nature of the condition, and assisting caregivers with safety and management issues (Table 34-2).

BEHAVIORAL ISSUES

Management of patients with dementia involves matters of self-care, safety, and communication. Individuals with dementia are characteristically disorganized, forgetful, and inefficient in many of their activities, making it difficult and unsafe for them to function independently. Complicating this, they may be impulsive, have limited insight into their abilities, and fail to learn from experience.

Neuropsychiatric symptoms are common, and almost all persons with dementia will experience them at some point during the course of their illness. Providers should inquire about them with patients and caregivers at each visit. Specifically, they may be labile and unstable, irritable, or anxious; they may be fearful, easily frustrated, or apathetic and withdrawn. They may wander at night or endorse paranoid thoughts or delusions. Because of

Table 34-2. Overall principles of dementia management.

- Periodically assess safety and self-care function
- Assess caregiver each visit
- Address advance directives early
- Educate patient and caregivers about condition
- Refer to Alzheimer's Association and supportive community organizations
- Treat secondary disorders (anxiety, depression)
- "Fine-tune" comorbid illnesses (e.g., congestive heart failure)
- Consider a trial of cholinesterase inhibitors for mild-to-moderate AD
- Consider a trial of memantine for moderate-to-severe AD

circadian rhythm disturbances, patients with AD may tend to be awake and wandering during the night, leading to sleep deprivation in caregivers.

These traits create special problems in managing and caring for patients with dementia, and many interactions with family and caregivers therefore focus on day-to-day management issues and behavioral problems. The following sections provide some general guidelines for addressing these issues. It is useful in many situations to refer patients and their families to groups that can provide counseling, home evaluations, and case management.

In general, nonpharmacological strategies for behavior management should be attempted first, and if unsuccessful, medication trials may be indicated. In practice, many distressing symptoms, such as agitation, prompt providers to try medications concurrently.

SELF-CARE

The best approach to managing self-care activities such as bathing and dressing is to provide sufficient structure and guidance so tasks can be accomplished, while allowing some preservation of independence and choice. Individuals with MCI often get by with prompts and reminders. For individuals with more severe impairment, caregivers should offer a limited choice of clothing, food, or activities; use signs or pictures to identify important objects and locations; and emphasize routine and predictability. Breaking down complex and potentially overwhelming activities such as bathing into simple one-step tasks may keep these activities manageable well into the course of the illness. The caregiver may need to modify clothing, for example, by incorporating sweatshirts to avoid buttons, and using shoes with Velcro closures rather than laces. Incontinence often develops. Protective garments in clothing and timed toileting (e.g., having the patient go every 2 hours while awake) may prevent frequent accidents.

SAFETY ISSUES

Individuals with dementia are at increased risk for accidents because of their problems with attention, perception, and judgment. They are also at increased risk of abuse, including physical, emotional, and financial.

To assess risk of accidents, ask caregivers and patients about the home environment, how often the patient is left alone, and whether he/she wanders, cooks, or self-administers medications. Where safety is unclear, more detailed information can be provided by a home safety evaluation, often done by an occupational therapist.

The following guidelines are designed to minimize the risk of household accidents:

- Carefully supervise use of medications.
- Keep the home relatively free of clutter and keep passageways clear.
- Install railings and other safety equipment, such as shower chairs and tub rails.
- Use a night-light where necessary.
- Remove stove and oven controls if necessary.
- Remove firearms from the home, or store them in a locked cabinet.
- Use safety gates or install keyless locks on exterior doors if wandering is a problem.
- Make sure patients wear medical and personal identification bracelets. Registering the patient in the Safe Return program via the Alzheimer's Association is a common way to obtain identification bracelets or necklaces (see "Websites").

Driving poses another important safety issue. Deficits in attention, reaction time, visual spatial abilities, and judgment typically impair the ability of individuals with marked cognitive deficits to operate a motor vehicle safely. Individuals with dementia who continue to operate a car seriously endanger others as well as themselves. Unfortunately, patients with dementia may insist on driving because of their lack of insight into their problems, and caregivers may be reluctant to press the issue. Because driving is symbolic of independence, this often becomes an emotional issue. It is best addressed early in the cognitive impairment trajectory, so the patient and family can plan ahead and determine alternative transportation modes before driving cessation must occur.

Confidentiality must be weighed against issues of competency, safety of the public, and the duty to warn. Legal requirements vary considerably between states. For example, in California, physicians are required by law to report patients with a diagnosis of AD or other related dementias. In the case of accident or injury, physicians who have failed to make such a report may be legally liable. Clinicians should inform themselves of the legal requirements in their own state regarding this issue.

Advance care planning should be addressed as early as possible. Evidence has shown that patients are more likely to have their care preferences followed at the end of life with these in place, and routine documentation of these preferences helps that occur. Similarly, referral to social workers and specialized legal agencies can help ensure that the patient has adequate financial and personal protections legally and medically. It may be helpful to know of legal resources for patients and families in the local community.

COMMUNICATION

Individuals with cognitive impairment may have specific deficits in language comprehension and expression similar to the various forms of aphasia that occur in stroke patients. More common may be a generalized difficulty in communication secondary to a short attention span, memory problems, or confusion. Some guidelines

Table 34-3. Tips for communicating with the cognitively impaired.

- Make sure you have patients' attention when you speak with them. Keep distractions, such as television, radio, or other conversations, to a minimum by meeting with patients in a quiet place.
- Keep communications brief, simple, and concrete. Break more complex information down into smaller pieces.
- Give patients several options to choose among, or phrase questions in multiple-choice format.
- Have patients paraphrase back the information to make sure they have understood what was said.

for communicating with the cognitively impaired are presented in Table 34-3.

Another factor affecting communication may be hearing or vision impairment, which is highly prevalent and often minimized by the patient. Therefore, we recommend asking about vision loss and if necessary referring to an ophthalmologist for a full evaluation. Hearing loss compounds cognitive difficulty profoundly and can also worsen auditory hallucinations if present. When speaking with someone with dementia, portable amplifiers, called "pocket talkers," help ensure that the person can hear the conversation. These can be kept in the clinic for regular use. Trying a pocket talker, even if the patient denies significant hearing impairment, often reveals undercorrected hearing loss and improves communication tremendously.

Drug Therapy

Cholinesterase inhibitors may confer mild benefits for some patients with AD, vascular dementia, and DLB. Anecdotal evidence suggests that a subgroup of patients may achieve clinically important improvements. The decision to initiate therapy with an acetylcholinesterase inhibitor should be based on evaluation of benefits and risks associated with an individual patient. A beneficial effect is considered to be an improvement in or stabilization of target symptoms, which would generally be expected within 6 months of initiation of therapy. Evidence is insufficient to determine the optimal timing or duration of therapy. Common side effects of acetylcholinesterase inhibitors include nausea, anorexia, diarrhea, weight loss, syncope, agitation, distressing dreams, and urinary frequency. An ECG should be checked after dose increases to monitor for bradycardia. Starting doses, respectively, of donepezil, galantamine, and rivastigmine, are 2.5 mg orally once daily, 4 mg orally twice daily, and 1.5 mg orally twice daily. The doses are increased every 2–4 weeks as tolerated. It is advisable to see the patient several times during dose titration to check for adverse reactions, but efficacy should not be assessed until a 6- to12-month trial has been completed. If an adequate trial has been completed and there is no improvement in cognitive testing or report of behavioral symptoms, then the person should be deemed a "nonresponder" and the medication discontinued with titration.

Memantine, an *N*-methyl-D-aspartate (NMDA) antagonist may be helpful in patients with moderate-to-severe AD or vascular dementia, with or without concomitant use of an acetylcholinesterase inhibitor. Clinical trials have shown a statistically significant, but minimally clinically significant, improvement on standard tests of cognition. Some studies have also demonstrated improvements in behavior and quality of life with use of memantine. The starting dose is 5 mg daily; the dose may be increased by 5 mg in weekly intervals up to a maximum of 20 mg per day. Again, if there is no improvement on cognitive testing or behavioral symptoms after 6 to 12 months, the drug should be discontinued with titration.

Behavioral Interventions and Medication for Severe Behavioral and Psychiatric Symptoms

Behavioral symptoms, including hallucinations, delusions, paranoia, anxiety, and others, are common in dementia. New behavioral symptoms should prompt an evaluation for delirium, infection, or other medical illness. If no culprit is found, nonpharmacological strategies should always be the first-line approach for management of behavioral symptoms in dementia.

"Agitation," which could mean restlessness, wandering, perseverative yelling, picking at clothes, or many other behaviors deserves careful evaluation. New agitation may represent delirium, undertreated pain, depression, a distended bladder, fecal impaction, itching, or many other conditions.

Caregiver involvement is essential to managing behavioral symptoms of dementia without medications. Common strategies for behavioral problems are maintaining and promoting adequate daytime physical and social activity, avoiding confrontational approaches by redirecting questions or topics of conversation, and consistently using reassuring and calming responses to a patient's behaviors instead of anger or frustration. The Alzheimer Association has 24/7 telephone support for caregivers who are confronted with behavioral symptoms. Useful resources for caregivers can be found in the "Websites" section.

If no culprit is found for behaviors and nonpharmacological approaches are inadequate, an empiric trial of analgesics such as acetaminophen, an antidepressant medication, or a mood stabilizer may be worthwhile. Analgesics should be dosed on a scheduled rather than as needed basis if patients are unable to communicate their level of pain. However, any empiric trial should be time limited, and the medication stopped if there has been no appreciable benefit in symptoms.

When behaviors are severe and may lead to harm for the patient and caregiver, medications may be indicated. There is no clear consensus about pharmacological approaches to treatment of behavioral problems in patients who have not benefited from nonpharmacological therapies. The target symptoms—depression, anxiety, psychosis, mood lability, or pain—may suggest which class of medications might be most helpful in a given patient. Benzodiazepines should be avoided as they have significant potential for causing sedation, confusion, ataxia, and falls.

If nonpharmacological interventions and safer medications are not effective and behaviors are causing harm to the patient or caregivers, it is possible that a short trial of an antipsychotic will be necessary. The newer atypical antipsychotic agents (e.g., risperidone and quetiapine) may be better tolerated than older agents (e.g., haloperidol), but they confer an excess risk of stroke, weight gain, and hyperglycemia. Both typical and atypical antipsychotics are associated with an increased risk of death compared with placebo when used to treat patients with dementia and behavioral disturbances. When the choice is made to use these agents, patients and caregivers should be carefully warned of the risks. It is prudent to check an ECG prior to beginning antipsychotic therapy, and to seriously consider other alternatives when a patient is found to have a prolonged QTc. Starting and target dosages should be much lower than those used in schizophrenia (e.g., haloperidol, 0.5–2 mg orally; risperidone, 0.25–2 mg orally). Federal regulations require that if antipsychotic agents are used in treatment of a nursing home patient, drug reduction efforts must be made at regular intervals. If the problem continues, consider another agent or obtain consultation with a psychiatrist, preferably one specializing in geriatric psychiatry.

Cholinesterase inhibitors and memantine gave mixed evidence for effectiveness in treating behavioral symptoms of dementia. However, if they are being considered for cognition, it is reasonable to see if they have an impact on behavior as well. If possible, we recommend delaying the prescription of a second agent (e.g., antipsychotic or other psychoactive medication) until the impact of the cognitive medication can be evaluated.

Cognitive Rehabilitation

For patients in the early stages of dementia, cognitive rehabilitation offered by a trained therapist can be in an invaluable tool. It offers a variety of enjoyable activities designed for general mental stimulation to improve cognition, concentration, and memory and compensate for cognitive deficits. It is usually performed in a small group setting. The aim is to utilize strategies to help patients optimize memory and cognitive function. Activities include memory training, using external cues, and organizational aids. A 2012 systematic review revealed that research to date does demonstrate improved cognition with cognitive rehabilitation, though more studies are needed to glean the effects due to lack of randomized controlled trials.

CARING FOR CAREGIVERS OF PERSONS WITH DEMENTIA

Caring for cognitively impaired individuals is often exhausting and stressful, especially in the presence of neuropsychiatric symptoms. Primary care providers should ensure that caregivers also attend to their own needs and guard against fatigue and burnout. Ideally, primary care providers will assess caregiver needs at every visit with the person with dementia. Caregiver-specific inventories can be administered, such as the Revised Memory and Behavior Problems Checklist, to quantify the patient's behaviors and assess the caregiver's emotional burden. A number of organizations, such as the Alzheimer Association and Family Caregiver Alliance, offer education, support groups, and information about resources (see "Websites"). Specialized case management and home consultation services can also be very helpful in assessing patient and family needs and locating additional services. Respite-care and day-activity programs may be invaluable in allowing stressed families and caregivers time off and providing needed stimulation and increased structure for the patient.

LONG-TERM CARE PLACEMENT

It is often not possible for persons with dementia to remain at home with family and/or caregivers. This is an area fraught with strong feelings on the part of patients and caregivers alike, and it is often difficult to make objective decisions. Major predictors of nursing home placement include the presence of behavioral problems, safety issues, dementia severity, and extent of caregiver burden. Some important considerations related to nursing home admission are as follows:

- Can the necessary level of supervision and care required by the patient be realistically and dependably supplied at home? Such issues as wandering and the potential for neglect and abuse should be considered here.
- Is sufficient assistance available to caregivers for them to continue to care for the patient without becoming overstressed and burned out?
- What financial resources are available for the patient's care?

Many patients and caregivers prefer to remain in their own home. However, desirable this goal, it must be carefully weighed against issues of safety and practical limitations. In the advanced stages of dementia, when the patient becomes mute, bedbound, and incontinent, very often the services of a skilled care home are required to ensure that the patient receives proper care. Long-term care homes should be investigated carefully with both cost and quality in mind. Information about both complaints and compliance with state regulations can be found through government agencies, advocacy groups, and published reviews. Memory care homes may reduce behavioral disturbances and use of restraints. Some patients do better in structured environments such as memory care homes or day care programs than in less structured home settings.

Dementia is a terminal disease, and in late stages the patient may become bedbound, unable to recognize family, and have difficulty swallowing. In these instances, hospice care is often appropriate (see Chapter 42).

DELIRIUM

Delirium, sometimes referred to as acute metabolic encephalopathy or acute confusional state, is one of the most common neuropsychological disorders faced by older adults and is often the first sign of medical illness. Defined by a grouping of symptoms rather than a specific disease state, delirium is a subacute (within days) to acute (within hours) development of disorientation and attention disturbance with concurrent altered level of consciousness or disorganized thinking. It is not uncommon for patients with delirium to be mistaken for having dementia with behavioral disturbance; however, delirium is distinguished by rapid onset and fluctuating symptom severity whereas dementia onset is usually insidious and follows an expected course (Table 34-4). Up to half of all hospitalized older adults and approximately three-quarters of those who pass through an intensive care unit will experience delirium, which may lead to higher health care costs and doubled odds of in-hospital death. The effects of delirium can be enduring, if not permanent to some degree, extend weeks to months beyond discharge, and result in cognitive and functional complications that culminate in a loss of independence and a higher risk of mortality (40% at one year).

Table 34-4. Delirium versus dementia: signs and symptoms.

Delirium	Dementia
• Rapid onset; short duration	• Insidious onset; progressive deterioration
• May show heightened autonomic arousal	• No impairment in autonomic arousal
• Clouded consciousness or gross confusion	• Alertness retained in early stages
• Prominent waxing and waning	• Consistently impaired mentation except in late-stage dementia
• Often restless, agitated, hypervigilant, or lethargic	• Agitation less prominent; varies with stress
• Gross perceptual distortions and hallucinations common	• If psychotic, usually vague paranoid ideas

Delirium is categorized into hyperactive, hypoactive, or mixed hyper- and hypoactive variants. The majority of all cases are of the hypoactive type in which patients often exhibit slowed psychomotor responses, listlessness, withdrawn or blunted affect, apathy, and increased somnolence. Hyperactive delirium may present with increased psychomotor activity and restlessness (frequently noted as "agitation"), hypervigilance, aggression, combativeness, and unsafe behaviors. Visual hallucinations, perceptual distortions, paranoid and persecutory delusions, and fluctuating awareness of the environment may be seen among all three variants. Even though the pathogenesis is not entirely understood, it is hypothesized that dopaminergic, cholinergic, and other neurotransmitter pathways are likely at play in the development of delirium. Risk factors for delirium include underlying dementia, depression or other psychiatric disorders, functional impairment, history of falls, sensory impairments, alcohol and drug abuse, and polypharmacy. History of stroke, fractures and other traumas, heart failure, and chronic kidney disease are among the medical conditions that predispose older adults to delirium. The most common causes of delirium in older patients are infections (usually of the respiratory or urinary tract although other sites are not excluded) and medications. Specifically, drugs with anticholinergic properties, antihistamines, benzodiazepines, antispasmodics, sedative hypnotics, skeletal muscle relaxants, antiemetics, and anesthetic agents are frequently associated with delirium. In patients with dementia, inadequately treated pain, constipation, and urinary retention can cause rapid changes in mental status and behavior that look like superimposed delirium.

Since some changes in alertness and new onset confusion may be at first subtle or easily dismissed, many cases of delirium initially go unrecognized. This highlights the need for communication between health care providers across settings, outpatient establishment of baseline mentation, and collateral information from family, friends, and caregivers, all of which can be critical in a timely delirium diagnosis. Providers and nurses should serially screen every older adult at risk for delirium, especially those who are currently or have recently been hospitalized. A validated, time-friendly, and free screening tool is the Confusion Assessment Method (CAM) which asks the user to assess confusion onset and course, attention, thinking organization, and level of consciousness. Another validated method for quickly predicting the presence of delirium with greater than 90% sensitivity is to ask the patient to state the day of the week and recite in reverse order the months of the year.

Prevention of delirium is far more effective than treatment. Basic principles of prevention and management focus on knowing the patient's baseline cognitive and functional statuses, adapting the environment, and treating underlying and causative factors through the following:

- Avoiding potentially inappropriate and high-risk medications as well as unnecessary tubes, lines, catheters, and devices.
- Reinforcing the patient's usual sleep–wake cycle with melatonin, adjustment of medication administration and procedure times, and minimizing nighttime disruptions and noise.
- Promoting daytime wakefulness with social interaction, cognitively stimulating activities, and ambulation.
- Allowing family, friends, and caregivers to be present as much as possible and encouraging them to bring in pictures, comfortable clothes or sleepwear, a favorite blanket, etc.
- Ensuring glasses, hearing aids, dentures, assistive devices, and other personal items are readily available and routinely utilized.
- Adequately treating acute and chronic pain using a multimodal approach that likely includes ambulation, progressive mobility, scheduled acetaminophen and topical agents, and age-appropriate doses of opioids if necessary.
- Recognizing and addressing constipation or urinary urgency and retention.

Pharmacological therapy should be restricted to only those cases in which combativeness, aggression, and nonredirectable behaviors interfere with critical or life-sustaining care or compromise physical safety. Although there are no medications approved by the Food and Drug Administration (FDA) for the prevention and treatment of delirium, low doses of second-generation antipsychotics like quetiapine (6.25–25 mg every 6 hours), risperidone (0.5–1 mg every 12 hours), and olanzapine (2.5–5 mg every 6 hours) are first-line agents of choice if the patient is willing and able to take oral medications. Haloperidol, an older antipsychotic, is available in both oral (0.5–1 mg every 4 hours) and intravenous/intramuscular (0.25-0.5 mg every 4 hours) formulations; however, intravenous haloperidol is associated with increased risk of *torsades de pointes*, a potentially lethal arrhythmia. Providers should cautiously consider risks and benefits as all antipsychotics come with an FDA "black box warning" regarding increased risk of death associated with cerebrovascular events in addition to carrying risk for extrapyramidal symptoms, tardive dyskinesia, neuroleptic malignant syndrome, and QT prolongation. The lowest dose and shortest therapy duration necessary to achieve effect should be employed, and providers should routinely attempt to taper antipsychotics, as prolonged use of them often leads to metabolic syndrome among other longer term complications. Younger patients or those with primary psychiatric illness may require higher doses or alternate therapies. Physical restraints should always be an absolute last resort for maintaining safety, since their use has been found to increase risk for patient and family psychological trauma, physical injury, falls, ADL-dependence, cognitive impairment, and death. Lastly, delirium frequently entails patient, family, and caregiver emotional distress, and clinicians should be prepared to educate, provide empathic support, and refer to institutional and community resources for ongoing assistance.

DEMENTIA & DELIRIUM SUMMARY

Dementia is an increasingly common syndrome characterized by a progressive loss of cognition and functioning. Given the aging of the population, it is essential that clinicians become comfortable with diagnosis, counseling, community and specialist referral, and treatment. Early diagnosis may allow for identification of reversible causes, improved symptom management, and planning for the future.

When patients present with cognitive complaints, the clinician must consider differential diagnoses, including dementia, delirium, depression, and psychosis. Diagnostic workup includes a careful history from patient and family, physical examination, mental status examination, laboratory work, brain imaging, and, on occasion, referral for neuropsychological testing or other specialized assessment.

Treatment and management consist of ruling out treatable conditions, treating secondary disorders such as anxiety or depression, providing information to patients and families, and assisting caregivers with safety and management issues. Use of medications may modestly slow the rate of cognitive decline or help with management of severe psychiatric symptoms, but interventions also consist of adjusting the environment to make the patient as comfortable and safe as possible and providing support for caregivers.

CASE DISCUSSIONS

CASE ILLUSTRATION 1

Mrs. A is a delightful 82-year-old woman brought to a medical clinic by her daughter. Her husband died 6 months ago. The daughter reports increasing "forgetfulness" over the last 2 years that she thinks has worsened since her father died. She notices Mrs. A quickly forgets conversations and has had trouble learning how to pay the bills since her husband died. More recently, she has started neglecting her housework, and has started to look a little disheveled. She takes hydrochlorothiazide, a daily multivitamin, and occasional diphenhydramine for insomnia. She denies falls or mobility problems and still walks regularly. She was initially very sad over the death of her husband, but now has "come to terms" with her grief. She has never smoked and rarely drinks. She studied Romance languages in college and still practices Italian once a week with a friend. On exam, she is disheveled and mildly hard of hearing. She has a nonfocal neurological exam and her gait is normal. On SLUMS testing, she is partially oriented, names nine animals in 1 minute, recalls one of five items correctly, has trouble with her clock draw and misses items on the story for a total score of 16/30. A CT scan of her head shows only mild cerebral atrophy. Routine lab testing, including thyroid and vitamin B12 tests, is normal.

Mrs. A has early Alzheimer dementia. Her diphenhydramine should be stopped, and nonpharmacologic sleep strategies implemented. It is important to speak with Mrs. A and her daughter about home safety issues, cessation of driving, and to start planning for a time (which might not be far off) when it will no longer be feasible for Mrs. A to continue living independently. Mrs. A and her daughter should be referred to the Alzheimer Association. Mrs. A and her daughter may need to come back for several visits to consider treatment with donepezil or other medications, complete advance care planning and ensure the daughter has sufficient caregiver resources.

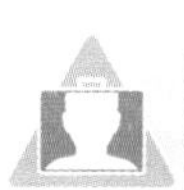

CASE ILLUSTRATION 2

A 75-year-old man is brought to the office by his family because he complains of seeing hallucinations of children and small animals when he is alone in a room. At times he has been disturbed and agitated by these hallucinations. His family also notes that he is having more difficulty walking and has had several falls. They also think his memory is not as good as it used to be, though they can't give specific examples of memory deficits. They have noticed that when they take him to a restaurant he has an extremely difficult time choosing what he wants to eat and will often ask for their help. He has stopped driving because he states he was getting lost trying to find his way to familiar places. Examination is unremarkable except for cogwheel rigidity and a wide-based gait. SLUMS exam is 20/30, with points missed in executive function, attention, and abstraction.

This patient has Lewy Body Dementia, and is exhibiting all three key characteristics of this disease, including cognitive impairment, parkinsonism, and visual hallucinations. While a clinician might feel pressed to treat his disturbing hallucinations with an antipsychotic medication, an acetylcholinesterase inhibitor, such as donepezil, is the first-line treatment for Lewy Body Dementia and has a good chance of improving his hallucinations and his cognition. He and his family should be counseled on ways to reduce fall risk, and they should be referred to the Alzheimer Association.

ACKNOWLEDGMENTS

David M. Pope, PhD, Alicia Boccellari, PhD, William Lyons, MD, Anna Chodos, MD, MPH, Bree Johnston, MD, MPH, and Kristine Yaffe, MD, were authors of prior editions of this chapter.

WEBSITES

Alzheimer's Association. http://www.alz.org. Accessed September 2019.

Alzheimer's Association Safe Return Program: https://www.alz.org/help-support/caregiving/safety/medicalert-safe-return. Accessed September 2019.

Alzheimer's Disease Education and Referral Center. https://www.nia.nih.gov/health/about-adear-center. Accessed September 2019.

American Association of Geriatric Psychiatry. www.aagponline.org. Accessed September 2019.

American Geriatrics Society. www.americangeriatrics.org. Accessed September 2019.

American Geriatrics Society Health in Aging Foundation: Caregiver Self-Assessment Questionnaire. http://www.healthinaging.org/resources/resource:caregiver-self-assessment/. Accessed September 2019.

AUDIT C: https://www.integration.samhsa.gov/images/res/tool_auditc.pdf. Accessed September 2019.

Confusion Assessment Method (CAM). https://consultgeri.org/try-this/general-assessment/issue-13.pdf. Accessed September 2019.

Cornell Scale for Depression in Dementia. http://www.scalesandmeasures.net/files/files/The%20Cornell%20Scale%20for%20Depression%20in%20Dementia.pdf. Accessed September 2019.

Mini Cog. http://mini-cog.com/wp-content/uploads/2018/03/Standardized-English-Mini-Cog-1-19-16-EN_v1-low-1.pdf. Accessed September 2019.

Montreal Cognitive Assessment (MoCA): https://www.mocatest.org/. Accessed September 2019.

St. Louis University Mental Status Exam (SLUMS). https://www.slu.edu/medicine/internal-medicine/geriatric-medicine/aging-successfully/assessment-tools/mental-status-exam.php. Accessed September 2019.

U.S. Preventive Services Task Force: Cognitive Impairment in Older Adults: Screening. https://www.uspreventiveservicestaskforce.org/Page/Document/UpdateSummaryFinal/cognitive-impairment-in-older-adults-screening. Accessed September 2019.

SECTION VI
Special Topics

Integrative Medicine

Selena Chan, DO & Frederick M. Hecht, MD

INTRODUCTION

The term, "integrative medicine" (IM) defines an approach to healing that explores the whole person, including individual values and lifestyle, while making use of all appropriate and evidence-informed therapeutic modalities, health care professionals, and disciplines to promote optimal well-being. Behavioral medicine is uniquely situated to implement an IM framework for several reasons. First, a central component in behavioral medicine is the biopsychosocial model. This model encompasses an assessment of the unique biological, psychological, social, cultural, and environmental influences on the whole person. Biological contexts include age, sex, genetic vulnerabilities, medications, substances of abuse, physical injuries, and medical illnesses. Psychological contexts include traumatic experiences, psychological defenses, and traits. Social contexts include community support, social skills, major life transitions, employment, cultural beliefs, values, spirituality, and access to health care. Second, both IM and behavioral medicine appreciate that healing occurs on multiple levels and that there is a bidirectional relationship between the mind and body. Last, IM and behavioral medicine share an emphasis on the therapeutic alliance and partnership between patients and those who contribute to their care.

THE EVOLUTION OF CONVENTIONAL MEDICINE & INTEGRATIVE MEDICINE

While pharmaceutical and surgical therapies have been central to advances in medical treatment, there has been a growing awareness of therapies used in place of conventional medicine, or "alternative medicine." The United States' National Institutes of Health (NIH) addressed this interest by establishing the Office of Alternative Medicine in 1991. In 1998, the center's name changed to the National Center for Complementary and Alternative Medicine (NCCAM). The term, "complementary medicine" was added to reflect non-mainstream modalities used together with conventional medicine, rather than in place of conventional medicine, and five domains were classified (Table 35-1). In 2014, the center's name changed again to the National Center for Complementary and Integrative Health (NCCIH) as "complementary approaches have grown in use to the point that Americans no longer consider them an alternative to medical care." The term "integrative medicine" emphasizes the concept of integrating elements of what has been thought of as complementary or alternative medicine, particularly those with evidence to support their use, into health care.

USE OF COMPLEMENTARY & ALTERNATIVE MEDICINE

For over 60 years, the U.S. National Health Interview Survey (NHIS) has served as an important source of information to monitor the health of the nation. Data from NHIS consistently show that one-third of U.S. adults have reported complementary and alternative medicine (CAM) use in the previous year. These results align with finding of a 1993 study published in the *New England Journal of Medicine* by Eisenberg and colleagues that 34% of adults in the United States used at

Table 35-1. Five domain system for classifying complementary and alternative medicine modalities.

Domain	Examples
Biologically based therapies	Dietary interventions, vitamins, minerals, supplements, herbal/botanical medicines
Mind–body interventions	Meditation, relaxation and breathing techniques, guided imagery, hypnosis, biofeedback, yoga, tai chi, qigong, expressive arts therapies, spiritual practices, and other forms of "directed" attention
Manipulative and body-based methods	Osteopathic manipulative therapy, chiropractic spinal manipulation, massage therapy, physical therapy
Alternative or whole medical systems	Traditional Chinese medicine, ayurveda, naturopathic medicine, homeopathy, Polynesian medicine, Unani-Tibb medicine, traditional African medicine, traditional Mayan medicine
Energy therapies	Acupuncture, tai chi, qigong, reiki, therapeutic or healing touch, bioenergetic therapy, and other methods that affect the body's "bioelectric" field

least one unconventional form of health care during the previous year.

In a 2013 publication, Purohit and colleagues analyzed 2007 NHIS results to assess the prevalence of CAM use in 23,393 U.S. adults in relationship to neuropsychiatric symptoms. Neuropsychiatric symptoms surveyed included depression, anxiety, insomnia, attention deficits, headaches, excessive sleepiness, and memory loss. CAM use was more prevalent in adults with at least one neuropsychiatric symptom (43.8%) as opposed to adults without neuropsychiatric symptoms (29.7%). The higher the number of neuropsychiatric symptoms, the higher the prevalence of CAM use, particularly mind–body therapies. Over one-half of all adults with neuropsychiatric symptoms did not report CAM use to a conventional provider. One-fifth of patients used CAM because standard treatments were either ineffective or costly. One-fourth of patients used CAM due to recommendation by a conventional provider. Additionally, CAM use is common among children with mental health conditions. According to 2012 NHIS data, anxiety, stress, attention-deficit/hyperactivity disorder, and insomnia were among the top six conditions for which CAM was used in children.

NONDISCLOSURE & COMMUNICATION IN INTEGRATIVE MEDICINE

The common use of CAM approaches within both the general and mental health population, limited disclosure of CAM use to health care providers, and potential safety risks of lack of shared information underscore the importance of exploring an individual's personal preferences, lifestyles, and background. Because most patients do not spontaneously offer information on CAM use, clinicians may have a falsely low perception of patient usage and therefore do not pursue discussing the topic. Jou and Johnson analyzed 2012 NHIS data and identified 7493 respondents who both used CAM and had a primary care physician. Approximately 42.3% of respondents did not disclose CAM use to their primary care physician. Nondisclosure was *least often* due to past discouragement or potential discouragement of CAM use by physicians (2.0% and 2.8%, respectively). Instead, nondisclosure was most often related to physicians not asking about CAM use (57%) or a belief that physicians did not need to know about their CAM use (46.2%). Surprisingly, only 7.6% reported nondisclosure of CAM use was due to belief that the physician was less knowledgeable about CAM.

Clinicians may fear that if they ask about CAM, they need to be well versed in all forms of CAM. On the contrary, providers can have varying levels of involvement in IM coordination, ranging from more conservative to more active roles. For example, the clinician could refer out to an IM specialist, serve as an integrative medicine navigator who makes appropriate referrals to CAM providers, or directly provide all integrative modalities "under one roof." Regardless of the role chosen, it behooves the clinician to be curious about the factors influencing a patient's decision-making process about treatment.

INTRODUCTION TO INTEGRATIVE MEDICINE ASSESSMENT: AN ANALOGY TO CREATING THE GOURMET MEAL

Integrative medicine assessment parallels vital principles in conventional medical treatment including informed consent and assessment of patient capacity to convey a thorough understanding of treatment. It may be helpful for clinicians learning features of an IM assessment to use an analogy of key components needed to create a gourmet meal. In the same way that a gourmet meal tailors to individual tastes, an IM assessment involves asking a patient about treatment preferences. A gourmet meal depends on access to specific ingredients influenced by season, local availability, and cost. Likewise, cultural background, financial constraints, and accessibility to services inform patient treatment options. Considering essential dietary needs is akin to considering medical indications. Just as meals change, medical indications and patient needs change. Asking about food allergies and intolerances is analogous to evaluating contraindications, safety risks, and treatment interactions. Determining the track record of how ingredients interplay to form a tasty meal is similar to using an evidence-informed decision-making process, while following a recipe with specific measurement of ingredients is analogous to implementing a treatment protocol. Reflecting on who is eating together and meal location exemplifies foundational elements in behavioral medicine and IM: learning about patient relationships, communication patterns, environment, and psychosocial influences.

One component in creating a gourmet meal is surveying a "buffet" of ingredients, including unfamiliar ingredients. Similarly, IM assessment involves exploration of a wide array of healing modalities. Patients may have sought out different providers with conflicting perspectives and methods of healing leading to confusion about a long list of treatments. The clinician may facilitate the patient in clarifying treatment timelines, effects, and barriers to adherence. Last, the "farm to table" concept involves a multidisciplinary team, including those who cultivate and harvest ingredients, those who transport ingredients to the grocery store or restaurant, those who prepare or cook the meal, and those who serve the meal. Similarly, IM appreciates coordination across disciplines and respects the unique talents and diverse lenses that each practitioner brings to the table.

Suppose a clinician is prescribing an oral contraceptive pill (OCP) and an antidepressant to a female patient. The clinician remembers to ask about CAM use. The patient reveals interest in the use of St. John's wort (SJW), an herbal medicine purported to have antidepressant effects. The clinician reviews the patient's motivations in considering SJW. She describes a strong preference for natural products and shares that researching this potential remedy promoted a sense of autonomy. She asks the clinician about effectiveness and any risks. The clinician shares that while there is some evidence SJW may improve depression, well-designed studies fail to show it is more effective than placebo. The clinician also alerts her to several safety concerns related to drug interactions. SJW induces the cytochrome P450 enzyme system in the liver, which is responsible for metabolizing many medications. SJW may increase clearance and lower activity of drugs that go through this pathway (e.g., certain anticonvulsants, oral contraceptives, HIV medications, warfarin, immunosuppressants, and cardiovascular medications). Conversely, seemingly benign foods, such as grapefruit, may inhibit metabolism of many drugs and increase drug levels, conferring risk for side effects and toxicity. In this case, SJW would induce the metabolism of OCPs, resulting in reduced efficacy of the OCP and increased risk of contraceptive failure. As the patient is also taking an antidepressant, concurrent use of SJW could also increase risk of serotonin syndrome, a medical emergency. Providing this information can help such a patient make more informed choices about SJW.

OVERVIEW OF CAM/IM DOMAINS & RESEARCH

As noted earlier, NCCAM previously classified CAM modalities into five primary domains (see Table 35-1). These five domains remain a useful framework for organizing thoughts on various CAM approaches and practices. The following sections aim to introduce these domains and provide several example therapies within each domain relevant to behavioral medicine. Note that a CAM modality may have features that fit into more than one domain. Particularly relevant to behavioral medicine, many therapies overlap in mind–body effects. This overlap in domains influenced the NCCIH decision to streamline complementary health approaches into two broader categories: mind and body practices or natural products.

It may be helpful for the clinician to organize domains on a spectrum, noticing how close an approach fits into a scientific paradigm. Typically, approaches falling closer to a biological, scientific model are a more natural fit for double-blind, randomized controlled trials (RCT) and thus more widely accepted into conventional medical practice. Approaches deviating from a rigorous, scientific model are more likely to be considered less conventional in Western medicine. However, the World Health Organization (WHO) estimates that over one-fourth of modern medical drugs stem from traditional healing knowledge. The WHO Traditional Medicine Strategy 2014–2023 report notes that traditional and complementary medicine is an underestimated part of global health care, often used for accessibility, affordability, and cultural congruence (see Chapter 8). The WHO estimates 70–95% of the population in developing countries (e.g., Asia, Africa, Latin America, and the Middle East) rely on traditional healing methods for primary health care. Industrialized nations are also using traditional medicine, with the WHO approximating use in 70–90% of populations in Canada, France, Germany, and Italy.

RESEARCH CONSIDERATION FOR CAM/IM APPROACHES

In assessing the evidence base for CAM/IM therapies, several methodological research challenges may be helpful for health care practitioners to understand. Some of these challenges apply to behavioral medicine more broadly. Most research on conventional therapies use drug treatment that can easily be blinded, and defining the primary outcome is straightforward as there is a single therapeutic goal (e.g., benzodiazepines to reduce anxiety). In contrast, most IM therapies (similar to many behavioral interventions) have multiple components, need to be implemented by a skilled practitioner, and aim to influence multiple symptoms. For example, mindfulness-based cognitive therapy (MBCT) involves an 8-week course with multiple components led by an expert facilitator. MBCT aims to prevent depression relapse but may also improve anxiety and other outcomes. To address these challenges, researchers studying an intervention like MBCT will develop an extensive outline of specific program components to improve consistency ("manualization"), check program implementation ("fidelity checks"), and define more than one outcome. Other challenges include blinding a practitioner or participant to the treatment assigned in a trial and selecting an appropriate control group.

One method to address concerns about nonspecific effects of an intervention, such as the benefit of group attendance for depression rather than exposure to the specific content of MBCT, is to use an active or attention control group. Similar to use of a placebo to control for expectancy effects in a pharmaceutical trial, attention control conditions are intended to determine the active component of the CAM/IM/psychological interventions by balancing nonspecific effects. An example of an attention control condition for MBCT might be providing an education group without the content of an MBCT program. However, for a patient and provider, the most relevant question may be a more pragmatic one. For example, the benefits from MBCT likely come from both the participation in a group and the content of the group. Patients and providers may be more concerned with the overall benefit of attending an MBCT group compared to using antidepressants, rather than figuring out which component of MBCT confers what benefit. Trials comparing real-world alternatives often fit into pragmatic clinical trials. Such studies may be just as scientifically valid as a study with an attention control group but aim to answer different questions.

BIOLOGICALLY BASED THERAPIES & NATURAL PRODUCTS

Dietary Supplements

Several dietary supplements are marketed for conditions such as anxiety, depression, or insomnia, and are therefore relevant for behavioral medicine practice. The U.S. Food and Drug Administration (FDA) mandates that before releasing pharmaceuticals to the public for sale, they must pass several rigorous phases of testing to show evidence of safety and efficacy. The **Dietary Supplement Health and Education Act (DSHEA)** was enacted in 1994 to standardize how natural products are regulated, sold, and marketed in the United States. Under DSHEA, dietary supplements are considered foods, not pharmaceuticals. DSHEA provides "grandfathered status" for any supplement marketed before 1994; that is, these supplements are not required to prove safety or efficacy before marketing. In contrast, newer supplement ingredients introduced after 1994 require a reasonable review of evidence for safety before marketing, and the FDA is responsible for post-marketing surveillance and action.

Kava (*Piper methysticum)* is a commonly cited example where botanical quality and preparation make a difference. Kava is an herbal anxiolytic postulated to target the same neurotransmitter as benzodiazepines, gamma-aminobutyric acid. Several case reports of liver toxicity surfaced in the 1990s leading to an initial ban of kava in Europe. However, further studies questioned if the raw material used in kava had changed, as case reports related to concentrated extracts manufactured in Germany or Switzerland. Additionally, many case reports of suspected kava hepatotoxicity involved concurrent use of several medications. Kava inhibits the liver cytochrome P450 system; thus, kava used concurrently with other medications metabolized through this system could cause these medications to rise in the blood to toxic levels. Traditional or "noble" forms of kava indigenous to many Pacific Island cultures have been used in social gatherings for centuries. Noble kava typically matures in the ground for several years before harvesting, and its preparation involves using the peeled root with water as the solvent for extraction. To expedite production and increase kava potency, some manufacturers began to use a different cultivar type, *Piper wichmanii*, to create "two-day" or "tudei" kava. Two-day kava is concentrated via the use of ethanol or acetone–water mixes and may use nontraditional plant parts such as nonpeeled parts and leaves or stem (as opposed to peeled kava root).

Dietary Interventions

Most studies concluding unhealthy diets worsen depression, or healthy diets improve depression, are observational or survey-based studies. However, an RCT called the "SMILES" trial studied the effects of directly applying a dietary intervention to treat depression in participants with poor diet quality. The study included 67 participants with moderate to severe depression who also engaged in conventional treatment for depression at baseline. The intervention group attended dietary support sessions with a nutritionist and ate a modified Mediterranean diet (no caloric restriction, low in refined carbohydrates, low in processed oils, and a focus on whole foods). The control group received no dietary intervention but attended social support sessions. At 3 months, the dietary intervention group achieved significant improvement in depression.

A larger RCT, the PREDIMED study, compared a low-fat diet to two different variants of a Mediterranean diet and examined the incidence of depression in a subset of 3923 participants without depression at baseline. This study found a trend toward decreased incidence of depression in participants assigned to a Mediterranean diet supplemented with nuts, but this was not statistically significant (multivariate hazard ratio 0.78; 95% confidence interval 0.55–1.10). There was a statistically significant decrease in depression in the subgroup with type 2 diabetes. Taken together, these results provide modest support for encouraging a healthy diet using a Mediterranean dietary pattern in patients with depression, particularly in those with poor diet quality.

MIND–BODY INTERVENTIONS

Mind–body practices enhance health by facilitating interactions among the brain, mind, body, and behavior. Mental state may affect physical health (e.g., depression worsening coronary artery disease outcomes), and the physical body can affect mental state (e.g., aerobic exercise improving mood). Examples of mind–body therapies are breathing exercises, meditation, guided imagery, biofeedback, hypnosis, progressive muscle relaxation, yoga, tai chi, and qigong.

Meditation & Mindfulness

Meditation and related contemplative practices involve various methods to self-regulate attention and have been used for centuries to achieve states of emotional calm and self-understanding (see Chapter 7). While meditative practices are often derived from various spiritual traditions, they can be used without a religious context, and they are increasingly used within health care settings to address mental and physical health conditions. Three well-studied mindfulness-based interventions used to address regulation of anxiety, depression, or substance use are mindfulness-based stress reduction (MBSR), MBCT, and mindfulness-based relapse prevention (MBRP). Some forms of psychotherapy also incorporate elements of mindfulness, such as dialectical behavioral therapy (DBT) and acceptance and commitment therapy (ACT) (see Chapter 26).

In the words of Jon Kabat-Zinn, the creator of MBSR, mindfulness practice is rooted in "paying attention in a particular way: on purpose, in the present moment, and nonjudgmentally." Meta-analyses studying the efficacy of MBSR programs on mood disorders appear to vary based on populations studied. One systematic review found robust intergroup effect sizes in patients with anxiety and mood disorders who participated in MBSR, while another review of 15 studies did not find a clear benefit of MBSR programs for patients with mood disorders or patients with a combination of depression and medical conditions.

By combining mindfulness with elements from a validated treatment for depression, cognitive behavioral therapy (CBT), MBCT was created in the 1990s to reduce depression relapse. MBCT focuses on allowing distressing thoughts, emotions, and sensations to pass by, without the need to suppress, escape, or fight them. Most studies suggest that MBCT may be used as preventive maintenance for patients in remission from depression. Some studies suggest that MBCT programs may be useful as adjunctive therapy to conventional antidepressant treatment but may not be sufficient as monotherapy in treating depression. A 424-person RCT found MBCT as effective as continuing antidepressant therapy in the prevention of depression relapse in persons with three or more prior depressive episodes, and MBCT has become a standard therapy offered by the United Kingdom National Health Service.

MBRP has similar features to MBCT but is intended for relapse prevention of substance use disorders. A large RCT compared MBRP with treatment as usual, which included a 12-step program and psychoeducation. At 6-month follow-up, MBRP participants reported significantly lower risk of relapse to substance use and significantly fewer days of substance use among those who still used substances.

Yoga

Yoga is considered a mind–body approach because of three principal components: meditation, pranayama (breath regulation), and asanas (postures). There are a wide variety of ways yoga can be practiced that range in physical exertion level and primary intention (e.g., increasing self-awareness or examining conduct with self and others). Thus, it is helpful to learn the type of yoga a patient is practicing and look into tailored classes or instruction for specific conditions. In general, restorative yoga and hatha yoga are forms that employ gentle, mindful movement with a focus on body awareness and stillness.

Meta-analyses suggest benefits of yoga as adjunctive therapy for depression, while data on yoga as monotherapy are more limited. However, a recent RCT found that implementing an 8-week hatha yoga intervention resulted in statistically and clinically significant reductions in depression severity, and a subanalysis showed yoga participants were more likely to achieve remission. Another RCT assessed the use of a 10-week weekly trauma-sensitive yoga program as an adjunctive treatment for women with chronic treatment-resistant posttraumatic stress disorder (PTSD), compared to a supportive therapy group. Yoga was found to significantly reduce PTSD symptoms, with effect sizes comparable to well-researched approaches for PTSD, including psychopharmacology and psychotherapy.

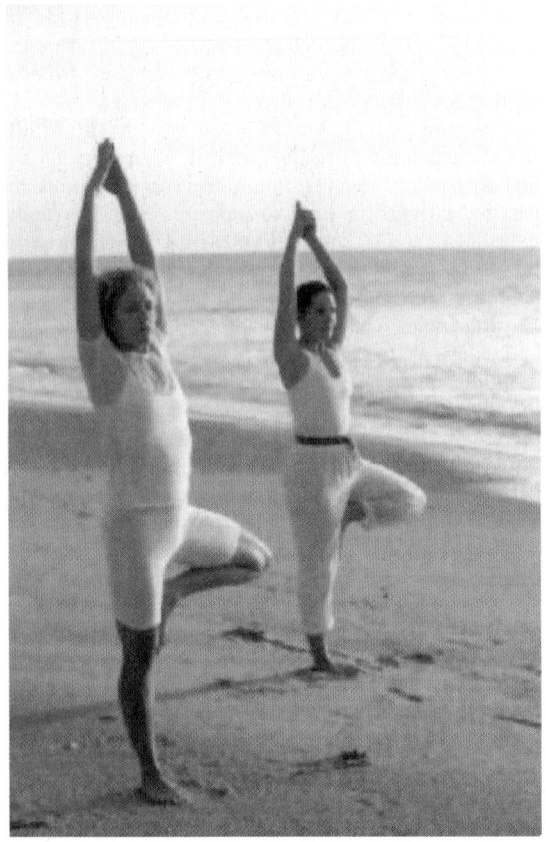

Tai Chi & Qigong

Tai chi and qigong are ancient forms of body movement practices. Both tai chi and qigong apply slow, intentional meditative movements that rely on self-awareness of body positions to adapt energy flow in the mind and body. A meta-analysis of regular tai chi practice showed significantly improved psychological outcomes including reduced stress, anxiety, and depression.

Biofeedback

The practice of biofeedback involves connection to sensors that receive feedback information about the body. These sensors monitor psychophysiological changes in brainwaves (electroencephalogram [EEG]), breathing patterns, heart rate, skin temperature, sweat gland activity, and muscle tension. A primary goal of biofeedback is to balance autonomic activity, typically helping a patient reduce sympathetic overflow. While biofeedback can address multiple health conditions, the best-supported applications of biofeedback are for pain syndromes, anxiety disorder, major depressive disorder, and attention deficit. Two guiding factors toward recommending biofeedback are patients who value self-control and patients who have medical conditions where stress is a significant component. A stress thermometer is a simple and low-cost way to implement biofeedback through a daily practice of hand-warming, a sign of relaxation.

MANIPULATIVE & BODY-BASED METHODS

Massage Therapy

Massage therapy is widely used by patients to promote a sense of relaxation and reduce muscle tension. Despite the widespread use of massage by patients in the community to manage anxiety, there are few rigorously controlled studies examining the efficacy of massage for psychiatric conditions. A 2016 RCT was one of the first monotherapy studies to address this gap, finding that Swedish massage therapy may be an effective treatment for generalized anxiety disorder (GAD).

Osteopathic Medicine & Osteopathic Manipulative Therapy

Doctors of Osteopathic Medicine (DOs) are fully licensed physicians who receive additional training on the neuromuscular system. Osteopathic physicians are taught to look beyond symptoms of illness and consider how lifestyle and environment impact well-being. Osteopathic manipulative therapy (OMT) is a set of hands-on techniques aimed to treat structural, muscle, and tissue abnormalities; relieve joint restriction and misalignment; and promote circulation. OMT involves a physician manually applying pressure or resistance to specific regions of the body.

A 2017 review article suggests that an osteopathic approach may complement CBT in reducing fear avoidance of pain while improving confidence in movement. Another 2018 systematic review analyzed 16 RCTs for the effects of osteopathic treatment on psychosocial factors in patients with persistent pain. This review found that osteopathic treatment may be beneficial for anxiety, fear avoidance, quality of life, and general health status in patients with persistent pain. However, it is difficult to draw concrete conclusions about OMT itself providing the psychosocial benefits, as a biopsychosocial assessment is integral to osteopathic training and practice.

ALTERNATIVE OR WHOLE MEDICAL SYSTEMS

Traditional Chinese Medicine & Acupuncture

Traditional Chinese medicine (TCM) is a system of medicine practiced for thousands of years. In TCM, illness is understood as a disruption in the flow of qi or one's life force energy. To restore homeostasis, TCM uses an individualized combination of acupuncture, herbal medicines, and specific recommendations for optimal diet, physical activity, lifestyle, and emotional/spiritual connection. Acupuncture is one component of TCM treatment that involves placing thin needles on particular sites on the body in a specific way. Using functional magnetic resonance imaging (fMRI) studies of healthy subjects, Hui and colleagues found that acupuncture stimulation affects the emotional brain through primary deactivation of the amygdala and hypothalamus.

Meta-analyses of acupuncture for depression show conflicting results. Some reviews find no difference in depressive symptoms reduction, and other reviews suggest that acupuncture is as effective as antidepressants. The National Acupuncture Detoxification Association (NADA) protocol is a type of auricular acupuncture that may lessen the severity of withdrawal symptoms when used adjunctively with detoxification treatment. The NADA protocol is typically administered in group settings to improve adherence and involves bilateral needle insertion at five specific acupoints located on the ear. A 2011 prospective trial by Carter and colleagues compared adjuvant NADA acupuncture plus conventional treatment with stand alone conventional treatment at a 28-day residential treatment program. The study found that NADA acupuncture plus conventional treatment related to statistically significant improvement across all symptom measures.

NAVIGATING A COMPLEX CASE OF "TREATMENT RESISTANT" INSOMNIA

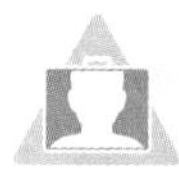

CASE ILLUSTRATION

A 70-year-old European American woman presents with "treatment-resistant" insomnia for over 20 years. Medical history includes major depressive disorder (in remission), fibromyalgia, hypothyroidism (stable without medications), obstructive sleep apnea (adherent to continuous positive airway pressure treatment), hypertension (controlled with losartan), remote history of breast cancer (in remission), and type 2 diabetes mellitus (diet-controlled). Psychotropic treatments to address fibromyalgia, depression, and insomnia include amitriptyline, duloxetine, and zolpidem.

The clinician invites the patient to discuss the impact of health care issues on her life, her intuition of what contributed to her illnesses, and her definition of health and joy. The patient describes fibromyalgia flares as flu-like with widespread body aches. Physical and cognitive limitations of having fibromyalgia influence the patient's self-efficacy, energy, and motivation. Having witnessed both parents go through dementia, she worries about aging and feels she has been accumulating illnesses. Insomnia and fatigue significantly affect her cognition. Neurologic examinations for cognitive impairment are unremarkable. She identifies good sleep quality, energy to engage in her favorite activities, and strong connections with others as vital components of overall health and well-being.

The clinician asks the patient about her experience with complementary and alternative treatments. The patient reveals that she consistently takes vitamin D_3 to replete a deficiency, D-ribose for fatigue, omega-3 fatty acids for cardiovascular protection, and occasionally melatonin for sleep. Weekly acupuncture treatments alleviate fibromyalgia flares. She has a morning practice of meditation and qigong and applies sleep hygiene techniques learned through CBT for insomnia: deconditioning the bed as a source of anxiety about sleep, avoiding naps, and switching to decaffeinated coffee.

Further assessment reveals that the patient consumes hidden sources of caffeine equating to 200 mg daily via decaffeinated coffee, dark chocolate, and sodas. The patient is surprised to discover that only 97% of caffeine must be removed from the coffee bean to bear the label of decaffeinated coffee and some forms may retain up to 30 mg of caffeine per cup. Through motivational interviewing, the clinician learns that the patient enjoys decaffeinated coffee for soothing qualities of a warm beverage. The patient self-identifies herbal teas as a suitable replacement and limits dark chocolate consumption to one ounce at lunch.

The clinician advises the patient to gradually taper off caffeine over a period of several weeks to avoid caffeine withdrawal symptoms. The patient experiences restful sleep and consequently a significant improvement in energy, cognition, and motivation. Amitriptyline, zolpidem, and D-ribose are eliminated eventually without decompensation in mood or energy. The patient also resonates with psychotherapy themes of dimming the spotlight on activities that do not match her values while brightening focus on activities that support her authentic desires.

This case demonstrates a shared goal in integrative and behavioral medicine: being attentive to an individual's narrative, directly asking about a wide array of therapies, and carefully teasing apart whether treatment is ineffective, or a cause of illness remains unaddressed. Rather than seeing each disease, symptom, and treatment as a separate entity, the clinician first expanded into a bigger-picture framework. Having a whole-person and whole-system viewpoint aided the clinician in revealing root causes and minimizing unnecessary or harmful interventions.

Many components of this patient's history may contribute to insomnia (i.e., depression, sleep apnea, fibromyalgia, hypothyroidism, vitamin D deficiency, and diabetes). However, a better understanding of this patient's story identified hidden sources of caffeine as an underlying cause of ongoing insomnia, previously labeled as "treatment resistant" illness. The seemingly basic intervention of tapering off caffeine improved sleep and facilitated eventual elimination of unnecessary medications with dangerous potential adverse effects in an older adult (e.g., risk for delirium from a tricyclic antidepressant or a benzodiazepine receptor agonist). The patient also began to decrease emphasis on thoughts and behaviors that were no longer useful and place more focus on thoughts and behaviors that enhanced joy and fulfillment in her life. While it is tempting to address a constellation of symptoms with complex treatments, careful attention to root causes and streamlining interventions may yield better patient outcomes.

CONCLUSION

The field of IM is rapidly evolving and becoming more mainstream, as evidenced by the widespread use of integrative therapies by patients, the growth of research in this area, and by an increasing number of conventional practitioners seeking additional training in IM. Behavioral medicine, with its inherent awareness of the relationship between mind, body, and spirit is a field particularly amenable to incorporating the practices of IM. The future of IM ideally combines the strengths of both conventional medicine and appropriate complementary modalities to facilitate healing.

SUGGESTED READINGS

Cramer H, Lauche R, Langhorst J, Dobos G. Yoga for depression: a systematic review and meta-analysis. *Depress Anxiety* 2013;30(11):1068–1083.

Frank DL, Khorshid L, Kiffer JF, Moravec CS, McKee MG. Biofeedback in medicine: who, when, why and how? *Ment Health Fam Med* 2010;7(2):85.

Fryer G. Integrating osteopathic approaches based on biopsychosocial therapeutic mechanisms. Part 2: clinical approach. *Int J Osteopath Med* 2017;26:36–43.

Hofmann SG, Sawyer AT, Witt AA, Oh D. The effect of mindfulness-based therapy on anxiety and depression: a meta-analytic review. *J Consult Clin Psychol* 2010;78(2):169–183.

Kuchta K, Schmidt M, Nahrstedt A. German kava ban lifted by court: the alleged hepatotoxicity of kava (*Piper methysticum*) as a case of ill-defined herbal drug identity, lacking quality control, and misguided regulatory politics. *Planta Med* 2015;81(18):1647–1653.

Kuyken W, Hayes R, Barrett B, et al. Effectiveness and cost-effectiveness of mindfulness-based cognitive therapy compared with maintenance antidepressant treatment in the prevention of depressive relapse or recurrence (PREVENT): a randomised controlled trial. *Lancet* 2015;386(9988):63–73.

Leo RJ, Ligot JS Jr. A systematic review of randomized controlled trials of acupuncture in the treatment of depression. *J Affect Disord* 2007;97(1-3):13–22.

Rapaport MH, Nierenberg AA, Howland R, et al. The treatment of minor depression with St. John's Wort or citalopram: failure to show benefit over placebo. *J Psychiatr Res* 2011;45(7):931–41.

Sanchez-Villegas A, Martinez-Gonzalez MA, Estruch R, et al: Mediterranean dietary pattern and depression: the PREDIMED randomized trial. *BMC Med* 2013;11(1):208.

Wang C, Bannuru R, Ramel J, et al. Tai chi on psychological well-being: systematic review and meta-analysis. *BMC Complement Altern Med* 2010;10(1):23.

WEBSITES

Academic Consortium for Integrative Medicine. https://imconsortium.org. Accessed July 2018.

National Center for Complementary and Integrative Health (NCCIH). https://nccih.nih.gov. Accessed July 2018.

National Institutes of Health Office of Dietary Supplements. https://ods.od.nih.gov. Accessed July 2018.

Natural Medicines. https://naturalmedicines.therapeuticresearch.com. Accessed July 2018.

Stress & Disease

36

John F. Christensen, PhD

INTRODUCTION

Human history is replete with dramatic stories of the connection between stress and disease. John Hunter (1728–1793), a surgeon and medical educator at St. George's Hospital in London, reportedly stated publicly, "My life is at the mercy of any rogue who chooses to provoke me," and soon afterward died following a contentious meeting with hospital administrators.

A review of coroners' records in Los Angeles in 1994 revealed a marked increase in deaths, including sudden death, related to atherosclerotic cardiovascular disease on the day of the 1994 Northridge earthquake. In 1999 during a 7.3 magnitude earthquake in Taiwan, patients on Holter monitors showed heart rate variability derangement due to withdrawal of parasympathetic activity and increase in sympathetic arousal. In the quarterfinal of the 1996 European football championships between the French and Dutch teams, a draw at the end of overtime resulted in a sudden death penalty shootout, which was won by the French. An analysis of mortality in the total population of Dutch men and women aged 45 years or more revealed a relative risk of death from acute myocardial infarction (MI) or stroke of 1.51 among the men on the day of the match, compared with the 5 days on either side. There was no such effect on French men. This gave new meaning to the term "sudden death penalty."

The psychological sequelae of exposure to life-threatening stressors are also problematic and disruptive to people's lives. The terrorist attacks on the World Trade Center and the Pentagon on September 11, 2001, were witnessed directly by an estimated 100,000 people and vicariously by millions of Americans and others worldwide. In the period of time between October 16 and November 15, 2001, it is estimated that 7.5% of Manhattan residents south of 110th street were suffering from posttraumatic stress disorder (PTSD) and 9.7% were suffering from depression. In a representative sample of the American population surveyed 3–5 days following the attacks, 44% reported one or more symptoms consistent with acute stress disorder (ASD). Refugees and prisoners of war who have been exposed to torture are also likely to develop symptoms of PTSD, anxiety, and depression.

Less dramatically, research since the late 1960s has demonstrated correlations between significant changes in individuals' lives and the subsequent onset of various types of physical and psychological illness. A consistent relationship has even been found between daily hassles and the onset of illness.

The interrelationship between mental stress and physical disease is complex and multifactorial. As a result, the study of stress and disease embraces a wide range of behavioral, emotional, cognitive, physiologic, hormonal, biochemical, cellular, environmental, and even spiritual interconnections, not easily understood or encapsulated in the controlled clinical trial.

It has been estimated that up to 70% of primary care visits are for problems related to stress and lifestyle. Most clinicians, however, have not been trained to extend their diagnostic workup and treatment interventions into the psychosocial context of these illnesses. Adequate treatment and prevention, however, require that providers regard their patients' illnesses and suffering in the context of their life struggles. This perspective allows the clinician to intervene at multiple points along the continuum from mind to molecule.

The ***biopsychosocial model*** of medicine regards illness as multidetermined—by biochemical alterations on the molecular level and by psychological and social events on the molar level. This model encourages clinicians to move conceptually up and down the hierarchy from patients' genetic susceptibilities and pathophysiologic processes to their unique life circumstances, stressors, and psychological meanings by which they construct their reality, to understand fully the origins of disease and the most appropriate therapies.

This chapter offers a framework for clinicians to think broadly and clinically about the stress–illness connection and suggests some approaches to assessing and treating stress-related illness. It offers a brief background of the research base for this perspective; provides a conceptual framework to guide diagnosis and treatment; suggests methods for communicating with patients about stress; and offers some options for stress assessment, prevention, and intervention.

CASE ILLUSTRATION 1

History: *A 54-year-old woman with a history of chronic migraine headaches, hypertension, hypercholesterolemia, mild obesity, and smoking presented to a new primary care physician. She was treated by her previous physician with sumatriptan for the migraines, and she routinely called in halfway through the month for extra refills. Other medications included atenolol for blood pressure elevation and migraine prophylaxis, as well as over-the-counter antacids for occasional heartburn.*

Patient Interview: *The patient appeared angry and complained that the medication was not helping her pain. The new physician listened to her complaints and agreed at the end of the visit to refill her medications but told her he would not prescribe more than the previous doctor. He asked her to return for her annual Pap smear, at which time he would take a history and do a physical examination.*

This case is a common occurrence in primary care medicine, and the patient's chronic complaints pull for efforts by the new physician to ease her symptoms, especially with pain medication. Many physicians might regard this as a "difficult patient" (see Chapter 4). Her new physician refrains from developing a treatment plan until after a complete history and physical, scheduled for the next visit. He provides a pain medication refill to meet the patient's immediate needs and elicits her agreement to return for the subsequent evaluation. That next visit will offer an opportunity, in addition to the physical examination, to explore the psychological and social stress pathways that contribute to the patient's symptom constellation. We will return to this case later, but first we will review the history and meaning of "stress," its research background, and the rich array of assessment and intervention tools available for the physician to help this patient steer a new course to health.

DEFINITIONS

The concept of stress was borrowed by physiology and psychology from physics, where it generally refers to a force acting against some resistance. In materials science, stress is what is imposed on a material by the outer world; strain is the reaction of the material to the stress.

Hans Selye is generally credited with introducing the concept of stress into physiology. He defined stress loosely as "the rate of wear and tear in the body" and more rigorously as "the state manifested by a specific syndrome which consists of all the nonspecifically induced changes within a biologic system." In this specific syndrome, termed by Selye the **general adaptation syndrome** (GAS), glucocorticoids are secreted by the adrenal cortex in response to adaptational demands placed on the organism by such disparate stressors as heat, cold, starvation, and other environmental insults—hence the expression "nonspecifically induced changes."

A distinction is usually made between "stress" and "stressors." Although **stress** is sometimes loosely used to refer to the environmental sources of threat to the organism, the term **stressor** is more appropriate in reference to these agents, whereas "stress" refers to the organism's response.

More recent definitions of stress in humans emanate from a transactional model that takes into account the interactions between persons and their environment. In this view, stress occurs when a situational demand presents a call for action that the individual perceives as exceeding available resources. I have proposed the following working definition: "**Stress** is a process of interchange between an organism and its environment that involves self-generated or environmentally induced changes that, once they are perceived by the organism as exceeding available resources (internal or external), disrupt homeostatic processes in the organism–environment system." This definition includes the traditional notion of stress as originating with an external demand (environmentally induced change) that exceeds the coping resources of the organism. It also includes, however, those expectations of events that arise from within (self-generated), that are seen as essential to one's survival or well-being, and that cannot be accommodated by the environment or the individual's capacity (exceeding available resources). The disruption of homeostasis in the organism–environment system can have its primary manifestation as a pathological end state in the organism (illness or tissue damage) or as a destructive alteration of the environment (violence as a stress response).

RESEARCH BACKGROUND

Psychoneuroimmunology

Psychoneuroimmunology (PNI) involves the study of the interactions of consciousness, the central nervous system (CNS), and the immune system (involving the body's defense against infection and aberrant cell division). The compelling evidence of these studies is that the CNS influences immune function and that, conversely, the immune system can influence the CNS. The brain is normally part of the immunoregulatory

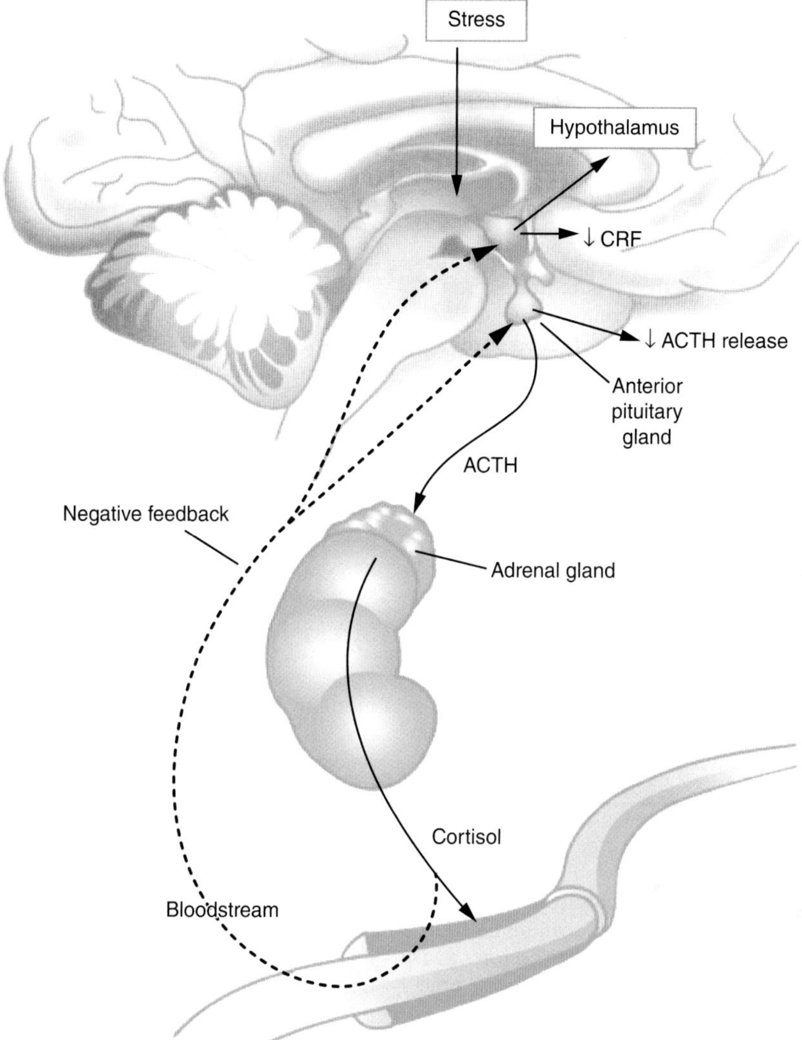

Figure 36-1. Hypothalamic–pituitary–adrenal (HPA) axis. (Reproduced with permission from Molina PE. Adrenal gland. In: *Endocrine Physiology*. 3rd ed. New York, NY: McGraw-Hill; 2009.)

network. Specifically, stimulation of the hypothalamic–pituitary–adrenal (HPA) axis leads to downregulation of immune system function in response to stress (Figure 36-1). Stressful thoughts and emotions may reach the hypothalamus by axons projecting from the limbic system (primarily the amygdala) or from the forebrain. Corticotropin-releasing factor (CRF), produced in the hypothalamus under conditions of stress, acts on the anterior pituitary to release adrenocorticotropin hormone (ACTH), which in turn stimulates the production of corticosteroids in the adrenal cortex. Under conditions of acute stress, corticosteroids have immunosuppressive effects on the lymphoreticular system and marked antiallergic and anti-inflammatory effects.

In addition, CRF leads to release of catecholamines, which themselves may produce changes in lymphocyte, monocyte, and leukocyte functions. Endogenous opiates (endorphins) are also elevated with stress, and they are generally thought to be immunosuppressive. Finally, growth hormone and prolactin, which are immunoenhancing factors, are initially elevated at the onset of acute stress, but under conditions of prolonged stress their secretion is inhibited. Thus, the combined effect of elevated corticosteroids, catecholamines, and endorphins, along with inhibition of growth hormone and prolactin, is to dysregulate the immune system.

Psychological stress can lead to increased production of proinflammatory cytokines, particularly interleukin-6

(IL-6), which is also triggered by infection and trauma. Proinflammatory cytokines have been implicated in a range of diseases in older adults that can be traced to inflammation, including cardiovascular disease, osteoporosis, arthritis, type 2 diabetes, certain lymphoproliferative diseases or cancers (including multiple myeloma, non-Hodgkin lymphoma, and chronic lymphocytic leukemia), depression, Alzheimer disease, and periodontal disease. Another development in stress research involves the concept of "allostatic load," which is the wear and tear on organisms that results from chronic overactivity or underactivity of allostatic systems. *Allostasis* refers to the body's ability to produce hormones (e.g., cortisol) and other mediators (e.g., cytokines) that help it to adapt to novel situations or challenges. These systems, which include the autonomic nervous system (Figure 36-2), HPA axis (see Figure 36-1), and the cardiovascular, metabolic, and immune systems, protect the body by responding to internal and external stress in an attempt to achieve stability through change.

The Brain–Gut–Microbiome Axis

Recent research has illuminated the interactive pathways between the brain and the gut microbiome. "Human microbiota" is the term used to describe all the microorganisms (bacteria, eukaryotes, archaea, and viruses) within the human body, while the "microbiome" is defined as the complete catalog of these microbes and their genes. There are trillions of microbiota inhabiting the human body, particularly the intestines, and they slightly outnumber human cells. The total weight of these microbiota (1–2 kg) is equivalent to that of the human brain. The bidirectional communication between the brain and gut microbiota has been termed the brain–gut–microbiome (BMG) axis, and this communication can occur across numerous physiologic channels, including neuroendocrine and neuroimmune pathways and the autonomic nervous system. The vagus nerve is the most important neural pathway for this bidirectional communication.

Disruptions to the BMG axis can originate in the brain or in the gut. Psychological stress disrupts homeostasis in the organism, including the ecosystem within the gastrointestinal (GI) tract. This disruption is mediated by the HPA axis described above. An example of such a disruption in the BMG axis is inflammatory bowel syndrome (IBS), in which HPA axis activation persists much longer than in healthy people. Interventions aimed at psychological stress reduction can have a beneficial effect on IBS symptoms (see section later on GI disorders). Likewise, disruptions to the gut microbiota, such as bacterial infections, may lead to inflammation, which is implicated in major depressive disorder (MDD) and increased responsiveness to stress. Another connection between mood disorders and the gut lies in the serotonin and tryptophan metabolism. Mucosal cells in the gut and the enteric nervous system (ENS) neurons produce 95% of serotonin within the body. Peripherally serotonin is involved in GI secretion, motility, and pain perception, whereas in the brain it regulates mood and cognition.

Interventions that may directly impact the gut microbiota are emerging. These include the use of *psychobiotics*, which can alter gut microbiota to promote a positive effect on mood, cognition, and stress response. Another feature of gut metabolism being investigated is the diversity of microbiota in the gut. Diversity is often an indicator of an ecosystem's health, and research has shown that the variety of species in Western microbiomes is typically much less than those of hunter-gatherers and people who consume rural agrarian diets. Although most studies on the BGM axis have been done with animals, clinical research with humans is beginning to show promise of treatments that will become available to target both brain and gut in restoring equilibrium and relieving distress.

Stress, Food, & Inflammation

Inflammation is a common link for diseases high in mortality risk, including cardiovascular disease, cancer, and diabetes. Stress and depression, as well as dietary intake, can promote inflammation through proinflammatory cytokine production. Diet influences cytokine-induced inflammation by means of the balance between omega-3 (n-3) polyunsaturated fatty acids (PUFA) and omega-6 (n-6) PUFA, with n-6 (refined vegetable oils) promoting the production of proinflammatory cytokines and n-3 (fish, fish oil, walnuts, flax seed) mitigating their production. The link between depression and inflammation interacts with dietary balance, with higher n-6/n-3 ratios showing a relationship with depression. In epidemiologic studies, greater fish consumption has been associated with a lower prevalence of depression. A diet with higher n-6/n-3 ratio can also increase vulnerability to inflammatory responses to stress. Stress, in turn, promotes unhealthy food choices that promote inflammation, with higher stress associated with decreased fruit and vegetable consumption and increased consumption of sweets and fast food. Higher stress is also associated with higher peaks in postprandial lipidemia and delayed gastric clearing of these compounds, both associated with atherogenesis.

Effect of Psychological Interventions on the Immune System

A meta-analytic review showed that three classes of interventions could reliably alter immune function. *Hypnosis with immune suggestions* showed a positive influence on total salivary immunoglobulin A (IgA)

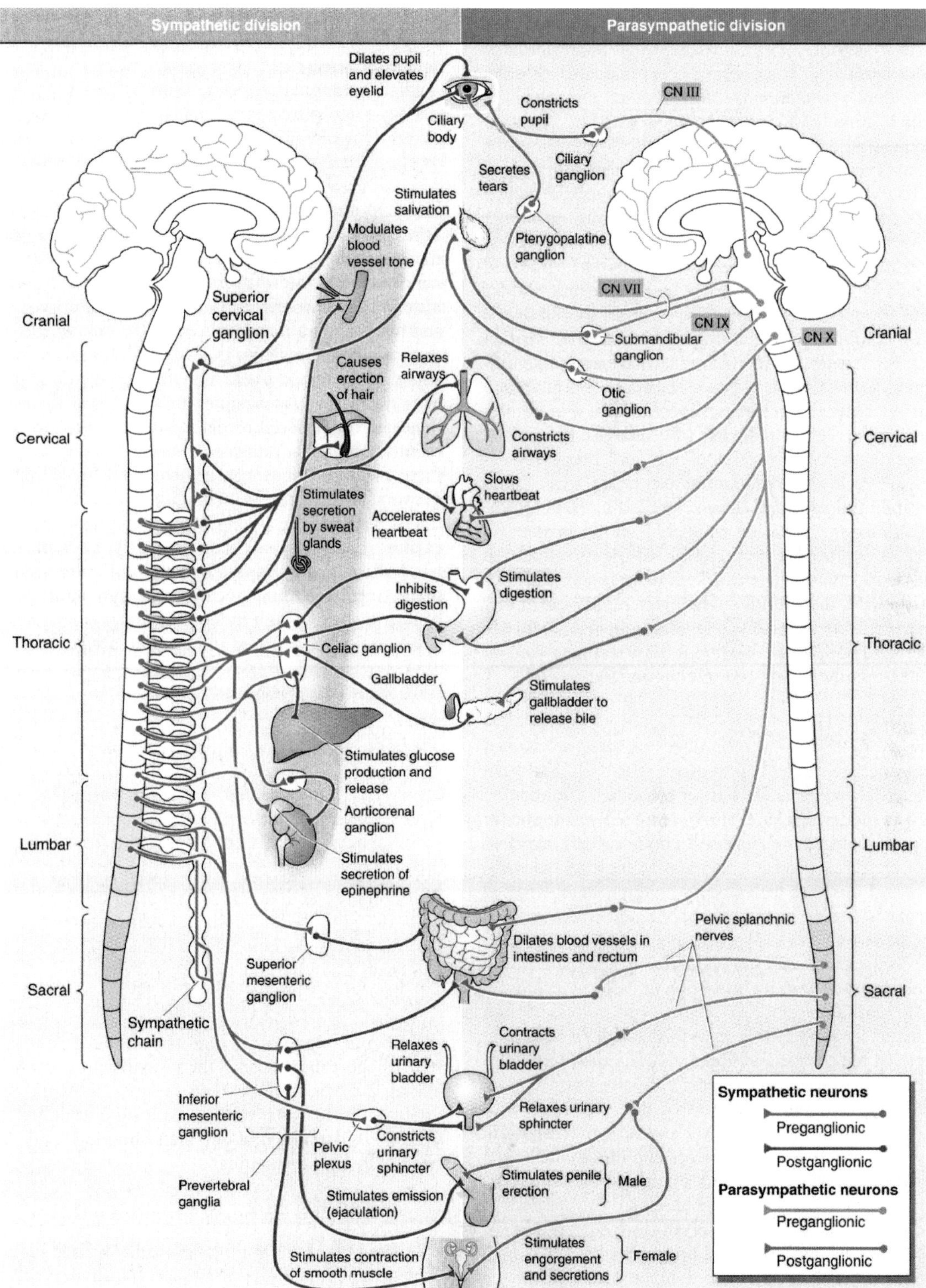

Figure 36-2. Autonomic nervous system. (Reprinted with permission from Boron WF, Boulpaep EL. *Medical Physiology*. Philadelphia: Elsevier, 2012.)

concentration and neutrophil adherence, along with a modest suppression of intermediate-type hypersensitivity erythema. These effects were mediated through relaxation. *Conditioning interventions*, in which a neutral stimulus is initially paired with an immune-modulating stimulus and later elicits the immune changes on its own, were able to enhance natural killer (NK) cell cytotoxicity. *Disclosure interventions*, which encourage patients to write essays about previously inhibited stressful experiences, have shown some success in reducing antibody titers to Epstein–Barr virus and enhancing the body's control over latent herpes simplex virus production. Another meta-analysis looked at the effect of mind–body interventions on gene transcription factors. Among the interventions that showed significant downregulation of genes related to proinflammatory cytokines were transcendental and mindfulness meditation, Tai chi, qigong, the relaxation response, mindfulness-based stress reduction, and breath regulation. A review of randomized controlled trials found that mindfulness interventions reduced markers of pro-inflammation, including circulating blood markers of C-reactive protein, interleukin 6, and the stress-induced inflammatory skin flare response. It also examined studies showing that mindfulness interventions can buffer declines in or increase CD4+ T-lymphocyte counts in stressed HIV-positive adults at posttreatment and at follow-up time points up to 9 months later.

Stressful Life Events

Retrospective studies have shown a relationship between recent life change and a host of pathological outcomes, such as sudden cardiac death, onset of MI, occurrence of fractures, pregnancy and birth complications, aggravation of chronic illness, tuberculosis, multiple sclerosis, diabetes, onset of leukemia in children, and onset of mental disorders such as depression and schizophrenia. Prospective studies have predicted future illness based on life change scores and subsequently verified the accuracy of those predictions by inspection of medical records.

Recent attention has focused on individual and situational variables that may mediate the relationship between life change and illness. Among the psychological variables that seem to mediate the stress response are locus of control (including the extent to which individuals prefer control in their lives and how much control they perceive they have over specific life events), need for stimulation, openness to change, stimulus screening, self-actualization, the use of denial, the presence of social supports, and emotional self-disclosure. Studies of *resilience* have focused on the neurochemical and hormonal feedback systems that dampen or switch off the stress response (HPA axis and sympathetic nervous system response described above). Among these resilience chemicals are *DHEA* (dehydroepiandrosterone), which lessens the effects of cortisol, and *neuropeptide Y*, which counters the effects of CRF at the anterior pituitary. These stress inhibitory mechanisms may be more prevalent in people who show a greater resiliency or hardiness in response to stressful events.

Technostress

Increased use of smartphones and the Internet has established new norms for work and connectivity in industrialized countries. Although allowing broader and more rapid access to information than ever before in human history, as well as increasing flexibility for work location and hours among many workers, these technologies also exact a toll on human health. In a Swedish study of young adults, high mobile phone use was a predictor of stress, sleep disturbance, and depression at a 1-year follow-up. Increased use of social media to interact frequently with friends near and far presents a paradox. On the one hand, these media facilitate engagement with social support networks, which are a well-established stress buffer. Chatting and texting are among the high-frequency activities of those in Generation Y (born after 1980). On the other hand, these media also lead to communication overload, the taxing of working memory through multitasking, distractibility, and guilt induced by the social expectation of immediacy of response and constant availability.

Stress in America Survey

The Stress in America survey, published annually by the American Psychological Association (APA), revealed that those who serve as caregivers—providing care to both the aging and chronically ill—report higher levels of stress, poorer health, and a greater tendency to engage in unhealthy behaviors to alleviate that stress than the population at large. The 2018 survey showed generational differences in overall self-reported stress (on a scale of 1–10), with Older Adults reporting the lowest (3.3), Boomers 4.1, Generation X 5.1, Generation Z 5.3, and Millenials 5.7. One cause of stress is the current political climate, which more than 6 in 10 Americans (62%) report is a significant stressor. When asked to consider the nation's future, more than two-thirds of Americans (69%) report that it causes them significant stress. Generation Z (those born between the mid-1990s and mid-2000s) reported gun violence as a significant stressor, with 75% concerned about mass shootings and 72% stressed by school shootings.

Work-Related Stress & Burnout

The demands of the workplace in industrialized societies are a persistent and intense stressor. Job strain is defined as a combination of high job demands and low perceived control. In a prospective study of healthy young adults (Cardiovascular Risk in Young Finns Study), job strain was associated with increased carotid atherosclerosis among the men, but not the women.

In another prospective study, the degree of job stress overtime increased the risk of the metabolic syndrome in a linear fashion, with subjects at lower grades of employment at greater risk.

Chronic work stress, defined as high demands and low control, was associated with cardiovascular disease events in a study of 10,308 middle-aged London-based civil servants. Associations were found between work stress and negative behaviors, such as low physical activity and poor diet, and pathophysiologic consequences, such as decreased heart rate variability and an increase in morning cortisol.

Burnout is a syndrome associated with unrelenting stress and has been studied extensively as a phenomenon in a variety of work settings and professions, including physicians. It includes symptoms of emotional exhaustion, depersonalization, and a decreased sense of personal accomplishment. In a prospective study, burnout was associated with an increased risk of type 2 diabetes in apparently healthy individuals.

In Japan, the concept of **karoshi**, or death from overwork, has received government attention in recent decades. Rapid growth in industrialization following World War II led to production efficiencies placing pressure on Japanese workers, who often worked overtime without additional compensation. A new phenomenon of sudden death among high-level businessmen who were previously healthy brought attention to these stressful work environments.

The Role of Acute & Chronic Stress in Cardiac Disease

Acute stress activates the sympathetic nervous system (see Figure 36-2), which leads to increases in heart rate and blood pressure, coronary vasoconstriction, and decreased myocardial electrical stability. Several behavioral and emotional events have been implicated as probable triggers of acute coronary syndromes (MI and sudden cardiac death) in vulnerable individuals, especially events within a 1- to 2-hour period before the onset of symptoms.

Behavioral triggers include physical exertion (more common in men than women), sexual activity, sleep disturbance, and heavy consumption of alcohol. Well-studied emotional triggers include earthquakes, sporting events, war, high-pressure deadlines at work, and anger. In one study, the relative risk of acute MI in the 2 hours following an anger episode was 2.3, and in comparison with a control period 24 hours earlier, it was 4.0. The risk of anger triggering an MI was inversely related to socioeconomic status. In a large-scale study, the relative risk of anger triggering an MI was 9.0 compared to usual levels of anger, but when limiting the analysis to patients who had no premonitory symptoms the relative risk increased to 15.7.

Takotsubo cardiomyopathy (TCM) is an interesting example of emotional stress causing physical illness. This condition mimics acute coronary syndrome and is accompanied by reversible left ventricular apical ballooning in the absence of angiographically significant coronary artery stenosis. In Japanese, "tako-tsubo" means "fishing pot for trapping octopus," and the left ventricle of a patient diagnosed with this condition resembles that shape. TCM, which is transient and typically precipitated by acute emotional stress, is also known as "stress cardiomyopathy" or "broken-heart syndrome." The disease is associated with excessive sympathetic stimulation, microvascular dysfunction, coronary artery vasospasm, and abnormal myocardial tissue metabolism. An excessive release of catecholamines seems to have a pivotal role in its development. Almost 90% of cases occur in postmenopausal women. TCM is a reversible cardiomyopathy with a generally favorable outcome. It is a relatively recently described phenomenon that needs to be considered early in any patient that presents with acute dyspnea, chest pain or collapse after an acute episode of grief, shock, or stress.

In addition to promoting unhealthy behaviors, *chronic stress* activates and reactivates the sympathetic nervous system. Repeated sympathetic stimulation increases heart rate and blood pressure, and autonomic nervous system dysregulation leads to decreased heart rate variability and baroreflex dysfunction, which has been associated with cardiovascular disease events. Depression increases levels of inflammatory markers, including fibrinogen, C-reactive protein, IL-6, and tumor necrosis factor. Chronic stressors also activate the HPA axis producing hypercortisolemia, which in turn promotes central obesity and insulin resistance, risk factors for cardiovascular disease.

In the Caregiver Health Effects study, 400 caregivers showed a 63% higher mortality rate than non-caregiving control subjects over a 4-year period. The increased mortality was particularly evident in caregivers who already had known cardiovascular disease. In a series of physiologically oriented studies, the San Diego Caregiver study examined possible pathways between caregiving and cardiovascular disease. Distressed caregivers had an increased risk for developing hypertension when followed over a 6-year period. Caregivers also had increased levels of D-dimer (a circulating procoagulant factor), more sleep disruption, and higher levels of circulating inflammatory cytokines.

Personality Influences on Cardiovascular Disease

Research has examined the relationship between heart disease and a personality constellation that includes hostility, anger, cynicism, suspiciousness, and excessive self-involvement. Hostility is conceptualized as comprising three elements: the emotion of anger, its expression, and cognitions of cynical mistrust. Using well-validated measures of the cognitive aspect of hostility, studies have linked higher hostility scores with subsequent coronary events like hospitalizations for angina, nonfatal MI, stroke, and congestive heart failure. Higher hostility has also been associated with coronary risk factors, such as increased plasma homocysteine levels, triglycerides, body mass index, waist-to-hip ratio, glucose levels, alcohol consumption, and smoking. In a study of middle-aged women, each 1-point increase in hostility scores predicted a significantly higher intimal–medial thickening in the carotid arteries.

Marital Quality & Health

Marriage and divorce can lead to immune alterations that have an impact on health. In troubled relationships depression provides a central pathway to immune dysregulation, inflammation, and poor health. Sleep disturbance and obesity can simultaneously feed off depression as they promote it. There tends to be a convergence of gene expression patterns in cohabiting partners, who exhibit noteworthy transcriptional similarity. In one study, couples living together had 50% less immunologic variation than between unrelated pairs. Furthermore, cohabiting couples' gut microbiotas are also more similar to each other than unrelated partners. This may account for the fact that serious mental or physical illness in one partner tends to increase risk in the other partner for illnesses such as depression, asthma, allergies, peptic ulcer disease, diabetes, metabolic syndrome, hypertension, arthritis, cancer, and cognitive functioning. One meta-analysis of the links between marital quality and health in 72,000 subjects from several countries found that greater marital quality was related to better physical health. There was also clear evidence that greater marital quality was related to lower cardiovascular reactivity during marital conflict.

Personality Factors & Longevity

One personality factor that has emerged in various studies as a strong predictor of health and well-being is **conscientiousness**. Individuals who are conscientious—that is, prudent, dependable, well organized, and persistent—stay healthier, thrive, and live longer. The size of this effect is equal to or greater than that of many known biomedical risk factors. Extensive research has revealed that conscientiousness is a very strong and reliable lifelong predictor of healthy pathways and of longevity. Individuals who live longer and have a higher quality of life with minimal disease burden tend to have the following characteristics throughout their lifespan: (1) They have good ties to social networks and are well-integrated into their communities; (2) they are physically active; and (3) they are conscientious, live and work with purpose, and are involved with helping others.

Positive Cognitive Styles

Evidence is accumulating from a variety of studies that optimism, perceptions of personal control, and a sense of meaning are protective of physical health. These cognitive resources assume special significance in helping people cope with intensely stressful events. Even unrealistically optimistic expectations appear to slow down the progression of disease in men infected with HIV. In a study of healthy older adults, a sense of coherence (one indicator of resilience) moderated the association between anticipation of moving and reduced NK cell lysis, with a low sense of coherence associated with poorest levels of NK cell lysis. In a study of the cognitive and psychological sequelae of the 2011 Japanese earthquake and tsunami among survivors in the primary disaster area, posttraumatic stress had a major impact on self-perceived quality of life 3 months after the disaster. The study authors concluded that reducing negative cognitions would have a greater impact than positive reappraisals on lowering depression and anxiety in this early stage of response. It was expected that positive reappraisals leading to *posttraumatic growth* (PTG) would occur over longer time frames. Similar to the time course of recovery from other disasters, it was expected that PTG would include enhanced relationships with others, a sense of new possibilities, self-perceived personal strength, a sense of purpose in life, the concept of *ikigai* (meaningfulness), and a deepened spirituality.

Religion & Spirituality

Several studies have shown a relationship between religious or spiritual practice and health outcomes. "Religion" can be considered a collection of beliefs and practices that are external expressions of spiritual experience. These expressions can be organizationally based or private but are usually grounded in a collective tradition. "Spirituality" can be considered an orientation toward or experiences with the transcendent, existential, or sacred dimensions of life. That which is transcendent or sacred is considered as something beyond oneself, whether it be conceptualized as a divine being, higher power, nature, spirit, or the ultimate ground of being. It is possible for people to engage in religious activities independent of having spiritual experiences, just as some people consider themselves intensely spiritual without being religious. Some consider their religious practice to be a pathway toward spirituality.

Types of studies on the religion–health connection have included cross-sectional as well as prospective and retrospective studies where participation in religious or spiritual practice is correlated with some health outcome measure, as well as intervention studies in which subjects were randomized into treatment and control groups. Correlational studies of religious or spiritual involvement and health outcomes have shown a positive association with longer life; less cardiovascular disease; less hypertension; more engagement in health-promoting behaviors; decreased risk of depression, anxiety, substance abuse, and suicide; better coping with illness; and better health-related quality of life. Among the intervention studies the best evidence for efficacy with health outcomes has been with religiously oriented cognitive therapy, meditation, 12-step fellowships, forgiveness therapy, and intercessory prayer.

A meta-analysis of the effects of religion and spirituality on the self-reported health of 32,000 adult cancer patients found a significant association between religious/spiritual practice and physical well-being, functional well-being, and physical symptoms.

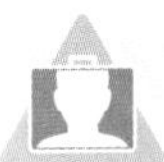

CASE ILLUSTRATION 1 (CONTD.)

Social History: *At the follow-up appointment, the physician took a social history, which revealed that the patient had been smoking a pack of cigarettes every day for the last 35 years but did not use alcohol or street drugs. Although never married, she had been involved in a 10-year relationship with her boyfriend, who suffered from severe emphysema and was dependent on oxygen. Three years previously this man had assumed responsibility for raising his two granddaughters (ages 8 and 11 years) because his daughter, the girls' mother, was a drug addict serving time in prison. The patient was not consulted about this custody decision. She accepted the stressor out of love for her partner, who was also dependent on her. The oldest granddaughter was now age 14 and had become unruly, rebellious, sexually active, and aggressive. She had asked the patient for help obtaining birth control. Although the patient wanted to leave this demanding social situation, she saw it as her responsibility to care for her partner and the two children. The history correlated these recent life events with increased frequency of migraines and initiation of daily use of Imitrex.*

Physician Facilitation of Emotional Self-Disclosure: *The physician actively listened to the patient's self-disclosure, which was accompanied by crying. At the end of the interview, the patient thanked the physician, who noted that she had not complained of migraines during that visit.*

In allowing the patient to disclose her psychological and social stressors, the physician was able to gain relevant information within a biopsychosocial perspective of patient care. Relevant stressors potentially contributing to this patient's medical symptoms included caregiving for a disabled partner, having to assume a parenting role of grandchildren, and a self-expectation of a way of loving her partner that allowed no escape for her from an uncontrollable situation. In allowing the patient's emotional self-disclosure, there was an immediate effect on mitigating migraine symptoms. Going forward from this interview, it was important for the physician to have a pathway to navigate and orchestrate the various biological, psychological, and social interventions relevant to this patient's condition.

A STRESS MODEL FOR MEDICAL CARE

The etiology of illness and its waxing and waning course are multifactorial. Any given illness episode is determined by many circumstances. The complex pathway by which stress influences the outcome of illness is subject to the ongoing accumulation of data and elaboration of heuristic and clinical models. A model of stress that can aid diagnosis, prevention, and intervention is shown in Figure 36-3. Adapted from an optical model first proposed by Rahe and Arthur, it depicts stressors as light rays filtered through successive lenses representing the individual's **perception** (threat appraisal), **coping**, **physiologic processes**, and **arousal reduction** activities, and then projected onto **illness outcome** screens. Each lens either augments or diminishes the intensity of light (heavy bold lines or dotted lines, respectively) on its pathway to illness outcome, and represents a potential focal point for the clinician's diagnosis of a stress influence or risk factor for patient illness. Each lens also represents a potential focus of preventive health care or intervention.

Perception refers to the person's appraisal of the threat involved in various stressors. Several personal variables that may affect the degree of perceived threat are shown in Figure 36-3. For example, the degree of openness to change or the extent to which one values change influences whether a particular life change, such as a child leaving home, is perceived as a threat to the self or an opportunity for growth. The degree of control individuals *prefer* to have in their lives, as well as the amount of control they *perceive* they have over specific stressors, also influence their perception of threat. Thus, a parent with a high need to control an adolescent child's outside activities experiences more stress when the child struggles toward emancipation than does a parent who has less of a need for control and who trusts the child's judgment.

Coping refers to methods one uses to mitigate the influence of stressors perceived as threatening. One

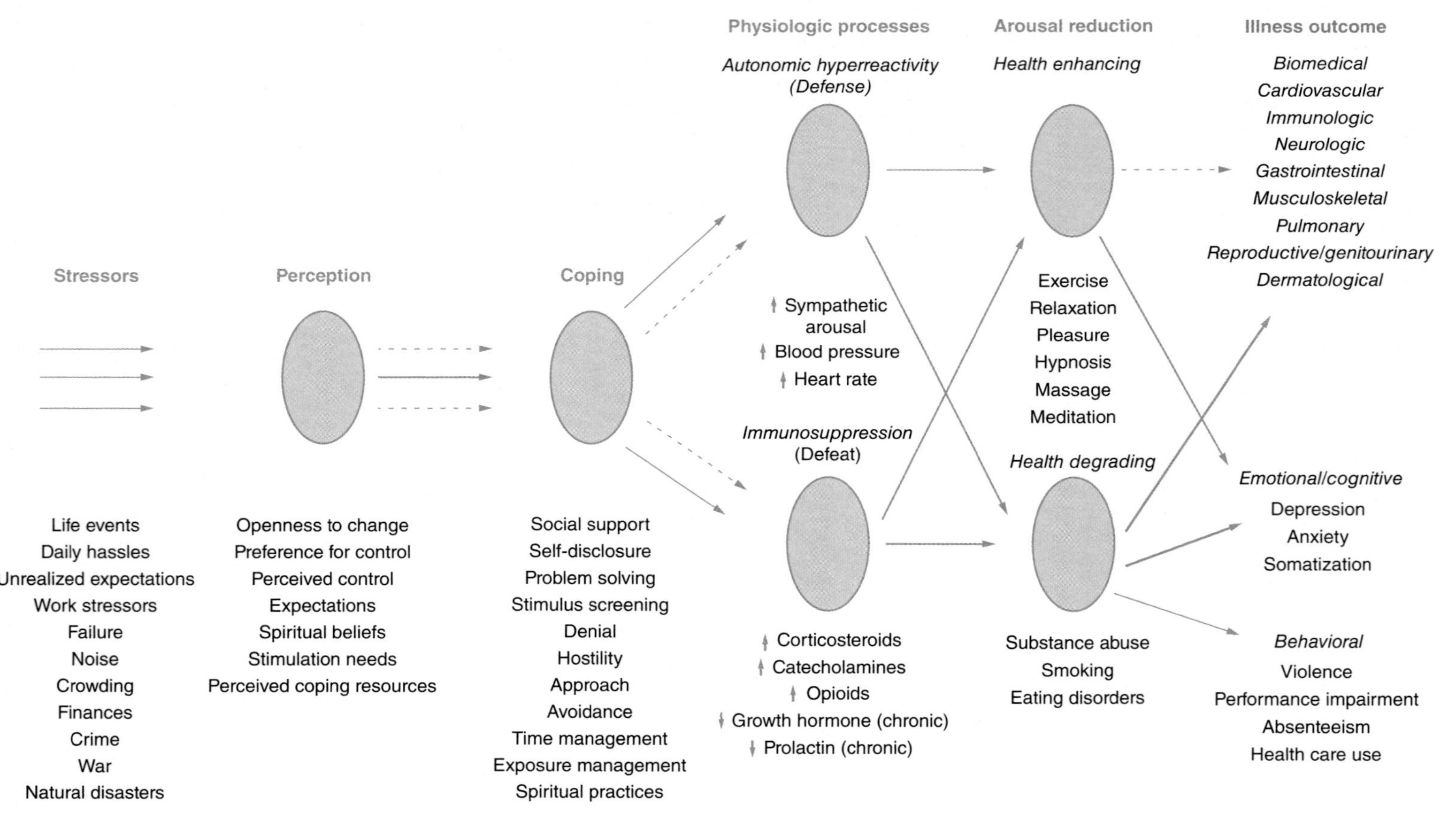

Figure 36-3. An optical model of stress pathways.

approach to coping is "exposure management," or attempts to increase or decrease the amount and intensity of stressors encountered. Thus, an overworked, overcommitted manager might attempt to mitigate stress by withdrawing from some commitments, by reducing work hours, and by delegating more responsibility to subordinates. Social supports are an important stress buffer, and successful coping with stressors may involve both developing confiding relationships and increasing the amount of one's self-disclosure about the effect of stressors in one's life. There is some evidence that emotional self-disclosure about stressors enhances immune functioning. "Stimulus screening" involves techniques to focus attention on relevant stimuli and to regulate the overall flow of stimulation to one's optimal level of functioning.

Two major classes of **physiologic response** to stressors that lead to target organ pathology are autonomic hyperreactivity and immunosuppression. Both are cortically mediated through the individual's perceptions and methods of coping. ***Hyperreactivity*** in the presence of stress, sometimes called the **defense reaction**, has been shown to be a factor in disease processes specific to vulnerable organ systems in persons with established disease. Thus, exaggerated pressor responses in hypertensives, increased electromyelogram responses in those suffering from tension headaches and chronic back pain, disturbances in glucose metabolism in insulin-dependent diabetics, and bronchoconstrictive responses in asthmatics are all examples of hyperreactivity in the presence of a definable stressor. In the case of hypertension, hyperreactivity is present in normotensives at risk for the disorder and in some studies has predicted future blood pressure levels. Other examples are increased levels of serum cholesterol seen in studies of tax accountants in the 2 weeks prior to April 15 and of fighter pilots landing on aircraft carriers compared with pilots on long commercial airline flights.

One of the adaptive functions of sympathetic activation (see Figure 36-2) is to prepare the organism for large-muscle movement to either attack or flee a threat. In twenty-first century human society, these somatomotor responses are often voluntarily suppressed or sublimated, leading to delayed elimination of released glucose and fatty acids and often bringing more powerful and prolonged increases in blood pressure. In addition, the relative absence of skeletal muscle exertion in affluent societies (without compensatory aerobic exercise) prevents the activation of endorphins that normally accompanies muscle exertion. Because these endorphins dampen mental arousal and sympathetic activity, in the absence of skeletal muscle exertion these arousal and activation states are prolonged.

Immunosuppression, as discussed previously, occurs through the mechanisms of increased levels of circulating corticosteroids, catecholamines, and opioids and decreased levels of growth hormone and prolactin under conditions of chronic or prolonged stress. Sometimes referred to as the **defeat reaction**, this response pattern occurs when patients are exposed to long-term stressful situations that tend to overwhelm ordinary coping mechanisms, thus leading to despair or deep sorrow in situations that appear to be beyond all hope and rescue. Rather than working directly on target organ systems as in the case of hyperreactivity, downregulation of the immune system in the defeat reaction increases vulnerability to external invasive organisms and endogenous neoplasms.

Several **arousal reduction** strategies are available to individuals to mitigate physiologic activation and disruption of homeostatic processes in conditions of stress. These include both **health-enhancing** and **health-degrading** activities. Among the health-enhancing arousal-reduction strategies are exercise, which expends accumulated corticosteroids and dampens sympathetic activation through the release of endorphins, and various approaches to stimulating the parasympathetic nervous system (see Figure 36-2). This latter category includes relaxation exercises, abdominal breathing, self-hypnosis, meditation, soothing music, massage, and contact with nature.

Health-degrading activities, which may be attempts at physiologic arousal reduction but that actually magnify the stress response and lead to target organ disease, include substance abuse, tobacco use, and eating disorders. Intensification of all of these behaviors may coincide with stressful life episodes. An example is the mediating role of increased alcohol intake in the relationship between occupational stress and hypertension seen in studies of air traffic controllers.

Various **illness outcomes** of stress include **biomedical disease** manifested in specific organ systems, such as cardiovascular, immune, and neurologic disorders; **emotional and cognitive disorders,** such as depression, anxiety, and somatization; and **behavioral disorders,** such as violence, performance impairment, absenteeism, and overuse of health care resources. These stress outcomes are the usual focus of medical and mental health intervention, but the larger model of the stress pathway provides primary care clinicians with potent opportunities for comprehensive preventive health care.

HEALTH OUTCOMES OF STRESS

Each organ system has a unique susceptibility to stress. The following is a brief overview of some of the stress and treatment implications in specific diseases.

Cardiovascular

Cardiovascular disease is the leading cause of mortality in the United States. As reviewed above, stress contributes to all expressions of heart disease, including coronary artery disease, congestive heart failure, and sudden cardiac death. Because a third of sudden cardiac deaths and MIs cannot be fully explained by the severity of the standard cardiac risk factors—family history, hypertension, dyslipidemia, diabetes, or tobacco use—stress may explain some of this variance. As mentioned above, there is a connection between hostility and cardiac disease. It has been shown that hostility contributes independently of other risk factors to the pathogenesis of heart disease through lipid accumulation, increased blood pressure, and heart rate and platelet physiology.

Mind–body therapies show promise in the treatment of coronary artery disease. A meta-analysis of the use of psychoeducational interventions (health education and stress management) as a component of cardiac rehabilitation showed an overall 34% reduction in mortality, a 29% reduction in recurrent MI, and positive effects on dietary and exercise habits, weight, smoking, cholesterol, and blood pressure.

Immune

Clinical expressions of immune deficiencies are in part the result of stress. They range from the common cold to some forms of cancer. Although research on the relationship between stress and cancer is still inconclusive, there is some evidence that stress and surgical excision of the primary tumor can promote tumor metastasis by suppression of cell-mediated immunity. The perioperative period is a particularly important window during which psychological or pharmacological interventions to prevent or reduce stress may offer a reduced risk of metastasis. Other immune-mediated diseases, such as rheumatoid arthritis and systemic lupus erythematosus, may show a pattern of exacerbation brought on by stress.

HIV

More rapid disease progression in people infected with HIV has been associated with greater concealment of homosexual identity, more cumulative stressful life events, and less cumulative social support over a 5-year period. Alternatively, more deliberate cognitive processing about the death of a close friend or partner has been associated with greater likelihood of finding positive meaning in the loss, less rapid decline in CD4+ cell levels, and lower rates of AIDS-related mortality over a 9-year period in HIV-seropositive men.

Neurologic

All forms of stroke show a circadian expression in their presentation, with peaks during the early morning hours when catecholamines are highest. Dizziness, vertigo, and other balance disorders often have stress as a causative or contributing factor. One of the most common neurologic expressions of stress in clinical practice is headache. Both tension headache and migraine headache are substantially influenced by patient stressors. Meta-analysis has shown behavioral interventions (relaxation training and skin temperature biofeedback) to be as effective as medication in treatment of migraine headaches. Hypnosis with hand-warming imagery is an effective method to reverse the progression of migraine headache, especially early in the prodromal stage (see Chapter 5).

Gastrointestinal

Peptic ulcer disease may have an association with stress. Gastric hyperacidity and excess pepsin production are hallmarks of the sympathetic arousal that occurs during stress. IBS, which is characterized by abdominal pain with altered bowel habits (constipation or diarrhea) in the absence of a definable lesion or structural abnormality, frequently correlates with periods of emotional stress. The human “defense reaction” (fight-or-flight response) promotes activation of the cardiovascular system along with inhibition of gastric motility. The role of stress in promoting proinflammatory cytokines is a probable mechanism in the etiology of this disorder. Inflammation is also associated with depression, which is frequently a comorbidity with IBS. A review of psychological interventions for IBS and inflammatory bowel diseases (IBDs) found strong evidence for the effectiveness of the three most commonly used evidence-based treatments: cognitive behavioral therapy (CBT), hypnotherapy, and mindfulness-based therapy. There is a large body of literature now supporting the use of these modalities with IBS, which has more associated emotional and psychological components, and a smaller body of literature supporting their use with IBD.

Musculoskeletal

Some forms of arthritis show stress-related exacerbations. Complex syndromes such as fibromyalgia seem to have a psychosocial trigger. Temporomandibular joint (TMJ) dysfunction and its related pain syndrome are frequently associated with mental stress. Chronic pain tends to correlate with stress in a person’s life. Persistent pain and psychological symptoms frequently seen after motor vehicle accidents (MVAs) may involve the impact of acute stress interacting with past experience, post-MVA behavior, and cognitive/psychological consequences to alter activity in brain pathways that process pain.

Pulmonary

Asthma and chronic obstructive pulmonary disease appear to be worsened by stress. Conversely, one of the more powerful, self-regulatory, stress-control techniques is relaxed abdominal breathing. Asthmatics who participate in stress reduction programs have shown improved physical activity and decreased medical visits. Hypnosis has helped some asthmatics decrease their use of bronchodilators (see Chapter 5).

Reproductive & Genitourinary

The neurohormonal, vascular, and immunologic effects of stress significantly impact the reproductive and genitourinary systems. Changes in estrogen and testosterone levels can show marked association with environmental and psychological stressors. Amenorrhea frequently occurs during stressful times in the lives of women. Fertility also can be affected by stress. Dysmenorrhea, dyspareunia, endometriosis, and erectile dysfunction all have substantial stress and strain connections.

Dermatological

A variety of skin lesions and rashes have been associated with the stress response. Stress-induced vasomotor changes may aggravate inflammatory dermatoses. Vasodilation is considered to be responsible for the thermal aggravation often expressed as pruritus. This lowering of the itch threshold by vasodilation may account for the pruritus seen with many dermatological syndromes. Emotional stress, fear, and pain are all accompanied by substantial drops in skin temperature of the fingers.

Wound Healing

Psychological stress has measurable negative consequences for production of proinflammatory cytokines, and stress-related delays in wound healing have ranged from 24% to 40% with effect sizes between 0.30 and 0.74. These effects on wound healing are consistent with other studies that have shown that greater fear or distress prior to surgery is associated with poorer outcomes, including longer hospital stays, more postoperative complications, and higher rates of rehospitalization.

Frailty in the Elderly

Elevated serum levels of the proinflammatory cytokine IL-6 have predicted future disability in older adults. These cytokines slow muscle repair after injury and accelerate muscle wasting. IL-6 and C-reactive protein play a pathogenic role in several diseases associated with disability among the elderly, including osteoporosis, arthritis, and congestive heart failure.

DIAGNOSIS

Given the multivariate, multiple-pathway nature of the stress response, clinical diagnosis of stress assumes a multifactorial approach. Traditional medical diagnosis and treatment occur at the point of illness manifestation in target organ systems. From the broader perspective of stress medicine, however, each of the lenses in the optical model (see Figure 36-3) is a potential focus of diagnosis.

The Medical Interview

The richest source of data concerning stressors, perception, coping, and arousal reduction strategies is the medical interview (see Chapter 1). Having the stress model in mind allows the clinician to inquire about current and recent life stressors and to make note of significant clusters of stressors that precede illness onset. A careful history should uncover whether life stressors are temporally related to the onset of chronic disease and to periods of disease exacerbation.

During the interview, the clinician can ask patients about their beliefs, expectations, self-perceptions, and needs that influence how stressors are perceived. For example, asking patients how much control they *prefer* in their lives and how much control they *perceive* that they have over specific life events can determine whether there is congruence or incongruence between preferred and perceived control. Incongruence tends to amplify the effect of stressors. It is also helpful to ask patients how they view their own resources (internal and external) for coping with stressors, since the more the perceived threats exceed the perceived personal resources, the greater the stress involved.

Patients' approaches to coping with stressors should also be probed in the interview. The presence or absence of social supports as well as the ability of patients to access these supports through self-disclosure are critical data for facilitating stress management. The perceptual and coping styles uncovered in the interview have implications for management of the patient's health, both in prevention and intervention.

It is also important to assess patients' approaches to arousal reduction and to ascertain the balance of health-enhancing and health-degrading strategies. The following questions can be helpful in this regard: "What are the signs indicating that you are experiencing stress?" "What are your physical symptoms?" "What happens in your emotional life?" "How do you act differently when you are stressed?" Methods used to mitigate this arousal can then be ascertained: "When you notice these signs of stress, what do you do to reduce the intensity of the physical symptoms?" It is also important to elicit the short-and long-term outcomes of these strategies: "How does this strategy work for you?" "How does it affect the way you feel immediately? . . . several hours later? . . . the next day?" Sometimes it is helpful to ask about specific arousal reduction techniques: "Do you practice a form of meditation or relaxation exercise?" "Do you get regular physical exercise?" When questioning patients about substance use or tobacco use, it is helpful to ask whether their use is associated with periods of stress.

Self-Report Questionnaire

A multitude of self-report questionnaires and inventories have been developed for research purposes that measure stressors and many of the variables listed in Figure 36-3 related to perception and coping. Given the limitations of physician and support staff time, it is recommended that any questionnaire be simple, brief, and provide data that can be used by the clinician in counseling patients in the area of stress management. An example of such an instrument is the Life Stress Inventory shown in Appendix 36-A. Borrowing from the life event scaling studies and the critical role that perceived control plays in mediating stress, this inventory asks patients in an open-ended way to list the major events (and expected nonevents), changes, and stressors that have occurred during the previous year. They are asked to check those stressors that are current, ongoing problems. In addition, patients are asked to rate each stressor on a scale of 1–10, indicating the extent of perceived control they had over these events. The provider can take the mean of the control ratings and place that number (1–10) in the "control score" blank. This instrument provides both qualitative and quantitative data on the nature of patients' stressors, those that are a current source of struggle, and patients' perceived control over these events. The higher the external control score, the more at risk the patient is for adverse consequences of stress. Examining with patients those stressors that seem under their control can allow the clinician to suggest lifestyle changes in those areas. In some instances, patients can be counseled to adjust their perceptions of no control in the direction of greater control. For example, a patient who perceives that she/he has no control over her/his work hours can be helped to see areas in which limits can actually be set. In other cases, patients can be led to consider changing their expectations and accepting areas that are truly beyond their control.

CASE ILLUSTRATION 1 (CONTD.)

Having reviewed the optical model of stress prior to the patient's second appointment, the physician had a number of options to recommend after eliciting her psychosocial history. In the ***coping*** *category, an obvious first step was to intervene in the dysfunctional family relationships that were a major stressor for the patient. Increasing support from her boyfriend and enlisting professional support in managing the hormonal challenges of the adolescent grandchild seemed an obvious starting point, so referral to family therapy was high on the agenda for that visit.*

Brief Counseling and Referral for Family Therapy: *The physician counseled the patient to realize that she was not isolated. He validated her efforts to work with the situation, even though she had the real option of leaving. He recommended family therapy, to which the patient agreed. Further medical treatment was deferred until after the family had engaged in therapy. The patient made no mention of pain medication during this visit.*

Change of Medication and of Lifestyle: *Prior to the next visit there were no further calls for pain medication refills. At that visit the patient stated that the migraines, although still present, were not as disabling. The focus of the visit was on improving management of hypertension, high cholesterol, and migraines. They discussed starting an exercise program, initiating a low-fat diet and weight loss, and quitting smoking. The physician remarked that the patient appeared to be gaining control over the life events involving her family.*

Disposition: *After several months of family therapy the patient had established a primary care relationship with a pediatrician to help her with the medical and hormonal issues of the grandchildren. Her boyfriend had increased his level of help. She had lost 8 lbs over 4 months, started walking 4 days a week for 30 minutes, and began a low-fat diet, all without pain medication. She agreed to start a smoking cessation program. The patient demonstrated a marked change in attitude and treatment of office staff, and the primary care provider developed a changed perception of her and an appreciation of the healing potential in "drug-seeking patients."*

PREVENTION & INTERVENTION

Stress Management in the Intensive Care Unit

The immune system of many patients in the intensive care unit (ICU) is suppressed due to trauma, sepsis, or profound physiologic and psychological stress. Increases in cortisol levels have been found to correlate with severity of injury in minor and moderate trauma immediately after injury and hours later. Sepsis often begins as a local process of inflammation involving cytokine upregulation. These cytokines eventually, however, may move into circulation, leading to inflammatory processes systemically. Psychological stressors reported by ICU patients include pain, sleep deprivation (due to noise, disturbances by health care staff, and pain), and fear or anxiety (which may manifest in the extreme as delirium, confusion, and other unreal experiences), each of which is associated with decreased immune functioning. The implications for the ICU team are that intervening to reduce these psychosocial stressors may help prevent nosocomial infection. Feelings of anxiety and isolation can be buffered by a nurse providing a nurturing presence. Anxiety can be decreased through the use of benzodiazepines, which may also aid sleep. Nurses can attempt to minimize noise levels as much as possible and decrease the number of times patients are disturbed. Although many analgesic drugs used in the ICU can suppress immune function, alternative approaches to reducing pain should be attempted, since pain itself is immunosuppressive.

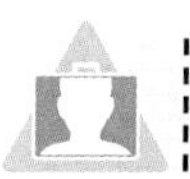

CASE ILLUSTRATION 2

Deborah Jones, an ICU nurse with 10 years' experience in critical care, joined a process improvement team (PIT) to examine an increased trend in nosocomial infections among ICU patients over the previous 12 months. Having recently completed a continuing education course in PNI, she was sensitized to the effect of stressors in the ICU environment on patients' immune functioning. Deborah shared this information with the team, and the group (including a physician critical care specialist, a pharmacist, the ICU nurse manager, a pulmonologist, and the chief medical resident) came up with some suggested modifications in the environment and administration of care. Staff entering the ICU were reminded verbally and with a posted sign to speak softly near patient beds. A review of all mechanical noise sources was conducted, and it was determined that a few changes could reduce ambient noise by 30%. Rounding on patients was coordinated to cluster around certain times of the day, and an attempt was made to have greater predictability to staff disturbance of patients when resting. Different staff members, regardless of discipline, were assigned to specific patients for brief visits of a nonmedical nature to provide support and nurturance, either verbally or through appropriate touch. A palliative care specialist was consulted to develop a menu of pain medications and doses to minimize the risk of immunosuppression, and alternative procedures such as acupuncture were sometimes ordered in collaboration with the patient. Within 3 months it was noted that the rate of infection in the ICU had dropped by 40%. In the face of that data, Deborah was delegated by the PIT to make a formal presentation to hospital administration, and the changes became hospital policy.

Stress Management in Primary Care

The model of stress, shown in Figure 36-3, offers the clinician various foci for illness prevention and intervention, just as it does for diagnosis. The clinician familiar with this model should be able to tailor specific psychological, social, behavioral, and pharmacological strategies to the unique needs of individual patients. This is preferable to referring the patient for "stress management," since this generic term does not address the multiplicity of stress-related variables and pathways discussed earlier.

Communicating With Patients About Stress

A primary component of stress prevention and treatment involves the way stress is discussed with patients. Avoiding the implication that "it's all in your head" is of great importance. Equally important is avoiding the message that "you are responsible for your illness," which implies greater personal control over somatic processes than is realistic. Here the risk is inducing guilt in patients who become ill and who feel they have failed at being a "better person." Avoiding negative emphases, for example, "Your hectic pace is going to kill you," in favor of a positive framing of the health benefits of stress management is more likely to have a positive influence (see Chapter 5). For example, the clinician can express optimism about the patient's ability to influence health as follows: "Fortunately there are many avenues available for examining and changing your habits of thought and ways of responding to life challenges. I'd like to give you an overview of some strategies that we can discuss now and in future appointments." Showing the patient a model such as that in Figure 36-3 can be helpful as part of this discussion.

It is also important to frame beneficial lifestyle changes as the patient's choice. Rather than using the stress model to assume more responsibility for patients' lives, the primary care provider can act as a consultant and coach, clearly giving feedback to patients about the patterns of stress revealed by the diagnostic workup and offering concrete strategies for health promotion along with likely consequences for adherence and nonadherence (see Chapters 19 and 20).

Counseling About Perception & Coping

The perception and coping variables listed in Figure 36-3 represent potential topics for primary care counseling with patients. Depending on the clinician's expertise, inclination, and time, this could be done during a portion of several primary care visits. For example, a parent who is feeling stressed because of a teenager's oppositional behavior could be invited to reflect on how much parental control is needed and coached on ways of setting realistic limits. With an accountant feeling overwhelmed about a recent promotion to senior management, the clinician could elicit the patient's recollections of previous adaptations to challenging life changes to help him become cognizant of his own resources.

Referring a parent of a child with recently diagnosed leukemia to a support group of other parents is an example of a coping strategy. Encouraging a widower to confide feelings of sadness to close friends is an example of helping a patient improve his use of social supports.

Table 36-1. Nonpharmacological interventions related to perception and coping.

1. Improve time management.
2. Improve sense of humor.
3. Pursue personal and vocational activities consistent with life values.
4. Explore the meaning and purpose of life.
5. Cultivate spiritual and transcendent activities:
   a. Prayer
   b. Communal religious observances
   c. Spiritual retreat
   d. Seasonal ritual celebrations
6. Increase emotional self-disclosure.
7. Pursue short-term psychotherapy.
8. Clarify values.
9. Cultivate social support network.
10. Increase assertiveness.
11. Reduce exposure to unnecessary stressors.
12. Monitor sensory input.
13. Help others.

Referring a teacher with a chronically explosive temper for short-term anger management therapy would potentially reduce a cardiac risk factor.

Counseling patients about time management offers a rich opportunity for clinicians to raise questions concerning the patients' values and missed opportunities for personal renewal. For example, the clinician can ask the patient to reflect on those important but nonurgent activities that can contribute to personal well-being (e.g., time spent playing with a child), but which are consistently postponed in favor of more urgent but less important tasks (e.g., keeping track of the performance of stocks). A list of potential nonpharmacological strategies related to perception and coping that can be suggested to patients is shown in Table 36-1.

Arousal Reduction Strategies

For patients showing a high degree of autonomic hyperreactivity, the clinician can provide or suggest several arousal reduction strategies that can work synergistically with perception and coping skills, as well as with pharmacological interventions. These strategies are listed in Table 36-2. Mindfulness meditation in particular is an effective method of stress reduction that not only activates the parasympathetic response but builds a mental habit of staying present to the task at hand while assuming a nonjudgmental stance toward the progression of one's thoughts and emotions (see Chapter 7). Referring patients to introductory books on mindfulness meditation, such as those listed at the end of this chapter, or encouraging them to take a meditation class, can provide them with a powerful stress management resource. One study showed that 16 weeks of transcendental meditation improved components of the metabolic syndrome (blood pressure, insulin resistance, and heart rate variability) among patients with stable coronary heart disease.

Table 36-2. Health-enhancing arousal reduction techniques.

1. Meditation
2. Self-hypnosis
3. Relaxation exercises
4. Time in nature
5. Massage
6. Abdominal breathing
7. Singing
8. Tai-chi
9. Listening to soothing music
10. Yoga

Referral for Psychotherapy

The clinician may choose to refer patients for psychotherapy or to educational groups to achieve some of the desired outcomes in the areas of perception, coping, and arousal reduction techniques. These referrals are more effectively targeted to the unique needs of patients if the clinician uses the multifactorial model in Figure 36-3. This model can also aid the primary care clinician in communicating with the psychotherapist about possible foci for treatment. Psychotherapy may be more effective than primary care counseling for altering dysfunctional belief systems (e.g., a perception of no control in one's life) or coping habits (e.g., excessive need for achievement) that amplify stress. In addition, it may offer focused training in the acquisition of arousal reduction skills such as meditation and self-hypnosis.

CONCLUSION

The relationship between stress and disease is well established, although the specific pathways are complex and multifactorial. Clinicians increasingly are asked to examine the cost-effectiveness of the time spent with their patients with a view to improving outcomes within the constraints of available financial and human resources. Attention to the function of stress in patients' illnesses creates the potential for improving treatment outcomes and preventing or delaying the onset of costly target organ disease or the exacerbation of chronic illness. Applying a multidimensional stress model that includes patients' perceptions, coping strategies, physiologic arousal mechanisms, and arousal reduction strategies offers the health care professional multiple opportunities for influencing the ecology of disease.

SUGGESTED READINGS

Allen AP, Dinan TG, Clarke G, Cryan JF. A psychology of the human brain-gut-microbiome axis. *Soc Personal Psychol Compass* 2017;11:e12309.

American Psychological Association. Stress in America: Generation Z. Stress in America™ Survey. 2018. www.stressinamerica.org.

Ballou S, Keefer L. Psychological interventions for irritable bowel syndrome and inflammatory bowel diseases. *Clin Transl Gastroenterol* 2017;8:e214.

Buric I, Farias M, Jong J, et al. What is the molecular signature of mind–body interventions? A systematic review of gene expression changes induced by meditation and related practices. *Front Immunol* 2017;8:670.

Christensen JF. The assessment of stress: environmental, intrapersonal, and outcome issues. In: McReynolds P, ed. *Advances in Psychological Assessment*. Vol. 5. San Francisco, NC: Jossey-Bass; 1981.

Cohen S, Janicki-Deverts D, Doyle WJ, et al. Chronic stress, glucocorticoid receptor resistance, inflammation, and disease risk. *PNAS* 2012;109:5995–5999.

Creswell JD. Mindfulness interventions. *Annu Rev Psychol* 2017; 68:491–516.

Foster JA, Rinaman L, Cryan JF. Stress and the gut-brain axis: regulation by the microbiome. *Neurobiol Stress* 2017;7:124–136.

Friedman HS, Kern ML. Personality, health, and well-being. *Annu Rev Psychol* 2014. 65:719–742.

Jim HSL, Pustejovsky JE, Park CL, et al. Religion, spirituality, and physical health in cancer patients: a meta-analysis. *Cancer* 2015;121:3760–3768.

Kiecolt-Glaser JK. Marriage, divorce, and the immune system. *Am Psychol* 2018;73:1098–1108.

Kiecolt-Glaser JK. Stress, food, and inflammation: psychoneuroimmunology and nutrition at the cutting edge. *Psychosom Med* 2010;72:365–369.

Kyutoku Y, Tada R, Umeyama T, et al. Cognitive and psychological reactions of the general population three months after the 2011 Tohoku earthquake and tsunami. *PLoS One* 2012;7:e31014.

Nishiyama K, Johnson JV. Karoshi—death from overwork. *Int J Health Services* 1997;27:625–641.

Robles TF, Slatcher RB, Trombello JM, McGinn MM. Marital quality and health: a meta-analytic review. *Psychol Bull* 2014;140:1–80.

Schuster MA, et al. A national survey of stress reactions after the September 11, 2001, terrorist attacks. *N Engl J Med* 2001; 345:1507.

Spickard A, Gabbe SG, Christensen JF. Mid-career burnout in generalist and specialist physicians. *JAMA* 2002;288:1447–1450.

Steptoe A, Kivimaki M. Stress and cardiovascular disease. *Nat Rev Cardiol* 2012;9:360–370.

Thomee S, Harenstam A, Hagberg M. Mobile phone use and stress, sleep disturbances, and symptoms of depression among young adults—a prospective cohort study. *BMC Public Health* 2011;11:1–11.

SUGGESTED READINGS FOR PATIENTS

De Mello A. *The Way to Love: The Last Meditations of Anthony de Mello*. New York, NY: Doubleday; 1991.

Kabat-Zinn J. *Full Catastrophe Living: How to Cope With Stress, Pain and Illness Using Mindfulness Meditation*.15th anniversary ed. London, UK: Piatkus Books; 2004.

Kabat-Zinn J. *Wherever You Go There You Are: Mindfulness Meditation in Everyday Life*. New York, NY: Hyperion; 1994.

Thich Nhat Hanh. *The Miracle of Mindfulness: A Manual on Meditation*. Boston, MA: Beacon Press; 1987.

Thich Nhat Hanh. *Peace Is Every Step: The Path of Mindfulness in Everyday Life*. New York, NY: Bantam; 1991.

WEBSITES

Center for Mindfulness in Medicine, Health Care, and Society. http://www.umassmed.edu/cfm/. Accessed April 2019.

PsychoNeuroImmunology Research Society. http://www.pnirs.org/. Accessed April 2019.

Appendix 36-A. Life stress inventory.

In the blanks below, list the major events, changes, or stressors that have happened to you within the last year. Also, list those events that you expected but that failed to occur. In the next column, place a check next to those stressors that are current, ongoing problems. In the last column opposite each stressor, indicate the degree to which this event has been under your control by writing a number corresponding to the scale at the top.

Life Event or Stressor	Current Problem	Within Your Control	Outside Your Control
		1 2 3 4 5 6 7 8 9 10	
1. ________	________	________	
2. ________	________	________	
3. ________	________	________	
4. ________	________	________	
5. ________	________	________	
6. ________	________	________	
7. ________	________	________	
8. ________	________	________	
9. ________	________	________	
10. ________	________	________	

Control Score________(mean of ratings)

John F. Christensen, PhD

HIV/AIDS

37

Elizabeth Imbert, MD, MPH & Mitchell D. Feldman, MD, MPhil, FACP

INTRODUCTION

Primary care for individuals at risk for human immunodeficiency virus (HIV) and people living with HIV (PLWH) requires an understanding of the epidemiology of HIV, risk factors for HIV, prevention and screening guidelines, as well as ongoing care that tends to the psychosocial needs of PLWH. This chapter reviews how to provide preventative care for those at risk for HIV as well as guidance on disclosure, adherence and retention, and neuropsychiatric manifestations of PLWH, including chronic pain, mental illness, substance use, and HIV-associated neurocognitive disorders.

EPIDEMIOLOGY

Approximately 36.9 million people are living with HIV worldwide. Most (75%) people living with HIV know their HIV status, and of these, the majority are accessing treatment and are virally suppressed. More than 1.1 million in the United States are living with HIV. Of those, about 15% are unaware of their HIV status. Young people are the most likely to be unaware of their HIV status with an estimated half of those aged 13–24 years not aware of their HIV status. Among all people living with HIV (including diagnosed and undiagnosed HIV infections), about one-half are in care and about one-half are virally suppressed. In the United States, there are approximately 40,000 new infections annually with about two-thirds occurring in gay and bisexual men; heterosexual contact accounts for about one-quarter. African Americans and Latinos are disproportionately affected by HIV. For example, while African Americans represent about 13% of the US population, they account for almost one-half of the new HIV diagnoses, and while Latinos represent 18% of the population, they account for 26% of new HIV diagnoses. Close to 300,000 women are living with HIV in the United States today. Women of color are particularly affected, and black women account for the majority of new HIV diagnoses among women.

ACQUISITION

In the United States, HIV is most commonly transmitted through anal or vaginal sex or sharing syringes and other injection equipment with someone who has HIV. Receptive anal sex is the highest-risk sexual behavior. Being the insertive partner in anal sex or having vaginal sex (insertive or receptive) is less risky, though either partner can get HIV. HIV is also acquired through sharing needles or syringes, rinse water, or other equipment used to prepare drugs for injection. Less commonly, HIV may be spread from mother to child during pregnancy, birth or breast-feeding, or via a contaminated needle or sharp object.

PREVENTION

There are several prevention strategies for HIV. *Treatment as prevention* refers to the concept that taking antiretroviral therapy (ART) and getting and keeping an undetectable viral load helps prevent transmission to others through sex or syringe sharing and from mother to child during pregnancy, birth, and breast-feeding. People with HIV who take ART as prescribed and are virologically suppressed have effectively no risk of transmitting HIV to their HIV-negative sexual partners and is the foundation of the public health campaign U=U or undetectable (i.e., undetectable HIV viral load) equals un-transmittable. We don't have enough data to know if being undetectable prevents HIV transmission among persons who inject drugs, but it is likely reduced. In addition, postexposure prophylaxis (PEP) with an antiretroviral-based regimen is an effective strategy to reduce the risk of infection for those who have a high-risk exposure to HIV within 72 hours. For individuals who are at ongoing high risk for HIV infection, preexposure prophylaxis (PrEP) is an effective strategy to reduce HIV infection (see section on PrEP). Condoms, if used consistently, decrease the risk of sexual HIV transmission and acquisition. For persons who inject drugs, opioid substitution, buprenorphine-naltrexone, and needle exchange programs are useful strategies to decrease risky behavior and, likely, HIV acquisition. Male circumcision reduces risk of HIV infection among heterosexual men; however, it has not been demonstrated to have a substantial benefit among men who have sex with men (MSM).

SCREENING

According to Centers for Disease Control and Prevention (CDC) guidelines, screening for HIV infection should be performed routinely in all health care settings for all patients aged 13–64 years. Patient should be retested at least annually if at high risk: persons who use injection drugs and their sex partners, persons who exchange sex for money or drugs, sex partners of HIV-infected persons, and MSM or heterosexual persons who themselves or whose sex partners have had more than one sex partner since their most recent HIV test. HIV testing should be offered to those with symptoms consistent with acute or chronic HIV as well those with possible exposure to HIV. Clinicians should maintain a high level of suspicion for acute HIV infection in all patients who have a compatible clinical syndrome and report recent high-risk behavior. In addition, HIV testing is recommended for those seeking evaluation or treatment of a particular sexually transmitted infection (STI), those starting TB treatment and those considering starting PrEP. In addition, all pregnant women should be tested for HIV including those who present in labor who are untested and whose HIV status is unknown.

TESTING

Patient should be informed verbally or in writing that an HIV test will be performed unless they decline ("opt-out screening"). In addition, they should be given an explanation of HIV infection and the meaning of positive and negative test results and an opportunity to ask questions.

A fourth-generation antigen/antibody combination HIV-1/2 immunoassay plus a confirmatory HIV-1/HIV-2 antibody differentiation immunoassay is recommended for HIV testing. Most rapid tests are antibody only tests and provide results in less than 20 minutes. They can be performed in the laboratory, in community based settings, or at home using whole blood or oral secretions. The accuracy of rapid tests for chronic infection is high; however, rapid antibody tests may miss about 10–15% of acute HIV infections and up to 8% of HIV-infected people can have a false-negative result when oral home tests are used. If a rapid test is positive, this is only a preliminary result and should be followed by a laboratory-based antigen/antibody test, and if positive, a confirmatory antibody differentiation immunoassay. When acute retroviral syndrome is suspected, a plasma RNA test should be used in conjunction with fourth-generation antigen/antibody combination HIV-1/2 immunoassay plus a confirmatory HIV-1/HIV 2 antibody differentiation immunoassay to diagnose acute HIV infection.

UNDERSTANDING RISK FACTORS FOR HIV

Sexual History

When seeing patients who are HIV positive as well as those who may be candidates for PrEP, it is of utmost importance to understand their sexual history and risk factors. When taking a sexual history, acknowledge that these questions are personal, reassure patients that you ask these questions to all your patients, and discuss the importance to their overall health. One author suggests that taking a sexual history should be like "peeling an onion." Starting at the outermost layer, the provider should progress through each layer of questioning with a nonjudgmental individualized approach. Negative responses may suggest that the provider should stop and not progress to the next layer. Know your patient's gender identity and their preferred pronouns. Ask all patients about their sexual identity (if they identify as gay, bisexual, lesbian, queer or straight), sexual attraction (who they are attracted to), and sexual behavior (who they have sex with). Remember the axes of sexual identity, sexual attraction, and sexual behavior are distinct. Ask about number of people they have had sex with and when was the last time they had sex. Then explore more specifics about their sexual behavior, for example gender of their partners, kinds of sex (genital, anal, oral, etc.), sex with drugs or alcohol, and exchanging sex for money or goods. Inquire about how they keep themselves safe (condoms, PrEP, etc.). Inquire about prior STIs and symptoms. Inquire about pregnancy, if they desire pregnancy and if not, how they are going to protect from pregnancy. Inquire about satisfaction with sex life. Ask about safety in relationships. Inquire about concerns regarding sexual health. (See Chapter 33.)

ALCOHOL & DRUG USE

It is also important to ask nonjudgmentally about alcohol and drug use. You should ask permission to discuss alcohol and drugs. Perform screening for alcohol and drug use and, if they screen positive, assess the quantity and pattern of use and assess for substance use disorder and other consequences. Adopting a harm reduction approach that promotes methods of reducing physical, social, emotional, and economic harms associated with drug and alcohol use and other harmful behaviors is key. (See Chapters 24 and 25 for further guidance.)

Preexposure Prophylaxis

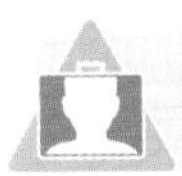

CASE ILLUSTRATION 1

Tom, a 28-year-old cis-gender man presents to his primary care doctor for an annual evaluation. On sexual history, the patient reports he identifies as gay, is attracted to men, and has had anal insertive and receptive sex with several male partners without using condoms. He often has sex when using methamphetamine, which he smokes and uses IV. He has had gonorrhea and chlamydia in the past but denies any symptoms today.

Daily oral PrEP with the fixed-dose combination of tenofovir disoproxil fumarate (TDF) 300 mg and emtricitabine (FTC) 200 mg has been shown to be safe and efficacious in reducing the risk of HIV acquisition (Figure 37-1). While PrEP uptake has been increasing since it was approved by the Food and Drug Administration (FDA) in 2012, we are still far off from the estimated 1.1 million individuals in the United States that could benefit from PrEP. Moreover, pharmacy data suggest that despite the fact that 44% of African Americans and 25% of Latinos would benefit from PrEP, only 1% and 3% of were prescribed PrEP, respectively (Figure 37-2).

PrEP should be offered to sexually active adult MSM, adult men who have sex with women, adult women who have sex with men, and adult persons who inject drugs who are at substantially high risk of HIV acquisition. The CDC Web site lists a number of factors to consider assessing risk of acquiring HIV: sex or injecting partner with HIV; recent bacterial STI, high number of sex partners, history of inconsistent condom use, commercial sex work, or sharing injection equipment. PrEP has also been studied for sex-driven use, where patients take two pills 2–24 hours before first sex act and then one pill 24 hours after and then 48 hours after sex act. Even though high efficacy rates have been demonstrated for both daily and on-demand PrEP among MSM, the FDA at this time has not approved oral PrEP for coitally timed or other noncontinuous daily use.

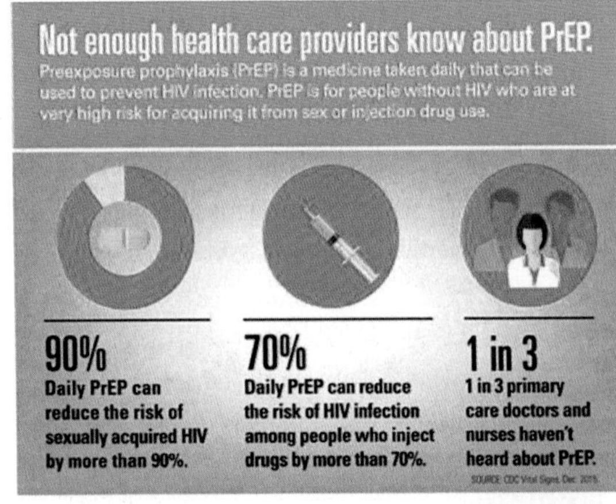

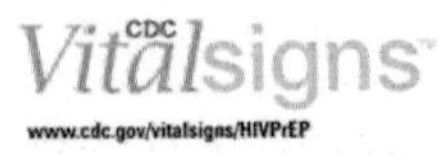

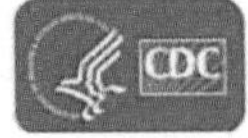

Figure 37-1. PrEP facts.

Prior to starting PrEP, conduct a thorough medical history to determine if the patient has any relative or absolute medical contraindications to PrEP, including history or current kidney or liver disease; current or chronic hepatitis B; and osteoporosis or other bone disease or symptoms of acute HIV infection. Order the following laboratory tests: HIV Ag/Ab test within 7 days *and* HIV viral load testing within 7 days if possible; serum creatinine; hepatitis B testing; hepatitis A and C testing if not previously documented; STI testing; and pregnancy testing for women of reproductive age if appropriate. Provide patients with the basic information on PrEP, including possible adverse effects, patient-centered risk reduction counseling, and condoms and medication adherence counseling. Prescribe less than or equal to a 90-day supply.

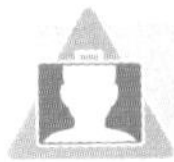

CASE ILLUSTRATION 1 (CONTD.)

You prescribe Tom a 3-month supply of PrEP, and he comes for his follow-up appointment. He reports that he takes PrEP most days but is still not using condoms during receptive and insertive anal sex and is using meth occasionally.

Patients on PrEP should be seen for follow-up at least every 3 months to provide HIV testing, medication adherence counseling, behavior risk reduction support, side-effect assessment, and STI symptom assessment. Upon initiating PrEP, providers may choose to see patients for a 1-month follow-up (in-person or via phone) to assess for acute HIV and STI symptoms, side effects, and adherence, and order HIV testing. HIV testing and assessing for signs or symptoms of acute HIV should be done every 3 months. Bacterial STIs should be tested every 3 months for asymptomatic MSM and at least every 6 months for other sexually active adults. Renal function should be checked at least every 6 months. Hepatitis C should be checked annually for persons who inject drugs and those with ongoing risk of hepatitis C exposure. For women of reproductive age, order a pregnancy test every 3 months if appropriate. You should also assess for clean needles and drug treatment services.

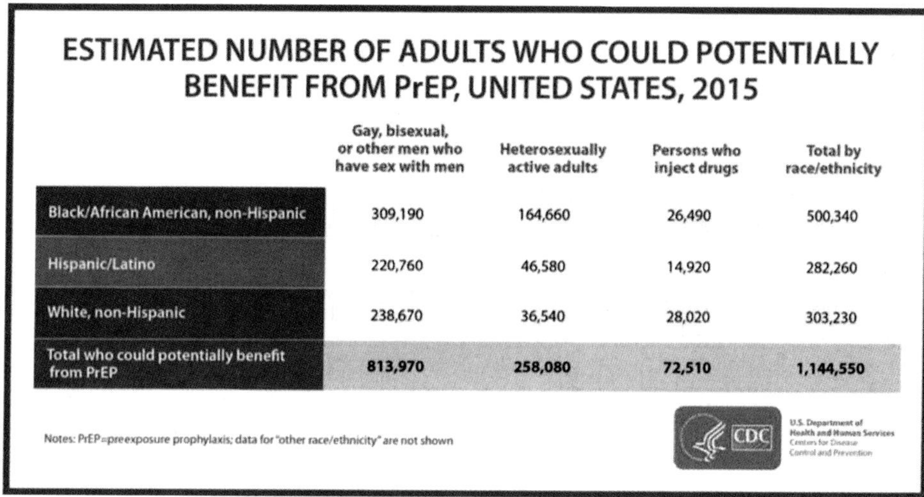

ESTIMATED NUMBER OF ADULTS WHO COULD POTENTIALLY BENEFIT FROM PrEP, UNITED STATES, 2015

	Gay, bisexual, or other men who have sex with men	Heterosexually active adults	Persons who inject drugs	Total by race/ethnicity
Black/African American, non-Hispanic	309,190	164,660	26,490	500,340
Hispanic/Latino	220,760	46,580	14,920	282,260
White, non-Hispanic	238,670	36,540	28,020	303,230
Total who could potentially benefit from PrEP	**813,970**	**258,080**	**72,510**	**1,144,550**

Notes: PrEP=preexposure prophylaxis; data for "other race/ethnicity" are not shown

CDC
U.S. Department of Health and Human Services
Centers for Disease Control and Prevention

Figure 37-2. Who Could Benefit from PrEP?

The CDC suggests several strategies for the clinical management of persons prescribed PrEP. (1) Interactive, patient-centered counseling where the conversation is tailored to a patient's sexual risk behaviors and the situations in which risks occur in combination with goal setting strategies for HIV prevention. (2) Elicit barriers to and facilitators to consistent condom use as well as barriers to and facilitators of reducing substance use. Help patient identify one or two feasible acceptable incremental steps toward risk reduction and identify and address barriers to accomplish next steps. You may say, "It is great that you are taking PrEP to reduce your risk of getting HIV. What else are you doing to keep yourself safe? What might you do differently?" (3) Acknowledge the effort required for behavioral change, reinforce success, and if not fully successful, identify factors interfering with accomplishing action plans and help identify next steps. (4) Provide access to drug treatment and relapse prevention services (i.e., methadone or buprenorphine-naltrexone for people who use opiates). (5) If the patient is not motivated to engage in drug treatment, provide access to unused injection equipment through needle exchange programs or prescription where legal. (6) Referral for cognitive or behavioral counseling and indicated mental health or social services may help reduce risky injection practices.

Psychosocial Impact of HIV/AIDS

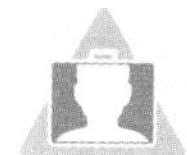

CASE ILLUSTRATION 2

Nick, a 23-year-old cis-gender man presents to urgent care after falling off a ladder and sustaining a calcaneal fracture. He identifies as bisexual and has condomless anal receptive and insertive sex with men and insertive vaginal sex with women. He had a negative HIV test 1 year ago. He does not recall flu-like symptoms, fever, rash, sore throat, or chills in the past year. Last sexual encounter was 1 week ago. You order an HIV Ag/Ab test that comes back positive, and the confirmatory test is pending. You ask the patient to return to clinic today to discuss this further. His HIV Ab confirmatory test later returns positive for HIV-1 Ab.

Counseling Patients Who Test Positive

If your clinical setting uses HIV Ag/Ab testing, this will come back prior to the HIV confirmatory Ab test result. When this occurs, share with patients based on their risk factors how concerned you are that they have HIV and that you are awaiting the confirmatory test. See Tables 37-1 and 37-2 for further guidance on discussing a new HIV diagnosis. (See Chapter 3.)

Table 37-1. Sharing an HIV diagnosis: starting the conversation.

Step 1	Share that you have the results of their lab work and their HIV test came back positive meaning that they have HIV.
Step 2	Allow a moment for patient to have their reaction to this (anger, surprise, sadness).
Step 3	Acknowledge their reaction.
Step 4	Ask permission to share more information (see Table 37-2)

Table 37-2. Sharing an HIV diagnosis: having the conversation.

Ask patients what they know about HIV and provide brief factual information. Tailor the information you share to the patient's medical literacy, knowledge, and readiness to hear this information.
Ask what they have heard about HIV meds. Discuss starting antiretroviral therapy, ideally even beginning today, and share that if they take their medications, their virus will be undetectable so they will not be able to transmit it.
Acknowledge that while this diagnosis changes things for them, that HIV is treatable with daily medications, and that many people lead long, fulfilling lives with HIV.
Suggest that they notify partners so they can get tested. If they don't want to or don't know their partners, the public health department can help with contact tracing without disclosing their identity.
Address practical needs of the patient. Ask if they need to help to take a medication every day. Ask about housing needs, financial help, and food resources.
Make it clear that you and your team are here to support them.
Most importantly, lay the groundwork through rapport building to ensure that they come for follow-up.

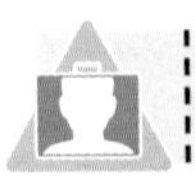

CASE ILLUSTRATION 2 (CONTD.)

Nick returns to clinic, and you inform him that his HIV test is positive, meaning he has HIV. You tell him that he can live a long life, and you can start him on medication today to treat his HIV. He reports that he is in between work and doesn't have a stable housing *situation. You let him know that you can help look into housing options and perform a warm handoff to your social worker in clinic to assist with this. In choosing ART, he states that he wants as few pills as possible because he is not good at remembering to take medications.*

Starting Antiretroviral Therapy

ART is recommended for all HIV-positive patients regardless of immune status. A collaborative approach in which the patient is closely involved in selecting an ART is recommended. Before choosing a regimen, providers should assess what HIV antiretroviral drugs (ARVs) are expected to be fully active against the patient's virus, have a good safety profile, and be convenient for the patient. Then, elicit the patient's preferences, ideas, concerns, and expectations about medications, and evaluate for barriers to adherence. Discuss pill size, pill number, dosing frequency, and possible side effects. Lower pill burden and once-daily regimens are associated with improved adherence. Encourage patients to let you know if they experience side effects or are otherwise struggling with adherence.

Adherence

It is important to categorize the nature of nonadherence (How often are they missing their medications? And for how long?) as well as nonjudgmentally explore what is the underlying cause. There are many strategies for addressing nonadherence. Simplify therapy to combination, single-pill formulations whenever possible. Ask pharmacies (ideally HIV-specialized pharmacies) to package medications in bubble packs, medi-sets, or wellness packs to reduce dosing errors, a strategy that has been associated with improved and persistent adherence. Link medication taking to existing routines using cues or reminder aids. At each visit, ask patients whether they are having side effects or otherwise struggling to take their ARVs consistently. Use nonjudgmental questions like, "Sometimes patients take medication differently than prescribed. Do you ever have to skip or forgo your HIV medication?" If a patient is nonadherent, consider switching to one of the alternative optimal regimens (this should be done in consultation with an HIV expert as it is important to take into account patient's prior regimens, prior resistance testing, viral loads, CD4 response, and patterns of adherence). If the barrier to nonadherence is mental illness, substance abuse, or homelessness, refer patients to a social worker to address these barriers and link them to additional resources. If their housing situation is unstable or there are other issues that make it hard for patients to pick up medications every month, or to keep them in their possession, dispense medications weekly from the clinic, if possible. (See Chapter 20 for more details.)

Improving Engagement & Retention in Care

Retention in care is associated with improved viral suppression, especially among those with low CD4 counts, improved survival rates, and greater increases in CD4 counts. Patients often cycle in and out of care. Common barriers reported by those not retained in care include competing priorities like child care and work, transportation difficulty, stigma, and insurance issues. Poor retention in care is associated with stigma, younger age, female gender, African American race, stimulant and alcohol use, heterosexual orientation, and low level of social support. Structural and clinic factors associated with poor retention in care include homelessness and a poor patient–provider relationship.

A strong patient–provider relationship defined by trust and collaboration has been demonstrated to promote engagement in care as does a care model in which social and financial barriers are addressed and mental health and substance abuse services are integrated.

Multiple interventions have demonstrated some success in mitigating barriers to care, including text messaging, peer navigation, and provider training to reduce stigma. It is important to revisit retention strategies with patients on a regular basis to address their changing perspectives on HIV and the role providers can play in helping patients continue to be engaged in care. Engagement in care is a lifelong process that requires the provider and team to respond to a patient's needs overtime.

SPECIAL ISSUES & POPULATIONS

Hepatitis B & C

For patients with chronic hepatitis B infection, you should choose 2 nucleoside reverse transcriptase inhibitors (NRTIs) active against hepatitis B. All individuals with hepatitis C should be offered curative treatment in consultation with an expert in treating HIV-positive patients with hepatitis C. For patients already on ART, a regimen switch may be indicated if components of the ART regimen cannot be used with the planned HCV antiviral agents.

Chronic Pain

Chronic pain is common among PLWH and is associated with significant morbidity. Approximately half of chronic pain in PLWH is neuropathic due to nervous system damage from HIV, infection with other pathogens, medication side effects, or other causes other than HIV-related conditions. Historically, pain has been undertreated in PLWH, particularly among those with low socioeconomic status, women, and persons who inject drugs.

PLWH should be screened for chronic pain by inquiring how much pain they have had in the last week and if the pain has lasted for more than 3 months. If patients screen positive, use a biopsychosocial approach to evaluate pain onset, duration, intensity, character, exacerbating and alleviating factors, past and current treatments, underlying or co-occurring disorders, and effect of pain on physical and psychological function. Conduct a physical examination, psychosocial evaluation, and a diagnostic workup to determine potential causes. (See Chapter 38.)

Early initiation of ART is recommended for prevention and treatment of HIV-associated distal symmetric polyneuropathy. For chronic neuropathic pain in PLWH, gabapentin is recommended as first-line therapy. If there is an inadequate response to gabapentin, consider a trial of selective noradrenaline reuptake inhibitors (SNRIs), tricyclic antidepressants (TCAs), or pregabalin. Capsaicin is recommended as a topical treatment for chronic HIV-associated peripheral neuropathic pain. Medical cannabis may be an effective treatment in certain patients. Alpha lipoic acid can also be used for chronic HIV-associated peripheral neuropathic pain. Opioid analgesics should not be prescribed as first line for long-term management of chronic neuropathic pain; providers may consider a time-limited trial for patients who do not respond to first line therapies. Acetaminophen and nonsteroidal anti-inflammatory drugs (NSAIDs) are recommended first line for the treatment of musculoskeletal pain.

Fatigue

Fatigue is a decreased capacity to initiate or maintain physical activity. Fatigue is common among PLWH and is often due to both physiologic and psychosocial factors. Providers should assess the severity and impact, search for underlying medical or psychiatric causes, review medications, review sleep patterns, and treat the underlying cause when present. For hypogonadal men, testosterone may help, but it should be weighed with risks of testosterone treatment. If the patient is able to tolerate it, moderate exercise is reasonable. A trial of a psychostimulant may be considered; however, this should be undertaken with caution and with consideration of underlying psychiatric illness, substance use disorders, and medical conditions.

Stigma

Stigma is a common, pervasive barrier to prevention and treatment for PLWH. Enacted stigma is the experience of prejudice or discrimination based on HIV status, and internalized stigma is internal endorsement of the external process of stigma. Stigma can manifest in several ways. First, stigma can take the form of discrimination against those living with or at risk of HIV preventing individuals from accessing services and leading to psychological and physical trauma. Second, it may take the form of anticipation of discrimination, which can lead to fear or testing, hesitancy to adopt prevention strategies, and unwillingness to seek care. Third, it may manifest as low self-worth, making it harder for a person to take action to prevent or treat HIV. Prior research has documented stigmatized beliefs and attitudes by health care providers and discriminatory practices including breaks in confidentiality, increased physical distance, and testing without consent. Perceived stigmatization in medical settings can lead to psychological distress, decreased patient satisfaction, low motivation to stay healthy, low self-esteem, and the feeling that one is undeserving of the care. However, positive interactions between health care providers and PLWH lead to improved adherence and health care–related quality of life. Providers and staff should be welcoming to patients in their clinic. They should assure patients of confidentiality, ask questions nonjudgmentally, and provide empathetic patient-centered care.

Women

Compared to men, women living with HIV report higher levels of negative self-image related to HIV status and higher fear or anticipation of HIV-related discrimination. One study found that depressive symptoms have been shown to mediate the relationship between internalized stigma and poor adherence to ART among women. Another study reported that women with chronic depressive symptoms were twice as likely to die as those with mild or no depressive symptoms, after controlling for clinical features and treatment. Providers need to recognize and provide appropriate and individualized intervention to improve emotional wellbeing and overall outcomes in women living with HIV.

NEUROPSYCHIATRIC COMPLICATIONS

There is a high prevalence of neuropsychiatric disorders among PLWH. The etiology of these conditions is complex and due in part to direct effects of the HIV virus, preexisting psychiatric and affective disorders, addiction, and responses to marginalization that can be associated with HIV diagnosis. The most prevalent psychiatric disorder is depression, followed by substance use disorder, anxiety, psychosis, adjustment disorder, and bipolar affective disorder. Neurocognitive impairment is also common. Recognition and effective treatment are necessary to maximize quality of life, HIV treatment, and life expectancy.

Table 37-3. CNS toxicity of ARVs.

ARV class	Neuropsychiatric effects
NNRTIs	Neuropsychiatric events: Efavirenz (EFV) > Rilpivirine (RPV) > Doravirine (DOR) > Etravirine (ETR) EFV: Somnolence, insomnia, abnormal dreams, dizziness, impaired concentration, depression, psychosis, and suicidal ideation. Symptoms usually subside or decrease after 2–4 weeks. Bedtime dosing may help reduce symptoms. Risk factors include known psychiatric illness, concurrent use of agents with neuropsychiatric effects, and increased EFV concentrations because of genetic factors or increased absorption with food. RPV: Depression, suicidality, sleep disturbances DOR: Sleep disorders and disturbances, dizziness, altered sensorium; depression and suicidality/self-harm
Integrase inhibitors	Insomnia, depression, and suicidality, primarily in patients with known psychiatric illness

Data from U.S. Department of Health and Human Services: AIDS Info (located at: https://aidsinfo.nih.gov).

Depression

Depression is prevalent among PLWH, and its relationship with HIV is complex. Depression can precede HIV infection and may be associated with risk factors for HIV. It can also be triggered by an HIV diagnosis and the stress associated with managing HIV as a chronic illness. Stigma may also contribute to the development of depression. In addition, the medical sequelae of HIV are associated with depression as are some ARVs (Table 37-3). In addition, disease progression of HIV has been associated with depressive symptoms. For PLWH, depression negatively impacts ART adherence, viral suppression, quality of life, and long-term survival, and it has been associated with risk behavior for sexual HIV transmission.

Providers should identify and treat depression in PLWH as depression is often underdiagnosed, untreated, or undertreated. Depression has typical clinical features of those not living with HIV; however, impaired concentration, hopelessness, guilt, fatigue, and loss of appetite and weight are more common in PLWH. PLWH are at high suicide risk. As with most patients, selective serotonin reuptake inhibitors (SSRIs), SNRIs, bupropion, and mirtazapine are recommended as first-line agents. Providers should be aware of drug-drug interactions between antidepressants and ARVs and should check for drug-drug interactions. It is worth noting that adherence to ART is higher in depressed patients who are prescribed and are adherent to antidepressants compared to those neither prescribed nor adherent. Mindfulness-based stress reduction and mindfulness-based cognitive therapies have psychological benefits in HIV-infected patients. Cognitive behavioral therapy (CBT) is effective at improving quality of life and depression in the short term and adherence in the long term. Furthermore, integrating CBT for adherence with CBT for depression has been shown to improve adherence and depression. (See Chapter 26.)

Substance Use & Substance Use Disorders

PLWH have a high prevalence of substance use and substance use disorders. Substance use is associated with HIV progression, poor adherence, detectable viral load, HIV transmission risk behavior, low perceived quality life, depression, and low social support. It is important to utilize a harm reduction approach and use nonjudgmental language that respects the patient's dignity and avoids perpetuating stigma. Partner with patients in setting their own health goals and help them take incremental steps to reduce substance use and unsafe practices. Let patients know that relapses or periods of return to unsafe health practices are not conceptualized as "failure of treatment." (See Chapters 24 and 19.)

Anxiety

PLWH have higher anxiety levels compared to the general population. Like depression, anxiety can precede HIV infection and can also be triggered by HIV diagnosis and the stresses that emerge. Anxiety can impair concentration, making individuals less likely to adhere to their medication. For the treatment of anxiety in HIV-positive individuals, psychological interventions are generally more effective than pharmacological interventions. (See Chapter 27.)

PTSD

Posttraumatic stress disorder (PTSD) is more prevalent among HIV-positive individuals than in the general population. PTSD exacerbates HIV risk behaviors and worsens health outcomes. HIV risk behaviors may increase exposure to trauma associated with increased likelihood of developing PTSD, and likewise, PTSD from prior trauma predisposes individuals to engage in behaviors that may place individuals at risk for HIV.

Schizophrenia

HIV leads to greater morbidity and mortality in patients with schizophrenia because they are more likely to have trouble explaining symptoms to providers, less likely to receive attention from providers for medical complaints, and more likely to have difficulty adhering to treatment plans. Reports suggest that new-onset psychosis in PLWH generally responds well to antipsychotics; however, PLWH are more susceptible to antipsychotic side effects like tardive dyskinesia and extrapyramidal symptoms. Schizophrenia in PLWH is managed similarly to schizophrenia in other patients.

CNS Toxicity of ARVs

Some ARVs are associated with neuropsychiatric symptoms and other CNS manifestations, and an individual's prior psychiatric illness should be considered when choosing an ARV.

HIV-Associated Neurocognitive Disorder

HIV-associated neurocognitive disorder (HAND) encompasses a spectrum of cognitive impairments that are not explained by another cause and range from asymptomatic impairment to severe impairment that interferes with daily functioning. Risk factors include low CD4, age, and other comorbidities. Early indicators of HAND include impairments in psychomotor function, attention and concentration, and mental agility and flexibility. Language, by contrast, is often preserved. HAND also leads to personality changes, like apathy and irritability, and changes in behavior, like social withdrawal and impaired activities of daily living. Neurologic manifestations include tremor, loss of balance, and poor coordination. ART is the mainstay of treatment of HAND. Management of HAND should be done in conjunction with HIV expert consultation.

CONCLUSION

In order to provide outstanding care for those at risk of HIV and patients living with HIV/AIDS, it is important to understand who is at risk, when to screen and how, how to prevent HIV as well as how to care for a patient who is living with HIV positive including psychosocial and psychiatric comorbidities.

SUGGESTED READINGS

Bruce RD, Merlin J, Lum PJ, et al. 2017 HIVMA of IDSA clinical practice guideline for the management of chronic pain in patients living with HIV. *Clin Infect Dis* 2017;65(10):e1–e37.

Centers for Disease Control and Prevention: US Public Health Service: Preexposure Prophylaxis for the Prevention of HIV Infection in the United States—2017 Update: A Clinical Practice Guideline. https://www.cdc.gov/hiv/pdf/risk/prep/cdc-hiv-prep-guidelines-2017.pdf. Published March 2018.

Imbert E. Antiretroviral Medication Adherence and Retention in Care. http://HIVinsite.UCSF.edu\InSite?page=md-ward86-adherence-retention. November 9, 2017.

Knights M. HIV Infection and its psychiatric manifestation: a clinical overview. *BJPsych Advances* 2017;23:265–277.

Panel on Antiretroviral Guidelines for Adults and Adolescents. Guidelines for the Use of Antiretroviral Agents in Adults and Adolescents Living With HIV. Department of Health and Human Services. http://www.aidsinfo.nih.gov/ContentFiles/AdultandAdolescentGL.pdf.

WEBSITES

http://www.unaids.org/en

https://www.cdc.gov/hiv/

https://www.hiv-druginteractions.org

PATIENT BIBLIOGRAPHY

cdc.gov/hiv/. Accessed August 23, 2019.

HIV.gov. Accessed August 23, 2019.

Pain

38

Michael W. Rabow, MD; Gregory T. Smith, PhD; Ann C. Shah, MD; & Steven Z. Pantilat, MD

INTRODUCTION

Most pain is acute and short lived. Acute pain is primarily a symptom of a pathological process or injury. Typically treating the illness or injury will reduce or eliminate acute pain symptoms. Analgesic medications are often used in this setting for comfort during the healing process. For the most part, treatment of the underlying pathology or injury and medication management are effective in the treatment of acute pain. Many resources exist for assisting clinicians with acute pain management strategies.

Despite even the best efforts, *acute pain* evolves into *chronic pain* in approximately one out of five patients. The management of chronic pain is complex and often involves both pharmacological and nonpharmacological interventions. Because chronic pain is also modulated by psychological status (e.g., depression and anxiety), environmental consequences (e.g., stressors or reinforcers), and prior conditioning history, a comprehensive, multidisciplinary approach to management of this condition is of critical importance.

Management of patients with chronic pain is often challenging and can lead to complex patient–physician relationships. Often these relationships engender strong reactions from primary care providers. This chapter focuses on helpful strategies for the management of chronic pain and approaches for facing the particular challenges of caring for patients with chronic pain.

CHRONIC PAIN PREVALENCE/ BACKGROUND DATA

The International Association for the Study of Pain (IASP) defines pain as an "unpleasant sensory and emotional experience associated with actual or potential tissue damage." The transition from acute to chronic pain is defined by duration. Acute pain may last up to 3 months at most, whereas chronic pain is any pain that lasts more than 3 months. Although pain from untreatable malignancies often lasts many months and is progressive, the terminal nature of the underlying condition leads most to consider *cancer-related pain* separately from *chronic noncancer pain*. Roughly 20% of the patients with acute pain will eventually seek treatment each year for chronic noncancer pain. Of these, 62% will report having pain for longer than 1 year; 57% report that their pain is episodic (e.g., migraine and neuropathy), whereas 43% will report having constant pain.

Chronic noncancer pain accounts for more than 70 million office visits per year in the United States, with annual direct medical costs of $125 billion and more in lost productivity at work. The cost of treating low back pain alone averages almost $86 billion annually. Although the diagnosis of low back pain represents only 5–10% of all disability claims, these claims account for 80–85% of the costs of disability. The cost of pain in the United States is greater than the combined cost of cancer and diabetes.

CLINICIAN–PATIENT RELATIONSHIP/ GOALS OF THERAPY

Taking care of patients with chronic noncancer pain can be problematic for the primary care provider. Even the most experienced practitioners occasionally find the clinical relationship with a patient with chronic pain to be challenging and frustrating. Some patients with chronic pain are engaged in living active lives with modest and stable doses of medication. Others are inactive and passive, seeking to rely only on escalating doses of medication, and often put their lives on hold as a result of pain. Primary care providers can find themselves in an oppositional relationship with the latter group of patients, which can lead to feelings of inadequacy, frustration, and anger for both the clinician and the patient.

Chronic pain typically has no cure and is poorly managed by medications alone. Although the etiology of chronic pain varies with each patient, there are usually comorbid psychological, social, and functional variables that contribute to the difficulty of managing patients with chronic pain. These comorbid conditions often need clinical attention as well. Treatment strategies limited to pharmacological interventions usually fail.

The effectiveness of the clinician–patient relationship is defined largely by the clinician's ability to acknowledge the patient's problem, address the patient's goals, and establish a collaborative management strategy on which both the physician and the patient can agree. Because the primary concerns of the clinician and the patient can be different, there is marked potential for miscommunication. An important first step for clinicians is to seek *patients' expectations of treatment* before sharing their own approach and philosophy of chronic pain treatment. Establishing a clear clinician–patient relationship is central to successful management of chronic noncancer pain.

Patients dealing with chronic pain present for medical attention with a number of possible feelings and goals:

1. They may simply want to discover the cause of the pain to allay fears about an underlying serious disease.
2. They may be interested only in relief from the pain.
3. They may want to regain impaired function to return to normal work, social, or recreational activities.
4. They may want medical and social acknowledgment that the pain is preventing normal activities.

The "three-function model of the medical interview" (Table 38-1) can be utilized as a format for the ongoing evaluation and reevaluation of patients with chronic pain (see Chapter 1).

Pain management is based on a number of basic guidelines.

1. Obtain a description of the pain and the meaning or impact the pain has on the patient's life and the life of others around the patient.
2. Assess for comorbid psychiatric conditions such as depression and anxiety.

Table 38-1. The three-function model of the medical interview.

1. *Data gathering*: Elucidate the physical and psychological etiology of pain. Arrive at a tentative working diagnosis even while considering alternative hypotheses.
2. *Relationship building*: Using empathy skills and active listening, determine the meaning the pain has in the patient's life, including the role of "pain behaviors" and pain dysfunction, both physical and social.
3. *Management*: Explain the role of pain medications, including the duration of their use, the importance of time contingency, and an expectation of the degree of relief.
    a. Plan the use of physical and other therapies designed to improve function.
    b. Acknowledge the roles and limitations of rest periods.
    c. Establish the value of return to normal work and recreational activity to overcome pain behavior and dysfunction

3. Perform a focused physical examination based on pain history.
4. Review or obtain diagnostic studies that might rule in treatable physical pathology.
5. Use communication and empathy skills to discuss pain treatment.
    a. Explain rationale for avoiding opioid analgesics for chronic noncancer pain.
    b. Provide nonpharmacological alternatives in context of Prochaska's "stages of change" model.
    c. Negotiate goals of treatment as restoring function and quality of life versus only eliminating nociception.
6. Provide relief and comfort through medication and reassurance.
7. Use multiple management modalities.
8. Assess for change in pain behavior and overall function.
9. Reinforce improvement in function and reduced pain (the goals of treatment) and discontinue ineffective treatments that do not achieve these goals.

In general, all interventions to manage chronic noncancer pain must be assessed repeatedly to determine the *balance between the benefits and harms of the treatment.* Patients and physicians should partner is making these assessments over time, with the focus on improved functioning as the primary goal.

BEHAVIORAL MEDICINE THERAPIES

Cognitive behavioral therapy (CBT) has been proven as a primary evidence-based approach in the treatment of chronic pain in multiple randomized controlled studies. Cognitive behavioral therapy is a form of psychological treatment that focuses on thinking as having an important role in determining how we feel and what we do. CBT and other therapies that have been demonstrated to be effective in the treatment of chronic pain include: Biofeedback Therapy, Hypnosis, Mindfulness Therapy, Acceptance and Commitment Therapy (ACT) and relaxation therapies. Table 38-2 summarizes behavioral therapy approaches used in treatment of chronic pain.

There are also patient self-help resources to which the clinician can refer patients who are literate and motivated to take an active role in managing their pain (Table 38-3).

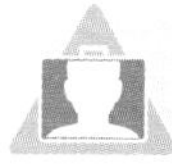

A CASE OF THE USE OF CBT

Michael is a 50-year-old concrete construction crew leader who experienced an injury on the job resulting in lumbar disc herniation with a multiple-level nerve root compromise and was treated with fusion

Table 38-2. Behavioral treatment methods for pain.

1. Cognitive behavioral therapy	This approach often involves the monitoring of automatic thoughts that are negative; recognizing the connections between thoughts, affect, and behavior; and alternatively replacing dysfunctional thoughts with more reality-oriented interpretations. Recent advances in CBT for the treatment of chronic pain have resulted in behavioral and cognitive methods to challenge dysfunctional beliefs about pain and the impact that pain has on normal functioning and replace them with more accurate reality-based beliefs.
2. Biofeedback	Computer-assisted measurement of physiologic changes previously thought to be involuntary, for the purposes of training the patient to bring them into voluntary control. Measurements often include surface electromyelography, skin temperature, galvanic skin response, respiration, heart rate, pulse time, distal plethysmography, and electroencephalogram.
3. Autogenic and relaxation training	A series of mental exercises designed to produce relaxation imagery that may be guided by a practitioner through suggestion or can be coupled with relaxation and exercise.
4. Progressive muscle relaxation	A systematic approach to relaxation with exercises involving the tensing and relaxing of muscle groups from head to foot.
5. Mindfulness	In this context, a type of CBT that emphasizes bringing nonjudgmental attention to the patient's present experience at each moment, with a focused awareness of thoughts, emotions, and sensations, including pain. In this way, the patient can develop an observing mind, to be aware of thoughts or judgments and emotional reactions to the changes in physical pain and to notice that one can respond in different ways that allows for a more complete or satisfying physical and emotional life together with acceptance of pain.
6. Hypnosis	A state of enhanced focus or awareness that can lead to increased levels of suggestibility. This can be helpful in the blocking of painful sensations (hypnoanalgesia).
7. Acceptance and Commitment Therapy	This approach combines the cognitive therapies of acceptance and mindfulness with behavioral change strategies. Central to the therapy is diffusion of thoughts from associated emotional reactions and to move toward valued behavior and learn not to over react or avoid painful situations.

including instrumentation with a quick recovery and return to work within 6 weeks. Six months later Michael experienced a reoccurrence of low back pain. Imaging studies revealed a solid fusion with no other abnormalities, and he was referred for injection therapies.

Table 38-3. Patient self-help resources.

1. Caudill M. *Managing Pain Before it Manages You*, revd ed. New York, NY: Gillford Press; 2002.
2. Catalano E, Hardin KN, eds. *The Chronic Pain Control Workbook: A Step-by-Step Guide for Coping with and Overcoming Pain*, 2nd ed. Oakland, CA: New Harbinger Publ.; 1999.
3. Butler DS, Moseley GL. *Explain Pain.* Adelaide, Australia: Noigroup Publications, 2010. www.noigroup.com/en/Store. Accessed September 2018.
4. American Pain Foundation. www.painfoundation.org. Accessed September 2018.
5. Internet support group. www.chronicpainsupport.org. Accessed September 2018.
6. Dahl, T.-Lundgren, T. "Living Beyond Your Pain" New Harbinger Publications, 2006.
7. Thorn, B. "Cognitive Therapy for Chronic Pain: A Step By Step Guide;" 2nd ed. Guilford Press, 2017.

Michael has a strong work ethic and is in need of continued full-time employment to support himself and his family. He has few easily transferable skills; concrete is all he knows. He benefited from steroid injections every 3 months and remained on the job. In between injections he used oral opioids, gradually requiring increasing amounts to provide a measure of pain relief. After 5 years he was found to be totally disabled by his doctors and referred for CBT to assist with his adjustment to disability.

After an initial period of anger toward his doctors, he began to take steps to manage his pain. He realized in treatment that his initial goal of total pain relief was unrealistic. He learned to observe his pain, his reactions of anger and fear to his pain, and how he made himself anxious and depressed by concluding that he was severely and permanently functionally impaired. He decided what level of pain was acceptable to him and learned what functional activities he wanted to pursue regardless of the pain. He learned self-management skills to reduce the pain without using medications or procedures when it was elevated. He then returned to work full time, less than a year after being declared disabled, in a less physically demanding job, armed with skills to live with his pain.

Mindfulness training is a primary modality for the treatment of chronic pain. Mindfulness is the practice of bringing complete attention to one's present experience. It recognizes the primacy of the present moment, whereas memories of the past and anticipated future events are mere mental constructs. As such, living only in the present moment is critical. Mindfulness also teaches that although thoughts are useful tools, they alone do not define an individual. Often pain as a private sensory experience is *reified* (made into a static thing), analyzed, and reacted to by our thinking. Our analysis and reaction to the sensory experience of pain is called "suffering" and is entirely in our control. The practice of mindfulness allows us to "relax into the pain" and to observe or even alter our reactions to the sensory experience of pain. In this way, patients learn to accept the pain as a natural part of their experience and limit or reduce reactions to it. This technique also emphasizes the need to make decisions about present and future activities or life plans despite the pain.

Acceptance and commitment therapy is an approach to treating chronic pain that uses mindfulness training as well. It combines mindfulness with *cognitive defusion* (the process of separating or defusing thoughts and images from emotions and memories). It teaches acceptance, which in this context is allowing painful thoughts, images, and memories to come and go without struggling with them. In this therapy, a values exploration is pivotal in helping each person discover what is most important. This approach promotes the individual's ability to accept pain, as well as thoughts and reactions to the pain.

Biofeedback is a computerized audio and visual feedback system that uses physiologic measures to amplify the individual's awareness including muscle contraction (through electromyography (EMG), sympathetic arousal, skin temperature change, heart rate variability (HRV), and brain activity (through electroencephalogram [EEG]). With this increased awareness individuals are taught to increase and decrease the physiologic feedback to gain greater control over their physical function and levels of arousal. Biofeedback has been shown to be quite useful in the treatment of headache and has also been shown to be useful in conjunction with active physical therapy for musculoskeletal back pain, as well as assisting with stress management training.

Relaxation and **stress management** have been shown to be useful in reducing comorbid anxiety and report of pain (see Chapter 35). **Hypnosis** can also be utilized through imagery and relaxation to focus attention and assist with reduced pain and improved sense of well-being (see Chapter 5).

When patients present with comorbid psychiatric conditions, such as depression or anxiety, a referral to a clinical psychologist or psychiatrist who works with chronic pain patients should be considered. In addition, behavioral medicine therapies have been shown to assist patients in reducing pain and suffering, as well as improving function and coping skills and can be provided in collaboration with other rehabilitative and medical techniques.

Pain Rehabilitation

Physical therapy treatment for acute pain is typically passive at first (hot packs, ultrasound, myofascial techniques, etc.) but then becomes more active (stretching, strengthening and endurance techniques, etc.) over a 6- to 12-week period. Physical therapy is useful for musculoskeletal pain complaints. Active physical therapy has been shown in combination with the behavioral medicine therapies and education to be effective in the treatment of chronic low back and musculoskeletal pain.

Occupational therapists often evaluate and treat dysfunction in the activities of daily living and daily functioning, both at home and in the work setting. Work site and home modifications, improved posture and body mechanics and use of adaptive equipment can be established by an occupational therapist to increase independent functioning.

Transcutaneous electrical nerve stimulation (TENS) units provides an electrical current topically and are commonly used for pain relief. The TENS unit can be beneficial in the treatment of neuropathic pain and when provided within an interdisciplinary pain treatment program.

Interdisciplinary Pain Programs

Interdisciplinary pain rehabilitation programs (IPRPs) utilize the services of a pain physician, pain psychologist, physical and occupational therapist, nurse, biofeedback therapist, and others often employ several healing modalities, including hypnosis, mindfulness, and ACT. These professionals work together on interdisciplinary teams to provide coordinated and collaborative care. These programs often involve primary behavior change and rehabilitative strategies together while adjusting medications and increasing function. The efficacy for the use of these programs with chronic pain conditions is evidenced based and well documented. In fact, the combination of CBT with rehabilitation in IPRPs has shown the best outcomes in the treatment of chronic pain.

Multidisciplinary pain procedure programs utilizing primarily injection therapies, medications, implantable pumps and stimulators, together with physical therapy and psychological treatment, work collaboratively to provide pain relief and to assist with improved mobility and coping skills.

Complimentary Medicine Therapies

Complimentary therapies for pain include acupuncture, chiropractic care treatment, massage, nutrition, and homeopathy. These therapies when provided as a series of treatments have shown to be useful in reducing pain.

Acupuncture has been shown to be an effective treatment for back and neck pain, osteoarthritis, chronic headache, and shoulder pain. Chiropractic care has also been shown to be effective for the treatment of chronic low and upper back pain. Nutrition as a primary intervention to reduce pain, has had growing acceptance both in reducing the inflammatory processes, as well as in improving diet for maximal function. The Nutrition Pain Management Certification course is available through the Association of Integrative Pain Management. Movement therapies, such as Feldenkris or Alexander Technique, can be useful in specific circumstances such as in fear of movement.

Treatment outcome can be improved when combined with behavioral medicine therapies to assist in both sustained pain reduction, increased function, and with improved mood and coping skills (see Chapter 35).

Community Pain Programs

Community pain programs utilize specific complementary medicine therapies within a behavioral medicine therapy framework to provide explicitly nonopioid treatment that is financially accessible to most people. These programs were developed recently in response to the growing national concern over the increased consumption of opioids. Community pain programs can combine any of the complimentary medicine therapies with CBT or ACT behavior change strategies together with activating therapies such as occupational therapy or yoga. In this way, these programs help people address everyday pain challenges without the use of opioids.

PHARMACOTHERAPY

Pharmacotherapy is often the first technique employed by the primary care provider for the management of chronic noncancer pain. It is an important technique in the treatment of pain, but *should not be the mainstay of treatment*. For mild-to-moderate pain, acetaminophen, aspirin, and nonsteroidal anti-inflammatory drugs (NSAIDs) may be sufficient. For moderate-to-severe pain, these agents combined with opioids may be helpful. Severe pain may require full opioid agonists.

Acetaminophen & NSAIDs

Acetaminophen and NSAIDs are in many cases the first-line pharmacotherapy for chronic noncancer pain. Appropriate doses of acetaminophen may be just as effective an analgesic and antipyretic as NSAIDs, but without the risk of gastrointestinal bleeding or ulceration. Hepatotoxicity is of particular concern because of how commonly acetaminophen is also an ingredient in various over-the-counter medications. Total acetaminophen doses should not exceed 3 g/d long term or 2 g/d for older patients and for those with liver disease.

Aspirin is an effective analgesic, antipyretic, and anti-inflammatory medication. Gastrointestinal irritation and bleeding are side effects, which are lessened with enteric-coated formulations of aspirin and concomitant use of proton pump inhibitor medication. Bleeding from other sources, allergy, and an association with Reye syndrome in children and teenagers further limit its use.

Commonly used NSAIDs and their dosages are listed in Table 38-4. Like aspirin, the NSAIDs are antipyretic, analgesic, and anti-inflammatory. NSAIDs increase the risk of gastrointestinal bleeding by 1.5 times normal. The risks of bleeding and nephrotoxicity from NSAIDs are both increased in elders. Topical formulations of diclofenac (patch or gel) result in lower blood levels of the NSAID and may be associated with decreased systemic side effects. NSAID gastrointestinal bleeding and ulceration may be prevented with the concurrent use of proton pump inhibitors or with cyclooxygenase (COX)-2 selective NSAIDs. Celecoxib is the only COX-2 inhibitor available and should be used with caution in patients with cardiac disease. The NSAIDs, including COX-2 inhibitors, can lead to fluid retention and exacerbations of congestive heart failure and should be used with caution in patients with that condition.

Opioid Medications

In general, opioid therapy should not be used routinely for chronic noncaner pain as the harms will generally outweigh the benefits. Opioids alone will rarely be sufficient to adequately manage the pain and, in this clinical setting, if they are used, it should be used in conjunction with the other management strategies outlined in this chapter. Opioids are the source of serious morbidities, diversion, and overdose deaths from opioids in the United States constitute what has been called an "epidemic." The mortality from opioids doubled in the United States between 2000 and 2016. Generally, patients on chronic opioids for chronic noncancer pain should have their doses decreased and potentially eliminated to limit these harms.

After very careful assessment of the potential benefits and harms, selected patients may be treated with opioids. Opioid medications are listed in Table 38-5. Full opioid agonists such as morphine, hydromorphone, oxycodone, methadone, fentanyl, hydrocodone, and codeine are used most commonly. Hydrocodone and codeine are typically combined with acetaminophen or an NSAID. Short-acting formulations of oral morphine sulfate, hydromorphone, or oxycodone are useful for acute pain not controlled with other analgesics. For chronic stable pain, long-acting medications are preferred, such as oral sustained-release morphine, oxycodone, or methadone. Methadone is inexpensive, available in a liquid formulation, and may have added efficacy for neuropathic pain due to NMDA antagonism. However, equianalgesic dosing is complex because

Table 38-4. Acetaminophen, aspirin, and useful nonsteroidal anti-inflammatory drugs and COX inhibitors.

Medication (alphabetic order)	Usual Dose for Adults ≥ 50 kg	Usual Dose for Adults < 50 kg[1]	Cost per Unit	Cost for 30 Days[2]	Comments[3]
Acetaminophen (Ofirmev)	1000 mg intravenously every 6–8 hours		$45.02 per vial of 1000 mg	$5402.40	
Acetaminophen or paracetamol[4] (Tylenol, Datril, etc.)	325–500 mg orally every 4 hours or 500–1000 mg orally every 6 hours, up to 2000–4000 mg/d	10–15 mg/kg every 4 hours orally; 15–20 mg/kg every 4 hours rectally, up to 2000–3000 mg/d	$0.02/500 mg (oral) OTC; $0.43/650 mg (rectal) OTC	$3.60 (oral); $77.40 (rectal)	Not an NSAID because it lacks peripheral anti-inflammatory effects. Equivalent to aspirin as analgesic and antipyretic agent. Limit dose to 4000 mg/d in acute pain, and to 3000 mg/d in chronic pain. Limit doses to 2000 mg/d in older patients and those with liver disease. Be mindful of multiple sources of acetaminophen as in combination analgesics, cold remedies, and sleep aids.
Aspirin[5]	325–650 mg orally every 4 hours	10–15 mg/kg every 4 hours orally; 15–20 mg/kg every 4 hours rectally	$0.02/325 mg OTC; $1.51/600 mg (rectal) OTC	$7.20 (oral); $271.80 (rectal)	Available also in enteric-coated oral form that is more slowly absorbed but better tolerated.
Celecoxib[4] (Celebrex)	200 mg orally once daily (osteoarthritis); 100–200 mg orally twice daily (RA)	100 mg orally once or twice daily	$4.37/100 mg; $7.58/200 mg	$227.40 OA; $454.80 RA	Cyclooxygenase-2 inhibitor. No antiplatelet effects. Lower doses for elderly who weigh < 50 kg. Lower incidence of endoscopic gastrointestinal ulceration than NSAIDs. Not known if true lower incidence of gastrointestinal bleeding. Celecoxib is contraindicated in sulfonamide allergy.
Choline magnesium salicylate[6] (Trilasate, others)	1000–1500 mg orally three times daily	25 mg/kg orally three times daily	$0.46/500 mg	$124.20	Salicylates cause less gastrointestinal distress and kidney impairment than NSAIDs but are probably less effective in pain management than NSAIDs.
Diclofenac (Flector)	1.3% topical patch applied twice daily		$13.43/patch	$805.80	Apply patch to most painful area

(Continued)

Table 38-4. Acetaminophen, aspirin, and useful nonsteroidal anti-inflammatory drugs and COX inhibitors. (*Continued*)

Medication (alphabetic order)	Usual Dose for Adults ≥ 50 kg	Usual Dose for Adults < 50 kg[1]	Cost per Unit	Cost for 30 Days[2]	Comments[3]
Diclofenac (Voltaren, Cataflam, others)	50–75 mg orally two or three times daily; 1% gel 2–4 g four times daily		\$0.95/50 mg; \$1.14/75 mg; \$0.52/g gel	\$85.50; \$102.60; \$249.60 gel	May impose higher risk of hepatotoxicity. Enteric-coated product; slow onset. Topical formulations may result in fewer side effects than oral formulations.
Diclofenac sustained release (Voltaren-XR, others)	100–200 mg orally once daily		\$2.70/100 mg	\$162.00	
Diflunisal[7] (Dolobid, others)	500 mg orally every 12 hours		\$2.07/500 mg	\$124.20	Fluorinated acetylsalicylic acid derivative.
Etodolac (Lodine, others)	200–400 mg orally every 6–8 hours		\$1.32/400 mg	\$158.40	
Fenoprofen calcium (Nalfon, others)	300–600 mg orally every 6 hours		\$3.40/600 mg	\$408.00	Perhaps more side effects than others, including tubulointerstitial nephritis.
Flurbiprofen (Ansaid)	50–100 mg orally three or four times daily		\$0.78/50 mg; \$1.18/100 mg	\$93.60; \$141.60	Adverse gastrointestinal effects may be more common among elderly.
Ibuprofen (Caldolor)	400–800 mg intravenously every 6 hours		\$20.08/800 mg vial	\$2410.00	
Ibuprofen (Motrin, Advil, Rufen, others)	400–800 mg orally every 6 hours	10 mg/kg orally every 6–8 hours	\$0.28/600 mg Rx; \$0.05/200 mg OTC	\$33.60; \$9.00	Relatively well tolerated and inexpensive.
Indomethacin (Indocin, Indometh, others)	25–50 mg orally two to four times daily		\$0.38/25 mg; \$0.64/50 mg	\$45.60; \$76.80	Higher incidence of dose-related toxic effects, especially gastrointestinal and bone marrow effects.
Ketoprofen (Orudis, Oruvail, others)	25–75 mg orally every 6–8 hours (max 300 mg/d)		\$1.12/50 mg Rx; \$1.24/75 mg Rx	\$134.40; \$148.80	Lower doses for elderly.
Ketorolac tromethamine	10 mg orally every 4–6 hours to a maximum of 40 mg/d orally		\$2.16/10 mg	Not recommended	Short-term use (< 5 days) only; otherwise, increased risk of gastrointestinal side effects.
Ketorolac tromethamine[8]	60 mg intramuscularly or 30 mg intravenously initially, then 30 mg every 6 hours intramuscularly or intravenously		\$1.45/30 mg	Not recommended	Intramuscular or intravenous NSAID as alternative to opioid. Lower doses for elderly. Short-term use (< 5 days) only.

(*Continued*)

Table 38-4. Acetaminophen, aspirin, and useful nonsteroidal anti-inflammatory drugs and COX inhibitors. (*Continued*)

Medication (alphabetic order)	Usual Dose for Adults ≥ 50 kg	Usual Dose for Adults < 50 kg[1]	Cost per Unit	Cost for 30 Days[2]	Comments[3]
Magnesium salicylate (various)	325–650 mg orally every 6 hours		$0.25/325 mg OTC	$60.00	
Meclofenamate sodium[9] (Meclomen)	50–100 mg orally every 6 hours		$7.74/100 mg	$928.80	Diarrhea more common.
Mefenamic acid (Ponstel)	250 mg orally every 6 hours		$17.41/250 mg	$2089.20	
Meloxicam (Mobic)	7.5 mg orally every 12 hours		$3.16/7.5 mg	$189.60	Intermediate COX-2/COX-1 ratio similar to diclofenac
Nabumetone (Relafen)	500–1000 mg orally once daily (max dose 2000 mg/d)		$1.30/500 mg; $1.53/750 mg	$78.00; $91.80	May be less ulcerogenic than ibuprofen, but overall side effects may not be less.
Naproxen (Naprosyn, Anaprox, Aleve [OTC], others)	250–500 mg orally every 6–8 hours	5 mg/kg every 8 hours	$1.29/500 mg Rx; $0.09/220 mg OTC	$154.80; $8.10 OTC	Generally well tolerated. Lower doses for elderly.
Oxaprozin (Daypro, others)	600–1200 mg orally once daily		$1.50/600 mg	$90.00	Similar to ibuprofen. May cause rash, pruritus, photosensitivity.
Piroxicam (Feldene, others)	20 mg orally once daily		$4.39/20 mg	$131.70	Not recommended in the elderly due to high adverse drug reaction rate. Single daily dose convenient. Long half-life. May cause higher rate of gastrointestinal bleeding and dermatologic side effects.
Sulindac (Clinoril, others)	150–200 mg orally twice daily		$0.98/150 mg; $1.21/200 mg	$58.80; $72.60	May cause higher rate of gastrointestinal bleeding. May have less nephrotoxic potential.
Tolmetin (Tolectin)	200–600 mg orally four times daily		$0.75/200 mg; $3.98/600 mg	$90.00; $477.60	Perhaps more side effects than others, including anaphylactic reactions.

[1]Acetaminophen and NSAID dosages for adults weighing < 50 kg should be adjusted for weight.
[2]Average wholesale price (AWP, for AB-rated generic when available) for quantity listed. *Source:* IBM Micromedex Red Book (electronic version) IBM Watson Health. Greenwood Village, CO, USA. Available at https://www.micromedexsolutions.com, accessed March 12, 2019. AWP may not accurately represent the actual pharmacy cost because wide contractual variations exist among institutions.
[3]The adverse effects of headache, tinnitus, dizziness, confusion, rashes, anorexia, nausea, vomiting, gastrointestinal bleeding, diarrhea, nephrotoxicity, visual disturbances, etc, can occur with any of these drugs. Tolerance and efficacy are subject to great individual variations among patients. Note: All NSAIDs can increase serum lithium levels.
[4]Acetaminophen and celecoxib lack antiplatelet effects.
[5]May inhibit platelet aggregation for 1 week or more and may cause bleeding.
[6]May have minimal antiplatelet activity.
[7]Administration with antacids may decrease absorption.
[8]Has the same gastrointestinal toxicities as oral NSAIDs.
[9]Coombs-positive autoimmune hemolytic anemia has been associated with prolonged use.
OA, osteoarthritis; OTC, over the counter; RA, rheumatoid arthritis; Rx, prescription.
Reproduced with permission from Rabow MW, et al. *Palliative Care & Pain Management.* In: Papadakis MA, McPhee SJ, Rabow MW. eds. *Current Medical Diagnosis & Treatment 2019,* New York, NY: McGraw-Hill; 2019.

Table 38-5. Opioids.

Medication	Approximate Equianalgesic Dose (compared to morphine 30 mg orally or 10 mg intravenously/subcutaneously)[1]		Usual Starting Dose				Potential Advantages	Potential Disadvantages
			Adults ≥ 50 kg Body Weight		Adults < 50 kg Body Weight			
	Oral	Parenteral	Oral	Parenteral	Oral	Parenteral		
Opioid Agonists[2,3]								
Buprenorphine parenteral (Buprenex)		380 mcg		300 mcg intravenously slowly once, may be repeated after 30–60 minutes once; or 600 mcg intramuscularly once; $18.20/300 mcg				
Buprenorphine transdermal (BuTrans)	Not available	Not available	Not available orally. Transdermal doses available: 5, 10, and 20 mcg/h. Initiate 5 mcg/h patch for opioid-naïve patients (may currently be using nonopioid analgesics); $114.77/10 mcg/h	Not available	Not available	Not available	7-day analgesia; may be initiated in opioid-naïve patients with 5 mcg/h. Can titrate up dose by 5 mcg/h after 72 hours, to a maximum dose of 20 mcg/h.	Concomitant use of other opioids for acute pain could be difficult due to strong receptor binding of buprenorphine, although this is often not found in clinical practice. QT prolongation.

Buprenorphine sublingual (Belbuca)	Sublingual strip approved for pain		In opioid-naive or opioid-intolerant patients, individualize dose every 12 h. Start: 75 mcg buccally every 12–24 h for at least 4 days, then increase to 150 mcg buccally every 12 h, then may increase by no more than 150 mcg buccally every 12 h no more frequently than every 4 days. Maximum: 900 mcg/12 h; \$6.07/75 mcg.					Used by pain management specialists. Do no cut, chew, swallow strip. Taper slowly to discontinue. Use lowest effective dose, shortest effective treatment duration. Titrate slowly in patients age > 65 yrs. See footnote[4] for dosing in opioid-experienced patients.
Fentanyl	Not available	100 mcg	Not available	50–100 mcg intravenously/intramuscularly every hour or 0.5–1.5 mcg/kg/h intravenous infusion; \$1.51/100 mcg	Not available	0.5–1 mcg/kg intravenously every 1–4 hours or 1–2 mcg/kg intravenously × 1, then 0.5–1 mcg/kg/h infusion	Possibly less neuroexcitatory effects, including in kidney failure.	

(*Continued*)

Table 38-5. Opioids. (*Continued*)

Medication	Approximate Equianalgesic Dose (compared to morphine 30 mg orally or 10 mg intravenously/subcutaneously)[1]		Usual Starting Dose				Potential Advantages	Potential Disadvantages
			Adults ≥ 50 kg Body Weight		Adults < 50 kg Body Weight			
	Oral	Parenteral	Oral	Parenteral	Oral	Parenteral		
Fentanyl oral transmucosal (Actiq); buccal (Fentora)	Not available	Not available	200 mcg transmucosal; 100 mcg buccal; \$18.80/200 mcg transmucosal; \$81.60/200 mcg buccal	Not available	Not available	Not available	For pain breaking through long-acting opioid medication.	Transmucosal and buccal formulations are not bioequivalent; there is higher bioavailability in buccal formulation.
Fentanyl transdermal	Conversion to fentanyl patch is based on total daily dose of oral morphine:[2] morphine 60–134 mg/d orally = fentanyl 25 mcg/h patch; morphine 135–224 mg/d orally = fentanyl 50 mcg/h patch; morphine 225–314 mg/d orally = fentanyl 75 mcg/h patch; and morphine 315–404 mg/d orally = fentanyl 100 mcg/h patch	Not available	Not available orally 12.5–25 mcg/h patch every 72 hours; \$14.43/25 mcg/h	Not available	12.5–25 mcg/h patch every 72 hours	Not available	Stable medication blood levels.	Not for use in opioid-naïve patients. Minimum starting dose is 25 mcg/h patch in patients who have been taking stable dose of opioids for at least 1 week at the equivalent of at least 60 mg/d of oral morphine.

Hydrocodone, extended release (Zohydro ER)	30 mg[1]	Not available	10 mg every 12 hours; $11.11/10 mg	Not available	Not available	Not available	Available as an extended-release formulation without acetaminophen.	
Hydromorphone[5] (Dilaudid)	7.5 mg	1.5 mg	1–2 mg every 3–4 hours; $0.48/2 mg	1.5 mg every 3–4 hours; $1.80/2 mg	0.06 mg/every 3–4 hours	0.015 mg/kg every 3–4 hours	Similar to morphine. Available in injectable high-potency preparation, rectal suppository.	Short duration.
Hydromorphone extended release (Exalgo)	See package insert	Not available	8 mg every 24 hours; $16.73/8 mg	Not available	Not available	Not available	Similar to morphine.	Taper dose 25–50% every 2–3 days to 8 mg/d to discontinue.
Levorphanol (Levo-Dromoran)	4 mg	Not available	4 mg every 6–8 hours; $53.40/2 mg	Not available	0.04 mg/kg every 6–8 hours	Not available	Longer acting than morphine sulfate.	
Meperidine[6] (Demerol)	300 mg	100 mg	Not recommended	100 mg every 3 hours; $2.72/100 mg	Not recommended	0.75 mg/kg every 2–3 hours	Use only when single-dose, short-duration analgesia is needed, as for outpatient procedures like colonoscopy. Not recommended for chronic pain or for repeated dosing.	Short duration. Normeperidine metabolite accumulates in kidney failure and other situations, and in high concentrations may cause irritability and seizures.

(Continued)

Table 38-5. Opioids. (*Continued*)

Medication	Approximate Equianalgesic Dose (compared to morphine 30 mg orally or 10 mg intravenously/subcutaneously)[1]		Usual Starting Dose				Potential Advantages	Potential Disadvantages
			Adults ≥ 50 kg Body Weight		Adults < 50 kg Body Weight			
	Oral	Parenteral	Oral	Parenteral	Oral	Parenteral		
Methadone (Dolophine, others)	Varies[7]	Varies[7]	5–20 mg every 6–8 hours; $0.31/10 mg	2.5–10 mg every 6–8 hours; $21.00/10 mg	0.2 mg/kg every 6–8 hours	0.1 mg/kg every 6–8 hours	Somewhat longer acting than morphine. Useful in cases of intolerance to morphine. May be particularly useful for neuropathic pain. Available in liquid formulation.	Analgesic duration shorter than plasma duration. May accumulate, requiring close monitoring during first weeks of treatment. Equianalgesic ratios vary with opioid dose. Risk of QT prolongation at doses >100–150 mg/d. Baseline ECG recommended.
Morphine[5] immediate release (Morphine sulfate tablets, Roxanol liquid)	30 mg	10 mg	4–8 mg every 3–4 hours; used for breakthrough pain in patients already taking controlled-release preparations; $0.52/15 mg tab; $0.84/20 mg liquid	10 mg every 3–4 hours; $11.90/10 mg	0.3 mg/kg every 3–4 hours	0.1 mg/kg every 3–4 hours	Standard of comparison; multiple dosage forms available.	No unique problems when compared with other opioids. Active metabolite accumulates in kidney dysfunction.

Morphine controlled release (MS Contin, Oramorph)	30 mg	Not available	15–60 mg every 12 hours; $1.50/30 mg	Not available	Not available	Not available		
Morphine extended release (Kadian, Avinza)	30 mg	Not available	20–30 mg every 24 hours; $5.69/30 mg	Not available	Not available	Not available	Once-daily dosing possible.	
Oxycodone (Roxicodone, OxyIR)	20 mg	Not available	5–10 mg every 3–4 hours; $0.48/5 mg	Not available	0.2 mg/kg every 3–4 hours	Not available	Similar to morphine.	
Oxycodone controlled release (Oxycontin)	20 mg	Not available	20–40 mg every 12 hours; $9.00/20 mg					Physical and chemical pill formulation to deter misuse (injection or intranasal administration).
Oxymorphone[5,8] oral, immediate release (Opana)	10 mg	Not available	5–10 mg every 6 hours; $2.95/5 mg	Not available				Taking with food can increase serum levels by 50%. Equianalgesic dosing conversion range is wide.
Codeine[9,10] (with aspirin or acetaminophen)[11]	180–200 mg	130 mg	60 mg every 4–6 hours; $0.64/60 mg	60 mg every 2 hours intramuscularly/subcutaneously; not available in the United States	0.5–1 mg/kg every 3–4 hours	Not recommended	Similar to morphine.	Closely monitor for efficacy as patients vary in their ability to convert the prodrug codeine to morphine.

(*Continued*)

Table 38-5. Opioids. (*Continued*)

Medication	Approximate Equianalgesic Dose (compared to morphine 30 mg orally or 10 mg intravenously/subcutaneously)[1]		Usual Starting Dose				Potential Advantages	Potential Disadvantages
			Adults ≥ 50 kg Body Weight		Adults < 50 kg Body Weight			
	Oral	Parenteral	Oral	Parenteral	Oral	Parenteral		
Hydrocodone[8] (in Lorcet, Lortab, Vicodin, others)[11]	30 mg	Not available	10 mg every 3–4 hours; $0.54/5 mg	Not available	0.2 mg/kg every 3–4 hours	Not available		Combination with acet-aminophen limits dosage titration.
Oxycodone[10] (in Percodan, Tylox, others)[11]	20 mg	Not available	10 mg every 3–4 hours; $1.37/5 mg	Not available	0.2 mg/kg every 3–4 hours	Not available	Similar to morphine.	Combination with acet-aminophen and aspirin limits dosage titration.
Combination Opioid Agonist–Norepinephrine Reuptake Inhibitor Preparations								
Tapentadol (Nucynta)	Not known	Not known	Start 50–100 mg once, may repeat dose in 1 hour. Can increase to 50–100 mg every 4 hours. Maximum daily dose 600 mg; $11.89/100 mg	Not available		Not available		Avoid in severe kidney or liver impairment.
Tapentadol, extended release (Nucynta ER)	Not known	Not known	Start 50 mg orally every 12 hours. Can increase by 50-mg incre-ments twice daily every 3 days to dose of 100–250 mg twice daily; $15.20/100 mg	Not available		Not available		Avoid in severe kidney or liver impairment.

Tramadol (Ultram)	300 mg	100 mg	Start 25 mg orally daily. Can increase by 25 mg every 3 days to 25 mg orally 4 times daily, then may increase by 50 mg/d every 3 days to 100 mg orally 4 times daily. Limit of 300 mg/d in patients > 75 years old; $0.83/50 mg	Not available	Not available	If creatinine clearance less than 30, limit to 200 mg/d; with cirrhosis, limit to 100 mg/d.

[1]Published tables vary in the suggested doses that are equianalgesic to morphine. Clinical response is the criterion that must be applied for each patient; titration to clinical efficacy is necessary. Because there is not complete cross-tolerance among these drugs, it is usually necessary to use a lower than equianalgesic dose initially when changing drugs and to retitrate to response.

[2]Conversion is conservative; therefore, do not use these equianalgesic doses for converting back from fentanyl patch to other opioids because they may lead to inadvertent overdose. Patients may require breakthrough doses of short-acting opioids during conversion to transdermal fentanyl.

[3]Several significantly more potent formulations of buprenorphine are available but generally reserved for the treatment of opioid use disorder with or without comorbid constant pain, most often by pain management specialists: a sublingual tablet (Subutex and others); a sublingual film (Suboxone and others) in which the buprenorphine is combined with naloxone; a subdermal implant of buprenorphine alone (Probuphine); and a subcutaneous depot injection (Sublocade). Each of these is used in maintenance treatment to reduce problematic use of other opioids. See text.

[4]In opioid-experienced patients, taper current opioids to 30 mg/d oral morphine equivalent prior to starting buprenorphine. Thereafter, buprenorphine dosing schedule depends on prior current oral morphine equivalent:

< 30 mg/d, 75 mcg buccally every 12 h;
30–89 mg/d, 150 mcg buccally every 12 h;
90–160 mg/d, 300 mcg buccally every 12 h;

In all patients, use same dose escalation and maximum dose as shown for opioid-naïve patients.

[5]*Caution:* For morphine, hydromorphone, and oxymorphone, rectal administration is an alternative route for patients unable to take oral medications. Equianalgesic doses may differ from oral and parenteral doses. A short-acting opioid should normally be used for initial therapy.

[6]Not recommended for chronic pain. Doses listed are for brief therapy of acute pain only. Switch to another opioid for long-term therapy.

[7]Methadone conversion varies depending on the equivalent total daily dose of morphine. Consult with a pain management or palliative care expert for conversion.

[8]*Caution:* Recommended doses do not apply to adult patients with kidney or liver impairment or other conditions affecting drug metabolism.

[9]*Caution:* Individual doses of codeine above 60 mg often are not appropriate because of diminishing incremental analgesia with increasing doses but continually increasing nausea, constipation, and other side effects.

[10]*Caution:* Doses of aspirin and acetaminophen in combination products must also be adjusted to the patient's body weight.

[11]*Caution:* Monitor total acetaminophen dose carefully, including any OTC use. Total acetaminophen dose maximum 3 g/d. If liver impairment or heavy alcohol use, maximum is 2 g/d. Available dosing formulations of these combination medications are being adjusted to reflect increased caution about acetaminophen toxicity. Acetaminophen doses in a single combination tablet or capsule will be limited to no more than 325 mg.

Note: Average wholesale price (AWP, generic when available) for quantity listed. *Source:* IBM Micromedex Red Book (electronic version) IBM Watson Health. Greenwood Village, CO, USA. Available at https://www.micromedexsolutions.com, accessed March 12, 2019. AWP may not accurately represent the actual pharmacy cost because wide contractual variations exist among institutions.

Reproduced with permission from Rabow MW, et al. *Palliative Care & Pain Management.* In: Papadakis MA, McPhee SJ, Rabow MW. eds. *Current Medical Diagnosis & Treatment 2019,* New York, NY: McGraw-Hill; 2019.

it varies with the patient's opioid dose, and caution must be used at higher methadone doses because of the risk of QT prolongation. Consultation with a pain or palliative care specialist may be appropriate.

A useful technique for opioid management of chronic pain is equianalgesic dosing (Table 38-5). The dosages of any full opioid agonists used to control pain can be converted into an equivalent dose of any other opioid. In this way, 24-hour opioid requirements and dosing regimens established using shorter-acting opioid medications can be converted into equivalent dosages of long-acting medications or formulations. *Cross-tolerance is often incomplete, however, so less than the full calculated equianalgesic dosage is generally administered initially when switching between opioid formulations.* Equianalgesic dosing for methadone is more complex and varies by dose and duration of use.

Although some clinicians and patients inexperienced with the management of severe chronic pain may feel more comfortable with combined nonopioid–opioid agents, full agonist opioids are typically a better choice in patients with severe pain because the dose of opioid is not limited by the toxicities of the acetaminophen, aspirin, or NSAID component of combination preparations. There is no maximal allowable or effective dose for full opioid agonists; however, one should also be aware of opioid-induced hyperalgesia that may present in patients on higher opioid doses.

As opioids are titrated upward, increasing difficulty with side effects can be expected. Constipation is common at any dose of opioid, and tolerance to this side effect does not develop over time. Opioid-induced constipation should be anticipated and prevented in all patients.

Although there is limited evidence for their efficacy, a number of strategies are used to try to limit the potential harms of opioids. Strategies include opioid risk assessment tools, limiting the total daily amount of opioids prescribed, conducting urine drug testing to assess for misuse, nonadherence and diversion, use of state electronic opioid prescription monitoring programs (registries), distributing opioid antidotes (naloxone), and the use of opioid agreements. The agreement aims to thoughtfully establish the goals of management prior to the initiation of any therapy. Key elements of a chronic pain management agreement are included in Table 38-6. Both the physician and patient should sign the agreement prior to therapy initiation and both individuals should retain a copy. Violation of the agreement by the patient can be met initially with a single written warning, but any subsequent violation should be met with the cessation of opioid therapy, after a brief taper to avoid opioid withdrawal. It is critical to make clear to the patient that care with other management strategies and interventions can continue even if opioids will no longer be prescribed (see Chapter 25).

Table 38-6. Key elements in a typical pain contract.

Establish goals of treatment, particularly that (1) pharmacotherapy is only one part of therapy, and that (2) medication is not expected to completely eliminate pain.
Only one provider will write prescriptions for pain medication.
Patient agrees to use a single pharmacy for all opioid and nonopioid analgesics.
Refills for pain medication are not provided for lost or stolen medications and are only provided during regular business hours with appropriate lead time.
Random urine drug screening is to be performed without prior notice.
Patient agrees not to give or sell medications to others.
Warnings regarding sedating effects and long-term side effects of medications.
Warnings to avoid any and all illicit substances.
Breaking one or more of the elements in the contract will result in discontinuation of opioid prescriptions after an appropriate taper; however, all other elements of care will continue.

Source: Adapted from publicly available contracts, including from www.dora.state.co.us/medical/policies/10-14SampleContract.Doc. Accessed November 20, 2011.

Neuropathic Pain

It is essential when taking a patient's history to listen for descriptions such as burning, shooting, pins and needles, or electricity, and for pain associated with numbness. Such a history suggests neuropathic (as opposed to nociceptive) pain, which is treated with some medications not typically used for other types of pain. A number of nonopioid medications have been found to be effective in randomized trials (Table 38-7).

The calcium channel $\alpha 2$-δ ligands gabapentin and pregabalin are considered first-line therapy for neuropathic pain. Both medications can cause sedation, dizziness, ataxia, and gastrointestinal side effects but have no significant drug interactions. Both medications require dose adjustments in patients with kidney dysfunction. Both medications are relatively safe in accidental overdose and may be preferred over tricyclic antidepressants (TCAs) for a patient with a history of congestive heart failure or arrhythmia or if there is a risk of suicide. When combined, gabapentin and morphine are more effective at lower doses of each medication compared to required doses when each is used as a single agent.

The selective serotonin norepinephrine reuptake inhibitors (SSNRIs), duloxetine and venlafaxine, are also considered first-line treatments for neuropathic pain. These should not be combined with other serotonin or norepinephrine uptake inhibitors due to concern for serotonin syndrome, but it can be combined

Table 38-7. Pharmacological management of neuropathic pain.

Drug[a]	Starting Dose	Typical Dose
Antidepressants[b]		
Nortriptyline	10 mg orally at bedtime	10–150 mg orally at bedtime
Desipramine	10 mg orally at bedtime	10–200 mg orally at bedtime
Calcium channel a2-d ligands		
Gabapentin[c]	100–300 mg orally once to three times daily	300–1200 mg orally three times daily
Pregabalin[d]	50 mg orally three times daily	100 mg orally three times daily
Selective serotonin norepinephrine reuptake inhibitors		
Duloxetine	30 mg orally daily or 20 mg orally daily in elders	60 mg orally daily
Venlafaxine[e]	75 mg orally daily divided into two or three doses	150–225 mg orally daily divided into two or three doses
Opioids	(see Table 38-5)	(see Table 38-5)
Other medications		
Lidocaine transdermal	5% patch applied daily, for a maximum of 12 hours	1–3 patches applied daily for a maximum of 12 hours
Tramadol hydrochloride	50 mg orally four times daily	100 mg orally two to four times daily

[a]Begin at the starting dose and titrate up every 4 or 5 days.
[b]Begin with a low dose. Pain relief may be achieved at doses below antidepressant doses, thereby minimizing adverse side effects.
[c]Common side effects include nausea, somnolence, and dizziness. Take medication on a full stomach. Do not combine with serotonin or norepinephrine uptake inhibitors, or with TCAs.
[d]Common side effects include dizziness, somnolence, peripheral edema, and weight gain. Must adjust dose for kidney impairment.
[e]*Caution*: Can cause hypertension and ECG changes. Obtain baseline ECG and monitor.
Reproduced with permission from Rabow MW, et al. *Palliative Care & Pain Management*. In: Papadakis MA, McPhee SJ, Rabow MW. eds. *Current Medical Diagnosis & Treatment 2019*, New York, NY: McGraw-Hill; 2019.

with gabapentin or pregabalin. Because venlafaxine can cause hypertension and induce ECG changes, patients with cardiovascular risk factors should be carefully monitored when starting this medication.

The TCAs may be used as well. They usually have an effect at lower doses than are needed for an antidepressant effect. Desipramine and nortriptyline are good first choices because they cause less orthostatic hypotension and have fewer anticholinergic effects than amitriptyline. Start with a low dosage and titrate upward every 4 or 5 days.

The 5% lidocaine patch is effective in postherpetic neuralgia (PHN) and may be effective in other types of localized neuropathic pain. A new patch is applied to the painful region daily for up to 12 hours.

Successful management of neuropathic pain often requires the use of more than one effective medication, as well as a foundation of behavioral treatments (see Case Illustration 4).

Other Pharmacologic Treatments

Ketamine has some evidence for its use in pain management. There is limited evidence for high-CBD medical cannabis in the treatment of neuropathic pain.

Interventional Pharmacotherapy

Injection Therapies: Injections include trigger point injections, epidural injections, and nerve blocks. Trigger points are localized areas of muscle tenderness and pain, and are often injected with local anesthetics in the treatment of myofascial complaints for temporary short-term relief. In conjunction with physical therapy, they may provide longer-term relief. Epidural injections utilize local anesthetics or steroids into the epidural space and can be used for both diagnostic purposes as well as to provide short-term relief. Epidural steroid injections may be repeated to provide longer-term relief, but providers need to monitor for long-term effects of chronic steroid use. Selected chronic pain patients may benefit from trigger point and epidural injections. Peripheral nerve blocks are typically used for peripheral neuropathy for short-term relief of pain. Nerve blocks may be provided in a series of three injections over a period of 3–18 weeks. In general, evidence is limited for long-term pain management with injections, but may be part of multimodal treatment in an effort to limit opioid use.

Implantable Pumps: Intraspinal infusion of opioids or other medications into the intrathecal area through an implanted pump is available. Because of increased proximity to pain receptors in the dorsal horn of the spinal cord, less than 1% of the oral opioid dose may be equianalgesic in the intrathecal space. In cancer patients, randomized clinical trials have shown better analgesic and toxicity profiles compared with systemic medication management. However, the efficacy of intrathecal therapy for noncancer pain is controversial. *Spinal Cord Stimulator:* Neurostimulation is provided by an implanted pulse generator through electrodes that are targeted to the spinal cord with the intent of blocking the pain signal. There is some evidence for the use of spinal-cord stimulators for complex regional pain syndrome and failed back surgery syndrome. However, in the context of the opioid epidemic, there is renewed interest in spinal cord stimulation as an alternative to systemic opioid therapy.

CHRONIC PAIN CASE EXAMPLES

The following case illustrations highlight major issues related to chronic pain management.

CASE ILLUSTRATION 1

Chronic Headache Pain

Lisa is a 39-year-old woman who sought care for her long-standing headaches. These headaches first appeared at the age of 18 years, at which time they were characterized by severe left orbital and temporal pain associated with nausea, nasal stuffiness, and photophobia. They were often preceded by a scintillating scotoma in the right temporal/visual field. Her workup included a normal lumbar puncture, several normal EEGs, computerized tomography (CT) scans, and blood chemistries. She was virtually headache-free for 1 year following a pregnancy in her early 20s. Headaches gradually recurred but remitted again for a year after a hysterectomy for endometriosis in her early 30s. She now reports that the headaches have increased in frequency, duration, and severity over the past 2 years with more photophobia, nausea, and vomiting.

Treatment modalities have included analgesia (aspirin, acetaminophen, NSAIDs, opioids), abortive agents (sumatriptan and topiramate), prophylactic medications (amitriptyline, cyproheptadine, phenytoin, valproic acid, propranolol), and vitamins, all of which have had only transient benefit. Dietary and activity prescriptions have also been of minimal success. Her main source or relief over the past year has been repeated emergency room visits for oral opioids. She has seen multiple internists, neurologists, anesthesiologists for trigger point injections and nerve blocks, allergists, and emergency room physicians.

Long-standing, recurrent, incapacitating, nonmalignant pain creates a number of challenges in management:

1. Seeking assistance from a series of caregivers without resolution.
2. A clear fluctuation in the frequency and intensity of the headache seemingly due to physiologic changes, but without an exploration of the possible behavioral or social changes associated with these fluctuations.
3. Failure to explore the impact the headache has had in the patient's life.

A pain history revealed that Lisa's headaches in early adulthood were infrequent (several per year) and were managed conservatively. Her single severe attack resulted in a hospitalization that was a source of embarrassment to her and her husband. During the early years of her marriage she continued to have infrequent but more severe headaches. During a period of 6 months of treatment with oral contraceptives her headaches became more frequent and severe. As her daughter grew older and her job responsibilities increased, the frequency and severity of the headaches grew. She further reported that she was best able to control her pain by being alone in a quiet room, reading, or listening to quiet music.

The patient is now identifying what may be a relationship between marital or social stress and her headache complaint. The headache can provide "time-out" from the conflicts at hand, and she can ease the pain by listening to music or reading. She further indicates that the headaches did not have a significant impact in her early life.

The headache pattern remained unchanged until 1½ years ago. At that time Lisa and her husband relocated as a result of her husband's work and they moved into a home that required major remodeling, the responsibility of which was largely the patient's. She had difficulty replacing her former employment and considered a new career. Although she reported enthusiasm for the remodeling and the relocation, Lisa also reported a marked increase in the frequency of the headaches. She was unable to work around the house remodeling or participate in family discussions when she had the headache, but was otherwise able to prepare meals, do housework, and drive as far as 30 miles one way for social and medical visits. She reported that when she retreats to her room with a headache her husband and children attend to her until she starts to improve. She also indicated that her husband returned home early from work during times of a severe headache. She has seen a cascade of physicians in various specialties with a variety of unremarkable diagnostic tests and specialty workups. Her average length of treatment with any one physician was five visits. She reported with embarrassment that she had been unable to keep up with her diet and exercise program and was increasingly overweight. Otherwise, she was in good health with no other medical problems.

Although the headache event is likely to have muscle contraction, endocrine, and vascular components, there appear to be a number of social situations or conditions that accompany its onset and severity. Moreover, it is clear that as life stress has increased, Lisa's headaches have also increased in severity and frequency. There seem to be behavioral factors that reinforce the headache complaint: (1) avoidance of stress and (2) increased attention.

The following treatment course of action was undertaken:

1. *The physician explained to the patient that she wanted to work with her to ease her headaches. She reassured Lisa that she thought that by working together and taking a broad view they could ease the frequency and severity of headaches and improve her quality of life overall.*
2. *It was agreed that the best course of treatment was to use as little opioid medication as possible. Even though opioids were found to be useful by the patient, she recognized that ultimately they were not changing the overall pattern of her headaches and decided to use them only for severe headaches that did not resolve with other measures. Patient and physician medication management responsibilities were outlined in the medication agreement, which specified the number and frequency of opioid medications.*
3. *It was agreed that the patient would not seek additional medical evaluation or treatment without discussing it with her primary care physician first.*
4. *The primary care physician agreed that she or her designee would be available within a 12-hour period of being contacted about a headache to discuss the headache and the possible situation surrounding it. It was agreed that these conversations would generally be brief and not longer than 5–10 minutes.*
5. *The physician discussed a comprehensive approach to the headaches, including a course of biofeedback training and instruction for neck exercises in physical therapy. Lisa agreed to participate actively in these treatments.*
6. *The physician also referred Lisa for CBT.*
7. *It was agreed that Lisa would take a more active role to self-manage the headache using behavioral and physical techniques primarily.*
8. *If this plan did not show significant reduction in headaches within 3 months, referral to a multidisciplinary pain rehabilitation program would be considered.*
9. *Finally, the physician would attend to all of Lisa's medical needs, including preventive care, which had been somewhat neglected due to a singular focus on the headache and the frequent changing of doctors.*

In this way, the primary care physician helped Lisa *redefine* the headache treatment regimen: it does not need immediate or intensive medical care; it does not need further diagnostic evaluation (because a detailed medical evaluation had already been done); and it does not need further multiple/different medication trials (these have also been tried). By creating an effective relationship with the patient, acknowledging the severity of her complaint, setting expectations for how to respond to symptoms, explicitly stating a desire and intent to help, and securing the patient's commitment to work within this setting, a productive patient–physician partnership was established to address Lisa's pain complaint.

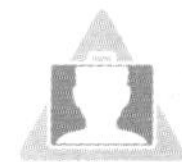

CASE ILLUSTRATION 2

Chronic Intractible Pain: Chronic Low Back Pain

Michael is a 45-year-old man with controlled hypertension who presented with low back pain. He reported that while working on a farm two years ago he experienced a motor vehicle accident that resulted in a herniated disc in his lumbar spine. A lumbar laminectomy and discectomy followed with some relief of pain for approximately 3 months. Since that time he had 6 weeks of passive physical therapy (hot packs, ultrasound, massage, gentle stretching) and was receiving oral opioids and NSAIDs from his surgeon. He had low back pain and no other complaints. He had not returned to work since the day of the injury and was currently involved in a vocational rehabilitation plan.

On physical examination, the patient was tender to palpation across his low back bilaterally. Passive straight leg raising was normal. Sharp, dull, and light touch sensations were intact throughout, with symmetric reflexes in both the lower extremities. The CT scan of the lumbar and sacral spine revealed old surgical repair of a herniated disc without other abnormalities. Recent nerve conduction studies were unremarkable for nerve slowing. The patient's surgeon, who had "nothing more to offer," referred him back to his primary care physician for continued treatment. The primary care physician referred him for a series of three epidural injections. The first injection resulted in partial pain relief for 2 weeks. The last two injections produced no relief of pain.

Chronic low back pain often has the following characteristics:

1. Subjective complaint of pain with minimal objective findings.
2. Use of "passive" rather than "active" physical therapy.
3. Continuous use of opioid medication in escalating dose to manage the pain.

The patient reported that he spends much of the day sitting in his reclining chair, either watching television or reading except when he attends the vocational training. He moves from the chair two or three times each day, primarily for meals. He frequently naps during the day and reports disrupted sleep at night, averaging 5–6 hours. He feels depressed and hopeless about his recovery and believes that unless his pain is relieved he will be unable to return to work. He acknowledges that his spouse and children are angry with him and his inability to return to work.

On further questioning it was discovered that the social "cost" of the pain is high. Michael's daily activities are greatly impaired. His self-esteem and affect have plummeted, and he is further emotionally isolated from his family. In a circumstance in which a patient's chronic pain is associated with the patient belief that pain relief is necessary to return to a degree of normal living, the doctor must accurately establish expectations for recovery and the probable outcomes of treatment. Because the patient is usually still focused on the pain as a continuation of the original precipitating injury, it becomes necessary to identify and deal with the patient's pain beliefs while focusing on improving function.

Although Michael reported feelings of depression, it is inaccurate to say that the pain is caused by the depression or vice versa, but rather it is *comorbid* to the pain. It has been shown, however, that the intensity of pain often diminishes with a trial of antidepressant medication, which can improve sleep as well.

The goals of treatment for chronic low back pain are primarily focused on improving the patient's activity level; diminishing their reliance on medications because, as in this case, they have not improved functioning despite escalating doses; and reducing pain behaviors (e.g., changing the focus of treatment from decreasing pain to increasing activity level for meaningful tasks). In this way, the doctor assists in "managing" the pain behavior.

At the same time the doctor should challenge the commonly held belief that increased opioid medication is necessary for increased activity. Whereas this is often the case for acute pain conditions, the same is not true for chronic noncancer pain conditions, and in many cases increasing opioid dose is associated with worse overall functioning and possibly leading to hyperalgesia. The doctor also should help the patient recognize that increases in pain with activity do not mean that the underlying medical condition is getting worse. The doctor should also reinforce the use of nonpharmacological methods of pain control while the patient is increasing his functional activity levels.

After a careful explanation by the doctor of the anatomy, physiology, and possible/probable causes of Michael's low back pain, a collaborative discussion followed, leading to an agreement on the following treatment plan:

1. *A course of physical therapy using primarily active exercises (e.g., aerobic exercise, walking, strengthening, and stretching). In addition, the patient agreed to take progressively longer walks each day. It was expected that with increased activity there would be an initial increase in pain.*
2. *Although there was no evidence of addiction or abuse of opioids, it was also clear that increasing opioid doses and as needed use had not improved the patient's pain or function. The physician recognized that the sole reliance on opioids for management was not working. The patient and physician agreed that reducing opioid use was a goal and would be done gradually over time. The physician reassured the patient that he would continue opioids for a short time but expected that a more comprehensive approach would lead to improvement that would obviate the need for opioids. Oral opioid medication was managed with a long-acting preparation with no short-acting or "breakthrough" dosing. This approach avoided linking the patient's pain with the timing and amount of dosing. The physician wrote monthly prescriptions. It was agreed that any request for change in his medication regimen would be directed only to the primary care physician and not to emergency rooms or other physicians. This was outlined and signed in a patient medication agreement.*
3. *The patient would be seen once a month by the doctor. A primary focus of future visits would be discussion about daily activities or return-to-work goals, if appropriate, rather than pain interferences with life.*
4. *Progress toward increased functional activities and reduced reliance on medications was monitored monthly through a brief activity-oriented questionnaire filled out at each doctor's visit.*
5. *Michael was referred for pain psychology treatment with Michael's approval.*

The doctor has now, in collaboration with the patient, established the parameters of treatment, clarified the expected outcomes in terms of function, developed a more rational plan for the use of opioids, and progressed toward meaningful employment goals if appropriate, all in the context of reassuring the patient that the physician was invested in helping him and would work with him. This approach is a far cry from the previous message of "there is nothing more to do" and provides hope to the patient. These steps define the treatment effort to reducing pain perception and pain behaviors and changing beliefs about pain impact. Patients who respond favorably to this treatment of chronic pain usually report either that the pain is significantly reduced or that it does not bother them as much as it used to. When pain behavior is more entrenched (the patient is unresponsive to treatment due in part to beliefs about pain impact or secondary gain or both), referral to an interdisciplinary pain rehabilitation facility is recommended.

Cognitive-behavioral therapy and other behavioral approaches (see Table 38-2) are often useful therapies independent of the multidisciplinary pain rehabilitation programs and would be reasonable adjuncts for this patient.

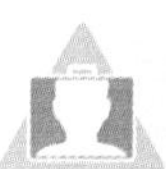

CASE ILLUSTRATION 3

Fibromyalgia

Kim is a 46-year-old woman with a known history of gastroesophageal reflux disease (GERD), who presented with total body pain. She reported that while lifting some baked goods in her kitchen 20 years ago she felt an acute snap coming from her right shoulder. She was later diagnosed with thoracic outlet syndrome and underwent removal of her first rib. She experienced pain relief for approximately 8 months with a recurrence of symptoms followed by an additional supraclavicular surgery. She continued to report having neck and shoulder pain. She was then diagnosed with cervical spondylosis and underwent a cervical laminectomy 5 years later with good benefit. Thereafter, she was tapered from her pain medications and returned to normal life, including work as a baker. For approximately 10 years following her surgery she reported essentially no recurring symptoms. She then had an onset of "achiness" in her shoulders and upper extremities bilaterally.

Kim now presents with pain in all four quadrants of her body and was positive for increased sensitivity for 16 of 18 tender points when applying 9 lbs of pressure. Kim also reports having an increased sensitivity to pain especially in her neck and shoulder.

Fibromyalgia is a clinical syndrome or cluster of symptoms for which there is little agreement as to cause or etiology. Complaints of total body achiness in all four quadrants of the body plus tenderness in 11–18 tender points when applying 9 lbs of pressure are sufficient to make a diagnosis according to initial diagnostic criteria. New criteria were developed in 2010 that do not use tender points but rather emphasize widespread pain and associated sleep problems, fatigue, and cognitive issues. Report of symptoms of fibromyalgia can occur with no known traumatic event or illness.

On physical examination, sensation was intact throughout with symmetric reflexes without evidence of clubbing, cyanosis, or edema. She had full range of motion in the bilateral upper and lower extremities with no motor deficits identified. An MRI of the cervical spine showed old cervical repair with no abnormalities. Kim was then referred to a pain relief specialist (anesthesiologist) at a multidisciplinary pain procedure program.

A detailed history taken at the multidisciplinary pain procedure program documented pain symptoms, together with chronic fatigue, sleep disturbance, intermittent headaches, loss of weight, subjective feelings of weakness, intermittent report of irritable bowel, and anxiety. The multidisciplinary evaluation included a psychological evaluation, which diagnosed comorbid depression and anxiety with an above-normal arousal response to stress.

The multidisciplinary evaluation identified a number of other symptoms that are commonly seen with fibromyalgia, including fatigue, sleep disturbance, intermittent headaches, weight loss or weight gain, complaints of weakness, irritable bowel, and anxiety and depression. Not uncommon with fibromyalgia is an abnormal startle response as well as decreased coping in the presence of increased stress or stimulation.

Kim reports that she is a single mother of three teenage daughters, two of whom are living at home. She reports her ex-husband to be estranged from her and her children. He has not provided child support, requiring that Kim work full time as the sole support of the family. As her daughters grew to their mid-teen years, an increasing number of conflicts occurred between them. Kim reports that she is most worried about her eldest, 17-year-old daughter, who has recently dropped out of school and is living with a boy. Kim fears that she is using recreational drug. Kim reports having missed several days of work due to her pain and has been warned by her employer on two occasions that further absences might lead to disciplinary action. Finally, she reports that she is involved romantically with a man who seems to like her daughters and has been responsive to her needs for support as her pain problems seem to worsen.

While it is unknown if stress is one of the triggers of fibromyalgia, it is not uncommon to find comorbid environmental or personal situations that promote symptoms of anxiety and depression.

Treatment initiated at the multidisciplinary pain procedure clinic included SSRI antidepressant medication, gabapentin, a trial of muscle relaxant medication, and a series of myofascial trigger point injections. She was also seen for a course of CBT designed to improve problem-solving capabilities and teach stress management techniques. She also engaged in passive physical therapy modalities (such as ultrasound, massage, and gentle stretching). Kim reported improved mood and greater relaxation in response to the passive physical therapy techniques and muscle relaxant medications. There was no benefit from the trigger point injections. Finally, it was reported by the psychologist that her decision making about her 17-year-old daughter was improving, with evidence of better coping skills. She also had scheduled relaxation into her daily routine. Kim decided to take a leave of absence from her employer on short-term disability.

In the absence of a true etiology, the tendency is to treat the symptoms of pain. The symptoms are often vague and transient and do not respond well to an acute pain treatment approach. Though Kim does benefit from treatments that are designed to reduce arousal and improve coping skills, she continues to report the symptoms of pain leading to increased disability.

Kim was discharged from the multidisciplinary pain procedure program and returned to the care of her primary care physician. In collaboration with her doctor, Kim agreed to continue with her use of the antidepressant medication and to gradually reduce and discontinue her use of muscle relaxant medications. Consideration was given to use of low-dose NSAIDs. She continued physical therapy that now included walking in the swimming pool three times a week for 1 month, followed by light aerobic exercises three times a week, and, finally, active physical therapy for muscle fitness. It was agreed that she would use hot packs and massage for temporary relief in lieu of the opioid or muscle relaxant medication. She was to continue her relaxation practice throughout the day and agreed to continue CBT to assist with coping.

The doctor agreed to meet with Kim once a month to review progress. Kim agreed to keep records of her daily exercises and her medication use. Kim also agreed in her medication contract that any flare-ups or changes in her medication would be managed by her primary care physician, who agreed to be responsive to her within 24 hours of initial contact between monthly visits.

After 4 months of treatment Kim was able to improve her function and daily activity sufficiently to return to work on a full-time basis. She was able to plan for her future wedding with her now fiancé and reported that her total body pain had reduced substantially, but "waxed and waned" intermittently.

CASE ILLUSTRATION 4

Postherpetic Neuralgia

Lynn is a 63-year-old woman with well-controlled hypertension and elevated cholesterol. Lynn works as a social worker and also volunteers with social service agencies. Twelve years ago, she developed a vesicular rash on her left frontal scalp and forehead. The area was severely painful. She presented to her general medicine physician 4 days after the rash appeared, having thought it was a reaction to a new shampoo.

She was diagnosed with varicella zoster virus infection (shingles). A careful evaluation was conducted to make sure she did not have any ocular involvement. Despite the delay in her presentation, she was treated with acyclovir and a 10-day course of prednisone.

For her acute pain, she was treated with hydrocodone/acetaminophen and ibuprofen. She received moderate control of her pain but felt somewhat dizzy with the hydrocodone/acetaminophen medication and experienced gastrointestinal upset with the NSAID.

Five weeks after onset and after complete resolution of the lesions, Lynn returned to her primary care physician with the complaint of continued pain on her scalp and forehead. The pain was described as "burning" and "searing." The patient was most aware of the pain at night, in bed before sleep and it sometimes kept her awake. When she was more active, she reported that she had less pain. However, sometimes the pain was so severe it was difficult for her to go about her usual activities. Lynn was diagnosed with postherpetic neuralgia (PHN).

PHN is an unfortunate complication of varicella zoster infection that is more likely to develop in patients older than 60 years. It can last for months or years or be permanent. The actual cause of the PHN is not known and, therefore, treatment is directed at managing the pain symptoms. People with PHN benefit from an honest explanation of the disorder, the typical course of the condition, and a multidisciplinary approach to management.

Lynn tried gabapentin but experienced little benefit. Moreover, she was burdened by severe sedation at a dose of 900 mg three times daily. Pregabalin was ineffective. She refused a trial of the lidocaine transdermal patch due to cosmetic concerns. Capsaicin cream was difficult to use on her scalp. Nortriptyline up to 150 mg nightly had only a modest effect. Other TCAs, SSRI, and SNRI medications were tried. Duloxetine proved most helpful among these. She continued to use hydrocodone/acetaminophen when the pain was incapacitating; however, she did not like the idea of using an opioid medication regularly and also reported some dizziness even at low doses. Pain relief was only partial at best. The mainstay of her pharmacological treatment was ibuprofen 400 mg two to three times daily. She added a proton pump inhibitor to help with stomach upset.

The side effects of analgesic medications often require management with other medications. Even patients who wish to limit their use of medications may soon find that their pharmacological regimen has become complex and burdensome. Moreover, as in this case, medications alone may not adequately treat the pain and behavioral medicine approaches should be considered.

Lynn tried acupuncture without success as well as a mindfulness-based stress reduction practice, with some benefit. She noted that her Mindfulness exercises were especially useful to her at night when she was going to sleep. She was referred to physical therapy, where modalities including contrast heat/cold treatments were used, followed by a trial of the transcutaneous nerve stimulator (TENS), all with only temporary benefit. She was referred for CBT where she learned to accept her pain, be mindful of her life with pain, and to live a normal life despite the pain.

In cases such as these, where pain is refractory to multiple medications, the focus is on chronic pain management. Chronic pain typically has no cure and is poorly managed by medications alone. Combining CBT techniques with physical rehabilitation and medications has shown the best outcomes in the treatment of neuropathic chronic pain.

After 6 months of managing her symptoms, Lynn settled into a regular medication regimen of ibuprofen, omeprazole, and duloxetine, and needed hydrocodone/acetaminophen only rarely. She recognized that being as active as possible at work and at home greatly improved her quality of life, including the management of her pain. After 12 weeks of CBT and 6 weeks of physical therapy, she now a has an active life despite the pain, a number of self-management approaches that she employs as needed, and an acceptable pharmaceutical regime with few side effects—all of which enhance her well-being and resilience.

SUMMARY

In this chapter, we presented several approaches to the treatment of persons suffering various types of chronic noncancer pain, which emphasize the evaluation and treatment of not only the biological but also the psychological and social implications of the problem. The primary care provider is encouraged to make good use of the three-function model for interviewing and ongoing communications with his or her patient (see Chapter 1). The following key factors should be attended to in the treatment of chronic pain:

- **Identifying pain as an issue:** Deal with it in a comprehensive medical, social, and psychological way at onset, instead of when it becomes a problem.
- **Pain behaviors:** Whereas the patient may be quick to understand the pain largely as derived from the precipitating event or factors, the treating physician must always attend to the social causes and consequences of the pain and its implications in the life of the patient at work, at home, and during play.
- **Meaning and impact of the pain:** Cultural influences may dictate differing attitudes and roles in the expression of pain. Changes in lifestyle or work can have a profound effect on the quality of life.
- **Doctor as "change agent":** In addition to providing direct treatment and advice, the doctor, through the patient/doctor relationship, can improve adherence to treatment.
- **Function, not dysfunction, oriented:** The interests and attention of the doctor influences greatly the thoughts and behaviors of the patient. By commenting on improving function as an indicator of healing, the doctor can redirect the patient's attention away from the pain and toward increased functioning.

SUGGESTED READINGS

Beal BR, et al. An overview of pharmacologic management of chronic pain. *Med Clin North Am* 2016;100(1):65–79.

Bonakdar R, Cotter, N. Certification Program in Nutritional Pain Management. *Academy of Integrated Pain Management.* 2017.

Catalano E, Hardin KN, eds. *The Chronic Pain Control Workbook: A Step-by-Step Guide for Coping with and Overcoming Pain*, 2nd ed. New Harbinger Publications, Oakland, CA; 1999.

Centers for Disease Control and Prevention (CDC). CDC guideline for prescribing opioids for chronic pain. 2017 August 29. http://www.cdc.gov/drugoverdose/prescribing/guideline. html.

Chapman CR, et al. The transition of acute postoperative pain to chronic pain: an integrative overview of research on mechanisms. *J Pain* 2017;18(4):359.e1–38.

Chou R. Diagnosis and treatment of low back pain. A joint clinical practices guideline from the American College of Surgeons and the American Pain Society. *Ann Intern Med* 2007;147:478–492.

Cordier Scott L, et al. JAMA patient page. Opioids for chronic pain. *JAMA* 2016;315(15):1672.

Dart RC, et al. Trends in opioid analgesic abuse and mortality in the United States. *N Engl J Med* 2015;372(16):1573–4.

Deer TR, et al. Dorsal root ganglion stimulation yielded higher treatment success rate for complex regional pain syndrome and causalgia at 3 and 12 months: a randomized comparative trial. *Pain* 2017;158(4):669–81.

Dowell D, et al. CDC guideline for prescribing opioids for chronic pain—United States, 2016. *JAMA* 2016;315(15):1624–15. http://www.cdc.gov/drugoverdose/prescribing/guideline.html.

Fornasari D. Pharmacotherapy for neuropathic pain: a review. *Pain Ther* 2017;6(Suppl 1):25–33.

Frank JW, et al. Patient outcomes in dose reduction or discontinuation of long-term opioid therapy: a systematic review. *Ann Intern Med* 2017;167(3):181–91.

Gatchel RJ, Okifuji A. Evidenced-based scientific data documenting the treatment and cost effectiveness of comprehensive pain programs for chronic nonmalignant pain. *J Pain* 2006;7:779–793.

Henschke N, et al. The epidemiology and economic consequences of pain. *Mayo Clin Proc* 2015;90(1):139–47.

Manchikanti L, et al. Responsible, safe, and effective prescription of opioids for chronic non-cancer pain: American Society of Interventional Pain Physicians (ASIPP) guidelines. *Pain Physician* 2017;20(2S):S3–92.

Qaseem A, et al. Clinical Guidelines Committee of the American College of Physicians. Noninvasive treatments for acute, subacute, and chronic low back pain: a clinical practice guideline from the American College of Physicians. *Ann Intern Med* 2017;166(7):514–30.

Rabow MW, Pantilat SZ, Shah A, Poree L. *Palliative Care & Pain Management*, 59th ed. *Current Medical Diagnosis and Treatment.* New York, NY: Lange Medical Books/McGraw-Hill; 2020.

Ray WA et al. Prescription of long-acting opioids and mortality in patients with chronic noncancer pain. *JAMA* 2016; 315(22):2415–23.

Sharan A, et al. An overview of chronic spinal pain: revisiting diagnostic categories and exploring an evolving role for neurostimulation. *Spine (Phila Pa 1976)* 2017;42(Suppl 14):S35–40.

United States Surgeon General, "Facing Addiction in America." https://www.surgeongeneral.gov/library/2016alcoholdrugshealth/index.html.

Vickers AJ, et al. Acupuncture for chronic pain: Individual patient data meta-analysis. *Arch Intern Med* 2012;172(19):1444–1453.

Errors in Medical Practice

39

John F. Christensen, PhD

The most fruitful lesson is the conquest of one's own error. Whoever refuses to admit error may be a great scholar but is not a great learner. Whoever is ashamed of error will struggle against recognizing and admitting it, which means that he struggles against his greatest inward gain.

Goethe

INTRODUCTION

Errors are inevitable in the practice of medicine. The most obvious causes are failures in individual performance related to attention, memory, knowledge, judgment, skill, and motivation. Errors also result in part from the nature of medical work, such as the complexity of medical knowledge, the uncertainty of clinical predictions, and the need to make timely treatment decisions in spite of limited or uncertain knowledge. Mistakes are also caused by system factors that influence working conditions and processes. Although much attention has been focused on the harmful effects of errors on patients, it must be understood that these incidents can be correspondingly distressing for health care providers, evoking shock and feelings of remorse, guilt, anger, and fear.

If dealt with effectively, errors can provide powerful learning experiences for health professionals and organizations; however, difficulty in dealing with mistakes may impede both learning and efforts to prevent future errors. Professional norms that assume physician infallibility and treat mistakes as anomalies or personal failures pose significant barriers to learning. Judgmental institutional responses and fear of litigation are further disincentives to the open discussion of mistakes and reduce the potential for wider learning.

Definitions

It is useful to define several terms related to what are commonly referred to as errors or mistakes. The Institute of Medicine (IOM) defines an **error** as "the failure of a planned action to be completed as intended (i.e., error of execution), or the use of a wrong plan to achieve an aim (i.e., error of planning). An error may be an act of commission or an act of omission." An **adverse event** is an injury due to health care. Errors differ from adverse events because they do not necessarily cause harm. They differ from **negligence** or **malpractice**, which require both preventable harm and violation of the standard of practice.

Prevalence

Most studies of medical errors have focused on adverse events in the hospital setting. Although the overall prevalence of errors is uncertain, it appears that they are common. Studies conducted in multiple states and countries suggest that the rate of adverse events may be as high as 10%. The Canadian Adverse Events Study reported that the incidence of adverse events among hospital patients in Canada was 7.5 per 100 hospital admissions (7.5%).

It is estimated that at least half of adverse events are preventable. One study used a Global Trigger Tool (GTT) to systematically review medical records for specific clues or triggers suggesting that an adverse event has taken place and concluded that more than 400,000 deaths per year are associated with preventable harm to patients. Globally the WHO estimates that adverse events in hospitals are the 14th leading cause of morbidity and mortality. The cost associated with medication errors is estimated to be US$42 billion annually.

The prevalence of errors in outpatient practice is less well studied. Diagnostic errors are thought to affect about 1 in 20 U.S. adults in outpatient settings. One study documented a prescription error rate of 7.6%; another study suggests errors in at least one-quarter of encounters, with a rate of adverse drug events of 27 per 100 patients. A literature synthesis found that the median preventable adverse drug events prevalence rate was 16.5% in ambulatory care-based studies. A study of ambulatory oncology care found that medication reconciliation resulted in 31 changes per 100 prescriptions.

A survey of patients attending primary care clinics found that nearly one in three reported experiencing a mistake or diagnostic error by a physician in the previous 10 years, with 14% of patients having changed physicians as a result.

Types

Mistakes occur in every aspect of medical practice—diagnosis, decision making (often because of ignorance of facts), the pace of evaluation or its timing, prescribing medications, and performing tests and procedures. Common examples of medical errors include missing a diagnosis, prescribing an incorrect dosage of a medication, inappropriate or premature discharge of a patient from the hospital, accidentally cutting an artery during surgery, and failure to convey vital information when handing off a patient to another team. In the Harvard Medical Practice Study, the most common adverse events involved performance or follow-up of a procedure or operation (35%). Failure to take preventive measures (e.g., failure to guard against accidental injury) was the next most common error (22%), followed by diagnostic errors (e.g., failure to use indicated tests, act on test results, or avoid delays in response) (14%), errors involving drug treatment (9%), and system errors (2%).

Cognitive Errors

Cognitive errors may result from failures in perception, faulty pattern recognition, and common biases in thinking. Two broad areas of cognitive functioning are relevant in these errors: the schematic and attentional control modes. In the ***schematic control*** mode of functioning, which is typical of the expert, sequences of thinking and acting are embedded in unconscious subroutines that allow more mental energy to be available for other activities. Examples would be speaking one's native language or driving a vehicle. In medicine, some procedural skills as well as pattern recognition skills (such as an intuitive appreciation of a patient's condition or hunch about a diagnosis) are under schematic control. When an anomaly occurs, or when the physician is fatigued or stressed, a shift occurs to the ***attentional control*** mode, which is more energy intensive and requires more deliberate thinking and action. This model is more prevalent in the novice learning any new skill (a foreign language, a new procedural skill). The attentional control mode can more quickly degrade over time. Errors can occur in each of these cognitive modes. A momentary break in a skilled routine in surgery, or a lapse in attention that leads to missing data are common examples.

These two modes of cognitive functioning are related to Kahneman's distinction between "fast and slow thinking." The *schematic control* mode is an example of what Kahneman calls "system one" thinking, which is fast, automatic, frequent, and unconscious. The *attentional control* mode is "system two" thinking, which is slow, effortful, infrequent, calculating, and conscious.

Other cognitive errors result from *biases inherent in human thinking*. Among these are thinking tendencies such as the "availability" bias, in which the first diagnosis that comes to mind is deemed most likely; the "confirmatory" bias, in which only data supportive of the first hypothesis is entertained; the "recency" bias, in which the last serious diagnosis managed looms large in probability estimates; and the "gambler's fallacy," in which a series of similar diagnoses leads the clinician to expect that the next presentation will be of a different disease.

Procedural Errors

Procedural errors occur in both surgical and nonsurgical settings. One study suggested that major complications occurred in 3.4% of surgical operations. Wrong site surgeries and retained foreign bodies are rare, but they can have devastating consequences for patients. Causes include individual errors—such as surgical technique (including slips and fumbles), judgment errors, inattention to detail—and incomplete understanding of the case. Other causes occur at other levels of the system, including poor communication among members of the perioperative team, poor planning (e.g., surgical implant not available on the day of surgery), lack of teamwork, and surgical site infection. Contributions to error in nonsurgical procedures (e.g., endoscopy, lumbar puncture, and line placement) include fatigue and disruptions. Many procedural errors might be prevented by use of the Joint Commission Universal Protocol or by simulation training.

System Errors

Errors occur throughout the health care system, many arising from the inherent fallibility of human beings working within systems not primarily designed for safety. Errors occur at the level of patient, task, individual practitioner, team, unit, organization, and beyond. They also occur in multiple locations, such as in the clinical diagnostic laboratories, the pharmacy, and the preparation and maintenance of medical devices. Identification errors, which involve confusing one patient, test, or treatment for another, are a common element in some adverse events. Another common occasion for errors is in the handoffs between different health care providers and locations of care. Communication problems are at the root of many adverse events as are problems with team functioning.

Medication Errors

Medication errors are very common. In the United States, more than four out of five adults take at least one medication in a given week, and almost one-third of adults take at least five different medications. The goal of safe and effective medication use is referred to as "the five rights": the right drug, right dose, right route, right time, and right patient. However, errors can occur with any drug product at any point in the medication use process.

Causes

A combination of human and system-related factors can lead to adverse events. Human error, which occurs at what is sometimes referred to as the "sharp end" of adverse events, happens close to the patient and includes deficits in skill (attention, memory, and execution), knowledge, decision making, and following of rules. System errors, the "blunt end" of adverse events, occur at multiple levels, including at the levels of patient, task, individual provider, team, unit environment, department, and institution. Examples of system errors include team members who are unfamiliar with one another, inadequate communication at change of shifts, understaffed units, inadequate equipment, long work hours, and production pressures.

Individual clinicians report a variety of reasons for their mistakes and frequently attribute the mistakes to more than one cause. These include lack of essential knowledge about a particular clinical issue and an overload of tasks to perform in a limited time. Fatigue can interfere with the clinician's ability to rely upon the "schematic control" mode of cognitive functioning, leading to more reliance on the less efficient "attentional control" mode, which is more vulnerable to decay. The common cognitive biases mentioned above also contribute to diagnostic and decision-making errors by the individual clinician.

Many errors are caused by conditions in the workplace and organizational processes largely independent of clinician attributes. Studies of system factors demonstrate the predictive power of these organizational factors. One study of an inpatient medical service found cross-coverage to be a significant predictor of preventable adverse events. Recent studies suggest that staffing ratios tend to be related to patient outcomes. Similarly, the incentives offered by third-party payers to order fewer diagnostic tests and to limit the number of referrals to subspecialists can lead to errors of omission.

An overlooked contributor to the prevalence of medical errors is the culture of medicine itself. Historically the "hidden curriculum" in medical training has held up an ideal of perfectionism that is heroic in fantasy but unattainable in practice. This perspective views mistakes as a failure of character, often leading to a "blame and shame" response to error. Over-focusing on individual perfection has led to an unrealistic reliance on error-free performance. It underplays the "blunt end" of system errors and overemphasizes the "sharp end" of clinician error. These cultural biases tend to drive discussion of mistakes underground, thus avoiding the reporting and discussion of error that can lead to meaningful change.

A systems-oriented view acknowledges that errors are expected even in the best of organizations. Lucian Leape, a leading scholar of medical error, has suggested, "*Any system that relies on error-free performance is doomed to fail. We need to build systems that assume errors will occur, but that can identify and absorb them before they become catastrophes.*"

Circumstances

Mistakes seem to occur particularly frequently during residency training, possibly because interns and residents are learning new skills, honing their clinical judgment, and accepting new responsibilities. Many mistakes happen in the inpatient or emergency department setting. The surgical specialties and intensive care units have also been identified as areas of high risk for patient safety. Severely ill patients require rapid assessment of a complex clinical picture as well as multiple procedures, evaluations, and decisions, thus affording many opportunities for mistakes to occur. One study found that patients in intensive care units had on average 178 activities performed on them, with 1.7 errors observed per day.

Patient characteristics can also increase the risk of mistakes. The risk of adverse events increases with increased age, severity of illness, length of hospital stay, and number of drugs prescribed. Older patients, for example, are likely to have advanced disease and comorbid conditions and are more likely to be taking numerous medications. These factors increase both the risk of errors and the likelihood that these errors will cause harm.

Serious medical mistakes also occur in office practice. In the United States the main source of medical care for patients is in ambulatory settings. Due to the decentralized structure and diverse nature of events, medical errors can be common. Three top patient safety concerns are diagnostic errors, medication adverse events, and surgical errors. A study of malpractice claims showed that the former two errors are of concern for outpatient diagnosis and treatment of cancer.

THE OUTCOMES OF MEDICAL MISTAKES

Consequences for Patient & Family

Some errors may have no major consequences for patients. In such cases, clinicians may not even be aware that an error has occurred. Often, however, errors have significant consequences for the patients involved, such as physical discomfort, emotional distress, need for additional therapy or procedures, increased and prolonged hospital stay, worsening of disease, permanent disability, or death. Mistakes can also cause distress for family members, including worry, anger, and guilt, particularly if they were involved in making treatment decisions.

Consequences for Health Care Providers

An error leading to patient harm (preventable adverse event) has negative consequences for patients and their families, who are the "*first victims*." The health care professionals involved can also become victims in the sense that they are traumatized after the event (*second victims*), and often experience significant personal and professional distress. It is estimated that nearly half of health care providers experience the impact of an error as a second victim at least once in their career. Colleague and organizational support for these "second victims" is critical and will be discussed further below.

Physicians

Physicians may experience emotional distress in reaction to a medical mistake, often reporting a variety of emotional responses such as remorse, anger, guilt, feelings of inadequacy, shame, and fear—particularly the fear of negative repercussions, such as malpractice suits. After a fatal mistake involving a young patient, one resident wrote, "This event has been the greatest challenge to me in my training."

Self-perceived errors have been associated with decreased quality of life, depression, and burnout among physicians. Some physicians report persistent negative psychological effects and impact on their career from mistakes that they have made. After a mistake caused the death of a patient, one resident commented, "This case has made me very nervous about clinical medicine. I worry now about all febrile patients, since they may be on the verge of sepsis." For another resident, a missed diagnosis made him reject a career in subspecialties that would involve "a lot of data collection and uncertainty."

Advanced Health Practitioners, Nurses, & Other Clinical Staff

Until recently not much attention has been focused on the impact of medical errors on non-MD clinicians, nurses, and the health care team. One literature review examined the characteristics of the work environment that played a significant role in how nurses responded to medical errors. If the work environment was punitive toward error, nurses experienced decreased confidence and increased anxiety after a medical error event. The nurse manager was identified as a key person in creating a climate for dealing with errors. The type of support provided to nurses included the following: discussing the error; offering advice, sympathy, and verbal support; being respectful and discreet; and expressing trust in the nurse. If supported, nurses reported feelings of restored personal integrity and were more likely to make constructive changes.

Consequences for the Clinician–Patient Relationship

In some cases, depending on the severity of the outcome for the patient and the quality of communication between clinician and patient, their relationship may be harmed by a mistake. For the clinician, feelings of guilt and shame or shaken confidence may lead to avoidance of the patient or to a diminution of open and frank discussion. One physician, for example, reported that his guilt from the death of a patient led him to act like an indentured servant to the patient's family, attempting to expiate his "crime" over a prolonged period of time by spending more time with the family and reducing his fees.

For the patient, learning about a mistake may cause alarm and anxiety, destroying the patient's faith and confidence in the physician's ability to help. There may be anger, erosion of trust, decreased respect, or feelings of betrayal that diminish openness. Patients may become disillusioned with the medical profession in general, causing them to reduce their adherence to beneficial treatments or habits.

If the doctor and patient can discuss their emotions directly and with mutual understanding and acceptance, the relationship is likely to endure; it may even deepen with time. The negative effect of a mistake on the doctor–patient relationship may also be mitigated if there is a history of shared decision making, which diffuses the responsibility of the physician, especially when there has been uncertainty about treatment.

RESPONDING TO MEDICAL MISTAKES

The way in which physicians respond to mistakes can turn these experiences into powerful opportunities for learning and for personal growth. Figure 39-1 outlines a strategy for handling a mistake, whether made by oneself or by a colleague.

Individual Responses

After recognizing that a mistake has occurred, the first step is to take any corrective action possible. Other important steps include beginning one's own coping process, disclosure to the patient and family, disclosure to colleagues and the health organization's risk management department (sooner if there is a serious adverse outcome), and attempting to learn from the incident.

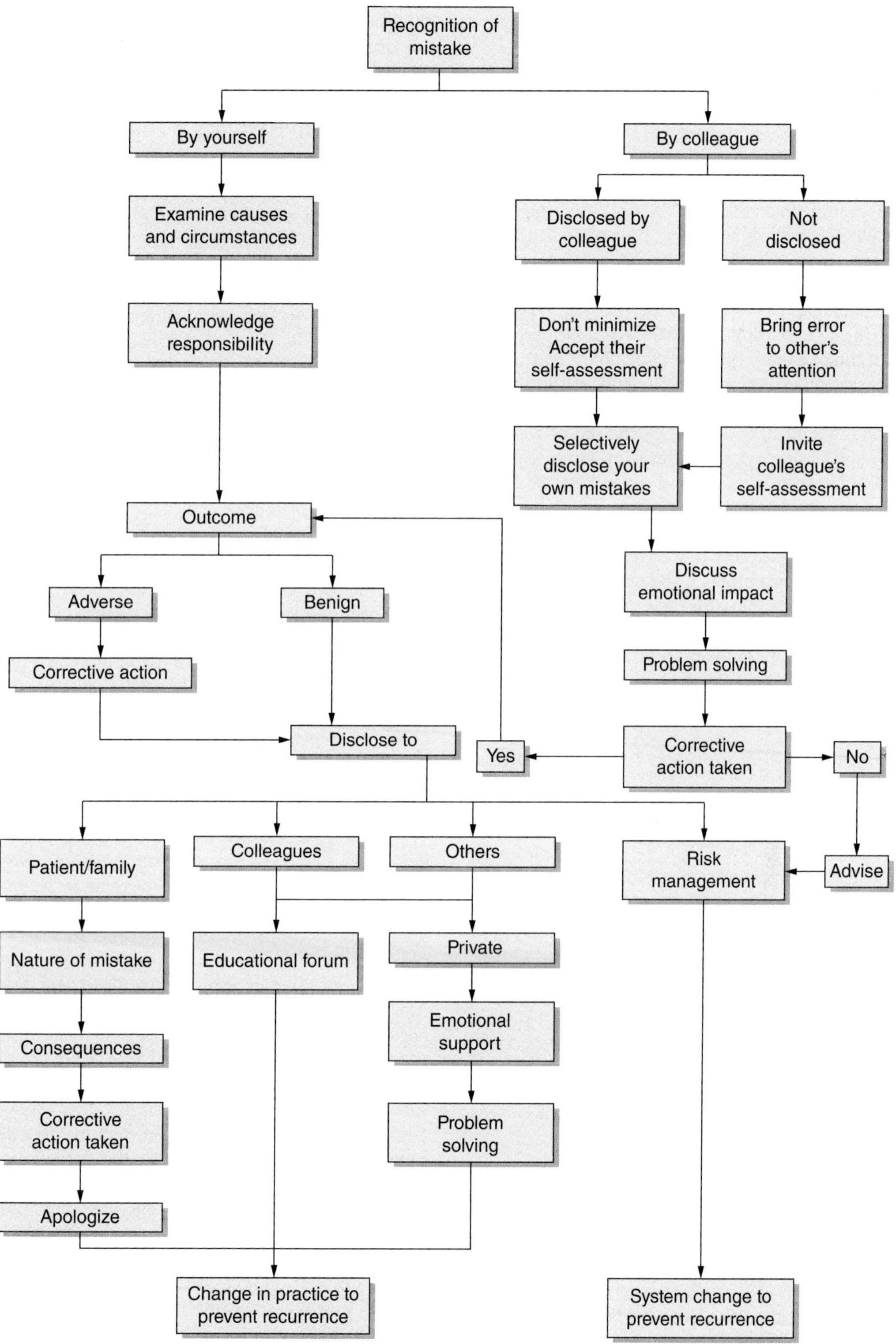

Figure 39-1. Strategy for handling mistakes.

Individual Coping With Mistakes

Two major modes of coping are *problem focused*, in which coping is directed at the problem causing the distress, and *emotion focused*, in which coping is directed at managing the emotional distress caused by the problem. Effective coping can prevent unhealthy responses such as denial, cynicism, and excessive concern. The use of effective coping strategies can also play a role in modulating physician stress and increasing physician work satisfaction.

Table 39-1 briefly summarizes some of the many possible strategies for coping with medical mistakes. Among these, accepting responsibility and problem-solving techniques may be those most often used. As an example, accepting responsibility would include statements such as "I made a promise to myself that things would be different next time"; "I criticized or lectured myself"; and "I apologized or did something to make it up." Seeking social support and controlling emotions may be somewhat less frequently employed, and escape/avoidance and distancing are used even more rarely.

Accepting responsibility is a prerequisite to an individual learning from a mistake, and physicians who cope by accepting responsibility for their mistakes seem to be more likely to make constructive changes in practice. They may also be more likely to experience emotional distress, however, as in the case of the resident who described persistent feelings of guilt and shame after realizing that inappropriate management of a diabetic patient's foot ulcer led to an amputation.

Table 39-1. Potential strategies for coping with medical mistakes.

Approach	Strategy
Problem focused	Acceptance of responsibility Consultation to understand nature of mistake Consultation to correct mistake Planned problem solving (e.g., obtaining extra training)
Emotion focused	Pursuance of social support Reframing of mistake (e.g., recognizing it as inherent in practicing medicine) Disclosure to colleague, friend, or spouse Disclosure to patient Emotional self-control (e.g., repressing one's emotional response) Escape/avoidance Distancing

Data from Wu AW, Folkman S, McPhee SJ, et al. How house officers cope with their mistakes: doing better but feeling worse? *West J Med* 1993;159:565–569; Christensen JF, Levinson W, Dunn PM. The heart of darkness: the impact of perceived mistakes on physicians. *J Gen Intern Med* 1992;7:424.

Disclosure to Patients & Families

It is difficult to disclose mistakes to patients or their families, and several reports suggest that physicians are reluctant to tell patients about mistakes. Studies suggest that physicians and trainees have conflicting feelings of responsibility to the patient, colleagues, institution, and themselves. These feelings are complicated by fears, anxieties, and an uncertain self-efficacy and outcome expectancy. There are many barriers to disclosure, including fear of damaging one's reputation as well as fear of disciplinary action and litigation. Even the National Practitioner Databank, designed to improve quality of care, provokes fear and resentment among physicians.

Professional societies, including the American Medical Association and American College of Physicians, as well as legal and ethical experts suggest that in general physicians should disclose errors to those involved. The Canadian Disclosure Guidelines state that "when a harmful incident occurs, the patient should be told what happened. Disclosure acknowledges and informs the patient, which is critical in maintaining the patient's trust and confidence in the healthcare system." Disclosure of a mistake also fosters learning by compelling the physician to acknowledge the error truthfully. In addition, when there are serious adverse consequences, disclosing a mistake to the patient may be the only way for the clinician to achieve a sense of absolution.

In the past, clinicians have been unaware of the guidelines that exist on disclosing adverse events to patients, leaving them to develop their own approach to each case. Disclosure and discussion of an error with the patient or family can be made easier by several techniques. First, clinicians should try to acknowledge their own emotions. Before approaching the patient or family, it may be helpful for clinicians to center themselves (perhaps with diaphragmatic breathing for relaxation) and to remind themselves that the adverse event and present feelings do not define them as either a healer or a person. Second, rehearsing a few simple, direct statements ahead of time can provide a road map in this awkward moment. Finally, when meeting the patient or family, the clinician should make a brief, direct statement, accompanied by a genuine apology. Such directness may help avoid the kind of long and rambling discussion that often increases anxiety for both clinician and patient.

For example, if a medication was mistakenly prescribed without checking the patient's allergies, the clinician might tell the patient: "Mr. Jones, I've discovered what made you sick last week. I regret to say that I failed to check whether you were allergic to the antibiotic before I prescribed it. You are allergic to it, and that information is clearly in your medical record. I feel awful that my not checking has caused you so much distress. I am truly sorry." It would then be appropriate to pause and allow the patient to respond. Reflecting and accepting the patient's feelings can help to heal the relationship more effectively than overwhelming the patient with information. The clinician–patient relationship can be enhanced by honesty and empathy in this difficult and sensitive moment (see Chapter 3).

It is possible that disclosure of an error of which the patient had been unaware may lead to a lawsuit, particularly if there was serious harm. It is certain, however, that the risk of a lawsuit is multiplied when a cover-up comes to light. Limited evidence suggests that risk may be reduced if disclosure is made promptly, if the patient appreciates the clinician's honesty, if it is part of an ongoing dialogue about the patient's care, and if there is a sincere apology. In the event of serious injury, a prompt and fair settlement may be essential.

Several organizations have reduced costs and litigation as a result of a policy of full disclosure. For example, one academic health center adopted guidelines for full disclosure that emphasizes five principles, including effective and honest communication to patients and families, a sincere apology and rapid compensation for inappropriate care, learning from mistakes, quick disciplinary action for recklessness, and proper support for physicians and staff. There are seven pillars of their guidelines: (1) All cases require patient safety incident reporting. (2) In the case of an incident, they launch an immediate, standardized investigation. (3) A risk manager or patient safety officer aids physicians in communication and full disclosure. (4) If there is harm as a result of unreasonable care, there is early compensation, apology, and remediation. (5) Prompt system improvement follows a root cause analysis. (6) There is data tracking and performance evaluation of the system improvement. (7) All personnel receive education and training on the system improvement. These guidelines have not led to increase in litigation or compensation. Another result was increased recognition of provider stress leading to peer support. These guidelines emphasize the crucial importance of timeliness in responding to any patient safety incident.

Disclosure to Colleagues & the Institution

It may be important for colleagues to know about a mistake, particularly if they are also participating in the care of the patient as a supervisor or other member of the team. Knowing about a mistake can also benefit the institution, enabling it to provide assistance in handling the mistake, to help individuals appreciate the causes or significance of the incident and learn from it, and to prevent future occurrences. Physicians, however, seem reluctant to tell their colleagues about mistakes. Some physicians report that they find this kind of discussion both threatening, because of the fear of judgment by colleagues, and unhelpful, because of the tendency of colleagues to minimize the event. Discussing mistakes with colleagues, however, serves the purpose of problem-focused coping: correcting the situation that led to the mistake. Sharing mistakes with colleagues can also provide emotion-focused coping by preventing isolation and starting the necessary healing process of remorse and learning.

Changes in Practice

Table 39-2 summarizes changes in practice that often follow an error. These changes can either be constructive or they can be defensive and/or maladaptive. Constructive changes cited by physicians include paying more attention to detail, confirming clinical data personally, changing protocols for diagnosis and treatment, increasing self-care, changing methods of communication with staff, and being willing to seek advice. Additional constructive action includes attempting to effect institutional change to prevent future incidents.

Physicians also report making defensive changes. These include an unwillingness to discuss the mistake, avoidance of similar patients, and—in some circumstances—ordering additional tests. Defensive changes in practice are more likely to occur if the institutional response to a mistake is punitive or judgmental.

Table 39-2. Common changes in practice following mistakes.

Constructive Change	Defensive Change
Increasing information seeking • Asking advice • Reading Increasing vigilance • Paying more attention to detail • Confirming data personally • Changing data organization • Ordering additional tests as appropriate • Improving screening for disease Improving communication with patients Improving self-pacing Improving communication with staff Supervising others more closely	Being unwilling to discuss the error Avoiding patients with similar problems Ordering additional but unnecessary tests

Learning From Errors

Several factors may determine the extent to which physicians learn from mistakes. When negative emotions such as shame, guilt, or humiliation follow from the mistake, the clinician's energy may focus on the emotional aspects of coping. Addressing these negative emotions directly can enhance the clinician's ability to learn new information or new approaches to the problem. Failure to appreciate these emotions can lead to denial. The cause to which the clinician attributes the mistake can also affect learning. Physicians in one study were more likely to report constructive changes if the mistake was caused by inexperience or faulty judgment in a complex case; they were less likely to do so if they believed that the mistake was caused by job overload. Physicians who responded to the mistake with greater acceptance of responsibility and more discussion were also more likely to report constructive changes.

Responding to Colleagues Who Make Mistakes

When responding to a colleague who discloses an error, it is important to elicit or accept the colleague's self-assessment and not to minimize the importance of the incident. At this point, a selective and discreet disclosure of one's own past mistakes can reduce the colleague's sense of isolation and legitimize the discussion. It is then appropriate to inquire about the emotional impact of the mistake and how the colleague is coping with it. An important consideration here is that negative emotions are not necessarily problems to be solved, and they can often be mitigated by acknowledging them. The clinician should return to the content of the mistake and help the colleague to correct it with problem-solving techniques, making the necessary changes in practice and incorporating the new lessons that have been learned.

Providing a safe setting in which clinicians can share mistakes and their emotional impact can correct the culture of perfectionism and provide a mutually supportive approach to learning from these experiences. One of the authors (JFC) has developed a workshop format in which physicians from various specialties have reflected in small groups on their mistakes. After writing a brief narrative of the mistake, they discuss in a confidential setting the emotional impact the mistake had on them, how they coped with these emotions, whether they disclosed the error to anyone, the personal beliefs underlying their emotional responses, and the changes in clinical practice that ensued. Many participants have shared afterward that this was the first time they had shared their experience of the error with anyone. Learning from others' stories and being listened to in a nonjudgmental format facilitated their healing.

One institutional approach to supporting clinicians suffering emotionally in the wake of errors is the development of a "second victim" support team. In this approach, a team of clinicians is trained to provide emergency peer support to clinicians involved in a traumatic patient-related event. Additional levels of support are then offered in the days and weeks following the event, depending on the clinician's needs.

Witnessing Mistakes by Others

A clinician who sees an error made by another clinician has several options: waiting for the clinician to disclose to the patient, advising the clinician to disclose the mistake, actively telling the patient oneself, or arranging a joint meeting to discuss the mistake. Although some clinicians may feel an obligation to report mistakes they have seen, most are reluctant to say anything. There are many barriers to such a discussion, including fear of eliciting anger and threatening relationships with colleagues or referral sources.

The simplest option is to wait for the clinician who made the mistake to report it. There is no assurance, however, that the patient will actually be informed. Telling the patient directly may be awkward, particularly if the observing clinician does not know the patient, and doing so may interfere with the existing provider–patient relationship. Advising the clinician who made the error to tell the patient may fulfill the observing clinician's responsibility for disclosure, but the patient may still not be informed. Simultaneously advising the clinician and the hospital or clinic quality-assurance or risk-management personnel increases the likelihood that the patient will be told. Arranging a joint conference can satisfy the observer that appropriate disclosure is made while preserving the primacy of the relationship between the patient and the treating clinician (see Figure 39-1).

INSTITUTIONAL RESPONSES

Hospitals & Clinics

A goal for institutions is to develop a "safety culture" that allows learning from adverse events. A safety culture encourages clinicians to be aware of the potential for error and to include system thinking in their everyday practices, and it provides adequate data regarding errors to managers. Physicians sometimes feel that a climate of judgment inhibits them from talking about their mistakes. To avoid a vicious circle of blame, denial, and repeated problems, it is crucial for senior health system leadership to assume a blame-free attitude that encourages the reporting and handling of errors. Some institutions have formal settings for discussing mistakes, such as morbidity and mortality conferences. However, important issues such as a discussion of the physician's feelings about the mistake and disclosure by colleagues of how they coped with their own mistakes are commonly avoided in these conferences. The risk management departments of health centers could take a leading role in this area—promoting comprehensive, supportive forums for discussing mistakes and using emotion-focused coping to maximize problem-focused learning and to minimize future errors.

Graduate Medical Education

In spite of fears of public disclosure of mistakes, there is growing consensus that patient safety, physician fallibility, and methods of handling medical errors are appropriate topics for medical school, residency, and fellowship training. Although they may experience initial reluctance, physicians sometimes find that discussing a mistake is a positive experience: "Presenting this case at interns' report was difficult—I felt under a lot of scrutiny from my peers. In the end, I felt as though I had gotten more respect from presenting this kind of case rather than one in which I had made a great diagnosis."

Mistakes can be discussed in attending rounds, at morning report, or at morbidity and mortality conferences. In these venues, it is important to address issues such as overwork, burnout, shared responsibility with other physicians (e.g., consultants and attending physicians), and appropriate protocols for communicating with staff. These discussions also present a good opportunity to expose cognitive biases and explain strategies to reduce them. In addition, although ensuring that everyone involved learns from the mistake, care should be taken that errors are seen as an unfortunate inevitability in the practice of medicine and that there are appropriate ways of coping with them and of responding to colleagues who make them. To address variability in faculty response and local culture, training institutions can disseminate clear, accessible algorithms to guide behavior when medical errors occur.

Disclosing clinical errors to patients and families is a teachable skill. Several medical residency training curricula have incorporated modules to enhance trainees' skills in this very difficult kind of communication. One review of such curricula found that most consisted of a brief, single encounter, combining didactic lectures, or small group discussions with role-play. Several studies described learners' self-reported improvements in knowledge, skills, and attitudes toward disclosure.

Greater attention should also be given to practicing physicians in the outpatient setting. Evidence shows that a short formal curriculum improves attitudes and comfort toward full disclosure of medical errors, allowing cultural change in patient safety. Future work could focus on identified themes such as learning from errors and near misses, learning and teaching in emotionally charged situations, and balance between individual and systems responsibility.

Primary Care Practice Groups

Collegial support should be an explicit rule, providing a safe and confidential setting for discussion of the mistake (see the guidelines discussed earlier for responding to a colleague's mistake). It would also be wise for the practice group to formalize—and thus legitimize—periodic discussions about mistakes; these could broaden the scope of the emotion-focused support, allow members to learn from colleagues' mistakes, and address system flaws that contribute to the mistakes. A bonus of this approach is the gain in personal well-being of the group members—a nonspecific yet significant contribution to the practice climate.

PREVENTING MISTAKES

Reducing the frequency and severity of mistakes is the highest priority. There are several ways to help clinicians learn from their mistakes and to make constructive changes in practice. The majority of improvements, however, need to occur at the system level.

Individual Clinician

As noted earlier, clinicians should be encouraged to accept responsibility for their mistakes. Although those who do so seem more likely than those who do not to make constructive changes in practice, accepting responsibility for mistakes can engender emotional distress. It is therefore important for colleagues and supervisors to respond with sensitivity to the distress of practitioners acknowledging their mistakes. The probability of future mistakes can be reduced if the current error can be reviewed in a way that decreases emotional distress, invites disclosure of uncertainty in diagnosis and management, and leads to a discussion of appropriate changes in practice.

Many medication errors are caused by poor communication or misunderstandings about the use of medication. Physicians should place greater emphasis on reconciling their own lists with their patients and informing patients about appropriate medication use. They can also encourage patients to become more active members of the health care team. For example, patients should maintain lists of their own medications and allergies and take every opportunity to share these with their clinicians.

Developing self-awareness can be a vital corrective to the cognitive biases mentioned above. Both in medical training and continuing medical education, learning the skills of mindfulness (see Chapter 7) can help clinicians be aware of the emotional and contextual conditions in which they are more likely to engage in cognitive shortcuts (low-level decision rules) that lead to diagnostic errors. They can learn to default to high-level decision rules, for example, looking beyond early hypotheses, when they perceive themselves as impatient, fatigued, or anxious for a quick resolution.

System

Simple, easily implemented safety strategies to prevent errors include consistent use of a reliable method to verify patient identity, use of metric measurements, and adequate workplace illumination and organization. Other strategies include elimination of abbreviations and acronyms, provision of up-to-date information at the point of care, and partnering with patients regarding their own safety. At the level of individual tasks, thoughtful standardization can enhance patient safety. Reading back laboratory results during telephone calls is a cost-effective way of reducing miscommunication. Using auto racing and Formula 1 pit stops as a model, standardizing handoffs of patients can reduce technical errors, improve information handoffs, and reduce the duration of handoffs in an easy to teach protocol.

Administration

Efforts to forestall errors must begin at the highest administrative levels. Making patient safety an explicit priority is crucial in helping institutions learn from mistakes. Clinically, more active supervision may prevent some mistakes or mitigate their adverse effects. Senior clinicians should be more available to their less experienced colleagues for help in making critical decisions, especially in complex cases that require more mature clinical judgment. Group practice administrators and training program directors should address problems in staffing, scheduling, and nature of work—which may all contribute to mistakes. Optimizing communication during handoffs between different providers and care locations is an important goal.

Sleep deprivation has been shown to be a source of errors; job overload and fatigue can also lead to mistakes. Working under these conditions may lead residents to tolerate and rationalize errors; in addition, it may make them less likely to seek the corrective information that could help prevent future mistakes. Senior clinicians are also vulnerable to the effects of sleep deprivation.

Using protocols, standardizing procedures, and employing checklists can help physicians do the right thing. Examples of such protocols include a "Sign Your Site" protocol for surgeons to eliminate the risk of wrong-site surgery, the WHO Safer Surgery Checklist to reduce other problems in surgical care, a "central line cart" providing needed supplies to reduce catheter-related bloodstream infections, and a simple checklist to improve medication reconciliation as patients move from surgical recovery room to the ward.

Changes in staffing can also improve safety. Having a dedicated nurse for discharge facilitations in close cooperation with residents and primary care physicians can increase hospital discharges, increase patient satisfaction and medication reconciliation, and reduce work hours for residents. The addition of specialist nurses and specialist support roles such as dietary assistants can also have an important impact on positive patient outcomes. Decreasing the patient-to-nurse ratio can decrease mortality rate, although it increases hospital costs. Hospital administrators need to carefully balance costs with workloads and allow nurse supervisors more control in setting staffing levels to ensure patient safety. A 10% rise in occupancy has been shown to increase the risk of adverse events by up to 15% in hospitals that are continually overcapacity.

Identifying & Reporting Errors

Investigation and root cause analysis to elucidate the causes of adverse events often suggest specific strategies for preventing future harm. This is aided by routine mechanisms to identify adverse events, such as anonymous reporting by physicians and nurses or computerized feedback about adverse drug reactions, which are beginning to prove useful in providing information about the frequency and nature of mistakes.

Workplace Design

Interventions can be applied at the level of specific tasks and clinical microsystems. A "human factors" approach seeks to optimize the relationship between humans and systems by studying human behavior, abilities, and limitations and using this knowledge to design systems for safe and effective human use. Assuming that the human component of any system will inevitably produce errors, human factors engineers design human/machine interfaces and systems that are tough enough to reduce both the rate of errors and the effects of the inevitable error within the system.

Changes can be made to the physical design and layout of work areas to improve safety. Some of these changes are intended to overcome barriers to following good practice. For example, compliance with hand hygiene guidelines can be improved by optimizing design features of alcohol hand gel dispensers.

Computerized Systems

Computerized systems can detect and avert medication errors, including overdoses, incorrect routes of administration, drug interactions, and allergies. Computerized order entry systems, automated medication-dispensing machines, and bar coding of medications, blood products, and patients have been shown to reduce the incidence of adverse events.

It is essential, however, that new technology be introduced in a way that acknowledges the risks as well as benefits of such change. Health care workers must receive sufficient preparation and training so that technologies are not disruptive or that they themselves do not become inadvertent sources of error. There are risks, however, when clinicians, hospitals or health systems become over-reliant on technology to the extent that vigilance about errors may become dulled.

SUMMARY

Individual physicians, leaders, and institutions should make whatever changes in practice are warranted to prevent new mistakes and to prevent the recurrence of similar events. Providing emotional support to clinicians in the wake of a mistake can reduce distress and increase the likelihood of meaningful learning that leads to constructive changes in practice. The training of health care clinicians should include confidential, nonpunitive opportunities for discussing mistakes and their emotional impact on both clinician and patient. Recognizing and dealing with mistakes honestly and directly can improve the quality of patient care and lead to more rewarding practice.

ACKNOWLEDGMENT

Stephen J. McPhee, MD and Albert W. Wu, MD, MPH contributed to this chapter in the fourth edition and some material from that chapter has been retained here.

SUGGESTED READINGS

Christensen JF, Levinson W, Dunn PM. The heart of darkness: the impact of perceived mistakes on physicians. *J Gen Intern Med* 1992;7:424–431.

Gillies R, Speers S, Young S, et al. Teaching medical error apologies: development of a multi-component intervention. *Fam Med* 2011;43:400–406.

Graber ML, Kissam, S, Payne VL, et al. Cognitive interventions to reduce diagnostic error: a narrative review. *BMJ Qual Saf* 2012;21(7):535–557.

Helmchen L, Richards M, McDonald T. How does routine disclosure of medical error affect patients' propensity to sue and their assessment of provider quality? *Med Care* 2010;48:955–961.

Institute of Medicine. *Preventing Medication Errors.* Washington, DC: National Academies Press; 2006.

James JT. A new, evidence-based estimate of patient harms associated with hospital care. *J Patient Saf* 2013;9:122–128.

Kachalia A, Kaufman SR, Boothman R, et al. Liability claims and costs before and after implementation of a medical error disclosure program. *Ann Intern Med* 2010;153:213–221. PMID: 20713789.

Kohn LT, Corrigan JM, Donaldson MS, et al, eds. Committee on Quality of Health Care in America, Institute of Medicine. In: *To Err is Human. Building a Safer Health Care System.* Washington, DC: National Academy Press; 2000.

Lewis EJ, Baernholdt M, Hamric AB. Nurses' experience of medical errors: an integrative literature review. *J Nurs Care Qual* 2013;28:153–161.

Patient Safety Advisory Group. Health care worker fatigue and patient safety. The Joint Commission Sentinel Event Alert 2011; 2018 Addendum; 48:1–4. https://www.jointcommission.org/sea_issue_48/.

Seys D, Wu A, Gerven EV, et al. Health care professionals as second victims after adverse events: a systematic review. *Eval Health Prof* 2012;36:135–162.

Stroud L, Wong BM, Hollenberg E, Levinson L. Teaching medical error disclosure to physicians-in-training: a scoping review. *Acad Med* 2013;88:884–892.

West CP, Huschka MM, Novotny PJ, et al. Association of perceived medical errors with resident distress and empathy: a prospective longitudinal study. *JAMA* 2006;296:1071–1078.

Wu AW, Cavanaugh TA, McPhee SJ, et al. To tell the truth: ethical and practical issues in disclosing medical mistakes to patients. *J Gen Intern Med* 1997;12:770–775.

OTHER RESOURCES

Barnett P. Dialogue about unwanted and tragic outcomes. Web-based learning module in *DocCom: an Online Communication Curriculum.* American Academy on Communication in Healthcare. https://doccom.org/. Accessed August 2019.

WHO Multi-professional Patient Safety Curriculum Guide. https://www.who.int/patientsafety/education/mp_curriculum_guide/en/. Accessed August 2019.

WHO 10 Facts on Patient Safety. https://www.who.int/features/factfiles/patient_safety/en/ Updated March 2018. Accessed August 2019.

VIDEO

Video 39-1. Disclosing Medical Errors (9 min, 39 sec) Access by scanning the QR code above or visit mhprofessional.com/feldman5evideos.

Intimate Partner Violence

40

Mitchell D. Feldman, MD, MPhil, FACP & Gina Moreno-John, MD

INTRODUCTION

Intimate partner violence (IPV) is defined as any intentional, controlling behavior consisting of physical, sexual, or psychological assault, or stalking by a current or former intimate partner. IPV affects men and women from all socioeconomic strata, professions, locations, and cultural backgrounds. Women visiting outpatient medical and obstetric/gynecologic clinics as well as the emergency department (ED) are often there for complaints directly attributable to IPV. Because they are frequently misdiagnosed, they may return time and time again, often with increasingly severe trauma. In addition to increased morbidity and mortality of victims, IPV confers a tremendous financial burden in the United States. The total annual costs related to IPV are estimated to be between $2 and $7 billion, and the CDC estimates that the lifetime costs are up to $36 trillion, including medical expenditures, lost productivity among victims and perpetrators, criminal justice costs, and property loss or other damage.

Despite its magnitude in society and in medical settings, IPV is sometimes described as a "silent epidemic." Considered a private family problem by the government, and a social problem by the medical establishment, victims often have nowhere to turn. This predicament has gradually improved. Intimate partner violence is now acknowledged to be an important public health problem, and medical practitioners have a variety of diagnostic and treatment guidelines available to them. All clinicians must be knowledgeable about and comfortable with the evaluation and care of patients who are subjected to IPV (also see Chapter 41).

EPIDEMIOLOGY

Recent information from the CDC-sponsored National Intimate Partner and Sexual Violence Survey (NIPSVS) found that 37% of women have experienced sexual or physical violence or stalking by an intimate partner in their lifetime, with up to 23% of women and 14% of men reporting severe physical violence by an intimate partner (including acts such as being hit with something hard, being kicked or beaten, or being burned on purpose). This type of violence is more prevalent during a woman's lifetime than diabetes, depression, or breast cancer. In addition, an estimated 19.3% of women and 1.7% of men in the United States reported having been raped, and cross-sectional studies from outpatient primary care clinics and ED settings have found even higher rates in primary care, emergency departments, obstetrics and gynecology clinics, and mental health and addiction practices. Pregnancy has been found to double the risk of IPV. IPV accounts for more than half the murders of women in the United States every year. Unfortunately, prevalence rates have remained essentially unchanged since 2010.

Most studies ask about violence exclusively in the context of heterosexual relationships. However, a similar prevalence of IPV appears to exist in LGBT (Lesbian, Gay, Bisexual, Transgender) relationships, with the same physical and emotional consequences. In fact, the NIPSVS shows that the highest prevalence of lifetime physical violence, rape, and stalking is among bisexual women (61%). Most bisexual women report having only male perpetrators (90%). In addition, the NIPSVS found rates of 44% for IPV among lesbian women and 26% among gay men. Primary care providers should be aware that it may be more difficult for LGBT patients to disclose that they are in an abusive relationship for social and legal reasons, and they are less likely to actively seek help compared with heterosexual victims. In addition, the commonly held bias that violence does not occur in these relationships further lowers detection rates.

Men report being physically abused by their female partners at rates just below those reported by women. The NIPSVS shows that 29% of men have experienced rape, physical violence, and/or stalking by an intimate partner in their lifetimes. Up to 14% of men report severe physical violence. Unfortunately, there are fewer research studies focusing on men than women, in part because the prevalence of serious consequences of violence is higher among women than among men and serious injury is more likely for women. Nearly two-thirds of men affected by IPV, however, do not receive the services needed.

DIAGNOSIS

Many women seek medical care both for the direct and indirect consequences of IPV, but only a small percentage of them are diagnosed and treated appropriately. The following case is illustrative of the type of patient commonly seen in medical settings.

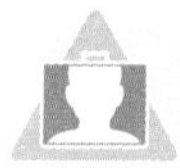

CASE ILLUSTRATION 1

A 40-year-old nurse presents to the ED with a chief complaint of a headache. She reports having been in a motor vehicle accident 3 days earlier and striking her head on the dashboard. She says that her friends encouraged her to come in, and she is accompanied to the ED (but not the office) by her partner. On physical examination she appears tense and sad, with bilateral, periorbital ecchymoses.

History

A thorough history is the cornerstone of the diagnosis of IPV. Because the presentation is often subtle, with few dramatic injuries, detection requires a high index of suspicion. There are many clues in the medical history, as shown by the case illustration, that should prompt the physician to evaluate the patient for IPV (Table 40-1). Patients who have been assaulted often delay seeking medical attention, in contrast to accident victims who generally seek out medical attention immediately. Injuries that are attributed to a mechanism that seems illogical should always raise concern. For example, periorbital ecchymoses ("black eyes") generally are not caused by a motor vehicle accident, a "doorknob," or anything other than a fist.

Table 40-1. When to screen for IPV.

- Delay in seeking care
- Illogical explanation of injury
- Multiple somatic complaints
- Depression, anxiety, and other mental disorders
- Pregnancy
- Substance use
- Recent diagnosis of HIV
- Family history of IPV
- Overbearing partner

Chronic Conditions

The CDC's Behavioral Risk Factor Surveillance System (BRFSS) survey highlights the increase in chronic conditions among people who experience IPV. These conditions include diabetes, asthma, arthritis, hypertension, hyperlipidemia, and cardiovascular disease. This survey is the largest nationally representative telephone survey of health conditions in the United States and indicates that health care providers should look beyond physical injuries when assessing patients who may be at risk for partner violence.

Multiple Somatic Complaints

Some persons present with vague somatic complaints as their only symptom of IPV. Fatigue, sleep disturbance, headache, gastrointestinal complaints, abdominal and pelvic pain, genitourinary problems such as frequent urinary tract and genital infections, chest pain, palpitations, and dizziness are just some of the complaints with which women present. IPV should be considered as a sole or contributing cause of these problems.

Depression, Anxiety, And Other Mental Disorders

Depression, eating disorders, and anxiety disorders such as posttraumatic stress disorder (PTSD) and panic disorder are more common among victims of IPV than among the general population. If these conditions are present, the clinician should always screen for IPV, and, if IPV is known to be a factor in a patient's history, screening for mental health disorders is essential. These mental and behavioral disturbances should be thought of as a consequence, not a cause, of IPV. Some patients may feel hopeless and turn toward suicide as a way out. Studies show that 10% to 31% of battered women have attempted suicide in their lifetime; of those, 50% try more than once.

Pregnancy

Unintended pregnancy can be associated with IPV. Factors associated with this outcome can include forced or coerced sex, a partner's refusal to use condoms, or sabotaging a woman's contraception. Other studies have demonstrated that women are at increased risk of physical and sexual abuse during pregnancy. Clues to be alert for include delay in seeking prenatal care, depressed or anxious mood, injuries to breasts or abdomen, frequent spontaneous abortions, and preterm labor. In addition to the physical and emotional trauma to the pregnant woman, these assaults can result in preterm birth, low birth weight, placental separation, fetal fractures, and fetal demise.

Substance Use

Although violence and substance use may coexist, it is inaccurate and generally not helpful to frame IPV as secondary to the substance use. Although the perpetrator, and at times the survivor him or herself, often asserts that violence is a consequence of altered behavior from drugs or alcohol, in fact the violent behavior must be addressed as a separate issue and is unlikely to end even if the substance use does.

Conversely, some studies have found an increased rate of substance use in victims of IPV. At times, this may take the form of increased use of pain medications, anxiolytics, or other substances in an effort to cope with the assaults. It is even more imperative in this instance that clinicians not attribute the IPV to the substance use; it is precisely this mentality of "blaming the victim" that has often prevented the appropriate evaluation and treatment of IPV in all medical settings.

HIV AND STIs

Among women of reproductive age, partner violence is associated with poor sexual health outcomes, including recurrent sexually transmitted infections and human immunodeficiency virus (HIV) infection. Some women report an initiation or escalation of IPV after informing their partner of their HIV seropositive status. Although every attempt should be made to notify sexual partners of HIV-positive results, practitioners should assess their patient's risk of violence while discussing the issues surrounding notification. Discussion of IPV and review of a safety plan should always be part of post-test counseling (see Chapter 37).

RISK FACTORS

FAMILY HISTORY OF IPV

Patients who report a family history of IPV, particularly those who witnessed parental violence as a child or adolescent, are at increased risk themselves even if they are not presently in an abusive relationship. Such women should, therefore, be educated and screened more carefully.

OVERBEARING PARTNER

An overbearing partner who, for example, insists on accompanying the patient into the examining room, acts overly solicitous or concerned (sometimes to the point of knocking on the examining room door to inquire about her well-being), or is hostile to the health care team may be a clue to the presence of IPV. Never probe about IPV if the perpetrator is in the examining room, as this may unintentionally escalate the violence and put the patient in extreme danger.

SOCIOECONOMIC OR ETHNIC STATUS

Many health care providers mistakenly believe that IPV disproportionately affects persons from certain ethnic or socioeconomic groups; in fact, it cuts across all groups and all economic strata. Although some studies have found that women who are uninsured or on medical assistance are at increased risk of IPV, this is most likely due to selection bias in the studies. Women from lower socioeconomic status (SES) groups may be overrepresented in some statistics, because those from higher SES groups have more resources available to them and the abuse is therefore more likely to remain hidden. Women with fewer resources are forced to take refuge in shelters or county hospital EDs, for example, whereas their middle-class counterparts may flee to a hotel or their offices and are therefore underrepresented by some of the surveys.

CASE ILLUSTRATION 2

A 28-year-old postdoctoral fellow presents to her primary care practitioner (PCP) complaining of new-onset insomnia and headache. On physical examination, the PCP discovers bruising on her chest and back and inquiries about IPV. The patient breaks down and reports that her partner, a professor at the university, has been emotionally and physically abusing her for years and that only one friend was aware of this history. When the abuse escalated, the patient would seek refuge in her laboratory, sometimes conducting experiments all night.

PHYSICAL EXAMINATION

The physical examination may provide the first clues of the presence of IPV. These include what appears to be "inappropriate" behavior, multiple injuries, central pattern of injury, and injuries at different stages of healing (Table 40-2).

INAPPROPRIATE BEHAVIOR

Behavior that appears to be inappropriate at the time of the physical examination may be a sign of IPV. Fright, inappropriate embarrassment or laughter, anxiety, passivity, shyness, and avoidance of eye contact may all be clues of IPV.

MULTIPLE INJURIES

Intimate partner violence victims are more likely to have multiple injuries than most accident victims. Patients

Table 40-2. Physical examination clues to the presence of IPV.

- Inappropriate behavior
- Multiple injuries
- Central pattern of injury
- Injuries at different stages of healing

who have been subjected to IPV, for example, typically have injuries to the head, neck, face, abdomen, and chest, whereas accident victims often present with less widespread trauma. The common emotional reactions to an IPV assault—denial, confusion, and withdrawal—may also lead to more extensive injuries.

CENTRAL PATTERN OF INJURY

Victims of IPV often experience injuries such as bruises, lacerations, burns, bites, and more severe injuries secondary to assaults with a deadly weapon or repeated beatings that cause massive internal injuries and fractures. Injuries are most commonly seen in the central areas of the body—the head, neck, chest, abdomen, breasts—and occasionally upper arms from fending off blows.

INJURIES AT DIFFERENT STAGES OF HEALING

As with child abuse, multiple injuries at different stages of healing should always prompt an inquiry about IPV.

In summary, medical providers must be alert to the signs and symptoms of IPV. It is important to remember that most IPV victims do not present with injuries that require emergency treatment or lead to hospitalization. In fact, for many patients, even in EDs, the presenting complaint is often medical or psychological, rather than a physical injury. For this reason, detection of IPV will increase only if clinicians include it on the differential diagnosis and actively screen for it during the medical encounter.

SCREENING FOR IPV

Screening for IPV is broadly recommended. The 2018 U.S. Preventive Services Task Force (USPSTF) recommendation is to screen for IPV in all women of reproductive age. Other expert groups such as the Joint Commission on Accreditation of Healthcare Organizations, the American Medical Association, and the Institute of Medicine also advocate for screening women in clinical settings to increase detection rates. Since the potential benefits of screening appear to outweigh the potential harms, and since research has demonstrated that most abused and nonabused patients favor routine screening by their health care practitioners, questions about IPV should be incorporated into the routine history and physical examination for all female patients. Some practitioners also screen men, particularly men in intimate relationships with other men, although no data are currently available on the screening of men.

The optimal method of screening, whether by including questions about abuse on the electronic health record (EHR) or intake medical history questionnaire, or verbally as a part of the social or past medical history, or both, is a subject of ongoing research. The HITS screening instrument is widely used and consists of four questions ("Have you been **h**it, **i**nsulted, **t**hreatened, or **s**creamed at?) on a 5-point Likert scale from "never" to "frequently"; it is available in several languages and has been validated for use with men and women. Some patients may feel more comfortable revealing IPV by screening with the following questions that seek to normalize the problem:

> **Doctor**: "Because abuse and violence are so common in women's lives, I've begun to ask about it routinely. At any time, has a partner hit or otherwise hurt or threatened you?" (See Table 40–3 for suggested screening questions.)

If the answers are vague or evasive, more direct questions must be asked to determine if abuse is taking place. If this is done in a supportive, nonjudgmental manner, most patients will feel comfortable and respond honestly.

Table 40-3. Screening questions.

- We all fight at home sometimes. What happens when you or your partner fight or disagree?
- Do you feel safe in your home and in your relationship?
- Do you ever feel afraid of your partner?
- Because abuse and violence are so common in women's lives, I've begun to ask about it routinely. At any time, has a partner hit or otherwise hurt or threatened you?
- Does your partner ever force you to engage in sex that makes you feel uncomfortable?
- Does your partner threaten, hit, or abuse your children?

TREATMENT

Multiple studies show that screening alone, without intervention, does not improve a woman's health outcomes. Instead, an empathetic response by the health care provider, coupled with a multicomponent interventional approach, has shown benefit in patients who experience IPV. When IPV is detected, five basic tasks must be accomplished (Table 40–4). First, **validate the problem** by making a clear statement to the patient that violent behavior is unacceptable and illegal, and that nobody has the right to abuse him or her. The physician's acknowledgment of the IPV as a real issue may be the first step in helping to free the patient from the abuse.

Table 40-4. After detection: five tasks to accomplish.

1. Validate the problem.
2. Assess the patient's safety, and review an emergency escape plan.
3. Document clearly and completely.
4. Provide information and appropriate referral.
5. Be aware of reporting and other legal requirements.

Under all circumstances, avoid language that could be interpreted as blaming the victim for the violence.

Because most people are not ready to leave the relationship when the IPV is detected, a main task for the primary care provider is to build the relationship with the patient. Statements that express empathy can be an effective way to accomplish this task, for example: "I really respect the way you have been dealing with this" and "we can work on this problem together." Research has shown that even brief discussions with clinicians can be therapeutic for the patient, and health outcomes are improved when the conversation is conducted in a concerned way. It is important to help the patient set short-term goals (e.g., to obtain the skills required for a particular job) so that they are not distressed when it takes time to realize the long-term goal of ending the abuse and/or the relationship. Above all, avoid recapitulating the power and control dynamics that so often characterize the patient's abusive relationship. Never insist that they leave the relationship and always allow them the autonomy to make their own decisions.

Second, it is essential to **assess the patient's safety**. Is it safe to go home? Other options (such as friends, shelters, and so on) should be explored and an emergency escape plan reviewed. For patients not returning home, advise them to inform one or two coworkers about the situation, as the perpetrator may attempt to find them at work. It is important to ask if there are children who are potentially at risk. Risk factors for escalating violence such as an increase in the frequency and severity of assaults, an escalation in threats, and the availability of a firearm should be carefully assessed.

Third, it is imperative that practitioners **document clearly and completely** when they uncover IPV. The medical record should include a complete description of the assault with quotes, if possible, from the patient's own account. Include relevant details in the past medical history and social history. Be sure to document clearly; successful prosecution should never be compromised by sloppy recordkeeping. Injuries should be described and visually documented, either with a body chart or with photographs if the patient consents (include the patient's face in at least one photograph). If the police are called, always include the name of and any actions taken by the investigating police officer.

Fourth, the patient must be provided with **information and appropriate referrals**. Studies indicate that women experiencing violence want providers to offer tangible medical and social resources, in keeping with the 2018 USPSTF recommendation for providers to refer women to ongoing support services. No study has identified an optimal treatment plan, however, studies also show that only offering brief interventions or information about referrals is generally ineffective. Health care providers should be familiar with multicomponent social and legal services available in their area. Information about shelters should be offered even if the patient intends to return home (though it is important to understand that discovery of such information by the perpetrator may lead to an escalation of the abuse). All patients should be assessed for the presence of psychiatric or substance use problems that would benefit from treatment or referral. Practitioners should have a basic understanding of legal options, such as restraining orders, so that they can help advise patients who wish to take immediate action to ensure their safety.

Finally, understand the IPV **reporting requirements** in your state. Health practitioners often are required to report to the police all incidents of IPV that result in an injury. The usual doctor–patient privileged communication is explicitly preempted by this law. Providers should work with their ED, hospital, or clinics to be sure that information about reporting requirements as well as other patient education literature is freely available and in multiple languages.

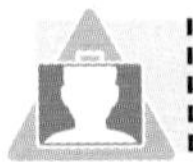

CASE ILLUSTRATION 3

A 32-year-old man was admitted to the hospital for treatment of injuries and bleeding after reporting that he "fell through a glass door." He required an emergency operation to repair lacerations to internal organs and had to receive 2 units of packed red blood cells. Five days postoperatively, he was visited in the hospital by his male partner, who became belligerent when the surgical residents attempted to obtain additional history. Later that day, the patient revealed that he had been in a long-term abusive relationship, and that the abuse had been escalating over the past 6 months, and in fact he had been pushed through the door by his partner. The hospital social worker was called to speak with the patient and told him that she would report his case to the domestic violence hotline. The patient said that he had finally made the decision to leave the relationship and was intending to press charges and was grateful for the support of the hospital doctors and staff.

What to Avoid?

There are four pitfalls to avoid when caring for victims of IPV:

1. Do not insist that the patient terminate the relationship, even if you believe that this is the most appropriate action. Only the patient can make that decision. Trying to control the patient's behavior, albeit subtly, recapitulates the same negative dynamic that is taking place in the abusive relationship.

2. Recommend couple counseling *only* when the perpetrator acknowledges the problem, wants to change his or her behavior, and both partners want to preserve the relationship.
3. Do not use the word *alleged* in the medical record. It implies that you do not believe the patient's story, and you may inadvertently impede his or her ability to bring the case to court.
4. Do not ask what the victim did to bring on the violence.

BARRIERS

Physician Barriers to Detection

Many studies have revealed that physicians and other health care practitioners do a poor job of detecting IPV, with detection rates rarely exceeding 10% for women. Several factors are responsible for this dismal record. First, many practitioners lack the appropriate knowledge and training to effectively detect and treat victims of IPV. The first step in improving their ability to do so is to disseminate information more widely about its prevalence and consequences and to include IPV in medical school, residency, and continuing medical education curricula.

Lack of institutional support is a second important barrier. Despite the enormity of the problem and the increasing requirements that all health care institutions have IPV protocols in place, most hospitals and clinics have few, if any, adequately trained support staff, accessible guidelines for practitioners, or information for patients. In addition, with growing pressure to see more patients and use fewer resources, issues such as IPV may be overlooked. Many of the physicians interviewed in one study identified time constraints as the major deterrent to opening the "Pandora's box" of IPV.

The diagnostic and treatment strategies outlined here, however, are not particularly time intensive. Inquiry about IPV adds less than 1 minute to the typical new patient evaluation; if widely employed, it could yield enormous savings through the prevention of injury, decreased health care usage, and the prevention of physical and emotional harm to patients and their families.

The third barrier to detection of IPV arises from practitioner discomfort. Many practitioners feel uncomfortable addressing issues that do not fit neatly into the traditional medical model. Numerous studies have shown that many do a poor job discussing issues with their patients having to do with sex, violence, mental disorders, and substance use. Delving into the cause of a suspicious injury may make them uneasy: it is often not amenable to a straightforward solution and may raise embarrassing or uncomfortable feelings. All practitioners must reflect on the feelings that IPV raises in them to be effective in caring for these vulnerable patients.

Patient Barriers to Terminating an Abusive Relationship

Providers often have difficulty understanding why more patients do not terminate their abusive relationship. Why they remain in these relationships is complex. Some of the reasons include the following:

1. *Fear.* Fear for their own safety or for their children. Patients often are not at home when the assault takes place, so it is clear that leaving is no guarantee of safety.
2. *Economic.* Many IPV victims lack employment skills or experience and would find it very difficult to support themselves and/or their children outside of the relationship.
3. *Psychological.* Some may find it difficult to leave because of the "psychological dependence" the years of repetitive abuse have created. Survivors are told overtly and covertly that they are "worthless"; some eventually internalize this and come to believe that they are incapable of surviving on their own.
4. *Social support—or the lack thereof.* Survivors are often encouraged by well-meaning friends and family members to "try to work things out," or they are advised to stay "for the children's sake."
5. *Lack of other options.* Shelters are often full, friends and family unavailable, and legal counsel not accessible.
6. Not all survivors want the relationship to end, just the violence.

PERPETRATOR PROGRAMS

In some cases, a patient in a health care setting may self-disclose being a perpetrator of violence. These patients may be more amenable to behavior change. However, very few studies have looked at interventions for perpetrators of violence. Few evaluation studies have been done on outcomes, and recent reviews show only a small effect size for prevention of future abuse. Most interventions are ordered by the criminal justice system and, unless mandatory, have very high dropout rates.

NEWER TECHNOLOGIES

Patients find computer-based IPV screening methods acceptable, and IPV screening done on a computer leads to substantially higher rates of IPV detection compared with usual care. Computer-based screening methods may help to detect IPV in emergency and primary care settings. One research group was able to build a model based on symptoms that can predict the risk of future diagnoses of abuse. Next steps might be a warning system for clinicians through the EHR for such high-risk patients.

Videoconferencing-based health interventions such as telemedicine have been shown to help trauma and abuse victims by providing psychological services via telemedicine. Rates of symptom improvement (reductions in depressive and PTSD symptoms) are comparable to effect sizes documented for traditional cognitive behavioral therapy and appear to be a viable future option for underserved populations.

From an institutional standpoint, some practices are now using system-level approaches and performance improvement measures to revise their system-wide interventions with success. The National Health Resource Center on Domestic Violence (https://ipvhealthpartners.org) has sponsored a tool, available to health care institutions to track their progress in improving the organizational response to IPV victims.

CONCLUSION

Along with the criminal justice system, physicians and other health care providers are most likely to come into contact with victims of IPV. Health care providers have a professional and ethical obligation to recognize IPV and intervene appropriately as well as to exert their influence on a broader level. This may be to lobby for more funding for shelters or to advocate for teaching about IPV at all levels of medical education. Screening for and treating IPV should be a routine part of the practice and training of medicine. We all have the obligation to confront the epidemic of IPV and strive to lessen its impact as one of the most important public health issues of our time.

SUGGESTED READINGS

Miller E, McCaw B. Intimate partner violence. *N Engl J Med* 2019;380:850–857.

Miller E, McCaw B, Humphreys B, Mitchell C. Integrating intimate partner violence assessment and intervention into healthcare in the United States: a systems approach. *J Womens Health* 2015;24:92–99.

Sugg N. Intimate partner violence: prevalence, health consequences, and intervention. *Med Clin North Am* 2015;99:629–649.

US Preventative Services Task Force. Screening for intimate partner violence, elder abuse, and abuse of vulnerable adults: US preventive services task force final recommendation statement. *JAMA* 2018;320(16):1678–1687.

WEBSITES

https://www.loveisrespect.org. LoveIsRespect.org is an organization that empowers youth to prevent and end dating abuse, sponsored by the National Domestic Violence hotline. Accessed March 2019.

https://www.thehotline.org. The National Domestic Violence Hotline is a resource to help victims get help and stay safe. There are also opportunities for volunteers to get involved. Accessed March 2019.

https://ipvhealthpartners.org. Online toolkit for Community Health Centers. Includes information for identifying and responding to IPV cases, and for developing community partnerships. Accessed March 2019.

Trauma

41

Coleen Kivlahan, MD, MSPH; Edward L. Machtinger, MD; & Nate L. Ewigman, PhD, MPH

INTRODUCTION

Recognizing and addressing trauma offers a powerful opportunity to improve the experience and outcomes of primary care for both patients and clinicians. For clinicians, understanding that trauma underlies and perpetuates many common health conditions helps clarify why certain conditions often remain refractory to standard medical treatment. This understanding, in turn, can lead to deeper and more compassionate connections with patients and more effective treatment plans. For patients, understanding the connection between the experience of trauma and their current health issues can lead to greater self-acceptance, engagement in care, healthier coping mechanisms, and improved health outcomes.

WHAT IS TRAUMA?

The Substance Abuse and Mental Health Services Administration (SAMHSA) defines trauma as "an event, series of events, or set of circumstances that is experienced by an individual as physically or emotionally harmful or threatening and that has lasting adverse effects." Examples of these events and circumstances include childhood and adult physical, sexual, and emotional abuse; neglect; loss; intimate partner violence; community violence; war; and structural violence such as racism, sexism, xenophobia, homophobia, and transphobia, among many others. Repeated exposure to trauma (e.g., witnessing the ongoing physical abuse of one's mother, experiencing serial sexual abuse) is known as "complex trauma" and is associated with particularly harmful consequences to physical and emotional health and well-being.

HEALTH IMPACT OF TRAUMA

Childhood and adult trauma are associated with many common causes of adult illness, death, and disability in the United States. The seminal Adverse Childhood Experiences (ACE) study documented remarkably high rates of serious childhood physical and sexual abuse, neglect, and household dysfunction among 17,000 predominately white, middle-class adults. The study calculated an ACE score (0–10) based on how many categories of childhood events adults had experienced: 64% reported at least one ACE category, and one in six reported four or more. Notably, 25% of women and 16% of men reported having experienced childhood sexual abuse. The study revealed a strong dose–response relationship between childhood trauma and adult heart, lung, and liver disease; depression; substance abuse; obesity; diabetes; sexually transmitted infection risk; and intimate partner violence (IPV). Individuals who reported four or more ACE categories had 2 times the rates of lung and liver disease, 3 times the rate of depression, 3 times the rate of alcoholism, 11 times the rate of intravenous drug use, and 14 times the rate of attempting suicide than those who reported ACE scores of 0.

Similarly, trauma in adulthood is common and associated with poor health outcomes. It is also frequently undiagnosed. More than one-third of U.S. women experience stalking, physical violence, and/or rape from an intimate partner during their lifetimes. One in five men experiences sexual violence in their lifetimes. Adult experiences of trauma are also strongly correlated with many of the same illnesses and unhealthy coping strategies as childhood trauma. In addition, these data are likely to underestimate the impact of trauma, since most studies do not account for the chronic toxic stress associated with pervasive structural violence such as racism and xenophobia (see Chapter 40).

Primary care clinicians have an obligation to recognize and respond to the impact of trauma on health. They can improve health outcomes across an array of common, difficult-to-treat conditions such as substance use, depression, chronic pain and obesity by understanding patients' trauma and providing care that includes opportunities to better cope with it and ultimately to heal from it. As will be described in the next sections of this chapter, adopting a trauma-informed approach also has the promise to transform the caregiving experience for primary care clinicians to one that is more satisfying and meaningful.

Identifying Risk Factors for Trauma

Primary care clinicians are likely to identify patients who have experienced childhood and/or lifetime exposure to trauma, as well as those at risk for future exposure. There are a number of known risk factors that can inform screening, education, and treatment of patients. Early life exposure to trauma is a known risk factor for experiencing trauma later in life. It is also important to note that not all people respond to trauma in the same way; some people are more prone to have lasting negative impacts. Risk factors that are more likely to result in lasting impact from trauma include prior personal or family history of mental or behavioral disorders, life-threatening events, intensely negative emotional responses following the trauma, and dissociative experiences.

Most of the research on risk factors for exposure to trauma is in children. Some risk factors are known to be modifiable; some are not. Examples of nonmodifiable risk factors include prior history of exposure to trauma, stressful life events, preexisting mental illness/depression, family history, and metabolic and genetic vulnerability. Demographic factors such as female gender, age, socioeconomic status, and African American race often are thought of as nonmodifiable risk factors, but it is increasingly clear that societal response to race, gender, or age, and the resultant chronic stress, may create the actual risk in these populations.

As primary care clinicians, we also know that the experience and impact of trauma is affected by potentially modifiable environmental factors (e.g., poverty, stressful neighborhoods), social factors (e.g., family instability), biological factors (e.g., lower cognitive functioning, emotional dysregulation), and occupational exposure (e.g., firefigthers, police personnel).

Modifiable risk factors for the development of PTSD include patients' cognitive styles, maladaptive thoughts (e.g., rumination), coping styles (e.g., wishful thinking), psychological traits (e.g., behavioral disengagement, impulsivity), and level of social support. Many of these modifiable factors appear more commonly in people with poor access to support such as health care, medications, and mental health treatment and in those who experience a lifetime of discrimination. The risk of PTSD also increases with the number and severity of traumatic events.

Asking Patients About Trauma

Inquiring about current and past trauma in the setting of a busy primary care clinic can seem like a daunting task. With a little practice, however, doing so can build deeper, more satisfying, and more effective relationships. It is helpful to set the stage for this inquiry by preparing both the primary care practice and yourself.

Preparing Your Practice

One of the chapter authors (ELM) and colleagues have described four basic steps to prepare a primary care practice to inquire about recent and past trauma.

First, recognize that **trauma is common**. Understanding the impact of traumatic experiences on behavior and health can clarify why some conditions remain refractory to traditional therapies and why some patients can appear reactive, chaotic, or adversarial. This understanding can help reduce clinician frustration, help maintain a compassionate and patient-centered approach, and inform more effective interventions.

Next, adopt **trauma-informed principles**. Trauma can damage one's sense of safety and can adversely affect relationships with others. To provide a healing environment for both patients and the health care team, integrate trauma-informed principles into your practice. These principles include safety, trustworthiness, collaboration, peer support, empowerment, and cultural humility and responsiveness.

Then, offer **education and resources** for patients, providers, and staff. Educate all patients and the entire health care team about the connection between trauma, health, and health-related behaviors. Examples of patient education include: posters and flyers in the waiting area, brief informational pamphlets given to patients when taking their vital signs, and invite conversations as part of routine practice and/or when trauma-related conditions are discussed. Understand that patients may not disclose trauma for many reasons, including fear and shame.

Finally, establish **referral processes** for patients who want additional services and/or treatment. Knowing the options for additional support helps clinicians be more comfortable engaging patients about trauma, and ensures that patients are "matched" to onsite or community-based services most appropriate for their desires, needs, and stage of readiness for change. Integrating behavioral health clinicians into primary care greatly facilitates this process.

Preparing Yourself

Techniques described by Dr. Leigh Kimberg as the "Four C's" can help prepare you to inquire about, and respond to, recent or past trauma:

1. Stay **Calm.** Your ability to stay calm when caring for a patient who has experienced trauma can make your visits more productive and healing for your patient and yourself. Practice brief breathing and mindfulness techniques to use with your patients.
2. **Contain** the interaction. You do not need to elicit a detailed trauma history to offer help. Provide information, resources, and referrals to trauma-specific care, without necessarily asking for disclosure of trauma details (see options for trauma inquiry below). This reduces the risk of overwhelming you or the patient.

3. **Care** for yourself and the patient compassionately. Destigmatize the adverse sequelae of trauma such as substance use, overeating, and depression. One way is to shift the way you think about illness from "What's wrong with you?" to "What happened to you?" Recognize and address the traumatic life experiences and vicarious trauma of health care staff and providers. Vicarious trauma, also called secondary traumatic stress, is an occupational risk for people working in fields such as law enforcement, emergency medical services, and health care due to exposure to victims of trauma and violence. Use employee support services and interdisciplinary teams to reduce staff and clinician isolation.
4. Focus on **Coping**. Emphasize resilience and strength. Solicit and incorporate the skills and strategies the patient has used in the past to overcome current difficulties. Ask about and reinforce practices that help the patient feel better (e.g., exercise, music, volunteering, structured groups, supportive friends or family, and prayer/spirituality).

Inquiry about Recent Trauma

The patient's immediate safety is the top priority when inquiring about trauma. For example, IPV is a common form of violence in patients presenting to primary care. IPV has a strong evidence base for effective screening and response, and screening can be done conversationally or with standardized tools. Screening should always be done in private and, if required, with professional translation. Some settings may choose to emphasize universal education, in which providers use informational materials to educate patients about IPV, provide resources, and facilitate discussion before direct inquiry. For details about inquiry and response to IPV see Chapter 40.

Inquiry about Past Trauma

Machtinger and colleagues describe four general approaches for inquiry about past trauma (Table 41-1). The choice of approach depends on the resources, expertise, and patient population of the practice.

Option 1: Assume a history of trauma instead of asking
All patients can be approached using a "trauma lens" that assumes that difficult life experiences may have contributed to current illnesses and coping behaviors. Universal patient education can be provided about the connection between trauma and physical and emotional health. Regardless of whether or not a patient chooses to disclose their trauma history, referrals can be offered to onsite or community-based interventions that address experiences and consequences of past trauma.

Option 2: Screen for impact of past trauma instead of the trauma itself
Screen for common conditions that are highly correlated with traumatic experiences, such as anxiety, posttraumatic stress disorder, depression, suicidality, substance use disorder, chronic pain, and morbid obesity. These conditions are often "markers" for past trauma and are highly stigmatized. Patients with these conditions benefit greatly from a nonjudgmental, compassionate, trauma-informed approach and by offering referrals to onsite or community-based treatments that are trauma-informed.

Option 3: Inquire about trauma using open-ended questions
In contrast to structured tools, open-ended questions allow patients to disclose any form of trauma they choose. Clinicians can use an open-ended question: "Difficult life experiences, like growing up in a family where you were hurt, or where there was mental illness or drug/alcohol issues, or witnessing violence, can affect our health. Tell me about any of your past experiences that may affect your physical or emotional health?" Followed by "I am so sorry that happened to you. Past traumas can sometimes continue to affect our health. If you would like, we can talk more about services that are available that can help."

Option 4: Use a structured tool to explore past traumatic experiences
If a structured screening tool is used, it is necessary to consider when, how, and by whom it will be administered, as well as who will have access to the information. Some clinics use a previsit screening tool administered via electronic tablet, paper, or small "wipe-off" board. In other settings, nonclinical staff administer the tool, or clinicians may conduct the standardized screening in the exam room. Regardless of what tool is used and how it is administered, it is essential that the patient have the opportunity to discuss their responses with the clinician in private.

Table 41-1. Four steps to inquire about trauma.

1. Assume a history of trauma instead of asking.
2. Screen for impact of past trauma.
3. Inquire about trauma with open-ended questions.
4. Use a structured tool.

Examining Patients With Trauma

Key Points:

- Establish a safe environment for your patient
- Provide choices and options to increase control
- Seek informed consent at each step
- Respect the personal space at all times
- Be aware that some procedures may trigger trauma with procedures

In the course of treatment, primary care clinicians are likely to perform physical examinations on trauma survivors. The first and most important principle is the patient's perception of personal safety. In this setting, it is essential that the patient be protected from real and perceived threats of injury or harm. Many trauma survivors are hesitant to seek medical care, be touched by strangers, and may live in unsafe situations. Patients can experience repeat traumatization in clinical settings, which may manifest as difficulty trusting medical staff, challenges managing their own emotional processing and internal states, and needing more time and explanation for basic procedures. Many experience fear and anxiety before medical appointments. In addition, the process of undressing, putting on gowns, being exposed to gels and lubricants with exams or invasive procedures, or lying on exam tables in small rooms with closed doors is highly stressful. Patients may cancel or no show appointments, dissociate, appear uninvolved in the visit, show excessive modesty, and leave against medical advice. In emergency room and hospital settings, the excessive noise, multiple strangers, unclear rules, and inadequate time for complete explanations put trauma survivors at risk for anxiety, fear, acute delirium, and confusion.

Emotional self-regulation is a challenge for most trauma survivors. In the examination room, this may present as anxiety, minimization, dissociation, unwillingness to undress, extraordinary fear, concern about being judged, shame, and reenactment of traumatic events. Slow movements on the part of the clinician with continuous reassurance are helpful. In addition, seeking consent for each part of the examination and providing an ongoing narrative for the patient about the next steps in the evaluation is essential. While the extent of the trauma history may be unknown, the physical examination should begin with body parts which have reportedly not been injured or hurt, and slowly move toward areas most likely to trigger retraumatization. Patients may be especially sensitive to procedures such as having blood drawn or having their mouth or genitalia examined. The patient should be given the option to stop the examination at any point if they grow uncomfortable, to ask for a clinician of a different gender or ethnicity (one not resembling a perpetrator), or to take a break or reschedule. Respecting the personal space of the trauma survivor is central to achieving safety, and observing the patient's responses during the interview and examination will provide clues about their comfort with your physical distance. The clinical environment, examination room, and the staff should be welcoming and flexible, with the goal of minimizing retraumatization.

Trauma can range from an acute, single event to repeated and recurrent events lasting years. Patients' responses to the medical system will vary based on risk factors previously discussed, as well as frequency and severity of traumatic events. Some populations of patients present with highly challenging histories and examination findings. Trauma as a result of torture (defined as "any act by which severe pain or suffering, whether physical or mental, is intentionally inflicted on a person . . . by or at the instigation of or with the consent or acquiescence of a public official or other person acting in an official capacity") is especially challenging and demands specialized clinical training. Patients may experience serious and life-threatening events as children, others experience torture during wars or while detained for political or social reasons. Another population requiring special care are people with disabilities who have been traumatized. This group is far more likely to experience repeated episodes of personal violence compared with people without disabilities and have limited skills to verbalize their trauma histories.

Patients with trauma exposure commonly present to primary care and other settings with seemingly unrelated acute or chronic physical and mental health conditions at much higher rates than patients without trauma exposure. Trauma and PTSD survivors have a higher prevalence of chronic cardiac, digestive, musculoskeletal, nervous system, and endocrine conditions. Somatization symptoms in these patients can result in unnecessary tests and hospitalizations. It is critical for primary care clinicians to consider the possibility that some of our most challenging patients may have extensive trauma histories. The opportunity for deep healing in primary care settings is directly related to our knowledge of, and compassion for, the impact of trauma in the lives of our patients.

Screening for Posttraumatic Stress Disorder in Primary Care

While exposure to trauma is common among primary care populations, only some go on to develop clinical psychopathology. Most community-based samples estimate that 5–12% of patients demonstrate a clinical level of posttraumatic symptoms at some point in their lifetime. The most common forms of posttraumatic psychopathology include acute stress disorder (ASD) and posttraumatic stress disorder (PTSD). While both ASD and PTSD involve a cluster of symptoms including hyperarousal, negative cognitions, reexperiencing, and avoidance, ASD is a reaction that occurs 3 days to 1 month after the traumatic exposure, while symptoms persist for more than 1 month after exposure in PTSD.

Detection rates of PTSD in primary care are low, and effective treatments are available for symptoms appearing after trauma exposure. Thus, screening for PTSD is an important skill for primary care clinicians and practices. While the United States Preventive Services Task Force (USPSTF) recommends screening for IPV, depression, and alcohol in adults in primary care, screening for past trauma exposure has not specifically been addressed. USPSTF notes that "screening should be implemented with adequate systems in place to ensure accurate diagnosis, effective treatment and appropriate follow-up." While there is currently no national guideline mandating universal screening for past trauma exposure, we suggest that using any one of the four options discussed above provide a proactive strategy for addressing the high prevalence of lifetime trauma in primary care.

The five-question Primary Care PTSD (PC-PTSD-5) screen is a widely used tool to detect PTSD in primary care within the Veterans Health Administration (Table 41-2). While the generalizability of this tool outside of older veterans seeking primary care is not well known, it represents one of the few brief, primary care-oriented screening tools for PTSD.

A score of 3 or more on the PC-PTSD-5 confers a high likelihood of trauma-related psychological distress and/or PTSD. For patients who score 3 or greater on the PC-PTSD-5, additional screening and/or referral is recommended. Options for additional evaluation include referral to community behavioral health resources or, ideally, collaborating with integrated behavioral health clinicians onsite in the primary care clinic. Research shows that primary care clinics with integrated behavioral health clinicians are much more likely to detect patients who have previously undiagnosed PTSD. For clinics without these resources, traumatized patients are more likely to be incorrectly diagnosed or sometimes labeled as "noncompliant" or "difficult" because trauma symptoms often interfere with adherence. The presence of integrated behavioral health clinicians reduces the stigma of mental health treatment as well as barriers to care, making it more likely that accurate diagnoses and treatment plans will be deployed.

Table 41-2. The Primary Care PTSD Screen for DSM-5.

Sometimes things happen to people that are unusually or especially frightening, horrible, or traumatic. For example: a serious accident or fire, a physical or sexual assault or abuse, an earthquake or flood, a war, seeing someone be killed or seriously injured, having a loved one die through homicide or suicide.

Have you ever experienced this kind of event? YES/NO.

If yes, please answer the questions below. **In the past month, have you...**

1. Had nightmares about the event(s) or thought about the event(s) when you did not want to? YES/NO
2. Tried hard not to think about the event(s) or went out of your way to avoid situations that reminded you of the event(s)? YES/NO
3. Been constantly on guard, watchful, or easily startled? YES/NO
4. Felt numb or detached from people, activities, or your surroundings? YES/NO
5. Felt guilty or unable to stop blaming yourself or others for the event(s) or any problems the event(s) may have caused? YES/NO

Reprinted by permission from Prins A, et al. The Primary Care PTSD Screen for *DSM-5* (PC-PTSD-5): development and evaluation within a veteran primary care sample. *J Gen Intern Med* 2016; 31:1206–1211.

Consulting behavioral health clinicians are likely to use tools such as the PTSD Checklist (PCL) (https://www.ptsd.va.gov/professional/assessment/adult-sr/ptsd-checklist.asp) and/or the Clinician-Assisted PTSD Scale for DSM-5. (https://www.ptsd.va.gov/professional/assessment/adult-int/caps.asp) for further assessment, diagnostic clarity and treatment planning.

When referrals are not available for your patients, primary care clinicians can be reasonably confident in their diagnosis of posttraumatic symptomatology and need for trauma-focused treatment referral when a patient:

1. Is exposed to, directly or indirectly, trauma that involved actual or perceived death, injury, or sexual violence
2. Reexperiences the trauma (e.g., nightmares, unwanted memories) with negative emotional and/or physical reactivity
3. Avoids situations or thinking/talking about the trauma
4. Has a lot of negative thoughts and feelings after the trauma
5. Is experiencing hyperarousal (e.g., edgy, always "on the lookout," irritable, easily startled, jumpy, having difficulty sleeping)
6. Screens positive on the PC-PTSD-5 (score 3 or greater)

Many patients exposed to trauma will share only some of these symptoms and experiences, so the primary care clinician's threshold for referral to behavioral health should be low. While the criteria above are suggested as signs that should raise suspicion for posttraumatic psychopathology, the trigger to PTSD must be an exposure to actual or threatened death, serious injury, or sexual violation. PTSD symptoms are grouped into four distinct clusters: re-experiencing the trauma (memories, nightmares, flashbacks), avoidance (emotional/cognitive vs. situational), negative changes in thinking/mood (not remembering aspects of the trauma, changes in beliefs about self/others/the world, self/other-oriented blame, persistent negative emotions, anhedonia, isolation, difficulty experiencing positive emotions), and arousal (sleep disturbances, irritability/anger outbursts, exaggerated startle, hypervigilance, attentional disruption, self-destructive behavior). PTSD results in clinically significant distress or impairment in the social interactions, capacity to work, or other important areas of functioning (American Psychiatric Association, *Diagnostic and Statistical Manual*, Version 5, PTSD).

Trauma-Informed Primary Care

Research consistently finds that patients exposed to trauma are higher utilizers of health services overall, and this is also true for patients with comorbid mental health and substance use disorders who often seek care in primary care settings. Thus, primary care clinicians have an important role to play in addressing trauma and the impact on many common behavioral and physical health conditions. Recognizing the impact of these conditions on patients' lives and on primary care practices, some clinics evolve to become a trauma-informed primary care (TIPC) practice. The process can be facilitated by resources designed to help practices make this transition over time.

According to the U.S. Department of Health and Human Services Substance Abuse and Mental Health Services Administration (SAMHSA) concept of a trauma-informed approach, "A program, organization, or system that is trauma-informed:

Realizes the widespread impact of trauma and understands potential paths for recovery

Recognizes the signs and symptoms of trauma in clients, families, staff, and others involved with the system

Responds by fully integrating knowledge about trauma into policies, procedures, and practices; and

Seeks to actively resist retraumatization

The five core components of TIPC are described below and depicted in the accompanying graphic. (See Figure 41-1 adapted from Machtinger et al 2018. See suggested reading for full citation.)

Practice Environment

A TIPC practice is calm, safe, and empowering for both patients and staff, and is designed to reduce triggers and promote healing. The first step includes the training of all staff and clinicians about how trauma impacts health, the use of trauma-informed skills to use with patients and one another, and how to access trauma-specific services onsite and in the community. Clinicians work as an interdisciplinary team to help create services that are well-coordinated and are able to effectively care for traumatized patients without the experience becoming overwhelming for the patient, clinician, or staff.

Education

Education should be provided in a variety of formats to all patients and staff about the relationship between trauma, health, and health-related behaviors.

Inquiry

Just as many practices have normalized routine screening for interpersonal violence or child abuse, routinely providing the opportunity for patients to disclose past trauma is a core component of a trauma-informed practice. Ideally, this inquiry occurs in the setting of an ongoing relationship. The prior section, "Asking Patients About Trauma" describes a variety of methods to inquire about recent and past trauma most appropriate to the clinical setting, clinician, and patient.

Responding to Disclosure of Trauma

For patients, a disclosure of recent or past abuse is, on its own, potentially therapeutic. Responses to disclosures of trauma are supportive, empathetic, and validating of patients' experiences, choices, and autonomy. Responses can also solicit and build on the strengths and wisdom patients have used in the past to overcome adversity.

Disclosures of some forms of recent trauma such as IPV require an immediate response. This response has become more standardized and simple by the availability of consultation at any time by local and national domestic violence hotlines (National Domestic Violence Hotline 1-800-799-SAFE 7233). An appropriate response to recent IPV affirms that the patient does not deserve to be treated in this way and expresses concern for his/her safety. It also typically also includes a "warm handoff" to a domestic violence agency by telephone and/or to an onsite psychosocial team member who can construct a safety plan; lethality assessment, referrals for safe housing, legal, police, and other community resources; individual and/or group therapy; and peer support.

Unlike recent trauma, disclosures of past trauma do not require an immediate intervention. Rather, clinicians can express empathy ("I'm so sorry that happened to you. You didn't deserve that") and provide information about the availability of services to help cope with and heal from past trauma ("I am available to talk more with you about that. We have access to services that can help you cope with this experience"). In general, primary care clinics respond to lifelong trauma and its consequences (e.g., substance abuse, mental illness, chronic pain, obesity) by ensuring that onsite services are trauma-informed and by building strong community partnerships to facilitate referrals to trauma-informed services. Clinicians play a crucial role by linking patients to onsite or community-based psychosocial staff members who are skilled in providing this treatment. Practices should also engage in strategies to reduce the impact of vicarious or secondary trauma response based on exposure to traumatized patients. Self-care is vital for caregivers.

The Foundation of TIPC

TIPC includes a core set of trauma-informed values that inform the clinic's physical setting, activities, relationships, use of clinic champion(s), "buy-in" from organizational leadership, interdisciplinary team-based care, partnerships with trauma-informed community organizations, and robust support for clinicians and staff.

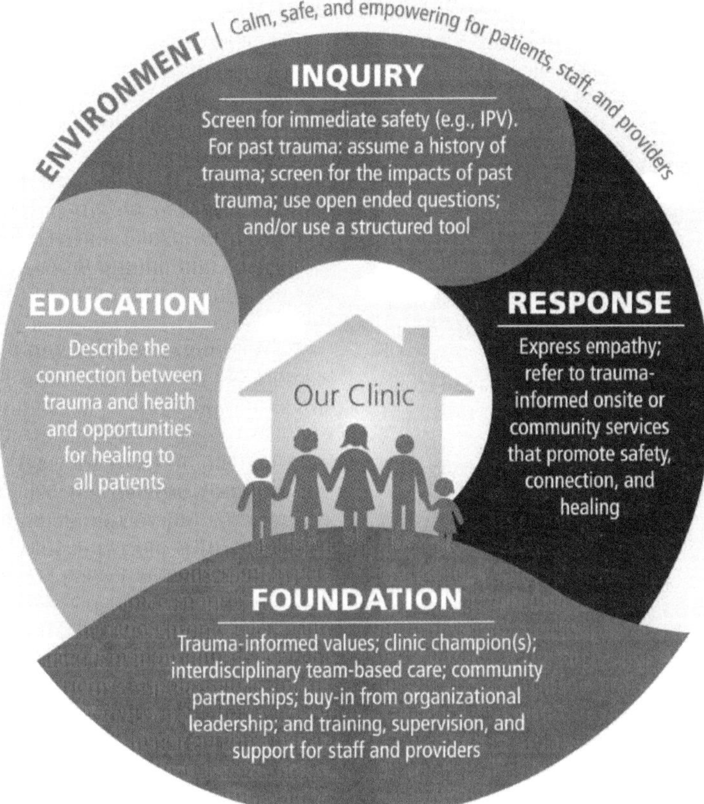

Figure 41-1. Trauma-informed health care. (Reprinted from Machtinger EL, Davis KB, Kimberg LS, et al. From treatment to healing: inquiry and response to recent and past trauma in adult health care. *Womens Health Issues* 2019;29(2):97–102.)

It is possible, and may be beneficial, to implement these elements incrementally (Table 41-3). Steps may include training all practice staff and clinicians about the impact of trauma on health and behavior and about trauma-informed communication skills to use with patients and with each other. Over time, clinic champion(s) may emerge, partnerships can be formed with local trauma and service organizations, and protocols for education, screening, and response can be developed. High quality, practical resources, and technical assistance are available to guide each element of TIPC. Consider integration of mental health services within your primary care practice so that the entire primary care team develops better skills to diagnose and treat patients who experience trauma and PTSD. It is hard to overstate the beneficial impact of creating a team structure within which clinicians

Table 41-3. First steps to trauma-informed primary care.

1. Think about the connection between trauma and health in your patients. Realize that trauma exposure can changes who people are and how they behave.
2. Put educational materials about the impact of trauma on health in your waiting room. It sends a powerful message.
3. Get expert training for you and your staff on the impact of trauma on health.
4. Practice talking with your patients about trauma. Determine the best approach for you and your practice.

Over time, clinic champions will emerge in your practice; protocols for screening can be used; and responses to trauma can be developed in partnership with local organizations.

do not individually shoulder the burden of caring for highly traumatized patients. Implementing TIPC provides a powerful opportunity to change the caregiving experience for clinicians and staffs. For both patients and clinicians, moving toward TIPC has the potential to transform the experience and efficacy of primary care from the treatment of symptoms and diseases to genuine healing.

Treatment of PTSD

Evidence-based treatments are available for patients with PTSD. While the primary care clinician will usually not be providing trauma-focused therapies, basic knowledge about which treatments are most effective is helpful to facilitate effective referrals.

The Department of Veterans Affairs (VA) has long been a leader in the treatment of PTSD and has developed guidelines based on expert review of the best evidence. VA guidelines strongly recommend individual, trauma-focused psychotherapy as first-line treatment over pharmacological treatments. Effective psychotherapies for PTSD involve an element of reprocessing the trauma (through guided, gradual exposure) and helping change posttraumatic, unhelpful thought and behavioral patterns (such as isolation). These therapies are adapted from cognitive behavioral therapy and specifically target posttraumatic psychopathology. The most common types of evidence-based, trauma-focused therapy are prolonged exposure (PE) therapy, cognitive processing therapy (CPT), eye movement desensitization and reprocessing (EMDR), and cognitive behavioral therapy for PTSD. Such treatments are best delivered by therapists with specialties in trauma (such as psychologists, licensed clinical social workers, and licensed counselors). Typically, homework is part of treatment, and treatments may extend to 10–15 weekly sessions of 50–90 minutes each. Armed with this basic knowledge about trauma-focused therapy, primary care clinicians can be confident in their ability to provide high-quality referrals and help with the expectations of their patients.

For primary care practices with integrated behavioral health clinicians, therapy may be available within the practice. Recent evidence has shown that trauma-focused psychotherapy can be adapted to the fast-paced environment of primary care. For example, PE therapy has been adapted to the primary care setting (PE for primary care [PE-PC]) and shows promising evidence for symptom reduction within four sessions. The presence of integrated mental health professionals increases the likelihood that primary care patients with PTSD will initiate treatment within their trusted primary care setting.

When trauma-focused psychotherapy is not available, national guidelines recommend pharmacotherapy, in particular sertraline, paroxetine, fluoxetine, or venlafaxine as first-line monotherapies. There is not currently adequate evidence to recommend for or against the use of prazosin for PTSD-related nightmares, despite its prevalence in clinical practice. The following medications are contraindicated either because of lack of efficacy or potential for harm: divalproex, tiagabine, guanfacine, risperidone, benzodiazepines, ketamine, atypical antipsychotics, hydrocortisone, or D-cycloserine as mono- or augmentation therapies.

PTSD often presents with psychiatric comorbidities such as depression, anxiety, and substance misuse disorders. Comorbid treatment of depression and anxiety is recommended. While conventional practice held that substance misuse should be treated first, there is evidence that PTSD can successfully be treated simultaneously.

In addition to the misuse of substances, another common comorbidity of PTSD is insomnia. Insomnia may be the result of hypervigilance/hyperarousal, avoidance of experiencing nightmares, or simply unhelpful sleep behaviors. Insomnia tends to improve in about one-half of patients with PTSD who undergo successful trauma-focused psychotherapy; however, for those who have longer-term insomnia, cognitive behavioral therapy for insomnia (CBTi) is recommended. CBTi, as other evidence-based psychotherapies for common comorbid conditions, is also a good initial treatment choice for individuals with PTSD who are not yet ready to engage in trauma-focused psychotherapy.

Chronic pain, smoking, and obesity are also common comorbidities with PTSD. For such patients, it is important to keep in mind that improving health behaviors is much more challenging in the context of actively symptomatic PTSD. Patients may need psychotherapeutic approaches that combine treatments (e.g., prolonged exposure + smoking cessation, integrating behavioral pain management within a trauma-focused psychotherapy) or may need their PTSD adequately managed before attempting to improve other health behaviors (e.g., losing weight, quitting smoking).

As with all conditions, there are a number of patients who do not respond to first-line treatments. It is important to stay patient-centered and honor treatment preferences of trauma survivors. Moreover, many trauma survivors will not be ready for formal trauma-focused treatment. In this case, the primary care clinician can confidently recommend social, community, and religious engagement. Trauma survivors often feel isolated and disconnected from loved ones and positive emotions. Thus, advising social reconnection and identifying a person with whom the trauma survivor can safely discuss the details of their trauma can be highly therapeutic. Additionally, recommending mindfulness, yoga, acupuncture, and regular moderate to vigorous exercise can improve insomnia and other hyperarousal symptoms that are common to trauma survivors (see Chapter 35).

Preventing Trauma

The profound impact of violence and trauma on individuals and communities demands that we practice prevention at all levels. The identification and treatment of trauma in adults also serves as a primary prevention method for trauma in children as a substantial portion of trauma in children is related to the emotional and physical health of parents and caregivers; effectively treating the impact of parental trauma is key to the prevention of inter-generational trauma in families and children. Other primary prevention strategies for primary care practices include support for new parents, support for home visiting programs, and universal preschool options, and firearm access reduction.

Secondary prevention approaches include screening for recent and past abuse using a trauma-informed framework, developing a deep awareness of the consequences of trauma, and early treatment and intervention including referrals for your patients with trauma histories. Prevention goals include the reduction of trauma reexposure, as well as the improvement of current trauma symptoms and the development of resilience.

In addition to risk reduction strategies, characteristics that promote resilience in survivors such as self-esteem, trust, humor, internal locus of control, secure attachments, and social relationships, as well as a personal sense of safety, religious affiliation, strong adult role models, and use of existing resources can be reinforced by primary care clinicians.

CONCLUSION

There are untapped opportunities to use our understanding of the health impacts of trauma to improve the experience and efficacy of primary care for both patients and the health care team. When we are able to more deeply appreciate the stories of our patients, we are reminded of the meaning of our work, and curiosity and generosity blossom. Patients with undetected trauma histories are often seen as "difficult" or "hostile," frequently are late or miss appointments, are often in crisis, have poor self-care, and chronic pain. Such patients also may be labeled as "noncompliant," with seemingly intractable health behavior problems. Committing to a trauma-informed approach provides clinicians and staff with a framework to better understand patient behavior, and to care for patients in a more compassionate, effective, and satisfying way. Primary care practices can start with a few simple steps outlined in this chapter as we transform our practice to one that is trauma-informed.

CASE STUDIES

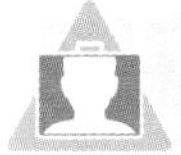

CASE ILLUSTRATION 1

Scott is a 34-year-old man seeking primary care and requesting medications for his insomnia and chronic pain. His problem list includes smoking, subdural hemorrhage following being hit by a city bus, unwitnessed seizures, traumatic brain injury, autism, PTSD, and depression.

He has pressured speech, disorganized tangential thinking, agitation, memory changes, and states that he is in excruciating chronic "insomnia" pain. He uses opioids and benzodiazepines daily. He often feels like the walls are closing in when he is in the primary care office. He smokes 2 ppd of cigarettes.

He has been unable to work, has had repeated episodes of being a victim of domestic violence with prior roommates, has been banned from his Al-Anon group for violent speech, and describes his parents as even more addicted to substances than he is. He uses the emergency room regularly for care, then leaves against medical advice when physically touched. He describes periodic suicidal thoughts. He revealed that he "has PTSD from childhood sexual and physical abuse" from his elder brother, who also broke his legs as a young child. The brother is now incarcerated.

Scott was terminated from, and he himself "fired," several primary care practices. He is currently stable in a primary care practice as a result of clear boundaries and expectations with a new clinician and staff who have an understanding of the impact of trauma on his behavior. The clinician approached Scott with curiosity and compassion, and the health plan ensured the presence of his care manager during all visits. Scott is not prescribed any controlled substances, his depression is treated, and he has now completed specialty follow-up visits in neurology and pain management. He has not insulted or threatened his medical home staff in the past 6 months, despite his continued demanding number of phone calls. The practice has instituted a case conference where Scott's behavior and needs are discussed, and staff can support each other in their caregiving.

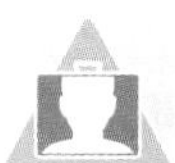

CASE ILLUSTRATION 2

Devon is a 62-year-old man engaged in primary care with a history of poorly controlled diabetes, chronic pain, advanced liver failure, daily smoking (cigarettes and marijuana), and alcohol misuse.

He is mostly home-bound lying in bed, drinking alcohol, and alternately smoking cigarettes and marijuana throughout the day. Despite his close relationship with his primary care clinician, he feels that there is no point in taking care of his health as he is "going to die soon anyway." He has been hospitalized numerous times because of liver disease and poorly controlled diabetes. When hospitalized, he consistently yells at and threatens other patients and clinicians. He has left the hospital against medical advice on several occasions when he feels "triggered."

He has been unable to work for decades, and witnessed the murder of several close family members as a child. He denies that he is addicted to any of the substances he uses.

At the primary care clinician's recommendation, he consulted with a psychologist to discuss his substance use and trauma. After multiple sessions of engagement- and substance-oriented Motivational Interviewing, Devon was ready to start trauma-focused psychotherapy (Cognitive Processing Therapy, or CPT). After 8 sessions of CPT, Devon no longer met criteria for PTSD and had quit smoking and drinking. Throughout treatment, close coordination with the primary care clinician allowed a unified message to Devon and helped him feel that "finally I have my team."

Unfortunately, he was soon diagnosed with metastatic laryngeal cancer. He no longer displayed behavioral difficulties or threatened to leave the hospital against medical advice. Before he died, he expressed gratitude to his integrated primary care team about the peace he had been able to find near the end of his life.

CASE ILLUSTRATION 3

Pebbles is a 51-year-old woman with HIV and a long history of substance abuse. She was a teenage prostitute who experienced serial sexual and physical abuse throughout her life. Pebbles eventually married her pimp, who controlled most of her life activities. When Pebbles was 50, her husband died.

Over the next 4 years, Pebbles' substance abuse and HIV medication adherence worsened. She sought out primary care only at times when her health greatly deteriorated. At those visits, efforts were made to refer her to inpatient substance abuse treatment. Each time, she thrived in the inpatient setting, and regained her health and lovely demeanor, only to relapse almost immediately when she was discharged to the community. This cycle continued repeatedly and included a number of hospital stays for HIV-related pneumonia and bacteremia.

The primary care clinic at which Pebbles received care worked to become a trauma-informed primary care clinic. Part of this entailed educating all staff and providers about the consequences of trauma, including substance abuse and PTSD. As a result, her clinician administered a PTSD screening tool for the first time. The result was strongly positive. Pebbles was referred to a newly integrated psychiatric nurse practitioner who diagnosed her formally with PTSD. She was treated with medications for her PTSD-associated nightmares and anxiety and referred to a community-based therapist with expertise in trauma and substance abuse. She also goes regularly to Narcotics Anonymous.

With appropriate therapy for both her substance abuse and PTSD, Pebbles has stayed abstinent from drugs for over a year. Her stability allowed her to fulfill a lifelong goal: she brought her adult child (who had been born with a cognitive impairment while Pebbles was in her addiction) into her apartment and began providing full-time care for her. She has also been fully adherent to her HIV medications.

SUGGESTED READINGS

American Psychiatric Association. PTSD. In: *Diagnostic and Statistical Manual of Mental Disorders*. 5th ed. Arlington, VA: American Psychiatric Publishing; 2013.

Bohnert, KM, Sripada RK, Mach J, McCarthy JF. Same-day integrated mental health care and PTSD diagnosis and treatment among VHA primary care patients with positive PTSD screens. *Psychiatr Serv* 2015;67(1):94–100.

Cigrang JA, Rauch SA, Mintz J, et al. Moving effective treatment for posttraumatic stress disorder to primary care: a randomized controlled trial with active duty military. *Fam Syst Health* 2017;35(4):450.

Department of Veterans Health Affairs. VA/DOD Clinical Practice Guideline for the Management of Post-traumatic Stress Disorder and Acute Stress Disorder (v. 3.0, 2017). https://www.healthquality.va.gov/guidelines/MH/ptsd/VADoDPTSDCPGFinal012418.pdf. Accessed January 16, 2019.

Felitti VJ. Adverse childhood experiences and adult health. *Acad Pediatr* 2009;9(3):131–132.

Impact of adult trauma: Centers for Disease Control and Prevention Division of Violence Prevention. U.S. Department of Veterans Affairs National Center for PTSD, 2014.

Kimberg L. Trauma and trauma-informed care. In: King, TE Wheeler, MB eds. *The Medical Management of Vulnerable and Underserved Patients: Principles, Practice and Populations*. New York, NY: McGraw-Hill Professional; 2016:chap 36.

Liebschutz J, Saitz R, Brower V, et al. PTSD in urban primary care: high prevalence and low physician recognition. *J Gen Intern Med* 2007;22(6):719–726.

Machtinger EL, Cuca YP, Khanna N, Rose CD, Kimberg LS. From treatment to healing: the promise of trauma-informed primary care. *Womens Health Issues* 2015;25(3):193–197.

Machtinger EL, Davis KB, Kimberg LS, et al. From treatment to healing: inquiry and response to recent and past trauma in adult health care. *Womens Health Issues* 2019;29(2):97–102.

Substance Abuse and Mental Health Services Administration. SAMHSA's Concept of Trauma and Guidance for a Trauma-Informed Approach. SAMHSA's Trauma and Justice Strategic Initiative. July 2014. Rockville, MD. http://www.traumainformedcareproject.org/resources/SAMHSA%20TIC.pdf.

Palliative Care, Hospice, & Care of the Dying

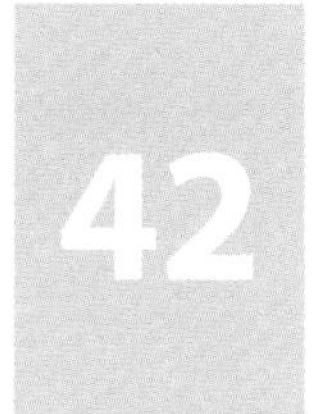

Bethany C. Calkins, MS, MD; Michael Eisman, MD; & Timothy E. Quill, MD, MACP, FAAHPM

INTRODUCTION

The goals of medical practice based exclusively on cure and restoration of function are frequently called into question when patients are irreversibly ill and potentially dying. New goals, such as pain and symptom management, enhancing quality of life, and finding meaning in the face of death may take precedence, becoming an increasingly important part of the treatment plan. Some clinicians may wonder if death is something to be fought at all costs, but no matter what the overarching goal of treatment, relieving suffering should always be a central part of our responsibility as clinicians.

Enhancing the quality of life for those afflicted with serious chronic illness is the cornerstone of the rapidly developing specialty of palliative care. As illustrated in Figure 42-1, palliative care can be provided alongside aggressive treatment of a patient's underlying disease, but as the patient becomes sicker and closer to death, palliation often becomes the primary objective.

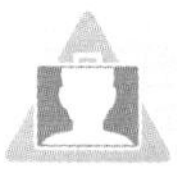

CASE ILLUSTRATION 1

Ella, a 71-year-old woman, develops pains in her lower chest for a month before visiting her personal physician. When a chest film shows several nodular masses suggestive of widespread lung cancer, the physician phones Ella and tells her there is a problem, making an office appointment for the next day. At this visit, the doctor discusses the results of the chest film with the patient and her son. Ella, having long suspected she might get lung cancer from smoking heavily, weeps openly upon hearing the results. Bronchoscopy is recommended, and she is referred to a pulmonologist. Bronchoscopic biopsies show a small-cell lung cancer. The pulmonologist refers Ella to an oncologist who recommends chemotherapy.

The patient and her son return to her primary care doctor to discuss her options. Ella says she would like to proceed with chemotherapy but wants to stop it if she becomes too ill from the treatments. A Roman Catholic, she has discussed with her priest the morality of refusing extraordinary treatment, including feeding tubes, if she were to have a terminal condition. She has appointed her son as her health care proxy and discusses her desire not to undergo cardiopulmonary resuscitation (CPR). The physician gives Ella a living will and a do-not-resuscitate (DNR) document; she and her son complete them with her doctor. She wants to try all other potentially effective disease-directed treatments, and she also agrees to have her pain and shortness of breath treated aggressively as well. She also knows that cure is very unlikely with this treatment, so she begins to work with a financial planner to get her affairs in order.

Ella undergoes chemotherapy for several months but gradually grows thinner and weaker. She and her son visit her doctor, and they are told that treatment is not controlling the disease and that the only options left for cancer treatment are experimental. She is referred to a home hospice program and agrees to a plan that is now directed exclusively at relieving her suffering. Ella lives alone and does not want to die in her apartment. Neither does she want her son to have to provide home care for her when she becomes too dependent to live alone. She also wants to know whether she could move to a hospice house or a nursing home for the very last phase of her illness when she is unable to care for herself at home. Her doctor and her son agree to find other placement when the need arises.

When she becomes confused 1 month later and is unable to stay at home, she is admitted to a comfort

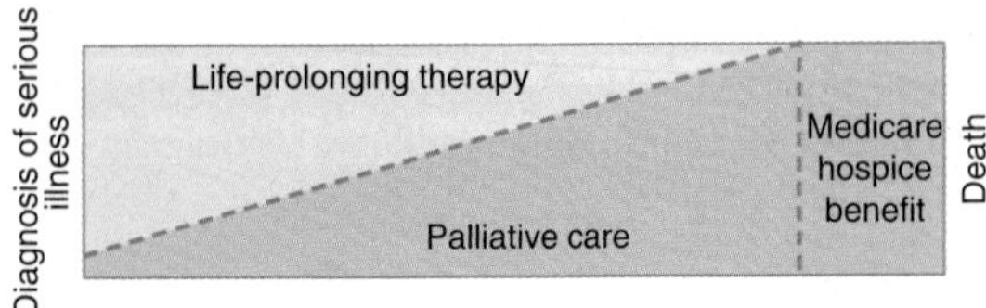

Figure 42-1. The place of palliative care in the course of illness. (Adapted from *The National Consensus Project's Clinical Practice Guidelines for Quality Palliative Care,* 4th edition. Copyright 2018. Available at: https://www.nationalcoalitionhpc.org/ncp/.)

care floor at a local nursing home. An intensive palliative treatment regimen is initiated, and she dies 2 weeks later with her son at her bedside, 6 months after the initial diagnosis.

Early after this patient's initial diagnosis, she received palliative care alongside aggressive treatment of her disease. Withholding aggressive pain and symptom management until referral to hospice is misguided and unfair, depriving patients of optimal treatment of their suffering from the beginning of their illness. This "both/and" approach has been one of the most important conceptual breakthroughs for palliative care, for it allows quality-of-life issues to be addressed for all seriously ill patients, not just those who are referred to hospice. It also allows patients simultaneously to "hope for the best" (that even improbable or experimental treatment might affect their disease and prolong their life) and "prepare for the worst" (make sure that financial affairs are settled and consider religious or existential issues should they wish to do so). It may be easier for some patients to make the transition to hospice if they have had this "both/and" conversation with their physician from the start of their illness.

KEY ISSUES

Nonabandonment

When a patient is given the diagnosis of a life-threatening illness, a wide spectrum of feelings may emerge, including denial, anxiety, fear, sadness, and anger. If practitioners are surprised by the diagnosis, feel as though they missed a clue to the diagnosis earlier on, or are discomfited by death, they may feel inclined to withdraw from the patient's care or to minimize the meaning and impact of the diagnosis. The commitment not to abandon the patient requires that clinicians learn to work through their own feelings, become knowledgeable about palliative care as well as all reasonable disease-directed treatment options, and recognize that the process of dying can be a unique spiritual and personal experience for both doctor and patient. The goal should be to form a partnership that will help the patient face the future with courage and dignity.

The goals of partnership and shared decision making are sometimes limited by strong emotional reactions as well as long-standing personality traits that can isolate the patient from the clinician, friends, and family. In addition, physicians may be unable to commit the time and energy needed to develop close personal contact with the seriously ill and dying patient. Clinicians need to realize that extraordinary effort is sometimes required to be a partner with patients and their families through what initially may be a vigorous fight against disease, but eventually may end in the patient's death.

The goal of palliative care is to provide the best possible quality of life for patients and their family. Palliative care addresses the biological, psychosocial, and spiritual dimensions of suffering, emphasizing state-of-the-art pain and symptom management, as well as a fresh look at patient goals and prognosis. Unlike Medicare-sponsored hospice programs, palliative care does not require patients to give up on aggressive treatment of their underlying disease, to accept a prognosis of less than 6 months, or to accept palliation as the central goal of therapy. Thus, it allows "hospice-like" treatments to be made available to those seriously ill patients who want to continue some or all disease-directed treatments. For example, patients who are highly likely to die but want to try improbable experimental therapy in hopes that it might prolong their lives, should receive palliative care, but they would not qualify for a Medicare-sponsored hospice program. Hospice programs enroll patients with a terminal disease who are more likely than not to die within the next 6 months' time once they agree to forgo curative treatments for their disease and focus only on improving quality of life. Palliative care allows better pain and symptom management, careful attention to quality of life, an examination of the goals of treatment, and an opportunity to provide a much broader range of patients' reflection on issues of life closure at the same time they received desired disease-directed treatment. Unfortunately, the medical infrastructure that supports the patient and family receiving palliative care at home is much less comprehensive than the medical infrastructure supporting hospice.

Patients confronting a severe illness may opt for an all-out, disease-oriented medical treatment, or a trial of aggressive medical care with set limits (such as a DNR order). Optimally, both of these patient pathways would also receive palliative care consultation from the time of diagnosis. When undergoing time-limited trials of aggressive care, patients have the opportunity to gauge and discuss with their provider whether the suffering involved with the treatment, given the odds of success, is worth it. If and when treatments begin to fail, or if supposedly curative treatments become too burdensome, patients can stop at any time and consider a transition to an approach that emphasizes pure palliation with their palliative care provider. This would be the time to consider referral to hospice, where relieving symptoms and alleviating suffering take precedence over attempts to treat the underlying disease.

Hospice

Hospice programs provide comprehensive care to dying patients, with a multidisciplinary team of nurses, physicians, social workers, clergy, and volunteers. These programs, which accept only patients who are more likely than not to die in the next 6 months and are willing to forgo disease-directed therapies and hospitalizations, help patients and their families live as fully as possible by providing quality palliative care. In the United States, only about 30% of deaths occur in hospice programs, and many of these patients are referred to hospice too late in the course of their illness to take full advantage of the resources and supports available to them. The palliative care philosophy underlying hospice can be applied in a range of settings including acute-care hospitals, skilled nursing facilities, and within the homes of patients. The advantage of hospice programs is the expertise brought to techniques of palliative care by the multidisciplinary staff, as well as the added support for patient and family at home, including payment for palliative medications and medical equipment. In most outpatient hospice programs, the primary care physician and the hospice team form a partnership to care for the patient. The primary care provider, with whom the patient may have a long-term relationship, should be intimately involved in both the decision for hospice referral and the patient's ongoing care. Once distressing symptoms are controlled, the hospice team may then help the patient find new avenues for hope, meaning, and ways of saying good-bye.

Dealing With Grief

At times it may be difficult to distinguish normal grief reactions to the dying process from pathologic states that may require consultation and special treatment. There is a natural sadness that human beings experience with regard to death. This sadness, which may be a way of preparing for death, has been called **preparatory** or **anticipatory grief**. Grieving over the loss of physical abilities, social position, and contact with pleasurable routines—whether one's own or those of a loved one—is a natural reaction. The absence of grief over these losses may indicate denial and emotional numbing. Sharing and exploring the grief can help both the patient and the clinician enter into a relationship that acknowledges each other's humanity. Having the courage to explore these feelings assists the patient in coming to terms with death and may prevent the isolation and subsequent clinical depression to which some patients are prone.

Depression

Distinguishing clinical depression from the natural grieving process that accompanies a terminal illness may be difficult, as they share many common symptoms. The vegetative symptoms of depression—fatigue, changes in appetite, sleep disorders, decreased sexual drive—are all common in serious illness. As many as 80% of the psychological symptoms that occur in cancer patients go untreated simply because it is difficult to diagnose depression in this population. Providers should have a high index of suspicion for depression in patients with serious disease. The affective and cognitive signs of depression, such as loss of interest, withdrawal, sadness, inability to concentrate, and hopelessness may be realistic assessments in the face of severe suffering, fear of a loss of dignity, and the expectation of death. Major depression should be considered when the cognitive symptoms of dysphoria, shame, guilt, isolation, or suicidal ideation seem out of proportion to the patient's situation (see Chapter 26). Depression in the terminally ill can be very responsive to pharmacotherapy as well as counseling, even when it is part of a normal reaction. Depending on the expertise of the physician and other members of the multidisciplinary team, more challenging cases of depression and anxiety should be referred to a mental health professional. Psychotherapists who are familiar with the dying process and are experienced with medically ill patients can provide an invaluable resource, both diagnostically and therapeutically, in the care of the terminally ill.

Transitions

In terminal illness, patients frequently decline in health in a stepwise fashion. These transitions near the end-of-life result in feelings of loss for patients and their families and provide the potential for personal growth and the acceptance of death. Progressive declines initially may be treated as another form of bad news, but they also potentially provide the opportunity for enhanced meaning and control in the dying process. Physicians caring for terminally ill patients must explore and work through these transitions with their patients. Questions that clinicians can ask their patients in exploring their views on end-of-life issues are listed in Table 42-1. These can be asked as hypothetical questions to explore the patient's beliefs about life and death. In patients with more advanced illness, the questions and their answers may be highly relevant to immediate treatment decisions.

Table 42-1. End-of-life issues to be discussed with patients.

Life support
• Do you have an advance directive (a living will or health care proxy)? • Do you know what CPR is? It may not work very well for people in your condition, and it is very painful. Should you choose to forego CPR, we can focus our treatments on anything that has a good chance of helping you without harming you. • In the event an illness led to your being unable to eat or drink on a permanent basis, would you want to be fed with feeding tubes? • Do you want your medical care primarily geared to prolonging your life, or is improving or maintaining your quality of life more important?
Personal beliefs
• What life experiences have you had around death and dying? • How have these experiences affected your own attitudes about death? • What are your worst fears about dying? What are your biggest hopes? • What would be a "good death" for you? • What do you believe happens to you when you die? • If you were to die sooner rather than later, what would be left undone?
Long-term care and support systems
• If you become too ill to take care of yourself, who will take care of you? • Who would you want to make health care decisions for you if you became unable to do so? • If you were dying, would you prefer to be at home or in an institution such as a hospital or nursing home? • Do you know what hospice care is? Would you want that kind of care if you were terminally ill? • Who would you want to be present at the time of your dying and death? • Is there anything you need to get done before you die?

CASE ILLUSTRATION 2

Carlos, a 70-year-old man, has been diagnosed with advanced hepatocellular carcinoma. In exploring the treatment options with his physician, he is clear about wanting only palliative measures, and referral to a home hospice program is initiated. Carlos is not a verbal man, and discussions about death and dying are met with little response.

At first, periodic nursing visits are all that is needed. He has an antique tool collection and spends countless hours labeling and ordering the tools. His nurse talks to him about this process, which has come to symbolize his anticipatory grief. As he deteriorates, nursing visits become more frequent, and home health aides come to help with his personal care. Carlos gradually becomes bed bound. Although his family initially feels uncomfortable with his dying at home, a family meeting with the physician and hospice nurse sets up a rotation of visits to provide for both company and supervision. Children who had been estranged are in the rotation, and it becomes a time of family healing. Although little is explicitly said about his approaching death, the presence of family and talk about the tools provide a vehicle for saying good-bye. Carlos dies quietly at home with his family present.

Patients' willingness and ability to enter into deep discussions about death and dying vary considerably; clinicians need to be flexible in their expectations about how much exploration is desirable or even possible. It is unusual for a lifelong pattern of behavior to be altered by the dying process; therefore, those who lived very private lives may not be able to "open up" significantly at the end of life. For some, dying may be a time for personal growth, reflection, and meaning, but for others, personal factors and emotional reactions block an acceptance of death. The most frequently encountered of these reactions are denial, anger, depression, fear, and anxiety. These reactions may be present in different degrees and at different times in the dying process. Clinicians need to acknowledge, explore, and eventually understand what function the reaction is serving for the patient. Exploration and empathy where possible, rather than withdrawal, are the ways to deepen the patient–clinician relationship and create an atmosphere in which personal growth is more likely to occur (see Chapter 2).

CASE ILLUSTRATION 3

At 68 years old, Albert has severe end-stage emphysema from years of smoking, severe mitral regurgitation, congestive heart failure, cardiac arrhythmias, and alcoholism. He lives with his wife, whom he has bullied and dominated throughout their 40-year marriage. He has been on home oxygen and has had multiple hospital admissions for shortness of breath.

Admitted to the emergency room with severe shortness of breath, Albert is found to have pneumonia and heart failure. He had previously decided not to have CPR and wanted "no part of any of those damned machines." He is admitted to the hospital and treated with aggressive medical means but is not put on a respirator. Albert regularly yells and curses at the respiratory therapists, nursing staff, physicians, and his family for not taking care of him, for making him suffer, and for not being prompt enough with meals, medicines, and treatments. He insists that the only thing wrong with him is that the medicines are making him sick.

Efforts to engage Albert in a dialogue that explores his feelings are met first with an unwillingness to talk and then a life history of feeling abandoned, powerless, betrayed by employers, and subject to bad luck. He describes himself as an "ornery son of a bitch." He fears lingering and suffering in the hospital, and although he hopes he will die quickly, he is also afraid to die. One of Albert's fears is of being buried alive, a phobia fed by a television program he had seen about the difficulty of determining when someone was dead and the possibility of being sent to the undertaker while still alive. The anxiety of being trapped in a "tight" place is overwhelming to him.

Albert's physicians had initially resisted placing him on anxiolytic drugs or narcotics out of fear they would compromise his breathing. The palliative care consultant recommended that both be started and reassured both the treating physicians as well as the patient and family of the safety and effectiveness of these treatments in this circumstance as long as they are started at low doses. Low-dose opioids and anxiolytic medications are eventually started around the clock, and his dyspnea and anxiety are dramatically improved. Placed in a room with a large picture window to the outside, he spends long periods of time staring out the window. His complaints diminish, and he seems much more relaxed. He allows the hospital chaplain to visit and to pray with him, though he does not otherwise want to talk about the nearness of death or any regrets he has about his life. He eventually tells his wife he has suffered enough and does not want to live any longer. He gradually becomes more confused as a result of the rising carbon dioxide levels and dies several nights later.

Patients with difficult personality traits who are experiencing the dying process can be especially challenging to caregivers. The use of multidisciplinary specialties to brainstorm potential approaches and to share expertise may facilitate providers' commitment not to abandon these particularly challenging patients and families.

Information, Prognosis, Alternatives

Clinicians need to provide the patient with information about the disease, the prognosis, the treatment options, and the anticipated course of the illness. Most patients and their families want to know how much time is left when a terminal diagnosis is made. Providing ranges of survival times and allowing for outliers on either end is better than predicting an exact amount of time. ("The average person with your illness will live two to six months. It could be longer, and we will try to make that happen, but it could also be shorter, so you may want to make sure everything is prepared just in case things don't go as we hope.") Refusing to give time estimates or withholding other grim information to protect the patient is usually not productive and may not allow the patient and family to prepare for death. The possibility of a miracle or an exception to the usual course of the illness ("it could be longer…") allows a glimmer of hope for some patients. However, clinicians giving prognostic information must discipline themselves to also discuss the possibility that death may come sooner than expected, so that patients are not unprepared for this possibility as well. In general, the physician should be guided by patients and their families in determining how much prognostic information is desired. ("Would you like to hear what we are thinking about in terms of prognosis?")

Alternative healing methods may offer hope to some patients when traditional methods are not working, have proven too burdensome, or are not consistent with the patient's preferences. Patients who are interested in pursuing alternative methods of treatment should be supported in doing so, particularly if those treatments are noninvasive and are therefore unlikely to harm. There is nothing to preclude combining nontraditional treatments with traditional treatments as part of an individually tailored plan. Improbable aggressive therapeutic alternatives offer some patients a degree of hope, but clinicians and patients should explore the tradeoffs of this type of hope together. Examining the risks and benefits of both traditional and nontraditional therapies is frequently enough to begin the dialogue, which can then continue by exploring the probabilities of improvement, the specific risks and benefits of the treatment, and by distinguishing false hope from a meaningful alternative (see Chapter 35).

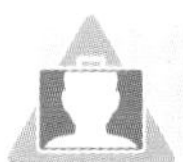

CASE ILLUSTRATION 4

Max, a 63-year-old, recently retired, and previously healthy man, develops abdominal pain and is found to have widely metastasized colon cancer. He goes to a physician and is advised that no treatment would be beneficial and that he has approximately

6–12 months to live. He is given acetaminophen and codeine for pain and told to come back when the combination no longer relieves the discomfort. Max and his wife cannot bear the thought of just waiting for him to die and decide to cast a wider net in seeking a cure—or at least some kind of treatment. They hear of a cancer treatment clinic out of the country and go there for a 6-week program of intensive vitamin and herbal treatments, coffee enemas, a variety of teas, and dietary supplements. Max is also given a long list of treatments to follow when he returns home; this keeps him busy trying to "beat" the cancer. The clinic is supposed to provide follow-up by mail or telephone; however, several months go by and there is no contact from the clinic.

Discouraged, Max and his wife go to another physician in their hometown when the abdominal pain intensifies and ascites and jaundice set in. The physician and the couple discuss the available options and agree on purely palliative care measures. Max is referred to a home hospice program and dies 4 weeks later, approximately 9 months from the time of diagnosis. His family feels he received superb care for his last 4 weeks; however, they feel abandoned and betrayed with regard to his prior treatment. His wife never receives any follow-up information from the overseas clinic, nor does anyone from the original physician's office call to offer condolences on her husband's death.

The patient in case illustration 4 has been abandoned twice. The first treating physician failed to explore all treatment alternatives (such as a second opinion, experimental therapy, and guidance in exploring nontraditional treatments) and then offered inadequate follow-up (asking him only to come back when his pain is uncontrollable at home). The alternative clinic offered the patient an active treatment approach which he and his wife desperately sought, but then deserted him by failing to follow through after the treatment was completed. The third physician finally helped the patient and family come to grips with the reality of his condition and arranged for a program that provided care and follow-up for his final weeks. Nonabandonment is always a key element in the care of the dying patient.

Hope & Meaning

Throughout the dying process, the search for hope and meaning is always present, even if it is not dominant. Hope aids patients and their loved ones in enduring suffering when faced with a terminal illness. It comes in many forms, not simply through cure or recovery: to hope for a peaceful death, to hope for more time to "finish business," to find new meaning and the possibility of personal growth, and to hope for more emotional closeness with loved ones or with God. None of these hopes are dependent on cure of the body.

CASE ILLUSTRATION 5

Rhea, a 64-year-old woman with metastatic breast cancer, is on high-dose long-acting morphine because of bone pain. She has fractures of her clavicle and both femurs and has requested no resuscitation in the event of cardiac or pulmonary arrest. She hopes to be able to die at home, where she has very close family support, without more painful episodes or fractures. She is enrolled in a home hospice program, and her sister moves in with her to serve the role as primary care provider.

Rhea eventually shows signs of increasing confusion and dehydration. She expresses the strong wish not to die yet, because her children and their families are arriving in 2 weeks. She wants not only to see them but also to be as alert and pain free as possible while they visit. Blood work is done to see if she has anything that might be easily reversible, and hypercalcemia is found. Because she wishes to die at home with only palliative measures taken, she remains at home for another day. She knows that she will likely die from the effects of the untreated hypercalcemia, but that she then would likely not get to see her children. Despite attempts at oral treatment, she becomes progressively less alert, and is brought to an acute hospice unit when her oral intake stops.

In hope of having her alert for her family's upcoming visit, treatment is initiated with intravenous fluids, diuretics, and bisphosphonates. The hypercalcemia is corrected, her confusion clears, and she is able to go home after a week. By the time her children arrive, Rhea is alert and able to communicate coherently. She is quite elated that she can have last words with them and her grandchildren. Despite the need for increased doses of morphine and multiple other medications to control her symptoms, she is not readmitted to the acute hospice unit when her hypercalcemia and the associated confusion recur. She dies quietly at home several days later.

Fortunately, the hope for more time in case illustration 5 could be achieved because the patient was willing to be admitted for intravenous fluids, and the hospice program allowed flexibility to meet her short-term goals. Invasive interventions that exceed the usual boundaries of hospice care but that extend meaningful life and improve quality of life are sometimes appropriate even within a hospice approach, as long as the patient consents. Remaining flexible in the face of changing, difficult situations and allowing the patient's goals to guide the treatment as much as possible permit the clinician to hope along with the patient for a death with as little meaningless suffering as possible.

Trying to find and maintain hope when the patient's goal of recovery is futile often calls for personal and spiritual exploration. It may be necessary to probe in depth the patient's feeling of hopelessness before possible new avenues for hope and meaning can be uncovered. It is important not to provide false hope through simple or formulaic solutions to complex problems; hopeful solutions are often uniquely personal and may be discovered through the patient's continuing exploration with family, friends, health care providers, and clergy.

PLANNING FOR THE FUTURE

Advance Directives

Advance directives are formal documents that direct health care decisions should patients lose the capacity to speak for themselves in the future. There are two types of advance directives: living wills and health care proxies (also called durable powers of attorney).

A **living will** allows a patient to direct the kinds of treatments wanted if the capacity to make decisions is lost. Some living wills focus on general goals, whereas others specify exact treatments (cardiopulmonary resuscitation [CPR], artificial ventilation, artificial hydration, and nutrition) and explicit circumstances (terminal illness, persistent vegetative state, unable to make decisions for oneself). Living wills become operative only when patients are unable to communicate for themselves, and when the circumstances specified in the document are realized.

A **health care proxy** or **durable power of attorney** allows patients to designate a person to make healthcare decisions on their behalf should they become unable to do so. These directives allow much more flexibility than do living wills, as it is difficult to anticipate all possible medical conditions and treatment options that might be in question for a particular patient.

Many people complete both documents: a living will to represent an overarching philosophy to guide care and a health care proxy to designate a person to help interpret that philosophy when the patient can no longer do so. For healthy persons, discussing a living will or a health care proxy may be the first time they have had to face their own mortality. For those with terminal illness, completing an advance directive may be seen as another indication of their inevitable deterioration.

Involving family members in the discussions of advance directives is useful. A proxy who is uninformed about the values and wishes of the patient has an arduous job when difficult care decisions must be made on behalf of a now incapacitated patient. Although they cannot cover every situation, living wills with clear statements about goals, values, and directions help the clinician and the designated proxy formulate a care plan. In addition, having a form to fill out helps many patients and their families discuss death- and disability-related issues. For severely ill patients, the advance directive decisions can provide a starting point for discussions about limitations on care and the burdens of suffering as well as orders not to resuscitate.

Do Not Resuscitate

The "do-not-resuscitate" (DNR) order refers to the withholding of CPR, specifically closed-chest cardiac massage, defibrillation, and artificially supplied respiratory support. For most patients with a terminal disease, CPR is ineffective, and its harshness makes it a cruel, expensive, technological death ritual. Many studies have shown that CPR provides no increase in out-of-hospital survival for patients with progressive multisystem disease, particularly patients with advanced cancers and renal failure.

Unfortunately, many patients and their families equate DNR with abandonment or "giving up" and agonize over its issuance. This is in part due to the way medical personnel emphasize what will be withheld rather than what will be done. When alternative treatment strategies are not explained, patients and families think that a DNR order means nothing will be done to treat potentially reversible conditions or to relieve uncomfortable symptoms. They sense that second-class treatment will be given—which may indeed happen if clinicians and the institutions they work in are not knowledgeable about the narrow focus of a DNR directive. It should be understood that agreement to a DNR order in no way limits other treatment options. A way of articulating this is to say: "We want to do everything possible to help you, but we also do not want to harm you. CPR would not work given your condition, and it is very harsh. I would recommend that you set that limit while we continue to provide any and all treatments that will help you."

DNR orders do, however, signal that things are different. The notion that being resuscitated from cardiopulmonary arrest will not add appreciably to the quality and/or quantity of life is an open acknowledgment that death might be near—and that reversing the dying process is not within the power of medicine. Although some patients are initially frightened by this discussion, many feel relieved and appreciate the opportunity to avoid treatment that would not help them.

Emergency rescue crews are obligated to attempt cardiopulmonary resuscitation unless they have specific instructions not to proceed. DNR orders that are valid in the inpatient setting may not be valid in the outpatient setting unless special forms, which vary by locality, are completed. These issues should be addressed with terminally ill patients who want to remain at home, as resuscitation may be carried out in times of crisis if the proper documentation is not on hand. In New York and other states, the Medical Orders for Life Sustaining Treatment (MOLST) has been accepted as a legal document that must be honored by emergency medical technicians and first responders in all settings.

Restricted Interventions

Patients at the end of life, or patients with a high degree of suffering, may elect through their advance directives not to undergo treatments that may be considered routine under other circumstances. Patients have the right to forgo therapies such as intravenous fluids, nasogastric feeding, and supplemental oxygen, among others. Documentation of these choices is vital if the patient does not wish to undergo treatments and can be done on the MOLST form. Restricted intervention forms are also available in other states to augment the advance directives (it is critical to know which forms and what restrictions exist in one's own state to ensure that desired treatments and limitations are honored in all settings).

Pain & Symptom Relief

An important goal in palliative care is to keep patients as free of pain as is possible. Long-acting opioid preparations, when given in sufficient quantity in a regular dosing schedule with proportionate supplemental doses as needed, are effective in alleviating most chronic pain without significantly compromising quality of life (see Chapter 38). Knowing that they can control their own pain is reassuring to patients, especially those who have seen painful deaths. Both realistic and unrealistic concerns about addiction from patients, families, and caregivers should be anticipated and addressed, as these worries often present a major obstacle to adequate pain relief. Withholding narcotics in the seriously ill because of unrealistic fears is unwarranted and cruel. On the other hand, care must be taken to prevent misuse of opioids in patients with substance abuse problems and serious illness through prescribing contracts and clear consequences for violation.

Delirium & Coma

Many patients die in profoundly altered states of sensorium. There are also an increasing number of patients with dementing illnesses in whom cognitive and affective life may have diminished significantly prior to the terminal episode. Terminally ill patients with delirium present the physician and the patient's family with a dilemma. Delirium may be due to reversible factors that, if treated, could extend life. The extent to which reversible causes of delirium are searched for and treated depends on the patient's current goals, previous directives, and concurrent discussions with the family in light of the underlying medical condition. The prior degree of suffering and the patient's wishes should largely determine what should be done.

CASE ILLUSTRATION 6

Caleb, a 101-year-old rugged dairy farmer, has become partly deaf and then blind in the last 5 years of his life but remains alert and communicative. He develops a cough and fever and, despite treatment for pneumonia, becomes progressively more dyspneic. He tells his physician that he does not wish to be resuscitated. He says he is "ready to die and does not want to be saved in any way." Because his elderly wife cannot care for him at home, Caleb is hospitalized where he is referred to hospice and managed with "comfort measures only." He becomes progressively more confused and withdrawn, and his deafness and blindness further confound communication. He lies still in bed for long periods of time. Efforts by physicians and nurses to engage him in conversation are usually met with short responses such as yes, no, or okay. His physician asks him one morning what experiences he is having, and he replies that he is flying over fields of golden wheat on a sunny day. Then, in a voice of wonderment, he asks if he is still alive or if he has died. His physician replies that he is still alive. Caleb dies later that day.

The internal, subjective experience of a person dying with altered mental status may vary significantly from the outside perception. Patients who recover from delirium and coma sometimes report experiences that range from nightmarish, terrifying visions, on the one hand, to very pleasant out-of-body travel or visions of light and angelic beings on the other. Some may not be able to remember anything about the experience. Occasionally, the disorientation becomes profound and the sense of the world is lost.

Patients who experience delirium at the end of life need supportive treatment. If not already done in advance by the patient, decisions about artificial hydration and feeding should be made and formalized through the designated health care agent. The agent or the family, taking into consideration the patient's condition, prognosis, and prior stated wishes, must make a "substituted judgment" as to what they believe the patient would want if he were able to understand the nuances of his condition. If the patient's own preferences cannot be determined, the physician's decision should be based on a consensus among family and providers about what is in the "best interest" of the patient.

Providing nutrition and hydration through feeding tubes and intravenous lines when the dying patient can no longer eat or drink may appear compassionate, but such practices may inadvertently prolong dying and aggravate suffering. When a person with a terminal illness is actively dying, acceptance of this fact should guide all treatments in the direction of decreasing the suffering, enhancing the quality of remaining time, and respecting the patient's dignity.

The Wish to Die

Sometimes, even with the best methods of palliative care, suffering cannot be alleviated to the patient's satisfaction. If this occurs, the patient may feel that dying is the only way out. The patient may no longer be able to tolerate the pain, humiliation, loss of control, increased dependency, or burden the illness places on the family. Such patients often actively begin to contemplate ending their lives.

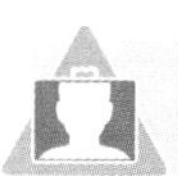

CASE ILLUSTRATION 7

Marvin is a 63-year-old man with amyotrophic lateral sclerosis who has been on a respirator at home for one year. He has lost the ability to use his arms and legs and requires total care. He increasingly resents his life on the respirator and requests that it be removed and that he be permitted to die. He makes this request repeatedly over the course of a month. His primary care physician sees him several times on home visits and discusses the request with Marvin's family. They agree that the respirator should be stopped. A psychiatrist visits the patient and indicates that he finds Marvin competent, not depressed; he concurs with the patient, family, and primary care physician on removing the respirator. Past attempts to remove the respirator led to air hunger and feelings of suffocation, so prior to removing the respirator a morphine drip is instituted, and the dose is adjusted to keep him comfortable as the respirator is turned off. The patient dies comfortably several minutes later, attended by his family and physician.

The **double effect** of providing medications intended to relieve suffering while taking the risk that they may unintentionally shorten the patient's life is an accepted part of medical practice and palliative care, provided the patient's suffering is proportionately severe. Withdrawing life-sustaining but burdensome treatments, even though the withdrawal leads to death, is also an accepted part of practice based on the patient's right to bodily integrity. These practices have widespread legal, ethical, and medical acceptance and should not be confused with the controversy surrounding assisted suicide and voluntary euthanasia. In this case, the patient's wish to die can be acceded to provided it is fully informed and not based on inadequate palliation. In such circumstances, treatments that are life-sustaining but very burdensome could be removed in conjunction with the provision of proportionate doses of narcotic intended to lessen suffering (Table 42-2).

Some patients, however, may ask the clinician, sometimes in an off-hand way as if testing the water, about more direct assistance in dying through either assisted suicide or euthanasia. This subject has both ethical and legal repercussions, and physicians are often as reluctant as their patients to discuss it.

If the patient has terrible suffering but does not have a life-sustaining treatment that can be withdrawn (e.g., respirator, dialysis, feeding tube) or the kind of pain that can justify high doses of narcotics, the request for help in dying would put the clinician in a more difficult position legally and ethically. **Voluntary active euthanasia** is the act of intentionally intervening to cause the patient's death, at the explicit request of, and with the full informed consent of, the competent patient. The physician administers a lethal agent, with the intent of both alleviating suffering and causing death. Although voluntary active euthanasia was recently legalized in all of Canada and is legal is several western European countries, it is clearly illegal everywhere in the United States and would lead to prosecution if discovered. In **assisted suicide**, the physician provides the means (such as a prescription for barbiturates) at the request of the patient, but the patient must eventually take (or not take) the potentially lethal medication by his or her own hand. Assisted suicide is legal in Oregon, Washington, Montana, Vermont, Hawaii, California, Colorado, Maine, New Jersey, and Washington DC, but it is explicitly illegal or legally very uncertain in other U.S. states. There is probably an underground practice in these other states, but its extent remains uncertain as it is conducted in secret with no open documentation or oversight. There are now data about the legalized practice in Oregon and Washington that can allow for comparison of utilization patterns of assisted dying and other last-resort palliative care practices with other states. In Oregon, for example, 1 in 6 terminally ill patients talks with their families about it, 1 in 50 talks with their doctors, but it accounts for only 1 in 300 deaths.

Table 42-2. Last resort interventions: definitions.

Term	Definition	Legal Status in the United States
Double effect	Administering drugs that are intended to relieve suffering but may unintentionally shorten life. The risk of shortening life must be proportionate to the degree of suffering. The clinician can foresee that life might be shortened, but it is not intended.	Legal
Withholding or withdrawing life-sustaining treatment	Withholding or withdrawing life-sustaining care that might result in the patient's death with the consent of the patient or surrogate. Justification based on the right to bodily integrity.	Legal with the proper consent
Palliative sedation to unconsciousness (also called terminal sedation)	With consent from the patient or surrogate, the patient is sedated to unconsciousness to relieve otherwise intractable suffering, and then food and fluids are withdrawn. Generally viewed as a combination of double effect and withdrawal of treatment, but not without moral controversy if viewed in aggregate.	Legal with the proper consent
Physician aid-in-dying (also called physician-assisted suicide)	Physician provides, at the patient's request, the means for the patient to end his or her own life. The patient then takes or does not take the overdose at a future time.	Illegal in most U.S. states except for Oregon, Washington, Montana, Vermont, Hawaii, California, Colorado, Maine, New Jersey, and Washington DC
Active euthanasia	Physician administers an intentional lethal overdose of medication with the competent patient's informed consent. The physician is the direct agent causing death at the patient's request.	Illegal, and likely to be successfully prosecuted in the United States if discovered

CASE ILLUSTRATION 8

Sara, a bedridden 84-year-old woman with end-stage congestive heart failure, is seen on rounds. She is on multiple medications, including morphine, to relieve her dyspnea and pulmonary edema. Despite intensive treatment, even eating causes her to be dyspneic. She looks up from her bed and asks to be given a lethal dose of medicine so that she can die. When asked why she wants to die now, Sara replies that she has lived long enough—through the deaths of her husband, two of her children, three of her brothers, and both of her sisters. Her one remaining son is dying of leukemia and has only weeks to live. She wants to die before him so that she will not have to grieve his death. Her request for lethal medication is not granted. Sara leaves the hospital with public health nurses and family to look after her. Her physician agrees to make home visits as Sara is too weak to travel to the office. A few days later, Sara is found dead in bed by the visiting nurse. The physician, called to the house to pronounce the patient dead, notices several empty pill bottles, including those from the morphine, at the bedside. The physician thinks that this may have been a suicide but decides not to pursue it and simply completes the death certificate as for a natural death.

A patient's request to hasten death should be explored in detail. At first, it should be considered a cry for help. It may represent the wish to escape from depression, anxiety, uncontrolled physical pain, shame of dependency, and other psychosocial issues. Once the underlying reasons for the request are fully understood, the problem(s) can usually be ameliorated through appropriate techniques of palliative care, and the request is frequently withdrawn. If the request is ignored, minimized, or belittled, the patient is left to deal with these feelings alone, and may (as in case illustration 8) take an overdose because of suffering that might have been dealt with by other means.

There are times, as in our example, when protracted pain and other debilitating symptoms might make choosing death a plausible alternative to continued suffering. The relationship between the physician, patient, and family as well as the physician's own values and the status of the law where the patient and physician live frame the response to such requests. Clinicians who refuse to participate in assisted suicide where it is legally permitted because of their own moral positions should make this clear to the patient who inquires. In this event, they have an obligation to seek common ground with the patient and to continue to search for other avenues to relieve suffering. Usually such intractable suffering can be addressed with symptom management, withdrawal of potentially life-sustaining therapies, and terminal sedation as a last resort.

In this particular case, if the patient's request was found to be rational and all reasonable alternatives had been explored, the patient could have stopped all of her heart failure medicines except for her morphine, which could have been titrated upward to control emerging shortness of breath. Those clinicians who are considering any last-resort options (legally permitted, and especially if legally prohibited) should fully explore the potential personal, professional, and legal consequences and get second opinions from experienced clinicians before proceeding. Guidelines for assisted suicide have been published, and clinicians confronted with a reasonable request to end life should refer to these, as well as to colleagues experienced in palliative care, for help. In almost all cases, legally permissible and clinically preferable alternatives can be found.

ACCEPTANCE

Some patients are not afraid of dying and come to accept death as a natural step in completing the life cycle. Many such persons are able to die with grace and ease, demonstrating that death does not always have to be feared or denied. Furthermore, some patients experience profound personal growth in the process of dying. For some highly independent persons, this becomes a time to be more accepting and appreciative of the love and care of others.

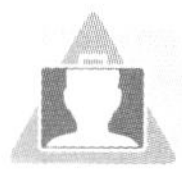

CASE ILLUSTRATION 9

A 64-year-old veterinarian, Richard, develops headaches so severe that he can no longer carry on his surgical practice. Within 3 months, he is diagnosed with an inoperable brain tumor. Over the ensuing 6 months, despite aggressive disease-directed treatment, he loses the ability to walk and swallow. Because of recurrent aspiration, he is placed on a home ventilator and fed through a gastrostomy tube. In the face of his overwhelming losses, he decides he wants relatives, friends, colleagues and members of his church to come to his home and tape a description of his life and journey to the point at which he is now. When this process is complete, Richard says good-bye to his wife and family and requests that the respirator and fluids be withdrawn. With his physician's consent and instructions to family members, he is given regular doses of morphine and the respirator is turned off. He dies with his loved ones in attendance. His life and death leave a legacy of courage and acquiescence to fate that touches the hearts of those he knew.

The search for love, a connection to others, and a sense of meaning are essential in helping patients through the dying process. The ability to experience love and meaning can ameliorate considerable suffering. If love and purpose can be found, fears usually lessen, and dying may be accepted as an end to one adventure and entry into the next phase of existence.

CARE OF THE FAMILY

Terminal illness can help resolve or intensify family conflict. Issues of power, money, allegiances, previous losses, and grief may surface along with unforeseen courage and the noblest sacrifices that family members may ever have made for each other. Paradoxical feelings of anger and love, fear and bravery, anxiety and compassion, depression and transcendence never seem to be far removed from dying patients and their caregivers.

The physician can be a healing presence in this volatile mix by including the patient's family and other caregivers as part of the treatment team. Such collaboration broadens the patient's network of support, enlisting new allies and more widely distributing the burden of care.

The clinician needs to communicate clearly with the family members regarding plans for care, prognosis, complications, and who will make decisions should the patient be unable. Establishing advance directives with the patient and the proxy is essential when it is likely the patient will lose capacity during the illness. The selection of a proxy forces the patient to choose among family members and may trigger old family wounds over who was favored and who has more power. The patient's wishes and choices should take precedence over what family members may want, although in actual practice this is sometimes difficult to achieve. When the patient loses mental capacity, the family becomes the focus of decision making, and processes are brought into play that may create conflict. Family pressures may even influence the decisions of a competent patient. The clinician may need to remind family members that whether the patient is competent or not, the patient's values, beliefs, and preferences need to be honored.

When a family has many members, the clinician may want to meet regularly with a small group and at critical times with more members. The family can be asked to designate representatives who can stay in close touch with the physician. If patients have lost the capacity to express their wishes and family members are in conflict about a certain plan, it is best to focus on what the patient would have wanted, applying the ethical principle of substituted judgment. If the patient's wishes are unknown, efforts should be initiated between the clinicians and the patient's family to determine the patient's best interests under the current circumstances. Views on what is truly in the patient's best interest may vary widely between family members and clinicians (see Chapter 11).

Unexpected Death

An unexpected death puts a particular strain on the family and the clinician. Sudden or traumatic death sends a shock through the family and, when it occurs in a medical facility, may elicit strong doubt about competence in clinicians. Meeting with the family, expressing sympathy, and answering questions in as straightforward a way as possible may be helpful. Family members should be allowed to view and stay with the deceased; when possible, the eyes and mouth should be closed and the limbs arranged peacefully. Strong emotional reactions should be anticipated and the tears of grief encouraged.

The clinician should recognize each family member present and solicit each person's reaction. Cultural norms may vary widely in the emotional behaviors displayed. The normal strong emotional reactions to grief in some cultures may seem histrionic or frightening to those from less demonstrative backgrounds, whose stoic reactions to extreme loss may seem equally incomprehensible to others (see Chapter 15). Only through experience with various manifestations of grief can the clinician judge what "normal" grief should look like. Physicians and nurses may want to call in clergy and social workers; each may have something to offer a family that is trying to integrate the shock and loss.

When an unexpected death occurs in the context of ongoing medical care, the practitioner should critically examine what, if anything, could have been done to prevent its occurrence. Self-recrimination and blame may initially be part of this process for the clinician, especially if a possible medical misjudgment was involved. Learning from the experience, discussing it with trusted colleagues, and disclosing it to the family are often appropriate. It is important that clinicians not bear the burdens of these experiences alone (see Chapter 39).

Unresolved Grief

Of all the causes of unremitting grief, one of the most overwhelmingly difficult for families and practitioners is the death of a child, especially when the death is unexpected. The parents' grief must be followed closely for signs of becoming pathological. The physician should not try to ameliorate the pain of the loss prematurely. Supportive listening, acknowledging and legitimizing the suffering, and expressing empathy may be the best initial approach. Follow-up visits to elicit stories and memories give the parents a chance to talk about the deceased if they choose. Discussing and expressing anger, guilt, and sadness can assist in the bereavement process. In many other cases, survivors are unable to deal with the loss of a parent, a sibling, a spouse or partner, or a long-time friend. Grief that is unresolved may lead to clinical depression, social isolation, and emotional numbing as well as multiple physical symptoms. Social problems such as drug abuse, marital and work conflicts, and feelings of hopelessness and abandonment may also appear. If the clinician cannot help the family resolve the grief, referral should be made to an appropriate support group or a therapist for counseling.

Under the Medicare Hospice Benefit, hospices provide bereavement support for at least a year to families of patients they have served. They also provide bereavement services to partners and close friends. Often, hospices provide this support to people in their community even if the death did not occur with hospice care.

SELF-CARE

How health care workers take care of themselves when involved in work related to death and dying has not received a great deal of attention. Burnout is common among physicians and nurses who work with patients who are suffering with a terminal illness. Having responsibility for dying patients' care and management in a society that denies death only exacerbates the problem. From the initial delivery of bad news about a new serious diagnosis, to discussions about disease recurrence, to the transition to hospice, to decisions about whether to attend the funeral, clinicians are confronted with thoughts and feelings that enmesh them with the patient and the family. How closely the patient's family resembles their own family dynamics or illness experience may determine how emotionally involved they become. The grief that follows the death of a close patient may be quite profound and requires time and reflection to heal. Unfortunately, most institutions do not have an organized way for caregivers to get and give support during these times. The feelings of loss need to be recognized and discussed. Support or bereavement groups may help in this process. Hospital morbidity and mortality committees review the decedent's medical care, but they rarely reflect on how caregivers felt about the death, or what effect it has on the staff. Setting aside time to review the death from this perspective is likely to be helpful for staff morale, cohesiveness, and healing (see Chapter 6).

Taking care of the dying patient enables clinicians to view death at very close range. Feelings of compassion and love as well as loneliness and vulnerability are frequently stirred up in providers. Healing responses may include turning to music, art, religion, literature, nature, humor, or psychotherapy for solace and understanding. Spiritual questions of purpose and meaning in life become more immediate in the face of impending death. Not only do workers in the realm of death and dying midwife patients through the dying process, but also the dying patient midwives us into a fuller experience of life.

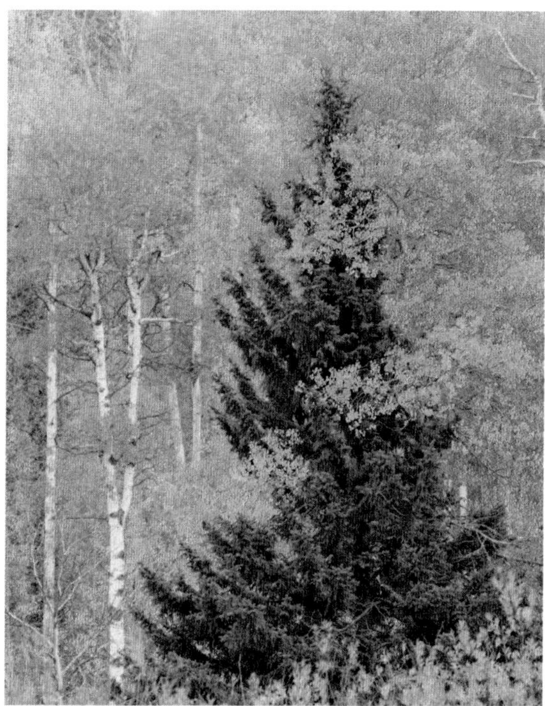

Photo by Hank Christensen (www.hankchristensen.com).

SUGGESTED READINGS

Back AL, Arnold RM, Quill TE. Hope for the best, and prepare for the worst. *Ann Intern Med* 2003;138:439–443.

Block SD. Psychological issues in end-of-life care. *J Palliat Med* 2006;9:751–772.

Casarett DJ, Quill TE. "I'm not ready for hospice": strategies for timely and effective hospice discussions. *Ann Intern Med* 2007;146:443–449.

Clinical Practice Guideline: Management of Cancer Pain. Agency for Health Care Policy and Research. Publication No. 94–0592. Available through the National Cancer Institute.

Meier DE, Back AL, Morrison RS. The inner life of physicians and the care of the seriously ill. *JAMA* 2001;286:3007–3014.

Quill TE. *Caring for Patients at the End of Life: Facing an Uncertain Future Together*. New York, NY: Oxford University Press; 2001.

Quill TE, Bower KA, Holloway R, et al. *Palliative Care Primer*. 6th ed. Chicago, IL: American Academy of Hospice and Palliative Medicine; 2014.

Quill TE, Ganzini L, Truog RD, Pope TM. Voluntarily stopping eating and drinking: clincial, ethical and legal aspects. *JAMA Intern Med* 2018:178(1):123–127.

Quill TE, Lo B, Brock DW. Palliative options of last resort: a comparison of voluntarily stopping eating and drinking, terminal sedation, physician-assisted suicide, and voluntary active euthanasia. *JAMA* 1997;278:2099–2104.

Snyder L, Quill TE, eds. *Physician Guide to End-of-Life Care*. Philadelphia, PA: ACP-ASIM Publishing; 2001.

Sulmasy DP. Spiritual issues in the care of dying patients: ". . . it's okay between me and god." *JAMA* 2006;296:1385–1392.

UP-TO-DATE CHAPTERS

Okon TR. Overview of Comprehensive Assessment in Palliative Care.

Meier, DM, McCormick E, Langman RL. Hospice: Philosophy of Care and Appropriate Utilization in the United States.

Hauer PC. Pediatric Palliative Care.

Bailey FA, Harmen SM. Palliative Care: The Last Hours of Life.

Kumar S. Palliative Care and Hospice Outside of the United States.

Rosenstein DL. Challenging Interactions With Patients and Families in Palliative Care.

WEBSITES

American Academy of Hospice and Palliative Medicine. www.aahpm.org. Accessed September 2019.

Center to Advance Palliative Care. www.capc.org. Accessed September 2019.

Compassion and Choices. www.compassionandchoices.org. Accessed September 2019.

Death with Dignity National Center. www.deathwithdignity.org. Accessed September 2019.

Education in Palliative and End-of-Life Care. www.epec.net. Accessed September 2019.

Hospice Foundation of America. http://www.hospicefoundation.org/. Accessed September 2019.

National Consensus Project for Quality Palliative Care (2013). *Clinical Practice Guidelines for Quality Palliative Care*. 3rd ed. http://www.nationalconsensusproject.org. Accessed September 2019.

National Hospice and Palliative Care Organization. www.nhpco.org. Accessed September 2019.

National Palliative Care Research Center. www.npcrc.org. Accessed September 2019.

Medical Orders for Life-Sustaining Treatment (MOLST). www.molst.org. Accessed September 2019.

Physician Orders for Life-Sustaining Treatment (POLST). http://www.polst.org/. Accessed September 2019.

SECTION VII
Teaching and Assessment

Competency-Based Education for Behavioral Medicine

Jason M. Satterfield, PhD & Eric S. Holmboe, MD

Wendy is a second year internal medicine resident currently struggling to feel "competent" as an outpatient primary care provider. Over the course of her internship year, her competence and confidence with inpatient care grew. However, her outpatient clinics were infrequent in comparison, and she feels like she hasn't learned to be a "good primary care doctor." She shares her frustrations with her mentor—in part fueled by the breadth of skills required, the lack of benchmarks to measure her progress, and the lack of validated assessment tools. Her mentor attempts to help Wendy develop an individualized learning plan with formative assessments.

Medical education has recently undergone a transformation from process-oriented measures of success to more outcomes-oriented assessments that gauge what a learner can actually do and not only to what they have been exposed. Although the notion of competencies is not new, more recent conceptualizations move far beyond simple listings of skills and include multi-dimensional, dynamic, contextual, and developmental elements. This movement has been particularly transformative in the realm of graduate medical education (GME) with the advent of the Accreditation Council for Graduate Medical Education (ACGME) competencies and has become increasingly common as medical schools begin to embrace competency-based medical education (CBME) and translate the GME competencies for medical students "further upstream." Learning objectives and related competencies are now more frequently articulated and tend to be more commonly linked to specific assessment tools that measure achievement of that specific competency. However, the practice of medicine is inherently complex and often requires subtle, nuanced skills that are both difficult to teach and challenging to quantify. In particular, competencies that fall within the realm of the Behavioral and Social Sciences (BSS) have proven particularly difficult to articulate, teach, and assess.

This chapter will first provide a brief overview of CBME that articulates common advantages and limitations of this approach. We then offer a summary of BSS curricular thinking within medical education, including the work of the Association of American Medical Colleges (AAMC) BSS Expert Panel, the BSS Curriculum Consortium (funded by National Institutes of Health [NIH]), and the behavioral science subcommittee of the MCAT 5th Revision (MR5) Committee. This chapter presents a careful melding of the concepts and processes of CBME with the content of BSS by offering a synthesis of the innovative work emerging on both undergraduate medical education (UME) and GME levels. Specific assessment methods and evaluation tools for BSS competencies are described in Chapter 45.

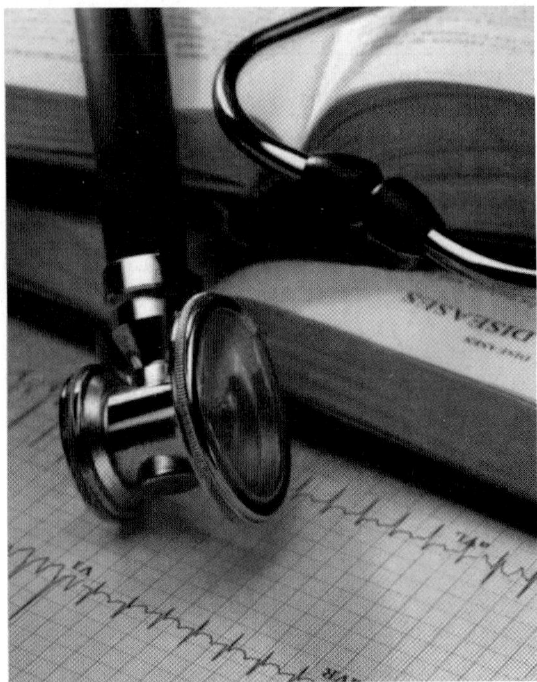

PEDAGOGICAL BUILDING BLOCKS FOR CBME

The International Competency-based Medical Education (ICBME) consortium defined CBME as "an outcomes-based approach to the design, implementation, assessment and evaluation of an education program using an organizing framework of competencies." CBME is intended to focus on outcomes, emphasize abilities, de-emphasize time-based training, and promote greater learner-centeredness. Epstein defines professional competence as "the habitual and judicious use of knowledge, technical skills, clinical reasoning, emotions, values, and reflection in daily practice for the benefit of the individual and community being served." More simply, Ten Cate defines competence as "the threshold level in the development of expertise that permits unsupervised practice."

A number of classic pedagogical and learning theories have helped medical education move from an expert-centric, apprenticeship model to a more evolved, evidence-based approach emphasizing adult learning and professional development. Medicine is perhaps unique in the number of disciplines, the quantity of knowledge, and the integrative capacity required to achieve even minimal competence. Miller's Pyramid offers a useful rubric in considering the progression of skill acquisition moving from "Knows" to "Knows How" to "Shows How" to "Does" as learners progress in their training. Dreyfus and Dreyfus created a stage model of professional development that represents a continuum ranging from novice at one end, then progressing to advanced learner, competent, proficient, and expert. It is notable that in the Dreyfus model "competent" does not lie at the end of the continuum but precedes proficient and expert implying that competence is a stage, an important benchmark, on the way to becoming an expert.

In each of these important models and definitions, it is clear that competence is thought to progress in a developmental fashion in response to direct (and indirect) intervention from the educational system and the learning environment. Recognizing this developmental aspect to competence, an international group developed a set of definitions to help clarify the confusion often engendered by the terms competencies, competence, and competent. Competencies are best viewed as "abilities" that integrate knowledge, skills, attitudes, and behaviors. Competence and competent represent states of being that can be further subdivided into three categories:

- Competent: Possessing the required abilities in all domains at a specified stage of medical education or practice.
- Dyscompetent: Relatively lacking in one or more domains of required abilities at a specified stage of medical education or practice.
- Incompetent: Lacking the required abilities in all domains in a certain context at a defined state of medical education or practice.

Competence is acquired by the learner and not necessarily imparted by the faculty. Peers, patients, allied health professionals, the learner himself or herself, and others may be considered teachers capable of assisting a learner in acquiring competence. Once competent, learning and growth continue well into the professional years and perhaps for the rest of one's career. Competence is multidimensional and includes knowledge, procedural skills, metacognition, emotional management, social relationships, and communication. To best grasp how such breadth can be meaningfully captured and assessed to assist the faculty and learner in our opening vignette, it is helpful to review the history and evolution of CBME.

History of CBET and CBME

CBME is not a new concept and represents an amalgam of educational theories, with origins in the work of Thorndike and Dewey. The earliest conception of competency-based training actually arose in the United States during the 1920s as educational reform became linked to industrial and business models of work that centered on clear specification of outcomes.

Table 43-1. The competency-based education and training.

CBET Principles	CBET Characteristics
1. Competencies are role derived, specified in behavioral terms, and made public 2. Assessment criteria are competency based and specify what constitutes mastery level of achievement 3. Assessment requires performance as the prime evidence but also takes knowledge into account 4. Individual learners progress at rates dependent on demonstrated competency 5. The instructional program facilitates development and evaluation of the specific competencies	1. Learning is individualized 2. Feedback to the learner is critical 3. Emphasis is more on the exit criteria than on the admission criteria 4. CBET requires a systematic program (approach) 5. Training is modularized 6. Both the learner and the program have accountability

However, the more recent conception of CBME had much of its genesis in the teacher education reform movement of the 1960s. This interest was spurred by a U.S. Office of Education National Center for Education research grant program in 1968 to 10 universities to develop and implement new teacher training models that focused on student achievement (outcomes). Elam laid down a series of principles and characteristics of competency-based education and training (CBET) in 1971 that still inform CBME today (Table 43-1). In 2002, Carraccio and colleagues noted that some sectors in medical education explored competency-based models in the 1970s, but except for one study, no comparisons between competency-based and the traditional structure/process-based curricula were undertaken. The World Health Organization (WHO) commissioned a paper published in 1978 that strongly recommended the adoption of competency-based educational models for medical education, noting, "The intended output of a competency-based programme is a health professional who can practise medicine at a defined level of proficiency, in accord with local conditions, to meet local needs." The driving force behind this WHO report was to better connect medical education to public health needs.

In the few studies within medical fields that have investigated competency-based models, there appear to be some benefits to trainees in the CBET model. For example, The University of Toronto employed a competency- and mastery-based approach in its orthopedics residency, with success in accelerating competency in specific surgeries and even in graduating some residents earlier than the typical 5 years.

In 2002, the ACGME Outcome Project changed the accreditation focus from a program's process and structure (e.g., rotations, written curricula) to actual learner/program outcomes. Programs had to rigorously document that their residents achieved competence in six general domains of practice (i.e., competencies)—Medical Knowledge, Patient Care and Procedural Skills, Communication and Interpersonal Skills, Professionalism, Practice-Based Learning and Improvement, and Systems-Based Practice. In phase 1 of the Outcome Project, programs defined objectives to demonstrate learning in the competencies. In phase 2, they integrated the competencies into their curricula and expanded their evaluation systems to assess actual performance. The first two phases informed a substantial change in the design of accreditation in GME in 2012. Called the Next Accreditation System (NAS), the NAS incorporated more of a quality improvement focus by introducing the Clinical Learning Environment Review (CLER) program, the self-study visits and the Milestones (Table 43-2).

In addition to the ACGME, a number of international competency frameworks have been developed to guide UME and GME curricula and assessment. Each provides a useful contrast to the ACGME approach but, like ACGME, is not specific to the social and behavioral sciences. Table 43-3 provides a side-by-side comparison of these different competency frameworks.

Table 43-2. ACGME competencies and assessment tools.

ACGME Competency	Recommended Assessment Tools
Medical knowledge	MCQ exam, oral exam, chart stimulated recall
Patient care and procedural skills	Standardized patient, objective structured clinical examination (OSCE), patient survey, multisource feedback (a.k.a. 360 degree assessment), simulation (procedures), direct observation
Communication and interpersonal skills	Standardized patient, OSCE, patient survey, multisource feedback (a.k.a. 360 degree assessment)
Professionalism	OSCE, patient survey, multisource feedback
Practice-based learning and improvement	Portfolio, medical record review, evidence-based practice review
Systems-based practice	MCQ exam, patient survey, multisource feedback, practice audit

Table 43-3. Medical competency frameworks.

ACGME (United States)	General Medical Council (Great Britain)	Scottish Doctor (Scotland)	CanMEDS Framework (Canada)
Six broad competency areas	Seven outcome categories for provisionally registered doctors	Twelve learning outcomes domains	Based on six physician roles and the integrative role of the medical expert
Medical knowledge	• Good clinical care	• Basic, social, and clinical sciences and underlying principles • Medical informatics	• Scholar
Patient care	• Good clinical care	• Clinical skills • Practical procedures • Patient investigation • Patient management • Decision making skills and clinical reasoning and judgment • Health promotion and disease prevention	• Health advocate • Medical expert
Interpersonal and communication skills	• Relationships with patients working with colleagues	• Clinical skills • Health promotion and disease prevention	• Communicator
Professionalism	• Health (self-care) • Probity (integrity)	• Attitudes, ethical understanding, and legal responsibilities • Role of the doctor in the health service • Personal development	• Professional
Practice-based learning and improvement	• Maintaining good medical practice		• Leader
Systems-based practice	• Working with colleagues • Teaching and training, appraising and assessing	• Patient management • Role of the doctor in the health service	• Collaborator • Leader • Medical expert (integration of all roles)

Competencies have been grouped by their approximate equivalence to the ACGME categories.

The ACGME, in collaboration with the 24 certification boards, sponsored the development of milestones for all residency and fellowship programs training using the Dreyfus stage model of development as the frame of reference for the milestones. The six general competencies are further subdivided into a variable set of subcompetencies (dependent on specific specialty needs) and broken into five levels of descriptive narratives guided by the stages of the Dreyfus model and the learner's level of training. For example, what represents competence in interpersonal communication and skills changes as the resident progresses through the training program. Milestones development has also been informed by nonphysicians and trainees to ensure key developmental milestones were not missed and were stage appropriate. A number of specialties are already working on Milestones 2.0 based on lessons learned in the first 5 years of the Milestones experience. The Milestones 2.0 working groups include trainees, public members and interprofessional expertise in the competencies of professionalism, interpersonal skills and communication, systems-based practice, and practice-based learning and improvement.

By the time a learner reaches competence, he or she has already progressed from simply applying rules to facts and features without context (novice) to considering the specific features of concrete situations (advanced beginner). The competent learner considers both context-free and situational elements but also hierarchically organizes and reduces them to a smaller set on which to base a decision. In addition, he or she becomes more intimately involved in the process and feels more responsible for the outcome. In the next stage, proficiency, learners solve problems with an intuition that usually derives from some time in unsupervised practice. Thus, although it is expected that some residents will achieve proficiency in many competencies, the ACGME and GME community have set "proficiency" as the desired goal but not a mandatory requirement. Most Milestones defined the level of competent in sufficiently robust terms that a resident deemed "competent" at graduation would be able to practice medicine effectively in an unsupervised clinical environment, a critical "entrustment" decision all training programs ultimately must make. All the ACGME competencies are listed in Table 43-2 and paired with recommended assessment tools.

CBME has been embraced by UME as it moves away from the classic Flexner model of classroom-based basic science in years 1–2 with little clinical experience until year 3. Many medical schools have adopted the ACGME competency framework for both conceptual reasons and expediency. More recently, AAMC created a core set of entrustable professional activities for graduation as meaningful preparation to effectively enter residency training (see below). Presumably all graduating students will continue on to GME, and so they will need to be familiar with the ACGME competencies. Conceptually, it is compelling to think of a full continuum of benchmarked competencies beginning with the first day of medical school and ending with achievement of competencies in residency. Of course, true CBME argues for a move away from time-based education, which could mean that some students (or residents) will achieve competence in less time whereas others may take longer. As with GME, UME BSS competencies are subsumed under the same rubric but perhaps less well articulated and more challenging to assess. Benchmarks for UME BSS competencies have not been developed, but helpful guidelines and tools have been provided by the Institute of Medicine (IOM) and AAMC (described below).

More recently, the concept of "entrustable professional activities" (EPAs) has emerged as a more practical and holistic approach related to competency assessment. In medical training, a teacher essentially wants to train and "entrust" a learner to perform a particular activity such as performing a cardiac examination or diagnosing depression. Once "entrusted," the learner may continue to deepen that particular skill but can do so as a self-directed learner. Additional activities are added throughout training and potentially throughout an entire medical career. Although newer models of CBME have added contextual and multidimensional factors, the EPA approach does this in a more robust, holistic, systematic, and measurable way that yields practical outcomes. As noted above, the AAMC is currently studying 13 core EPAs for entering residency. The purpose of these core EPAs is to help ensure graduating medical students have achieved sufficient competence in core activities to effectively transition to residency. For example, two of the core EPAs relevant to BSS are "gather a history and perform a physical examination" and "collaborate as a member of an interprofessional team."

Promises & Pitfalls of CBME

CBME represents a dramatic shift in the way we think about medical training and evaluation of medical learners at all levels. However, CBME is not without its critics. CBME, and particularly Milestones, struggle with the issue of granularity, or how atomistic one must be to reduce a complex skill into its constituent elements. Such reductions run the risk of becoming long, exhaustive lists of overlapping and sometimes redundant skills that still manage to be incomplete and may fail to capture the more subtle skills required in a complex interaction.

Particular "doctoring" skills, such as empathy or respect, and important skills like self-care or reflective capacity may prove particularly hard to benchmark and assess. Some have argued that the substantial assessment burden is amplified by the lack of psychometrically valid instruments and the lack of appropriately trained faculty evaluators. Beyond the obvious objections to the time, money, and resources required for CBME, some have argued that CBME focuses on the lowest common denominator rather than promoting learner excellence. As the level of learner advances, competencies become more specialized, requiring ever greater levels of detail and specificity by program directors and evaluators. Proponents argue that despite these challenges, medicine has and always will be required to "entrust" its trainees to deliver medical care. Greater attention to specific, contextualized competencies makes this inevitable process more valid, reliable, and safe.

Creating a BSS Competency Framework

Despite the substantive struggles bound to arise from CBME, the challenge of articulating a particular skill set, describing its developmental progression, and developing assessment methodologies has important implications for the field. Recent educational research has supported the reduction of complex skill sets into constituent foundational skills, and CBME consensus conferences have affirmed the relative value of CBME in contrast to past guiding approaches. Moreover, CBME holds special promise for nonbiomedical disciplines often overlooked in medical curricula or thought to be too difficult to assess. BSS leaders have been required to articulate, operationalize, and justify BSS competencies thought essential to the practice of medicine. These initial efforts can be found in the work of the NIH BSS Curriculum Consortium, the IOM BSS Report Committee, and the AAMC BSS Expert Panel (see below).

Few would argue that BSS do not have a place within medical education and practice, but BSS is not always in sync with the culture of medicine which is still dominated by biomedicine. The BSS umbrella includes specific clinical content (medical knowledge) such as understanding the relationship between smoking and cardiovascular disease. However, BSS also includes methods of inquiry (qualitative or survey research) and introduces a philosophy of science and knowledge that includes the interdependence of variables, nonlinear causal models, tolerance of ambiguity, and social contextual factors. BSS includes meta-processes such as habits of mind, reflective capacity, self-regulation, professional identity development, and emotional management. And, finally, BSS speaks of the sociopolitical aspects of medicine, including medicine's "contract" with society, social justice, health care equity, ethics, and morality. In ACGME competency terms, BSS falls within all six competency domains but is most heavily represented in the Professionalism, Communication and Interpersonal Skills, and Systems-Based Practice categories.

Although lists of key BSS topics and more focused BSS competencies are available, they are not universally accepted and are paradoxically seen as both bloated and incomplete. Rather than focusing on the exclusion or inclusion of favored topics, these lists can serve as important starting points to develop and evaluate BSS curricula and competencies. To date, work to further define and list BSS topics and competencies has included the foundational work of the Association of Behavioral Science and Medical Education (ABSAME), the IOM BSS report (2004), the NIH BSS Curriculum Consortium, and more recently, the MR5 group and the AAMC BSS report (2011). Highlights from these seminal reports are presented below, and links to the full reports are provided at the end of this chapter.

ABSAME sought to develop and promote the inclusion of the behavioral sciences in medical education. As part of that process, this AAMC-affiliated group (retired in 2017) developed one of the earliest and most comprehensive BSS content lists. Broad content categories included "Health, Illness, Sickness, and Disease," "Biological Components of Human Behavior," "Individual Behavior," "Interpersonal and Individual/Social Behavior," "Culture, Society, Institutions, and Organizations," "Epidemiology," "Clinical Reasoning," and "Psychopathology."

In 2004, the IOM released the report, *Social and Behavioral Sciences in Medical Education*. After a comprehensive review of BSS curricula across U.S. medical schools, this report included 5 recommendations to move the field forward and presented a listing of 6 essential BSS content areas and 20 high-priority topics (Table 43-4).

Table 43-4. IOM content areas and high-priority topics.

Core Content Area	High-Priority Topics
1. Mind–body interactions in health and disease	• Biological mediators between psychological and social factors and health • Psychological, social, and behavioral factors in chronic disease • Psychological and social aspects of human development that influence disease and illness • Psychosocial aspects of pain
2. Patient behavior	• Health risk behaviors • Principles of behavior change • Impact of psychosocial stressors and psychiatric disorders on manifestations of other illnesses and on health behavior
3. Physician role and behavior	• Ethical guidelines for professional behavior • Personal values, attitudes, and biases as they influence patient care • Physician well-being • Social accountability and responsibility • Work in health care teams and organizations • Use of and linkage with community resources to enhance patient care
4. Physician–patient interactions	• Basic communication skills • Complex communication skills
5. Social and cultural issues in health care	• Impact of social inequalities in health care and the social factors that are determinants of health outcomes • Cultural competency
6. Health policy and economics	• Overview of the U.S. health care system • Economic incentives affecting patients' health-related behaviors • Costs, cost-effectiveness, and physician responses to financial incentives

These core content areas and topic listings have since been corroborated with a national faculty survey.

In response to one of the report recommendations, NIH funded nine medical schools to develop and evaluate BSS curricular innovations. Innovations have included greater explication of the IOM content areas and improved pedagogical methods and more valid and reliable assessment tools for BSS competencies.

The MR5 Committee addressed the issue of BSS competencies even further upstream by specifying what BSS concepts, knowledge, and skills would be assessed for all medical school applicants taking the new MCAT. By setting the assessment standards, the MR5 committee essentially provided a road map to medical school advisors and applicants regarding what they should learn before applying to medical school. Table 43-5 lists the five core content areas and associated topics. As would be expected, these BSS areas represent the basic science of BSS, in contrast to the clinical applications of BSS described in the IOM report.

The report from the AAMC BSS Expert Panel, *Behavioral and Social Sciences Foundations for Future Physicians*, defines BSS within the context of medicine, illustrates the ways in which both BSS content and process influence teaching and clinical care, and provides a short list of sample BSS competencies. More importantly, this report provides a robust curricular tool that guides educators and learners in identifying and elaborating BSS content that arises in any clinical case. This tool, the BSS Matrix, uses the IOM content areas (see Table 43-4) and the CanMEDS professional roles (Table 43-6) as complementary rubrics to reduce complex clinical encounters into their foundational BSS competency units for further teaching and/or evaluation (Figure 43-1).

We resume our opening example to illustrate how the resident and preceptor could use the BSS Matrix to promote BSS competence.

Preceptor: *Wendy, thank you for bringing this up. It might take a long time and a lot of patience before you can really start to feel competent as a primary care*

Table 43-5. MCAT BSS content.

Foundational Concept 1 (ways that individuals perceive, think about, and react to the world)	Foundational Concept 2 (factors that influence behavior and behavior change)	Foundational Concept 3 (factors that influence how we think about ourselves and others)	Foundational Concept 4 (ways in which cultural and social differences influence well-being)	Foundational Concept 5 (ways in which social stratification affects access to resources and well-being)
A: Sensing the environment 1) Sensory processing 2) Vision 3) Hearing 4) Other senses 5) Perception	A: Individual influences on behavior 1) Biological bases of behavior 2) Personality 3) Psychological disorders 4) Motivation 5) Attitudes	A: Self-identity 1) Self-concept and identity 2) Formation of identity	A: Understanding social structure 1) Components of social structure 2) Theoretical approaches 3) Specific social institutions 4) Culture	A: Social inequality 1) Spatial inequality 2) Social class 3) Health disparities 4) Health care disparities
B: Making sense of the environment 1) Attention 2) Cognition 3) Memory 4) Language	B: Social processes that influence human behavior 1) Socialization 2) How the presence of others affects individual behavior 3) Group processes 4) Culture	B: Social thinking 1) Attributing behavior to persons or situations 2) Prejudice and bias 3) Processes related to stereotypes	B: Demographic characteristics and process 1) Demographic shifts and social change 2) Demographic structure of society	
C: Responding to the world 1) Emotions 2) Stress	C: Attitude and Behavioral change 1) Associative learning 2) Observational learning 3) Attitude and Behavioral change	C: Social interactions 1) Self-presentation and interacting with others 2) Social behavior 3) Discrimination 4) Elements of social interaction		

Table 43-6. CanMEDS physician competency framework (2015).

As *Professionals*, physicians are committed to the health and well-being of individuals and society through ethical practice, profession-led regulation, and high personal standards of behavior.
As *Communicators*, physicians effectively facilitate the doctor–patient relationship and the dynamic exchanges that occur before, during, and after the medical encounter.
As *Collaborators*, physicians effectively work within a health care team to achieve optimal patient care.
As *Leaders*, physicians engage with others to contribute to a vision of a high-quality health care system and take responsibility for the delivery of excellent patient care through their activities as clinicians, administrators, scholars, or teachers.
As *Health Advocates*, physicians responsibly use their expertise and influence to advance the health and well-being of individual patients, communities, and populations.
As *Scholars*, physicians demonstrate a lifelong commitment to reflective learning, as well as the creation, dissemination, application, and translation of medical knowledge.
As *Medical Experts*, physicians integrate all of the CanMEDS Roles, applying medical knowledge, clinical skills, and professional attitudes in their provision of patient-centered care. Medical Expert is the central physician Role in the CanMEDS framework.

provider. There are a lot of skills involved and they are probably best taught while immersed in the context of caring for real patients. Do you have a case you can share with me? We'll use the AAMC BSS Matrix to identify some key learning issues for your development plan.

Resident: *Well, my last patient was a 27-year-old man coming to see me after his second trip to the ED for a-fib following a night of heavy drinking. He was pretty shaken up by the experience and had no idea that binge drinking and atrial fibrillation could be related. He needed an INR check and warfarin adjustment, but I wanted to counsel him about binge drinking. I'm not sure if I did a very good job of it.*

Preceptor: *Terrific case and lots of important behavioral and counseling issues we can discuss. Let's map it onto the BSS Matrix and see what roles and what content jump out at us. First, identify what roles you might be required to fill as his primary care provider. Next, think about the BSS core content you need to know and the competencies you need to possess. Let's fill in the cells with learning questions for this case together. (See Figure 43-1.)*

Preceptor: *Great list! Now I'd like to ask you to circle the cell where you feel most competent already and the one to two cells where you feel least competent. Maybe we can start our conversation there and develop a learning approach to build your competence.* [The conversation continues....]

As can be deduced from the above examples and the various BSS competency and content lists, the process of developing CBME for BSS requires a high level of faculty and learner engagement, time, resources, and, most importantly, an institutional or organizational culture that supports this material. However, it is important to remember that even if those necessary conditions are not present, organizational transformation does occur and can be stimulated from both the bottom-up and top-down. In Chapter 44, the authors carefully detail the necessary and sufficient conditions to support BSS education and the steps to promote cultural shifts that ensure both the quality and sustainability of the resulting product.

Although BSS competencies may "set the bar," it is the assessment toward achieving those competencies that allows us to "entrust" the learner with those clinical activities. Assessments may be formative (i.e., used to shape learning plans) or summative (i.e., providing a grade or determining attainment of a particular skill level). Within the realm of CBME, most assessments measure skills or abilities rather than attitudes, since behavior and attitudes tend to be only weakly correlated. Direct observations of the learner are the most commonly used assessment methodology, but observations should occur frequently and require observer training and standardization. In Chapter 45, Carney and Milan describe a full menu of assessment and evaluation approaches, including the relative advantages and disadvantages of each approach. As they argue, regardless of the selected methodology, BSS competencies can and should be assessed frequently and in conjunction with other more biomedically based competencies.

Given the international convergence of competency-based models of medical education, ranging from medical school through medical residencies, it appears that CBME is here to stay for the foreseeable future. Although broad and including general "meta-skills" along with foundational scientific knowledge, the BSS fit within current CBME frameworks and can be measured with existing tools. As learners struggle to develop competence and teachers stretch to accommodate their needs, tools such as the AAMC BSS Matrix can identify the complex, interactive learning issues embedded in each case. Moreover, as the construct of EPAs further develops, perhaps BSS knowledge and skills can be seen as foundational to the practice of medicine in partnership with the biomedical sciences.

		CanMEDS Physician Roles					
		Professional	**Communicator**	**Collaborator**	**Leader and Systems Thinker**	**Health Advocate**	**Scholar**
IOM BSS Concepts and Evidence	**Patient behavior**		What are stages of change and how can I use motivational interviewing to help this patient?	How or when can I refer to a behavioral health counselor?	Are there quality indicators that track detection and intervention of binge drinking?		What are the evidence-based interventions for binge drinking?
	Mind–body interaction						Is stress a causal factor for binge drinking?
	Physician role and behavior	What are my ethical or legal responsibilities in this case?	What are my personal beliefs about binge drinking and do they influence my communication style?				
	Doctor–patient interaction	How can I assess drinking and educate the pt about risks without sounding judgmental?	How can I build rapport and strengthen our connection?				Does research support particular communication strategies for educating pts about risk?
	Health policy, economics, and systems (including population health)			How can I communicate more effectively with ED docs?	Can I tap local resources to support behavioral change for this pt?	Could I promote better pt education programs in the ED?	
	Social and cultural context	How can I be sensitive to his age, gender, culture, or socioeconomic status?					Is this problem more common in men?

Figure 43-1. The AAMC BSS matrix. Sample case: a 27-year-old man with atrial fibrillation following binge drinking episodes ×2.

SUGGESTED READINGS

Association of American Medical Colleges. The Core Entrustable Professional Activities (EPAs) for Entering Residency. https://www.aamc.org/initiatives/coreepas/. Accessed September 9, 2018.

Carraccio C, Wolfsthal SD, Englander R, Ferentz K, Martin C. Shifting paradigms: from Flexner to competencies. *Acad Med* 2002;77:361–367.

Epstein RM, Hundert EM. Defining and assessing professional competence. *JAMA* 2002;287:226–235.

Frank JR, Snell LS, Ten Cate O, et al. Competency-based medical education: theory to practice. *Med Teach* 2010;32:638–645.

Green ML, Aagaard EM, Caverzagie KJ, et al. Charting the road to competence: developmental milestones for internal medicine residency training. *J Grad Med Educ* 2009;1:5–20.

Holmboe ES, Edgar LE, Hamstra SJ. *The Milestones Guidebook.* https://www.acgme.org/Portals/0/MilestonesGuidebook.pdf?ver=2016-05-31-113245-103. Accessed September 9, 2018.

Nasca TJ, Philibert I, Brigham T, Flynn TC. The next GME accreditation system—rationale and benefits. *N Engl J Med* 2012;366(11):1051–1056.

Nousiainen MT, Mironova P, Hynes M, et al. Eight-year outcomes of a competency-based residency training program in orthopedic surgery. *Med Teach* 2018:1–13.

Satterfield J, Adler S, Chen CH, Hauer K, Saba G, Salazar R. Creating an ideal social and behavioral sciences curriculum for medical students. *Med Educ* 2010;44:1194–1202.

Ten Cate O, Snell L, Carraccio C. Medical competence: the interplay between individual ability and the health care environment. *Med Teach* 2010;32:669–675.

WEBSITES

AAMC Behavioral and Social Science Foundations for Future Physicians (2011). https://www.aamc.org/publications. Accessed May 2019.

CanMeds Competency Framework (2015). http://canmeds.royalcollege.ca/en/framework. Accessed May 2019.

IOM BSS Report (2004). https://www.ncbi.nlm.nih.gov/books/NBK10238/. Accessed May 2019.

MCAT (2011). http://aamc.org/mcatprep. Accessed May 2019.

Teaching Behavioral Medicine: Theory & Practice

Debra K. Litzelman, MA, MD; Mark DiCorcia, PhD; Ann Cottingham, MAR, MA; & Thomas S. Inui, ScM, MD, MACP

When one of my preceptors is running behind schedule during clinic hours he always pokes his head in the exam rooms of the patients who are waiting and apologizes for their wait. He also tells them that he hasn't forgotten about them and that he will be there to see them as soon as possible. I think that this is a great way to show respect for patients and their schedules and it helps prevent them from becoming angry and frustrated. This is a habit that I will definitely adopt when I am a physician.

Third-year medical student

One of my fellow students and I were on duty when there was a code called overhead. Everyone ran to assist in the code and the student was asked if she wanted to participate. This is something very neat for a third year because we never get to do that. However, the student spotted the wife of the coding patient at the end of the hall standing by herself with no one to comfort her. So instead of going to help in the code, the student went to talk to the patient's wife and explain to her what was going on. I thought that was very caring because no one else even noticed the wife standing there, and sometimes we get caught up in the chance to do something medical and forget about the families.

Third-year medical student

INTRODUCTION

Today it is widely recognized that health and wellness, promoting behavior change, and addressing disease states can only be accomplished through the delivery of high-quality patient care built on a foundation of knowledge and abilities in the basic, clinical, and behavioral and social sciences. Social and behavioral factors are estimated to contribute to more than half of all causes of disease and death in the United States, including cancer, heart disease, chronic obstructive pulmonary disease, and type II diabetes. Knowledge of the complex behavioral, social, and psychological contributors to disease has important implications for clinical practice and physician education, both formal and informal. Physicians must understand these factors and their interrelationships, and be able to apply this knowledge in the care of patients to optimize individual, local community, and national health outcomes and enhance their own sense

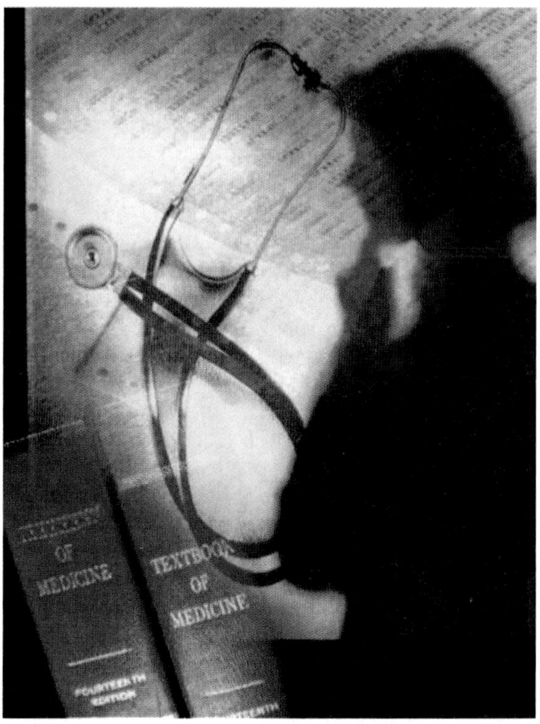

of well-being and personal and professional growth, while reducing feelings of cynicism and burnout.

Although most health training programs have increased behavioral and social science-related content throughout their curriculum, many behavioral and social science curricula remain fragmented, incomplete, and marginalized. Emphasis on formal curricular development may also overlook the importance of the informal curriculum (or learning environment)—the influence of physician and resident modeling of behaviors and attitudes on professional identity formation and practice patterns. Therefore, educators must be attentive to both influences in the preclinical and clinical years of student education and its impact on student attitudes toward the behavioral and social sciences in their role as future physicians. Using current theories of learning, this chapter illustrates innovative educational methods that integrate the formal and informal curricula to effectively teach social and behavioral science (SBS).

BACKGROUND

The IOM (now referred to as the National Academy of Medicine) report, *Improving Medical Education: Enhancing the Behavioral and Social Science Content of Medical School Curricula*, identifies 26 topics in six SBS domains that are important to the education of future physicians (Table 44-1). This table, while lengthy, is included in its entirety because it provides in detail specific topics for learning that could/should serve as specific objectives for SBS learning, in whatever form they are expressed in the core curriculum of medical schools.The demographic and social contexts contributing to the need for such training in the SBS have been well documented. Nevertheless, several decades of efforts to teach this content have resulted in mixed success. Medical education literature clearly identifies several types of difficulties specific to the teaching of SBS in the formal curriculum, including the marginalization of SBS content, lack of appropriately trained faculty, timing of teaching the SBS content, mismatch between teaching methods and context of use, and failure of social scientists and clinicians to work together to create effective learning experiences. It is not difficult to find examples. SBS content may be treated as an "add on" to the traditional basic science and clinical curricula. Medical training programs may lack support and incentives for faculty to include SBS content, and for career development programs in SBS. SBS topics may fit into available time slots rather than be taught at the appropriate times in the trainees' development and in the appropriate depth. For example, topics such as death and dying are often covered in small-group discussions in the first or second year and not revisited in any formal way in the clerkship years, yet research on knowledge use and acquisition concludes that there is little immediate transfer of learning from one context of use to another. Thus, students who discuss death and dying only in the early year or two of training (academic context) will be challenged to exhibit professional and humanistic behavior in the presence of real patients (practice context) without further formal training in the clinical context.

Although some gains have been made, there are additional well-documented structural impediments from a systems perspective to fully realizing the successful integration of SBS into the larger medical education curriculum. Medical education is by and large examination driven, quantitative in nature, heavily weighted toward the basic medical sciences (BMS), and competition among and between students is based on these numerical rankings. This system continues to perpetuate the marginalization of SBS to a supporting or secondary role in the minds of faculty and students in favor of more influential BMS curriculum. For example, on the national level, the Association of American Medical Colleges' Medical College Admission Test (MCAT) as well as other high-stakes examinations (e.g., USMLE Step 1) include SBS content but are still primarily multiple-choice, BMS-focused exams. These exams are not Pass/Fail despite sufficient evidence that, once a learner achieves a particular threshold of success on the examination, there is no difference in clinical performance based on achieving a greater numerical score. Despite this evidence, many institutions continue to use the specific scores to screen applicants for entrance to U.S. medical schools and residencies. School administrators are under pressure, and in some cases even rewarded, for only recruiting and admitting those with the highest test scores instead of developing criteria that would more heavily weigh such areas as the 26 topics in the six SBS domains as the discriminating factors.

In response to similar concerns, Canada's McMaster University developed the Multiple Mini-Interview (MMI) for use in the admissions process. Resembling an objective structured clinical examination (OSCE), the MMI consists of short-interview stations that focus exclusively on noncognitive domains. The open-ended interviewer–applicant interactions instead revolve around areas such as the ability to collaborate, communication skills, and moral reasoning. By focusing on these noncognitive professional abilities the MMI has consistently demonstrated greater reliability (i.e., around 0.75) than standard interview methods to accurately assess for these qualities, which are grounded in SBS and valued in clinical practice. It has also been established that the MMI has a significant and moderately large positive correlation in predicting clinical clerkship performance as well as a statistically significant positive correlation for those subsections of national licensing examinations assessing professional quality domains.

Despite the MMI findings, many evaluations of performance in the basic sciences in undergraduate medical education, including discipline-specific NBME Shelf

Table 44-1. SBS domains with priority topics and learning objectives.

Domain: Mind–Body Interactions in Health & Disease
Biological Mediators Between Psychological and Social Factors and Health
Describe how behavioral and social factors and stress alter physiology to make disease more likely and the interconnectivity of homeostatic systems. Explain the relationship between chronic stress, affective illness, social support, and health.
Psychological, Social, and Behavioral Factors in Chronic Illness
Understand the interrelationship between psychological, social, behavioral, and lifestyle factors and particular chronic medical conditions (e.g., diabetes, coronary artery disease [CAD], arthritis, and cancer). Understand and predict ongoing risky health behaviors. Describe how to recognize stress in chronically ill patients.
Psychological and Social Aspects of Human Development That Influence Disease and Illness
Recognize the various life cycle theories (Freud, Piaget, Erikson, Bowlby) in normal development and the Epigenetic Principle of Life Cycle Theory. Understand the interplay between stages of human development and disease states.
Psychological Aspects of Pain
Understand the wide range of psychosocial and cultural factors that influence the perception and expression of pain. Be familiar with the classic gate control and contemporary theories of pain. Perform a functional analysis of patients with chronic pain. Describe the multimodal treatments for pain control and the risk of addiction with opioid over use. Recognize the physician biases that influence the treatment of pain.
Psychological, Biological, and Management Issues in Somatization
Understand the definition, prevalence, common symptoms, and underlying affective illnesses associated with somatization. List the diagnostic criteria for somatoform disorders. Reflect on personal reactions to patients presenting with possible somatoform disorders.
Interactions Among Illness, Family Dynamics, and Culture
Understanding family and cultural influences on patient's interpretation of illness and treatment decisions and the importance of eliciting such information.
Domain: Patient Behavior
Health Risk Behaviors
Understand the psychological factors associated with the development and maintenance of behaviors associated with major causes of morbidity and mortality. Demonstrate the ability to assess patients for health risk behaviors. Understand key strategies for prevention and cessation of these behaviors. Reflect on the role of health care providers in instigating and maintaining changes in these behaviors. Apply principles of motivational interviewing and counseling for behavioral change to the patient care situations.
Principles of Behavior Change
Demonstrate the ability to apply the various models (classical conditioning, cognitive social learning theory, health belief model, theory of reasoned action, stage-of-change model) available for guiding behavior change. Understand how behaviors are acquired, maintained, and eliminated in the context of health risk. Understand patient, family, and sociocultural variables that impact motivation to change behavior.
Impact of Psychosocial Stressors and Psychiatric Disorders on Manifestations of Other Illness on Health Behavior
Recognize the association between, and co-occurrence of, chronic medical illness and mental disorders. Know and be able to discuss with patients the range of treatment options when medical and mental illness coexist. Know the role of a primary care physician and specialist in the treatment when medical and mental illness coexist. Demonstrate the ability to screen patients for depression. Understand the pathogenetic relationships between depression and comorbid conditions.

(*Continued*)

Table 44-1. SBS domains with priority topics and learning objectives. (*Continued*)

Domain: Physician Role and Behavior
Ethical Guidelines for Professional Behavior
Analyze ethical and professional dilemmas faced by health care professionals. Identify and apply guidelines of ethical decision making.
Personal Values, Attitudes, and Biases as They Influence Patient Care
Describe how the effect of family of origin, cultural background, gender, life experiences, and other personal factors may influence your attitudes toward emotional reactions to patients. Identify methods for processing the highly emotional encounters that regularly occur in medical care.
Physician Well-Being
Recognize risk factors and warning signs for mental health issues in yourself. Develop personal wellness strategies.
Social Accountability and Responsibility
Engage in activities that foster the development of socially responsible leadership skills. Recognize the ever-changing health care needs of the community, region, and/or nation you serve.
Work in Health Care Teams and Organizations
Recognize the contribution that each member of the health care team has to offer. Identify ways to work effectively as a part of the team.
Use of and Linkage With Community Resources to Enhance Patient Care
Identify available community resources in the patient's community. Demonstrate a working knowledge of the types of interventions offered.
Domain: Physician–Patient Interactions
Basic Communication Skills
Demonstrate basic communication skills including establishing rapport and building trust, eliciting adequate information to permit a robust differential diagnosis, understanding, and addressing patient. Understand how to engender (and potential barriers to development of) a therapeutic relationship. Demonstrate ability to express empathy, actively listen, elicit information about patients' lives and reasons for medical visit. Demonstrate motivational interviewing techniques and the 5A's counseling skills.
Complex Communication Skills
Demonstrate ability to communicate effectively in contextual (cultural, translator, family) and developmental (pediatric, adolescent, geriatric) interview situations. Demonstrate ability to communicate effectively in assessment and counseling situations. Practice basic skills in communicating effectively in challenging situations using principles of patient-centered interviewing. Practice basic skills in communicating effectively with colleagues using principles of relationship-centered communication.
Context of a Patient's Social and Economic Situation, Capacity for Self-Care, and Ability to Participate in Shared Decision Making
Demonstrate an awareness of the patient's ability to participate in decision making. Identify necessary resources available to ensure access to care.
Management of Difficult or Problematic Physician–Patient Interactions
Describe approaches to working with patients in difficult situations. Identify taxonomy of difficult interviews (including personal or sexual history taking; abusive relationships; patients with HIV; breaking bad news). Identify key characteristics of difficult patient encounters, including personality types and stressful situations. Identify and use basic skills of patient-centered interviewing to ask sensitive questions and listen respectfully and nonjudgmentally.

(*Continued*)

Table 44-1. SBS domains with priority topics and learning objectives. (*Continued*)

Domain: Social & Cultural Issues in Health Care
Impact of Social Inequalities in Health Care and the Social Factors That are Determinants of Health Outcomes
Analyze the intricate relationship that social factors (race, ethnicity, education, income, and occupation) have with patients' health. Reflect on the impact your (students'/physicians') own social views can have on the delivery of effective health care.
Cultural Competency
Describe the impact the cultural context of illness can have on a successful patient–physician relationship. Recognize ways that cultural competency encompasses language, customs, values, belief systems, and rituals.
Role of Complementary and Alternative Medicine
Describe complementary and alternative medicine treatments available in the local community and within local ethnic/cultural groups. Recognize and apply required skills for eliciting information from patients seeking or using alternative treatment methods. Describe to patients the efficacy and safety of alternative methods of treatment.
Domain: Health Policy & Economics
Overview of the U.S. Health Care System
Appreciate the magnitude of the investment in health care services made by individuals and organizations in the United States, the impact of these expenditures on individuals and on organizations, and the limited "return on investment." Explain why competition and other "market forces" may not work in health care. Use state-of-the-art utilization controls within the TBL scenario in an attempt to allocate financial resources to critical sectors of care.
Economic Incentives Affecting Patients' Health-Related Behaviors
Appreciate how patients' values and life circumstances may affect their motivations for health-supporting behaviors, health care utilization, and preference for outcomes of health care. Use this understanding to predict a patient's response to a complex and costly plan of care for several concomitant, chronic conditions, including the need to choose among therapeutic alternatives, adherence challenges, and patient-based assessments of risk. Outline potential physician actions in this situation that might preserve the essential ingredients of effective care.
Costs, Cost-effectiveness, and Physician Responses to Financial Incentives
Appreciate how "delivery system" income is allocated to sectors of cost, using a microsystem model as an exemplar. Apply this understanding, together with a statement of practice objectives, to develop the key elements of the practice in a financial context—staffing, services provided, in-office equipment, patients accepted, relationship to payers.
Variations in Care
Appreciate how large the variations in practice are, even in the presence of generally accepted evidence-based guidelines for care, and what some of the determinants of those variations might be. Apply this knowledge to a specific case example, decide what "unwanted" variation means in this situation, and design a plan of action to eliminate this variation.

SBS Domains with Priority Topics: Cuff PA, Vanselow NA, editors. Improving Medical Education: Enhancing the Behavioral and Social Science Content of Medical School Curricula. Washington (DC): National Academies Press (US); 2004.; Learning Objectives: Used with permission of the Office of Medical Education and Curricular Affairs, Indiana University School of Medicine, (IUSM) Indianapolis, Indiana.

Exams, lend themselves to "multiple choice" measures making the evaluation of SBS content difficult to evaluate objectively. SBS curriculum often requires additional time and resources in both teaching and evaluating. Therefore, even if SBS content is woven into all years of the curriculum, it is often not as heavily weighted or given equal focus in course examinations. This not only perpetuates the idea that SBS content is not as important to professional identity formation and role as a physician, but for the learner whose measure of success rests on quantitative success (i.e., to get into medical school, a residency, or pass an examination/clerkship), it creates a systems-induced survival strategy of "if it's not going to help me on the test then it's not important." This mentality or two-tiered system of valuing the objectively quantifiable over the more often subjectively qualitative SBS is as much a systems issue as the difficulties specific to the teaching of SBS in the curriculum noted above.

Finally, emphasis on discipline-based knowledge creates another barrier to integration of SBS content.

True integration of SBS content requires disciplinary communities to work closely together to establish joint responsibility for knowledge creation, development, and dissemination. With the exception of family medicine residency training programs, which have emphasized training in SBS, the same limitations and critiques directed toward undergraduate medical education hold true for graduate medical education as well.

Informal education in the SBS also has presented a challenge. Research indicates that it is the social environment of the medical school, the so-called "informal curriculum," that guides most aspects of a future physician's behavior. The role modeling that physicians and residents actually provide, much more than what they say, powerfully influences the beliefs, values, and role expectations of physicians-in-training. Patient care and clerkship experiences—where physical, emotional, behavioral, social, and cultural issues become embodied for learners in their patients—have the potential to be particularly important behavioral and social science learning opportunities. Here attending and resident teaching could seamlessly integrate SBS education into daily clinical activities. Unfortunately, studies show that attributes such as social-mindedness and interest in the psychosocial issues embedded in all illness decline rather than improve during this time, and many students experience a diminishment, not enhancement, of their moral values base.

Work must be done to raise faculty and resident consciousness of the power that their words and actions have in shaping students' perceptions of patients, their specialty and medicine in general. Students and faculty benefit alike from the opportunity to process and learn from their own experiences, making each more conscious of the relationship between their values, actions, and behavior, and better prepared to model and teach the SBS aspects of patient care and the practice of medicine.

INTEGRATING THE FORMAL & INFORMAL CURRICULA TO TEACH SOCIAL & BEHAVIORAL SCIENCE

Educational Learning Theories Foundational to Creating Social & Behavioral Science Curriculum

As medical training programs seek to integrate their formal and informal curricula to improve SBS education, current learning theories provide a useful underlying framework. Understanding the various theoretical orientations will allow educators to address concerns raised in the IOM report about incorporating the most appropriate teaching methodologies when teaching SBS. The five learning theories described in the adult learning literature include behaviorist, humanist, social learning, cognitivist, and constructivist orientations. An overview of these orientations, associated educational methods, and theoretical principles are briefly summarized in Table 44-2.

Table 44-2. Learning theories and orientations foundational to teaching and evaluating social and behavioral sciences.

Orientation	Educational Methods/Tools	SBS Abilities	Theoretical Principles
Behaviorist	Direct observation Standardized patients Checklists Rating forms	Clinical and psychomotor skills Other observable behaviors	Learning results from environmental factors and positive and negative reinforcement that shapes behavior
Humanist	Narrative reflection Problem-based learning	Self-awareness Autonomy Self-directedness	Learning results from the learners' desire to achieve their full potential
Social Learning	Role modeling Mentoring Collaborative/cooperative learning, for example, team-based learning	Social adaptability Teamwork	Learning results from the learners' interaction with and observation of others in a social context in which creative retrievable cognitive representations are used by learners when they are motivated to act
Cognitivist	Cognitive maps Reflective exercises	Insight Information processing	Learning results from relating new knowledge/experiences to existing knowledge/experiences
Constructivist	Reflective journaling Commitment to change statements Building portfolios	Ability to broaden one's perspective Critical reflection Ability to create meaning from experiences	Learning results from the learners' construction of meaning from experiences through critical reflection on their existing assumptions

Teaching Methods Foundational to Learning Social & Behavioral Sciences

The five Theoretical Orientations are presented as a frame for teaching SBS. A brief description of each of the suggested methods under each orientation is provided. Specific case illustrations applying the suggested methods in teaching and SBS are also included. In some cases, the examples provided by the authors could be categorized under more than one orientation. However, the main purpose of the illustrations is to provide a wide sampling of educational vignettes that integrate the formal and informal curricula as a foundation upon which to build an SBS curriculum for varying levels of medical trainees.

BEHAVIORAL ORIENTATION

The behavioral orientation is very useful for teaching technical, clinical, and psychomotor skills as well as other observable behaviors. Direct observation of trainees with real or standardized patients (SPs), particularly when trained observers utilize well-designed checklists and/or rating forms, provides valuable formative and summative assessment about trainees' social and behavior science competence.

Direct observation: Direct observation of trainees is an important way to foster medical trainees' basic clinical and communication skills as well as interpersonal and professional behavior; yet it is infrequently done. Here, resident or student patient care competency, contextualized in the everyday interactions of the informal curriculum, or institutional culture, is brought into the formal curriculum for purposes of formative feedback.

Direct observation is itself a skill that requires faculty training and practice. Faculty training should focus on standardizing, to the extent possible, the behaviors of interest and how to accurately identify such behaviors in the trainees. This is especially important for high-inference behaviors, such as those provided below (see case illustration 1). For example, in the behaviorist approach, what does nonjudgmental communication about a sexually transmitted disease actually look like? Faculty should spend some time discussing these issues as part of the standardization and calibration process.

Standardized patients: In an effort to standardize training of doctor–patient communication, physical examination skills, and other areas, medical schools, residency training programs, and the National Board of Medical Examiners (NBME) have progressively moved toward using SPs. Simulations can be videotaped and used for self or group reflection. Paradigmatic examples could also be used for faculty development in recognizing and developing intercoder reliability on behavioral evaluations. From these examples, skills in providing feedback and creating learning opportunities could be developed.

HUMANISTIC ORIENTATION

The humanistic orientation promotes learning activities that are autonomous and self-directed for learners to develop a deeper understanding of the path needed to reach their full potential and, in return, recognize the humanness in themselves as well as their patients. Problem-based learning (PBL) and exercises that promote self-assessment are educational tools for fostering humanistic-style learning.

Problem-based learning: Problem-based learning is a learner-centered method of small group learning usually built upon paper cases developed from real patient care vignettes. The case discussions generally evolve over several days or weeks with progressive disclosure of information to the students upon request or at critical times. Students identify their own learning issues and resources for finding solutions to their learning needs. A facilitator guides the process of the small group sessions but does not serve as a content expert for the learners. This process promotes autonomous, self-directed, lifelong learning skills and prompts learners to reflect on the cultural assumptions or observations that shape their list of learning issues and resources, providing an opportunity for integration of the informal curriculum.

CASE ILLUSTRATION 1

As part of the first-year medical students' Concepts of Health and Disease PBL course, SBS objectives addressing principals of behavioral change have been woven into a case covering medical and genetic risk factors for cardiovascular disease (CVD). Students meet Monday, Wednesday, and Friday during 1 week to cover serial aspects of the case of: "Robert Richardson's Achilles Tendon."

Sample excerpts from the case:

Day 1:

Mr. Robert Richardson, a 44-year-old male, visits his family physician, Dr. Roberts, for a follow-up of his myocardial infarct suffered several weeks ago. Mr. Richardson has been feeling well and continues his prescribed walking program. He is trying to follow his suggested diet and has begun a smoking cessation program. Mr. Richardson tells Dr. Roberts that he has been experiencing pain in his left Achilles tendon for the past several days. Mr. Richardson says that the pain had appeared several times during the past year. The pain usually resolved itself within several days without treatment.

Student instructions:

During the week the case is being presented, please make a commitment to change the following:

- *Engage in some form of aerobic exercise every day for at least 10 minutes.*

- *Take the provided pill twice a day. (Students are each given a packet of inert pills.)*
- *Diet—give up one thing that contributes to heart disease that you eat regularly.*

Suggestions: *salt, red meat, butter, cheese, milk, eggs, fried foods.*

At the end of each day write a paragraph or two about the experience of complying with these activities. Did it all go as planned? Rate the amount of effort necessary to do these things, with 1 being the easiest and 10 being the hardest. What happened if things did not always go as planned? What did you struggle with? What were your successes?

Facilitator Notes:

The facilitator might consider doing these things as well to be able to aid in the discussion.

Guided self-assessment: Self-assessment exercises can be built into a variety of educational activities stimulated by prompting questions posed by medical educators. Creating a forum for students to safely discuss their personal reflections on journal entries or information collected as part of self- and peer-assessment programs can promote self awareness, personal growth, and professional development in one-on-one and group settings and is another example of formal/informal curricular integration. Students are asked in the formal curriculum to reflect upon and assess their abilities and performance in both the formal and informal curricula.

To be effective, self-assessment is not performed by the student in isolation. The impact of self-assessment is most valuable when performed with *guidance*, which we define as either externally provided data (e.g., peer assessment, etc.) or in conjunction with an advisor or mentor.

CASE ILLUSTRATION 1 (CONTD.): ROBERT RICHARDSON'S ACHILLES TENDON (PBL)

Sample excerpts from case:

Day 2:

Dr. Roberts reports that Mr. Richardson's lipid and enzyme values are improved, that he should continue to follow the prescribed treatment and that his prognosis will remain improved as long as he follows the diet, exercise, and medication program. He should have semiannual checkups to follow his cholesterol and liver enzyme levels.

Facilitator Notes:

On the second and last day of the session, ask the following questions of the group.

Guided discussion of journals—prompting questions:

- *What was hardest?*
- *What was easiest?*
- *Any association with your lapses?*
- *How did you feel after you lapsed?*
- *How well did you comply with your journal writing?*

Thinking about Mr. Richardson and what you learned with your own exercise, how could you help Mr. Richardson and his children to comply with these lifelong issues?

A sample of one student's self-assessment logged in her personal dietary/exercise/medicine adherence journal as part of the PBL exercise above:

Overall, this exercise has shown me that it is all too easy for a physician to become annoyed and frustrated with noncompliant patients, and write them off as not caring about their own well being or progress. Adherence with diet, exercise, and medication is not as simple as it seems. I hope to remember those lessons in the coming years as I struggle with explaining to patients why it is so important, so they don't feel they are just doing something "because the doctor said to."

First-year medical student

SOCIAL LEARNING ORIENTATION

According to the social learning orientation, learners assimilate new information and assume new roles through role modeling, behavioral rehearsal, and attending to observed behaviors. This orientation is central to the importance of the informal curriculum on shaping the professional development of trainees. Identifying ways to make stories about role models within an academic community more tangible and visible will inevitably lead to a heightened awareness about the importance of role modeling. Educational methods that promote collaborative, cooperative learning such as team-based learning (TBL) also highlight the complexities and value of collective problem solving and resourcefulness.

Role modeling: Role modeling shapes the professional culture or informal curriculum of an organization and substantially impacts the professional identity of trainees. The window into the impact of medical educators' role modeling can be seen in the trainees' stories about their learning environment. How the faculty conduct themselves and live their values through their actions can be influenced by integrating trainees' stories into the "formal" content of faculty development programs.

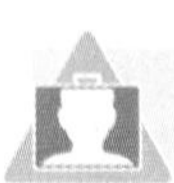

CASE ILLUSTRATION 2

Story of a negative role model from a student's professionalism journal maintained during her ambulatory block rotation.

During my second month I encountered a difficult patient that had chronic diarrhea as his primary diagnosis but also had a positive psychiatric history. During the course of his hospitalization the patient became very anxious and dramatic about every change that was being made to his care. We switched residents during this patient's hospitalization and our new resident was very aggressive. When we rounded together he hardly introduced himself to the patients before he asked direct and imposing questions or scolded them for behaviors like drinking if their diagnosis was pancreatitis. After seeing our difficult patient with diarrhea my resident pulled me aside and told me that he would give me some advice. He told me that I shouldn't be too nice to patients because it is not good to build a relationship. He said, "if you do this then it is very difficult to get them out of here." Considering this resident had been on service for only 2 days and barely knew any of the patients I felt his comment was offensive. I agree that there must be a line between being a patient's friend and a patient's doctor, but it is hard to imagine medicine without compassion and some empathy for those under your care. I understand hospitals are busy but because this resident didn't take the time to care I felt that our patients actually stayed longer because there was a lack of communication between our team and the patient about our goals and expectations.

Third-year medical student

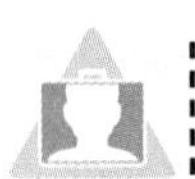

CASE ILLUSTRATION 3

Story of positive role modeling from a student's professional journal maintained during her medicine rotation.

One of the students on my team this month has had three patients back-to-back who have required palliative care. It had gotten to the point that several of us, including her, gently joked about her being a "bad omen" to the patients or a "black cloud." It was nothing mean or cruel, simply something to make her laugh or smile . . . something to keep her going and forget about the true impact of the situation. Her first two patients went home to die with their families. Her third patient presented with AMS and a terminal condition, and it was clear within hours of admission that the patient would die in the next few days. This student never spoke with the patient, as she was unresponsive, but she developed a relationship with the family. On the 3rd day, the student announced during rounds that the patient had passed away at 3:30 that morning. Her voice did not falter as she relayed the news, but we could all tell that it was difficult to get the words out. Our new attending, who had only been with us for 1½ days and had only moments before asked to make presentations quick, stopped rounds, looked directly at the student, and simply asked "How are you feeling?" It surprised most of us at the table, and at first, the student didn't know what to say. Our attending continued to speak with her and discuss the impact of this loss. He encouraged her to stop and consider what she was feeling as the bond between a physician and patient is unique and special in its own way. He reassured her that it is okay to feel disappointed; it only means you truly gave yourself to that patient's care and invested an interest in their health. For the first time, the student admitted to the pain that she was feeling. I was really impressed with our attending's actions. As physicians, I feel as though most faculties are focused solely on the health of the patients and the information/aid that we can bring to the table. It was unique to see this physician take time to teach us a valuable lesson about personal care and coping. He even offered to speak with this student at any time if she wanted to talk. It was a great learning experience, and we felt as if he really cared about our education and growth as medical students. This whole time, the rest of us were trying to make her laugh to keep her going. It never crossed our minds that the best thing for her would be to stop for a moment and reflect.

Third-year medical student

Team-based learning: Team-based learning has potential to be a major vehicle or education methodology for SBS. This methodology promotes active learning and effective team skills without requiring intensive faculty resources for tutoring sessions. TBL uses principles to develop small groups of students into effective learning teams who not only learn course content but also high-level content application, problem solving, and effective team interaction.

The three-part team learning instructional strategy puts these principles into action. Part I is the initial exposure to the concepts of an instructional unit through a Readiness Assurance Process. The Readiness Assurance Process begins with individual preclass work (through assigned readings, work on computer modules, and other modalities). It includes students completing an Individual Readiness Assurance Test (IRAT) during the first few minutes of class that covers the preassigned material. Immediately following the IRAT, the teams take the same test (a Group Readiness Assurance Test, or GRAT), which allows for peer discussion of important course content. The IRAT/GRAT tests are reviewed in class to ensure all students have thorough knowledge of foundational content. The instructor provides focused feedback and instruction on areas needing additional clarification. Teams have the opportunity to appeal and defend any answers marked incorrect. This allows teams an opportunity to further review and discuss difficult concepts.

Upon completion of the Readiness Assurance Process, teams are ready to begin work on team application assignments (Part II). Team assignments allow students to increase their understanding of the main unit concepts by using them to solve a problem. Assignments generally ask team members to reach a decision (rather than write a report) and thus stimulate a high level of team interaction. At a given point, all teams simultaneously reveal their decisions and begin cross-team feedback and discussion. Team assignments for a given instructional unit usually progress from the simple to the more complex. Individual team members prepare for team assignments outside of class and then work together with their team members in class to reach a consensus conclusion. After sufficient team application practice, the instructor reviews the major course content and application learning points and students are formally assessed on an individual basis on their ability to solve a final application problem (Part III).

These team-learning experiences provide a perfect opportunity for learners to move from "stage-to-stage" as part of the process of professional development and role recognition. The experience of being a member of a TBL group also directly addresses key SBS learning objectives, including "*identify ways to work effectively as a part of a team*" and "*engage in activities that foster the development of socially responsible leadership skills*" (refer to Table 44-1 under the Physician Role and Behavior Domain). TBL also formally includes Peer Assessment in the sessions and can incorporate Self-Assessment as well.

Student narratives describing their experiences in the informal curriculum can provide opportunities for TBL groups to integrate multiple SBS competencies/domains into a discussion that addresses key learning objectives and exploration of the science supporting these objectives. Used in this way, narrative has the potential to utilize personal experiences of the informal curriculum to enhance the relevance and enrich the content related to formal curricular objectives.

COGNITIVIST ORIENTATION

The cognitivist orientation suggests that learners use cognitive tools such as insight, information processing, perceptions, and memory to facilitate learning by assigning meaning to events. Use of cognitive maps and reflection exercises are educational methods for promoting the cognitivist orientation.

Concept mapping: Concept mapping exercises provide trainees with a tool to graphically depict their understanding of complex problems or systems. Concept mapping offers a way for learners to incorporate new information into existing knowledge frameworks by associating relationships. Concept mapping can be used longitudinally to visually represent the progressively more complex neural connections in the developing mind. One can readily see the increasing complexity, hierarchical layers, and growing complexity of cross-linking between the pre- and postfigures (Figures 44-1 and 44-2) and when learners' cognitive development is tracked across time.

Analysis and reporting of developmental changes in concept mapping within individuals across time and between groups can be performed. Qualitative analysis of phrases and terms entered onto maps can be performed using software packages along with some quantitative or semiquantitative measures based on scoring schemes reported elsewhere.

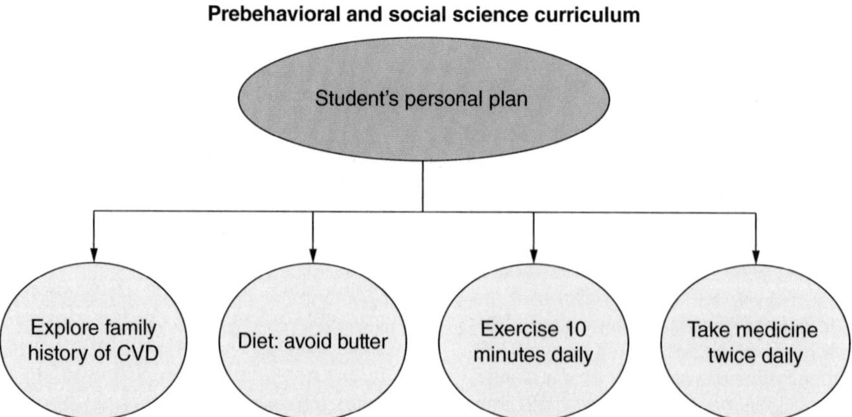

Figure 44-1. ***Concept maps:*** Understanding factors influencing cardiovascular disease (CVD) risk.

CASE ILLUSTRATION 4 (CONTD.)

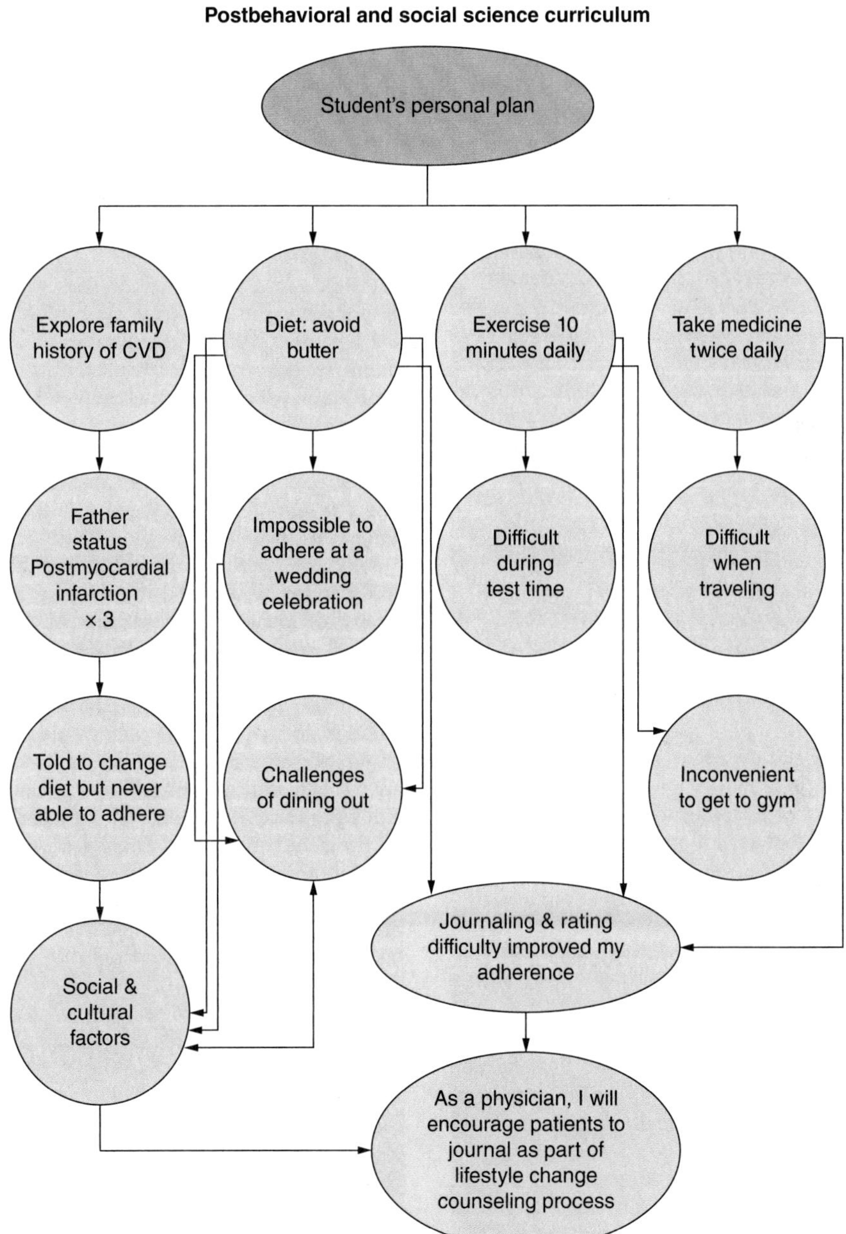

Figure 44-2. ***Concept maps:*** Understanding factors influencing CVD risk.

Reflective exercise: Medical training programs are increasingly incorporating 360-degree (multisource) evaluations for trainees. When accompanied by facilitated one-on-one reviews with mentors and advisors, these sessions offer the opportunity for learners to use a breadth of cognitive tools in an effort to assign meaning to these highly complex and personal data.

CASE ILLUSTRATION 5

A sample of one student's personal reflection stimulated by reviewing his self- and peer-assessment data during his annual meeting with his self-selected self- and peer-assessment advisor.

"... the ideal professional physician must be respectful, tolerant, patient, and a good listener. From my peer assessment, I realize I don't need to be the first to speak when I think an underdog is being exploited ... it is better to first listen to understand before making assumptions about whether a colleague is demonstrating tolerance ... this will help me be a better doctor."

Second-year medical student

CONSTRUCTIVIST ORIENTATION

The constructivist orientation supports the theory that knowledge is formed within the learner by integrating learning activities and experiences into knowledge and beliefs. The creation of meaning from these experiences emerges through critical reflection on existing beliefs and assumptions. Reflective journaling and active creation of learning or competency portfolios are examples of education methods used by educators to tap into constructivist learning styles.

Reflective journaling: Medical training institutions are including reflective journaling in their curricula. SBS constructs, such as identity, bias, privilege, social connections, and emotional management can be potent personal triggers requiring supported opportunities for reflection and growth. Reflection and reflective practice are essential habits of a good physician. (Although reflection is seen as a teachable skill with lifelong utility, it is especially important in the context of an intensive and challenging training environment.) Journaling exercises can range from brief informal invitations to write one's thoughts about a personal experience from the informal curriculum, to writing annual letters to one's self that are personally reviewed, to more extensive narrative writing exercises that are formally analyzed by faculty with expertise in "Narrative Medicine" (see Chapter 47). Reflective journaling can be solely for personal use and review, for one-on-one review with learner-selected and trusted mentors, for de-identified uses within small group seminars, or for required carefully evaluated narrative writing courses. Many guidelines for critical reflection exist. One example is the "LEAP" guidelines (LEAP = "**L**earning from your **E**xperiences as **A** **P**rofessional") that teach learners to write reflections similar to medical "SOAP" notes (i.e., the **s**ubjective experience, the **o**bjective data about the event, the learner's **a**ssessment of causes and **p**ossible learning points, and the learner's plan of what she/he will do next).

Reflective journaling serves to make more seamless the experience of the medical trainees regarding biomedical principles and social/behavioral principles in the context of patient care. Trainees' narratives can provide clear evidence of their ability to integrate these different dimensions of health and disease, in a more holistic manner than the knowledge measures or other quantitative measures of student performance. With permission, trainee's personal reflections (stories) can be used to generate new curricular materials linking informal and formal aspects of their training.

Commitment to change statements: Another approach to help learners integrate knowledge and experience is commitment to change (CtC) statements (see student journaling exercise on lifestyle change commitments above under case illustration 1). Research has shown the CtC method does enhance the probability of an individual making a change. At the end of an educational experience, the student is simply asked to write down a limited number of things they wish to change or accomplish as a result of the educational experience. In addition to writing what they would like to do differently, they can provide a rating on how motivated they are to make the change and how difficult they believe it will be to make the change. At a predetermined follow-up time, the student's CtC statements can be returned to them to reflect on whether they were successful in making the change and why. If they were not successful, they can also reflect on what the barriers were to making the change and lessons learned from the experience.

CASE ILLUSTRATION 6

Students select de-identified journal entries made by their cohort to discuss in small group, facilitated professionalism seminars during the medicine clerkship. In discussing their own narratives in a small group, the students are being professional as they talk and learn about professionalism. Reflection is stimulated by questions posed by the seminar facilitator such as: "What was it about this setting or these individuals that makes this possible?" As the students examine their experiences together, they are bringing their lived encounters—the informal curriculum—into the explicit, formal curriculum. Students report that the experience of being present to others' stories of professionalism helps them to feel less isolated and alone in their own experiences and also helps them to name professional issues that might otherwise go unacknowledged and unaddressed.

A sample from one student's professionalism journal entry made while on her third-year medicine rotation:

Today the fire alarms went off at the county hospital and all the elevators were stopped. I entered the stairwell on the sixth floor to go down stairs and encountered a hospital employee in a hair net coming up, four loaded food trays precariously stacked in her arms. Her breathing was loud and labored, and she implored Jesus with each exhalation. I ran down the few steps to her side and asked if she needed help. Between gasps and prayers she told me she was an asthmatic and really should not be climbing stairs, especially not six flights, and definitely not carrying four heavy trays. I relayed to her that a maintenance man told me it won't be long before the elevators are operating again, and maybe she could wait a few minutes. She replied, "we can't let the patients suffer just because the elevators are out and we've got a touch of asthma, now can we?" I was surprised by her dedication to her job and her care for the well-being of the patients. It reminded me how noble it is to be responsible at any level for the care of another human being, and how many important roles there are in providing that care to each patient.

Third-year medical student

Portfolios: Learning portfolios aggregate learning products review and analysis by trainees and/or course and residency program directors. Portfolios have been found to be of high utility in documenting evidence of performance in SBS areas, such as self-awareness, professionalism, ethical judgment, and moral reasoning. Trainees can populate portfolios with documented experiences or activities from the formal or informal curricula. Given the sensitive nature of some materials entered into trainees' portfolios, several institutions have created ways to allow learners to self-populate both "personal" and "academic" versions of their portfolios. For ease of handling data, electronic portfolio tracking systems are increasingly available.

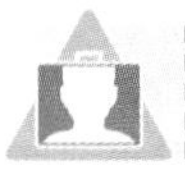

CASE ILLUSTRATION 7

As part of an electronic portfolio pilot program, 16 first-year medical students from IUSM's Terre Haute campus were asked to self-populate fields built to document students' performance in each of the core competency areas. Four students chose to populate their academic portfolios with their reflective narratives written following their observations of an autopsy. One student mapped his narrative into the "Using Science to Guide Diagnosis, Management, Therapeutics, and Prevention" competency, explaining that the experience helped him better understand the anatomy important for performing future procedures. One student added her story to the "Self-Awareness, Self-Care, and Personal Growth" competency stating, although she would never want to be a coroner, she now has a new appreciation for the important role these health care providers play as members of the larger health care team. Two students logged their entries into the "Moral Reasoning and Ethical Judgment" competency. One student reflected on the inappropriate behavior of the health care providers in handling human body remains of a deceased patient for whom some family members were likely still grieving. The second ethics entry included the student's reflection about how providers choose to deal with medical errors that resulted in a child's death. This demonstrates how a single curricular exercise can provide highly varied educational experiences for trainees uncovered through self-categorization based on the personal meaning these experiences had for the individual student. Portfolios can help document broad curricular exposure to all core competency areas as perceived by trainees.

Medical Education Methods Effective for Teaching Behavioral & Social Science

Educational methods found to improve student learning of traditional basic science or clinical content apply equally well to education in the SBS. Below are four examples.

ADULT LEARNING METHODS

The central tenet of teaching adult learners is recognizing and engaging their wealth of experience as an educational resource and creating "active" versus "passive" (e.g., lecture) learning activities. SBS lends itself to this approach because learners can often access the content through reflection on their own experience (e.g., racism, homophobia, caring for the elderly), in small group discussions or working together with peers on TBL cases. Students who participate in the learner-centered approach are more likely to go beyond passively absorbing the curriculum; they develop habits of inquiry, reflection, and teamwork as they move forward in the progressive development of a socially enlightened physician identity. In addition, activated learners participate in shaping the curriculum or delivering it to themselves and their peers. Further curricular enhancement can derive from interprofessional TBL experiences. Disciplines such as nursing and social work have a long history of SBS-focused patient care and curriculum, which can increase its salience and influence on physician problem solving and worldview. These students may be especially motivated to develop and support SBS teaching not only in their practice but as models for future generations of physicians.

HIGHLIGHT CLINICAL RELEVANCE

An important mission of all medical schools is to graduate learners who are prepared for medical practice, and SBS curricula are central to this mission. Emphasizing clinical relevance for preclinical and clinical students can counter the perception that SBS lacks practical utility in patient care. Although there is no national consensus framework for presenting SBS material, existing guidelines may prove useful in determining how SBS content can best be implemented into clinical care. Early exposure to longitudinal patient care can provide students with a "lived" experience from the patient's perspective of interacting with a health care system that the students will soon be in a position to impact clinically, economically, and perhaps in policy. It might now be possible to use published literature that emphasizes patient and/or doctor narratives to conduct clinicalpathological conference (CPC)-like discussions to explicate the SBS elements in the framework of biopsychosocial health stories. Although less factually based, a salient patient interview may prove far more memorable in illustrating the effects of poverty on health than a required journal article. Similarly, a well-crafted longitudinal patient care experience or PBL case that highlights issues such as substance abuse, social supports, and the value of the therapeutic relationships—while also integrating them with clinical and basic sciences—might more effectively convey those constructs compared to a didactic lecture.

INCLUDE A FOCUS ON QUALITY OF CARE

An emphasis on quality of care further maximizes clinical relevance for students. Teaching students about the social and behavioral determinants of health, the major impact that SBS problems have on mortality, and methods of addressing these health risks moves the issue beyond a matter of political correctness or social trends. Teaching students how to ask about health-related behaviors and how to facilitate behavior change has direct benefits for quality of care. Teaching about health systems, health care teams, and ways to avoid medical errors clearly relates to quality improvement (QI). If SBS concepts are framed as practical tools to help students become better doctors, the perceived value increases. Furthermore, creating opportunities for students to be involved in actual, small-scale QI projects takes the process from passive knowledge attainment to actively acquiring the skills and efficacy to facilitate a measureable impact on both patients' and doctors' lives as well as the health care system as a whole.

CREATE A SPIRAL CURRICULUM

Given the vast amount of information to teach, many educators make the mistake of trying to teach too much at one time. Stand-alone behavioral science courses are so overfull that little time is left to promote clinical application and improve trainee retention. A developmentally appropriate "repetition and elaboration" approach should be created that first introduces the materials on a beginner's level, and then revisits those same constructs later with greater complexity and learner demand. However, in some instances these SBS linkages may already exist in the formal and informal curriculum, but they are poorly mapped and rarely if ever explicitly identified to the student in a purposeful way. This lack of purposefulness further perpetuates the belief that SBS concepts and curriculum are "just common sense" and do not require the same focus or prioritization as the biomedical sciences. Mapping would help identify areas where SBS concepts occur naturally in the curriculum, which in turn helps educators better identify and elaborate on them in a meaningful way. Mapping would also help curriculum designers identify specific lacunae where SBS needs to be addressed.

CREATING A COMMUNITY THAT MODELS & SUPPORTS THE BEHAVIORAL & SOCIAL SCIENCE KNOWLEDGE & ABILITIES

The educational methods described above will be minimally effective unless grounded within a community that models and teaches these values, knowledge, and abilities. Serious attention to education in the behavioral and social sciences must, therefore, include attention to the informal curriculum of the institution that so strongly influences the developing professional identity and practice patterns of trainees. The educational methods described below are designed to foster the development of the medical training institution itself.

Promote Relational Practices Across the Organization

Teaching behavioral and social sciences in the informal curriculum requires institutional and faculty/staff development that promotes key behavioral and social science-informed (relational) behaviors in the everyday environment. Practices that build relationships include faculty development that enhances both individual and group communication skills. New practices in meetings can enable participants to get to know the person, not just the position, sitting next to them. These include an invitation for participants to "check in" at the start of a meeting and share some small piece of personal or professional information ("My son won his bike race yesterday!" or "My clinical research project was funded!") that enables a deeper level of interaction. Collaboratively and transparently establishing the meeting agenda at the start of a meeting, ensuring that everyone has the opportunity to speak, and actively seeing and valuing a wide range of perspectives on any particular topic help to create an organizational culture that models the values and behaviors students are taught in their formal education.

Take Time to Examine and Publicize What is Working Well

Traditional organizational development strategies often begin by identifying what is not working in the institution, the "problem," and focus on finding ways to avoid, decrease, or solve that problem. This deficit approach to change asks participants to address and study the question "what are we lacking?" In contrast, the organizational development method of Appreciative Inquiry (AI), grounded in positive psychology, challenges conventional approaches with the premise that people are more motivated to engage in change by finding what's working well and doing more of it. Described by its founder, David Cooperrider:

> *Appreciative Inquiry is the cooperative search for the best in people, their organizations, and the world around them. It involves systematic discovery of what gives a system "life" when it is most effective and capable in economic, ecological, and human terms. AI involves the art and practice of asking questions that strengthen a system's capacity to heighten positive potential. It mobilizes inquiry through crafting an "unconditional positive question".*

AI seeks to discover what members of a community are already doing well, and to hold those achievements up as an attainable standard of success. It can be used by medical training institutions to identity existing strengths in key behavioral and social science domains, such as the ability to effectively address mind–body interactions in health and disease; understanding patient behavior and motivating behavioral change; exemplifying a professional physician role and behavior; demonstrating effective, compassionate physician–patient interactions; modeling facility in addressing social and cultural issues in health care; and demonstrating approaches to care that take into consideration health policy and economics. With its focus on the positive work that the institution is already modeling, AI inspires and motivates the community to reach its full potential.

Create a Reflective Community

Self-reflection is important not only for individuals but for institutions as well. It enables members to intentionally examine the professional and learning environments that they and their institution foster and promote. Institution-wide conversations about positive and challenging critical incidents—published in weekly newsletters or other public format—can promote open reflection about an institution's learning and professional environment, allow acknowledgment of error, promote discussion of values, and provide an opportunity for the members of an institution to thoughtfully consider the moral ethos of their culture.

SUMMARY

Medical training programs have employed a variety of organizational and theoretical frameworks as vehicles for increasing education in the SBS. These efforts, while important, are an incomplete solution. Attention to trainees' learning environment, and their experiential learning in the informal curriculum, are also critical. The authors suggest that educators consider including learning experiences that draw upon and integrate both formal and informal curricular content and experiences. They provide examples of educational activities within a range of theoretical orientations that accomplish this integration. Examples illustrate how narratives, generated by trainees and other members of the academic community about personal experiences and perceptions of the organization's professional culture, can be creatively integrated into the formal curriculum in a variety of contexts. This strategy promotes personal and organizational reflection and mindfulness, and reinforces the importance of lessons learned in the informal curriculum. This cyclical process promotes awareness of the individual community members' roles in the creation of a culture conducive to learning and caring for patients.

ACKNOWLEDGMENTS

The authors acknowledge Drs. J Satterfield, A. Schickedanz, R. Salazar, S. Adler, H. C. Chen, K. Hauer, D. Hughes, and G. Saba for providing contributions to the "Medical Education Methods Effective for Teaching Behavioral and Social Science" section. Funded in part by NIH Award R25AR060994.

SUGGESTED READINGS

Charon R, Holmboe E, Holmes J, et al. *Behavioral and Social Science Foundations for Future Physicians.* Report of the behavioral and social science expert panel. Association of American Medical College, Washington, D.C., 2011.

Cooperrider DL, Whitney D. Appreciative inquiry: a positive revolution in change. In: Holman, P Devane, T eds, *The Change*

Handbook. San Francisco, CA: Berrett-Koehler Publishers, Inc.; 2005, pp. 245–263.

Frankel RM, Eddins-Folensbee F, Inui TS. Crossing the patient-centered divide: transforming healthcare quality through enhanced faculty development. *Acad Med* 2011;86:445–452.

Inui TS. *A Flag in the Wind: Education for Professionalism in Medicine*. Washington, DC: Association of American Medical Colleges; 2003.

Karnieli-Miller O, Vu TR, Frankel RM, et al. Which experiences in the hidden curriculum teach students about professionalism? *Acad Med* 2011;86:369–377.

Litzelman DK, Cottingham, AH. The new formal competency-based curriculum and informal curriculum at Indiana University School of Medicine: overview and five-year analysis. *Acad Med* 2007;82:410–421.

Reiter, HI, Eva KW, Rosenfeld J, Norman GR. Multiple mini-interviews predict clerkship and licensing examination performance. *Med Educ* 2007;41:378–384.

Satterfield JM, Adler SR, Chen HC, Hauer KE, Saba GW, Salazar R. Creating an ideal social and behavioral sciences curriculum for medical students. *Med Educ* 2010;44:1194–1202.

Suchman, AL, Sluyter, DJ, Williamson, PR. *Leading Change in Healthcare: Transforming Organizations Using Complexity, Positive Psychology and Relationship-Centered Care*. London: Radcliffe Publishing; 2011.

Suchman A, Williamson P, Litzelman D, et al. Toward an informal curriculum that teaches professionalism: transforming the social environment of a medical school. *JGIM* 2004;19:501–504.

Torre DM, Daley BJ, Sebastion JL, Elnicki DM. Overview of current learning theories for medical educators. *Amer J Med* 2006;119:903–907.

WEBSITES

Behavioral and Social Science Foundations for Future Physicians. https://www.aamc.org/download/271020/data/behavioralandsocialsciencefoundationsforfuturephysicians.pdf. Accessed August 2018.

Early Data on the Validity of the Psychological, Social, and Biological Foundations of Behavior Section of the New MCAT Exam.

https://www.aamc.org/download/448364/data/mcatpsbbvalidityresearch.pdf. Accessed August 2018.

Improving Medical Education: Enhancing the Behavioral and Social Science Content of Medical School Curricula. https://www.ncbi.nlm.nih.gov/books/NBK10238/. Accessed August 2018.

O'Sullivan P, Aronson L, Chittenden E, Niehaus B, Learman L. Reflective Ability Rubric and User Guide. MedEdPORTAL; 2010. www.mededportal.org/publication/8133. Accessed August 2018.

Team-Based Learning Collaborative: http://www.teambasedlearning.org/. Accessed August 2018.

Assessing Learners & Curricula in the Behavioral & Social Sciences

Patricia A. Carney, PhD; Felise Milan, MD; & Jason M. Satterfield, PhD

CASE ILLUSTRATION

In compliance with the recommendation for yearly alcohol screening for adults in primary care, a family medicine residency director wants to develop a curriculum to teach her residents how to use a validated alcohol-screening tool and provide brief alcohol counseling. Given competing educational demands, she wants this curriculum to be both efficient and effective. She plans to evaluate her residents and the curriculum....

INTRODUCTION

Health professional training programs are increasingly focused on assessing clinical competencies that demonstrate a learner's readiness for (or progression toward) independent practice. Training programs must track a multitude of competencies or "entrustable professional activities" (EPA's) that often include both concrete observable procedures and more nuanced but essential "doctoring" skills, such as empathy, cultural sensitivity, and professionalism. Although the general principles of learner and curricular assessment hold equally true for the behavioral and social sciences (BSS), these content areas can be more difficult to operationalize and evaluate. Moreover, high-quality BSS teaching and assessment tools often require explicit, robust institutional support that relies on careful programmatic evaluations that align with institutional goals, learning activities, and curricular performance. Although evaluations assess a learner and/or program, the results should also iteratively drive curricular and institutional evolution toward improvements often related to new or updated educational and clinical care features.

This chapter provides guidance on designing evaluation and assessment strategies for both health professional learners and curricular programs with an eye toward continuous improvement. In the section "Assessment & Evaluation Planning," we outline how to plan assessments including evaluation processes, methods, and tools for evaluation program design. In the section "Learner Assessment & Evaluation," we describe assessment methods and instrumentation that can ensure learners have the skills needed to address behavioral and social issues that influence health. In the section "Program Evaluation," we address how measurements can be used to assess curricular and program performance. Lastly, in the section "Educational Research & Scholarship," we underscore the importance of educational research and dissemination of best practices as a means to move the science of education and educational evaluation forward.

Fundamental principles have influenced the content of each section. First, evaluation is as important as the training curricula delivered. Evaluations should not be undertaken as an afterthought after the curriculum has already been delivered. Second, just as we urge our learners to practice evidence-based medicine, we urge educators to practice evidence-guided learning. Although educational science is young, there is a growing body of research to guide selection of educational interventions, curricular timing and "dose," and the choice of valid and reliable assessment tools. Educational tradition and convenience are not sufficient to guide efficient and effective uses of precious curricular hours. Finally, we assert that rigorously developed, delivered, and evaluated curricula should be published and shared as scholarly peer-reviewed works to advance both educators' skills and the science of learning.

ASSESSMENT & EVALUATION PLANNING

Evaluation designs are critical for determining the impact of curriculum or teaching approaches on learners' knowledge, attitudes/values, and skills. Selection of your evaluation design might also consider cost effectiveness, systems change, or the impact on patient or clinical outcomes. Implementing a design to test established or new curricular strategies takes careful planning and measurement considerations. The best approach for evaluation design is to develop the assessment(s) *as the curriculum or educational program is being developed,* rather than after so alignment of these areas can be undertaken so the most effective assessment is used. Too often, evaluations are planned at the end when opportunities to revise for meaningful assessment of learner and program outcomes have passed. Early evaluation planning will ensure that programmatic goals have been articulated and aligned with measurable learning objectives, best approaches and tools for evaluation have been identified, and processes for evaluation are timed for best results. Although the planning process will vary based on resources, expertise, and other contextual factors, the following four questions highlight common issues to be considered during evaluation planning.

1. What is the goal of the evaluation? All educators assume their training program "works" but the specific purpose of the education may vary. For example, does the intervention target changes in knowledge, attitudes, or skills? Does the program intend to demonstrate minimally sufficient competence or extraordinary talent and achievement? Will the results be formative or summative? How will the data be used? Will it influence institutional policy or identify strengths or weaknesses of the program?
2. Which theoretical models will best guide evaluation designs and specific curricular content? For example, an educator interested in determining "competence" could use the Dreyfus model of skill acquisition that starts at novice, and progresses to advanced beginner, competent, proficient, and expert. In this case, assessment tools that target a determined threshold for "competence" and benchmarked steps leading to competence would be needed. Other models that guide evaluation development include Miller's pyramid (knows, knows how, shows how, does), Kirkpatrick's hierarchy of evaluation (assesses level of impact of the curriculum ranging from learner satisfaction to changes in clinical outcomes), or Bloom's taxonomy (assesses recall/remember, understanding, applying, analyzing, evaluating, and creating). Models that guide educational content might include the Transtheoretical (Stages of Change) Model and motivational interviewing that matches behavioral counseling to patients' readiness to change (see Chapter 19). A demonstration of "competence" would require the use of the general Dreyfus model with specific assessment items relevant to motivational interviewing.
3. What are the available evaluation resources? Resources include time (for faculty and/or learners), money, faculty/evaluator skills, and buy-in from program leaders and learners. Assessments may range in time, cost, and labor-intensiveness, such as expensive, high-stakes standardized patient (SP) assessments, though peer role plays are quicker and cheaper observations. Careful attention must be given to the test characteristics of the assessment tools chosen and whether feasibility compromises the utility of the results.
4. What are the key methodological considerations? Even with clear goals and sufficient resources, critical decisions must be made that can affect the value of evaluations. As discussed below, psychometric properties such as reliability, validity, and fidelity of instruments must be considered. Standard setting, benchmarking, scoring, and remediation should also be determined. All four key considerations are applied to the opening Case Illustration in Table 45-1.

Creating Reliable & Valid Instruments

Concepts of reliability and validity are central to designing and implementing high-stakes assessments. The higher the stakes associated with the assessment (e.g., pass or fail a course/clerkship), the greater the need for the assessment to be valid and reliable. In very simple terms, validity refers to whether the assessment measures what it intends to measure. A common misconception is that assessment instruments can be considered universally valid, when, in fact, validity can only be shown for a given population and context. Validating an assessment consists of evaluating potential threats to validity to ensure that the assessment actually represents the intended construct as applied in the intended setting. Common threats to validity include construct underrepresentation (e.g., too few items or cases) and construct-irrelevant variance (e.g., flawed rating scales, poorly constructed items, inappropriate ordering of items, and poorly trained SPs).

Reliability in educational assessment is a measure of reproducibility. Statistical methods of measuring reliability determine the difference between the "true score" and the "observed score" or the amount of error in the observed score. The greater the measurement error, the less reproducible the assessment becomes. There are three different questions to be asked about the reproducibility of a given test score if it were given to the same group of students more than once: (1) Would the same students pass or fail? (2) Would the rank order from best

Table 45-1. Developing assessments for an alcohol counseling curriculum.

1. Goals of the Curriculum	2. Theoretical Model(s)	3. Resource Considerations	4. Methods: Tools	Methods: Timing
To produce lasting changes in resident knowledge and skills regarding alcohol screening and brief intervention.	-Miller's pyramid -National Institute on Alcohol Abuse and Alcoholism (NIAAA) clinician's guide to patients who drink to excess -Stages of change and motivational interviewing	-3 hours of large group didactic time -4 hours of small group discussion or role play -Use of three SP cases about alcohol use	-SP examinations -Written test -Survey -Focus groups	-Preknowledge test -Post-SP examination -Postwritten examination -Postsurvey and focus group

to worst score be the same? (3) Would all the students receive the same scores? Three different theories can be used statistically to assess reliability, including classical test theory (using Cronbach's alpha), generalizability theory, and item response theory. A psychometrics consultation can often answer these and many key evaluation development questions.

STANDARD SETTING & GRADING

Standard setting refers to the process of determining a cut score or passing score. For traditional assessments, such as multiple-choice examinations, standard setting techniques are well developed. For any performance-based assessments to be effectively used for summative decisions, setting defensible standards is necessary. Although standard setting may require attention to psychometrics, ultimately it incorporates consideration of institutional culture, policy, and resources.

Determining the passing score includes determining how many students are going to fail. The "stakes" or ramifications of failing an assessment (e.g., repeating a course, need for remediation, and ability to graduate) will play the largest role in determining how to set the passing score. Two broad categories of standard setting are normative (grading on a curve) and absolute or criterion referenced. Normative grading involves determining how a cohort of learners performed and then setting a cut-point as a multiple of standard deviations below the mean. Criterion-referenced standard setting is more work intensive but usually favored for performance-based assessment, as it is based on how each learner performs against a determined competency standard. Grading can be compensatory, allowing a learner to compensate for a low performance in one domain or case with higher performance on another, or noncompensatory. Noncompensatory grading will result in a greater number of students failing the assessment. For example, if students need to pass a certain number of cases to pass an Observed Standardized Clinical Examination (OSCE), they can compensate for poor history taking with outstanding interpersonal skills. If students must pass the history and interpersonal aspects of each case to pass an examination, passing will be more difficult.

LEARNER ASSESSMENT & EVALUATION

Ideally, learners (and programs) will be assessed at multiple points with performance data being used to iteratively drive improvements. In a competency-based model, a threshold is set that all learners must achieve; however, benchmarks or milestones on the path toward competence can be used to track learner progression toward more advanced skills over time. Programs should articulate skill development pathways that repeatedly assess learners and offer remediation, as needed.

A number of validated assessment tools are available for the BSS and a recent systematic review published by Carney et al. in 2016 identifies BSS tools rated highly for their validity and reliability (see "Suggested Readings" and "Websites"). Table 45-2 provides examples of specific tools that assess core BSS areas such as social attitudes and behavior change counseling. Evaluators may select validated tools or develop their own based on the specific assessment needs. Remember that assessment instruments are not universally valid or reliable. Although it is helpful to review the psychometric properties of tools as they have been previously studied, it will still be necessary to evaluate any tool's performance when used with learners in the context of your assessment. Assessment goals (e.g., changing attitudes, knowledge, or skills), available resources, and preferred methodologies all inform the selection of measurement tools.

Assessing Attitudes

Educational programs seek to instill particular values or attitudes in their learners (e.g., empathy, respect, nonjudgment, and equity). Educational activities, especially

Table 45-2. Examples of BSS assessment tools for learners.

Assessment Tool	Description	Where to Find It
1. Attitudes Toward Social Issues in Medicine	A 63-item Likert-type attitude survey with seven subscales including social factors, interprofessionalism, and prevention.	Parlow & Rothman. *J Med Educ* 1974;49:385–387.
2. Video Assessment of Simulated Encounters (VASE-R)	Three video-based case vignettes are used to assess learner skills in motivational interviewing.	John S. Baer, PhD VA Puget Sound Healthcare System-Seattle jsbaer@u.washington.edu http://adai.washington.edu/instruments/VASE-R.htm
3. Cognitive Behavior Survey	A seven-scale, 120-item questionnaire that profiles cognitive, meta-cognitive, and experiential aspect of learning for residents or students.	Dr. Rudolph Mitchell, Massachusetts Institute of Technology, (rudy@mit.edu). See *Acad Med* 2009;84:918–926.
4. Brief Negotiated Interview (BNI)	A 21-item checklist used to evaluate the quality of a brief negotiated interview for problematic substance use.	http://www.ihs.gov/nc4/documents/appendix_a_yale_bni_manual.pdf

those that are part of clinical clerkships or rotations, are often indirect or occur on an experiential level and can be highly influenced by institutional culture and the "hidden curriculum" (see Chapter 48). Attitudes are most commonly assessed with self-report surveys that are highly efficient but have fairly obvious demand characteristics. Respondents may know the socially desirable answer and may not answer honestly. Indirect testing measures, such as the Implicit Associations Test (IAT), attempt to tap unconscious bias by tracking milliseconds of reaction time to words paired with race, gender, or other demographic identifiers. Multisource feedback (also known as "360-degree evaluations") involve eliciting learner evaluations from peers, allied health professionals, patients, and others with first-hand knowledge of the learner's tone, emotion, and behaviors—all of which infer attitudes.

Assessing Knowledge

Educational or learning objectives are critical for both curriculum development and evaluation. Objectives should specify observable and measurable changes brought about as a consequence of curricular exposure. Even for objectives limited only to medical knowledge, the levels or content of knowledge expected can vary, ranging from simple recall to complex synthesis using foundational knowledge and principles (see Bloom's Taxonomy). Written tests are commonly used to assess medical knowledge, but their content and format should be determined by knowledge level expected. Because learning can occur at many levels, from simple recall to problem solving, multiple-choice questions (MCQs) should target the level of learning that aligns with the content taught. Characteristics of effective MCQs are related to the item, the question stem, and answer options. Poorly constructed MCQs will not produce accurate or meaningful test scores and could negatively affect learner pass rates. Tips for developing MCQs can be found on The National Board of Medical Examiners web site.

Although MCQs can be problematic in nearly any content area, they are especially difficult to develop for BSS content. MCQs commonly test recognition (choosing an answer) rather than recall (constructing an answer), allow guessing, and are time consuming to construct with choices that are neither intuitive nor unequivocally correct. Thus, case write-ups, critical essays, or innovative tools like concept mapping might better assess a learner's mastery of BSS content. For example, in the UCSF School of Medicine, medical students keep a "sociocultural skills tracker" that includes a longitudinal series of patient-based assignments to demonstrate progress toward competence working with patients of diverse backgrounds. "Tracker" entries are used to provide feedback and shape subsequent exercises.

Assessing Skills

Achieving behavioral science competency includes mastery of broad content as well as communication and interpersonal skills. Although relatively little has been studied about assessing students' behavioral science knowledge, a rich literature exists on performance-based testing to assess communication skills. Most of this work assesses learners at the "shows how" level of Miller's pyramid (know, knows how, shows how, does) and are stronger predictors of whether learners will demonstrate these skills in the clinical setting than written examinations. Using unannounced SPs in the clinical setting is an example of a performance-based assessment that evaluates learners at the "does" level of the pyramid, assuming they are unaware they are being assessed.

In the following section, we discuss several methods of performance-based assessments to evaluate communication and interpersonal skills. Many of these performance-based assessment methods can also be used to directly measure knowledge and indirectly measure attitudes.

Direct Observation

Direct observation of learners in health professions education is essential but underutilized, especially in clinical settings. Both the Liaison Committee on Medical Education (LCME) and Accreditation Council for Graduate Medical Education (ACGME) require ongoing assessment of trainees that includes direct observation of clinical skills. The Mini-Clinical Evaluation Exercise (mini-CEX) is the most studied format for performance evaluation using direct observation. Less formal observations are also commonly done using behavioral checklists, global rating scales, or other observational tools.

Inter-Rater Reliability

Several factors are important to consider when evaluating the quality and accuracy of assessments using direct observation. Overall assessments based on clinical observation generally have poor reliability. Variability in rater assessments has been attributed to measurement errors of leniency, threshold setting bias, and poor performance discrimination. Whereas case specificity is typically unavoidable and affects reliability, rater variability also plays a role in accuracy. Judgments made by raters can be extremely subjective, influenced by raters' moods and likely to be idiosyncratic.

Using interviews of faculty raters, Kogan and colleagues identified four themes that provide insight into how ratings form: (1) faculty rely on variable frames of reference during observations including their own performance, performance by others known to them at different levels of training, standards of performance considered necessary for patient care, and patient outcomes; (2) inference often plays a key role, including assumptions about learner motivations and attitudes; (3) faculty use variable approaches to synthesizing judgments into numerical ratings across or within different observations; and (4) contextual factors (complexity of the encounter, learners' level of experience, the faculty–resident relationships), and residents' responses to feedback play a role in faculty judgments. Thus, raters need both tools and training to improve reliability.

Observation Tools

Tools to guide observations and structure assessments come in different forms. Kogan and colleagues published a systematic review of tools for direct observations with students, residents, and fellows in clinical settings. Another review of tools to assess communication skills evaluated 15 instruments based on criteria from the Kalamazoo Consensus Statement. Global rating scales have been found to be the more efficient of these tools, and are as reliable as checklists when completed by expert faculty. Checklists have advantages for lesser-experienced raters such as students or SPs.

Both checklists and rating scales vary greatly in length and format based on the objective of the assessment, the aspects of performance being assessed, and who is doing the rating. Checklists typically measure a list of behaviors observed that can be scored dichotomously as "done" or "not done." This approach is not ideal for assessments of complex and nuanced behaviors such as empathy or respect. In general, rating scales measure implicit processes and offer a range of responses usually on either a numerical or Likert-type scale or a behaviorally anchored rating scale (BARS). A BARS specifically lists the learner behaviors that must be observed to achieve a particular score. For example, for the item, "*Allows the patient to tell their story,*" the behavioral anchors can range from the lowest level "*fails to let patient tell story or sets pace with closed Q&A style, not conversational*" to the highest level of "*encourages and lets patient tell story with open-ended questions and doesn't interrupt patient.*" Behavioral anchors can improve inter-rater reliability as they provide a more explicit definition of each level of performance. Global rating scales use fewer items but assess larger domains that may be difficult to reduce to a micro-skill set (e.g., empathy, cultural sensitivity). Global rating scales have been shown to be reliable when used by expert faculty or well-trained raters.

Observer Training

Despite the difficulties inherent in faculty raters, their assessments of learners' performance are essential for any educational program. Faculty training can improve their observation skills, which is far more important than choosing the "perfect" rating instrument.

Behavioral Observation Training (BOT) focuses on improving the ability of the observer to detect, perceive, and remember performance of learners. Strategies include practice by increasing the number of observations done, using a tool to record observations, establishing the learning objectives, and considering encounter logistics. Performance Dimension Training (PDT) is designed to familiarize faculty with the definitions and criteria for the competencies being observed. When faculty understand performance dimensions as a group, it is easier to achieve consensus on behaviors that constitute a superior versus inferior performance. Frame of Reference Training is an extension of PDT. It encourages faculty consensus and distinguishing minimum criteria for performance levels. Training includes several exercises where faculty work together to set criteria for satisfactory performance and create a BARS. Vignettes are viewed and rated using the scale, followed by feedback from the session trainer on the "true" ratings with explanations. Finally, Direct Observation of Competence training (developed by Holmboe and colleagues) incorporates elements of all the above rater training methods and adds relevant, practical exercises in direct observation. These exercises can be done in faculty development sessions and have been shown to lead to meaningful improvements.

Clinical Simulations

OSCE/Clinical Skills Examinations

Since direct observation by faculty in clinical settings does not have the reliability necessary for high-stakes assessments, most institutions now rely on structured performance testing. Clinical skills examinations, such as OSCEs or Clinical Performance Examinations (CPEs), are used by many programs to assess progression of learners to the next level of training. The United States and Canada both include a Clinical Skills Examination as part of their medical licensure requirements. These examinations often include a series of encounters with SPs who have been trained to portray patients with specific medical needs. By holding variables in the encounter constant, the reliability of these examinations is greater than observations with real patients. However, artificially creating and standardizing patient encounters does not fully eliminate threats to validity.

Standardized clinical examinations measure a learner's skills at the "show's how" level of Miller's pyramid; however, this occurs in an artificial situation. The key question for Clinical Skills Examinations is how well its scores predict learner performance in actual clinical settings (e.g., the "does" level of Miller's pyramid). Several studies support the predictive validity of CPE communication scores showing strong correlations between medical student CPE scores and later performance as residents. Although evidence supports the validity of CPE to assess communication, there are many aspects of communication in real clinical settings that are unmeasured, such as team communication and adaptability of communication styles in various clinical settings.

Contextual fidelity, or the extent to which the CPE can be affected by the learner, environment, task, or technical system, can threaten the validity of communication skills assessment. Also, the artificial context of the CPE may deprive the learner of contextual cues found in a real clinical environment and, therefore, stymie the learner's ability to communicate empathically. To consider these challenges to validity, some experts recommend the use of reflective practice, challenging cases, and rater training on how to give feedback to enrich the SP simulations in evaluating empathy. When the artificiality of the testing environment is further increased by "over standardization" in SP training, this can lead to encounters that lack fidelity and validity.

There is some debate about whether BSS skills can be reliably assessed using clinical cases or whether they are more accurately assessed when the explicit goal of the case is BSS focused, such as smoking cessation counseling. Some have also questioned whether general assessment of a learner's BSS skills can be measured across several cases or requires case specificity. Generally, each clinical case in a CPE has a separate and relevant content checklist for history and physical examination items, but the CPE may have only one global checklist (global rating scale) to evaluate the BSS skills across all cases. A study by Guiton of fourth-year medical students found high generalizability for seven communication skills across seven OSCE cases, supporting the ability to identify a set of generic communication skills across cases. However, they also found significant case-student variability in communication scores. This suggests that even though one communication skills checklist can be used across several cases, in any performance assessment of communication skills, several cases providing a variety of communication (or BSS) challenges should be used to achieve adequate reliability.

Although inter-rater reliability is generally greater in CPEs than in directly observed encounters with real patients, it is important to address this form of reliability when assessing BSS skills. There are inconsistent findings in the literature as to whether faculty and SP ratings correlate or if faculty are rating something different than SPs in assessments of communication and other BSS skills. Faculty are often looking for communication behaviors or skills that are known to be effective with patients, and SPs are reporting their experience from inside the interaction on the effectiveness of the skills observed. Some differences between expert faculty and SP raters have been found when global ratings are used in lieu of checklists. Training raters and using standardized tools (e.g., checklists) can reduce the number of raters needed for reliability and can increase inter-rater reliability.

High-Tech Simulation

Technically sophisticated mannequins and task trainers have been increasingly integrated into health professions education for both teaching and assessment of clinical skills. A growing literature demonstrates that the practice of high-risk procedures on computerized, highly technical mannequins that appear to blink, sweat, and breathe create enough realism or fidelity that the skills demonstrated in these scenarios carry over to real clinical situations. Psychological fidelity—or how "real" the situation feels—and whether it requires the same cognitive and emotional skill set as a real situation must also be considered. Although medical procedures are well suited for high-simulation mannequin assessments, they can also be used to test teamwork skills, clinical reasoning, and emotion/stress-management.

Patient-focused simulation training involves a combination of mannequins and real people within a simulated scenario to provide psychological and functional fidelity. These simulations allow learners to tap into conscious and unconscious responses that can provide opportunities to assess skills of delivering bad news, communication of medical errors, ethical decision making, and end-of-life care, to name a few.

Computer-based virtual patients are another emerging technology for BSS assessment. More can be learned about the use and development of virtual patients on the MedBiquitous web site (see "Websites").

Performance Portfolios

Assessment of learner attitudes, knowledge, and skills is complex and requires a robust toolbox of assessment instruments. For BSS skills the most valid evaluations use planned overlaps among SPs, case assignments, faculty observations, and other "real-world" tools such as multisource feedback or chart review. These diverse data elements are often integrated into "performance portfolios" where learners and mentors are given some latitude in selecting artifacts that demonstrate progression toward or achievement of competence. By drawing from a pool of validated assessment instruments and evaluation data (e.g., CPE, OSCE), portfolios ensure some level of standardization while still allowing sufficient flexibility for learners with different strengths and needs. Ideally, portfolios serve both summative and formative purposes.

PROGRAM EVALUATION

Accumulated learner assessment data inform how well a program is operating to develop knowledge, behaviors/attitudes, and skills of its graduates. However, program evaluations might also include institutional impact, cost, conformity with program objectives or goals, and unplanned impacts on other programs or schools. As with learner assessments, program evaluation should be designed concurrently with the program itself and not added after program completion. Moreover, program evaluation data hold great value as a summative process that drives curricular change. A simple program evaluation cycle is commonly used that begins with curricular planning and preparation then moves to teaching, data collection, reflection, analysis, and revision.

A hierarchy of evaluation (inspired by Kirkpatrick) is shown in Figure 45-1. Satisfaction surveys (the lowest level) are most commonly used but do not assess a program's success in impacting knowledge or skills. Ideally, medical educators could show that their training interventions affect learner behavior in the real world and ultimately influence patient outcomes.

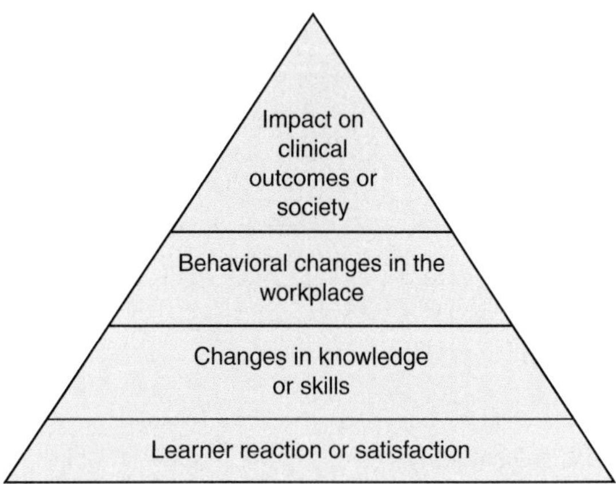
Impact on clinical outcomes or society
Behavioral changes in the workplace
Changes in knowledge or skills
Learner reaction or satisfaction

Figure 45-1. Hierarchy of evaluation.

The chosen evaluation level and matched assessment tools will depend on a variety of factors, including programmatic goals, resources, feasibility, audience, and preferred methodologies. In addition to the evaluation tools described under learner evaluations (e.g., CPE and MCQs), sources of evidence for program evaluation might include satisfaction surveys, graduation or exit interviews, focus groups, and ratings from expert/outside observers. Table 45-3 provides examples of BSS program assessment tools.

CASE ILLUSTRATION (CONTD.)

After collecting learner data from SP (CPE) examinations around alcohol screening and brief interventions, a satisfaction survey and focus group are administered as a final program evaluation tool. The family medicine residency director reviews the data to evaluate and improve the alcohol counseling curriculum. She first turns to mean composite scores for residents completing the CPE.

The CPE composite data presented in Figure 45-2 show that Relationship Development and Physical Examination skills are better developed in this class of family medicine residents than their history taking. It also shows that scores on alcohol screening and counseling (a more specialized skill set) are about the same as general history taking. These mean scores from all learners reflect how well the program is performing in teaching these skills. Typically, a benchmark above 85–95% demonstrates that the examination is developmentally appropriate for residents. With a benchmark score below 85–95%, the examination may not be not performing well, either because it is too hard, not well designed, or the curriculum was not effectively taught. Because history taking and

Table 45-3. Examples of BSS assessment tools for programs.

Assessment Tool	Description	Where to Find It
1. Tool to Assess Cultural Competence Training	A self-administered curriculum assessment tool used to identify gaps and redundancies in cultural competence curricula.	https://www.aamc.org/initiatives/tacct/
2. Communication, Curriculum, and Culture Instrument (C-3)	A 29-item tool used to assess the "hidden curriculum" of an institution.	Haidet P, et al. Characterizing the patient-centeredness of hidden curricula in medical schools: development and validation of a new measure. *Acad Med* 2005;80:44–50.
3. Association of American Medical Colleges (AAMC) Graduation Questionnaire (GQ)	An AAMC web-based survey. Administered to all graduating medical students including 24 potential BSS variables.	Carney PA, et al. Utility of the AAMC's Graduation Questionnaire to study behavioral and social sciences domains in undergraduate medical education. *Acad Med* 2010;89: 165–176. www.aamc.org.

alcohol counseling scores in this figure are lowest and the benchmark is low at 80%, both this portion of the examination and the curriculum addressing these skills should be reviewed. In Kirkpatrick terms, this CPE assesses changes in learner skills but is not able to address changes in actual clinical practice or changes in patient outcomes.

Resident satisfaction surveys and focus groups addressed the lowest Kirkpatrick level of learner reaction but still provided important formative feedback to shape future curricular iterations. Learners were generally satisfied with the curriculum and would recommend it to their peers. However, residents requested more training in learning how to access community alcohol treatment resources and more direct observations of their counseling skills with real clinic patients. Interestingly, residents also noted there was great preceptor variability in alcohol screening and counseling skills and suggested the inclusion of faculty preceptor training.

The above case illustrates how data generated from learner evaluation can then be used to improve both the curricular program and the faculty teaching in it. This comprehensive evaluative approach should be routinely used to make the most of the evaluation data collected.

EDUCATIONAL RESEARCH & SCHOLARSHIP

Research into the development and delivery of valid and reliable tools is a high priority and should be considered on par with other more traditional academic research

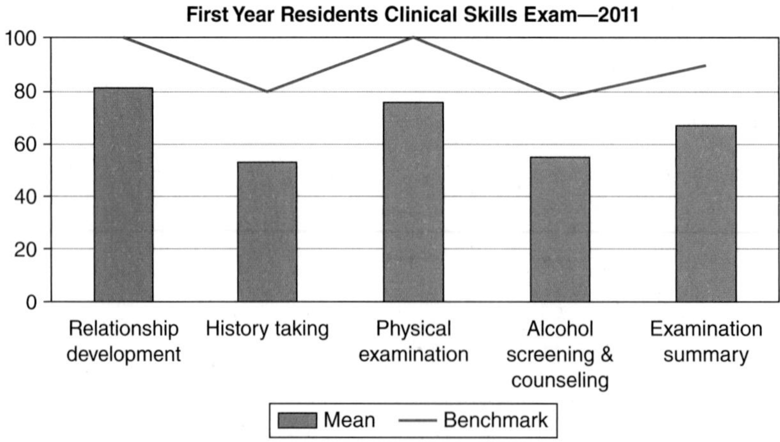

Figure 45-2. Mean composite scores for the resident Clinical Performance Exam.

pathways. It is the responsibility of deans, curriculum leaders, and educators to rigorously design and study their curricular innovations and to submit them to peer-reviewed journals for appropriate critique and dissemination.

Although educational funding streams pale in comparison to clinical research, organizations such as Agency for Healthcare Research and Quality (AHRQ) or Health Resources and Services Administration (HRSA) and foundations such as FIPSE, Harvard-Macy, and Stemmler regularly support educational research projects. Innovative programs to support faculty development in educational research skills are increasingly common as are Master's programs in education. As with any scholarly endeavor, adherence to ethical and practical guidelines regarding subject recruitment, data collection methods, and authorship is expected. In the end, "raising the bar" in BSS assessment and evaluation presents a "win-win-win" situation—learners receive higher quality feedback, programs and curricula constructively evolve, and contributions to educational science are recognized for academic advancement.

SUGGESTED READINGS

AAMC. Medical Simulation in Medical Education: Results of an AAMC Survey. https://www.aamc.org/download/259760/data/medicalsimulationinmedicaleducationanaamcsurvey.pdf. Accessed February 2014.

Carney PA, Palmer RT, Fuqua Miller M, et al. Assessment tools for behavioral and social science competencies in health care: a systematic review. *Acad Med* 2016;91(5):730–742.

Cook DA, Beckman TJ, Bordage G. Quality of reporting of experimental studies in medical education: a systematic review. *Med Educ* 2007;41:737–745.

Corbett E, Jr. Berkow R, Bernstein L, et al. *Recommendations for Clinical Skills Curricula for Undergraduate Medical Education.* Association of American Medical Colleges, Washington, D.C., 2008. https://www.aamc.org/download/163788/data/recommendations_for_preclerkship_skills_education_for_ugme.pdf. Accessed February 2014.

Downing S, Yudkowsky R. *Assessment in Health Professions Educations.* New York, NY: Routledge; 2009.

Duffy D, Gordon G, Whelan G, Cole-Kelly K, Frankel R, & All Participants in the American Academy on Physician and Patient's Conference on Education and Evaluation of Competence in Communication and Interpersonal Skills. Assessing competence in communication and interpersonal skills: the Kalamazoo II report. *Acad Med* 2004;79:495–507.

Epstein RM. Assessment in medical education. *N Engl J Med* 2007;356:387–396.

Epstein RM, Hundert EM. Defining and assessing professional competence. *JAMA* 2002;287:226–235.

Haidet P, et al. Characterizing the patient centeredness of hidden curricula in medical schools: development and validation of a new measure. *Acad Med* 2005;80:44–50.

Kneebone R, Nestel D, Wetzel C, et al. The human face of simulation: patient-focused simulation training. *Acad Med* 2006;81:919–924.

Kogan J, Holmboe E, Hauer K. Tools for direct observation and assessment of clinical skills in medical trainees: a systematic review. *J Am Med Assoc* 2009;302:1316–1326.

Schirmer J, Mauksch L, Lang F, et al. Assessing communication competence: a review of current tools. *Med Stud Educ* 2005;37:184–192.

Schuwirth L, Van Der Vleuten C. General overview of the theories used in assessment: AMEE Guide no.57. *Med Teach* 2011;33:783–797.

WEBSITES

AAMC Tool to Assess Cultural Competence Training. https://www.aamc.org/initiatives/tacct/. Accessed September 2018.

American Board of Internal Medicine Mini-CEX. http://www.abim.org/program-directors-administrators/assessment-tools/mini-cex.aspx. Accessed September 2018.

Brief Negotiated Interview. https://medicine.yale.edu/sbirt/curriculum/manuals/SBIRT%20training%20manual_2012_100719_284_13471_v3.pdf. Accessed September 2018.

MedBiquitous. http://www.medbiq.org. Accessed September 2018.

NBME MCQ Guide. http://www.nbme.org/publications/item-writing-manual.html. Accessed September 2018.

VASE-R. http://adai.washington.edu/instruments/VASE-R.htm. Accessed September 2018.

Evidence-Based Behavioral Practice 46

Bonnie Spring, PhD, ABPP & Stephen D. Persell, MD, MPH

RELEVANCE OF BEHAVIOR TO MEDICAL PRACTICE

Human behavior has a major impact on health and well-being. The patients that you see in medical practice are likely to have behaviors (e.g., smoking, drinking, and eating habits) that place them at risk of developing chronic disease. Equally likely, they may have psychological problems (e.g., depression) that impair their quality of life and undermine their motivation to follow your treatment recommendations. Moreover, if you treat families and see the same patients over many years, you may observe unhealthy behaviors long before you see the emergence of biological risk factors like hypertension, hypercholesterolemia, or hyperglycemia. By helping your patients to address unhealthy behaviors, you have the opportunity to help them prevent the onset or worsening of chronic diseases. Just as in evidence-based medicine, you should know how to find and appraise the evidence base for behavioral (nondrug, nonsurgical) treatments, so you can help your patients with the most appropriate behavioral treatment option. Below is a case you might encounter in the primary care clinic.

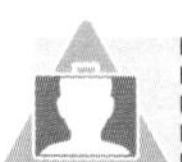

CASE ILLUSTRATION 1

A 43-year-old man presents for a preventive care visit. He has not had any preventive care in over 5 years but at an urgent care visit 4 months ago he was told he had high blood pressure. His past medical history is remarkable only for mild eczema. He is married, has two children, and works as an attorney. He says his work is sometimes stressful but denies a depressed mood or loss of interest in leisure activities. He has no difficulty sleeping. He recently cut back to about five cigarettes per day and has three to four alcoholic drinks almost every night. He does not exercise regularly, but walks about 5 minutes twice a day to the train. He does not follow any particular diet: breakfast is usually coffee and toast; lunch is fast food or a deli sandwich; he snacks on cookies or pastries at work. His wife cooks "healthy food" sometimes and they order from restaurants frequently. On physical examination his weight is 207 lbs with a body mass index of 29.7 kg/m^2. An average of three office blood pressures is 139/88 mm Hg. The rest of the examination is normal except for an eczematous rash on his arms. As you prescribe triamcinolone cream for his rash, you consider how best to counsel him about behavior change. The list of changes you think would be beneficial include: (1) stopping smoking; (2) reducing total calories; (3) following a diet low in sodium and high in vegetables, fruits, whole grains, and nonfat dairy products; (4) reducing saturated fat in his diet; (5) reducing alcohol use to no more than two drinks per day; and (6) increasing the amount of moderate-intensity physical activity he does by an additional 90–120 minutes each week.

APPLYING EVIDENCE-BASED PRACTICE IN PRIMARY CARE

This patient has several risk factors and behaviors that put his health at risk and that are potential targets for behavior change interventions. You are probably familiar with how to practice evidence-based care when making medical decisions about the use of medications or procedures. There is also a scientific evidence base about how to treat most unhealthy behaviors. For the purposes of this chapter, we use the broader term "evidence-based practice" (EBP) that includes both traditional evidence-based medicine and evidence-based behavioral practice.

EBP 5A's: Ask Questions

A practical way to approach EBP is by using a 5-step process better known as the "5A's": Ask, Acquire, Appraise, Apply, and Analyze & adjust (Figure 46-1).

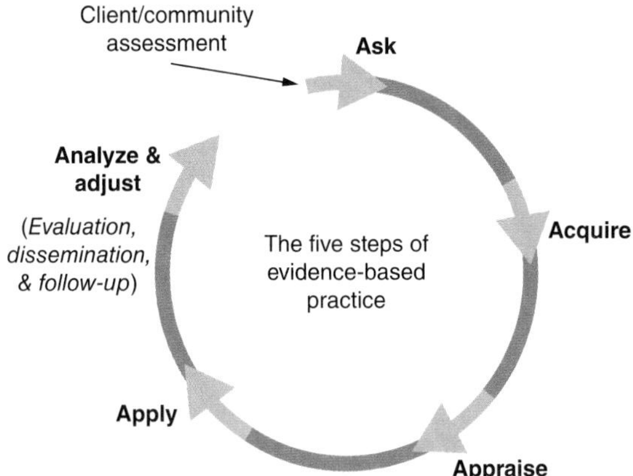
Client/community assessment
Ask
Acquire
Appraise
Apply
Analyze & adjust
(Evaluation, dissemination, & follow-up)
The five steps of evidence-based practice

Figure 46-1. Five steps of evidence-based practice. *Source:* Evidence Based Behavorial Practices. (www.ebbp.org.)

The first step is to ask focused questions that can be answered through review of the scientific literature. Two kinds of questions connect health care providers with the knowledge base needed to offer best preventive care. The first (prognostic questions), asks which factors (i.e., biomarkers, behaviors, environmental conditions) convey risk or protection with respect to the likelihood of developing a chronic disease. The second (treatment questions) asks which treatments are most effective at reversing disease risk factors and promoting health protection.

Early in their careers, most clinicians become familiar with the evidence base that evaluates which biomarkers warrant consistent clinical attention because they are risk factors for the development of chronic disease. They also learn to monitor and treat elevated cholesterol, blood pressure, and glucose to slow the patient's progression toward clinical disease. For disease prevention to be effective, it is important to recall that many unhealthy behaviors (e.g., substance use, physical inactivity, overeating) warrant as urgent attention as risk biomarkers. By asking prognostic questions and consulting the scientific literature, you can master the knowledge base that supports the contention that lifestyle behaviors are just as strongly associated as risk biomarkers with the onset of disease. With that awareness, you can then inquire about the best ways to treat unhealthy lifestyle behaviors.

EBP 5A's: Acquire & Appraise

Next steps in the EBP process are to acquire the evidence and critically appraise it for its quality and relevance to your patient. As a health care practitioner, you are a consumer of research; sometimes you will look for primary research evidence such as individual research studies, including clinical trials. More often you will turn to a secondary, synthesized evidence base that has been assembled in the form of systematic reviews or evidence-based guidelines.

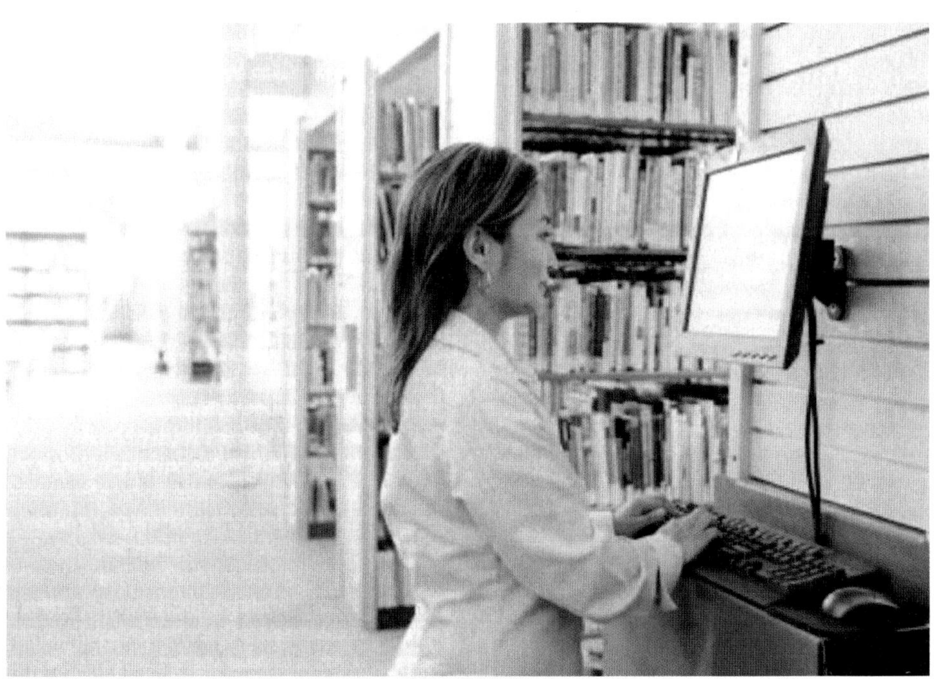

Much research exists about the lifestyle risk behaviors and treatment options for the patient described in the case. This evidence has often undergone systematic reviews to develop evidence-based treatment guidelines. For example, the *Guide to Clinical Preventive Services,* prepared by the U.S. Preventive Services Task Force (USPSTF), rigorously evaluates and makes recommendations about the merits of preventive measures, including screening tests, counseling, and preventive medications. Another guideline, *Treating Tobacco Use and Dependence,* prepared by the U.S. Public Health Services (USPHS), evaluates and makes recommendations about treating tobacco use. The National Heart, Lung, and Blood Institute sponsored systematic reviews that informed guidelines about obesity treatment issued jointly by the American Heart Association, American College of Cardiology, and The Obesity Society. Each review grounds interpretation of the evidence in an analytic framework that summarizes observational epidemiologic studies showing evidence of harms from the unhealthy behavior, as well as evidence of reduction in these harms when the behavior is stopped. These guidelines offer many recommendations relevant to your patient's smoking, unhealthy use of alcohol, obesity, and sedentary lifestyle.

Brief Versus Intensive Behavioral Interventions

The act of having a health care professional identify an unhealthy behavior, provide brief counseling to promote change, and follow up produces measureable improvement in several risk behaviors, including cigarette smoking. Usually, however, behavior changes are small and most patients do not respond. It is very important that the clinician not interpret this experience to mean that behavior cannot be changed. After all, most unhealthy habits were acquired over a period of many years and have become deeply ingrained. More intensive treatments (that involve more and longer counseling sessions with specially trained providers) produce larger behavioral improvements in a greater proportion of those treated. For example, the Diabetes Prevention Program and Look AHEAD established that multiple sessions of diet, exercise, and behavior change counseling could produce a 7–8% weight loss, improved glycemic control, delayed progression of diabetes, and improved cardiovascular risk factors. Similarly, many studies synthesized to develop the USPHS Tobacco Guideline show that providing a greater number of counseling sessions or offering counseling combined with quit smoking medications substantially improves the patient's odds of becoming smoke free for the long term.

Multiple Unhealthy Behaviors

Although the evidence supporting intensive health behavior change treatments is strong and derived from well-executed multisite randomized controlled trials, research is sparse in terms of indicating how to treat multiple co-occurring unhealthy behaviors and medical comorbidities. A majority of treatments directed at health behavior change address a single behavior, for example, excess alcohol intake, obesity, or risky sexual behavior. It has not been well studied how many behaviors are feasible to change at once, whether attempts to change multiple behaviors should be made simultaneously or sequentially, how to prioritize which behavior(s) to tackle first, or whether it is more effective to encourage patients to increase healthy behaviors or decrease unhealthy ones. If several behaviors in sequence will be changed, there is little research to guide the practitioner about how long to wait before tackling a new behavior and what sequence of behaviors will maximize the chances of success. The evidence base is particularly scant about whether patients' efforts to make healthy lifestyle changes will bolster, compromise, or have no effect on their simultaneous efforts to adhere to medical treatment of comorbid illness. These are important gaps in knowledge that clinicians and patients need researchers to fill.

EBP 5A's: Apply

Having asked key questions about the patient's health risks and treatment options, and having acquired and appraised the evidence, you have now reached the *apply* step in the EBP process. Deciding how to apply the evidence is the heart of how clinicians translate research into practice. As Figure 46-2 illustrates, making decisions about how to apply evidence requires integrating data from each of the three circles: best available research, patient characteristics (including preferences

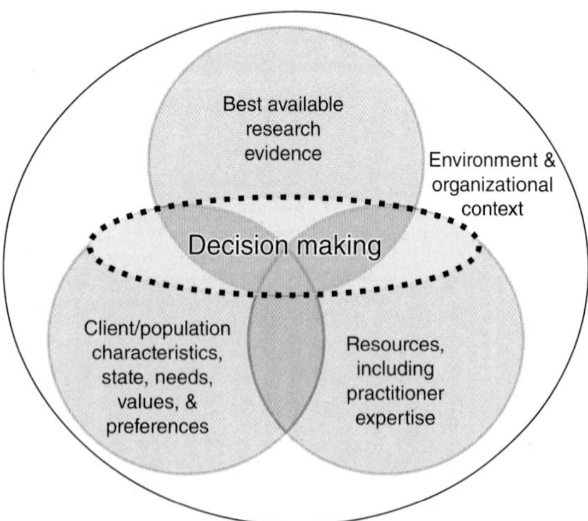

Figure 46-2. Elements that need integration in evidence-based practice. (*Source:* Spring B, Hitchcock K. Evidence-based practice in psychology. In: Weiner IB, Craighead WE, eds. *The Corsini's Encyclopedia of Psychology*, 4th ed. Wiley, 2009.)

and values), and resource considerations (including practitioner expertise or skills).

For this patient, there are a number of effective interventions, some brief and some intensive, to address his risk behaviors. With so many unhealthy behaviors, the real challenge is to know where to begin. To prioritize which behaviors to treat, you will want to consider all three circles. An important first step is to evaluate the magnitude and immediacy of risks associated with each of the patient's health behaviors. Research evidence informs you that, ordinarily, smoking and obesity top the list of risk factors that have the greatest harmful impact. For this patient, though, his alcohol use could pose a greater immediate risk of harm. You might also want to evaluate whether a coexisting mental health disorder like depression or anxiety is present that warrants treatment in its own right and that could complicate efforts at behavior change.

To address the patient's risk of drinking, you will probably want to start off with a procedure called SBIRT (Screening, Brief Intervention, and Referral for Treatment). Based on the patient's responses to a screening questionnaire, you would inform him about how his amount of drinking corresponds to a level of intake that confers a risk of significant health consequences. You would then assess his motivation or level of readiness to change. Depending on his readiness, you and the patient might collaboratively set a goal that falls somewhere between touching base about drinking at the next medical appointment, to reducing his number of drinks per week, to beginning intensive treatment with a substance abuse counselor. Alternatively, the patient may not be interested in changing his drinking, but motivated to become more physically active. The more the patient can be engaged in collaborating to formulate a behavior change goal, the greater the likelihood that he will follow through, thereby growing more confident and motivated to attempt new healthy changes (see Chapter 19).

Another key consideration arises from the third circle: resources. What assets are available to support your patient's behavior change? Financial resources will probably factor in, as may your team's time and professional skills. As practitioners acquire knowledge of evidence-based interventions to change behavior, they need to maintain self-awareness of their own skills, time, and resources. They need to be aware of their own limitations and understand when the evidence suggests that a behavior change intervention that they cannot provide is likely to be more effective than what they can offer. If they are unable to develop those services in their practice, they should refer patients to practitioners and programs in their community that can provide them. To adequately support health promotion, clinicians need to cultivate a professional referral network that includes experts in behavior change (psychologists), nutrition (dieticians), and exercise (exercise physiologists). To serve those without resources to pay for intensive behavioral treatments, the doctor will also want to keep on hand a roster of no- or low-cost resources, including free telephone counseling services (e.g., smoking quit line), community programs (e.g., training clinics that offer free or sliding scale billing, church-based programs, YMCA), internet or mobile treatment programs, and books.

EBP 5A's: Analyze & Adjust

At the end of the day, the best intervention is not necessarily the one supported by the highest quality clinical trial evidence, but rather the one that works for the particular patient. The treatment supported by the best available evidence is the best initial treatment to try, but decision making about intervention begins rather than ends when an initial treatment is selected and delivered. The important rest of the story unfolds by measuring and analyzing what benefits (positive behavior changes) and harms (side effects, distress, worsening of other health behaviors) accrue to the patient as a result of receiving the chosen treatment. If the balance of benefits and harms continues in an unfavorable direction, the provider will want to consider adjusting the type, dose, or administrator of the treatment.

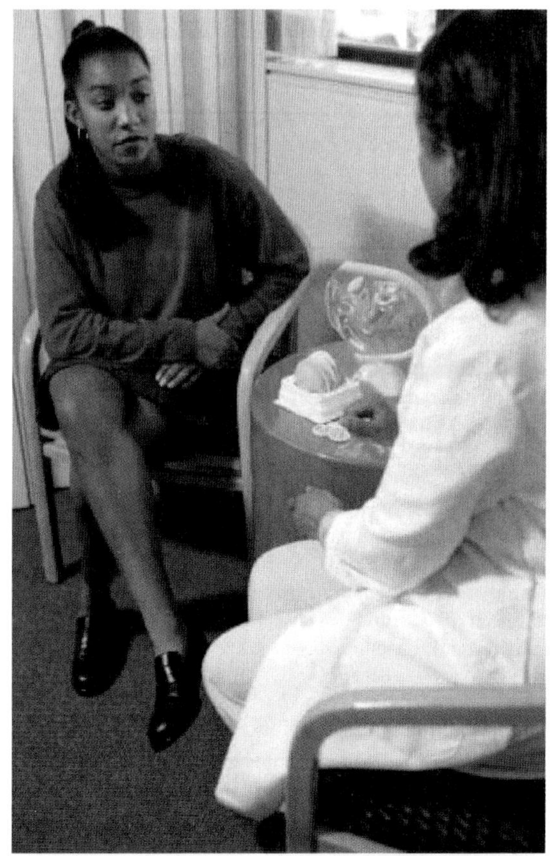

Clinicians should not be surprised if the benefits they observe from any treatment in actual clinical practice are smaller than those seen in research studies. There are many reasons for this discrepancy. Clinicians who provide an intervention in actual practice may be less well-trained, exert fewer checks on the quality of treatment delivery, and provide less intensive care because they have competing priorities. Cost may also be a barrier that constrains patients' full engagement in treatment; behavioral interventions may be expensive, and third-party coverage may be less generous or nonexistent for these services. Out-of-pocket costs to the patient can pose a real obstacle to full engagement with treatment.

SETTING UP A PRACTICE TO SUPPORT EVIDENCE-BASED BEHAVIORAL PRACTICE

Prospects for preventive medicine hinge upon making evidence-based behavioral practice a reality. Because lifestyle behaviors constitute the major preventable causes of chronic disease, monitoring and treating them effectively through the entire health care system and across the lifespan offers the greatest hope of real primary prevention. Useful tools that fit into the clinical workflow can help make it easier for clinical practices to systematically complete screenings for risky behaviors. Redistributing the roles played by care team members can take some of the burden off the physician and make the delivery system more efficient and reliable. Electronic health record tools like clinical reminders or checklists can encourage completion of standardized health behavior assessments that serve as screeners or that track progress over time. Tools like internet portals connected to patients' electronic health records can allow patients to complete assessments prior to a medical visit and allow the patient to self-monitor personal progress over time. Mechanisms that simplify and expedite the process of referring patients to expert interventionists also are needed so that the barriers to referral are reduced when patients require more than just brief behavioral treatment. Because we cannot manage what we do not measure, effective health promotion through lifestyle intervention would be enhanced by increased use of performance measures that assess screening for and treatment of risk behaviors. Some of these exist and are used to varying degrees (such as in reporting programs by entities like the Centers for Medicare and Medicaid Services).

Assessing and intervening with risk behaviors in a manner that integrates best available research, patient characteristics and resources is the pathway to integrative care that prevents illness in addition to managing disease.

SUGGESTED READINGS

Fiore MC, Jaen CR, Baker TB, et al. *Treating Tobacco Use and Dependence: 2008 Update.* Clinical Practice Guideline. Rockville, MD: U.S. Department of Health and Human Services. Public Health Service, May 2008.

Guyatt G, Rennie D, Meade MO, Cook DJ. *Users' Guides to the Medical Literature: A Manual for Evidence-Based Clinical Practice*, 3rd ed. New York: McGraw Hill Publishers; 2015.

Ryan DH, Kahan S. Guideline recommendations for obesity management. *Med Clin North Am* 2018;102:49–63.

Satterfield J, Spring B, Newhouse R, et al. Toward a transdisciplinary model of evidence-based practice. *Milbank Q* 2009; 87:368–390.

Spring B. Evidence-based practice in clinical psychology: What it is; why it matters; what you need to know. *J Clin Psychol* 2007;63(7):611–631.

Taggart J, Williams A, Dennis S, et al. A systematic review of interventions in primary care to improve health literacy for chronic disease behavioral risk factors. *BMC Fam Pract* 2012;13:49.

Tsai AG, Remmert JE, Butryn ML, Wadden TA. Treatment of obesity in primary care. *Med Clin North Am* 2018;102(1):35–47.

World Health Organization. Toolkit for delivering the 5As and 5Rs brief tobacco control interventions in primary care. Geneva: World Health Organization; 2014.

WEBSITES

Centers for Disease Control and Prevention. https://www.cdc.gov/tobacco/campaign/tips/partners/health/hcp/index.html. Evidence-informed advice to health care professionals about how to help patients quit smoking. Accessed December 17, 2018.

Duke and UNC Chapel Hill Introduction to Evidence Based Practice. https://guides.mclibrary.duke.edu/ebmtutorial/home. Brief online tutorial and resources about evidence based practice. February 2014. Accessed December 27, 2018.

Evidence-Based Behavioral Practice. www.ebbp.org. Free online modules that illustrate the EBBP process for both individual clinical practice and public health. Accessed December 27, 2018.

U.S. Preventive Services Task Force. https://www.uspreventiveservicestaskforce.org/Page/Name/recommendations. Preventive care recommendations for primary care practitioners to intervene on chronic disease behavioral risk factors, mental health and substance abuse based on systematic evidence reviews performed by Agency for Health Care Research and Practice Centers.

Narrative Medicine

47

Jonathan Amiel, MD; Anne Armstrong-Coben, MD; Melanie Bernitz, MD, MPH; Hetty Cunningham, MD; Julie Glickstein, MD; Deepthiman Gowda, MD, MPH, MS; Gillian Graham, MS, PMHNP-BC; Nellie Hermann, MFA; Constance Molino Park, MD, PhD; Delphine Taylor, MD; & Rita Charon, MD, PhD

A group of physicians, writers, and educators sits around a conference table in a busy medical school, eating hurried lunches, coordinating course materials for medical students, and reviewing with excitement or concern what just happened in their first-year medical interviewing courses. More people gather, and the room quiets. Today, the novelist on the faculty reminds them that they are reading "Aquarium," a personal essay written by writer Aleksandar Hemon who has lost his baby daughter to brain cancer. The mood in the room shifts from light camaraderie to an attentive sense of purpose. "I had such a hard time reading this," a seasoned family physician sighs. "It made me want to run home and pick up my baby," offers the hospitalist.

As the conversation develops, the novelist draws the group's attention to the essay's title and its governing image, an important metaphor for his experience with illness and loss. "The whole thing is about an aquarium," an internist and literary scholar offers. "You feel very much like an outsider reading this," admits a pediatrician.

After some discussion, the novelist offers a writing prompt: *Describe an aquarium that you yourself have been in.* The group members take out pen and paper and, heads bowed, write intently for 4 minutes. When the time is up, many offer to read their work. Some read aloud descriptions of experiences with literal aquariums, marveling at the foreignness of aquatic life. A psychiatrist and a general internist each read aloud what they wrote about—times when they felt isolated in family or work and unable to truly communicate with those around them. Some wrote about feeling that, as doctors, they are inside an aquarium; others wrote about the experience of being on the outside. "The whole patient experience is like being in a fishbowl," reflects a pediatrician, "and in the story, the doctors are in a fishbowl too." The internist and literary scholar replies, "But this story is like instructions about how not to be marooned. It gives a glimpse into that fishbowl but also says *and then you can write*. It opens up a way to talk about and then use the imagination and the power of words."

WHAT IS NARRATIVE MEDICINE?

This session is a typical example of the kind of work this group does every week. They are medical educators, the faculty of Foundations of Clinical Medicine (Columbia's "doctoring" course) who employ the techniques of narrative medicine to sharpen their clinical skills, deepen their teaching, and reflect on their work. Narrative medicine developed out of the integration of medicine and literary studies to fortify clinical practice with the narrative competence to recognize, absorb, metabolize, interpret, and be moved by the stories of illness. Its unifying tenet is that the giving and receiving of accounts of self are the central events in health care—whether the account is given by a patient, family member, student, clinician, or members of the lay public and whether it is received by a doctor in the office, a circle of peers in a teaching session, a multidisciplinary team meeting in a clinic, or a Congressional hearing about health reform. Although arising only in 2000 from earlier efforts in humanities and medicine and primary care medicine, narrative medicine has spread quickly first at its home at Columbia University and then throughout the United States and abroad. Synthesizing theories and methods from the humanities, the social sciences, and the behavioral sciences, narrative medicine models a bridge among disciplines and, more importantly, supports the interior integration of cognitive, behavioral, imaginative, aesthetic, and affective states to which the effective clinician aspires.

Narrative medicine unfolds in three broad and simultaneous movements—**attention, representation, and affiliation**. These movements conceptualize and then guide a clinical and teaching practice that can establish contact with self, patients, students, colleagues, and the public that medicine serves. We will first define these movements and then follow with real-life examples.

Attention is that state of receptivity whereby a listener or witness or reader can receive the account given by another. To attain the state of attention, the receiver focuses closely and deeply on the person giving an account, whether that person is a patient, a student, a novelist, a poet, or even a painter or a composer. The receiver does not efface himself or herself but rather offers the contours of the self as a container for what is given by the other. Combining mindfulness with curiosity, the receiver captures all that the other transmits, squandering no word or silence or gesture or mood from the evidence that emerges from the encounter.

Representation includes the means by which any attentive witness confers form on what is received. Typically this is done with language as one writes a story or a vignette or a progress note to capture that which has been received from the other. (Although visual representations can also be made, we restrict ourselves here to written representations.) What is represented can be read—by the writer, by the subject of the representation, or by others. Because, as psychoanalyst Hans Loewald suggests, writing is a sensorimotor act that transforms the immaterial into the material, it allows the writer to communicate what was not known until the writing to self and then to others.

Affiliation is the ultimate goal of any clinical act—affiliation between the patient and clinician, between the clinician and colleagues, between the clinician–teacher and student, and between health care professionals and the public we serve. Robust affiliation provides the grounds for any event of healing.

These movements intensify one another, attention fueling the capacity to represent, representation fortifying the capacity to attend, and both of them spiraling toward affiliation. Doctor and patient write their way through clinical events. Medical students write reflective essays about early clinical experience, and their teachers receive them with newly developed skills in close reading. Patients and clinicians share writing groups to write about their lived experiences with illness. Multidisciplinary teams meet on the wards or the clinics to develop their own capacity to collaborate and unite. These methods permit us to get under the distinctions that typically isolate us from one another and bring us, in common, onto the grounds of human suffering and the desire to lessen that suffering.

NARRATIVE MEDICINE IN CLINICAL PRACTICE

Querying all faculty of Columbia's Foundations of Clinical Medicine course, we compiled a table of goals that have been accomplished in clinical practice through the use of narrative methods (Table 47-1). Selections from our respondents' accounts of accomplishing some of these goals in practice thicken the descriptions of our listed goals. We categorize these goals according to the three movements of narrative medicine, although it is easily seen how these movements converge and occur simultaneously.

Table 47-1. The movements of narrative medicine.

Attention
Self-awareness and self-care Recognition of the patient Recognition of colleagues
Representation
Writing as discovery Writing in the shadow of texts Writing with patients
Affiliation
With patients Among colleagues Among human beings

Attention

CASE ILLUSTRATION 1: SELF-AWARENESS AND SELF-CARE

Several years ago, I cared for a retired health care professional whom I found to be enormously difficult to care for. . . . I was unsuccessful at bringing her attention to the likely undercurrent to her various somatic complaints—a long-standing and untreated depression and anxiety disorder. . . . [S]he expressed to me that she felt I was not providing adequate care. Ultimately, I felt frustrated and powerless, and in light of her impression about my care, I suggested that she switch to another physician. Soon after this clinical relationship ended, I reflected and wrote about this patient in our Narrative Medicine group and shared my writing with the others. Through the writing, I clarified the events that led to certain outcomes and I understood more deeply what I felt was at stake for me. As a clinician, I felt as though I had failed and had abandoned the patient. As an educator, I felt particular shame, given that I had unsuccessfully managed this clinical relationship, yet teach students how to navigate communication with "difficult patients." In the writing and telling, others were able to relate to my experience and normalize what was going on. I was able to forgive myself, and I reframed what had become an overly harsh self-judgment. I recognized my own humanity in the enterprise.

(Written by a general internist.)

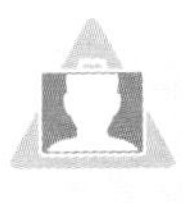

CASE ILLUSTRATION 2: RECOGNITION OF THE PATIENT

I had just spent some time doing intense narrative medicine work. . . . When I walked into my practice I felt more excitement than stress when I saw the box of charts. I looked upon this as opportunity to hear patient stories rather than feeling burdened by the workload. I saw a mother and son that afternoon. The child had a superficial cut that required little medical care. My "former self" (and the fact that there were numerous patients waiting) would have likely left it at that. . . . Superficial cut, antibiotic ointment, anticipatory guidance about keeping him away from scissors. However, my head began to ask more questions, and my eyes were more in tune to the Mom. I realized I had not heard the whole story. I probed more, listened more intently, and discovered why she was really there. The mother had taken boarders into her apartment who were HIV positive. These individuals had had a number of violent fights, which included cutting with scissors. She had asked them to move out. During the move, her son had found the scissors and cut his hand. This was her true fear. Using narrative attention, the desire to hear the story, enabled me to address what was really needed that day.

(Written by a general pediatrician.)

Representation

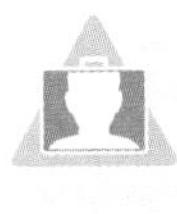

CASE ILLUSTRATION 3: WRITING AS DISCOVERY

We were asked to identify a difficult patient and write about them. I had never previously written about a patient in this manner, and never really taken the time to consider why I reacted in such a way to certain patients. It is always easy to identify the "heart sink" patients, the ones whose names you see on your schedule and who you hope will not come in that day. The patient I chose to write about on that day was one [with] few "real" medical issues, but [who] always tried to cloak her reason for the visit with a physical complaint. . . . When writing about her, I realized that I actually really did like her. . . . Subsequent to writing about her, I felt a lot less frustrated about the situation. I actually welcomed seeing her on my schedule. I felt empowered to know what my role was and what my duty was toward her. I felt like I did have something to offer, I realized that there was a reason why she chose to come back and see me again and again. I felt honored. And now that she has moved on and is no longer my patient, I actually miss her. . . . [M]y resentment turned to gratitude. Through writing that first time about a patient I have started on my own journey towards understanding the power of narrative on my own personal journey as a physician.

(Written by a family physician who practices in Student Health.)

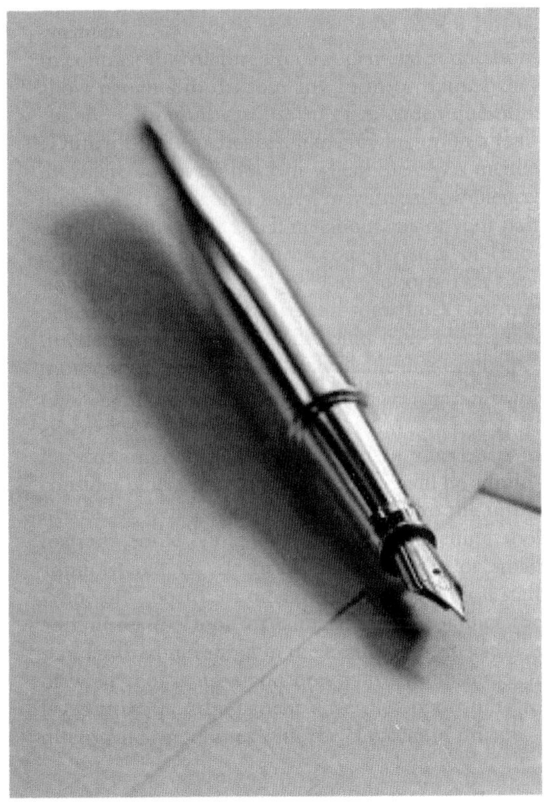

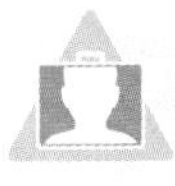

CASE ILLUSTRATION 4: WRITING WITH PATIENTS

A 53-year-old business executive, for whom I'd served as internist/endocrinologist for 10 years, suddenly and almost parenthetically said she sometimes thought of her long-deceased sister when she came to my office. . . . I silently wondered if the stressful time of menopause with possible thoughts of mortality had reawakened feelings of loss, especially of an older sister, and I suggested that perhaps she'd benefit from writing about why she might associate our visits with thoughts of her sister's death. A month later the patient returned having written on the topic and wanting to share thoughts and memories. She vividly recalled that ten years ago I'd been the first physician to have paused during the routine family history after she'd impassively recited yet again that her older sister had committed suicide when they were both teenagers 30 years earlier. She had even on occasion thought vaguely of exploring memories of her sister's early death with me and then perhaps a psychiatrist but only now, after writing about her sister and her own concerns about mood, did she have the courage to begin this.

(Written by an internist/endocrinologist in private practice.)

Affiliation

CASE ILLUSTRATION 5: AFFILIATION WITH PATIENTS

I run a narrative medicine seminar for a group of health care professionals at the hospital. It happens that three of the persons who attend the group are also my internal medicine patients. Every month, we gather to read together and then to write in the shadow of what we have read. Once, I chose a poem by Rachel Hadas, "Tenor and Vehicle," as the text. In it, the poet conveys the close relationship between ivy and the wall on which it climbs—the ivy dependent on the wall at the very time that it both adorns it and destroys it. The image implies, without specifying, the paradoxes of intimate personal relationships in which both participants play both roles. Some of the writers wrote about their own practice in the hospital, caring for very dependent and needy patients. One of my patients, who was undergoing an incredibly challenging health situation and finding great resilience and courage in the face of it, wrote of how this poem seemed to her to be her own vows for her upcoming marriage, turning the poem around to connote mutual courage and generosity. It was a stunning expressive act not only for the writer vis-à-vis her love relationship but also for all the other members of the group, able to see how vast was the reach of this short poem.

(Written by an internist who practices in the medicine clinic.)

CASE ILLUSTRATION 6: AFFILIATION WITH PATIENTS AND FAMILIES

The ultimate goal for the fetal cardiologist is to facilitate the best possible outcome for the fetus and the family. . . . During the patient encounter, the physician changes narrative perspective from the interpreter of the medical images and data, to the narrator of the diagnosis and prognosis for the baby, to the listener while the parents serve as narrator of their lived experience and support milieu, to a participant in the integration of all the above information in guiding the parents towards a final decision. During each process, the narrative techniques of empathy, imagination, and of entering the patient's presence with attuned concentration and observation allow the physician to adapt himself or herself to the individual needs of each patient and to form an individual bond that will be the foundation for the stressful journey upon which he or she is to embark with the parents.

(Written by a fetal cardiologist who practices in the fetal echocardiography unit.)

WHY WE READ & WRITE

These examples demonstrate some of the guiding goals and powers of narrative medicine. As a discipline based on textual practices, narrative medicine can train its students to do what close readers and writers do—enter alien narrative worlds, comprehend those worlds from others' points of view, co-create with the inhabitant of these worlds the substrate for meaning, and be nourished by the process. Adopting the policy that every word counts, close readers learn to take account of the formal features of a text—its genre, diction, temporal structure, metaphors, narrative strategies—so as to receive the full "message" of what is written. Whether reading Aleksandar Hemon's "The Aquarium" or a Stephen King thriller, the reader surrenders to the demands of the text, wondering why the story is told the way it is told or why it triggers particular moods or thoughts. Perhaps one reason that serious readers seek out opportunities to read with others or to read what others have written about a text is to learn how infinite are the potential interpretations of any stretch of text. Readers learn to honor the text as an entity unto itself as well as a powerful mirror for the self of the reader. When in the clinical setting, these readerly skills get transposed to powerful skills of attentive listening to patients' words and silences and bodies. The reader/listener enters the patient's world with openness and curiosity, able more effectively to imagine the whole, to raise consequential hypotheses about what goes on, to accept the strangeness of any alien world as plausible, and, ultimately, to make contact with the patient. The reader/listener seeks out groups of peers to work with, realizing how enriched is one person's interpretation by congress with others.

As is demonstrated in our clinicians' responses to our query, narrative medicine has developed many forms of writing in its practice. In all cases, the writer needs a reader. The faculty-participants in this project were trained in close reading as they wrote in concert with their peers. Always, what any of us wrote was read or listened to closely and skillfully by our peers. By developing the reading capacities of our faculty, we could ensure that when students are asked to write about their experiences, they will obtain close and skilled reading of their texts. We furnish faculty members with "readers' guides" instead of rating scales so that they can attend to what their students express, not to judge and rate the levels of reflection achieved but rather to read the text closely enough to be able to say what is seen.

Some reflective writing practices are practical means to concentrate attention on a particular clinical situation—write about a challenging patient; write about a patient you brood about; write about a patient you love. Other practices that engage clinicians and patients in writing seem farther afield from clinical practice, although these too circle back very directly to the writer's capacity to offer or receive health care. Often, the writing is encouraged by first reading a literary text with a group—a poem, a paragraph of a novel, a short story, a prayer. A narrative medicine group adopts close reading techniques in which one inspects the form, the metaphors, the tempo, the mood, and the movements of the text. You might feel like you were in English class for this part of the narrative medicine seminar. But unlike the English teacher, the narrative medicine teacher will offer a writing prompt that invites you to consider some aspect of your own experience. Creating the writing prompt is the hardest part of teaching narrative medicine, for it has to be an economical and compelling invitation to expand the mind of the learner toward both the "business" of the text and the interiority of the reader.

Here are a couple of examples.

the death of fred clifton
by lucille clifton
11/10/84, age 49

i seemed to be drawn
to the center of myself
leaving the edges of me
in the hands of my wife
and i saw with the most amazing
clarity
so that i had not eyes but
sight,
and, rising and turning,
through my skin,
there was all around not the
shapes of things
but oh, at last, the things
themselves.

The prompt used sometimes in teaching this poem is, "Write about the things themselves." One of us recently taught this poem using this prompt to a group of palliative care fellows. No matter how many deaths these doctors had accompanied, they wrote about "the things themselves" in their own lives. One intensivist wrote four words: "Love, Family, Work, Joy." Those of us hearing these words told him he had just written the words on his own family crest. It was as if he had found a direct line to those essentials within the edges of self, thereby bringing into immediate contact the dilemmas of his dying patients with his own search for meaning in his life.

A paragraph from a book on illness narratives offers the following story written by Eduardo Galeano. Arthur Frank heard it years ago and finds himself still brooding about the story and sharing it with others:

> Fernando Silva ran the children's hospital in Managua. On Christmas Eve, he worked late into the night. Firecrackers were exploding and fireworks lit up the sky when Fernando decided it was time to leave. They were expecting him at home to celebrate the holiday.
>
> He took one last look around, checking to see that everything was in order, when he heard cottony footsteps behind him. He turned to find one of the sick children walking after him. In the half light he recognized the lonely, doomed child. Fernando recognized the face already lined with death and those eyes asking for forgiveness, or perhaps permission.
>
> Fernando walked over to him and the boy gave him his hand.
>
> *"Tell someone, . . .* "the child whispered. *" Tell someone I'm here"*

The prompt we have used with this paragraph, taken from Art Frank's explanation of what stories can do to their readers is, "Write about a story that is working on you." This prompt can be met either with a clinical story still gripping the writer or, as likely, an event from childhood, a fairy tale, or an account from a sacred text.

These examples of writing prompts suggest, we hope, the function of the writing of narrative medicine. The learner is not asked to write "about" the text but, rather, from within the mood and train of thought of the text and the conversation the group has experienced about it. Writing in the shadow of the text suggests that powerful states of contemplation and reflection can be entered—oftentimes very quickly—by paying serious attention to well-written texts or works of art. Close reading might be a form of meditation, in which the reader concentrates on the text in its entirety—not only its linguistic freight but its music, its echoes to other texts, its balance, its jar, its form. Captivated, the reader can then be taken to places, in his or her writing, that might have been hard to achieve without first reading. Another way to say this is that the reader is quickly made permeable to the text, first, and then that permeability is extended to self. Such states, we know, are achieved when beholding great works of art or hearing great musical compositions. These findings fuel the recent trend in bringing medical students to art museums or symphony halls, not to civilize them but to confront them with the otherness of great beauty, a confrontation that invariably brings them closer to the world and to themselves.

These examples from narrative medicine practice hint at the pleasure and freedom available in simple reading and writing exercises. When a writer reads aloud to a group what he or she has written in the shadow of a text, the group members expand *their* minds toward the text as well as toward the writer. Writing as discovery, as Loewald describes it, these learners gain access to what they know but might not realize they know. They then accept the risks of exposing this "newly known" to self and listener, thereby intensifying both self-awareness and contact with peers. When a narrative medicine group is composed of persons unlike one another—nurses, social workers, patients, doctors, administrators might be in the same group—the reading and writing actions release them from the distinctions that typically separate them. They are equals in the reading and writing if not in the hierarchical structures that surround them.

NARRATIVE MEDICINE IN TEACHING

Armed with an understanding of the important clinical goals reachable through the use of narrative methods, we turn to ways in which we have used narrative medicine methods in our teaching practice. The educational goals parallel the clinical goals. Here, we display the educational experiences in a developmental sequence, starting with the premedical student and ending with the senior resident, suggesting which movements and specific goals have been reached in each example.

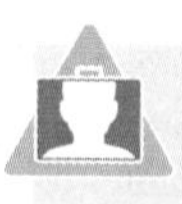

CASE ILLUSTRATION 7: PREMEDICAL STUDENT—REPRESENTATION (WRITING AS DISCOVERY)

A premed student was asked to witness my office hours. She had been an art history major who was embarking on a master's degree in international health. She wrote witness notes (similar to field notes an anthropologist might write) after observing in clinic, and I could see that she was "getting" what was going on between my patients and me, attentive to aspects of the encounters that I had not noticed myself. Her first personal statement for medical school applications was a smart crisp statement about international health movements and health care reform. Then, after her month of writing about what she witnessed in the office, she totally revised her statement. Her exposure to what patients said about themselves and the narrative routines in my practice transformed her view of what sick people really need and what doctors can to do help them.

CASE ILLUSTRATION 8: FIRST-YEAR STUDENT—ATTENTION (SELF-AWARENESS)

A student told a story [in class] last week about the experience of seeing a patient interviewed in front of the whole class. It sounded like an old-time "demonstrate the pathology" session, with the patient passive and seemingly clueless and the doctor all-powerful. The student cried when she related the story and the whole group resonated. When I ran into her on the subway yesterday, she told me she hadn't realized how upset she was. But articulating the experience helped her to realize and think about why this was so disturbing.

CASE ILLUSTRATION 9: FIRST-YEAR STUDENT—AFFILIATION (WITH PEERS)

[A first-year medical student] came into the standardized patient encounter eager and animated. She began well, introducing herself and setting the tone.

The patient was quiet and depressed, yet the student was unable to change her tone to respond to the patient's cues. She continued the interview, but her enthusiasm and energy pushed the patient further and further away.

The semester continued and her enthusiasm did not wane. She continues to grapple with managing her perky manner while interviewing a patient who was quieter, depressed, or troubled. She told me that her outward demeanor was actually covering up extreme anxiety about the patient interaction, and that her often almost manic interviewing skills were a result of her protecting herself from falling apart during patient interviews.

She wrote about her patient encounters, and often shared to the class what she wrote. She wrote about accepting the anxiety, and learning to read the physical manifestations, the clammy palms, the racing heart. She wrote that she has learned to just feel these sensations and not let them overshadow what she needs to say to the patient or do for the patient. She wrote that she has learned to let go of the anxiety surrounding the patient interview and instead feel the excitement of caring for the patient.

Although she has been writing about how it feels to interview, her objective ability to interview a patient, in a more controlled, dignified, professional way, has improved dramatically. The enthusiasm is still palpable, yet the energy is more controlled. I believe her ability to use narrative writing to express her feelings regarding the interview has allowed her to see herself in a way that she never would have, even with her preceptor or her peers commenting on her interview skills numerous times. The self-reflection that came from the narrative allowed her to undergo a truly transformative experience that will benefit her future career as a doctor.

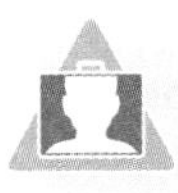

CASE ILLUSTRATION 10: SECOND-YEAR STUDENT—REPRESENTATION (WRITING AS DISCOVERY); ATTENTION (SELF-AWARENESS AND SELF-CARE)

After reading the paragraph from Art Frank's book about the dying child, I invited my students to write about a story that is working on them. One student had not disclosed in the context of our seminar complex events of her childhood related to the serious illness and death of a sibling. Until given this opportunity to write, the student had not disclosed the challenging role she herself had been asked to play in obtaining health care for her family. How did she benefit from writing about this? The permission to write let her acknowledge that these events, and her role in this story, had created who she is, and are part of the reason she is in medicine in the first place.

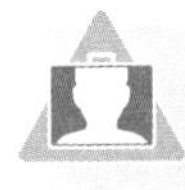

CASE ILLUSTRATION 11: THIRD-YEAR STUDENT—ATTENTION (SELF-AWARENESS); AFFILIATION (WITH PEERS)

While precepting third-year students on their internal medicine rotation, I devote one session a week to writing in the Parallel Chart, where I invite students to write about aspects of their patients that are critical to their care but that do not belong in the hospital chart. One student bristled at the idea of writing as discovery, saying she hated to write and, instead, just took long runs and did her contemplation and self-examination in that way. I invited her simply to bring in to class lists of things that went through her mind as she ran across the George Washington Bridge. She did so, and she created luminous texts filled with fragments of images that cohered into fragile meaning. I told her she was writing poems. She started bringing poems into our sessions. When she brought Dylan Thomas's "Do Not Go Gentle Into That Good Night" and read it with her classmates, she made a breakthrough in the care of a dying patient in her care, able for the first time to leave her own perspective on his care and to comprehend his and his family's continuing wish for aggressive care.

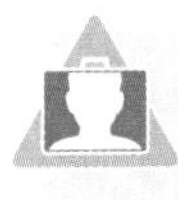

CASE ILLUSTRATION 12: FOURTH-YEAR STUDENT—ATTENTION (SELF-AWARENESS); AFFILIATION (WITH PATIENTS)

[During a fiction-writing workshop, I gave medical students a prompt to write of a complicated situation from a point of view other than their own.] One student said that imagining her patient as if she were he changed everything for her. He had made her cry, she said, this was years before, and she hadn't been able to forget him and his hostility. But when she wrote from his point of view, suddenly she felt she could understand him—understand why he was rude to her—even if it

were only her imagination of why. It was enough. She felt better. It wasn't about her after all.

CASE ILLUSTRATION 13: HOUSE OFFICER—ATTENTION (TOWARD PATIENT, SELF-AWARENESS)

I try not to interrupt the harried resident who is getting paged back on the floor, who has papers to be signed, and whose patient just wants to see the GI doctor, no matter that she had a normal colonoscopy last year in the Dominican Republic. "Strange," I say, after consciously not asking for clarifying details or asking for a differential diagnosis. "What do you think is going on here? Why is this 38-year-old woman so adamant about a referral?" The resident looks at me, lists the possibilities, appropriately including a concern for domestic violence or nonconsensual sex, and then stops and stares. "Why don't you ask her what she is concerned about?" With a shrug, she gets up and returns a few minutes later, now glowing: "Aha! Her mother-in-law—mother-in-law had colon cancer, and she's worried she could have it!" This patient-narrative approach does not discredit the physiologic or epidemiologic approach to diagnostic reasoning. It simply contextualizes it, and, I believe, saves a great deal of time and money. As a supervisor and teacher, if I use the same stance toward my learner, who indeed is telling me a story, allowing myself to be the receiver at first, not yet the coach, then perhaps I am modeling behavior I would hope they would adopt in their own clinical work.

WHAT IS NARRATIVE MEDICINE *FOR*?

We see a developmental sequence unfolding for learners in our school and teaching hospital. Since narrative work has been adopted as one of our teaching and practice methods, the students are exposed to it longitudinally while their own skills deepen and complicate. From the premedical and first-year students' early experiences of "seeing" what goes on either in office hours or in some lecture in the amphitheater, the students progress to more consequential telling of the self and claiming for oneself the formative force of autobiographical truths. They discover their peers to be valuable witnesses and confirmers of their own experiences. Their skills as readers of texts and spoken language come to represent valuable resources for their lives as doctors and as persons. More seasoned students write their ways through the inevitable assaults and sadnesses of ward medicine. By turning their developing writing powers to face actual conflicts or dilemmas with patients, they start to use these techniques to establish genuine contact with patients and then to solve clinical problems.

A short poem by Philip Larkin gives us courage to ask, "What is narrative medicine *for?*"

Days
What are days for?
Days are where we live.
They come, they wake us
Time and time over.
They are to be happy in:
Where can we live but days?

Ah, solving that question
Brings the priest and the doctor
In their long coats
Running over the fields.

The examples cited above, whether from clinical practice or in classroom or ward teaching, demonstrate the utility and gifts of narrative routines in health care. We hope you can trace the similarity of our work with patients and peers and our work with students. We fuel our own teaching of these skills with the benefits that these skills have given to us in practice. Our own clinical-narrative experience gives us a place from which to continue to develop these skills, to research their outcomes for other groups, and to convey them to learners who have entrusted us with their educations.

NARRATIVE MEDICINE OUTCOMES RESEARCH

To capture the longitudinal effects of students' narrative medicine work over time in order to strengthen reflective capacity, faculty at Columbia created a 4-year curriculum, which we call the Portfolio. Narrative texts paralleling the arc of students' medical school experiences are selected for congruence with the current themes in the curriculum, such as awareness of multiple perspectives in a clinical encounter. We strengthen this curricular space with an end-of-semester meta-reflection exercise during which students are asked to review their Portfolio entries and write to the prompt: "Think about your writings as a mirror; write about what you see." Because the raw material for this meta-reflection are students' own entries, which are written spontaneously in-class to open-ended prompts designed to stimulate creativity, the possibilities for attention and self-discovery are heightened, and students gain perspective on their development, both personal and professional.

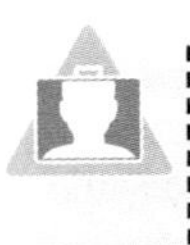

CASE ILLUSTRATION 14: MEDICAL STUDENT—REPRESENTATION (WRITING FOR DISCOVERY)

"It's really interesting to look back on my old writing and see it with the distance of time . . . I like the person who did the writing, even if I'm no longer exactly that person. I am not sure what kind of doctor that woman is going to become, I guess because I already feel a level of dissociation from her. I think she would have been a great doctor: a little naive, but incredibly optimistic. Concerned. Considerate. Hopeful."

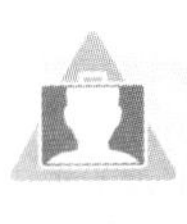

CASE ILLUSTRATION 15: MEDICAL STUDENT—ATTENTION (SELF-AWARENESS)

"A recurring theme in my writing this semester has been anxiety. I entered medical school like a kid running through the gates of Disneyland. Five months later, that excitement has been overwhelmed by a flood of uncertainty, insecurity, and second-guessing."

In addition to students themselves looking back on their writing, an attentive reader who can bear witness to discoveries that emerge through writing is crucial. Within our Portfolio curriculum, learning is deepened through each student's relationship with his or her longitudinal narrative medicine mentor, who reads their meta-reflections, as well as other entries selected by the student. Mentor feedback forms the basis for individual meetings and is explicitly not evaluative, relying rather on close reading methods of observation and description.

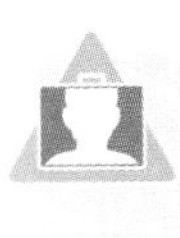

CASE ILLUSTRATION 16: MEDICAL STUDENT—AFFILIATION (WITH TEACHER), ATTENTION (SELF-AWARENESS)

"My earliest [meta-reflection], the first one we wrote, is much vaguer. The later ones are more about specific, often anxieties about what is to come which is probably more about my psyche than anything else. But getting to know my preceptor, who I think is fantastic, matters. And the knowledge that this person is going to read it, is going to respond, and knows you as a person—that makes a big difference to me."

Eager to understand the effect of the Portfolio on students' reflective capacity, a group of faculty members undertook a qualitative research project to study the meta-reflections of one cohort of medical students. Through a grounded-theory, constant comparison method of iterative reading and guided by a conceptual representation generated by the students' writings, the research team consensually developed codes and code families. Applying these codes to the reflections of 97 members of the class (73%), the team identified students' emphasis on themes of Recognition (empathy, self-awareness) and Grappling (internal change, dichotomies, wonder, questioning). This outcomes study enables us, together with our students, to refine the Portfolio structure and to respond all the more supportively to the joys and challenges of our students.

Not only the outcomes of narrative medicine methods in teaching but also their outcomes in clinical practice are being rigorously studied. As several of the cases presented in this chapter demonstrate, narrative medicine has great promise to improve numerous dimensions of clinical practice. Previous studies at Columbia and elsewhere have documented specific outcomes of narrative medicine techniques in a variety of in-patient settings, including improved team cohesion, improved perspective-taking, and decreased emotional exhaustion in clinicians.

We have implemented and evaluated narrative medicine interventions in ambulatory clinical settings as well to explore questions of feasibility, effective program design, and various outcomes. One such effort involved the implementation and evaluation of a 1-year narrative medicine program, funded by the Josiah Macy, Jr. Foundation, in three academic primary care clinics in New York City. When beginning this program, we spoke with clinic directors about the types of outcomes they were interested in achieving. Clinic leaders felt that narrative methods might have many dividends, including helping to improve interprofessional collaborative practice, reconnect clinical work with a sense of purpose, and provide opportunities to reflect on important clinical experiences.

In our program, we allotted 30 minutes per month to narrative medicine sessions during required interprofessional team meetings. All members of the staff attended the sessions, including attending physicians, residents, nurses, social workers, nursing assistants, and other staff. We asked the groups to engage with creative works (including poetry, art, and film), write to open-ended writing prompts, and share writings with one another.

CASE ILLUSTRATION 17: CLINIC HEALTH CARE TEAM—ATTENTION (RECOGNITION OF COLLEAGUES), REPRESENTATION (WRITING IN THE SHADOW OF A TEXT), AFFILIATION (AMONG COLLEAGUES)

We read the poem "The Ship Pounding" by Donald Hall during a narrative medicine session in a primary care clinic. The poem features a narrator who visits a sick wife in the hospital and likens the hospital (and perhaps one's journey of life) to a ship, with promise of visiting safe harbors. Yet by poem's end, we recognize that the ship has never left port.

Despite the poem's darkness, the group is captivated. A community health worker, who hadn't spoken during the earlier clinical meeting, volunteers to read the poem a second time to get a better handle on it. She posits that this "describes the daily lives in the hospital" and the "uncertainty" that patients grapple with. The group continues to explore the idea of uncertainty and how it affects one's clinical work. The research assistant taking field notes writes in her reflection, "Everyone spoke within the workshop session. Those who did not speak in the team meeting voluntarily participate in the discussion, possibly showing how the workshops offer a space for them to share."

We found that the program was feasible, even in busy urban primary care practices. Staff were engaged—interprofessional staff attended regularly and participated actively. Staff reported that the sessions were "meaningful" and even "restorative." Communication that occurred across professions and levels of hierarchy was also identified by staff as noteworthy. Program success was contingent on the support of administrative leadership and on availability of skilled facilitators. This mixed-methods feasibility study paves the way for continued implementation studies.

CONCLUSION

The field of narrative medicine is continuing its search for insight, for contact, and for affiliation. As health care delivery in the United States becomes more corporately controlled and bureaucratized, less and less time is allotted to hear fully the stories of patients. Pay-for-performance systems and revenue prioritization discourage clinicians from learning deeply about patients' lived experiences that influence their health. As more is learned about structural causes for health disparities, more activism and advocacy are called for to reach the over-arching goals of health care justice and health equity. We propose that narrative training will equip both seasoned and emerging clinicians with the wherewithal to see the suffering, to commit themselves to health care justice, to be available to peers and patients, to come to know the self, and to make that healing contact with patients and peers now so dangerously lacking in the care we give to our sick.

ACKNOWLEDGMENTS

We acknowledge our faculty colleagues in the K07 seminar and the students in the Foundations of Clinical Medicine course at the Vagelos College of Physicians and Surgeons of Columbia University. This work has been supported by NIH NHLBI R25 HL108014, "Enacting the Behavioral and Social Sciences in the Clinical Setting: Institution-Wide Teaching of Effective Team-Based Patient Care."

SUGGESTTED READINGS

Berthoff AE. Learning the uses of chaos. In: *The Making of Meaning: Metaphors, Models, and Maxims for Writing Teachers*. Montclair, NJ: Boynton/Cook Publishers; 1981:647–651.

Charon R. *Narrative Medicine: Honoring the Stories of Illness*. New York, NY: Oxford University Press; 2006.

Charon R, DasGupta S, Hermann N, et al. The principles and practice of narrative medicine. New York, NY: Oxford University Press; 2017.

Clifton L. *Blessing the Boats: New and Selected Poems 1988-2000*. Rochester, NY: BOA Editions; 2000:51.

Epstein R. *Attending: Medicine, Mindfulness, and Humanity*. New York, NY: Scribner; 2017.

Hemon, A. The aquarium: a child's isolating illness. *The New Yorker*, June 13 & 20, 2011:50–62.

Larkin P. Days. In: Thwaite A, ed. *Collected Poems*. London, UK: Farrar Straus Giroux and the Marvell Press; 1989:98.

Merleau-Ponty M. Cézanne's doubt. In: *Sense and Nonsense*. Chicago, IL: Northwestern University Press; 1964:9–25.

Santayana G. *The Sense of Beauty: Being the Outline of Aesthetic Theory*. New York, NY: Dover Publications; 1955.

Weil S. *Waiting for God*, translated by Craufurd E. New York, NY: Harper & Row; 1951.

Educating for Professionalism

48

Richard M. Frankel, PhD & Frederic W. Hafferty, PhD

KEY CHALLENGES IN EDUCATING FOR PROFESSIONALISM

Concerns about medicine's status as a profession have been growing for the past 80 years. By the late 1990s, many experts felt that medicine had become self-serving and insular, had violated its social trust, and was in danger of losing its vaunted professional status. The slowness of medicine's awakenings notwithstanding, the inaugural decade of the twenty-first century was marked by a flurry of actions deigned to define, assess, and institutionalize professionalism within the classrooms of medical education, the hallways of clinical practice and in terms of professional development for faculty. By 2000, for example, virtually every medical school and residency program had implemented some type of formal professionalism curriculum.

Medical professionalism faces a number of challenges. Perhaps the most important is the need to reconcile professionalism being taught in the "classroom" (which includes the professionalism embedded in the codes, charters, competencies, and curricula) with professionalism being observed and experienced by learners in the clinical settings modeled on a day-to-day basis by more senior clinicians and faculty. At root is a classic hidden curriculum problem of the gap between efforts to formalize professionalism instruction and the day-to-day or moment-to-moment lived experiences of trainees. In some cases, the gap has been great enough to cause trainees to "push back" against and disavow the formal professionalism curriculum. Successfully developing and implementing approaches to teaching professionalism that integrate elements of the formal and informal or hidden curriculum remain elusive.

Competency-based medical education has further defined, benchmarked, and assessed professionalism. The Accreditation Council for Graduate Medical Education (ACGME) professionalism competency emphasizes the development of professional character, high standards of accountability, humanism in all dealings with others, and altruism—putting the interests of the patient before self-interest. There are now a large number of readily available formal professionalism curricula, assessment tools, and literature (see Websites for Further Learning and Suggested Readings). Although the challenge of formal versus informal curricula remain, these resources identify important aspects of professionalism and point to areas for further curricular development.

Professionalism requires attention to several domains of physician behavior, including truth-telling, confidentiality, disruptive behavior, assuming responsibility, respectful communication with patients and colleagues, giving and receiving feedback, bullying, sexual harassment, personal appearance and attire, and others. In this chapter, we focus on three major professionalism issues: inappropriate use of social media, plagiarism, and boundary violations. We first define each challenge, then illustrate each with one or more cases. We end the discussion of each challenge with commentary regarding educational and institutional implications in four areas: (1) formal/informal curriculum; (2) faculty development; (3) institutional response; and (4) remediation.

Social Media

The explosive growth in information technology, especially the adoption of social media, presents a new challenge to professionalism. Concerns about sharing confidential patient information on public social media websites, posting of inappropriate personal information, using social media at inappropriate times such as on rounds or during lectures and other educational activities, and failure to maintain good professional boundaries by, for example, "friending" patients on social media sites, are among the problematic behaviors that have been noted among recent cohorts of medical students and residents. "Millennials," or Generation Y (those born between 1980 and 1994), which includes medical students, residents, and, to some degree, fellows and junior faculty, are almost constantly engaged in using social media. It is estimated that in the United States alone, there are over 170 million users of Facebook, and that number is growing rapidly. This method of communication has supplanted other forms of interaction, including the telephone and even email, which is more commonly used by older faculty. In the area of social media, faculty are what Prensky has termed "digital immigrants," whereas their younger charges who grew up with digital technology are "digital natives." Capitalizing on the benefits and understanding the risks inherent in social media remain a challenge for undergraduate and graduate training programs.

CASE ILLUSTRATION 1: "A CLICK IS ALL IT TAKES"

A Student Reports: I recently posted an offensive and tasteless "doctor joke" for my friends to see on Facebook. Another medical student who viewed it thought the posting was highly unprofessional and put the school in a potentially negative light so brought it to the attention of school administrators. As a result of my actions, I was required to make an appearance before the student promotions committee and face the possibility of dismissal for behavior unbecoming a medical student.

As a result of this experience, I have become acutely aware of the attractions and dangers of social networking and its potential to do harm. Since a case in which a student at Rutgers committed suicide after compromising information about him was circulated on social networking sites, I have come to realize that I have a responsibility to recognize that one click of the mouse is all it took to jeopardize my entire future as a physician. (MS II)

The essay above, written by a second-year medical student and president of his class, was published in SCOPE, Indiana University School of Medicine's weekly electronic newsletter that is distributed to the entire medical staff of some 2500 people on nine different campuses. It was written after the student had been cited for unprofessional behavior and only was permitted to stay in school contingent upon successful remediation with the school's competency director (RMF). The essay was voluntary, the result of a conversation between the student and two faculty members about alerting other students to the risks of posting information on social networking sites. The student volunteered to give a presentation based on his case to the entering freshman class.

Educational & Institutional Implications

1. Formal/informal curriculum
   - Many students and residents are unaware of the risks of using social media. For example, a study of online posting by medical students and residents found that only 37.5% made their Facebook pages private.
     - Education can be effective. One school that developed an educational intervention around Internet privacy saw an 85% drop in publicly available Facebook pages.
   - Modeling professional behavior in the informal curriculum
     - Engaging students in respectful dialogue and discovery about how and why they use social media can be helpful in bringing about behavior and culture change.
     - Enlisting student leaders who may have had experiences with professionalism issues relating to Internet usage may also help students recognize that the issue is serious and affects their peers and colleagues.
2. Faculty development
   - Inappropriate use of social media among faculty has increased as evidenced by a recent flurry of articles in the popular press and a study of the actions of state medical boards dealing with this issue.
     - Faculty development programs focusing on the use and abuse of social media by students and colleagues can be helpful in raising awareness of the risks involved.
     - Encouraging faculty to lead by example in the use of smart phones and other handheld devices can also be effective in addressing inappropriate usage.
3. Institutional response
   - The use of social media by medical trainees is growing.
   - Surveys by school administrators to determine the extent of social media use and its appropriateness/inappropriateness can help give the school a sense of the extent of social media practices among students, residents, and faculty, and help shape institutional policy.
   - Few schools have written policies that specifically deal with social networking. Evidence indicates that schools with such policies are better able to handle violations than schools without them.

- Developing written policies that take into account school size and the range of problem behaviors can be helpful in crafting institutional responses that are targeted and appropriate.
- Collaborative engagement of students, residents, and junior faculty in policy development facilitates implementation of the policies in question.

4. Remediation
   - There are currently no national standards for remediation of unprofessional behavior involving social media among medical students and residents. It falls to individual deans, course and clerkship directors, and faculty to come up with remediation procedures that are fair and fit the questionable behavior.
   - Apart from dismissal from school, remediation is best accomplished in the spirit of improvement and increased awareness of the risks associated with social media use. Personal research by students who have violated social media standards into what is known about millennials and their status as "digital natives" along with journaling and reflection is often useful.
   - Recruitment of student leaders who have had professionalism lapses and who share messages about the risks of inappropriate use of social media can be an effective method of "spreading the word" about expectations and appropriate behaviors.

Plagiarism

Another challenge in educating for professionalism is plagiarism. This problem may, in part, derive from the "digital divide" between generations and their knowledge and understanding of the rules that govern electronic, print, and written media. For example, evidence of plagiarism was found in 5.2% of the personal statements of residency applicants to a single institution by comparing them with readily available Internet sources. Likewise, in their undergraduate coursework some medical students believed that citing Internet sources such as Wikipedia or other websites was unnecessary because of the "open source" nature of these sites. Equally concerning is the trend among some faculty and trainees to "copy and paste" medical records in clinical care. Residents may observe their attending physicians engaging in this practice or get the message that it is okay to "copy and paste" a patient's history from day to day or from previous hospital admissions. Medical students, for whom there is typically no formal instruction in this area, learn to follow suit. The result is an "epidemic" of behavior that is a threat to both professionalism and quality of care.

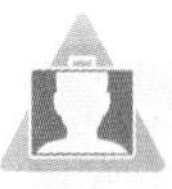

CASE ILLUSTRATION 2: PLAGIARISM

A. Residency Application	B. Internet Match http://csa-notes.com
"I am accustomed to working for long hours, making decisions under pressure and performing multiple tasks simultaneously. I possess a sound medical knowledge base and aspire to further my education. I am a team player who enjoys collaborating with others and can assume leadership when appropriate."	"I am accustomed to working for long hours, making decisions under pressure and performing multiple tasks simultaneously *and working independently.* I possess a sound medical knowledge base and aspire to further my education. I am a team player who enjoys collaborating with others and I can *communicate clearly* and assume leadership when appropriate."

The *Oxford English Dictionary* defines plagiarism as "the wrongful appropriation or purloining and publication as one's own, of the ideas, or the expression of the ideas . . . of another." The two samples above come from the personal statement of an application for residency at Harvard Medical School (Column A) and a popular website with examples of application essays (Column B). With the exception of two phrases deleted by the applicant and highlighted in italics, they are identical. Applicants must certify in writing that their essays are accurate and original. In the case of a residency application, the response to plagiarism is straightforward and involves rejecting the application and the applicant. With increasingly sophisticated tools available to prospective applicants as well as to faculty and administrators, the challenges of educating about, and monitoring for, plagiarism have become more pressing.

Educational & Institutional Implications

1. Formal/informal curriculum
   - Plagiarism may occur in many forms in preclinical and clinical contexts.
     - It is not safe to assume that students and residents will have learned about plagiarism in college. Consequently, formal instruction on the various types of plagiarism in medicine can help trainees be aware of what is and what is not considered plagiarism.

- Certification may be another alternative for teaching about plagiarism. In the same way that researchers must obtain human subjects certification to do their work, trainees would have to complete one or more modules on plagiarism and become "certified." This would ensure that subsequent plagiarism breaches could not be attributed to sheer lack of knowledge and would make clearer to students the consequences of such actions.
- Use of informal channels such as reviewing articles in a journal club format, brown bag discussions, or "Ethics at Lunch," led by students with input from faculty advisors, can be a useful avenue for raising awareness about falsification and plagiarism.

2. Faculty development
   - Many faculty members who suspect plagiarism in written reports are hesitant to invest the time and energy to prevent or "prove" these occurrences. Several automated programs are available to check for plagiarism (e.g., www.duplichecker.com, www.scanmyessay.com, and www.turnitin.com for admissions essays). In addition, faculty may not readily make the connection between activities like copying and pasting of notes in the electronic medical record and plagiarism.
     - Faculty development seminars on how to detect and respond to instances of plagiarism can be quite useful in addressing the problem.
     - Raising awareness of faculty about the risks (malpractice and otherwise) of cutting and pasting their own hospital notes and the fact that residents and students will do as they see their role models doing may help address this problem.
3. Institutional response
   - Clearly stated institutional policies, procedures, and consequences regarding plagiarism in the preclinical and clinical years are essential for students and residents to understand the risks involved in copying one's own or another person's words and ideas or falsifying records.
     - Academic policies as well as student promotions committees can be helpful in setting standards. Working together with student leaders to develop standards can facilitate their acceptance by the student body.
     - Using the honor code, if one exists, to clearly define the role of plagiarism can help students understand what is expected of them in this domain.
4. Remediation
   - Remediation depends in large measure on the type of plagiarism that has occurred. Serious cases involving the scientific integrity of a piece of work by stealing another's ideas and representing them as one's own should be dealt with by considering failure in a course, clinical rotation and in some cases, dismissal from school.
     - Plagiarism of any sort is a serious offense, whether premeditated or inadvertent. Remediation is often more successful if the trainee has a clear sense of what rule or norm has been violated and what its present and future impact may be. Using literary examples like the historian Stephen Ambrose whose otherwise unblemished career was sullied when it was discovered that he had plagiarized his own and others' works in his books are useful in bringing plagiarism issues to the forefront.
     - It may also be useful to bring attention to the link between unprofessional behavior of undergraduate medical students, including plagiarism, and risk of subsequent censure by state boards of medical practice.

Boundary Management

Another challenge for professionalism training is boundary management. Although there are dimensions of boundary management that touch upon the use of social media, for example, whether it is appropriate for physicians to be "friends" with their patients on Facebook, or First Amendment issues of whether schools or residency programs have the right or obligation to monitor their trainees' individual postings, students and residents also confront a range of boundary issues in their day-to-day work and roles. Little attention is paid to these issues in the formal professionalism curriculum because the issues are not recognized or do not fit well into the global categories of professionalism such as altruism, beneficence, or humanism. In addition, abstract discussions of professionalism often exclude issues of power and hierarchy which dominate many students' thinking and experience. A particular challenge in this regard is the transition from classroom learning, which typically takes place in the first and second year of medical school, to clinical rotations where classroom learning is disregarded or derided. Students are often left on their own to piece together the appropriate boundaries of their professional role in regard to patients, peers, allied health professionals, and teachers while realizing that they are often at the lower rungs of power and potentially vulnerable to negative evaluations should they incorrectly define their professional role.

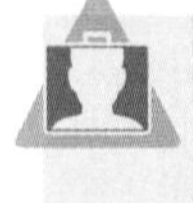

CASE ILLUSTRATION 3: MANAGING PROFESSIONAL AND PERSONAL BOUNDARIES

Scenario 1

An intern went out of his way to "warn" the members of our team that a particular . . . [professional] working with us was "an idiot" . . . I thought this was extremely disrespectful to the [professional], who was unaware of any of this . . . I wanted to say something but I wasn't sure if that was my place. I had no idea how to handle the situation. (Narrative written by a third-year medical student.)

Medical students frequently struggle with the concept of professional boundaries, especially as it relates to their role in hierarchical situations. On their clinical rotations, and in their role primarily as observers, students often witness behaviors in others which they perceive to be unprofessional but feel powerless to address. Fear of reprisal, loss of face among peers, and being labeled a "whistleblower" or a troublemaker are frequent reasons given by medical students for failing to act in the face of behavior perceived to be unprofessional. In these cases, as illustrated above, boundaries defined by power differentials may be particularly difficult for students to navigate. Especially troubling to medical students are situations that involve disrespect. Boundaries are not specifically included in the Association of American Medical Colleges (AAMC) professionalism categories, but can be considered proxy measures for concerns about personal and professional conduct.

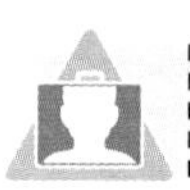

CASE ILLUSTRATION 3 (CONTD.)

Scenario 2

I was sitting in the conference room when the assistant came in and said, "You have a patient in the exam room who is going to make your day." I walked in and this woman is dressed in like a wet tee-shirt, no bra, very good looking and shapely. I started talking to her and she was giggling every other word and acting more inappropriately than I'm used to. . . . And it was very uncomfortable because I was sitting in that room looking at her and I couldn't divert my attention from looking at her breasts. I tried to spend a lot of time looking down at her chart, but every time I looked up my eyes zoomed in on her breasts. She was controlling my eyes . . . jiggling those things around so that her already prominent breasts were more prominent. . . . She was just too flirtatious for me. I was really uncomfortable. (Third-year resident)

Sexuality and sexual feelings are a normal part of being human. Sexual feelings between a doctor and patient are not abnormal, but they can sometimes be confusing and troublesome. When acted upon, they can be dangerous to the relationship and potentially exploitative. In previous research based on the narratives of students, residents, and practicing physicians, we found that the majority of situations in which providers' sexual feelings came into play involved boundary confusion on the physician's part. These situations typically involved their recognition of a sexual attraction or the potential for becoming aroused during the medical visit. Very infrequently, the feelings led to a boundary crossing where physician and patient mutually disclosed their feelings of attraction to one another. Much more frequently, the physician took steps to avoid the feelings by fleeing the encounter or skipping portions of the physical examination. Both male and female physicians described failing to do rectal, genitourinary (GU), and breast examinations to avoid boundary confusion. The above narrative from a third-year resident in internal medicine graphically illustrates the effect sexual feelings and assumptions about others' behavior can have on the medical encounter.

It is clear from this narrative that the patient's appearance and manner of interacting (inappropriately described by the assistant as "a patient who's going to make your day") led the resident to "sexualize" the situation and make some assumptions about the patient, her behavior, and her intentions. He then became caught and confused between the nature and boundaries of the doctor–patient interaction and those of an encounter between himself as a sexually interested man and an attractive woman. It is interesting to note that the resident did not recognize his own role in nonverbally encouraging the very behavior that made him so uncomfortable. He reported that each time he looked up, his eyes zoomed in on her breasts, the result of which he felt was to make her display them even more prominently. The resident was clearly stuck, attracted to his patient, and at the same time struggling to distance himself sufficiently to maintain an appropriate professional boundary. He knew something was wrong, but was not sure what it was, or what to do about it. This sense of helplessness and lack of clarity is typical of confusing boundary situations.

As it happens, our resident is not alone in feeling a confusing attraction to his patient. Prior research among psychiatry residents has found that most men and about half of the women reported sexual attraction to one or more patients, and 1% acknowledged sexual contact with patients. Another study found that 57% of medical students had sexual feelings about patients, and that males had them more frequently than female students. Twenty-one percent of the students surveyed thought it was okay to have sex with patients. The same study reported that there was no teaching in the undergraduate curriculum about sexual boundaries in medical care.

Educational & Institutional Implications

1. Formal/informal curriculum
    - Both students and residents find it difficult to act in the face of witnessing unprofessional behavior or experiencing sexual feelings that could threaten or cross boundaries.

- Curriculum offerings that focus on duty, responsibility, and accountability can help trainees define boundaries so that they have a clear understanding of the issues involved.
- Curricula should discuss physical and sexual boundaries with patients, peers, and faculty. Role-plays could address ways to respond to sexual confusion or boundary transgressions. Clear legal and ethical ramifications should be discussed.
- Communication skills for dealing with conflict, especially where there is an authority gradient, can be helpful in giving students and residents the requisite skill set to successfully address boundary crossings and violations.
- Curriculum content that reinforces the consequences of boundary confusion, crossing, or violations for patient safety and quality can help raise awareness of the larger issues that underlie professionalism. For example, using evidence to show that disruptive surgeons have worse complication rates and are more likely to be sued frames unprofessional behavior as a risk rather than a personality trait.
- Looking for positive examples of maintaining healthy sexual and other boundaries among students, residents, and faculty can also be helpful in terms of reinforcing desired norms in the informal curriculum.

2. Faculty development
   - Faculty members are often unaware of how their behavior affects students and residents. Strong emotions such as frustration, anger, and contempt are amplified among students and residents who view themselves in a "one down" position. Relational coordination and safety in the learning environment suffer when students feel intimidated or humiliated.
   - Faculty development programs that emphasize new rules and regulations with zero tolerance for disruptive behavior, mistreatment of trainees, or sexual boundary violations can help inform faculty members and raise awareness.
   - Opportunities to practice skills of maintaining healthy boundaries with peers can help surface personal and professional boundary issues that were never taught in medical school or residency. Working through cases with peers helps to create a culture of respect among faculty with a "trickle down" effect on residents and students.
   - Faculty development courses such as the ones put on by the Academy of Communication in Healthcare, use skill development and personal awareness together to teach faculty how to create a safe, satisfying learning environment for trainees and how to recognize and deal effectively with sexual and other boundary issues.
3. Institutional response
   - Clear institutional policies for dealing with boundary concerns and violations are critical to creating safe, supportive work environments.
   - Having personnel and procedures in place for faculty and trainees to present their concerns, have them investigated and hopefully resolved in a nonjudgmental way can help reinforce both the informal and formal curriculum.
   - Orientation programs for entering medical students, residents, and fellows with opportunities for small group discussion and role play can be helpful in putting the issues of healthy boundaries in a positive, constructive light. Similar programs are useful in orienting new faculty and staff.
4. Remediation
   - Remediation for students who have engaged in unprofessional behavior that threatens or crosses personal or professional boundaries should be handled on a case-by-case basis. Obviously, remediation will depend on the seriousness of the boundary issue in question. Consequences, too, will vary from dismissal from medical school or residency to learning about the risks of boundary confusion, boundary crossings, and boundary violations.
   - If it is determined that the boundary issue is one in which there is a deficit in performance, suitable remediation might include activities such as: coaching and role play; research on the causes and consequences of boundary issues in medical students and residents; developing and presenting a teaching module to peers on professional boundaries; counseling and psychotherapy; and close supervision by faculty during clinical rotations.
   - If it is determined that the boundary issue is due to an impairment, steps should be taken to alert institutional representatives who are prepared to deal with such issues.

SUMMARY & CONCLUSION

In this chapter, we have highlighted some of the most pressing professionalism issues that trainees encounter. Although global concepts like altruism, respect, and equity are enormously helpful in setting community or disciplinary standards of behavior, the lived experience of medical students and residents is much more tightly bound to the local cultures and contexts in which they live and work. One of the most important aspects of educating for professionalism is to build bridges between students' experiences in the informal curriculum and the aspirational concepts they represent.

One pedagogical and practical challenge is to remain nonjudgmental about the behaviors observed in, or reported by, students and residents. It is very easy to slip into the role of moral arbiter in situations in which unprofessional behavior is being discussed. The surgeon who yelled at a student or the attending who admonished a patient to lose weight may have had good reasons for doing so (e.g., the student was about to break the sterile field, and the patient had dangerously high blood pressure and was at imminent risk of a heart attack). Rather than acting on the student's or resident's behalf in the face of a reported boundary issue, helping trainees to develop their own skill set for dealing with the behavior, and closely monitoring their progress can be very fruitful. Obviously, if there is suspicion that the issue represents a boundary violation with potential for harm to the trainee, immediate action and fact finding may be required.

At the student level, professionalism challenges tend to be recurrent; caring, compassion and communication (especially across an authority gradient), respect, and teamwork tend to dominate the concerns. For residents, autonomy, conflicts of interest, and mistakes take on special importance. For both students and residents, boundary issues, albeit different for each group, tend to occur with great frequency in professionalism discussions.

Pedagogically it is helpful to start with trainees' lived experiences of professionalism and deepen reflection on them through small group discussion, use of student narratives, and facilitated faculty discussion. This approach optimizes the likelihood of making professionalism education salient and engaging for both students and faculty. Discussions of topics like medical mistakes, boundary issues, sexuality and professionalism, impaired physicians, quality and safety, and conflicts of interest can help highlight and deepen trainees' understanding of their own and others' behavior and reinforce the value of professionalism to the individual, community, and society. From a practical point of view, focusing on professionalism as a way of being rather than an abstract set of concepts helps trainees make connections between their existence in the real time environments in which they are training and their hopes, dreams, and aspirations for their lives in the profession of medicine.

SUGGESTED READINGS

Ginsburg S, Regehr G, Lingard L. The disavowed curriculum: understanding students' reasoning in professionally challenging situations. *J Gen Intern Med* 2003;18:1015–1022.

Hafferty FW, Levinson D. Moving beyond nostalgia and motives: towards a complexity science view of medical professionalism. *Perspect Biol Med* 2008;51:599–615.

Karnieli-Miller O, Taylor AC, Cottingham AH, Inui TS, Vu TR, Frankel RM. Exploring the meaning of respect in medical student education: an analysis of student narratives. *J Gen Intern Med* 2010;25:1309–1314.

Levinson WL, Ginsberg S, Hafferty F, Lucey CR. *Understanding Medical Professionalism*. New York, NY: McGraw-Hill Education; 2014.

Papadakis MA, Teherani A, Banach MA, et al. Disciplinary action by medical boards and prior behavior in medical school. *N Engl J Med* 2005;353:2673–2682.

Passi V, Doug M, Peile E, Thistlethwaite J, Johnson, N. Developing medical professionalism in future doctors: a systematic review. *Int J Med Educ* 2010;1:19–29.

Ziring D, Frankel RM, Danoff D, Isaacson JH, Lochnan H. Silent witnesses: faculty reluctance to report medical students' professionalism lapses. *Acad Med* 2018;93(11):1700–1706.

WEBSITES FOR FURTHER LEARNING

ABIM Project Professionalism. https://medicinainternaucv.files.wordpress.com/2013/02/project-professionalism.pdf. Accessed May 2019.

Academy of Communication in Healthcare. https://www.achonline.org/. Accessed August 2018.

AMA Position Statement on Medical Professionalism. https://ama.com.au/position-statement/medical-professionalism-2010-revised-2015. Accessed May 2019.

American College of Physicians. Medical Ethics and Professionalism Cases. http://www.acponline.org/running_practice/ethics/. Accessed May 2019.

Annals of Internal Medicine Physician Charter on medical professionalism. http://annals.org/article.aspx?volume=136&issue=3&page=243. Accessed May 2019.

Trainee Well-Being

49

John F. Christensen, PhD & Mitchell D. Feldman, MD, MPhil, FACP

Becoming a health professional is a challenging and complex process. Trainees frequently experience stressors that exceed their previous life experience and coping skills. These demands are proportionate to the responsibility and complexity of caring for patients in all their variability and vulnerability. These demands of professional training are enormous, and trainees often neglect their own physical, emotional, relational, and spiritual health; however, a central component of professionalism is awareness of one's own limits and mindfulness about the wise allocation of one's energy in providing quality patient care (see Chapters 6 and 7). Neglect of this awareness may sow the seeds of burnout and lead to poor quality care and medical error (see Chapter 39). Close attention to maintaining well-being, however, can enhance satisfaction with a health professions career and optimize the clinician–patient relationship. Given that trainees are vulnerable to pressures to postpone their own well-being until training is completed, it is paramount to include promotion of self-care in the formation of health professionals.

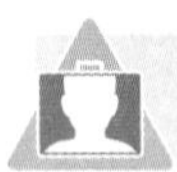

CASE ILLUSTRATION 1

Jill Rayburn had not slept much in 30 hours. She had been studying for her pathophysiology examination for a week, and still she felt ill prepared. As a second-year medical student, she was beginning to wonder whether she was cut out for medicine in spite of the fact that she was in the upper 20% of her class. Many of her classmates seemed to have mastery of the material for this examination; some had even gone for a hike yesterday afternoon. Last night Jill declined an invitation to play indoor soccer even though it was mid-January and cold outside, and she was tired of being stuck in the library. She was beginning to resent the professor who invited her to coauthor a paper, even though at the time she felt flattered that he had singled her out for this honor. Now she did not feel up to the task, and she wished she had started preparing for this examination earlier rather than working on the paper. She looked back to her days of high school and college, when she was consistently at the top of her class, and remembered many carefree days. She wondered what had happened to that other side of her with the sense of humor and the time to hang out with friends. As she looked ahead to the remainder of the year, all she saw were more deadlines and isolated days in the library without respite. She wondered if she would ever have fun again.

A common trait of physicians and other health professionals is compulsivity. Although many attributes of compulsivity—thoroughness, accuracy, second guessing, monitoring changes—are beneficial to patient care and success in medical training, this trait may also erode the personal health, satisfaction, and well-being of clinicians. Early in her training, Jill is manifesting many of the associated characteristics of compulsivity that if unchecked may lead to cynicism and burnout later in her career. She is beginning to question her competence, in spite of the fact that she is in the top fifth of her class. She is at risk of developing what has been labeled the "imposter syndrome," in which the individual feels that she has fooled others into thinking she is competent, but the threat of being unmasked as a fraud lurks at every turn. Jill is also feeling guilt about not having been wiser in her allocation of time. No matter how hard she has worked, it does not seem to be enough. In addition to self-doubt and guilt, Jill is also carrying a burden of responsibility for meeting all her obligations, and she feels alone with that burden. She thinks about her peers enjoying an outing together and envisions continued isolation for herself in the library. This triad of doubt, guilt, and an exaggerated sense of responsibility has been described in a classic paper by Glen Gabbard as constituents of the compulsivity that is a "normal" trait in most physicians.

Jill's discontent has its roots in the early conditioning of many bright young people in American society that implies that our value or worth as persons is linked to academic success or outward performance. Most of us have an inherent need for love and acceptance, and when children are repeatedly told that they are special and valued only when they are "exceptional," that is, at the top of their class in grades and stars in various performance endeavors, they begin to link their personal worth to meeting these standards of excellence. This high need for achievement collides with the reality that many of one's peers in medical school also came from the top of their class and consequently being smart and performing well are not so exceptional. They must work harder to stand out. Being less than outstanding is construed as having failed to meet an essential marker of their worth and value as a person. They are left with the dilemma of backing off from overwork and consequently carrying the self-stigma of being "second best," "ordinary," "mediocre," and unconsciously feeling less lovable; or of working harder to stand out. Paradoxically these efforts to excel and "stand out" can lead to the very isolation and loneliness from which they are trying to escape.

The personality factors of compulsiveness in combination with the reinforcement systems of the culture of perfectionism may contribute to a high prevalence of depression in medical students. A recent meta-analytic study found that about one-third of medical students were suffering from depression, which is two to five times the prevalence in people of similar age in the general population. The same study found an 11% prevalence of suicidal ideation in medical students. These findings were similar to a previous meta-analytic study that found a 30% prevalence rate of depression among resident physicians. Clearly, a systemic influence is at work in medical training when almost one-third of trainees are depressed.

Some trainees may have the nagging thought that overwork is not good for them, that taking care of themselves by getting enough sleep, exercise, eating well, having fun, and spending time with friends are all important, but in the "psychology of postponement," they think, "As soon as this exam is over, then I can unwind." In addition, their elevated expectation of themselves multiplies this self-bargaining: "As soon as I get into the residency I want, then I can relax;" "as soon as I get accepted for a fellowship, then I can start working out;" "as soon as I start my first real job, then I can have a life." Thus early in professional training, a habit of postponement can develop that if unchecked can lead to neglecting many of one's most valued relationships and activities throughout one's career. Sir William Osler in a commencement address to graduating medical students in 1889 had these words to say about postponement:

> Engrossed late and soon in professional cares … you may so lay waste that you may find, too late, with hearts given way, that there is no place in your habit-stricken souls for those gentler influences which make life worth living.

Jill's story also illustrates the way the system of medical education with its overt and covert rewards and punishments can reinforce the student's inherent compulsivity. Her exceptional performance has been noticed by one of her professors, who asked her to work with him as coauthor on a paper for publication. It is natural for teachers to ask top performers to do more, yet neither the teacher nor the student pause to reflect on the potential toxicity of rewarding overwork. Medical school traditionally is better at channeling students into ever-refined strata of academic and professional success than at mentoring them into building a career in which their professional endeavors unfold within a context of a healthy life well lived. Unless Jill were to encounter a mentor who has this broader grasp of personal and professional well-being, her role models and professors may continue unwittingly to provide a "hidden curriculum," which conveys the message that being a successful physician entails putting one's own life on hold.

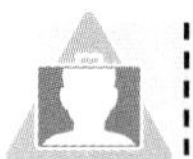

CASE ILLUSTRATION 1 (CONTD.)

Jill was walking across the quadrangle after her pathophysiology examination and failed to notice Dr. Ann Bennington, her teacher from the previous term in a class on the medical interview. Dr. Bennington noticed Jill's hunched over posture and drawn facial expression: "Jill, you look like you have the weight of the world on your shoulders and haven't slept in days. How are you doing?" Jill managed a smile and protested, "I'm fine. I just finished the pathophys exam." Ann confronted her mildly, "Well you look exhausted. When's the last time you had an evening off?"

When she noticed a tear forming in Jill's eyes, Ann replied, "Jill, I suspect you're carrying more of a burden than you let on to others. I'd really like to talk with you more about this." She then suggested they meet later that afternoon in her office. At the meeting later in Dr. Bennington's office, after some initial hesitation Jill opened up with the self-doubt, emptiness, fatigue, and isolation she had been feeling the last few weeks. After a pause Ann replied, "You know, Jill, you remind me of myself when I was a medical student." Noticing Jill's tears, she continued, "The fact that you are one of the brightest people in your class doesn't seem to matter to you now, and I think I know why. Like me you are perfectionistic, and there are reasons too numerous for us to go into now why we are that way. But one of the effects of that perfectionism is that we never feel we can get enough praise or external validation for our worth. That's because we weren't taught to value ourselves from within, that we are lovable and have immense worth before we ever set out to do great things." She paused to observe Jill's response. Since she was breathing more freely and seemed curious, Ann continued: "There's nothing wrong in striving for excellence. In fact, that's desirable. But what we mean by 'excellence' needs to be challenged. Your work as a physician, like your work as a student, will always occur within a real-world context of the various values you hold and commitments you have made, as well as the limitations of time, personal energy, and competing tasks. Bumping up against these limits can be humbling, but ultimately accepting those limits and allowing your excellence to be contextualized into your life will give you wisdom. Your body, mind, and spirit are giving you feedback that you should not ignore. Rather than anesthetizing yourself to this pain, let it teach you more about yourself and the full context of joy of which you are capable. To the extent you can let your awareness of the origin of this pain lead you to greater self-acceptance, you will be an excellent physician and a healing presence for others."

Jill's chance encounter with Dr. Bennington, along with Ann's willingness to mentor Jill about the importance of honoring life values in becoming a doctor, shows the powerful influence of senior clinicians, who have struggled themselves to attain life wisdom. In choosing mentors, students would do well to seek out clinicians who tolerate the tension of keeping their personal and professional lives in balance and who explicitly honor a variety of values beyond their professional lives, including family relationships, friendships, recreational pursuits, hobbies, and personal self-care.

Having a mentor is a critical component of career satisfaction and success in medicine. The mentoring relationship has been described as one of the most complex and developmentally important in a person's life. Mentors act as teachers, exemplars, and guides for their mentees. On a practical level, medical students and residents who have a mentor report better career preparation than do those without a mentor. Ideally, the mentoring relationship provides some benefits to both mentor and mentee, such as opportunities for collaboration, mutual teaching and learning, and the promotion of self-reflection as illustrated by the above vignette.

Among the perspectives worth cultivating is the awareness that becoming a health professional is a process that occurs over several years and that self-perceived imperfection is an inherent part of that process. It is helpful to think of ourselves as "becoming" rather than insisting on holding an image of what we have not yet become, then unfavorably comparing ourselves with that image. Given the continual pressures inherent in medical training to judge our own competence, it is important to cultivate the equally important capacity for "self-appreciation." When we respond to a sunset, to the first flower blooming in the garden in spring, or to the final movement of Beethoven's *9th Symphony*, this is typically not an act of judgment, but one of appreciation. It is impossible to engage the "judgment" and "appreciation" centers of our minds at the same time.

The exaggerated sense of personal responsibility that is part of the compulsive triad noted by Gabbard is often reinforced by the competitive climate of getting into medical school and advancing through training. This attitude is frequently carried into residency training and subsequent practice, in which the illusion is maintained that one is a self-sufficient professional, that asking for help is a sign of weakness, and that competency is distinguished by the ability to "go it alone." Nothing could be further from the actual process of delivering health care, in which systematic attempts to improve quality and reduce error now demand that teams of professionals from various disciplines work cooperatively to provide patient care and promote the health of the community. The best medical schools are beginning to train for this, and the Accreditation Council of Graduate Medical Education (ACGME) states that "systems-based practice," which largely involves working as part of a team, is one of the core competencies to be mastered during residency (see Chapter 43). Whether or not teamwork is reinforced by one's training as a health professional, cultivating the practice of working cooperatively with others and committing oneself to helping colleagues succeed can contribute enormously to one's personal and professional satisfaction.

CASE ILLUSTRATION 1 (CONTD.)

In April of her fourth year of medical school, Jill dropped by Dr. Bennington's office to let her know she would be going to a family medicine residency in the South. "How are you feeling about the match?" Ann asked. "Well, to tell you the truth," Jill replied, "my first choice was another program where I could have pursued some work in epidemiology based on that paper I coauthored a couple of years ago. Since the match, however, I've thought more about the program I'm going to, and especially about one physician on the faculty there who interviewed me. I was struck by the pictures he had on his wall of his wife and children, his children's poems and drawings, and what he shared with me about how much their training program valued both professionalism and the personal growth and life satisfaction of their residents." Ann smiled and nodded. Jill went on, "I have you to thank for reaching out to me at a critical moment a couple of years ago and helping me realize there was more to me than trying to be a star. You helped me realize the value of humility, which includes appreciation of my gifts as well as acceptance of my limitations. You also gave me the greatest gift, which was affirming my own capacity for appreciating my life and for letting that be the ground from which to appreciate others." In June, after graduation, Jill opened a card from Dr. Bennington, which contained this poem by Derek Walcott:

Love After Love

The time will come
when, with elation
you will greet yourself arriving
at your own door, in your own mirror,
and each will smile at the other's welcome,
and say, sit here. Eat.
You will love again
the stranger who was yourself.

Give wine. Give bread. Give back your heart
to itself, to the stranger who has loved you
all your life, whom you ignored
for another, who knows you by heart.
Take down the love letters from the bookshelf,
the photographs, the desperate notes,
peel your own image from the mirror.
Sit. Feast on your life.

CASE ILLUSTRATION 2

Bill Trimmell was shaking as he sat in the residents' room wondering why he had yelled at the patient he had just admitted to the hospital, scolding her about not doing enough to monitor her blood sugars, resulting in hyperglycemia and subsequent infection. As he reflected on the unpleasant conversation with her, he suddenly asked himself, "What am I doing?" This was only the second admission of the day, and already he could not wait to go home. He had had a busy morning caring for a patient he had admitted to the intensive care unit, leaving him only 10 minutes over the noon hour to eat a stale bagel left over from the morning conference. Bill was only a third of the way through his second year of internal medicine residency, and he found himself frequently resenting many of his patients and wondering what had happened to the altruistic dream of helping people that had led him into medical school. Why did he feel like he no longer cared?

Bill is showing the classic signs and symptoms of *burnout*, which consists of emotional exhaustion (including compassion fatigue and dissociation from feelings in general), depersonalization in relationships (treating oneself, patients, coworkers, and family members as objects), and a perceived clinical ineffectiveness. Burnout has been described as "an erosion of the soul," and it spreads gradually and continually over time, sending people into a downward spiral in which it is difficult to recover if one remains in the circumstances that generated it. Burnout has been associated with impaired job performance and poor health, including headaches, sleep disturbance, irritability, relationship difficulties, fatigue, hypertension, anxiety, depression, myocardial infarction, and chemical dependency. Cognitive performance as well can be compromised by burnout. A national U.S. study of internal medicine residents found that symptoms of burnout, which were associated with higher medical school debt, were also associated with lower In-Training Examination scores. For physicians the seeds of burnout may be sown in medical school and residency training, where fatigue and emotional exhaustion are often the norm. By mid-career, the momentum of this condition is maintained by the subtle reinforcements in the work setting for being a hard worker and placing service to others before self-care.

All too often residents are confronted with the reality of patients who for one reason or another are nonadherent to medical regimens, or who have chronic health problems that are refractory to interventions (see Chapters 4 and 20). Unremitting exposure to cases in which one's own efforts appear futile can engender frustration and cynicism. Without the opportunity to discuss these common experiences with their peers and faculty, trainees may begin to experience the early symptoms of burnout.

A large U.S. study of burnout among medical students, residents, and early-career physicians found that symptoms of depression, suicidal ideation, and low sense of personal accomplishment were most prevalent during medical school and then declined incrementally with each career stage. Another finding was that overall burnout, high depersonalization, and high fatigue were most prevalent during residency/fellowship and then improved for early-career physicians. Moreover, burnout is more prevalent among medical trainees than among the similarly aged U.S. population.

A frequent manifestation of burnout is "compassion fatigue," in which an overload of suffering threatens to run our emotional tank dry and lead to *dissociation*, characterized by a withdrawal of attention from emotions and somatic sensations as we focus cognitively and visually on complex patient care problems or get absorbed in our "to do" list. We become anesthetized to feelings and cannot relate to family and friends once we leave work. The cognitive correlate of dissociation is *decontextualization*. This involves a habit of thinking of others (and even ourselves) in a utilitarian way that abstracts and constructs persons into categories that have usefulness for our jobs and getting our tasks done in a timely way.

This habit of thinking ignores the full life context in which others (and we ourselves) are embedded. Thus, we relate to patients as diagnoses or appointments on the schedule, to coworkers as facilitating or impeding our work, to family and friends as intruding or placing unrealistic demands on our time, and to ourselves as task-processing machines.

Bill understandably feels a disconnect between the sense of vocation he once felt about medicine and the sense of futility about how he spends his working hours. In the absence of time to reflect on what is happening or discuss it with others, he finds himself slipping into disillusionment and cynicism. His job as a resident has begun to feel meaningless.

CASE ILLUSTRATION 2 (CONTD.)

In January of his second year, Bill attended a resident well-being retreat offered three times a year to all residents in his program. This particular retreat was focused on finding personal renewal in the work of caring for patients. During a small group discussion, one of the senior residents shared that she had felt burned out and uncaring by the middle of her second year. This led to a discussion about burnout and the vulnerability most residents have to this phenomenon. Another resident stated that what had helped him was observing an attending at the bedside of a dying patient showing considerable patience and compassion and asking him how he did that. This attending had replied that he kept a journal of memorable events from the day that gave him an opportunity for reflection. As the group talked, it became clear to Bill that he was not alone with this erosion of meaning and that there were personal and group strategies for renewing his enthusiasm for medicine.

Carl Rogers once said that "what is most personal is most universal." Nothing can be so personally isolating as the perception that one has lost one's way professionally. It is reminiscent of the poignant lament of Dante at the opening of the *Divina Comedia*:

> *In the middle of the road of my life, I awoke in a dark wood where the true way was wholly lost.*

Nothing can be so healing and reassuring as to know that others have traveled the same road and have emerged as colleagues to admire and emulate. Retreats, support groups, or even impromptu discussions during lulls in the pace of work to share common experiences and struggles can remind trainees that they are part of the human community and that they have the capacity for renewal and change.

Support groups are an especially valuable learning format in residency training programs to help residents navigate personal and professional developmental tasks, learn self-management and emotion management skills, build authentic community with their peers, and promote their well-being. Developmental challenges common to residents include establishing one's professional identity, developing professional confidence, coping with patient deaths, erosion of an idealized view of medicine, cognitive and behavioral management of stress, assuming the responsibility of a team leader, developing a reflective capacity for self-awareness, finding a career path, and learning self-acceptance and the limitations of personal control. Having a safe and confidential format for sharing these issues with one's peers is vital to a resident's professional development, and training programs would be wise to incorporate this into their curricula.

Emotional Intelligence

Among the strategies that trainees can use for restoring a capacity for compassion and enjoyment of work is the cultivation of "emotional intelligence." Developing self-awareness is essential to emotional intelligence. This is a challenge for clinicians who have been trained to dissociate from their feelings as a way of being "objective" in their professional role with patients. Since the quality of clinicians' relationships with their patients is a major component of the therapeutic process as well as a major contributor to their own well-being, developing self-awareness to maximize this process is essential (see Chapter 7). Emotional intelligence includes developing a language for one's emotions and a capacity for self-disclosure to others. The mirror of this process of self-awareness and self-expression is the capacity to recognize and understand emotions in others. We can use our own emotions to develop hypotheses about what the other is feeling. We can learn to check our feelings with others, reflect feelings, comment on what we are observing, and receive the emotional disclosure of others without judgment. It can be helpful to regard emotions as value-neutral information that is passing through our awareness like weather systems, which in themselves are neither right nor wrong. Thus, we can think of attending to the patient's feelings as getting a "weather report" and awareness of our own feelings as "checking the weather." Accepting our own emotions and those of others can be liberating and allow us to be fully present to others and ourselves (see Chapters 2 and 7).

Other components of emotional intelligence include controlling impulses, especially by delaying our response in conflict situations, delaying gratification for the sake of achieving goals, and using cognitive reframing and self-instructional statements to regulate our moods. We can enhance our emotional intelligence by naming internally what we are feeling at the moment, keeping a journal that captures the predominant feelings we have experienced on a given day, practicing emotional self-expression with friends and intimate partners, reflecting the feelings that others disclose to us, and, in some cases, by engaging in psychotherapy to enhance our emotional literacy.

Self-regulation of anxiety and situational stress is a skill that can be learned in the context of training. It is an essential prerequisite for the accurate perception of patients' distress, which facilitates the use of empathy skills (see Chapter 2). A Belgian study of resident physicians on an inpatient rotation found that their self-reported anxiety and physiologic measures of sympathetic nervous system arousal were inversely related to their ability to detect patients' distress.

Bill's feeling of futility in caring for patients who did not get better in spite of his best efforts emanated from his own beliefs and expectations about control. Gaining clarity about the extent to which control is possible in the events of our lives, and in the profession of medicine in particular, is essential to satisfaction with the work of being a clinician. Although people tend to be more satisfied when they perceive a greater control over the events that impact them, most of the outcomes of patient care are multidetermined and, to a large extent, dependent on many forces beyond the clinician's control, including patient choices as well as genetic and environmental variables. Thinking in terms of "influence" rather than "control" may be more realistic. Within the large array of factors that contribute to illness and health, clinicians can have enormous influence, but medical care is only one of several events that contribute to the eventual outcome. Assuming a Zen approach of focusing on "right action" in the moment—whether it is the exercise of empathy, conducting a careful physical examination, engaging clinical reasoning, or performing a procedure—and releasing the need to have the outcome be a marker of one's competence, can provide a helpful cognitive framework for self-assessment. Other strategies for inoculating ourselves against futility may include finding meaning in small victories, such as preventing a hospitalization for a patient with chronic emphysema; using a recurrent worsening of a condition, such as a patient repeatedly admitted for diabetic ketoacidosis, as an opportunity to learn more about clinical medicine; regarding "difficult patients" as visiting professors because of the learning they can provide about how to manage such patients; focusing on the quality of the relationship with the patient whose condition is worsening; and spending some reflective time recalling the positive connections with patients who appreciate the work we do.

Common to several of the unhealthy habits described above (compulsiveness, the psychology of postponement, dissociation from feelings, and tolerating conditions of burnout) is the notion of work as *energy depletion*. Hence many physicians, nurses, administrators, and other health professionals view weekends, vacations, and time with family as the opportunity to recharge and recapture a more expansive awareness. Some seek to expand the time available for recharging by working part-time. The converse of protected "personal time" is the intense compression of "work time" and the density of tasks to be processed in a given day. During this surreal pursuit of the processing of tasks in which "productivity" is equated with "being good," an altered state of consciousness emerges (see Chapter 5). This is a trance that one enters in the presence of certain ritualistic cues (the door to the office, turning on the computer, checking the schedule, retrieving voice mails) and may include running an incessant "to do" list, looking for brief tasks to complete in an illusory pursuit of "closure," a shortened attention span, irritability in the presence of lengthy or labored conversations, a habit of checking and rechecking one's work, stewing about difficult interactions in the past, and worrying about future events.

Renewal, Reflection, & Mindfulness

Steve McPhee has used the metaphor of solar-powered versus gasoline-powered automobiles to contrast different approaches to human energy in our daily lives. The notion of work as a locus of energy *depletion* (requiring a leaving of work to find energy *renewal*) is similar to the nonrenewable dependence of industrial societies on fossil fuels. In the long run, such a view of one's own energy is unsustainable. An alternative perspective is that *energy renewal* is continually available as one moves through the day, whether at work or away from work. This is analogous to a solar-powered car, which requires the opening of panels to draw on the renewable energy from the sun. Such a fundamental shift in our thinking about energy may entail reevaluating our notion of who we are. The fossil fuel model represents a view of oneself as an individual source of productivity and accomplishment, acting with agency upon the material world and upon people's lives to achieve outcomes. The solar panel model suggests a view of oneself as a medium of energy exchange, a self-organizing system much like a candle flame that gives off light in the process of continuous transformation, a system that is embedded within, and a part of, larger self-organizing systems such as a doctor–patient relationship, a health care system, a society, the earth itself.

Trainees should ask themselves: How can we open ourselves to renewal as we move through our days, both at work and at home? What is the psychological equivalent of "opening our solar panels?" One approach is the cultivation of *mindfulness*, which is the practice of being present to where we are and what we are doing. It is the discipline of living an intentional, conscious life (see Chapter 7). Our stream of consciousness often includes thoughts about the past, sometimes accompanied by regret or resentment, and thoughts and images of the future, sometimes threatening, sometimes escapist. Mindfulness is a counterweight to this enchantment with the "there and then" by increasing our skill at being present in the "here and now." Mindfulness involves nonjudgmental attention to our emotional and mental states as they pass through awareness. We learn to see ourselves as vessels through which the various feelings of joy, sorrow, anger, affection, peace, and agitation flow without defining who we are in any moment of intensity. Twenty minutes a day practicing mindfulness meditation can enhance our capacity for mindful attention. This practice can help clinicians be present to patients without interference from what happens before or after that encounter. Mindfulness is also the gateway to accessing opportunities for personal renewal in the midst of work, where in addition to expending energy, we are also receiving energy from personal interactions or the satisfaction of work well done.

The process of approaching each day with mindfulness and openness to the uncertainty of who will walk in the door next, and nonjudgmental attention to the "weather" of our own emotions and those of others, is captured in this poem by Rumi, the thirteenth-century Sufi mystic whose verses reach across the centuries and cultures to speak to our own experience:

The Guest House

This being human is a guest house.
Every morning a new arrival.

A joy, a depression, a meanness,
some momentary awareness comes
as an unexpected visitor.

Welcome and entertain them all!
Even if they're a crowd of sorrows,
who violently sweep your house
empty of its furniture,
still, treat each guest honorably.
He may be clearing you out
for some new delight.

The dark thought, the shame, the malice,
meet them at the door laughing,
and invite them in.

Be grateful for whoever comes,
because each has been sent
as a guide from beyond.

Incorporating a brief period of reflection at the end of each day is one way of conditioning ourselves to perceive the opportunities for personal renewal and meaning contained in various encounters of the day. Using a journal or simply reflecting back for a few minutes on the events of the day can offer a transitional time to let go of the day and absorb the gifts that came our way. Angeles Arrien suggests that we ask ourselves three simple questions: "What surprised me today? What moved me today? What inspired me today?" Sometimes we may find that there has been great meaning in our encounters with the full panoply of human experience, including suffering. A related practice is that of keeping a "gratitude journal," which can be done at the end of the week. This involves writing down a few things from the week for which one is thankful, from simple events like watching a particularly beautiful sunrise to more profound ones like a satisfying encounter with a patient with whom one had a previously troubling relationship.

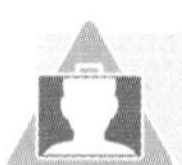

CASE ILLUSTRATION 2 (CONTD.)

In the weeks following the resident retreat, Bill experimented with keeping a journal. Gradually he found himself noticing sources of energy boost during his day—a joke shared with the nursing staff, the satisfaction of having been present to a patient's distress with compassion, learning a new way of working up patients for certain illnesses, being able to guide an intern in managing a difficult admission, observing a faculty preceptor facilitate a difficult family meeting about end-of-life care. He read a little each day in an introductory book on mindfulness meditation and on some days was able to take 5 minutes to practice meditation before his day began. Some days were incredibly busy, and he was still confronted with uncertain medical dilemmas and difficult patients, but he seemed to take it more in stride. He found himself more frequently centering himself before walking into the next patient's room by taking a couple of breaths and letting go of what went before, while embracing the unknown of the encounter awaiting him. Most helpful to him were some discussions with fellow residents in which he found himself more willing to share the stresses and uncertainties of his work and to enjoy the comradeship of knowing he was not alone.

Intimacy & Value Clarification

If our relationship commitments are consistently subordinated to work demands, a review and clarification of our values is in order. Although humbling, we can get a glimpse into our value hierarchy by examining how we actually spend our time and energy in any given week. We may find that what our practice reveals is at variance with what we tell ourselves and others about our deepest values. We also may find that much of the way we spend our time is in response to urgent demands that are not that important in the long run.

In addition to the challenge of nurturing our relationships with family and friends when constrained by professional demands, another barrier is posed by a fear of intimacy or the lack of skill in sharing our inner selves with others. Since clinicians spend much of their time on the receiving end of others' confidences and disclosures, they may have less practice in self-disclosure. It is in relationship with others, however, that we deepen our identity and sense of who we are as persons. This requires not only the presence of close relationships, in and out of medicine, but also time spent with them and the capacity for self-disclosure and intimacy.

- *Friends.* Given the general erosion of community in American life, we must actively seek connections with others. Sometimes opportunities for forming friendships will arise in the work setting, and there it depends on our willingness to take the initiative. We also can develop hobbies and interests outside of medicine that form natural settings for people with similar interests coming together, whether it is through the arts, volunteer work, political action, a faith community, sports, or engaging in outdoor activities. It is not sufficient to have a network of friends without developing our capacity for self-disclosure. Learning to confide in trusted friends is an essential counterbalance to long hours of receiving the confidences of patients in our professional roles.
- *Intimate partners.* A love relationship sustained over time can be one of the great spiritual paths to our growth and development as persons. A long-term and even lifelong journey with an intimate partner is a cauldron which both tests our identity and expands our capacity to embrace life and endure its stresses and challenges. It is in such a relationship that we can learn acceptance of ourselves with all our flaws and virtues. We also can learn the art of compassion through nurturing our beloved and seeking their well-being. Building and maintaining a successful partnership require scheduled time. Enhancing our interpersonal communication skills—especially the art of active listening, disclosure of feelings, and negotiating respectfully when there are differences and conflict—is central to an enduring relationship. Other vital intimacy skills include awareness of our family of origin influences on couple communication and expectations; learning to tolerate differences in tastes and preferences; clarifying mutual values as a couple; and negotiating time, sex, money, space, division of labor, and whether and how to raise children. Romance and sex may occur spontaneously in the early stages of a relationship but over time require our intentional planning to create the time and conditions for this vital component of a relationship to be a lasting source of mutual renewal. Sometimes couples get stuck in stagnating patterns or impasses in their communication, and at such times couple counseling can be a valuable resource.

Organizations & Trainee Well-Being

Although it is essential to engage in self-reflection, value clarification, and behavior change to move our own lives toward renewal and sustainability, viewing this solely as a personal project will not be enough to make meaningful changes. Well-being is not only an individual process but a systems and political process as well. With the best of intentions we may begin a practice of mindfulness, enhancement of our intimate relationships, and caring for ourselves physically—only to have those intentions evaporate at the next attending rounds or faculty meeting where overwork is reinforced and rewarded by the esteem of colleagues and the imperatives of meeting productivity expectations. For the well-being of trainees to thrive, the organizations in which they are trained and work (hospital systems, group practices, academic medical centers, and government institutions) must be sustainable enterprises that value the health and well-being of all their workers. Each of us has a responsibility not only to ourselves but to our colleagues and our profession to engage in the difficult work of changing our organizations—medical schools, residencies, health care systems, and practice settings—so that they allow time and energy for "those gentler influences which make life worth living."

CONCLUSION

The woodblock print seen below, *The Great Wave off Kanagawa*, by the artist Katsushika Hokusai, is from a series entitled "36 Views of Mt. Fuji." It captures several of the elements of personal and organizational well-being we have discussed above. The first and most obvious element is the waves, which are relentlessly chaotic and threaten to capsize the boats. The waves call to mind the ongoing challenges and uncertainty of clinical training and practice. The second element is the people in the boats, who require cohesion, teamwork, and ongoing communication to keep the boats headed into the waves and moving successfully forward on their journey. Our colleagues and team working alongside us are a vital resource for navigating each day of patient care and the developmental hurdles of professional formation. A healthy organization provides such a disciplined collaboration for its members, so that no one person bears the sole burden of responsibility. The third element is Mt. Fuji, at first indistinguishable from the waves, which in its deeply grounded stability provides the still point in the center of this painting around which the chaos revolves. Mindfulness and self-awareness can provide such an inner stillness, allowing us to rest at the deepest center of ourselves as we continually adjust our balance to catch the next wave.

Training health professionals in this complex, information-rich and choice-rich era of human history requires new skills that were not required of previous generations. At the same time, doing so in a way that sustains both educators and trainees as persons requires drawing upon the "practical wisdom" of previous generations. This practical wisdom, what Aristotle called *phronesis*, incorporates the cognitive, emotional, behavioral, and interpersonal skills to expand our capacity as persons and reduce or eliminate the nonimportant and unnecessary loads that erode our spirits. We also need to develop a practical wisdom of working within health care systems that is mindful of the factors that promote sustainability, such as expanding our capacity for service through teamwork, clarifying the organization's values, and establishing structures and processes that promote the well-being of health care workers. This perspective is the responsibility of trainees and faculty alike. Developing the practical wisdom to engage in this work in a sustainable way is our personal and collective challenge.

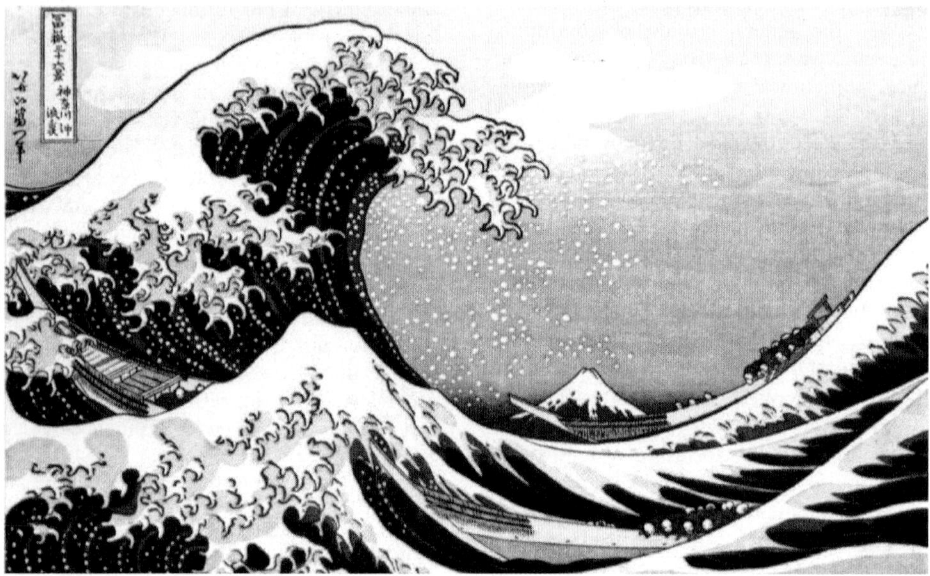

The *Great Wave off Kanagawa*, Katsushika Hokusai, c. 1830.

SUGGESTED READINGS

Barks C, trans. *The Essential Rumi.* Edison, NJ: Castle Books; 1997.

Christensen JF, Feldman MD, eds. Recapturing the spirit of medicine (Special issue on physician well-being). *Western J Med* 2001;174:1–80. http://www.ncbi.nlm.nih.gov/pmc/issues/116276/. Accessed April 2019.

Dyrbye LN, West CP, Satele D, et al. Burnout among US medical students, residents, and early career physicians relative to the general US population. *Acad Med.* 2014;89:443–451.

Gabbard GO. The role of compulsiveness in the normal physician. *JAMA* 1985;254:2926–2929.

Gabbard GO, Menninger RW. The psychology of postponement in the medical marriage. *JAMA* 1989;261:2378–2381.

Kabat-Zinn J. *Wherever You Go There You Are: Mindfulness Meditation in Everyday Life.* New York, NY: Hyperion; 1994.

Mata DA, Ramos MA, Bansal N, et al. Prevalence of depression and depressive symptoms among resident physicians: a systematic review and meta-analysis. *JAMA* 2015;314:2373–2383.

McPhee SJ. Letter from the abbey. *Western J Med* 2001;174:73–75.

Meunier J, Libert Y, Merckaert I, et al. How much is residents' distress detection performance during a clinical round related to their characteristics? *Patient Educ Counsel* 2011;85: 1880–1187.

Osler W. Address to students of the Albany Medical College, February 1, 1899. *Albany Med Ann* 1899;261:307–309.

Regehr C, Clancy D, Pitts A, LeBlanc VR. Interventions to reduce the consequences of stress in physicians: a review and meta-analysis. *J Nerv Ment Dis* 2014;202:353–359.

Rotenstein LS, Ramos MA, Torre M, et al. Prevalence of depression, depressive symptoms, and suicidal ideation among medical students: a systematic review and meta-analysis. *JAMA* 2016;316:2214–2236.

Satterfield JM, Becerra C. Developmental challenges, stressors, and coping strategies in medical residents: a qualitative analysis of support groups. *Med Educ* 2010;44:908–916.

Thich Nhat Hanh. *The Miracle of Mindfulness: A Manual on Meditation.* Boston, MA: Beacon Press; 1987.

Walcott D. *Collected Poems 1948–1984.* New York, NY: Farrar Strauss & Giroux; 1987.

West CP, Shanafelt TD, Kolars JC. Quality of life, burnout, educational debt, and medical knowledge among internal medicine residents. *JAMA* 2011;306:952–960.

OTHER RESOURCE

Christensen JF. Balance and self-care. *Web-Based Learning Module in doc.com: An Interactive Learning Resource for Healthcare Communication.* American Academy on Communication in Healthcare. http://doccom.org/. Accessed September 2019.

WEBSITES

American Medical Student Association. Resources on medical student well-being. http://www.amsa.org/well/. Accessed September 2019.

Clinician Well-Being Knowledge Hub. https://nam.edu/clinician-wellbeing/. Accessed September 2019.

Positive Psychology Center, University of Pennsylvania. https://ppc.sas.upenn.edu/. Accessed September 2019.

Index

Note: Page numbers followed by *t* indicate tables; those followed by *f* indicate figures.

D